Heart Failure

Basic Science and Clinical Aspects

FUNDAMENTAL AND CLINICAL CARDIOLOGY

1. *Drug Treatment of Hyperlipidemia*, edited by Basil M. Rifkind
2. *Cardiotonic Drugs: A Clinical Review. Second Edition, Revised and Expanded*, edited by Carl V. Leier
3. *Complications of Coronary Angioplasty*, edited by Alexander J. R. Black, H. Vernon Anderson, and Stephen G. Ellis
4. *Unstable Angina*, edited by John D. Rutherford
5. *Beta-Blockers and Cardiac Arrhythmias*, edited by Prakash C. Deedwania
6. *Exercise and the Heart in Health and Disease*, edited by Roy J. Shephard and Henry S. Miller, Jr.
7. *Cardiopulmonary Physiology in Critical Care*, edited by Steven M. Scharf
8. *Atherosclerotic Cardiovascular Disease, Hemostasis, and Endothelial Function*, edited by Robert Boyer Francis, Jr.
9. *Coronary Heart Disease Prevention*, edited by Frank G. Yanowitz
10. *Thrombolysis and Adjunctive Therapy for Acute Myocardial Infarction*, edited by Eric R. Bates
11. *Stunned Myocardium: Properties, Mechanisms, and Clinical Manifestations*, edited by Robert A. Kloner and Karin Przyklenk
12. *Prevention of Venous Thromboembolism*, edited by Samuel Z. Goldhaber
13. *Silent Myocardial Ischemia and Infarction: Third Edition*, Peter F. Cohn
14. *Congestive Cardiac Failure: Pathophysiology and Treatment*, edited by David B. Barnett, Hubert Pouleur, and Gary S. Francis
15. *Heart Failure: Basic Science and Clinical Aspects*, edited by Judith K. Gwathmey, G. Maurice Briggs, and Paul D. Allen

Additional Volumes in Preparation

Cardiovascular Disease in the Elderly Patient, edited by Donald Tresch and Wilbert Aronow

Coronary Thrombolysis in Perspective: Principles Underlying Conjunctive and Adjunctive Therapy, edited by Burton E. Sobel and Désiré Collen

Systemic Cardiac Embolism, edited by Michael Ezekowitz

Heart Failure

Basic Science and Clinical Aspects

edited by

Judith K. Gwathmey

Institute for Cardiovascular Disease and Muscle Research Inc.
Harvard Medical School
and Beth Israel Hospital
Boston, Massachusetts

G. Maurice Briggs

Sterling Winthrop Pharmaceuticals
Rensselaer, New York

Paul D. Allen

Harvard Medical School
and Brigham and Women's Hospital
Boston, Massachusetts

Marcel Dekker, Inc. New York • Basel • Hong Kong

Library of Congress Cataloging-in-Publication Data

Heart failure : basic science and clinical aspects / edited by Judith K. Gwathmey, G. Maurice Briggs, Paul D. Allen.
p. cm. — (Fundamental and clinical cardiology;15)
Includes bibliographical references and index.
ISBN 0-8247-8772-2 (alk. paper)
1. Heart failure—Pathophysiology. 2. Heart failure. I. Gwathmey, Judith K. II. Briggs, G. Maurice. III. Allen, Paul D. IV. Series.
[DNLM: 1. Heart Failure, Congestive—etiology. 2. Heart Failure, Congestive—physiopathology. W1 FU538TD v.15 1993 / WG 370 H4363 1993]
RC685.C53H433 1993
616.1'29—dc20
DNLM/DLC
for Library of Congress 93-15908
CIP

The publisher offers discounts on this book when ordered in bulk quantities. For more information, write to Special Sales/Professional Marketing at the address below.

This book is printed on acid-free paper.

Marcel Dekker, Inc.
270 Madison Avenue, New York, New York 10016

Current printing (last digit):
10 9 8 7 6 5 4 3 2 1

Printed in the United States of America

To discover and teach are distinct functions; they are also distinct gifts; and are not commonly found united in the same person.

On the Scope and Nature of University Education, Preface
John Henry, Cardinal Newman

To Thomas W. Smith, M.D., who exemplifies the rare combination of uncommon gifts: He is at once the physician-scientist, the clinician-educator, and the student-mentor. These abilities have enabled him to play a pivotal role in defining one of the most important areas of cardiovascular medicine, the basic science and clinical aspects of congestive heart failure. As he has influenced many of the contributors to this book, Dr. Smith continues to shape the progress of cardiovascular science.

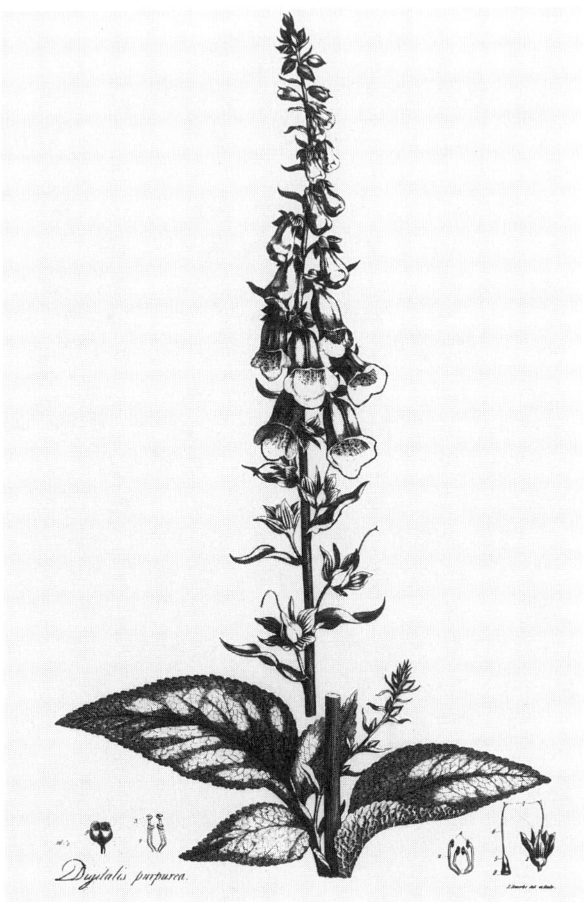

Series Introduction

Marcel Dekker, Inc., has focused on the development of various series of beautifully produced books in different branches of medicine. These series have facilitated the integration of rapidly advancing information for both the clinical specialist and the researcher.

My goal as editor of the Fundamental and Clinical Cardiology series is to assemble the talents of world-renowned authorities to discuss virtually every area of cardiovascular medicine. In the current monograph, *Heart Failure: Basic Science and Clinical Aspects,* Drs. Gwathmey, Briggs, and Allen have edited a much needed and timely book. Future contributions to this series will include books on molecular biology, interventional cardiology, and clinical management of such problems as coronary artery disease and ventricular arrhythmias.

Samuel Z. Goldhaber

Foreword

The past decade has seen dramatic advances in our understanding of the basic mechanisms of cardiac contraction and relaxation. These advances have led to a growing appreciation of cellular and molecular causes of heart disease. However, this rapid growth of knowledge has also created a widening gap in communication between physicians responsible for managing patients with heart disease and scientists working to advance the frontiers of knowledge.

Health care practitioners commonly view the heart as an organ that pumps blood and understand heart failure as a deficiency in cardiac pumping. Although the intricacy of the heart's machinery is appreciated by the clinician, the vast and growing body of new molecular understanding has become overwhelming in both volume and complexity. Basic scientists, on the other hand, while able to relate specific aspects of the heart's performance to precisely characterized features of specific molecules within myocardial cells, are often not well trained to understand the clinical challenges posed by the patient with heart failure. This book, which focuses on what is becoming the most important cause of heart disease in our aging population, seeks to bridge this gap by juxtaposing the latest knowledge of the mechanism and control of cardiac contraction with discussions of the pathophysiology and therapy of heart failure.

One consequence of our new understanding of the pathophysiology of heart failure is a blurring of the definition of this condition. At the beginning of this century, clinicians had no difficulty in defining heart failure simply as impaired pumping by a diseased heart. C. J. Wiggers, in his 1915 book *Circulation in Health and Disease,* stated that cardiac insufficiency occurs "when the heart fails to discharge as much blood as it receives." This definition was echoed in 1933 by Sir Thomas Lewis, who wrote in his *Diseases of the Heart:* "There is but one meaning to the term cardiac failure—it signifies inability of the heart to discharge its contents adequately." Sir James MacKenzie, in the third (1915) edition of his *Diseases of the Heart,* defined heart failure as the "condition in which the heart is unable to maintain an efficient circulation when called upon to meet the efforts necessary to the daily life of the individual."

Even at the beginning of this century, however, some physicians recognized that heart failure was more than a disorder of cardiac pumping. Sir William Osler, in the first (1892) edition of his classic *Textbook of Medicine,* recognized that while the initial hypertrophic response to a hemodynamic overload was compensatory, subsequent deterioration of the chronically hypertrophied heart overcame the compensatory effects of hypertrophy. In describing the latter phenomenon, which he called "broken compensation," Osler wrote:

> Broken compensation may come on suddenly during very severe exertion. Death may result from acute dilatation; but more commonly it takes place slowly and results from degeneration and weakening of the heart-muscle.

Osler's "broken compensation" was reproduced experimentally in the 1960s by F. Z. Meerson, who used aortic banding to subject canine and rabbit left ventricles to chronic pressure overload. In 1964, in the introduction to an NIH-sponsored review of the status of heart failure research, Louis N. Katz wrote:

> One thing seems certain, namely, that chronic overload of the heart does lead eventually to heart failure even when the myocardium is normal at the start. How this failure comes about is a question that needs settling. Perhaps the solution to this last problem, as much as anything else, will go far to advance our knowledge about heart failure.

More recently, I suggested that the molecular changes leading to the progressive degeneration of the overloaded heart could be viewed as a "cardiomyopathy of overload," and that these load-induced changes play a major causative role in the clinical deterioration and eventual death of patients with heart failure.

The theme of the present text was, in fact, heralded by MacKenzie, who wrote in the first (1908) edition of his *Diseases of the Heart:*

> The more I study the symptoms of heart failure, and the more I reflect on the part played by the heart muscle, the more convinced I am that heart failure can be summed up in the general statement that heart failure is due to the exhaustion of the reserve force of the heart muscle.

This remarkable statement is echoed by many of the following chapters, which define the concepts of "exhaustion" and "reserve force" in modern biochemical and molecular terms. These discussions illustrate the modern shift in emphasis of heart failure research from abnormalities of the circulation, which is really the victim of impaired pumping by a failing heart, to the culprit, which is, of course, the diseased heart itself.

The changing focus of our efforts to define heart failure illustrate the operation of a sequence of three paradigms, or archetypical models, that describe the development of our understanding of cardiac regulation during this century. These paradigms can be stated concisely as *organ, cell,* and *gene.* In seeking to understand the regulation of the work of the heart, for example, we have seen the focus of research move from organ physiology (Starling's law of the heart) through cell biochemistry (myocardial contractility) to altered gene expression (molecular biology).

As already pointed out, the early definitions of heart failure, which highlighted the clinical signs and symptoms arising from the interplay between the failing cardiac pump and the circulation whose needs it cannot satisfy, emphasized abnormal organ physiology. During the 1960s, characterization of the mechanisms regulating myocardial contractility, along with measurements of energetic abnormalities in failing myocardial cells, identified cellular changes that impaired the ability of the failing heart to meet the demands of the circulation. The result was a shift in emphasis from the first paradigm of abnormal organ function to the second paradigm of disordered cell biochemistry and biophysics. For example, it is now clear that abnormal calcium fluxes in the cells of the failing heart both depress contractility and impair relaxation. This text highlights the many abnormalities that alter both excitation–contraction coupling and relaxation. As noted in the final chapter, the failing heart is also an energy-starved organ, where declining levels of high-energy phosphate likely contribute to inotropic and lusitropic abnormalities in the failing heart. Details about these molecular abnormalities and how they influence both function and prognosis in patients with heart failure are still to be elucidated. Much remains to be written in this fast-moving and clinically important field.

It is my own prediction that as our understanding of heart failure continues to deepen, the clinical syndrome and its biochemical and biophysical causes (which represent the first and second of my three paradigms of knowledge of cardiovascular function) will be supplemented by new knowledge of the third paradigm of altered gene expression. I believe that the isoform shifts, altered membrane architecture, and other molecular abnormalities that contribute to the cardiomyopathy of overload provide yet another dimension in our efforts to understand the disordered cardiac contraction and relaxation, as well as the poor survival rates of patients with chronic heart failure.

In closing, I highlight the importance of this text for both clinical practitioners and basic scientists who seek to bridge the widening gap between these two vital aspects of our effort to understand and treat heart failure. The authoritative discussions on the following pages illustrate the value of the integrated approach to the clinical and investigative challenges posed by the patient with heart failure.

Arnold M. Katz
Professor of Medicine
Head, Division of Cardiology
The School of Medicine
University of Connecticut Health Center
Farmington, Connecticut

Preface

Unless they see signs and wonders they will not believe

Wesley H. Ketchum, M.D.

The major objective of this book is to address the scientific foundations of the principal clinical modalities in the treatment and management of heart failure. In addition, various clinical treatments of heart disease are discussed, and the basic aspects of excitation–contraction coupling in normal and diseased myocardium and vascular smooth muscle are reviewed. The goal of this text is to discuss clinically used agents as well as agents that may not be currently used or recognized as potential agents in the treatment of heart disease but may be of significant value.

Many physician/scientists believe that the primary defect in chronic heart failure is a reduction in myocardial contractile force. As a result, a search for potent inotropes has been undertaken, with the pharmaceutical industry focusing primarily on the development of such agents. However, the recent failure of the milrinone "Promise Trials" has raised an important question that must be answered by the scientific community and the pharmaceutical industry: Should the disappointing results of several clinical trials discourage further development of inotropic drugs? Also, do agents classified as "negative inotropes" (for example, afterload reducers, calcium channel blockers, and β-adrenergic receptor antagonists) warrant investigation?

The recent availability of human myocardium for study has begun to provide new and sometimes unexpected findings regarding the pathophysiology of human heart failure. As a result, views of the best management of heart disease must be reconsidered and, perhaps, altered. Physicians now wrestle with several treatment controversies on a daily basis.

Studies of the progression of myocardial disease should be directed toward identifying adaptive changes in diseased myocardium that are responsive to specific pharmacologic intervention. Neither clinicians nor the pharmaceutical industry can allow themselves to be mired in orthodoxy, but rather must be prepared to investigate all avenues of opportunity in order to reach their final goals.

The contributors to this text have been selected on the basis of their known expertise. The editors are very grateful for each contribution, and we heartily welcome the coming together of clinicians, scientists, and physician/scientists for such an important endeavor.

Judith K. Gwathmey

Contents

Part II: Smooth Muscle

Part III: β- and α-Receptors

Part IV: Protein Kinase C and Muscarinic Receptors

Part V: Sodium Potassium ATPase

Part VI: Phosphodiesterase Inhibitors

Contributors

Tai Akera, M.D., Ph.D. Vice President, Japan, Merck Research Laboratories, Division of Merck & Co., Inc., West Point, Pennsylvania

Paul D. Allen, M.D., Ph.D. Associate Professor of Anesthesia, Harvard Medical School, and Anesthesiologist, Brigham and Women's Hospital, Boston, Massachusetts

C. William Balke, M.D. Assistant Professor of Medicine, Assistant Professor of Physiology, and Director of Molecular and Cellular Cardiology, Departments of Medicine and Physiology, University of Maryland at Baltimore, Baltimore, Maryland

Joey V. Barnett, Ph.D. Instructor in Medicine, Cardiovascular Division, Department of Medicine, Brigham and Women's Hospital and Harvard Medical School, Boston, Massachusetts

G. Maurice Briggs, Ph.D. Research Investigator, Department of Cardiovascular Pharmacology, Sterling Winthrop Pharmaceuticals Research Division, Rensselaer, New York

Maurizio C. Capogrossi, M.D. Senior Investigator, Laboratory of Cardiovascular Science, Gerontology Research Center, National Institute on Aging, National Institutes of Health, Baltimore, Maryland

Jean-François Cloix, Ph.D. Faculté de Medicine-Broussais, Hôtel Dieu, Paris, France

Wilson S. Colucci, M.D. Associate Professor, Cardiovascular Division, Department of Medicine, Brigham and Women's Hospital and Harvard Medical School, Boston, Massachusetts

Pieter P. de Tombe, Ph.D. Assistant Professor of Medicine, Cardiology Section, Department of Internal Medicine, The Bowman Gray School of Medicine, Wake Forest University, Winston-Salem, North Carolina

Hans Armin Dieterich, F.E.S.C., F.A.C.C. Chief of Clinical Research and Procurist, Marion Merrell Dow Research, Rüsselsheim, Germany

D. A. Eisner, D. Phil. Professor, Department of Preclinical Veterinary Sciences, University of Liverpool, Liverpool, England

Arthur M. Feldman, M.D., Ph.D. Associate Professor, Division of Cardiology, Department of Medicine, Johns Hopkins University School of Medicine, Baltimore, Maryland

Hans-Reiner Figulla, M.D. Associate Professor of Medicine, Cardiology and Pulmonology Department, Medizinische Universitäts Kliniken, Göttingen, Germany

Richard M. Fleming, M.D. Division of Cardiology, Department of Medicine, University of Texas Medical School, Houston, Texas

Jonas B. Galper, M.D., Ph.D. Associate Professor of Medicine, Cardiovascular Division, Department of Medicine, Brigham and Women's Hospital and Harvard Medical School, Boston, Massachusetts

Richard A. Goldstein, M.D. Director, Cardiac and Vascular Diagnostic Center, Tower Imaging, Los Angeles, California

William Grossman, M.D. Dana Professor of Medicine, Harvard Medical School, and Chief, Cardiovascular Division, Beth Israel Hospital, Boston, Massachusetts

Judith K. Gwathmey, V.M.D., Ph.D. Director, Institute for Cardiovascular Disease and Muscle Research, Associate Professor of Cellular and Molecular Physiology, Department of Medicine, Harvard Medical School, and Research Associate in Medicine, Cardiovascular Division, Beth Israel Hospital, Boston, Massachusetts

R. W. Hadley, Ph.D. Assistant Professor, Department of Physiology, University of Maryland School of Medicine, Baltimore, Maryland

Roger J. Hajjar, M.D. Clinical Fellow, Medical Services, Massachusetts General Hospital, Boston, Massachusetts

Åke Hjalmarson, M.D., Ph.D. Professor, Division of Cardiology, Sahlgren's Hospital, University of Göteborg, Göteborg, Sweden

Joanne S. Ingwall, Ph.D. Professor of Medicine, NMR Laboratory for Physiological Chemistry, Brigham and Women's Hospital and Harvard Medical School, Boston, Massachusetts

Gregory J. Kaczorowski, Ph.D. Director, Department of Membrane Biochemistry and Biophysics, Merck Research Laboratories, Rahway, New Jersey

Ralph A. Kelly, M.D. Assistant Professor, Cardiology Division, Department of Medicine, Brigham and Women's Hospital and Harvard Medical School, Boston, Massachusetts

M. S. Kirby, Ph.D. Research Associate, Department of Physiology, University of Maryland School of Medicine, Baltimore, Maryland

Bernhard K. Krämer, M.D. Research Fellow, Cardiovascular Division, Department of Medicine, Brigham and Women's Hospital and Harvard Medical School, Boston, Massachusetts

Edward G. Lakatta, M.D. Chief, Laboratory of Cardiovascular Science, National Institute on Aging, National Institutes of Health, Baltimore, Maryland

W. J. Lederer, M.D., Ph.D. Professor, Department of Physiology, University of Maryland School of Medicine, Baltimore, Maryland

Howard R. Lee, M.D., F.A.C.C. Cardiologist, Heart Center of Salt Lake, Salt Lake City, Utah

Thomas Michel, M.D., Ph.D. Assistant Professor, Cardiovascular Division, Department of Medicine, Brigham and Women's Hospital and Harvard Medical School, Boston, Massachusetts

Matthew A. Movsesian, M.D. Assistant Professor, Cardiology Division, University of Utah Medical Center, Salt Lake City, Utah

Luigino Nascimben, M.D. Department of Medicine, NMR Laboratory for Physiological Chemistry, Brigham and Women's Hospital and Harvard Medical School, and Cardiovascular Division, Beth Israel Hospital, Boston, Massachusetts

Yuk-Chow Ng, Ph.D. Assistant Professor, Department of Pharmacology, The Milton S. Hershey Medical Center, Pennsylvania State University, Hershey, Pennsylvania

Edward D. Pagani, Ph.D. Research Fellow, Department of Cardiovascular Pharmacology, Sterling Winthrop Pharmaceuticals Research Division, Rensselaer, New York

John Pawlowski, M.D., Ph.D. Instructor in Anesthesia, Department of Anesthesia and Critical Care, Beth Israel Hospital, Boston, Massachusetts

Warren D. Rosenblum, M.D. Fellow, Division of Cardiology, Department of Medicine, Johns Hopkins University School of Medicine, Baltimore, Maryland

Johann Caspar Rüegg, M.D., Ph.D. Professor and Head, Physiology Department, University of Heidelberg, Heidelberg, Germany

Andre Ruzycky, Ph.D. Assistant Professor, Department of Obstetrics, Gynecology, and Reproductive Sciences, University of Pittsburgh School of Medicine, Pittsburgh, Pennsylvania

Michael C. Sanguinetti, Ph.D. Senior Research Fellow, Department of Pharmacology, Merck Research Laboratories, West Point, Pennsylvania

Heribert Schunkert, M.D. Klinik und Poliklinik für Innere Medizin II, Regensburg University, Regensburg, Germany

Peter K. S. Siegl, Ph.D. Director, Department of Cardiovascular Pharmacology, Merck Research Laboratories, West Point, Pennsylvania

Paul J. Silver, Ph.D. Director, Department of Cardiovascular Pharmacology, Sterling Winthrop Pharmaceuticals Research Division, Rensselaer, New York

Howard S. Silverman, M.D. Assistant Professor of Medicine, Division of Cardiology, Department of Medicine, Johns Hopkins University, Baltimore, Maryland

Randal A. Skidgel, Ph.D. Associate Professor, Departments of Pharmacology and Anesthesiology, University of Illinois College of Medicine at Chicago, Chicago, Illinois

R. John Solaro, Ph.D. Professor and Head, Department of Physiology and Biophysics, University of Illinois College of Medicine at Chicago, Chicago, Illinois

Michael D. Stern, M.D. Associate Professor of Medicine, Division of Cardiology, Department of Medicine, Johns Hopkins University, Baltimore, Maryland

James T. Stull, Ph.D. Professor and Chairman, Department of Physiology, University of Texas Southwestern Medical Center at Dallas, Dallas, Texas

Henk E. D. J. ter Keurs, M.D., Ph.D. Professor of Medicine, Department of Medicine and Medical Physiology, University of Calgary, Calgary, Alberta, Canada

Jochen Thormann, M.D. Professor, Department of Clinical Cardiology, Kerckhoff-Klinik der Max-Planck-Gesellschaft, Bad Nauheim, Germany

Finn Waagstein, M.D., Ph.D. Associate Professor of Medicine, Division of Cardiology, Sahlgren's Hospital, University of Göteborg, Göteborg, Sweden

Withrow Gil Wier, Ph.D. Professor, Department of Physiology, University of Maryland School of Medicine, Baltimore, Maryland

R. Ann Word, M.D. Assistant Professor, Division of Reproductive Endocrinology, Department of Obstetrics-Gynecology, University of Texas Southwestern Medical Center at Dallas, Dallas, Texas

Heart Failure

Basic Science and Clinical Aspects

1

Congestive Heart Failure: Role of Systolic and Diastolic Dysfunction

WILLIAM GROSSMAN

Harvard Medical School and Beth Israel Hospital
Boston, Massachusetts

The diagnosis of heart failure is most commonly made when a patient presents with congestive manifestations, such as peripheral edema, distended neck veins, ascites, dyspnea and/or orthopnea, and pulmonary edema. While any one of these clinical findings may result from abnormalities in systems other than the heart, the presence of two or more of these findings should certainly alert the clinician at least to consider a diagnosis of heart failure. As might be anticipated from the list of clinical findings just enumerated, the terms heart failure and congestive heart failure are often used interchangeably, which emphasizes the importance of congestive aspects in the clinical presentation of patients with heart failure. In fact, the traditional diagnosis of heart failure as a condition in which the cardiac output is not commensurate with the metabolic needs of the body is rarely useful to the clinician.

Another way to regard heart failure stems from a consideration of the heart's fundamental functions. The heart's primary functions are two: to receive blood into the cardiac ventricles under low pressure during diastole, and subsequently to propel blood into the great vessels during systole under sufficient pressure and in adequate amount to sustain the body's metabolic needs. Failure of the heart to receive blood into the cardiac ventricles at low pressure (i.e. $\leq$ 8 mmHg for the right ventricle and $\leq$ 12 mmHg for the left ventricle) constitutes *diastolic heart failure*. Failure of the ventricles to propel their contents into the great vessels under sufficient pressure ($\geq$ 15 mmHg for the right ventricle and $\geq$ 90 mmHg for the left ventricle) or in adequate amount ($\geq$ 2.8 L/min/m^2) during systole constitutes *systolic heart failure*. These concepts are reminiscent of the old subdivision of heart failure into "backward heart failure" and "forward heart failure." One difference between this newer approach to heart failure (i.e., categorizing heart failure as either systolic or diastolic) and the older approach (forward or backward heart failure) is that backward heart failure was commonly regarded as a consequence of forward failure rather than as an independent entity with its own unique pathophysiology. By regarding the heart has having two distinct primary functions, it is clear that systolic and diastolic heart failure can exist independently or together, and interact in a complex and variable fashion.

Many forms of heart disease affect the heart's ability *both* to fill and to eject; accordingly, systolic and diastolic heart failure commonly coexist. In fact, severe diastolic heart failure of necessity impairs the ability of the heart to function normally in systole. As pointed out by D.H. Lawrence in his Essay on Love, "So that the coming together depends on the going apart; the systole depends on the diastole; the flow depends upon the ebb. There can never be love universal and unbroken. The sea can never rise to high tide over all the globe at once. The undisputed reign of love can never be." (1).

I. SYSTOLIC HEART FAILURE

Systolic heart failure, defined as impaired ejection of blood into the great vessels under adequate pressure by one or both cardiac ventricles, is seen in a variety of disease states (Table 1). *Decreased myocardial contractility* develops acutely in the

Table 1 Causes of Systolic Heart Failure

Decreased myocardial contractility
Acute
Coronary occlusion with loss of myocardial contractility in a large segment of the left ventricle
Pharmacologic depression of contractility (e.g., high-dosage calcium blockers, ethanol, lidocaine, disopyramide, etc.)
Severe acidosis
Chronic
Myocardial infarction
Dilated cardiomyopathy
Myocarditis (may also be acute)
Toxin-induced cardiomyopathy (adriamycin, ethanol, etc.)
Advanced myocardial hypertrophy (i.e., chronic hypertension, ventricular pressure overload or volume overload, etc.)
Afterload mismatch
Acute
Malignant hypertension
Rapidly progressive aortic stenosis (e.g., thrombosis or calcification of a prosthetic valve)
Acute pulmonary embolism
Chronic: Aortic stenosis with inadequate hypertrophy (e.g., aortic stenosis in the elderly)
Valvular heart disease and other forms of cardiac overload
Acute
Mitral regurgitation
Acute ventricular septal defect
Acute aortic regurgitation
Chronic
Volume overload lesions (aortic, mitral or tricuspid regurgitation, ventricular or atrial septal defect, arteriovenous fistula, severe chronic anemia, etc.).
Pressure overload conditions (e.g., chronic systemic hypertension, primary pulmonary hypertension, recurrent pulmonary embolism, progressive aortic stenosis)

presence of myocardial ischemia. Occlusion of a coronary artery is followed by rapid and complete loss of contractile function of the affected myocardium. Contractile function ceases within seconds of coronary occlusion, and current evidence indicates that the rapid accumulation of hydrogen ion and inorganic phosphate in the ischemic myocardium is associated with desensitization of the myofilaments to calcium (2,3) even though ATP and creatine phosphate (CP) are relatively well preserved (4). This acute loss of contractile function will not lead to heart failure unless the mass of myocardium involved is sufficient to affect overall pump function adversely. Usually, this requires sudden loss of contractile function of 20% or more of the left ventricular myocardium. If 30–40% of the left ventricular myocardium is affected by the coronary occlusion, severe heart failure develops acutely, and the clinical picture of cardiogenic shock may emerge. Heart failure develops so promptly after the development of coronary occlusion that although one might think of this as heart failure in the setting of acute myocardial infarction, it is not necessary for myocardial necrosis actually to occur. In fact, profound heart failure may occur with obstruction of the proximal left anterior descending coronary artery, or the left main coronary artery, and relief of the obstruction will result in recovery from heart failure without any evidence of myocardial necrosis if the occlusion persists for 30 min or less. Heart failure can result from pharmacologic depression of myocardial contractility following the administration of an excessive dose of a calcium-blocking agent (e.g., verapamil, diltiazem, nifedipine), especially if this is delivered to the myocardium in high concentration, as with an intracoronary injection. Although acute alcohol intoxication results in some myocardial depression (5), the advanced systolic heart failure with low left ventricular ejection fraction seen in alcoholic cardiomyopathy is more complex than can be accounted for by this acute, reversible pharmacologic depression of myocardial contractility. Instead, chronic changes develop that may be associated with myocyte necrosis and dropout with hypertrophy of remaining myocytes, giving a picture of chronic dilated cardiomyopathy.

If coronary occlusion persists and acute myocardial infarction develops, heart failure may continue and worsen. However, hypertrophy of the noninfarcted regions of myocardium remote from the infarction develops promptly (6,7) and this hypertrophy, combined with ventricular dilatation and utilization of the Frank-Starling mechanism, tends to restore toward normal the left ventricle's ability to empty itself in systole, thus correcting systolic heart failure.

Afterload mismatch can also cause systolic heart failure. In this condition, the heart responds appropriately to an increase in afterload (increased systolic wall stress) by decreasing the extent of myocardial fiber shortening (8–10). This may be observed with any rapidly developing acute increase in ventricular afterload, such as malignant hypertension. For example, if a patient's systemic arterial blood pressure increases abruptly to 240/120 mmHg, the normal and previously nonhypertrophied left ventricle will eject a smaller stroke volume. The decreased stroke volume will result in increased left ventricular (LV) residual volume (LV end-systolic volume) and increased LV end-diastolic pressure; also, tachycardia will be required to maintain a normal cardiac output. A similar situation may occur in the presence of rapidly progressive aortic stenosis. This is seen clinically in the patient who develops thrombosis of a prosthetic heart valve in the aortic position, or in whom a porcine aortic valve prosthesis calcifies progressively and rapidly. Another example of acute afterload mismatch as a cause of systolic heart failure is seen in the patient with acute pulmonary embolism. If pulmonary emboli occlude more than 50% of the cross-sectional area of the pulmonary vascular bed, the normal right ventricle will fail to maintain ejection of a normal stroke volume. The right ventricle will dilate, right ventricular and right atrial pressures will become elevated, and tachycardia will develop in an attempt to maintain stroke volume. If the right ventricular systolic failure is severe, there will be a decrease in delivery of blood to the left ventricle with resultant systemic hypotension and/or cardiogenic shock. These examples of acute afterload mismatch, along with the systolic heart failure seen with abrupt coronary occlusion, may be regarded as relatively pure forms of systolic heart failure.

Valvular heart disease and other forms of overload may also lead to systolic heart failure. An example is the systolic heart failure resulting from sudden loss of integrity of the mitral valve apparatus. Acute mitral regurgitation, while not associated with any decrease in myocardial contractility or loss of the left ventricle's ability to eject blood, nevertheless is associated with a reduction in the left ventricle's ability to eject blood *into its great vessel* (i.e., aorta) under adequate pressure and in normal amount. Acute mitral regurgitation can occur as a result of bacterial endocarditis, ruptured chordae tendineae, or acute coronary occlusion with papillary muscle ischemia/necrosis. An additional condition that may lead to the abrupt onset of congestive heart failure is acute aortic regurgitation, as may be seen in the course of bacterial endocarditis or dissecting aneurysm of the aorta. Another condition in which abrupt overload can cause systolic heart failure is ventricular septal defect, which may develop acutely during the course of myocardial infarction. In this condition, the left ventricle ejects its contents simultaneously into the aorta and right ventricle, with the result that forward (aortic) output diminishes and pulmonary artery pressure increases. If the ventricular septal defect is sufficiently large, acute heart failure may result. In all the above listed conditions (acute mitral or aortic regurgitation, ventricular septal defect) left ventricular myocardial contractility is normal initially, and systolic heart failure develops as a result of a mechanical problem.

Chronic valvular heart disease may also result in congestive heart failure. Chronic aortic, mitral, or tricuspid regurgitation leads to progressive eccentric hypertrophy of the affected ventricular chamber. The hypertrophied myocardium provides adequate compensation initially, but with time myocardial contractility becomes depressed and systolic heart failure develops. Other forms of chronic volume overload (e.g., congenital ventricular or atrial septal defect, arteriovenous fistula, severe anemia) may lead to the same sequence of events. Finally, chronic pressure overload, as may be seen with chronic systemic hypertension, primary pulmonary hypertension, recurrent pulmonary embolism, or progressive aortic stenosis, results in concentric hypertrophy of the affected ventricular chamber. Initially, the concentrically hypertrophied ventricle will adequately maintain cardiac output and overall compensation; however, with time myocardial contractility may become depressed and heart failure will ensue.

II. DIASTOLIC HEART FAILURE

Diastolic heart failure, defined as increased resistance to filling of one or both cardiac ventricles, is also seen in a variety of disease states (Table 2). As can be seen from Table 2, diastolic heart failure may be the result of structural abnormalities

Table 2 Mechanisms of Diastolic Heart Failure

Condition	Mechanism of Diastolic Dysfunction
Mitral or tricuspid stenosis	Increased resistance to atrial emptying
Constrictive pericarditis	Increased resistance to ventricular inflow with decreased ventricular diastolic capacity
Restrictive cardiomyopathies (amyloidosis, hemochromatosis, diffuse fibrosis)	Increased resistance to ventricular inflow
Obliterative cardiomyopathy (endocardial fibroelastosis, Loeffler's syndrome)	Increased resistance to ventricular inflow
Ischemic heart disease	Impaired myocardial relaxation
Flash pulmonary edema, dyspnea during angina	Diastolic calcium overload
Postinfarction scarring and hypertrophy (remodeling)	Increased resistance to ventricular inflow (see hypertrophic heart disease)
Hypertrophic heart disease (hypertrophic cardiomyopathy, chronic hypertension, aortic stenosis)	Impaired myocardial relaxation Diastolic calcium overload Increased resistance to ventricular inflow due to thick chamber walls, altered collagen matrix Activation of renin–angiotensin system
Volume overload (aortic or mitral regurgitation, arteriovenous fistula)	Increased diastolic volume relative to ventricular capacity Myocardial hypertrophy, fibrosis
Dilated cardiomyopathy	Impaired myocardial relaxation Diastolic calcium overload Myocardial fibrosis/scar

As discussed in the text, diastolic heart failure is defined as increased resistance to filling of one or both cardiac ventricles.
Source: Grossman W. Diastolic dysfunction in congestive heart failure. N Engl J Med 1991; 325:1557–1564.

that increase resistance to ventricular inflow. These abnormalities may be extramyocardial, such as constrictive pericarditis, or intramyocardial, such as amyloidosis or diffuse fibrosis. For some conditions, such as advanced hypertrophy, the increased resistance to ventricular filling reflects both structural change (increased wall thickness, myocardial fibrosis) and dysfunction of myocardial diastolic relaxation of the hypertrophied myocardium.

The details of calcium cycling within the myocardial cell are reviewed elsewhere in this book. Calcium cycling provides the fundamental control of contraction and relaxation of the myofilaments. Calcium entry into the myocytes triggers release of calcium from the sarcoplasmic reticulum. This in turn is followed by a rapid rise in the concentration of ionized calcium within the cytosol, leading to a conformational change in troponin C. This conformational change removes the tonic inhibition provided by troponin C, allowing cross-bridges to form and cycle in the presence of adequate ATP stores. If ionized calcium concentration does not return to its normal low value following excitation–contraction coupling, myocardial relaxation will be impaired. Impaired myocardial relaxation is seen in a number of conditions, including myocardial ischemia (11–16) as well as in cardiac hypertrophy (17) and failure (18). Early diastolic filling is blunted in most patients with cardiac hypertrophy, especially concentric hypertrophy, and this results in increased dependence on late diastolic filling to achieve adequate end-diastolic sarcomere stretch. Accordingly, the development of atrial fibrillation is not well tolerated in such patients, since late diastolic filling results primarily from atrial contraction. Also, because coronary blood flow occurs primarily during diastole, impaired diastolic relaxation may also limit coronary perfusion.

There is controversy concerning the influence of myocardial ischemia on diastolic relaxation and distensibility. Current evidence suggests that myocardial relaxation is impaired in a setting of myocardial ischemia, as long as sufficient coronary blood flow persists to maintain myocardial pH and inorganic phosphate levels near normal. When myocardial ischemia is severe, the accumulation of hydrogen ion and inorganic phosphate causes marked depression of myofilament sensitivity, thus masking the development of diastolic dysfunction (19–22).

III. HYPERTROPHY AND DIASTOLIC HEART FAILURE

Chronic left ventricular hypertrophy is associated with increased passive diastolic stiffness, slowing of myocardial relaxation, and reduced ventricular distensibility. The increased passive diastolic stiffness results from changes in myocardial collagen (23–27) as well as an increase in wall thickness in patients with aortic stenosis. Hypertrophied myocardium exhibits intrinsic impairment in diastolic relaxation, but also shows increased susceptibility to ischemia-induced diastolic dysfunction (28,29). Patients with severe aortic stenosis but without obstructive coronary artery disease show an increase in left ventricular diastolic pressure relative to volume with tachycardia, indiacting a marked limitation in diastolic functional reserve. Patients with hypertrophic cardiomyopathy have markedly prolonged left ventricular relaxation and striking abnormalities in diastolic function (30). Recent studies (31) have shown that isolated cardiac muscle from patients with hypertrophic cardiomyopathy have marked impairment in calcium homeostasis, with prolongation of diastolic calcium decline and the development of a second or a plateau component (L_2), indicating elevated diastolic levels of cystosolic ionized calcium.

In patients with advanced heart failure from almost any cause (e.g., dilated cardiomyopathy, chronic ventricular overload, postinfarction remodeling), myocyte hypertrophy develops and is associated with impaired relaxation. The myocyte hypertrophy in these conditions is associated with impairment in internal calcium cycling, and it is common to see slow disappearance of calcium from the cytosol in patients with advanced heart failure from a variety of causes (32). The diastolic dysfunction as well as the abnormalities in intracellular calcium handling appear to be improved in vitro by the administration of agents such as forskolin, which increases cyclic AMP (33). There is evidence from a variety of sources to indicate that heart failure muscle is characterized by an increase in G_1, an inhibitory protein that regulates function of adenylate cyclase (34).

There is now firm evidence (35,36) that myocardium from patients with advanced heart failure exhibits a down-regulation of gene expression for the calcium ATPase pump of sarcoplasmic reticulum, as well as the regulatory protein of the sarcoplasmic reticulum, phospholamban. These abnormalities are consistent with other studies showing depressed function of sarcoplasmic reticular calcium uptake mechanism in advanced heart failure. Thus, there is an increasing body of evidence to suggest that diastolic dysfunction in advanced heart failure is commonly associated with impaired intracellular calcium homeostasis. While the mechanisms for this impaired calcium cycling are yet to be fully understood, altered gene expression of ion pumps and regulatory proteins appears to play an important role.

IV. CLINICAL IMPLICATIONS

Both systolic heart and diastolic heart failure may be present in the same patient, although each can be seen in isolation. While much has been written about systolic dysfunction, heart failure due to diastolic dysfunction has been of increasing interest in recent years. Diastolic dysfunction may be due to mechanical factors, biochemical alterations within heart muscle cells, or both in combination. The biochemical alterations may be the immediate consequence of impaired coronary blood flow (for example, decreased high-energy phosphates); in addition, changes in gene expression of critical ion pumps and regulatory proteins have now been demonstrated to occur in myocardium from patients with advanced heart failure. Thus, it appears likely that molecular biological research will add importantly to our understanding of heart failure in a variety of clinical conditions.

REFERENCES

1. Lawrence DH. Essay on love. In Herbert M, ed. Reflections on the death of a porcupine and other essays. Cambridge: The Cambridge Edition of the Works of D.H. Lawrence, p 7.
2. Koretsune Y, Corretti MC, Kusuoka H, Marban E. Mechanism of early ischemic contractile failure. Inexcitability, metabolite accumulation, or vascular collapse? Circ Res 1991; 68:255–62.
3. Kihara Y, Grossman W, Morgan JP. Direct measurement of changes in intracellular calcium transients during hypoxia, ischemia, and reperfusion of the intact mammalian heart. Circ Res 1989; 65:1029–44.
4. Momomura SI, Ingwall J, Parker JA, Sahagian P, Ferguson JJ, Grossman W. The relationships of high energy phosphates, tissue pH, and regional blood flow to diastolic distensibility in the ischemic dog myocardium. Circ Res 1985; 57:822–35.
5. Danziger RS, Sakai M, Capogrossi MC, Spurgeon HA, Hansford RG, Lakatta EG. Ethanol acutely and reversibly suppresses excitation–contraction coupling in cardiac myocytes. Circ Res 1991; 68:1660–8.
6. Anversa P, Loud AV, Levicky V, Guideri G. Left ventricular failure induced by myocardial infarction. I. Myocyte hypertrophy. Am J Physiol 1985;248:H876–H882.
7. McKay RG, Pfeffer MA, Pasternak RC, Markis JE, Come PC, Nakao S, Alderman JD, Ferguson JJ, Safian RD, Grossman W. Left ventricular remodeling following myocardial infarction: a corollary to infarct expression. Circulation 1986;74:693–702.
8. Ross J Jr. Afterload mismatch and preload reserve: a conceptual framework for the analysis of ventricular function. Progr Cardiovasc Dis 1976; 18:255–64.
9. Gunther S, Grossman W. Determinants of ventricular function in pressure-overload hypertrophy in man. Circulation 1979; 59:679–88.
10. Carabello BA, Green LH, Grossman W, Cohn LH, Koster JK, Collins JJ Jr. Hemo-

dynamic determinants of prognosis of aortic valve replacement in critical aortic stenosis and advanced congestive heart failure. Circulation 1980; 62:42–8.
11. McLaurin LP, Rolett EL, Grossman W. Impaired left ventricular relaxation during pacing-induced ischemia. Am J Cardiol 1973; 32:751–7.
12. Carroll JD, Hess OM, Hirzel HO, Krayenbuehl HP. Exercise-induced ischemia: the influence of altered relaxation on early diastolic pressures. Circulation 1983; 67:521–8.
13. Humphrey LS, Topol EJ, Rosenfeld GI, Borkon AM, Baumgartner WA, Gardner TJ, Maruschak G, Weiss JL. Immediate enhancement of left ventricular relaxation by coronary artery bypass grafting: intraoperative assessment. Circulation 1988; 77:886–96.
14. Serizawa T, Carabello BA, Grossman W. Effect of pacing-induced ischemia on left ventricular diastolic pressure-volume relations in dogs with coronary stenoses. Circ Res 1980; 46:430–9.
15. Momomura SI, Bradley AB, Grossman W. Left ventricular diastolic pressure-segment length relations and end-diastolic distensibility in dogs with coronary stenoses. An angina physiology model. Circ Res 1984; 55:203–14.
16. Aroesty JM, McKay RG, Heller GV, Royal HD, Als AV, Grossman W. Simultaneous assessment of left ventricular systolic and diastolic dysfunction during pacing-induced ischemia. Circulation 1985; 71:889–900.
17. Lecarpentier Y, Waldenström A, Clergue M, Chemla D, Oliviero P, Martin JL Swynghedauw B. Major alterations in relaxation during cardiac hypertrophy induced by aortic stenosis in guinea pig. Circ Res 1987; 61:107–16.
18. Grossman W, McLaurin LP, Rolett EL. Alterations in left ventricular relaxation and diastolic compliance in congestive cardiomyopathy. Cardiovasc Res 1979; 13:514–22.
19. Barry WH. Mechanical dysfunction of the heart during and after ischemia. Unraveling the causes. Circulation 1990: 82:652–4.
20. Bronzwaer JGF, de Bruyne B, Ascoop CAPL, Paulus WJ. Comparative effects of pacing-induced and balloon coronary occlusion ischemia on left ventricular diastolic function in man. Circulation 1991; 84:211–22.
21. Apstein CS, Grossman W. Opposite initial effects of supply and demand ischemia on left ventricular diastolic compliance: the ischemia–diastolic paradox. J Mol Cell Cardiol 1987; 19:119–28.
22. Ikenouchi H, Kohmoto O, McMillan M, Barry WH. Contributions of $[Ca^{2+}]_i$, $[P_i]_i$ and pH_i to altered diastolic myocyte tone during partial metabolic inhibition. J Clin Invest 1991; 88:55–61.
23. Weber KT, Brilla CG. Pathological hypertrophy and cardiac interstitium. Fibrosis and renin–angiotensin–aldosterone system. Circulation 1991; 83:1849–65.
24. Factor SM, Butany J, Sole MJ, Wigle ED, Williams WC, Rojkind M. Pathologic fibrosis and matrix connective tissue in the subaortic myocardium of patients with hypertrophic cardiomyopathy. J Am Coll Cardiol 1991; 17:1343–51.
25. Thiedemann KU, Holubarsch CH, Medugorac I, Jacob R. Connective tissue content and myocardial stiffness in pressure overload hypertrophy. A combined study of morphologic, morphometric, biochemical, and mechanical parameters. Basic Res Cardiol 1983; 78:140–55.
26. Hittinger L, Shannon RP, Bishop SP, Gelpi RJ, Vatner SF. Subendomyocardial exhaustion of blood flow reserve and increased fibrosis in conscious dogs with heart failure. Circ Res 1989; 65:971–80.
27. Douglas PS, Tallant B. Hypertrophy, fibrosis and diastolic dysfunction in early canine experimental hypertension. J Am Coll Cardiol 1991; 17:530–6.
28. Cuocolo A, Sax FL, Brush JE, Marion BJ, Bacharach SL, Bonow RO. Left ventricular hypertrophy and impaired diastolic filling in essential hypertension. Diastolic mechanisms for systolic dysfunction during exercise. Circulation 1990; 81:978–86.

29. Fifer M, Bourdillon PD, Lorell BH. Altered left ventricular diastolic properties during pacing-induced angina in patients with aortic stenosis. Circulation 1986; 74:675–83.
30. Lorell BH, Paulus WJ, Grossman W, Wynne J, Cohn PF. Modification of abnormal left ventricular diastolic properties by nifedipine in patients with hypertrophic cardiomyopathy. Circulation 1982; 65:499–507.
31. Gwathmey JK, Warren SE, Briggs GM, Copelas L, Feldman MD, Phillips PJ, Callahan M Jr, Schoen FJ, Grossman W, Morgan JP, et al. Diastolic dysfunction in hypertrophy cardiomyopathy. Effect on active force generation during systole. J Clin Invest 1991; 87:1023–1031.
32. Gwathmey JK, Copelas L, MacKinnon R, Schoen FJ, Feldman MD, Grossman W, Morgan JP. Abnormal intracellular calcium handling in myocardium from patients with end-stage heart failure. Circ Res 1987; 61:70–6.
33. Feldman MD, Copelas L, Gwathmey JK, Phillips P, Warren SE, Schoen FJ, Grossman W, Morgan JP. Deficient production of cyclic AMP: pharmacologic evidence of an important cause of contractile dysfunction in patients with end-stage heart failure. Circulation 1987; 75:331–9.
34. Feldman AM, Cates AE, Veazey WB, Hershberger RE, Bristow MR, Baughman KL, Baumgartner WA, Van Dop C. Increase of the 40,000-mol wt pertussis toxin substrate (G protein) in the failing human heart. J Clin Invest 1988; 82:189–97.
35. Mercadier JJ, Lompre AM, Duc P, Boheler KR, Fraysse JB, Wisnewsky C, Allen PD, Komajda M, Schwartz K. Altered sarcoplasmic reticulum (Ca^{2+}-ATPase gene expression in the human ventricle during end-stage heart failure. J Clin Invest 1990; 85:305–9.
36. Feldman AM, Ray PE, Silan CM, Mercer JA, Minobe W, Bristow MR. Selective gene expression in failing human heart. Quantification of steady-state levels of messenger RNA in endomyocardial biopsies using the polymerase chain reaction. Circulation 1991; 83:1866–72.

2

Excitation–Contraction Coupling in Mammalian Ventricle

WITHROW GIL WIER

University of Maryland School of Medicine
Baltimore, Maryland

I. INTRODUCTION

Excitation–contraction coupling (E–C coupling) in muscle consists of all the cellular processes that link electrical excitation of the surface membrane to development of force or shortening. In general terms, these cellular processes produce a transient rise in cytoplasmic free calcium ion concentration ($[Ca^{2+}]_i$-transient)(1,2) that activates contraction by increasing the binding of Ca^{2+} to contractile proteins. In considering E–C coupling in heart, it must be recognized that cells from different regions of individual hearts and cells from hearts of different species are diverse in both structure (3) and function. Since the main target of *inotropic interventions* is the human ventricle, mainly excitation–contraction coupling in the ventricular cells of mammals and humans will be considered here. In the most general terms, the physical or molecular elements of E–C coupling in mammalian ventricular cells are the surface membrane (sarcolemma; SL) including its transverse-tubules (t-tubules), the sarcoplasmic reticulum (SR), and the contractile proteins (myofilaments). Alterations in inotropic state are known to be effected by modulation of many of the diverse cellular processes taking place in these structural elements. Nevertheless, there seem to be only two *final* effectors in modulation of inotropic state: cytoplasmic free calcium ion concentration ($[Ca^{2+}]_i$), and the contractile proteins themselves. Function of some, at least, of the contractile proteins (e.g., troponin C,) may be modulated by phosphorylation (4), by nuclear control (e.g., shifts in myosin isoform content [5]), or by physical factors such as sarcomere length (6). In this chapter, however, I will focus mainly on the role of the $[Ca^{2+}]_i$-transient as a modulator of inotropic state. I will be concerned particularly with the cellular processes that link excitation in the sarcolemma to release of Ca^{2+} from the SR, since under most normal physiological conditions most of the Ca^{2+} that activates contraction (by binding to troponin C) is derived directly from the sarcoplasmic reticulum (7). The actual action of various inotropic

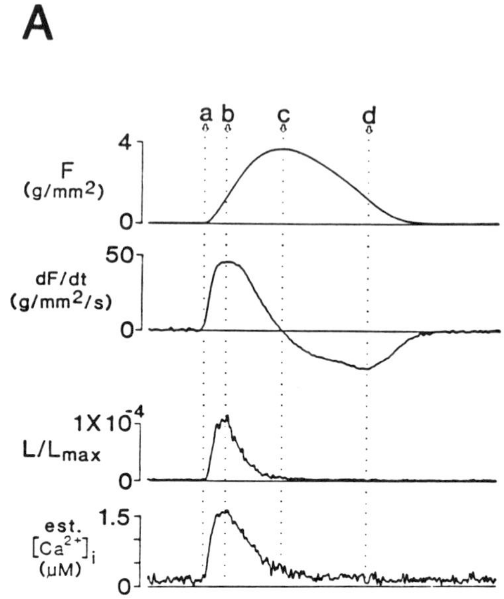

Figure 1 A. $[Ca^{2+}]_i$-transient and force of isometric contraction in a ferret right ventricular papillary muscle at 30°C. (Data from Ref. 13.) B. Action potential and $[Ca^{2+}]_i$-transient in a single isolated guinea-pig ventricular myocyte at 21°C. (Data from Ref. 57.) $[Ca^{2+}]_i$-transients recorded from papillary muscles contracting isometrically (A) are obtained under experimental conditions that are nearly physiological, but are subject to considerable quantitative uncertainty because of uncertainty in interpretation of the indicator signal (aequorin luminescence). A reasonably certain point is that $[Ca^{2+}]_i$ has declined to low levels by the time of the peak force of contraction. $[Ca^{2+}]_i$-transients recorded from single isolated cells using fluorescent Ca^{2+}-indicators (B) are subject to somewhat less quantitative uncertainty but are usually obtained under less physiological conditions: after enzymatic dissociation of the heart, at low temperature, and during unloaded shortening. The considerable difference between the time course of the two $[Ca^{2+}]_i$-transients may be related to the different indicators used or to the different experimental conditions.

agents on the sarcoplasmic reticulum and on the other molecules and cellular processes involved in E–C coupling is the subject of other chapters in this book.

Figure 1A illustrates a $[Ca^{2+}]_i$-transient, as calculated from aequorin luminescence (8), and force development in a mammalian (ferret) right ventricular papillary muscle at 30°C. Figure 1B illustrates the action potential and $[Ca^{2+}]_i$-transient of a single isolated guinea pig ventricular myocyte, at 21°C. As mentioned above, it is the rise in cytosolic $[Ca^{2+}]_i$ that links most directly excitation (action potential) of the sarcolemma (SL) to cell shortening or force development. A brief, introductory discussion of the theory of such $[Ca^{2+}]_i$-transients and their relation to force generation or shortening will be given, before the more detailed sections that follow. A detailed discussion of the theory and interpretation of $[Ca^{2+}]_i$-transients is available elsewhere (9,10).

A. Relationship Between $[Ca^{2+}]_i$ and Force

The relationship between $[Ca^{2+}]_i$ and force generation or shortening will not be discussed extensively in this chapter. For detailed information on this topic, the

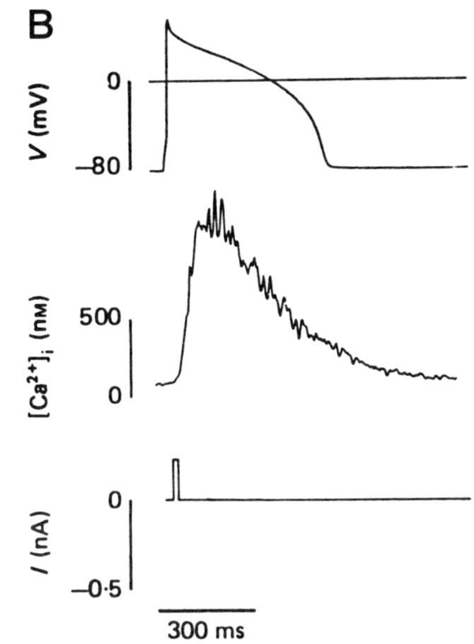

Figure 1 Continued

reader is referred elsewhere (11–16). Certainly the binding of Ca^{2+} to troponin C is the event that initiates the sequence of chemical and mechanical events leading to force generation or shortening. In cardiac muscle, it seems clear that it will be the binding of one Ca^{2+} to the one high-affinity Ca^{2+}-site on troponin C. Even in the steady state however, the relationship between $[Ca^{2+}]$ and force is complex; the steepness (16) and length-dependence of pCa-tension curves (17) in vivo and in skinned muscle may indicate co-operativity or force dependence in Ca^{2+} binding. The dynamic relationship between $[Ca^{2+}]_i$ and force (13) is expected to be yet more complex. Nevertheless, experiments in which $[Ca^{2+}]_i$ was measured with aequorin during contractions of ferret papillary muscle that covered the physiological range (i.e., from a closely coupled extrasystolic contraction to a highly potentiated postextrasystolic contraction) indicated a very close correlation between $[Ca^{2+}]_i$ and peak force development or peak rate of force development (Fig. 2).

B. The $[Ca^{2+}]_i$-transient

Many inotropic interventions are mediated by changes in the $[Ca^{2+}]_i$-transient during E–C coupling. Observations of $[Ca^{2+}]_i$-transients are often the first step in determining the mechanism of action of inotropic agents. Even when this formidable experimental task can be performed reliably, however, the mechanism of the inotropic agent may not be deduced easily because the $[Ca^{2+}]_i$-transient is determined dynamically by a large number of cellular processes. Also, present techniques for observing $[Ca^{2+}]_i$-transients do not reveal the subcellular spatial inhomogeneity of $[Ca^{2+}]_i$ that almost certainly exists in certain regions of the cell during E–C coupling. Nevertheless, observations of $[Ca^{2+}]_i$-transients are an important technique in the study of inotropic interventions and therefore I will present here a highly simplified theory of $[Ca^{2+}]_i$-transients. Despite the simplicity of this theory, it

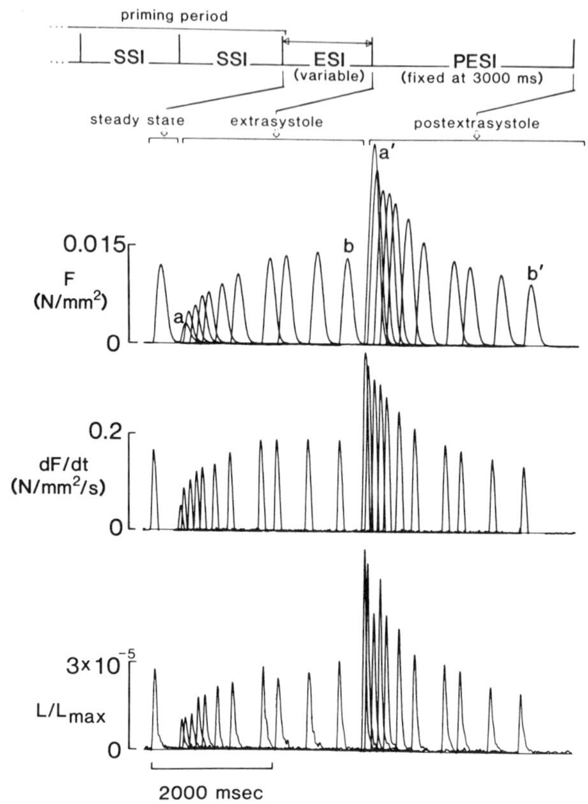

(A)

Figure 2 Relationship between amplitude of the $[Ca^{2+}]_i$-transient and force of isometric contraction in mammalian heart, over a large portion of the range of force production of which the papillary muscle is capable in a twitch contraction. A. Data from a ferret right ventricular papillary muscle contracting isometrically at 30°C. Superimposed tracing of isometric force development (F), rate of force development (dF/dt) (middle), and aequorin luminescence (L/L_{max}, bottom trace). The stimulus protocol (inset, above) was arranged so that the range of contractions produced was from a closely coupled extrasystolic contraction (a) to highly potentiated postextrasystolic contraction (a′). B. Graphs show a good (approximately linear) correlation between $[Ca^{2+}]_i$ estimated with aequorin luminescence and either peak force (F_{max}) or peak rate of force development (dF/dt_{max}). (From Ref. 15.)

can be useful in evaluating the contribution to the $[Ca^{2+}]_i$-transient of the various cellular processes that may be involved in an inotropic intervention. Such a simple theory is, in fact, the underlying assumption, whether or not it is stated (or even recognized), in most studies of $[Ca^{2+}]_i$-transients in heart.

C. Theory of $[Ca^{2+}]_i$-Transients in Mammalian Ventricle

The basic theoretical consideration is that for a small volume of the cytoplasm of a cardiac cell, the rate of change of $[Ca^{2+}]$ within it is determined by the sum of the fluxes (diffusional and transmembrane), and other movements (as from binding and unbinding to ligands), of free calcium ions (Ca^{2+}) into and out of that volume. The transmembrane fluxes are those occurring across surface or organellar mem-

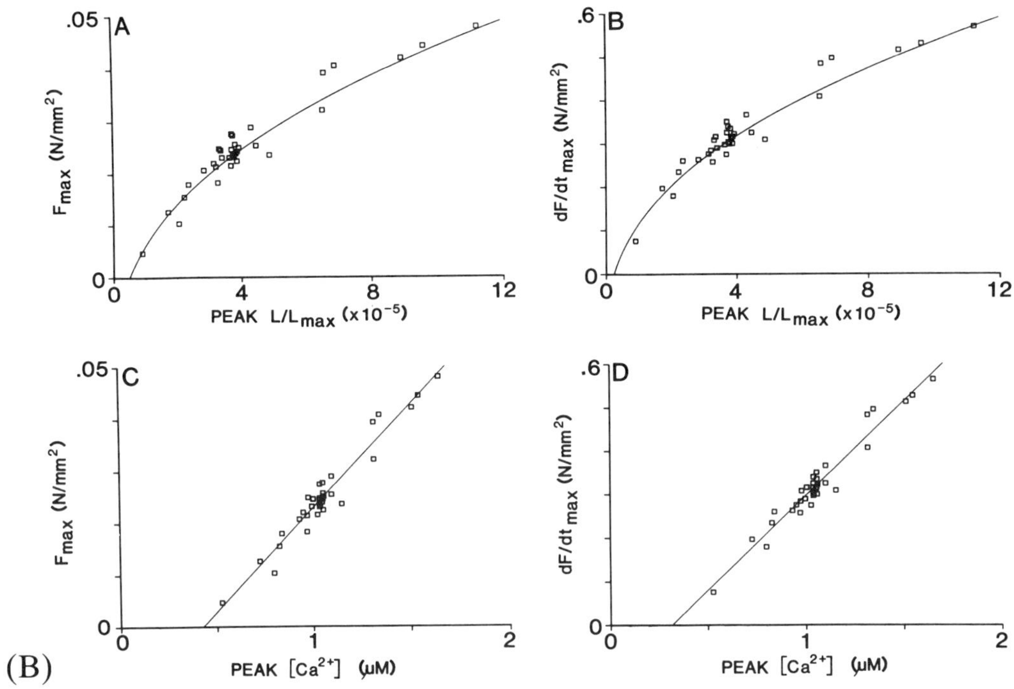

Figure 2 Continued

branes and the diffusional fluxes are those of Ca^{2+} from neighboring regions (elements, in finite element analysis) of cytoplasm, in which the $[Ca^{2+}]_i$ is different. Ca^{2+} also moves onto or off of binding sites (Ca^{2+}-ligands, such as troponin C) within the cytoplasm. A cardiac cell is highly heterogeneous with respect to the location of Ca^{2+}-binding ligands, organelles, or membranes that may bind, sequester, or release Ca^{2+}. An example of particular relevance to E–C coupling is the t-tubule–SR junction (discussed in detail below) in which Ca^{2+}-release channels of SR face a narrow gap (15 nm wide) between t-tubule membrane and SR membrane. In heart, L-type Ca^{2+}-channels may be located on the opposite side of the gap, in the t-tubule membrane. This juxtaposition of Ca^{2+}-channels, in a restricted space, makes it virtually certain that the $[Ca^{2+}]_i$ in the gap will be, at least for a time during Ca^{2+}-entry or Ca^{2+}-release, far different from that in other places in the cytoplasm. ($[Ca^{2+}]_i$-gradients are predicted from theory near the mouths of open Ca^{2+}-channels [18].) Ultimately, full understanding of E–C coupling must involve knowledge of $[Ca^{2+}]_i$ in this space, since Ca^{2+} is believed to bind to molecular sites located in this space and thereby modulate both its own entry through the L-type Ca^{2+} channels and its own release from SR (by binding to sites that activate and inactivate SR Ca^{2+}-release channels). $[Ca^{2+}]_i$ cannot be observed in spaces of these dimensions by any techniques now available. For most practical purposes, therefore, it is necessary to assume that the mammalian ventricular cell is a single homogeneous volume with respect to $[Ca^{2+}]_i$ during normal E–C coupling. This simplifies enormously the theory of the $[Ca^{2+}]_i$-transient because diffusional fluxes of cytoplasmic Ca^{2+} driven by concentration gradients need not be considered. The justification for this is that

$[Ca^{2+}]_i$-transients during E–C coupling *appear* to be spatially uniform, insofar as they can be observed with digital imaging fluorescence microscopy (19), and there is thus a lack of experimental evidence that would compel the consideration of $[Ca^{2+}]_i$ gradients; and that theory indicates that gradients of $[Ca^{2+}]_i$ within the myofilament space of each sarcomere may be small (the calculations did not consider regions as small as the t-tubule–SR junction). Experimental evidence and theoretical considerations suggest, therefore, that $[Ca^{2+}]_i$-gradients during normal E–C coupling are restricted to very small confined spaces or within molecular distances of membranes and channels. In order to proceed, there is little choice, therefore, but to make the (heuristic) assumption that there are no spatial inhomogeneities of $[Ca^{2+}]_i$ in a mammalian cardiac cell during normal E–C coupling. Of course, $[Ca^{2+}]_i$ can be observably nonuniform under some, abnormal, conditions in mammalian heart cells (19–21). In that case, the assumption of spatial uniformity would clearly not be justified or useful.

A mammalian ventricular cell will be assumed (Fig. 3) in which Ca^{2+} can move across surface membrane (SL) and sarcoplasmic reticulum membrane (SR). Mitochondrial membrane will be neglected, in accordance with recent results (22). SL is assumed to contain Na/Ca exchanger (23), L-type Ca^{2+}-channels (24), a Ca^{2+}-leak pathway (25), an ATP driven Ca^{2+}-pump (26), and low-affinity Ca^{2+}-binding sites (27). SR is assumed to contain Ca^{2+}-release channels (28), an ATP driven Ca^{2+}-pump (29) and Ca^{2+}-binding sites (SRb) (27). The Ca^{2+}-binding molecules (ligands) assumed to be in the cytoplasm (27) will be calmodulin (Cm), troponin C (TnC), and phosphate (phos). (The nth ligand is symbolized as "L_n".) Fluxes are denoted by "J," with the appropriate subscript, and have as units moles of Ca^{2+}/sec/cm^2 of membrane (SR or SL). Since it is assumed that $[Ca^{2+}]_i$ is uniform within the cell,

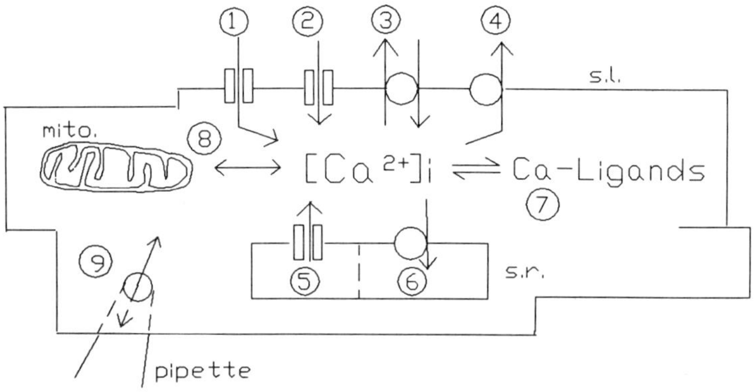

Figure 3 Simplified schema of excitation–contraction coupling. The various cellular processes that determine the $[Ca^{2+}]_i$-transient are indicated schematically and numbered according to the following key: 1. L-type Ca^{2+} channels in the surface membrane; 2. an unspecified "leak" pathway for Ca^{2+} entry into the cytoplasm; 3. the Na/Ca exchanger; 4. the Ca^{2+}-pumping ATPase of the surface membrane; 5. the Ca^{2+}-release channel of the sarcoplasmic reticulum (SR); 6. The Ca^{2+}-pumping ATPase of the SR; 7. the Ca^{2+}-binding molecules in the cytoplasm (ligands; troponin c, calmodulin, and others), 8. mitochondrial transport of Ca^{2+}; 9. the flux of Ca^{2+} that may occur from a micropipette electrode, when one is present in a typical experimental situation. The contribution of these cellular processes to the $[Ca^{2+}]_i$-transient is described mathematically by Equation (1).

there is no diffusional flux of Ca^{2+}. In this simplified, hypothetical mammalian cardiac cell, the rate of change of $[Ca^{2+}]_i$ at any instant in time will be given by Equation (1).

$$
\begin{aligned}
d[Ca^{2+}]_i/dt = {} & k_{SR} * (J_{SR_{rel}} + J_{SR_{pump}}) \\
& + k_{SL} * (J_{NaCa} + J_{I_{Ca}} + J_{Ca_{leak}} + J_{SL_{pump}}) \\
& - \text{Sum}\{d[CaL]_n/dt\}
\end{aligned} \tag{1}
$$

Flux out of the cytoplasm is considered a negative value.

where: $[CaL]_0 = [CaCm]$, $[CaL]_1 = [CaTnC]$, $[CaL]_2 = [Caphos]$, $[CaL]_3 = [CaSLb]$, $[CaL]_4 = [CaSRb]$, k_{SL} = (cell surface area)/(cell volume), k_{SR} = (SR surface area)/(cell volume), and $d[CaL]n/dt = k_{on} * [Ca^{2+}]_i * [L]_n - k_{off} * [CaL]_n$.

(A similar equation has been developed for describing $[Ca^{2+}]_i$-transients in skeletal muscle [30].) It will be shown later in this chapter that the release of Ca^{2+} from the SR, $J_{SR_{rel}}$, dominates Equation (1), under most normal circumstances in ventricular cells of the mammalian heart.

II. STRUCTURAL BASIS OF E–C COUPLING IN MAMMALIAN VENTRICLE

Evaluation of theories of E–C coupling is aided by knowledge of the location and physical characteristics (quaternary structure and dimensions) of the molecules involved. For example, "charge-coupled" mechanisms of release of Ca^{2+} from SR (31,32) in which electrically charged molecules in the SL move, with consequent mechanical effects on Ca^{2+} channels of the SR, require that such molecules exist in certain geometrical arrangements. In heart muscle, there is indirect evidence that Ca^{2+} channels may exist in SR that is far from any surface membrane (in addition to the SR Ca^{2+} channels at the t-tubule SR junction). The possibility for mechanical interaction of these channels with junctional SR channels is clearly unlikely. Thus, the information available on the structural basis of E–C coupling in mammalian cardiac muscle will be presented briefly.

Figure 4 illustrates schematically the general structure of a sarcomere of mammalian cardiac muscle. As represented here, a sarcomere is considered to consist of a segment of a cardiac ventricular cell that contains a single myofibrillar bundle (of myofilaments), bounded by Z discs, and containing invaginated portions of the sarcolemma (transverse tubules), sarcoplasmic reticulum, mitochondria, and other structures. All the cellular processes believed to be important in E–C coupling are contained within each sarcomere, as discussed briefly in each section below.

A. Surface Membrane

With regular spacing, the SL is invaginated, into transverse tubules (t-tubules) that contact sarcomeres in the region of the Z discs. As in skeletal muscle, the function of the t-tubules is probably to conduct the action potential into the interior of the cell and thus to make electrical excitation available to sarcomeres there. However, of all the vertebrates, only mammals have ventricular cells that possess t-tubules; atrial cells and Purkinje fibers of mammals do not (3). Aside from the ion-channels involved in the action potential, the major molecules contained in the SL that are known to be important on a beat-to-beat basis in E–C coupling are Ca^{2+}-pumping ATPase, sodium–calcium (Na/Ca) exchangers, and an unknown leak pathway for

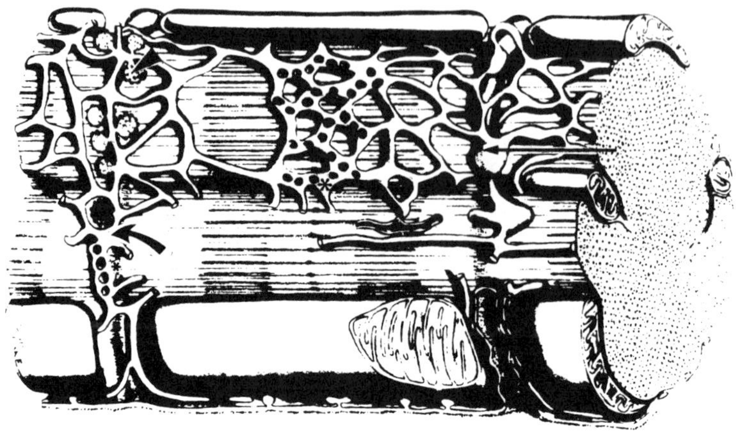

Figure 4 Schematic diagram of sarcomere of mammalian cardiac cell. Arrowhead indicates corbular SR. Curved arrow and straight arrows indicate junctional SR. Large and small asterisks indicate, respectively, fenestrations in the M and Z retes of the sarcoplasmic reticulum. (From Ref. 93.)

Ca^{2+}. (Other molecules located in the SL, such as adrenergic receptors, membrane-bound inositol phosphates, other phospholipids, other ATPases [Na/K], enzymes, and many others are certainly important in E–C coupling, but are not thought to be involved directly in the mechanism coupling t-tubule electrical depolarization to the change in $[Ca^{2+}]_i$ on each beat.) Judging from the D-600 sensitive charge movement in mammalian cardiac muscle (33), there must be many dihydropyridine (DHP) receptors in the SL of cardiac muscle, and it is not known whether these are all functional L-type Ca^{2+}-channels. In general terms, the contribution of these molecules to the generation of Ca^{2+}-transients is expressed mathematically in Equation (1), as discussed.

B. Sarcoplasmic Reticulum

In general, the SR is an internal membrane-bound compartment consisting of a network of flattened sacs and tubular regions that surround the myofibril. There is little doubt that it serves the functions of release and uptake of Ca^{2+} during E–C coupling. The SR contains several types of ion channels and other molecules, but the molecules believed to be most important in E–C coupling on a beat-to-beat basis are the Ca^{2+}-pumping ATPase, and the molecules at the t-tubule–SR junctions. According to a recent review (3) SR present in mammalian ventricular cells may be classified as two types; junctional sarcoplasmic reticulum (JSR) is that portion of the sarcoplasmic reticulum that contains junctional processes, whether or not these junctional processes occur at t–SR junctions, and *free* sarcoplasmic reticulum (FSR), which is that portion that does not contain junctional processes. Junctional processes are the structures that can be seen to span the gap between t-tubule membrane and SR membrane. Junctional processes may be the Ca^{2+}-channels through which Ca^{2+} is released from the SR, and thus their structure and localization within the cell are significant.

1. Free Sarcoplasmic Reticulum

According to Sommer and Jennings (3) this portion of the SR appears smooth in electron micrographs. It is presumed to be specialized for sequestration of Ca^{2+}, although it is known to contain small conductance Ca^{2+}-channels (34). The FSR forms "light" vesicles upon homogenization and sucrose density centrifugation. FSR contains several molecules that are, or could be, the target of inotropic interventions: Ca^{2+}-pumping ATPase, phospholamban, the small-conductance Ca^{2+}-channel, and others.

2. Junctional Sarcoplasmic Reticulum

The JSR has been classified as three distinguishable types (3). The SR that actually makes contact with t-tubular or sarcolemmal membrane will be referred to as JSR_j (Fig. 5). This is what is conventionally referred to as "junctional SR." JSR that does not make such contacts, but is otherwise indistinguishable from JSR_j, has been termed *extended junctional SR,* referred to here as JSR_e. JSR that has formed into "little baskets," particularly at Z-lines that lack transverse tubules, has been termed *corbular SR,* and will be referred to here as JSR_c (Fig. 6). As a final distinction, JSR_e has been noted to exist in two forms, that which is *continuous* with JSR_j, and that which is *discontinuous,* in that it is intercalated, particularly at Z-lines, into the FSR.

a. Junctional Processes. Junctional processes of cardiac muscle are defined as those structures that can be seen to span the gap between SR and SL (Fig. 5) (surface membrane to t-tubule). Junctional processes in cardiac muscle may be analogous to the "foot proteins" described in detail for skeletal muscle (35–37). In that tissue, foot proteins contain a ryanodine-binding site (38) and have Ca^{2+}-channel activity when reconstituted into lipid bilayers (39,40). According to Block and her colleagues (36) the foot protein actually consists, in its entirety, of a tetrameric intramembranous component (presumed to be the "Ca^{2+}-release channel", through which Ca^{2+} would be released from within SR during E–C coupling), and another tetrameric component (the foot), which spans the junctional gap between t-tubular membrane and SR membrane.

Vesicles made from "heavy SR" (presumed to be junctional SR) of both skeletal and cardiac muscle contain Ca^{2+} channels that are activated and inactivated by Ca^{2+} (more on this later) and are similarly affected by Ca^{2+}, Mg^{2+}, ATP, ruthenium red, and ryanodine (27,41–43). (Ryanodine is a specific marker for SR Ca^{2+}-channels.) Anderson and her colleagues (43) also used negative stain electron microscopy to show that the ryanodine receptor–Ca^{2+}-channel complex from cardiac SR had a fourfold symmetrical, four-leaf clover structure (30 nm × 30 nm) similar in appearance to the "junctional-associated foot structure" (i.e., junctional process). From this and the physiological effects of ryanodine in cardiac muscle (44) it seems clear that the ryanodine receptor isolated from cardiac SR is the Ca^{2+}-release channel of the SR, as it is in skeletal muscle. Furthermore, it has been shown (45) that the ryanodine receptors isolated from SR of cardiac muscle and skeletal muscle are similar at the molecular level in some respects; both are oligomers of a unique high-molecular weight polypeptide. The three-dimensional structure of the Ca^{2+}-release channel of skeletal muscle (but not cardiac muscle) has been revealed by computerized analysis of tilted and untilted negatively stained electron microscopic images of

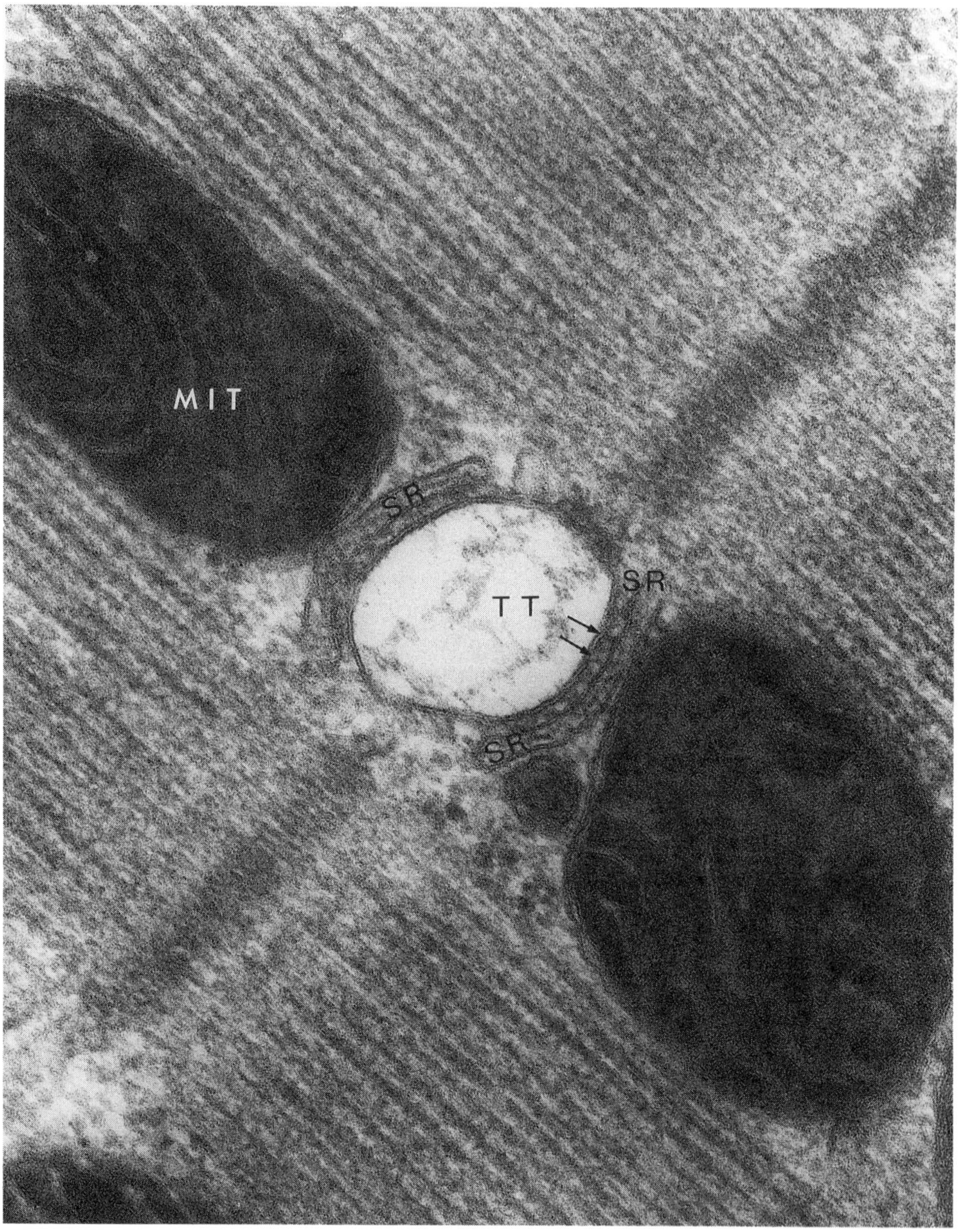

Figure 5 Thin section electron micrograph of t-tubule—SR junction in rat papillary muscle. Arrows indicate the junctional processes or "feet." TT, transverse-tubule; MIT, mitochondria; SR, sarcoplasmic reticulum. (From Ref. 46.)

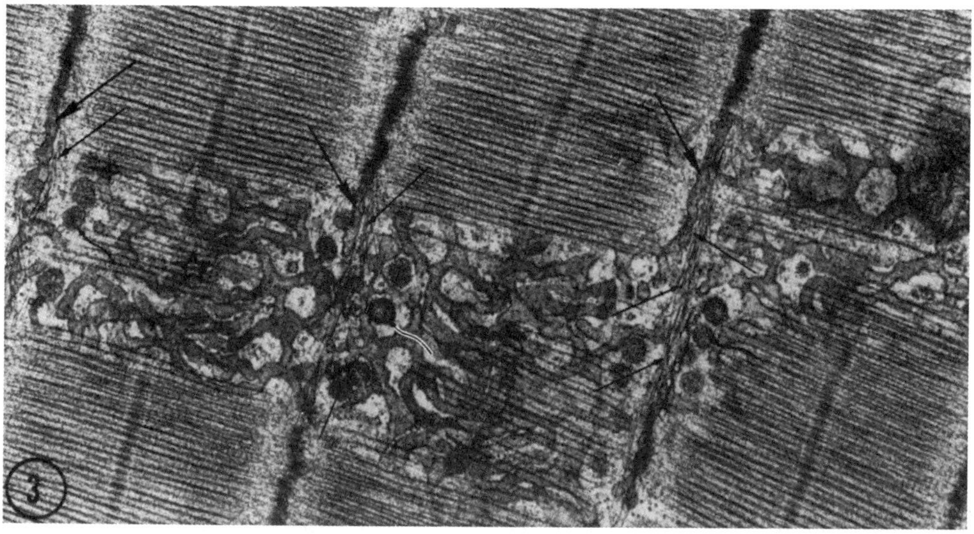

Figure 6 Corbular SR (JSR_c) in a primitive mammal (opossum). Corbular SR is indicated by the curved arrows. (From Ref. 92.)

isolated foot proteins (37). The images generated by the computer are complex, indicating a volume that contains a central channel with four channels radially branching off from it. These extend into vestibules in the peripheral regions of the volume. The function of these channels in conducting Ca^{2+} during E–C coupling has not been established yet.

The issue of whether junctional processes is extended junctional SR or corbular SR are Ca^{2+}-release channels is very important in a consideration of mechanisms of E–C coupling. If such junctional processes are Ca^{2+}-release channels, the mechanism of Ca^{2+} release from them cannot involve a charge-coupled mechanism. Jorgensen and her colleagues (90) have observed, through microprobe analysis of rat papillary muscle, that corbular SR stores Ca^{2+}, like junctional SR. These authors noted that their results were consistent with the idea that both the corbular SR and the (true) junctional SR (JSR_j) are potential sources of Ca^{2+} that could be released during E–C coupling.

In summary, cardiac and skeletal muscle both contain structures that span the junction between t-tubule and SR membrane. These structures appear similar in the two tissues. In heart, they have been termed junctional processes. In skeletal muscle, they have been termed foot proteins and the foot proteins are, at once, the Ca^{2+}-release channel of the SR and the ryanodine receptor. The SR of heart muscle also contains Ca^{2+}-channels and ryanodine receptors. On the molecular level, ryanodine receptors of skeletal and cardiac muscle are similar in many respects. It is not yet established however, that the junctional processes identified in cardiac muscle, particularly those (Fig. 6) found in SR away from true junctions (3) (Fig. 5) are, in fact, the same as or analogous to the foot proteins of skeletal muscle or the foot proteins of the cardiac t-tubule SR junction.

b. Structure of t-SR Junction. The detailed structure of the transverse tubule–SR junction in mammalian cardiac muscle is not known in great detail. The freeze-fractured and rotary shadowed images of t–SR junctions that have been so informative in revealing the detailed structure of the junction in skeletal muscle (36) are simply not available in cardiac muscle. Images of the t–SR junction in rat papillary muscle (46) (Fig. 5) obtained with transmission electron microscopy are similar in many respects to those in skeletal muscle and do not provide the basis to suggest specific differences between the structure of the t–SR junction in skeletal muscle and cardiac muscle. Ultrarapidly frozen, fractured, and etched images of the t-SR junction in cardiac muscle (46) reveal only the structures (junctional processes) that span the t–SR junction at highly regular spacing of 30 nm. Accordingly, the structure of the t–SR junction in skeletal muscle, which is known in more detail, will be reviewed briefly here. The assumption is that the junctional processes seen at the t–SR junctions of mammalian cardiac muscle are similar to the "foot proteins" that span the t–SR junction in skeletal muscle.

Block and her colleagues (36) have produced a putative three-dimensional reconstruction of the t–SR junction as it has been revealed in electron microscopy of skeletal muscle of various vertebrate species. The essential feature to note is the juxtaposition of ryanodine receptors (foot proteins) with "Jt–tubule tetrads" (DHP receptors). Only every other DHP receptor faces a SR Ca^{2+}-channel (foot protein). The close juxtaposition of the two molecules provides a basis, in theory, for a "charge-coupled" release mechanism (31). The DHP molecules are voltage-sensors, and are believed to move, revealed as charge movement (31), in response to changes in electrical polarization of the t-tubular membrane. By virtue of a possible connection between DHP receptor and SR Ca^{2+}-release channel, the SR Ca^{2+}-release channel could be opened. The structure of the t–SR junction also provides a possible basis for a Ca^{2+}-induced release of Ca^{2+} mechanism, both in skeletal and in heart muscle, as discussed extensively below.

III. PUTATIVE MECHANISMS OF RELEASE OF Ca^{2+} FROM SR

A. Ca^{2+}-Induced Release of Ca^{2+}

1. *Ca^{2+}-Induced Release of Ca^{2+} in Cardiac Cells*

Fabiato (47–49) has described a phenomenon in "skinned" mammalian cardiac cells in which Ca^{2+} is released from SR after the rapid elevation of free $[Ca^{2+}]$ at the outer surface of the SR. Through the use of an elegant experimental technique, Fabiato was able to change the $[Ca^{2+}]_i$ rapidly around the outer aspect of myofibrillar bundles, as shown in Figure 4. The intent of the experiments was to stimulate the change in $[Ca^{2+}]_i$ that might be provided in intact cells by the Ca^{2+} current, and to observe any subsequent release of Ca^{2+} from the SR.

Several features of the experimental technique deserve note before further discussion. The preparation Fabiato used was dog Purkinje fiber. These cells lack t-tubules. SR makes junctional contact with SL in "peripheral couplings." The preparations were fragments of single, mechanically skinned Purkinje cells and it seems reasonable to assume that the peripheral couplings were largely removed by the skinning procedure. The SR that remained must therefore have been FSR, JSR_e, or JSR_c, and not JSR_j. For reasons discussed later, it can be inferred that the extensive SR that did surround the myofibrillar bundle "shielded" the myofibrils from the imposed change in $[Ca^{2+}]_i$ of the bulk solution, by pumping Ca^{2+} from the bulk solution into itself (the SR) so rapidly that none of the Ca^{2+} in the bulk solution could reach the interior of the myofibril. This could occur because the volume of the solution around the skinned cell was reduced (by aspiration) rapidly after the change in $[Ca^{2+}]_i$, and thus it did not constitute an infinite source of Ca^{2+}. Consequently, it must also be concluded that the $[Ca^{2+}]$ of the bulk solution became rapidly reduced from its initial level to an unknown level.

In summary, the experimental method used by Fabiato provided the ability to change $[Ca^{2+}]_i$ rapidly (1 ms) only at the outer surface of extended junctional SR. At that surface, the $[Ca^{2+}]_i$ was not controlled precisely, after the solution was aspirated. Finally, the rate at which the change in $[Ca^{2+}]_i$ of the bulk solution was reached could be controlled by injecting a new bulk solution around the myofibrillar bundle at a controlled rate. The change in $[Ca^{2+}]_i$ of the bulk solution "induced" a release of Ca^{2+} from the SR, which did reach the myofibrils, as evidenced by force development. Ca^{2+} released from the SR reached the myofibrils because, presumably, it was released from the SR in such a way or at such a rate that the Ca^{2+}-pumps of the SR did not have immediate access to it. This technique yielded several major experimental results, three of which are discussed in detail below.

a. *Release of Ca^{2+} from SR: Dependence on $[Ca^{2+}]_i$.* The first major experimental result of Fabiato (48) was that the amount of Ca^{2+} released from the SR had a bell-shaped dependence on the $[Ca^{2+}]_i$ of the bulk solution used to "induce" the release of Ca^{2+} from the SR. The change in $[Ca^{2+}]_i$ in the bulk solution was made quickly (1 msec). Thus, when the $[Ca^{2+}]$ in the bulk solution was increased rapidly above an "optimum" level, the amount of Ca^{2+} released from the SR was reduced. $[Ca^{2+}]$ above 1×10^{-5}M in the bulk solution failed to induce release of Ca^{2+} at all. When $[Ca^{2+}]$ of 3.16×10^{-5} M was maintained in the bulk solution by not aspirating after injection, tension development was delayed by about 750 msec. This phenomenon was explained on the basis that high $[Ca^{2+}]_i$ inhibits, or inactivates, release of Ca^{2+} by the SR, and that the SR provides a barrier to diffusion of [Ca^{2+} from the bulk solution to the interior of the myofibril, as discussed above.

b. *Removal of Inactivation of Ca^{2+} Release.* Fabiato found that some inactivation of Ca^{2+}-release was present at normal, resting $[Ca^{2+}]_i$. After $[Ca^{2+}]_i$ of the bulk solution was suddenly lowered, without reduction of volume by aspiration, the amount of Ca^{2+} released by a subsequent induction of Ca^{2+}-release became progressively larger. This result suggested that inactivation of Ca^{2+}-release was being removed, at the lower $[Ca^{2+}]$. (This experiment is analogous in some ways to that showing removal of inactivation of an ion-channel after a depolarizing pulse.) The removal of inactivation appeared to occur as a single exponential process, with a time constant of about 1 sec, depending on experimental conditions, and the process had a Q_{10} of 1.68.

c. *Release of Ca^{2+} from SR Depends on the Rate of Change of $[Ca^{2+}]$.* The third major experimental result of Fabiato was that the amount of Ca^{2+} released from SR was dependent on the rate at which the final $[Ca^{2+}]_i$ of the bulk solution was reached. Thus, a $[Ca^{2+}]_i$ in the bulk solution of 1×10^{-6} M induced progressively larger releases of Ca^{2+} when that concentration was reached in 50 msec, 20 msec, 10 msec, 5 msec, and 1 msec.

d. Putative Mechanism of Ca^{2+}-Induced Release of Ca^{2+} from SR. Fabiato suggested (48) that results described above (and others) could be explained if Ca^{2+}-induced release of Ca^{2+} is through a Ca^{2+}-channel in the SR that is both activated and inactivated by Ca^{2+}. The fact that removal of Ca^{2+}-dependent inactivation is slow and first order suggested that Ca^{2+} binds to the inactivating site with high affinity, in a stoichiometric ratio with the site of 1:1.

More specifically, it was suggested that Ca^{2+} activated release by binding rapidly to a low-affinity site and inactivated release by binding less rapidly to a higher-affinity site on the Ca^{2+}-channel of the SR (now thought to be the intramembranous portion of the "foot protein," in skeletal muscle). It may not be immediately obvious that such a scheme can account, at least qualitatively, for the results described above. Mathematical modeling of such a scheme (Wier, unpublished data) confirms that the probability of the channel being open (and thus permitting release of Ca^{2+}) could indeed be dependent on the rate of change of $[Ca^{2+}]$. Thus, the molecular scheme proposed by Fabiato is plausible in explaining the results in skinned cardiac cells.

e. Putative Role of Ca^{2+}-Induced Release of Ca^{2+} in E–C Coupling. It might be noted that the molecular scheme described above is ideal for allowing the L-type Ca^{2+}-current to induce release of Ca^{2+} from SR, since Ca^{2+}-current represents the rate of entry of Ca^{2+} into the cytoplasm. On this view, Ca^{2+}-release from the SR would be "induced" by Ca^{2+} provided during the early fast change in $[Ca^{2+}]_i$ that occurs at the time of the peak of the sarcolemmal Ca^{2+}-current. Ca^{2+} entering the cell during the maintained component of the Ca^{2+}-current would not trigger release, because the accumulation of Ca^{2+} would tend to be slow, but would instead be taken up by the SR.

Membrane voltage has no direct role in Ca^{2+}-induced release of Ca^{2+}, as described in this scheme. Indeed Fabiato has shown that many of the features of E–C coupling that have been observed in intact cardiac muscle can be produced in preparations without a sarcolemma, but with a simulated Ca^{2+} current (49).

2. Activation and Inactivation of SR Ca^{2+}-Fluxes by Ca^{2+} in Skeletal muscle

Ca^{2+} both activates and inactivates release of Ca^{2+} from heavy SR vesicles (41,50), mechanically skinned frog skeletal muscle fibers (51), and single SR Ca^{2+}-channels (52). In the single channel studies of Smith and his colleagues (52), the $[Ca^{2+}]$ required for inactivation was very high, far above physiological levels. In the study by Best and Kwok (51), however, maximum inactivation occurred at a $[Ca^{2+}]$ of 1.26×10^{-7} M, well within the physiological range of $[Ca^{2+}]$. Recently, evidence has been obtained through several lines of experimentation (53,54) in frog skeletal muscle for Ca^{2+}-dependent inactivation of SR Ca^{2+}-release, and, in the presence of caffeine, Ca^{2+}-induced release of Ca^{2+}.

B. Current Theories on Release of Ca^{2+} in Skeletal Muscle

For skeletal muscle, a new theory of E–C coupling that incorporates Ca^{2+}-induced release of Ca^{2+} (47–49), charge-coupled Ca^{2+}-release (31), and the morphologic data on the t–SR junction (above) has been formulated by Rios and Pizarro (55). Ultimately, the mechanism of E–C coupling in mammalian cardiac muscle may be found to be similar.

In skeletal muscle, Rios and Pizarro (55) have postulated that two release mechanisms operate in parallel, one a voltage-gated Ca^{2+}-release that requires that a metal ion be bound, and a Ca^{2+}-induced release of Ca^{2+} that is activated by Ca^{2+} released from the SR. After t-tubule depolarization, the voltage-gated Ca^{2+}-release occurs first, via mechanical allosteric modification of SR Ca^{2+}-release channels by voltage sensors (nonfunctional Ca^{2+}-channels or DHP receptors) in the t-tubule membrane. Ca^{2+}-induced release of Ca^{2+} occurs via Ca^{2+}-activation of SR Ca^{2+}-channels that do not face voltage sensors. SR release channels are also inactivated by Ca^{2+}.

IV. REVIEW OF DATA ON E–C COUPLING IN MAMMALIAN VENTRICLE

In this section I will review the data from physiological experiments that are relevant to E–C coupling. First, $[Ca^{2+}]_i$-transients from experiments on normal intact mammalian ventricular cells will be discussed, with respect to understanding the cellular processes that produce them, within the theory of the $[Ca^{2+}]_i$-transient and the structural basis for it discussed above. Information on the contributions of Na/Ca exchange, L-type Ca^{2+}-current, and other processes to the $[Ca^{2+}]_i$-transient will be presented, but it will be shown that, under normal conditions, it is mainly Ca^{2+} release and uptake from the SR that determines the Ca^{2+}-transient. Some of these experiments have also yielded substantial information on the process of Ca^{2+}-induced release of Ca^{2+} in intact cells.

Second, information from "Ca^{2+}-jump" experiments will be considered. These are experiments in which, through the use of photolabile Ca^{2+}-chelators, $[Ca^{2+}]_i$ can be manipulated in intact cells in a way similar to that achieved by Fabiato in single-skinned cardiac cells. Third, I will discuss recent results on charge movement in cardiac muscle. These experiments have the potential to provide information that is relevant to charge-coupled release hypotheses of E–C coupling.

A. $[Ca^{2+}]_i$-Transients in Mammalian Ventricular Cells

Recent studies that have utilized fluorescent Ca^{2+}-indicators to observe $[Ca^{2+}]_i$-transients in voltage-clamped single cardiac cells have produced substantial new information on E–C coupling. Representative results are illustrated in Figure 7. In general, the following points of agreement have emerged from all these studies: the initial rapid increase in $[Ca^{2+}]_i$ elicited by depolarization into the physiological range of membrane potential arises primarily from Ca^{2+} released from SR; release of Ca^{2+} from SR has a bell-shaped dependence on membrane potential, declining to low levels at positive membrane potentials; Ca^{2+} can also be released from SR upon repolarization from positive membrane potentials (e.g., Fig. 7; depolarization to +90 mV); the slow rise in $[Ca^{2+}]_i$ upon depolarization to very positive membrane potential arises from Ca^{2+}-entry via the Na/Ca exchanger; the flux of Ca^{2+} provided by the calcium current makes only a small contribution ($< 20\%$) to the $[Ca^{2+}]_i$-transient under normal conditions (i.e., when SR is normally loaded with Ca^{2+}); most of the Ca^{2+} released from the SR is resequestered by the SR; the Ca^{2+}-pumping ATPase of SL contributes relatively little to Ca^{2+}-efflux; and the Na/Ca exchanger is the major route of Ca^{2+} efflux during each beat. Each of these points is discussed in more detail below.

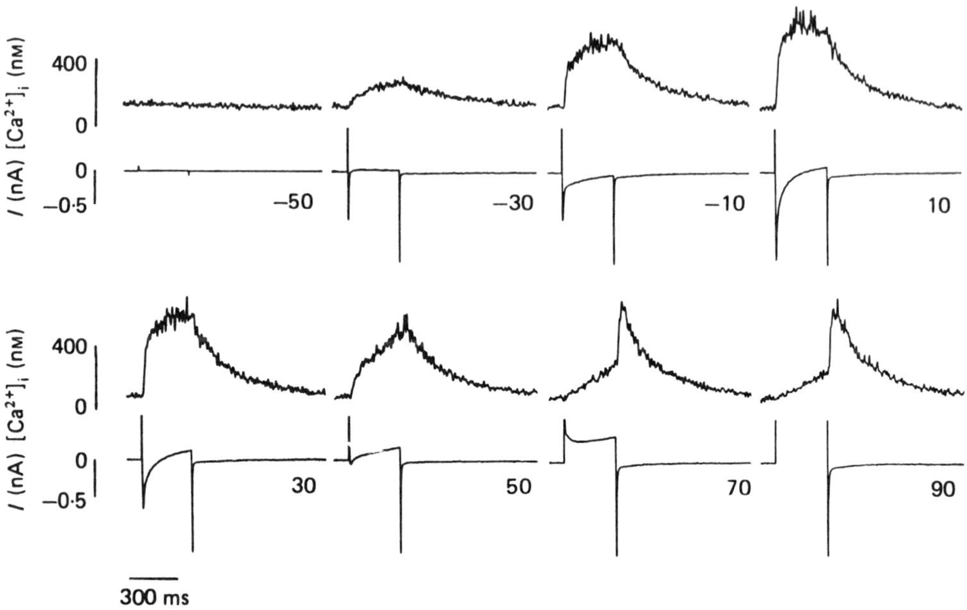

Figure 7 $[Ca^{2+}]_i$-transients and current during voltage clamp pulse depolarization from a holding potential of −68 mV. Voltage clamp pulses were to the membrane potentials indicated. Records are from a single isolated guinea pig ventricular myocyte at 21°C. (From Ref. 57.)

1. Sarcoplasmic Reticulum

A result common to all the recent studies is that depolarization into the range of the plateau of the action potential (+10 mV) elicits a large, rapidly rising $[Ca^{2+}]_i$-transient. This initial, rapid increase in $[Ca^{2+}]_i$ elicited by depolarization has been attributed primarily to Ca^{2+} released from the SR. The essential evidence in support of this is that in both guinea pig (56,57) and rat (58) ryanodine reduces this initial rise in $[Ca^{2+}]_i$ by up to 90%. Ryanodine is now known to "lock" the SR Ca^{2+}-release channel in a subconducting state. This seems to result in a more rapid loss of Ca^{2+} from the SR (60) and to interfere with the normal release of Ca^{2+} from the SR (44). Thus, depending on experimental conditions, the reduction of the $[Ca^{2+}]_i$-transient upon depolarization in the presence of ryanodine may arise either from depletion of Ca^{2+} in the SR or from interference with the release mechanism. In either case, however, the conclusion is valid that the initial rapid rise in the $[Ca^{2+}]_i$-transient upon depolarization results from Ca^{2+} released from the SR.

a. Ca^{2+} Release from SR on Depolarization. The use of single isolated cardiac cells and fluorescent Ca^{2+}-indicators has permitted the voltage dependence of the $[Ca^{2+}]_i$-transient, including release of Ca^{2+} from SR, to be studied more reliably than in the past. Before 1986, only one such study existed (61). The voltage-dependence of Ca^{2+} release from SR is expected to be of importance in identifying mechanisms of E–C coupling in mammalian cardiac muscle. The issue to be addressed is whether the voltage-dependence of the $[Ca^{2+}]_i$-transient reflects the voltage dependence of Ca^{2+}-current, as expected on the basis of Ca^{2+}-induced release of Ca^{2+}, or whether there is a direct influence of voltage, as expected from charge-coupled release mechanisms. If, as in skeletal muscle (62), Ca^{2+}-release from SR does not decline at positive membrane potentials, it is unlikely that Ca^{2+}-induced release of Ca^{2+} has a major role in E–C coupling, since Ca^{2+} current declines at positive membrane potentials, as Ca^{2+}-current approaches its reversal potential. In heart, the voltage dependence of the peak of the ryanodine sensitive $[Ca^{2+}]_i$-transient has been observed (57,58) as an indication of SR Ca^{2+}-release.

At least four studies (57,58,63,64) have now shown that the peak of the $[Ca^{2+}]_i$-transient in guinea pig or rat heart cells has a bell-shaped dependence on membrane potential. In all cases, these results have been interpreted to mean that release of Ca^{2+} from cardiac SR declines at positive potentials, a result that is distinctly different from that in skeletal muscle (62). All these studies have also shown that the voltage dependence of the peak $[Ca^{2+}]_i$-transient is shifted slightly to the left of that of L-type Ca^{2+}-current, but the significance of this finding in differentiating possible mechanisms of E–C coupling is not yet clear.

b. Ca^{2+} Release from SR on Repolarization. Increases in $[Ca^{2+}]_i$ *upon repolarization* (Fig. 7) have been observed in guinea pig ventricular cells (57,64) and in rat ventricular cells (58,63). Such $[Ca^{2+}]_i$-transients have been termed "repolarization transients" (63) or "tail transients" (57). The latter term will be used here since it reflects the putative connection between the $[Ca^{2+}]_i$-transient and the "tail" of Ca^{2+}-current that can occur upon repolarization from positive membrane potentials. Tail transients almost certainly arise from Ca^{2+} released from SR, since they are abolished by ryanodine (57,58). Since tail transients have never been observed in skeletal muscle and since their occurrence is not predicted by charge-coupled release mechanisms (65), their existence in heart muscle is potentially revealing of the mechanism of E–C coupling in heart muscle. In particular, their existence offers a unique opportunity to examine the relationship between Ca^{2+}-current and Ca^{2+} release from the SR, in the absence of depolarization *per se*. This relationship has been examined in detail (57) in order to test the obvious hypothesis that the release of Ca^{2+} from SR that underlies the tail transient is "triggered" via Ca^{2+}-induced release of Ca^{2+}.

The result of the study was that the amplitude of the tail transient does not correlate simply with the amplitude of the Ca^{2+}-current tail. Ca^{2+} current tails increase with increasingly negative repolarization voltage, but tail transients do not. Upon repolarization to very negative membrane potentials however, the Ca^{2+} current deactivates so quickly that the amount of Ca^{2+} entering during the tail is strongly reduced, and it was suggested that this could account for the reduction of the tail transient. This relationship needs to be examined further, and it was concluded that Ca^{2+}-induced release of Ca^{2+} could account for tail transients. It may be significant that the release of Ca^{2+} from SR *on repolarization* can be as large as that *on depolarization*. In rat heart cells particularly (58,63) the magnitude of tail transients upon repolarization can be similar to that elicited by depolarization.

c. Uptake of Ca^{2+} by SR. A variety of experiments have indicated that the SR is the major determinant of the decline of the $[Ca^{2+}]_i$-transient. The data discussed in the sections above lead to the conclusion that the Ca^{2+}-pumping ATPase (28) of the SR is the major determinant of the decline of the $[Ca^{2+}]_i$-transient. It is clear that when the SR is intact, but there is no Na/Ca exchange, cytoplasmic $[Ca^{2+}]_i$ falls much more rapidly than when the SR is inhibited by caffeine (c.f. 72 and 79). More information on the relative roles of SR and Na/Ca exchange in the normal decline of the $[Ca^{2+}]_i$-transient is presented below.

2. *NA/CA Exchange*

This section reviews briefly the role of Na–Ca exchange (23,66) in the $[Ca^{2+}]_i$-transient during each cardiac cycle. Mullins (67) was the first to point out that an electrogenic Na–Ca exchange could both bring Ca^{2+} into the cell during the action potential, making a direct contribution to the $[Ca^{2+}]_i$-transient, and also extrude Ca^{2+} from the cell when $[Ca^{2+}]_i$ is high and during the resting period (diastole). It has been suggested recently that release of Ca^{2+} from SR may also be triggered by the Ca^{2+} that accumulates secondary to Na^+_i-dependent Ca^{2+} influx ("reverse" or Ca^{2+}-influx mode) in which the rise in $[Na^+]_i$ is produced by the Na^+ current. These possible roles of the exchanger in E–C coupling are considered below.

a. Direct Contribution to $[Ca^{2+}]_i$-Transients. In evaluating the experimental data on this issue, two factors need special consideration: the chemical activity of intracellular Na^+ (a^i_{Na}), and the species of mammalian heart cell.

A brief discussion of intracellular Na^+ is necessary for this section. Intracellular Na^+ is critically important in determining Na–Ca exchanger activity because 3 Na^+ must bind, because the concentration of Na^+ required for half-maximal activation in heart is 20 mM (68), within the physiological range of $[Na^+]_i$, and because of the steep dependence of the reversal potential (E_{NaCa}) on $[Na^+]_i$ (23). Thus Ca^{2+} influx through the exchanger is steeply dependent on physiological $[Na^+]_i$. In experiments in which internally perfused cells are used, such as in many of those considered here, a^i_{Na} is presumed to be influenced by the $[Na^+]$ in the micropipette electrode. At physiological temperature and normal $[Na^+]_i$, a^i_{Na} is about 7 mM (69). This corresponds to $[Na^+]_i$ of 10 mM, on the assumption of an activity coefficient for Na^+ in the pipette filling solution of 0.7. The a^i_{Na} of ferret papillary muscle has been determined to be ~11 mM at 22–24°C (69) or $[Na^+]_i$ of 16 mM. Thus, the $[Na^+]$ in the micropipette electrode must be 16 mM and 10 mM to produce "physiological" a^i_{Na} at room temperature and normal mammalian temperatures, respectively.

In rat ventricular cells studied at 35°C, $[Ca^{2+}]_i$ did not increase during 100 msec depolarizing steps to +100 mV (63). The authors concluded that Ca^{2+} entry via Na–Ca exchange, which would be expected at +100 mV, was insufficient to activate Ca^{2+}-release from SR. In a recent review of Na–Ca exchange (70), it was concluded from this result that "under physiological conditions, any entry of Ca into the cell via Na-Ca exchange which is produced solely by depolarization is insufficient to materially affect $[Ca^{2+}]_i$." However, in the work cited (63), $[Na^+]$ in the micropipette electrode was far lower (3.75 mM in the form of Na-phosphocreatine) than required for physiological conditions (as discussed above). Similar results were obtained from rat heart cells (58) at room temperature (20–25°C) with $[Na^+]$ in the micropipette of 4.5 mM, in the form of 0.9mM Na_5 fura-2. Thus the $[Na^+]_i$ used in both these studies was substantially lower than that required to produce physiological levels inside the cell. Mitchell and her colleagues (71) observed a bell-shaped dependence on membrane potential of shortening in rat ventricular cells. In this case, a single-electrode voltage clamp was used, and the micropipette electrode contained no Na^+. Since perfusion of the cell is slow with this method compared to tight-seal recording with a low-resistance micropipette electrode, $[Na^+]_i$ is presumed to have been maintained close to physiological levels.

Components of physiological $[Ca^{2+}]_i$-transients attributable to Na–Ca exchange have been observed in guinea-pig ventricular cells. Barcenas-Ruiz and Wier (77) were the first to observe slowly rising $[Ca^{2+}]_i$-transients at positive membrane potentials (see record of depolarization to +90 mV, Fig. 7). In contrast to the rapidly rising component (depolarization to +10 mV, Fig. 7), and the "tail transient" (on repolarization from +90 mV, Fig. 7), this component of the $[Ca^{2+}]_i$-transient was resistant to SL Ca^{2+}-channel block (verapamil) and SR Ca^{2+}-release block (ryanodine). The initial rates of rise of such transients (which should reflect the initial net Ca^{2+} influx through the Na/Ca exchanger) were later shown by Beuckelmann and Wier (57) to have a nearly exponential dependence on membrane potential and to be increased by elevation of $[Na^+]_i$ (monensin) and blocked by Ni^{2+}, a putative blocker of Na-Ca exchange (68). Crespo and colleagues (72) have concluded that with normal $[Na^+]_i$ the rate of entry of Ca^{2+} through the exchanger is too slow to affect the upstroke of the normal Ca^{2+}-transient, a conclusion that is in agreement with the results illustrated in Figure 7.

Isenberg and colleagues (64) have examined the influence of the $[Na^+]$ in the pipette on the voltage dependence of the indo-1 fluorescence transient in voltage-clamped guinea pig ventricular myocytes. The cells had been loaded with indo-1 via exposure to indo-1/AM, so quantification of $[Ca^{2+}]_i$-transients was not attempted. Nevertheless, the studies demonstrate clearly that the absence of Na^+ in the pipette filling solution is associated with a bell-shaped voltage dependence of the fluorescence transient. In guinea pig cells voltage clamped with micropipette electrodes containing Na^+ at 10 mM, slowly rising fluorescence transients, which were not reduced at positive membrane potentials, were observed, as in the other studies cited. It has been reported (73) that Ca^{2+} influx via Na/Ca exchange is insufficient to activate contraction directly in rabbit ventricular muscle, unless a^i_{Na} is elevated.

Beuckelmann and Wier, from their study (74) of Na/Ca exchange in guinea pig cells, have pointed out that of the entities known to affect Na/Ca exchange, the two that change significantly during each cardiac cycle are $[Ca^{2+}]_i$ and membrane potential. Therefore, the Ca^{2+} fluxes through the exchanger can only be understood quantitatively by considering the relationship between $[Ca^{2+}]_i$ and exchange current (which is approximately linear in the physiological range of $[Ca^{2+}]_i$ [56,74,75]), and the effects of membrane potential on the exchanger (see Ref. 76 for thorough discussion of this).

The direct contribution of Ca^{2+} influx via Na/Ca exchanger to the $[Ca^{2+}]_i$-transient during E–C coupling is clearly dependent upon species and condition (membrane potential, $[Ca^{2+}]_i$, a^i_{Na}) dependent. A substantive contribution during the normal action potential seems likely, in the species studied so far, only in the guinea pig. On the other hand, when $[Na^+]_i$ is elevated and the membrane is strongly depolarized, slow contractions can be activated by Ca^{2+} entering via Na/Ca exchange.

Recently, Leblanc and Hume (78) have suggested that release of Ca^{2+} from SR can be triggered by Ca^{2+} that has accumulated secondary to the rise in $[Na^+]_i$ produced by the tetrodotoxin (TTX)-sensitive Na^+ current. This suggestion is based on the observation of a TTX-sensitive Ca^{2+}-release.

b. Ca^{2+} Efflux Through the Na/Ca Exchanger. In the absence of Na/Ca exchange, $[Ca^{2+}]_i$-transients decline only slightly more slowly than in its presence.

After repolarization, the time constants of the decline in $[Ca^{2+}]_i$ are increased only by about 20% (79) in the absence of external Na^+, compared to its presence (145 mM). Sudden exposure of ventricular myocytes to Na^+ leads to voltage-dependent relaxation (80), almost certainly reflecting Ca^{2+}-efflux through the Na/Ca exchanger. Sudden exposure to caffeine releases Ca^{2+} from the SR and is associated with an inward current that also reflects Ca^{2+} efflux through the exchanger (81). Similar conclusions have been reached by Crespo and colleagues (72).

3. *Surface Membrane*

The contribution of Ca^{2+} entering the cytoplasm via Ca^{2+} channels in the surface membrane has been the subject of extensive study. The subject is of interest from at least two major viewpoints. First, the direct activation of contraction by Ca^{2+} entering via the Ca^{2+} channels is of interest when one is thinking about inotropic mechanisms and therapies. Second, $[Ca^{2+}]_i$ transients attributable to Ca^{2+} entering across the surface membrane are of great interest when one is investigating the mechanisms of excitation-contraction coupling. It has recently been suggested that calcium fluxing across the sarcolemma can directly activate the myofilaments in human myocardium (85). As pointed out elsewhere in this chapter, the bulk of evidence favors the phenomenon of Ca^{2+}-induced release of Ca^{2+} as an important component of E-C coupling in mammalian heart. The salient features of that phenomenon, as observed in single skinned cardiac cells (47–49) is that it is the *rate of change* of free $[Ca^{2+}]_i$ resulting directly from the Ca^{2+} entering the cytoplasm via L-type Ca^{2+} channels that "triggers" release of Ca^{2+} from the SR. An important question to be resolved is whether in intact cells the Ca^{2+}-current can provide the type of signal required by the theory of Ca^{2+}-induced release of Ca^{2+}.

As is the case with the contribution of Na/Ca exchange to Ca^{2+} transients, the contribution of Ca^{2+} entering via Ca^{2+} channels cannot normally be observed directly. As will be shown below, however, it has become possible recently to isolate quite effectively a $[Ca^{2+}]_i$ transient attributable to Ca^{2+} entry via L-type Ca^{2+}-channels (84). The $[Ca^{2+}]_i$ transient obtained under the conditions used is certainly not representative in all ways of that component of the "normal" $[Ca^{2+}]_i$ transient due to Ca^{2+} entering via Ca^{2+} channels. As discussed below, however, the agreement between a theoretical $[Ca^{2+}]_i$ transient and that observed experimentally, albeit under nonphysiological conditions, means that the factors determining the relationship between Ca^{2+} current and $[Ca^{2+}]_i$-transient are understood adequately.

From the earlier studies done without intracellular Ca^{2+} indicators, a consensus arose on several points. First, the contribution of Ca^{2+} entry through Ca^{2+} channels to $[Ca^{2+}]_i$-transient is recognized to vary with the species, the type of heart muscle, and the situation, particularly the frequency of stimulation. It is believed that this contribution is least in rat and probably greatest in rabbit, with dog, cat, human, and others in between. In ventricular tissue, the rested state contraction is believed to result almost exclusively from Ca^{2+} entering via Ca^{2+} channels, since in this tissue the SR is depleted of Ca^{2+} by rest.

The earliest studies of $[Ca^{2+}]_i$-transients in mammalian cardiac Purkinje fibers revealed an early, rapidly recovering component of the $[Ca^{2+}]_i$-transient that was attributed to Ca^{2+} entry via Ca^{2+} channels (2). Later studies showed that this component was abolished by ryanodine (44), rendering this interpretation unlikely.

$[Ca^{2+}]_i$-transients attributable solely to entry of Ca^{2+} through L-type Ca^{2+} channels have been recorded under conditions in which both Na/Ca exchange and release of Ca^{2+} from the SR were eliminated (84). However, the change in $[Ca^{2+}]_i$ produced by the current under these conditions is not the same as under normal conditions, when many other cellular processes are contributing to the $[Ca^{2+}]_i$-transient. Finally, the agreement between theoretical $[Ca^{2+}]_i$-transient and recorded $[Ca^{2+}]_i$-transient does not exclude the possibility that a small amount of Ca^{2+} accumulates to much higher concentrations in a restricted space of small volume, such as near the junctional SR.

Recently, Cohen and Lederer (82) reported that in adult rat ventricular cells ryanodine shifted the steady-state inactivation of L-type Ca^{2+} current to the right by 13 mV. This effect was not blocked by buffering $[Ca^{2+}]_i$ with EGTA (or BAPTA), and the effect was not present in neonatal rat heart cells. It was concluded, therefore, that the effect was not mediated by $[Ca^{2+}]_i$ but was rather related to the presence of the SR in adult cells. It was suggested that ryanodine affected gating of Ca^{2+} current by virtue of the fact that the ryanodine binding site (on the SR Ca^{2+} release channel) has a physical connection to the SL L-type Ca^{2+} channel. In this scheme, gating of SL L-type Ca^{2+}-channels would serve not only to permit Ca^{2+} entry but also to control the SR Ca^{2+} release channel in some way. In adult guinea pig ventricular cells, however, ryanodine does not shift the inactivation curve of L-type Ca^{2+}-current (Balke and Wier, in preparation).

4. *Binding of Ca^{2+} to Intracellular Ligands*

Ca^{2+} ligands have a major role in the $[Ca^{2+}]_i$-transient. Recent studies indicate that the ratio of bound to free Ca^{2+} is about 50–100:1. The binding of Ca^{2+} to the intracellular ligands (L) can be calculated (83) directly from the measured free $[Ca^{2+}]_i$-transient, provided that the concentration and rate constants for Ca^{2+}-binding are known. In a recent study (84) the concentrations and rate constants assumed for this calculation were modified slightly from those tabulated originally by Fabiato (26). Troponin C bound the most Ca^{2+}, followed by fura-2, calmodulin, SR binding sites, SL binding sites, and phosphocreatine. At the peak of the $[Ca^{2+}]_i$-transient, the total $[Ca^{2+}]$ (bound plus free) was about 150 μM.

B. $[Ca^{2+}]_i$-Jump Experiments

The phenomenon of Ca^{2+}-induced release of Ca^{2+} can now be investigated in intact muscle cells by producing rapid increases (or even decreases) of $[Ca^{2+}]_i$ by the photolytic release (or complexation) of Ca^{2+} by certain Ca^{2+} chelators. $[Ca^{2+}]_i$ can also be manipulated in a known way through the use of voltage clamp and the fluorescent Ca^{2+} indicators.

1. *Ca^{2+} Release Induced by Flash Photolysis of Caged Calcium*

In intact rat ventricular cells, rapid increases (jumps) of $[Ca^{2+}]_i$ produced by flash hydrolysis of nitr-5 evoked twitch contractions in the presence of Ca^{2+} channel block (nickel ions) or low external $[Ca^{2+}]$ (no added Ca^{2+}, 1mM EGTA), but not in the presence of ryanodine (86). Similar results were obtained in guinea-pig ventricular myocytes (87), in which photolytic release of Ca^{2+} from DM-nitrophen (88) elicited twitch contractions under control conditions, but not in the presence of caffeine.

2. Inactivation of Ca^{2+} Release by Flash Photolysis of Caged Calcium

As described above, an essential component of the theory of Ca^{2+}-induced release of Ca^{2+} is that Ca^{2+} not only activates but also inactivates release of Ca^{2+} from the SR. Fabiato (47) found that a rapid increase of Ca^{2+} to 1.00×10^{-5} M could reduce a release of Ca^{2+} that had been induced just previously by a smaller increase in $[Ca^{2+}]$. In intact guinea pig ventricular cells however, photolytic release of Ca^{2+} from DM-nitrophen (87) always potentiated twitch contractions, irrespective of the time that the photolytic release was made to occur. No conditions could be found under which the photolytic release reduced the twitch contraction, as might be expected from the results obtained in skinned cardiac cells (47–49). As noted by the authors, this result could be explained by the failure to reach a high enough $[Ca^{2+}]_i$ for a sufficient period of time, as the $[Ca^{2+}]_i$ achieved by photolytic release was unknown. (According to the theory, the inactivating site has a high affinity for Ca^{2+}, but only binds Ca^{2+} slowly.)

3. Inactivation of Release of Ca^{2+} by $[Ca^{2+}]_i$

As described above, the effect of Ca^{2+} to inactivate release of Ca^{2+} from SR was also demonstrated in the steady state (i.e., the amount of Ca^{2+} released was dependent on the level of Ca^{2+} around the SR prior to the induced release). Since some inactivation was present at a $[Ca^{2+}]$ of 6.31×10^{-8} M, it was concluded that the inactivating site must have a relatively high affinity for Ca^{2+}. In physiological experiments (87) it is possible to elevate $[Ca^{2+}]_i$ measurably prior to inducing release via the Ca^{2+} current. Few experiments of this type have been reported, but elevation of $[Ca^{2+}]_i$ from 90 nM to about 110 nM failed to have any observable effect on the subsequent $[Ca^{2+}]_i$-transient. This result is equivocal, however, since the change in $[Ca^{2+}]_i$ was very small and the actual rate of release of Ca^{2+} from the SR was not calculated. Resolution of this issue will require that Ca^{2+} inactivation of Ca^{2+} channels be studied at the single-channel level.

C. Charge Movement in Cardiac Muscle

Nonlinear charge movement in skeletal muscle is usually interpreted as reflecting the movement of voltage sensors important in E–C coupling (see below). Recently, nonlinear charge movement has been recorded in mammalian ventricular cells (33,89). These studies have illustrated several similarities between charge movement in skeletal and cardiac muscle.

Bean and Rios (33) concluded that the D-600-sensitive charge movement is about 10 times larger than the Ca^{2+}-channel gating current that would be expected if the movement of channel gating charge were always accompanied by complete opening of the channel.

Gating charge does not seem to be related to the development of the SR, since gating charge is approximately the same in neonatal and adult heart cells, despite the great difference in the development of the SR and its connections with the SL. A recent study (90) concluded that calcium release is gated by calcium current and not by gating charge.

Finally, an elegant study (92) in which cardiac DHP receptors were expressed in dysgenic skeletal muscle indicated clearly that the cardiac DHP receptor could function as an L-type Ca^{2+} channel, but not as a voltage-sensor that controlled directly the release of Ca^{2+} from the SR.

Thus there seems to be no compelling reason, in heart muscle, to assume that the charge movement reflects anything other than the gating of Ca^{2+} channels. Nevertheless, the possibility that some of this charge movement is involved in E–C coupling cannot be eliminated.

V. SUMMARY: PLAUSIBLE MECHANISMS OF RELEASE OF Ca^{2+} FROM SR

In this section I will present several of the prevalent ideas on the release of Ca^{2+} from SR in cardiac muscle. I will attempt to integrate the information from the structural studies in heart and skeletal muscle and that from physiological experiments of various types in skinned and intact mammalian cardiac cells.

It now seems clear that Ca^{2+} can be released from SR of mammalian cardiac muscle, in a manner indistinguishable from that occurring physiologically, without depolarization, provided a change in $[Ca^{2+}]_i$ occurs. Ca^{2+} jump experiments produce twitches that are as large and fast as physiological twitches, presumably because the rate of release of Ca^{2+} produced is comparable to physiological. Ca^{2+} can be released from SR on repolarization, provided a tail of Ca^{2+} current occurs. The tail $[Ca^{2+}]_i$-transient elicited by *repolarization* can be as large and as fast as the $[Ca^{2+}]_i$-transient elicited by depolarization. All these phenomena are abolished by ryanodine, thus establishing that they do reflect release of Ca^{2+} from SR. The fact that "physiological" (large and rapid) SR Ca^{2+} release can be obtained in the absence of depolarization *per se* means that the hypothesis that Ca^{2+}-induced release of Ca^{2+} is the sole mechanism of release of Ca^{2+} from SR cannot be rejected.

From the ultrastructural studies, the possible occurrence of Ca^{2+}-activated SR Ca^{2+}-release channels (as junctional processes are presumed to be) in SR that does not make junctional contact with SL implies Ca^{2+}-induced release of Ca^{2+}. It is very important to determine if in fact these junctional processes are calcium release channels.

In cardiac muscle, depolarization *per se* is thus not a requirement for release of Ca^{2+} from SR. Apparently, most DHP receptors are regulated in such a way they are functional Ca^{2+}-channels. The rise in $[Ca^{2+}]_i$ produced by Ca^{2+} current is therefore adequate to cause release of Ca^{2+} by activating directly the SR Ca^{2+}-release channels. In mammalian cardiac muscle, the tSR junction is a structure that permits, in some unknown way presumably related to its geometry, the release of Ca^{2+} to be graded with Ca^{2+} current. The possibility that some feet proteins are connected to DHP receptors and that Ca^{2+} release can occur via mechanical allosteric modification is reduced because release of Ca^{2+} from cardiac SR has a bell-shaped dependence on membrane potential. If some Ca^{2+} release occurs via this mechanism at positive membrane potentials, it must be so small that Ca^{2+}-induced release of Ca^{2+} from neighboring feet proteins is not activated.

In *skeletal muscle,* depolarization *per se* is a requirement for release of Ca^{2+} from SR. The DHP receptors are regulated in such a way that the Ca^{2+} current is always very small, insufficient to cause release of Ca^{2+} by activating directly the SR Ca^{2+}-release channels. A sufficient number (half) of the feet proteins are connected to DHP receptors, so that depolarization results in sufficient Ca^{2+} release to supply contractile proteins with Ca^{2+} as well as to active further Ca^{2+} release via Ca^{2+} activation of those feet proteins that do not face DHP receptors. This would account for the characteristics of SR release, in which a component of the release seems to be inactivated by Ca^{2+}, and to be independent of membrane voltage. Another component is not inactivated until the membrane is repolarized (and charge moves back, closing Ca^{2+}-release channels).

A major problem with Ca^{2+}-induced release of Ca^{2+} as the mechanism of release of Ca^{2+} from cardiac SR is that physiological evidence for Ca^{2+}-dependent inactivation of Ca^{2+}-release has not been found. As noted, such evidence has been found in skeletal muscle. This is important, because Ca^{2+}-dependent inactivation of Ca^{2+} release is one way in which Ca^{2+} release could be graded with the Ca^{2+} current, which is the salient feature of E–C coupling in mammalian heart.

REFERENCES

1. Allen DG, Blinks JR. Calcium transients in aequorin-injected frog cardiac muscle. Nature 1978;273:509–13.
2. Wier WG. Calcium transients during excitation–contraction coupling in mammalian heart: aequorin signals of canine Purkinje fibers. Science 1980;207:1085–7.
3. Sommer JR, Jennings RB. Ultrastructure of cardiac muscle. In: Fozzard HA, ed. The heart and cardiovascular system. New York: Raven Press, 1986
4. Solaro RJ, Moir AGJ, Perry WV. Phosphorylation of troponin I and the inotropic effect of adrenaline in the perfused rabbit heart. Nature (Lond) 1976;262: 615–6.
5. Flink IL, Rader JH, Morkin E. Thyroid hormone stimulates synthesis of a cardiac myosin isozyme. Comparison of the two-dimensional electrophoretic patterns of the cyanogen bromide pepties of cardiac myosin heavy chains from euthyroid and thyrotoxic rabbits. J Biol Chem 1979;254:3106–10.
6. Hibberd MG, Jewell B. Calcium- and length-dependent force production in rat ventricular muscle. J Physiol (London) 1982;329: 527–40.
7. Sipido K, Wier WG. Net calcium flux of sarcoplasmic reticulum of guinea-pig cardiac ventricular cells during excitation–contraction coupling. Biophys. J. 1990; 57:173a.
8. Blinks JR, Wier WG, Hess PO, Prendergast FG. Measurement of Ca^{2+}-concentration in living cells. Prog Biophys Mol Biol 1982;40:1–114.
9. Wier WG. Cytoplasmic $[Ca^{2+}]_i$ in mammalian ventricle: dynamic control by cellular processes. Annu Rev Physiol 1990;52:467–85.
10. Wier WG. $[Ca^{2+}]_i$-transients during excitation-contraction coupling of mammalian heart. In: Fozzard HA et al, eds. The heart and cardiovascular system 2nd ed, ch 45, pp 1223–1248. New York: Raven Press, 1990.
11. Ruegg JC. Calcium. in: Muscle activation. New York: Springer-Verlag, 1988.
12. Bagshaw CR. Muscle contraction. New York: Chapman and Hall, 1982.
13. Yue DT. Intracellular $[Ca^{2+}]$ related to rate of force development in twitch contraction of heart. Am J Physiol 1987;21: H760–H770.
14. Fabiato A. Myoplasmic free calcium concentration reached during the twitch of an intact isolated cardiac cell and during calcium-induced release of calcium from the sarcoplasmic reticulum of a skinned cardiac cell from the adult rat or rabbit ventricle. J Gen Physiol 1981;78: 457–97.
15. Wier WG, Yue DT. Intracellular calcium transients underlying the short-term force-

interval relationship in ferret ventricular myocardium. J Physiol (Lond) 1986; 376:507–30.
16. Yue DT, Marban E, Wier WG. Relationship between force and intracellular [Ca^{2+}] in tetanized mammalian heart muscle. J Gen Physiol 1986;87:223–42.
17. Babu A, Sonnenblick E, Gulati J. Molecular basis for the influence of muscle length on myocardial performance. Science 1988;240: 74–6.
18. Smith SJ, Augustine GJ. Calcium ions, active zones and synaptic transmitter release. TINS 1988; 11(10):458–64.
19. Takamatsu T, Wier WG. High temporal resolution video imaging of intracellular calcium. Cell Calcium 1990;11:2/3:111–20.
20. Wier WG, Cannell MB, Berlin JR, Marban E, Lederer WJ. Cellular and subcellular heterogeneity of $[Ca^{2+}]_i$ in single heart cells revealed by fura-2. Science 1987; 235:325–8.
21. Takamatsu T, Wier WG. Calcium waves in mammalian heart: quantification of origin, magnitude, waveform and velocity. FASEB J 1990;4:1519–25.
22. Bond M, Moravec CS. Subcellular calcium redistribution during cardiac muscle contraction measured in situ by X-ray microanalysis. Circulation 1989;80, II-194 (abstr).
23. Blaustein MP. Sodium/calcium exchange and the control of contractility in cardiac muscle and vascular smooth muscle. J Cardiovasc Pharmacol 1988;12(5):S56–68 (suppl).
24. Reuter H, Porzig H, Kokubun H, Prod'hom B. Calcium channels in the heart. Properties and modulation by dihydropyridine enantiomers. Ann NY Acad Sci 1988; 552: 16–24.
25. Hilgemann DW. "Best estimates" of physiological sodium-calcium exchange function: calcium conservation and the cardiac electrical cycle. In: Zipes D, Jalife J, eds. Cardiac electrophysiology: from cell to bedside. Philadelphia: WB Saunders, 1989.
26. Carafoli E. Membrane transport of calcium: an overview. Methods Enzymol 1988; 157:3–11.
27. Fabiato A. Calcium-induced release of calcium from the cardiac s.r. Am J Physiol 1983;245, C1–C14.
28. Meissner G. Ryanodine activation and inhibition of the Ca^{2+} release channel of sarcoplasmic reticulum. J Biol Chem 1986;261(14):6300–6.
29. Inesi G. Mechanism of calcium transport. Annu Rev Physiol 1985;47:573–601.
30. Melzer W, Rios E, Schneider MF. A general procedure for determining the rate of calcium release from the sarcoplasmic reticulum in skeletal muscle fibers. Biophys J 1987;51: 849–63.
31. Schneider MF, Chandler WK. Voltage dependent charge movement in skeletal muscle: a possible step in excitation-contraction coupling. Nature (Lond) 1973; 242: 244–6.
32. Rios E, Pizzaro G. Voltage sensors and calcium channels of excitation–contraction coupling. NIPS 1989;3: 223–7.
33. Bean BP, Rios E. Nonlinear charge movement in mammalian cardiac ventricular cells. J Gen Physiol 1989; 94: 65–94.
34. Smith JS, Coronado R, Meissner G. Single-channel calcium and barium currents of large and small conductance from sarcoplasmic reticulum. Biophys J 1986; 50: 921–8.
35. Franzini-Armstrong C. Studies of the triad. I. Structure of the junction in frog twitch fibers. J Cell Biol 1970;47: 488–99.
36. Block BA, Imagawa T, Campbell KP, Franzini-Armstrong C. Structural evidence for direct interaction between the molecular components of the transverse tubule/sarcoplasmic reticulum junction in skeletal muscle. J Cell Biol 1988;107: 2587–600.
37. Wagenknecht T, Grassucci JF, Saito A, Inui M. Fleischer S. Three-dimensional architecture of the calcium channel/foot structure of sarcoplasmic reticulum. Nature 1989;338: 167–70.

38. Fleischer S, Ogunbunmi EM, Dixon MC, Fleer EAM. Localization of Ca^{2+} release channels with ryanodine in terminal cisternae of sarcoplasmic reticulum of fast skeletal muscle. Proc Natl Acad Sci USA 1985;82:7256–9.
39. Hymel L, Inui M, Fleischer S, Schindler HG. Purified skeletal muscle ryanodine receptor forms Ca^{2+}-activated multisubunit Ca^{2+}-channels in planar bilayers. Proc Natl Acad Sci USA 1987;85: 441–5.
40. Imagawa T, Smith JS, Coronado R, Campbell KP. Purified ryanodine receptor from skeletal muscle sarcoplasmic reticulum is the Ca^{2+}-permeable pore of the calcium release channel. J Biol Chem 1987;262: 16636–43.
41. Meissner G, Darling E, Eveleth J. Kinetics of rapid Ca^{2+} release by sarcoplasmic reticulu. Effects of Ca^{2+}, Mg^{2+}, and adenine nucleotides. Biochemistry 1986;25: 236–44.
42. Meissner G. Adenine nucleotide stimulation of Ca^{2+}-induced Ca^{2+}-release in sarcoplasmic reticulum. J Biol Chem 1984; 59: 2365–74.
43. Anderson K, Lai FA, Liu Q, Rousseau E, Erickson HP, Meissner G. Structural and functional characterization of the purified cardiac ryanodine receptor-Ca^{2+} release channel complex. J Biol Chem 1989;264:1329–35.
44. Marban E, Wier WG. Ryanodine as a tool to determine the contributions of calcium entry and calcium release to the calcium transient and contraction of cardiac purkinje fibers. Circ Res 1985;56:133–8.
45. McGrew SG, Inui M, Chadwick CC, Boucek Jr RJ, Junk CY, Fleischer S. Comparison of the calcium release channel of cardiac and skeletal muscle sarcoplasmic reticulum by target inactivation analysis. Biochemistry 1989;28:1319–23.
46. Frank J. Ultrastructure of the unfixed myocardial sarcolemma and cell surface. In: Langer GA, ed. Calcium and the heart. New York, Raven Press, 1990.
47. Fabiato A. Rapid ionic modification during the aequorin-detected calcium transient in a skinned canine cardiac purkinje cell. J Gen Physiol 1985;85(2):189–246.
48. Fabiato A. Time and calcium dependence of activation and inactivation of calcium-induced release of calcium from the sarcoplasmic reticulum of a skinned canine cardiac purkinje cell. J Gen Physiol 1985;85(2):247–90.
49. Fabiato A. Simulated calcium current can both cause calcium loading in and trigger calcium release from the sarcoplasmic reticulum of a skinned canine cardiac purkinje cell. J Gen Physiol 1985;85(2):291–320.
50. Rousseau E, LaDine J, Liu Q-Y, Meissner G. Activation of the Ca^{2+} release channel of skeletal muscle sarcoplasmic reticulum by caffeine and related compounds. Arch Biochem Biophys 1988;267(1):75–86.
51. Best PM, Kwok W. The sarcoplasmic reticulum calcium channel of skeletal muscle. Ann NY Acad Sci 1989; 401–402.
52. Smith JS, Imagawa T, Ma J, Fill M, Campbell P, Coronado R. Purified ryanodine receptor from rabbit skeletal muscle is the calcium-release channel of sarcoplasmic reticulum. J Gen Physiol 1989;92: 1–26.
53. Baylor SM, Hollingworth S. Fura-2 calcium transients in frog skeletal muscle fibers. J Physiol 1988;402:151–92.
54. Schneider MF, Simon BJ. Inactivation of calcium release from the sarcoplasmic reticulum in frog skeletal muscle. J Physiol 1988;405, 727–45.
55. Rios E, Pizzaro G. Voltage sensors and calcium channels of excitation-contraction coupling. NIPS 1989;3: 223–7.
56. Barcenas-Ruiz L, Beuckelmann DJ, Wier WG. Sodium-calcium exchange in heart: currents and changes in $[Ca^{2+}]_i$. Science, 1987;238:1720–2.
57. Beuckelmann DJ, Wier WG. Mechanism of release of calcium from s.r. of guinea-pig cardiac cells. J Physiol (Lond) 1988;405:233–55.
58. Callewaert G, Cleemann L, Morad M. Epinephrine enhances Ca^{2+} current-regulated

Ca^{2+} release and Ca^{2+} reuptake in rat ventricular myocytes. Proc Natl Acad Sci USA 1988;85:2009–13.
60. Hansford RG, Lakatta EG. Ryanodine releases calcium from sarcoplasmic reticulum in calcium-tolerant rat cardiac myocytes. J Physiol 1987;390:453–67.
61. Wier WG, Isenberg G. Intracellular [Ca^{2+}] transients in voltage clamped cardiac purkinje fibers. Pflugers Arch 1982;392:284–90.
62. Rios E, Brum G. Involvement of dihydropyridine receptors in excitation–contraction coupling in skeletal muscle. Nature 1987;325: 717–20.
63. Cannell MB, Berlin JR, Lederer WJ. Effects of membrane potential changes on the calcium transient in single rat cardiac muscle cells. Science 1987;238:1419–23.
64. Isenberg G, Spurgeon H, Talo A, Stern M, Capogrossi M, Lakatta E. The voltage dependence of the myoplasmic calcium transient in guinea pig ventricular myocytes in modulated by sodium loading. In: Clark WA, Decker RS, Borg TK, eds. Biology of isolated adult cardiac myocytes, Stowe: Elsevier Science Publishing Co., 1988.
65. Miledi R, Parker I, Zhu PH. Calcium transients studied under voltage-clamp control in frog twitch muscle fibres. J Physiol 1983;340:649–80.
66. Reeves JP. Sodium–calcium exchange. In: Bronner F, ed. Intracellular calcium regulation. New York: Alan R. Liss, 1989.
67. Mullins LJ. The generation of electric currents in cardiac fibers by Na/Ca exchange. Am J Physiol 1979;236(3): C103–C110.
68. Kimura J, Miyamae S, Noma A. Identification of sodium-calcium exchange current in single ventricular cells of guinea-pig. J Physiol 1987;384:199–222.
69. Blatter LA, McGuigan JA, Reverdin EC. Sodium/calcium exchange and calcium buffering in mammalian ventricular muscle. Jpn Heart J suppl. 1986;27:93–107.
70. Eisner DA, Lederer WJ. The electrogenic sodium–calcium exchange: In: Allen THA, Noble D, Reuter H (eds). Sodium–calcium exchange. Oxford: Oxford University Press, 1989.
71. Mitchell MR, Powell T, Terrar DA, Twist VW. Electrical activity and contraction in cells isolated from rat and guinea-pig ventricular muscle: a comparative study. J Physiol 1987;391:527–44.
72. Crespo LM, Grantham CJ, Cannell MB. Kinetics, stoichiometry and role of the Na-Ca exchange mechanism in isolated cardiac myocytes. Nature 1990;345:618–21.
73. Bers DM, Christensen DM, Nguyen TX. Can Ca entry via Na-Ca exchange directly activate cardiac muscle contraction? J Mol Cell Cardiol 1988;20:405–14.
74. Beuckelmann DJ, Wier WG. Sodium–calcium exchange in guinea-pig cardiac cells: exchange current and changes in intracellular Ca^{2+}. J Physiol (Lond) 1989; 414:499–520.
75. Berlin JR, Hume JR, Lederer WJ. $[Ca^{2+}]_i$-activated “creep” currents in guinea-pig ventricular myocytes. J Physiol (Lond) 1989;407:128 (abstr).
76. Hilgemann DW. Numerical approximations of sodium–calcium exchange. Prog Biophys Mol Biol 1990;51:1–45.
77. Barcenas-Ruiz L, Wier WG. Voltage dependence of intracellular $[Ca^{2+}]_i$ transients in guinea pig ventricular myocytes. Circ Res 1987;61:148–54.
78. Leblanc N, Hume JR. Sodium current-induced release of calcium from cardiac sarcoplasmic reticulum. Science 1990;248: 372–6.
79. Bers DM, Cannell MB, Lederer WJ. Intracellular Ca transients in rat cardiac myocytes: role of Na/Ca exchange in excitation–contraction coupling. Am J Physiol 1990; (in press).
80. Bridge JHB, Spitzer KW, Ershler PR. Relaxation of isolated ventricular cardiomyocytes by a voltage-dependent process. Science 1988;241:823–5.
81. Callewaert, GL, Cleemann L, Morad M. Caffeine-induced Ca^{2+}-release activates Ca^{2+}-extrusion via Na-Ca exchanger in cardiac myocytes. Am J Physiol 1989;257:C147–52.

82. Cohen NM, Lederer WJ. Changes in the calcium current of rat heart ventricular myocytes during development. J Physiol (Lond) 1988; 406: 115–46.
83. Robertson SP, Johnson JD, Potter JD. The time-course of Ca^{2+}-exchange with calmodulin, troponin, parvalbumin, and myosin in response to transient increases in Ca^{2+}. Biophys J 1981;34:559–69.
84. Sipido, KR and Wier, WG. Flux of Ca^{2+} across the sarcoplasmic reticulum of guinea-pig cardiac cells during excitation–contraction coupling. J Physiol 1991, 435:605–630.
85. Gwathmey JK, Slawsky MT, Hajjar RJ, Briggs GM, Morgan JP. Role of intracellular calcium handling in force–interval relationships of human ventricular myocardium. J Clin Invest 1990;85:1599–613.
86. Valdeolmillos M, O'Neill SC, Smith GL, Eisner DA. Calcium-induced calcium release activates contraction in intact cardiac cells. Pflugers Arch Eur J Physiol 1989;413: 676–8.
87. Naebauer M, Morad M. Ca^{2+}-induced Ca^{2+} release as examined by photolysis of caged Ca^{2+} in single ventricular myocytes. Am J Physiol 1990;258 C189–93.
88. Ellis-Davies GCR, Kaplan JH. A new class of photolabile chelators for the rapid release of divalent cations: generation of caged Ca and caged Mg. J Organ Chem 1988;53:1966–9.
89. Hadley RW, Lederer WJ. Intramembrane charge movement in guinea-pig and rat ventricular myocytes. J Physiol 1989;415:601–24.
90. Naebauer M, Callewaert G, Cleemann L, Morad M. Regulation of calcium release is gated by calcium current, not gating charge, in cardiac myocytes. Science 1989;244, 800–3.
91. Jorgensen AO, Broderick R, Somlyo AP, Somlyo AV. Two structurally distinct calcium storage sites in rat cardiac sarcoplasmic reticulum: an electron microprobe analysis study. Circ Res 1988;63:1060–9.
92. Tanabe T, Mikami A, Numa S, Beam KG. Cardiac-type excitation–contraction coupling in dysgenic skeletal muscle injected with cardiac dihydropyridine receptor cDNA. Nature 1990;344:451–3.
93. Sommer JR. The anatomy of the sarcoplasmic reticulum in vertebrate skeletal muscle: its implications for excitation–contraction coupling. Z Naturforsch 1982;37:665–78.

3

Pathophysiological Effects of Spontaneous Sarcoplasmic Reticulum Ca^{2+} Release on Myocardial Function

MAURIZIO C. CAPOGROSSI and EDWARD G. LAKATTA

National Institute on Aging, National Institutes of Health
Baltimore, Maryland

HOWARD S. SILVERMAN and MICHAEL D. STERN

Johns Hopkins University
Baltimore, Maryland

I. INTRODUCTION

The myocardium responds to an action potential with a synchronous release of Ca^{2+} from the sarcoplasmic reticulum (SR), which activates the myofilaments and produces a contraction (i.e., the twitch) (Fig. 1). However, the SR is also capable of spontaneous Ca^{2+} release, which occurs asynchronously within a cell and among the myocytes that form the tissue. The first report that can be found in the literature of the spontaneous asynchronous contractile motion is from experiments with cultures of chick embryo hearts done approximately 70 years ago (1). Subsequent reports of asynchronous contractions also appeared but it was not until two decades ago that this phenomenon began to be characterized in cardiac cells devoid of the sarcolemma (2–7) and in papillary muscles (8–10). More recently, spontaneous SR Ca^{2+} release has been observed also in myocytes with an intact sarcolemma, either by direct observation of the asynchronous contraction (11–13) or by determination of cytosolic $[Ca^{2+}]$, (Ca_i) changes in cells loaded with aequorin (14), or the fluorescent Ca^{2+} probes Fura-2 (15) or Indo-1 (16).

Spontaneous SR Ca^{2+} oscillations have been shown in all mammalian myocardial preparations studied (17), have a marked Ca^{2+} (10,12) and species (12,17) dependence (Fig. 2), and can be suppressed with ryanodine or by high concentrations of caffeine (18–20). It has been definitively established that spontaneous Ca^{2+} oscillations are dependent upon the extent of cell calcium loading, a functional SR, and sufficient energy supply. However, the mechanisms that initiate the release and those that are responsible for its propagation along the length of the cell have not been clearly identified (21). It is uncertain whether Ca^{2+} in the cytosol provides the trigger for opening the SR Ca^{2+} channel as it is likely to do during an electrically stimulated twitch, or

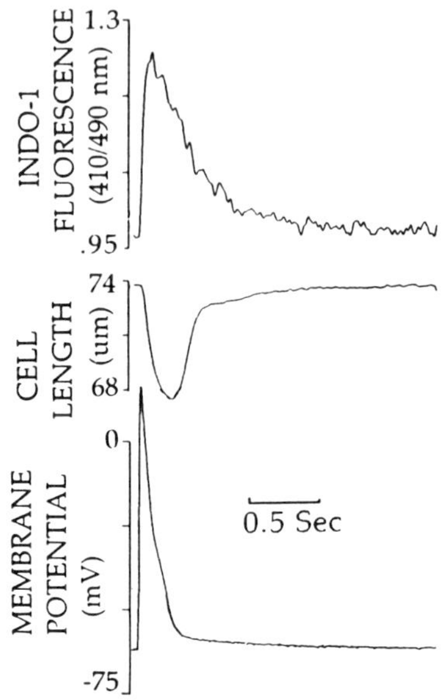

Figure 1 Transmembrane action potential, indo-1 fluorescence transient, and length changes during a rested-state contraction in a rat myocyte loaded with the ester derivative of indo-1 and bathed in 1.0 mM Ca_o. (From Ref. 16.)

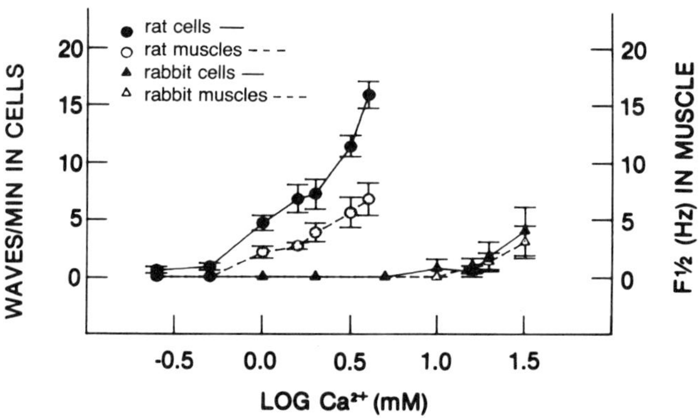

Figure 2 Species and Ca_o dependence of spontaneous SR Ca^{2+} oscillations. Spontaneous contractile wave frequency and scattered light intensity fluctuations expressed as $F_{1/2}$ (see text) were measured in unstimulated rat and rabbit myocytes and papillary muscles respectively. Wave frequency and F½ have been coscaled to facilitate comparison. While rat myocardial preparations exhibit spontaneous SR Ca^{2+} release at a Ca_o as low as 0.5 mM, in rabbit myocardium spontaneous Ca^{2+} oscillations are not observed at Ca_o lower than 10 mM. Following their appearance a further increase in Ca_o increases the frequency of oscillatory SR Ca^{2+} release regardless of the species. (From Ref. 12.)

whether the continuous accumulation of Ca^{2+} inside the SR reaches a threshold and succeeds in initiating the Ca^{2+} release without requiring Ca^{2+} as an outside trigger. In favor of the second possibility is the experimental evidence that Ca^{2+}-induced release of Ca^{2+} is maximal with an optimal Ca^{2+} trigger and that it is greatly inhibited by a supraoptimal Ca^{2+} trigger. This is in contrast to spontaneous SR Ca^{2+} release, which never shows inhibition but only enhancement by increasing bathing [Ca^{2+}], (Ca_o) (22). Once Ca^{2+} has been released from the SR into the cytosol, it reaches a concentration capable of releasing Ca^{2+} from the adjacent SR via Ca^{2+}-induced release of Ca^{2+} and causes the propagation of the Ca^{2+} wave along the length of the cell (21).

In single cardiac cells the mechanical manifestation of spontaneous Ca^{2+} release is readily visible as spontaneous sarcomere shortening, which begins locally and propagates along the cell as a contractile wave (11). Usually a single band of contracted sarcomeres originates at one end of the cell and propagates toward the other gap junction at a rate of approximately 100 μm/sec (19). This variety of spontaneous Ca^{2+} release has been termed "unifocal" (Fig. 3A), to differentiate them from "multifocal" oscillations (Fig. 3B) that originate either at both ends or in the center of the cell and propagate as two bands of contracted sarcomeres (23). An enhancement of the extent of cell Ca^{2+} loading increases both the frequency of spontaneous Ca^{2+} oscillations and the likelihood for them to be multifocal.

Spontaneous SR Ca^{2+} release causes a 1–3 mV depolarization due to Ca^{2+}-activated nonspecific cation channels (24), electrogenic Na/Ca exchange (25–27), or both. The peak of the Ca_i, the extent of cell shortening, and the amplitude of depolarization are all greater during multifocal than unifocal spontaneous Ca^{2+} release (Fig. 3C). Summation of the inward currents caused by multifocal Ca^{2+} oscillations can cause a depolarization of magnitude sufficient to reach threshold to trigger an action potential (Fig. 4). Another important sequela of spontaneous SR Ca^{2+} release is that its occurrence prior to a twitch has the effect of decreasing the amplitude of the electrically stimulated contraction and the duration of the associated action potential. These effects become more pronounced as the coupling interval between spontaneous Ca^{2+} release and twitch gets shorter (13).

II. SPONTANEOUS Ca^{2+} RELEASE FROM THE SR AS A MECHANISM FOR MAXIMUM INOTROPY IN THE MYOCARDIUM

In view of the experimental findings described above, we hypothesized that the occurrence of spontaneous Ca^{2+} release in the cardiac diastole might be a mechanism for the saturation of systolic contractile function upon exposure to inotropic perturbations that increase cell Ca^{2+} loading as well as for the increase in diastolic tonus and the occurrence of arrhythmias. To establish the validity of this hypothesis, the time when spontaneous SR Ca^{2+} release first occurs and its relationship to twitch saturation needed to be established.

A. Studies in Single Cells

In individual myocytes, we observed that regardless of whether contractility was enhanced by an increase in Ca_o (Fig. 5), by addition of cardiac glycosides or isoproterenol to the bathing fluid, or by permitting a period of rest following stimulation, which in rat myocytes leads to SR Ca^{2+} loading (Fig. 6), saturation of

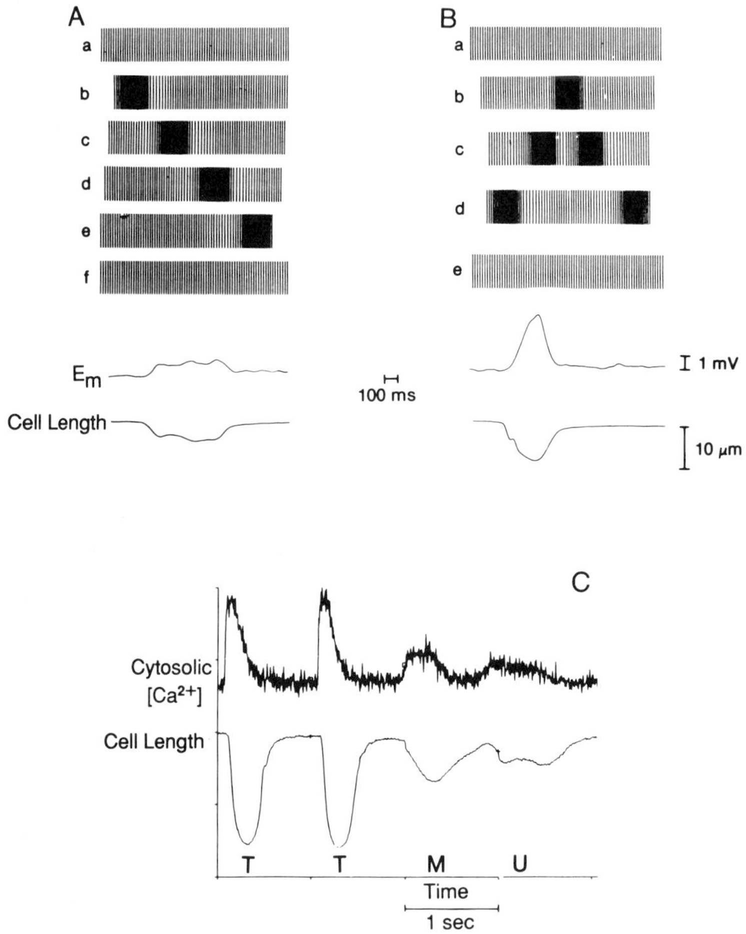
A
a
b
c
d
e
f
B
a
b
c
d
e
E m
Cell Length
100 ms
1 mV
10 μm
C
Cytosolic [Ca2+]
Cell Length
T
T
M
U
Time
1 sec

the twitch amplitude elicited by electrical excitation in a given myocyte occurred simultaneously with the onset of spontaneous SR Ca^{2+} release (28) (Fig. 7).

A concept that emerges from these experiments is that in multicellular tissues in which spontaneous Ca^{2+} release occurs asynchronously among cells, contractility never reaches the highest value of which the tissue is capable because some myocytes exhibit spontaneous diastolic SR Ca^{2+} release before others have achieved their maximum inotropic state. This concept is depicted in Figure 8 by averaging the twitch amplitudes in several single myocytes (the ensemble thus simulates a tissue) measured across a range of Ca_o. The average systolic shortening of an ensemble of cells can continue to increase, even though some cells begin to exhibit spontaneous Ca^{2+} release. Thus, it may be expected that in intact muscle excessive Ca^{2+} loading must be defined not by the presence of spontaneous Ca^{2+} release in some cells but as the state when the average magnitude of spontaneous Ca^{2+} release is sufficient to limit the average systolic function among the cells (i.e., to limit twitch amplitude).

B. Model Simulation of Muscle Behavior vs. Measured Muscle Behavior

1. Modeling of Data From Isolated Myocytes

To explore the effect of spontaneous Ca^{2+} release measured in individual cells on the contractility of the intact muscle and relate it to the behavior of papillary muscles, we constructed a schematic mathematical model (28). In this model the

---

Figure 3 Representation of spontaneous contractile waves in Ca^{2+} tolerant ventricular myocytes.

A. Diagrammatic representation of a unifocal spontaneous contractile wave: (a) the cell is at rest with uniform sarcomere length throughout; (b) a localized band of contracted sarcomeres arises at the left of the cell. This propagates through the cell (c, d, e) as a "contractile wave" and is followed (f) by the return to mechanical quiescence. The lower tracings in this panel represent the change in resting membrane potential and in cell length that occurred in a myocyte during a unifocal spontaneous contractile wave similar to that in the diagram. (From Ref. 23.)

B. Diagrammatic representation of a multifocal spontaneous contractile wave: (a) cell is quiescent; (b) localized band of contracted sarcomeres arises in the center of the cell and propagates in both directions; (c,d) to the cell ends; (e) the cell reaches the quiescent state in less time than in a unifocal wave. Note that two bands of contracted sarcomeres are simultaneously present (c,d) and that the change in cell length exceeds that observed during a unifocal wave as in A. The lower tracings in this panel were obtained from the same myocyte used for the traces in A and show that during a multifocal wave the change in membrane potential and cell shortening exceed those observed during the unifocal wave. (From Ref. 23.)

C. Changes in cell length (lower tracing) and in Ca_i (upper tracing) in an indo-1-loaded adult rat myocyte during electrically stimulated (T) and during spontaneous multifocal (M) and unifocal (U) SR Ca^{2+} release following the twitch. The signals are unfiltered and unaveraged signals. That the fluorescence underlying U and M is actually instantaneously present in only 10–20% of the cell (area within the contractile band) whereas fluorescence is measured from the entire cell indicates that the localized increase in Ca_i is of the order of magnitude of that during the stimulated twitch.

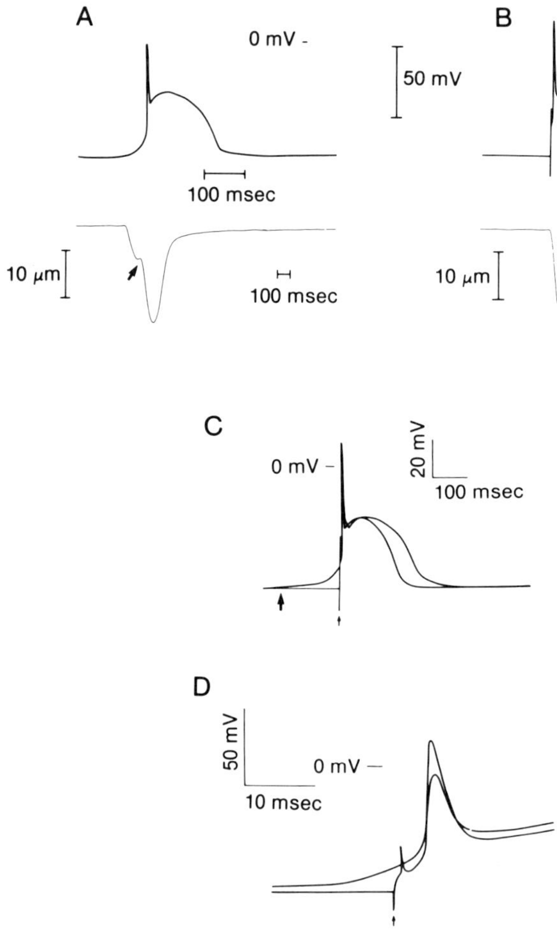
A
0 mV
50 mV
100 msec
10 μm
100 msec
B
0 mV
100 msec
10 μm
100 msec
C
0 mV
20 mV
100 msec
D
50 mV
0 mV
10 msec

"contractility" of the "muscle" is represented by the average releasable Ca^{2+} of an ensemble of cells, subject to spontaneous Ca^{2+} release (Fig. 9).

The model represents spontaneous Ca^{2+} release as a simple relaxation oscillator. When Ca^{2+} from a store is released during the twitch, some is temporarily "lost" from that releasable store. The Ca^{2+} reloading of that store is depicted as a monoexponential process, tending toward an asymptotic level, y_o, proportional to Ca_o, which, in our model, is defined as the "effective" Ca_o. The twitch amplitude in response to a test excitation at any time is proportional to the value of releasable stored Ca^{2+} at that moment, y(t). If y(t) exceeds a threshold value, y_m, the store is spontaneously released, resetting the system. It is important to note that this model is not intended as a complete model of force–interval relationship. In its schematic form it omits many phenomena. For example, because only a single "compartment" of stored Ca^{2+} is considered, the model has no memory for the effects of beats prior to the most recent one. In particular, the model does not consider explicitly the mechanism of spontaneous Ca^{2+} release, but makes use of one salient attribute: the fact that spontaneous release appears always to occur at a time when releasable stores have approximately the same level. As seen below, the qualitative explanatory power of this simple schematic model is considerable and shows that the phenomenon of spontaneous Ca^{2+} release can profoundly affect the behavior of whole muscle in ways not sensitive to the details of its mechanism.

In the schematic model, a single resting cell will execute periodic releases of Ca^{2+} with period

$$t_m = \log\left(\frac{y_0}{y_0 - y_m}\right), \tag{1}$$

and between releases the stored Ca^{2+} will be given by

$$y(t) = y_0(1 - e^{-t}), \tag{2}$$

Figure 4 A. Recording of spontaneous action potential and twitch resulting from multifocal spontaneous Ca^{2+} release. Arrow indicates cell edge displacement due to the occurrence of contractile activity due to the spontaneous Ca^{2+} release. B. Recording of an electrically driven action potential and the resultant contraction shown for comparison. C, D. Comparison of the action potentials shown in A and B at higher resolution. Note that while the threshold potential in the spontaneous vs. the driven action potentials is similar, the upstroke velocity of the spontaneous action potential (dV/dt = 45 V/sec) is less than that of the driven one (dV/dt = 120 V/sec). In D, the driven beat has a faster upstroke and overshoots zero potential. In C, the large arrow points to the beginning of the spontaneous depolarization that accompanies the contractile wave, and in both C and D the small arrow indicates the stimulus artifact of the driven beat. It is well known that with regular stimulation of rat myocytes the twitch amplitude markedly decreases and the action potential duration shortens compared with those following a long pause. The relatively large twitch and transmembrane action potential duration of the spontaneous events relative to the stimulated events in the figure arise because the latter were measured during the steady-state stimulation at 1 Hz, while the former occurred in the absence of regular stimulation. Thus, the design of this particular experiment precludes comparison of amplitudes of spontaneous with stimulated twitch amplitudes or of the duration of the transmembrane action potentials. Instead, the figure contrasts the take-off potential and the foot of the mechanical record in both types of events. (From Ref. 23.)

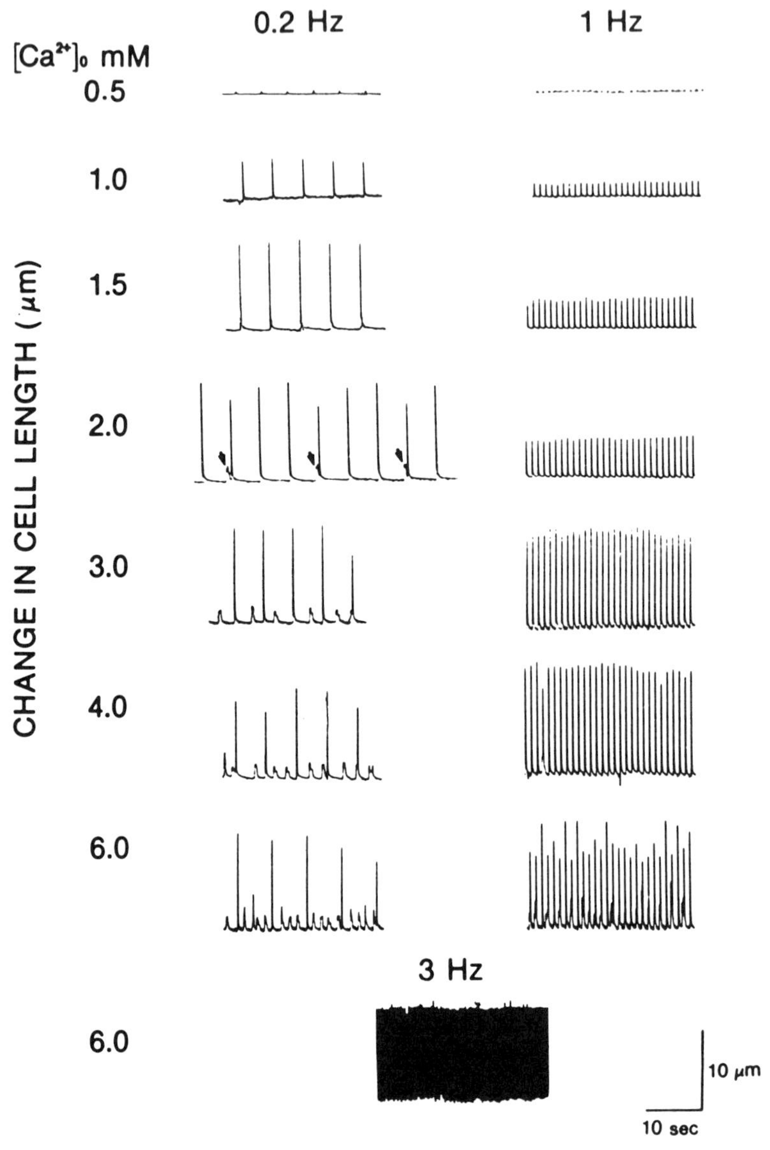

Figure 5 Tracing of cell displacement of a rat myocyte stimulated at different frequencies in varying Ca_0. The left-hand panels were obtained during stimulation at 0.2 Hz. The appearance of spontaneous contractile waves is indicated by arrows only in the tracing at 2 mM Ca_0. The right-hand panels were obtained during stimulation at 1 Hz. The bottom panel shows stimulation at 3 Hz in 6 mM Ca_0. (From Ref. 28.)

where we have taken the time constant for reloading of the store as the unit of time.

We now consider an ensemble of cells, whose Ca^{2+} stores are synchronously released by a stimulus at $t=0$. With time following this synchronous release SR Ca^{2+} reloading occurs. If y_0 is greater than threshold y_m, each cell will execute independent oscillations until the next stimulus. During this interval, there will be progressive dephasing of cells due to statistical variability in their oscillation frequencies. We represent this cell-to-cell variation (for computational purposes) as being due to a statistical distribution of the release threshold y_m, which, for simplicity, is assumed to be normally distributed about a mean value (variability of uptake rates or of y_0 would give similar dephasing effects). The aggregate twitch amplitude for a stimulus at time t is given by Equation (2), evaluated for the time elapsed since the last spontaneous release, and ensemble averaged over the distribution values of y_m. The time since the last release, for any given cell, will be that time since the last stimulus, less any whole multiples of the cell's oscillation period t_m. We find therefore, for the contractility at time t, in the presence of an effective Ca_o, y_0, the expression.

$$F(y_0, t) = y_0 \int_0^\infty \left(1 - \exp\{t_m(y_m, y_0)\ \mathrm{INT}[t/t_m\ (y_m, y_0)] - t\}\right) P(y_m)dy_m, \tag{3}$$

where INT means "integer part of" and $P(y_m)$ is the probability distribution of the cellular thresholds.

Another quantity of importance is the frequency R at which asynchronous spontaneous Ca^{2+} releases (contractile waves) occur throughout the muscle. A given cell will undergo its nth spontaneous release when $t=nt_m$. The cells undergoing their nth release between t and t+dt are therefore those with values of t_m between t/n and $(t+dt)$/n, whose number is given, using Equation (1), by

$$R_n dt = P[y_0(1 - e^{-t/n})]y_0/n\ e^{-t/n}dt. \tag{4}$$

Summing up over n, we find for the total number of release events per unit time

$$R(t) = \sum_{n=1}^{\infty} P[y_0(1 - e^{-t/n})]y_0/n\ e^{-t/n}. \tag{5}$$

Equations (3) and (5) are suitable for numerical evaluation, which are done using the modeling language MLAB.

In the model we considered first the macroscopic twitch amplitude of a muscle stimulated regularly at frequency f, as a function of Ca^{2+}. Figure 10 shows the model simulation for two stimulation rates. Initially the twitch amplitude rises with increasing Ca, to a degree inversely proportional to stimulation rate. Eventually, when the average spontaneous release frequency exceeds the stimulation rate, the twitch amplitude declines with further Ca^{2+} increases. Maximum contractility never reaches the peak value of which one cell is capable because some cells have spontaneous release before others reach maximum average force. Thus, regardless of the stimulation frequency, average contractility expressed as average Ca^{2+} release remains below its maximal value. However, because of the overdrive suppression of spontaneous Ca^{2+} release, the Ca_o at which peak contractility occurs is higher at 2

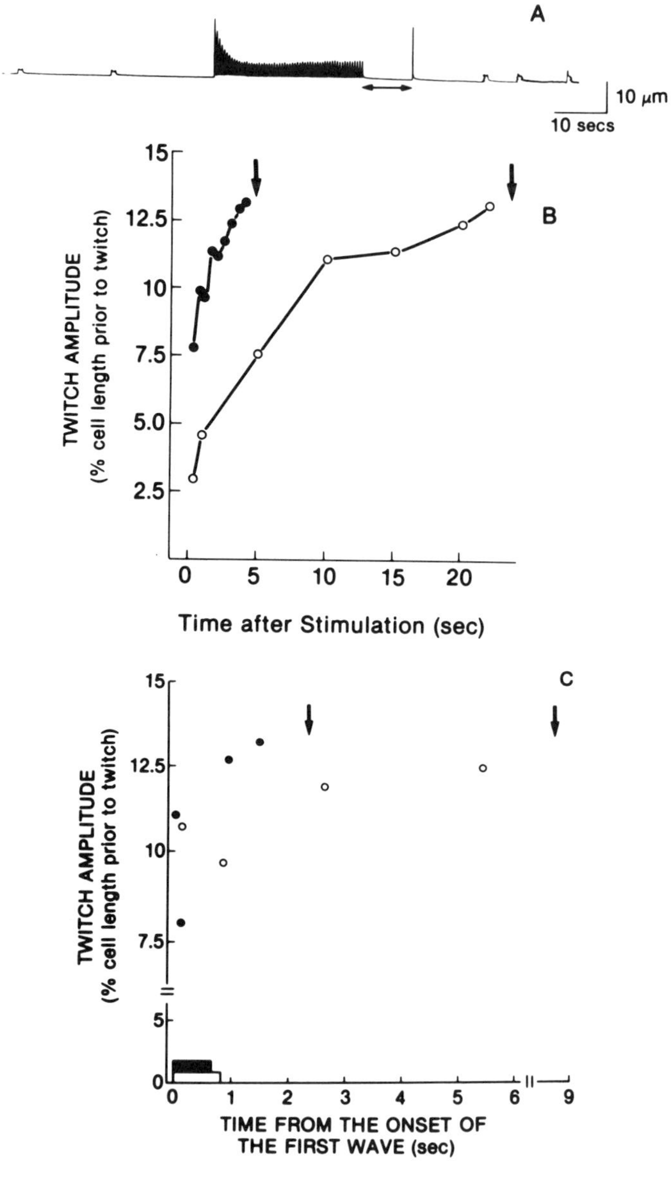
A
10 μm
10 secs
B
TWITCH AMPLITUDE
(% cell length prior to twitch)
15
12.5
10
7.5
5.0
2.5
0
5
10
15
20
Time after Stimulation (sec)
C
TWITCH AMPLITUDE
(% cell length prior to twitch)
15
12.5
10
7.5
5
0
0
1
2
3
4
5
6
9
TIME FROM THE ONSET OF
THE FIRST WAVE (sec)

Hz than at 0.5 Hz, a finding strikingly similar to the experiment with a single myocyte depicted in Figure 5.

Without adding any additional features to the model, we are at liberty to keep Ca_o fixed and vary *t*, the time elapsed since the last stimulus (i.e., as for the single myocyte in Fig. 6). It then becomes a model of time-dependent restitution of contractility with Ca^{2+} as a parameter (Fig. 11). In low Ca_o, restitution is a monotonic, roughly exponential process with the plateau contractility increasing in proportion to Ca_o. When Ca_o exceeds the average threshold for the onset of spontaneous Ca^{2+} release, the maximum contractility ceases to increase, and the pattern of restitution becomes oscillatory. A further increase in Ca_o shortens the period of the damped oscillation and lowers the plateau that occurs at long restitution time.

The frequency of asynchronous Ca^{2+} release as mentioned above may be indirectly observed by its contribution to diastolic tone, and more directly by laser scattering intensity fluctuations. Each release event will make a tiny brief contribution to the tension of the muscle; the aggregate of these will give rise to an active diastolic tension proportional to the instantaneous rate of release events in the muscle. Figure 12 shows the model simulation for restitution curves for twitch and resting force (taken to be proportional to the frequency of spontaneous Ca^{2+} release) in high and low Ca_o. As depicted in the figure, the model simulation of the onset of oscillatory restitution of twitch force is accompanied by the development of damped periodic after-contractions. The oscillations of twitch restitution lead the after-contractions in phase by about 90 degrees, because the peak contractility occurs when the largest number of cells are maximally Ca^{2+} loaded and have not yet undergone spontaneous release. Thus the present model interprets the after-contraction as a "storm" of asynchronous spontaneous Ca^{2+} release events, clustered in time because of the synchronizing influence of the previous stimulus.

Figure 6 Restitution of twitch amplitude after a train of stimulation in a representative rat cardiac myocyte. The protocol employed is given in A. The cell was stimulated at 2 Hz for 30 sec. The twitch amplitude in response to a test excitation at varying intervals after cessation of stimulation was then measured. After this measurement, the myocyte was stimulated again and the test interval was varied. At least 6 min were allowed to elapse between the stimulation trains to let any residual effect of stimulation on the cell dissipate. During these experiments, spontaneous contractile waves were present in the unstimulated state and did not occur during stimulation. In the example in A, Ca_o was 2 mM and the test interval is indicated by a longitudinal arrow. B. The effect of Ca_o on the restitution of twitch amplitude in 2 (○) and 4 (●) mM Ca_o. The abscissa indicates the time elapsed from the end of the stimulation train to the test stimulus, which in this panel always precedes the first contractile wave after stimulation. The arrow indicates the average time of occcurrence of the first spontaneous contractile wave in each Ca_o. This time was 24.9 ± 0.3 ($n = 4$) and 4.2 ± 0.9 sec ($n = 4$) in 2 and 4 mM Ca_o, respectively. C. The twitch amplitude of the test stimulus delivered either during the first or between the first and the second spontaneous contractile waves that occurred after stimulation in 2 and 4 mM Ca_o. Symbols are as in B. The abscissa indicates the time elapsed from the beginning of the first spontaneous contractile wave. The open and filled bars on the abscissa indicate the average duration of the spontaneous contractile waves in 2 and 4 mM Ca_o, respectively. The arrows indicate the average time of occurrence of the second contractile wave. (From Ref. 28.)

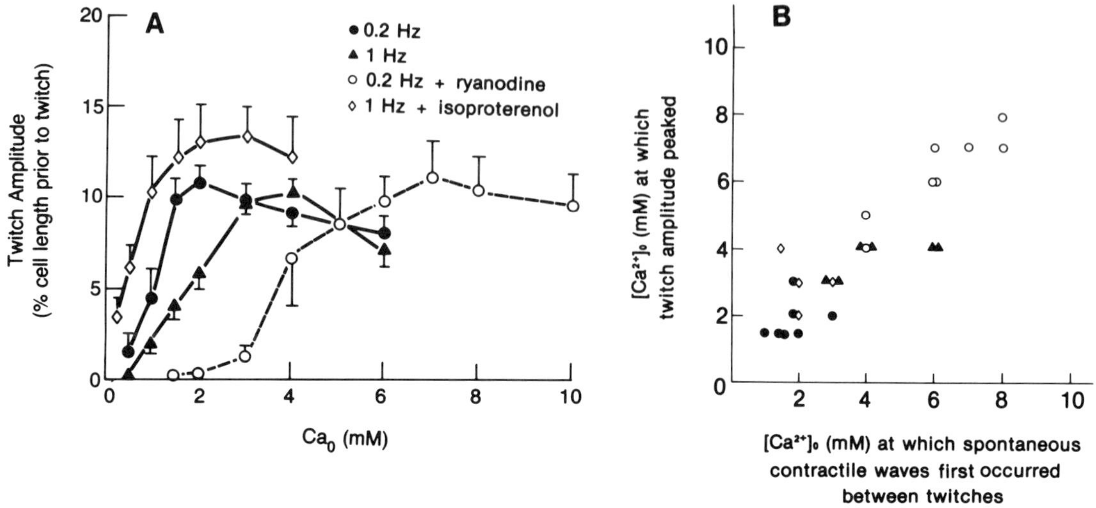

Figure 7 A. Twitch amplitude at varying Ca_0 in rat myocytes continuously stimulated at 0.2 Hz (●) and at 1 Hz (▲; n = 5), in the presence of isoproterenol at 1 Hz (◇; n = 5) and following a brief exposure to 1 μM ryanodine (○; n = 5). Maximum twitch amplitude is similar in the four groups. B. A unique relationship between the Ca_0 at which the twitch amplitude peaked and spontaneous contractile waves first appeared for all cells studied in four protocols, including all myocytes from A. Regardless of the drug or stimulation frequency, the Ca_0 at which the twitch saturated varied linearly with the Ca_0 at which spontaneous Ca^{2+} release first became manifest: $y = 0.70 + 8.83x$; $r = 0.90$, $p = <0.001$, $n = 25$. (From Ref. 28.)

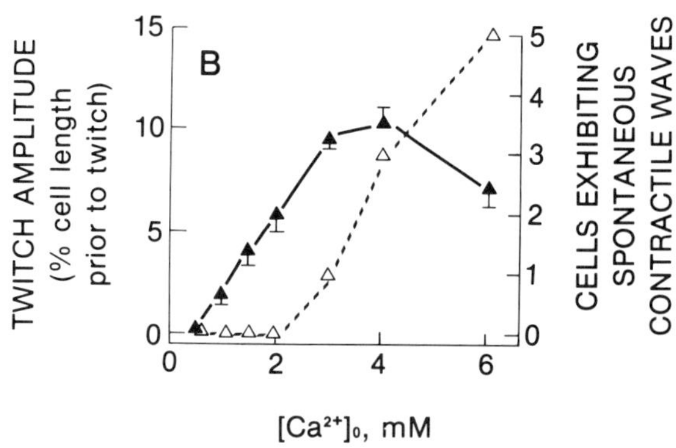

Figure 8 Average twitch amplitude in response to an increase in Ca_0 from myocytes stimulated at 1 Hz. The dotted line indicates how many of these cells exhibited spontaneous contractile waves in each Ca_0. (From Ref. 28.)

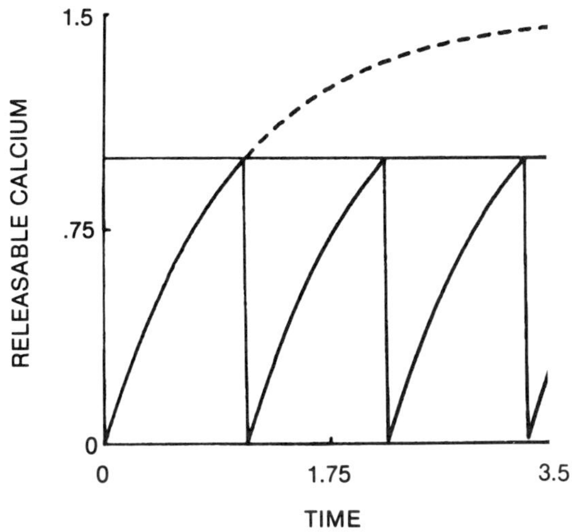

Figure 9 A heuristic model of Ca^{2+} release. At time zero "releasable Ca^{2+}" (ordinate) is depleted by stimulated release. It then increases monoexponentially towards an asymptote proportional to [Ca_o]. Before reaching the asymptote, releasable Ca^{2+} crosses the threshold for spontaneous release after which the process repeat itself causing diastolic oscillations. (From Ref. 21.)

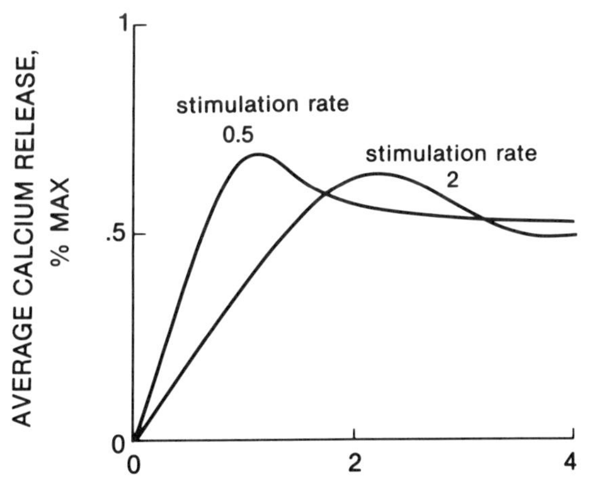

Figure 10 Average contractility of an ensemble of cells, calculated from the model (see text), expressed as average released Ca^{2+} during steady stimulation at two rates. The unit of time is the exponential reloading time of releasable Ca. The independent variable is "effective Ca_o," y_o defined as the asymptotic value that stored SR Ca^{2+} would approach if no spontaneous release occurred, expressed in units of the average threshold Ca^{2+} for spontaneous release. (From Ref. 28.)

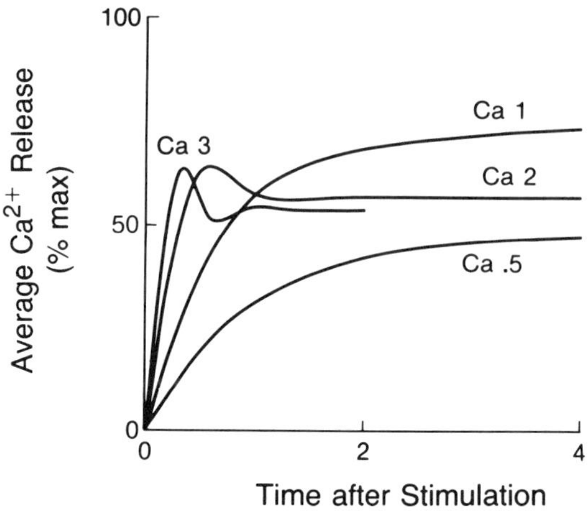

Figure 11 Restitution of "contractility" expressed as average Ca^{2+} release by a test stimulation as a function of time since the previous stimulus, for several values of "effective Ca_o" as defined in Figure 10. The units of time are the same as in Figure 10. (From Ref. 28.)

2. *Measured Behavior of Intact Muscle*

Studies in intact muscle sought to delineate the relationship between twitch or resting tension and spontaneous oscillatory SR Ca^{2+} release assessed as scattered light intensity fluctuations (SLIF) in a laser beam incident to the tissue. Measurements obtained during time-gated intervals following prior electrical stimulation or at rest in rat papillary muscles were used to determine whether the mathematical model derived from data in individual cells accurately predicted the behavior of intact tissue.

For the experiment to be described in this section, thin rat papillary muscles were mounted isometrically in series with a force gauge in a 3 ml glass chamber and were illuminated by a He–Ne laser beam. Light scattered from the muscle at a 30 degree angle was collected onto the photomultiplier. The resulting signal was analyzed by a digital autocorrelator. SLIF measurements are presented as $f_{1/2}$ (Hz)

$$f_{1/2} = \frac{1}{2\rho t_{1/2}}$$

where $t_{1/2}$ is the time (msec) for the autocorrelation function to decay to 50% of its baseline.

A biphasic Ca_o-twitch relationship similar to that depicted in single cells (Fig. 8) and in the model simulation (Fig. 10) is also observed in rat papillary muscles (29) (Fig. 13). In this representative experiment both SLIF and twitch tension were measured in a 2.5–5.5 sec window after stimulation at 1Hz and after a rested contraction. Peak twitch tension is achieved at different Ca_o, but at similar SLIF (2–3 Hz) under both conditions. As Ca_o increases further, SLIF increases but twitch tension declines. These observations raise the issue of what defines "excessive cell Ca^{2+} loading" at the intact tissue level. As shown in Figure 8, the average systolic shortening of an ensemble of cells can continue to an increase in peak force, even though some cells begin to exhibit spontaneous Ca^{2+} release. Thus, at the level of

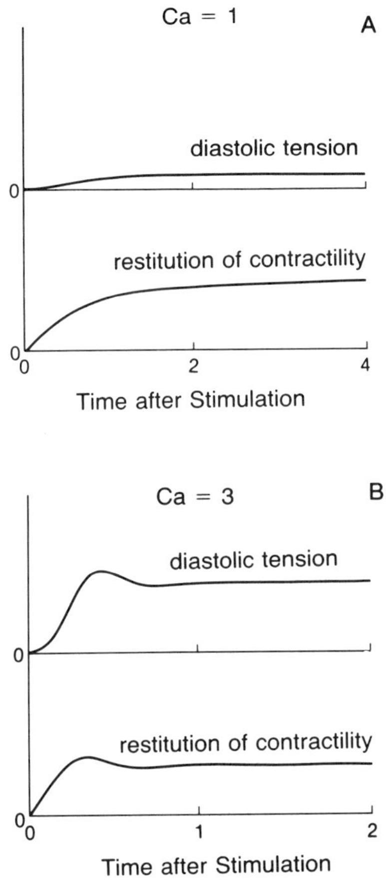

Figure 12 Restitution of average Ca^{2+} release in response to an action potential (contractility) and active diastolic tension (proportional to mean frequency of spontaneous release events) for two levels of "effective Ca_o" defined as in Figure 10. The units of time and Ca^{2+} are the same as in Figures 10 and 11. The vertical scales are arbitrary, but are the same for A and B (see text for details). (From Ref. 28.)

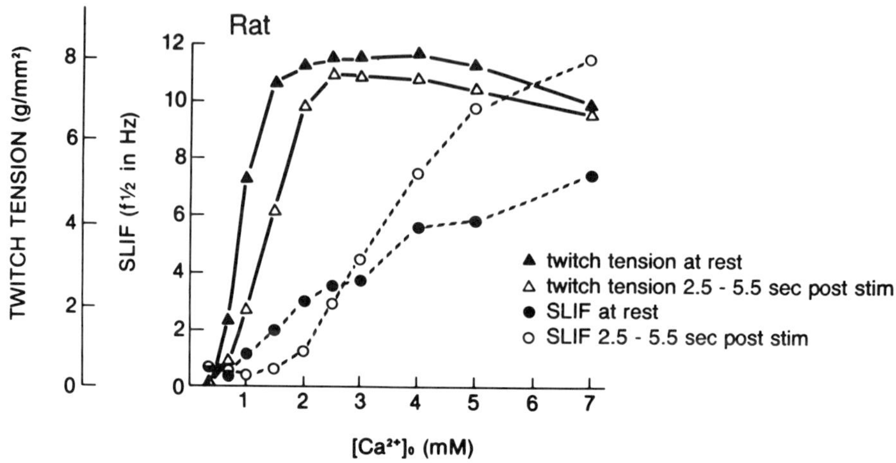

Figure 13 The effect of large variations of Ca_o on twitch tension and SLIF measured 2.5–5.5 sec poststimulation at 60 min^{-1} and at rest in a representative rat muscle. (From Ref. 30.)

the intact muscle excessive Ca^{2+} loading must be defined not by the presence of spontaneous Ca^{2+} release in some cells but as the state when the magnitude of spontaneous Ca^{2+} release is sufficient to limit the average systolic function among the cells, that is, to limit twitch force. Figure 13 also shows that in lower Ca_o, poststimulation SLIF values were lower than at rest and as Ca_o is increased a disproportionate enhancement occurs in SLIF poststimulation than at rest. This finding indicates that electrical stimulation can have opposite effects on the occurrence of oscillatory SR Ca^{2+} release, which can either be suppressed or enhanced according to the extent of Ca^{2+} loading of the myocardium. This is in agreement with the results of similar experiments in isolated myocardial cells (11,13), in which the restitution pattern of spontaneous contractile oscillations could be either temporarily enhanced or suppressed by varying the stimulation frequency and Ca_o. The greater degree of synchronization of restitution of spontaneous SR Ca^{2+} release achieved by enhancing Ca^{2+} loading in single cells may significantly affect resting tension and contractility in a multicellular cardiac preparation. If this interpretation is correct, then SLIFs, which are a manifestation of the microscopic motion due to these release events, should vary in phase with the restitution of resting tension and the occurrence of aftercontractions rather than with the restitution of contractility.

Figures 14 and 15 show in bulk rat cardiac muscle a Ca_o dependence of restitution phenomenon similar to that observed in single cardiac cells (Fig. 6) and simulated by the model in Figure 11. For 1–5 sec following stimulation of rat muscle bathed in 1.5 mM Ca_o, twitch and resting tension are depressed and SLIFs are transiently abolished. SLIFs and resting tension then recover simultaneously and monotonically but lag behind the restitution of twitch tension. In the absence of further stimulation, SLIFs persist and the rested state twitch amplitude remains potentiated. When Ca_o is increased above 2.5 mM the restitution of all parameters following stimulation is accelerated and becomes oscillatory. Figure 15 shows oscillatory patterns of restitution of SLIF, twitch tension, and resting tension within the 10 sec following stimulation in 3 mM Ca_o. Under these conditions of Ca^{2+} loading, SLIF

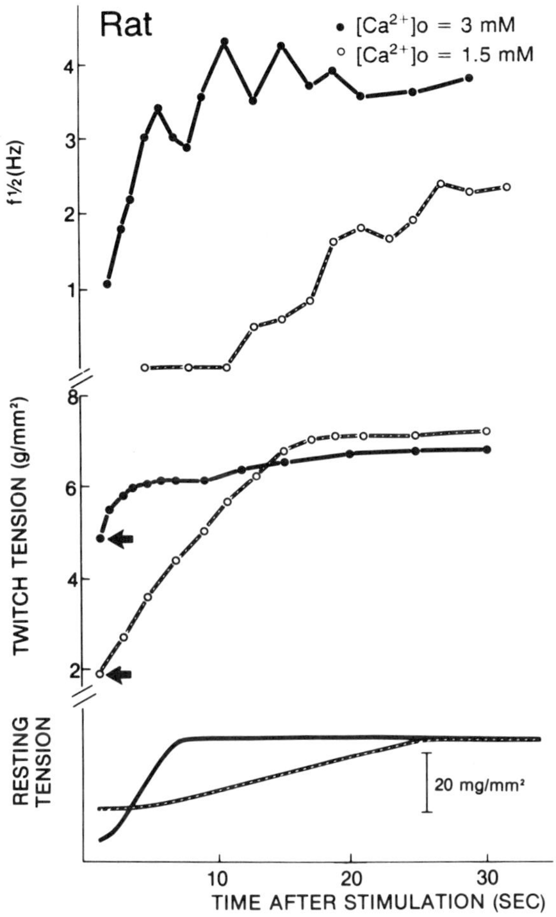

Figure 14 SLIF and tension restitution following stimulation at 40 min^{-1} in a representative rat muscle bathed in Ca_o of 1.5 mM or 3.0 mM. The recovery of SLIF and tension is accelerated in the higher Ca_o, but in both cases SLIF recovery occurs later than that of twitch tension. The arrows indicate the twitch tension during regular stimulation at 40 min^{-1}. The detection of the resting tension transient following a prior twitch in most muscles under this experimental condition requires recording at high sensitivity because the magnitude of the resting tension transient is relatively small. In this muscle the change in resting tension over the restitution interval was only about 20 mg (i.e., 2.5 orders of magnitude less than the steady-state twitch). The two resting tension curves were overlaid so as to have the same steady-state levels. This was necessary because the absolute resting tension decreases over the relatively long period required to implement this time-gating protocol. (From Ref. 30.)

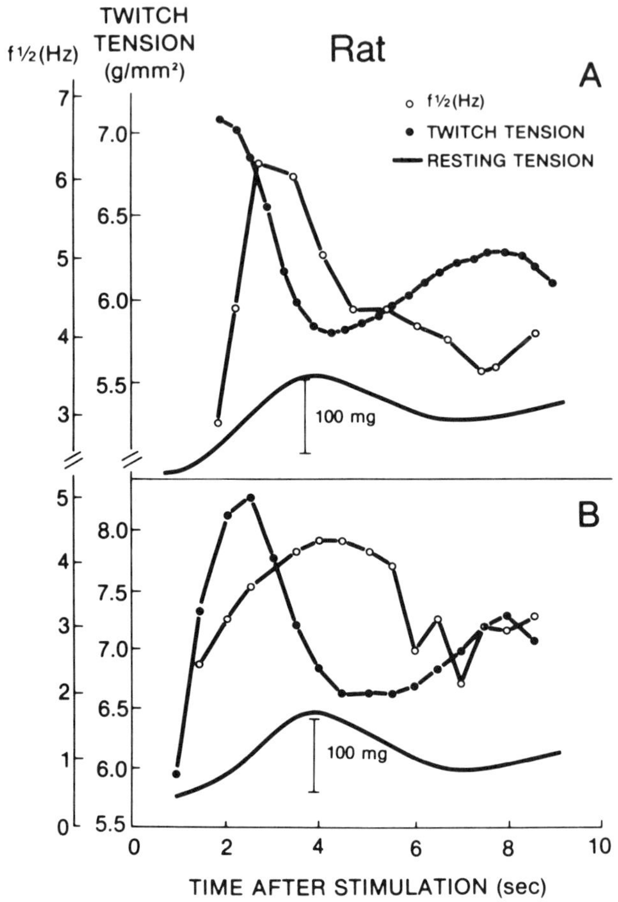

Figure 15 Oscillatory patterns of restitution observed following stimulation at 7 min^{-1} of rat muscles bathed in Ca_o of 3.0 mM. Both examples show that restitution of SLIF and resting tension is oscillatory but out of phase with the oscillatory recovery of twitch tension. (From Ref. 30.)

and resting tension restitution lag behind that of the twitch such that twitch amplitude increases, overshoots, and decreases to a nadir as SLIF and resting tension reach their initial maximum.

Thus, in a given muscle the maximum twitch amplitude occurs at an optimal level of SLIF: when this level is exceeded, either transiently during monotonic or oscillatory recovery following stimulation in a given Ca_o (Fig. 15) or in the steady rested state by an increase in Ca_o (Fig. 13), twitch tension plateaus and then decreases.

III. PATHOPHYSIOLOGICAL CONDITIONS

A. Acidosis

Acidosis is a clinically relevant condition that can be secondary to many pathologic states such as diabetic ketoacidosis (metabolic acidosis) or ventilatory disturbances with $C0_2$ retention (respiratory acidosis). In addition to these and other generalized disorders of acid–base equilibrium, it is also possible to have profound acidosis of a less generalized or focal nature, as occurs during myocaridal ischemia. The myocardial effects of a decrease in cytosolic pH, regardless of its cause, are marked and have a negative action on the inotropic state of the heart. The effect of acidosis is to decrease the affinity of troponin C for calcium, with resultant diminution in myofilament responsiveness to Ca^{2+} (31,32). In aequorin-loaded preparations there is an increase in the amplitude of the Ca_i transient associated with the twitch (33–35).

The effects of acidosis on calcium oscillations are complex, with several temporal phases, probably representing the influence of multiple antagonistic processes. Fabiato and Fabiato (31) investigated the direct effect of intracellular acidosis on calcium release from the sarcoplasmic reticulum, using mechanically skinned cardiac myocyte preparations. Lowering pH from 7.4 to 6.2, at constant pCa, caused a marked, reversible decrease in the frequency of spontaneous calcium release oscillations. They assessed the amount of calcium accumulated in the SR during 2 min at pCa 7.75 (determined by measuring the contraction produced by abrupt application of caffeine), and found that SR calcium loading also decreased steadily as pH was lowered. These studies, which showed purely negative effects of acidosis on SR loading and release, involved brief exposures to acidosis, so it cannot be excluded that there are slower polyphasic direct effects of pH on the SR.

Orchard et al. (35) studied the effects of acidosis on calcium oscillations in papillary muscles (monitored by SLIF and aequorin luminescence) and in isolated myocytes. In rat muscles and cells bathed in an elevated calcium concentration of 4 mM, they found a triphasic effect of acidosis produced by increasing the PCO_2 in a bicarbonate buffer system. Initially there was rapid, marked depression of SLIF frequency in papillary muscles, and of the frequency of spontaneous contractile waves in single myocytes. This was followed by an increase of oscillation frequency to 140% of control, which peaked at about 10 min. With continued acidosis, oscillation frequency again fell toward control. Measurement of aequorin light showed that, at the time of the enhanced oscillations, the twitch calcium transient was increased above control, even though the mechanical twitch was markedly depressed by the known depressant effect of acidosis on the myofilaments. The phase of increased oscillations was much less prominent when bathing calcium was less than or equal to 2 mM, but was still evident. In addition, the onset of the positive phase appeared to be delayed at normal calcium concentrations.

In this study, it was also observed that acidosis was associated with ~ 3 mv cell depolarization. This results in an increased likelihood for the transient depolarization caused by each spontaneous SR Ca^{2+} release to reach threshold and trigger an action potential (Fig. 16) and may represent a mechanism for the arrhythmogenic effect of acidosis. These authors hypothesized that the initial decrease in oscillation frequency was due to the direct effect of intracellular acidosis on the SR, as demonstrated by Fabiato and Fabiato (31). The secondary increase of oscillations was attributed to a presumed rise in Ca_i, of undetermined cause. A rise in Ca_i could, in fact, be demonstrated by resting aequorin luminescence in papillary muscles, but only in the presence of 5 mM Ca_o and ouabain. The rise in Ca_i was not detected in the presence of ryanodine. Increased "resting" Ca_i sufficient to be detected by aequorin was therefore a consequence of the increased oscillations. The decline of

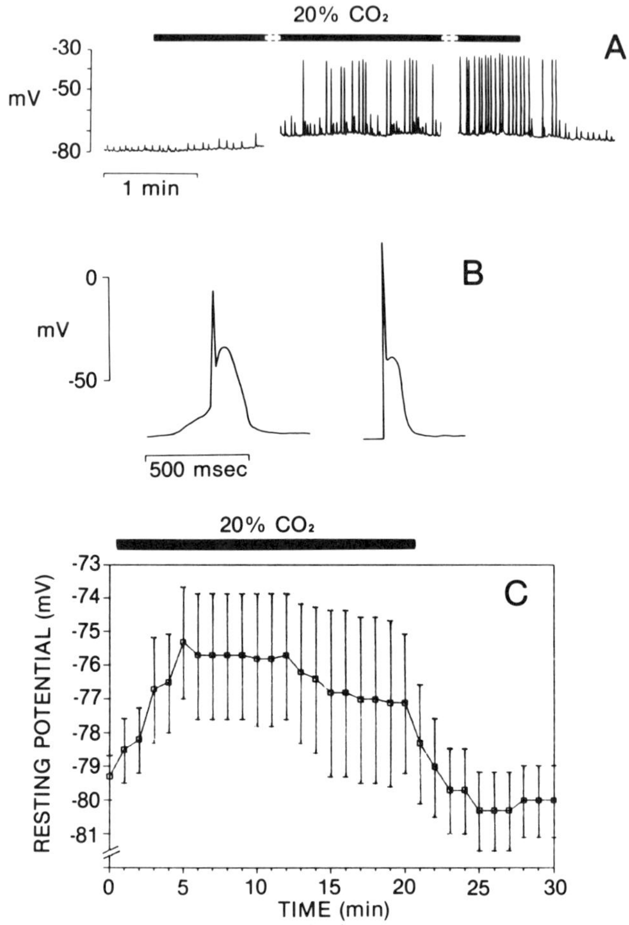

Figure 16 The effect of acidosis on spontaneous depolarizations of the cell membrane that accompany the spontaneous contractile waves. A. Records of membrane potential before and during the first minute of exposure to the acid solution (left), after 9 min exposure to the acid solution (middle), and during the 20th min of exposure to the acid solution and return to normal pH solution (right). The action potentials (large vertical lines) are truncated by the low-frequency response of the pen recorder. B. Reproductions of oscilloscope recordings of spontaneous transient electrical depolarization sufficient to trigger an action potential during acidosis. Left. Spontaneous depolarization that triggered the action potential. Right. An electrically stimulated action potential for comparison. C. Membrane potential measured between oscillations before, during, and after acidosis (mean ± SEM, n=4). All preparations depolarized on exposure to acidosis. (From Ref. 35.)

oscillations in the third phase was of unknown cause, when it was assumed, based on previous studies, that intracellular pH did not significantly correct toward normal during the period of application of 20% CO_2.

Recent studies of twitch contractility in guinea pig papillary muscles and sheep Purkinje fibers (36) found that there was a positive phase to the inotropic effect of intracellular acidosis in the presence of normal extracellular pH, but not when extracellular pH was simultaneously lowered. These studies were done with simultaneous monitoring of intracellular pH and sodium activity by ion-selective electrodes. It was found that the positive phase was associated with a rise in intracellular Na^+ activity, and that both were prevented by amiloride, a blocker of Na^+/H^+ exchange. It appeared, therefore, that the positive inotropic phase was due to entry of calcium by Na^+/Ca^+ exchange, in exchange for sodium that entered by Na^+/H^+ exchange, the latter process being inhibited by extracellular acidosis (37). In the light of these studies, it appears highly likely that the increase in Ca^{++} oscillations observed by Orchard et al. (35) during respiratory acidosis has a similar mechanism.

B. Ischemia and Hypoxia

During cardiac ischemia, contractile force rapidly declines, for reasons that are, as yet, incompletely understood. When the heart is reperfused following ischemia of moderate or prolonged duration, function does not, in general, return to normal, and after prolonged ischemia parts of the tissue do not survive after reperfusion. Chemical methods of analysis have shown a marked increase in total intracellular calcium following late reperfusion (38). Since calcium oscillations are indicative of the state of releasable calcium within the SR, and are increased in frequency in most states of "calcium overload," it is of great interest to know what happens to these oscillations during ischemia and during reperfusion. Since, as shown above, the oscillations themselves, occurring asynchronously throughout the myocardium, can affect macroscopic muscle function, it is also possible that these oscillations might play a role in the dysfunction accompanying ischemia or reperfusion.

One of the earliest clues to the effect of ischemialike states on calcium oscillations was the observation by Lakatta and Lappe (10) that the SLIF frequency declined when papillary muscles were deprived of oxygen and glucose, even while the resting tension of these muscles was rising (Fig. 17). The decline of SLIF frequency during this "ischemic" contracture was in striking contrast to the increase in SLIF associated with most "contractures" produced by calcium overload. Since the ischemic contracture was believed to be due to a rise in intracellular calcium (a point still under debate), this was particularly paradoxical. The effects of anoxia and reperfusion to decrease SLIF may relate to the finding that anoxia inhibits reperfusion and digitalis-induced ventricular tachyarrhythmias (39). It was subsequently shown by the same investigators that the mechanism for this effect of anoxia is a reduction of oscillatory potentials, and after-contractions (40), two events related to spontaneous SR Ca^{2+} release.

The papillary muscle preparation is not very suitable for studies of ischemia, since it is a superfused preparation and it is difficult either to achieve good hypoxia at the surface of the muscle or to limit the outward diffusion of metabolic products. To study actual ischemia, the SLIF technique was adapted to work in a backscatter mode, using laser light scattered off the epicardial surface of the heart. This technique is only applicable in species in which epicardial connective tissue is very thin or absent. Using this method, striking changes in SLIF frequency were found during ischemia and reperfusion (41). When an intact, Langendorff-perfused heart is made globally ischemic, SLIF frequency falls rapidly, reaching 50% or less of its

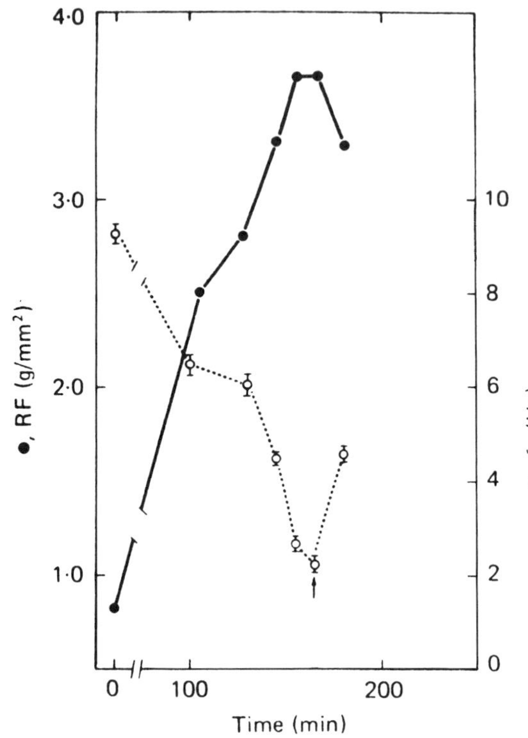

Figure 17 An example of the effect of prolonged superfusion with hypoxic and glucose-free bathing fluid on resting force (RF) and SLIF f½. At the time shown by the arrow, the perfusate was switched back to control. (From Ref. 10.)

control value within 5 min even at 30°C. This early decline parallels the decline in isovolumic contractile force observed in the same heart when stimulated at low frequencies (1–3 times/min, to permit the averaging necessary to record SLIF during diastole) (Fig. 18). Parallel experiments using nuclear magnetic resonance (NMR) of identically handled hearts indicate that neither the fall in intracellular pH nor the decline in high-energy phosphates is sufficiently rapid to account for these changes; however, the rapid rise of intracellular inorganic phosphate (P_i) might do so. Since SLIF frequency is roughly proportional to both the amplitude and frequency of the mechanical oscillations that occur as a consequence of cytosolic calcium oscillations, the early decline in SLIF could represent either a suppression of the calcium oscillations themselves or a depression of the mechanical myofilament response to them. Inorganic phosphate is known to depress myofilament isometric force. The direct effect of P_i on calcium oscillations has not yet been studied.

Within 30 min of global ischemia at 30°C, SLIF becomes undetectable in the majority of rat hearts (in contrast, perfused rat hearts always display SLIF at frequencies of several Hz or more). If ischemia is further prolonged, isovolumic resting pressure rises after about 45–60 min of ischemia ("ischemia contracture"). This rise is never associated with the redevelopment of SLIF (Fig. 18). When the heart is then reperfused, however, SLIF frequency rises rapidly to 3–5 times

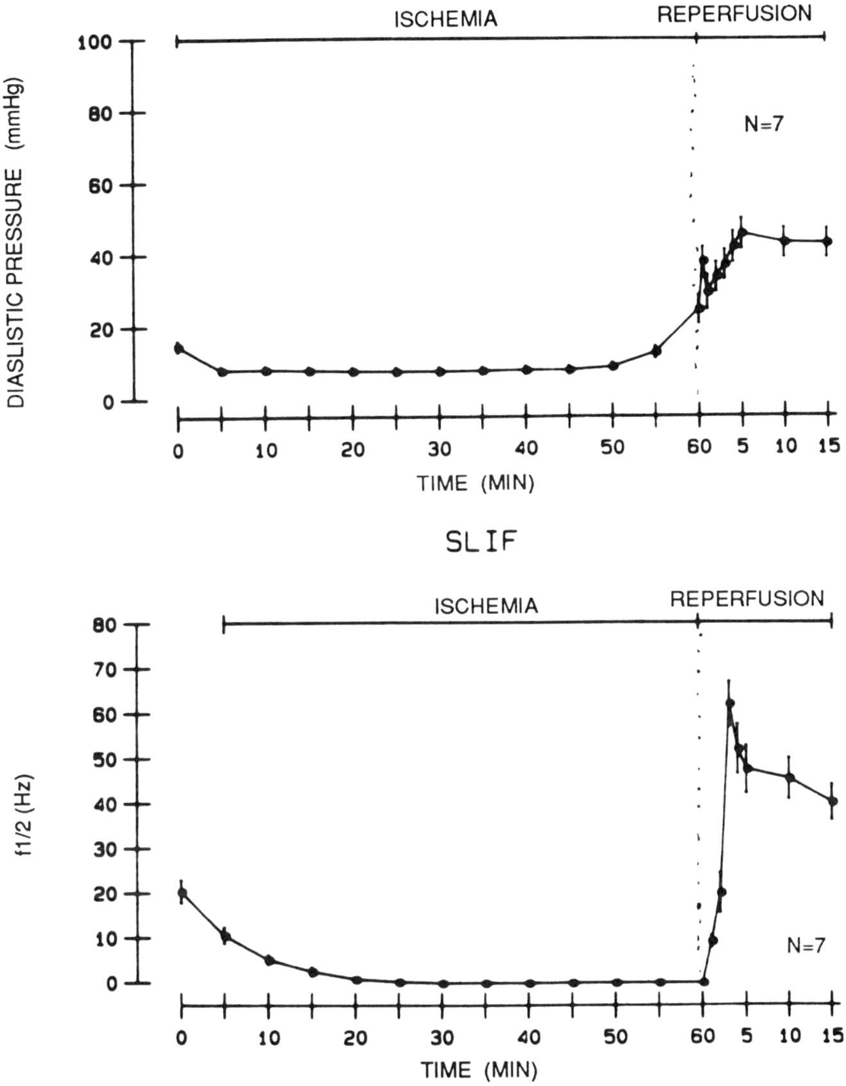

Figure 18 Average resting pressure (top) and SLIF f½ (bottom) from seven hearts subjected to global ischemia at 30°C, followed by reperfusion. (From Ref. 41.)

preischemic control within 3–5 min, and this is paralleled by a further rise in resting pressure ("reflow contracture"). At this period bulk calcium overload of the heart is known to occur; the fact that this contracture is a dynamic contracture, associated with spontaneous oscillations, suggests that at least some of this calcium overload is occurring in cells that are still potentially viable. During the postreflow period the frequency of SLIF is inversely correlated with the recovery of contractile function (42) (Fig. 19) and SLIF overshoots at a time when phosphorus 31 NMR spectra show that pH, ATP, PCr and, P_i have already recovered to a steady value. Reperfusion for the initial 10 min with 0.08 mM Ca_o before use of a perfusate with 1.5 mM Ca_o has significant beneficial effects. SLIF overshoot at 5–10 min was

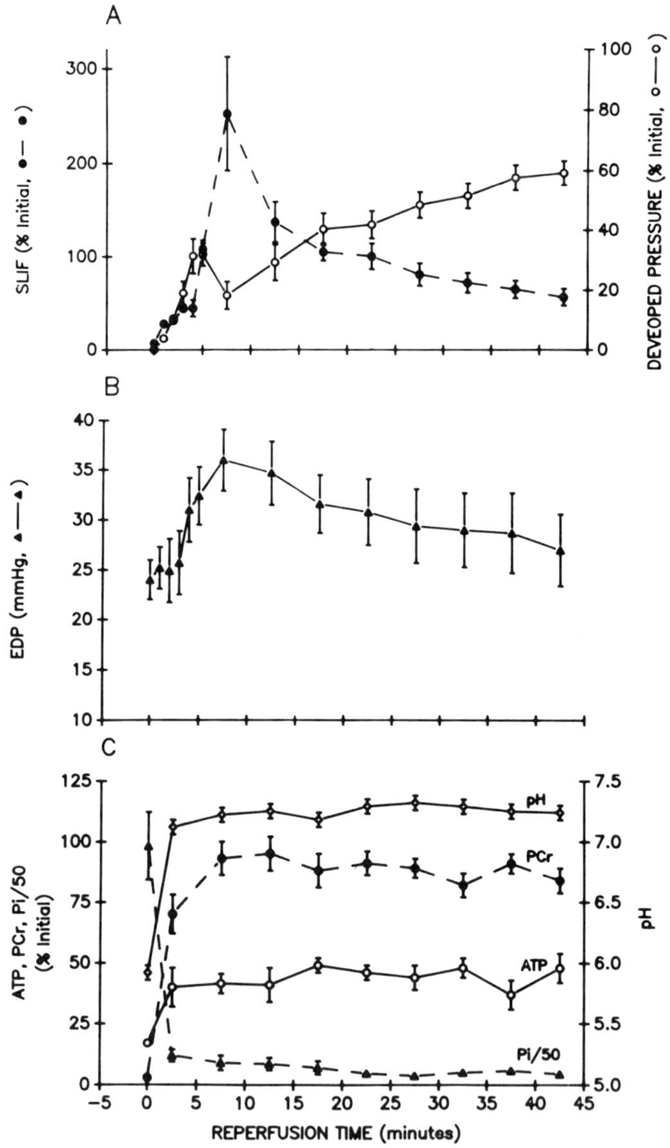
A
SLIF (% Initial, ●— ●)
DEVEOPED PRESSURE (% Initial, ○—○)
300
200
100
0
100
80
60
40
20
0
B
EDP (mmHg, ▲—▲)
40
35
30
25
20
15
10
C
ATP, PCr, Pi/50 (% Initial)
pH
125
100
75
50
25
0
7.5
7.0
6.5
6.0
5.5
5.0
pH
PCr
ATP
Pi/50
-5
0
5
10
15
20
25
30
35
40
45
REPERFUSION TIME (minutes)

prevented (Fig. 20A) and systolic function at 20 min of perfusion was enhanced; intracellular Ca^{2+} was decreased in comparison to heart that had been perfused only with buffer containing 1.5 mM Ca_o (Fig. 20B). These results are compatible with the hypothesis that the asynchronous Ca^{2+} oscillations may contribute, in part, to the depression of muscle function after reperfusion.

To acquire a more mechanistic understanding of the phenomena that underlie the pathophysiology of myocardial ischemia and perfusion and to define more precisely the effect of ischemic changes on calcium oscillations, it is necessary to study single myocytes. In isolated cardiac cells, the mechanism of excitation–contraction coupling can be more precisely measured under strictly controlled experimental conditions. Unfortunately, it is not possible to make a single myocyte ischemic. It is possible, however, to simulate the components of ischemia, namely hypoxia, substrate deprivation, acidosis, and the extracellular accumulation of metabolites, individually or in combination, with great precision. Most studies so far have concentrated on hypoxia combined with deprivation of glucose.

When isolated ventricular myocytes in suspension are made anoxic in the absence of glucose, they shorten, after a period of time that may vary from a few minutes to an hour or more, into a square form that is nearly completely depleted of ATP and probably represents a rigor state (43). When these cells are re-exposed to oxygen on a microscopic stage, they are noted to develop vigorous "spontaneous beating" within 1 min, following which they round up into structureless, blebbed "balls" (44). The latter appearance is exactly similar to that of cells destroyed by various forms of massive calcium overload.

To study this model of reoxygenation injury, Stern et al. (45,46) developed an apparatus permitting a single myocyte, under direct observation, to be subjected to extreme hypoxia (PO_2 < 0.02 torr). When rat myocytes were subjected to anoxia until they shortened into rigor forms, and were then reoxygenated, it was observed that they developed spontaneous SR Ca^{2+} oscillations. Moreover, it was observed

---

Figure 19 Contractile and metabolic recovery and diastolic Ca^{2+} oscillations (SLIF) during reperfusion (heart rate = 20 beats/min). Mean values of developed pressure (as percent initial, n=10), diastolic pressure (mm Hg, n=10), and SLIF (Hz, n=5) are plotted in A vs. reperfusion time (min). Developed pressure recovers during the first 5 min of reperfusion but then abruptly falls, reaching a nadir at 7.5 min. Thereafter, developed pressure increases slowly, attaining 60% of its initial value after 45 min of reperfusion. B. EDP climbs rapidly in the first minute of reperfusion, possibly because of the "garden hose" effect. EDP reaches a maximum at 7.5 min of reperfusion, which is significantly higher than that at 2 min of reperfusion ($p<0.01$) and occurs as developed pressure is falling. The EDP data during reperfusion are well fit by a third-degree polynomial ($p<0.008$) with an intercept of 23.4 and coefficients of 1.90, −0.92, and 0.001. C. PCr, ATP, and P_i are presented as percentage of initial, preischemic values. The mean preischemic values of PCr/ATP and P_i/ATP were 2.02±0.10 and 0.10±0.01, respectively. Metabolic parameters (n=5) recover to their full extent within 5–7.5 min of reperfusion and then plateau at a time when contractile function is falling. Diastolic Ca^{2+} oscillations, indexed by SLIF, increase from the end-ischemic value of zero and peak at a mean value of three times baseline at 7.5 min of reperfusion. This SLIF peak coincides with the transient fall in developed pressure and the peak in EDP. Subsequently, SLIFs decrease monotonically over the next 35 min of reperfusion while developed pressure recovers. (From Ref. 42.)

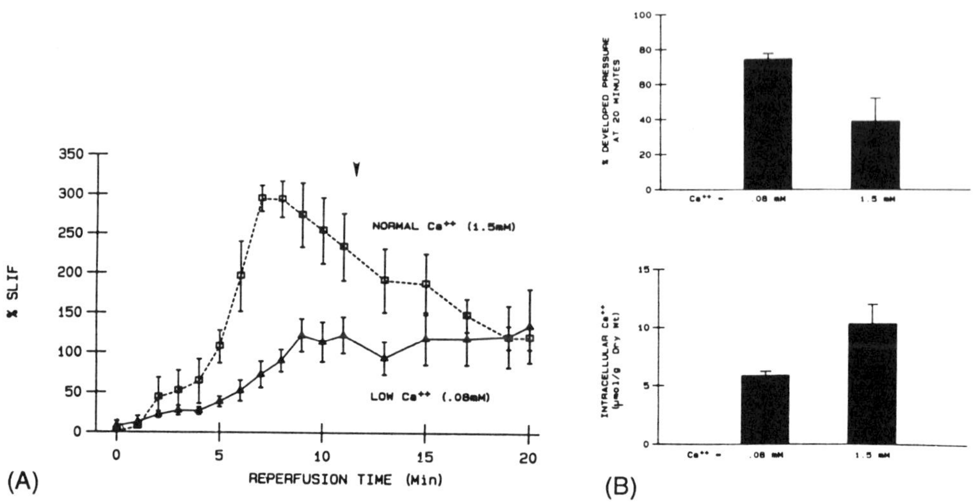

Figure 20 A. SLIF during reperfusion with low (0.08mM) and normal (1.5mM) Ca^{2+}-containing solutions. In hearts reperfused with low Ca^{2+} superfusate (n=4) after 65 min of no-flow ischemia, SLIFs increase slowly and do not "overshoot" to three times the baseline values as seen in hearts reperfused with normal Ca^{2+}-containing solution (n=4). SLIF levels are similar at 15 min of reperfusion in both groups. The arrow indicates when perfusate calcium of 1.5mM was restored in the low-calcium (0.8 mM) group. B. Developed pressure and cellular calcium following reperfusion with normal and low-calcium-containing perfusate. Hearts reperfused initially with 1.5mM Ca^{2+} have significantly higher cell calcium and lower developed pressure at 20 min than hearts perfused initially (0–10 min of reperfusion) with low (0.08mM) Ca^{2+}-containing solution. (From Ref. 42.)

that not all cells round up when reoxygenated. Rat myocytes that have spent a short enough time in the rigor state (less than about 15–20 min at 37°C) remain rectangular after reoxygenation. However, these cells also undergo a period of frequent calcium oscillations, beginning 1–3 min after reoxygenation, and lasting between 5–30 min before subsiding (see Fig. 22). Thus, the single myocyte reoxygenation model displays frequent calcium oscillations that seem to be analogous to the rise in SLIF frequency seen with reperfusion of the whole heart.

Because the myocytes can be observed directly, it is clear that there is a marked increase in the frequency of oscillations at the time of reoxygenation rather than just a change in their mechanical amplitude. However, it must be remembered that this model does not yet include the rapid shift in pH and extracellular potassium concentration that occurs upon reperfusion after actual ischemia. Therefore, one must be cautious in comparing the two models.

The single myocyte model sheds some surprising light on the apparent decline in calcium oscillations during ischemia. When myocytes displaying occasional contractile waves at rest are made anoxic, the waves disappear about 10 min before the onset of rigor (Fig. 21). However, if the myocytes are exposed to a small amount of oxygen (e.g., 1 torr), the opposite happens, and cells that did not display waves develop them de novo, and they become quite frequent, suggesting major calcium overload before the onset of rigor. In these hypoxic cells, shortly after the rigor state has fully developed there are no further spontaneous oscillations. This distinc-

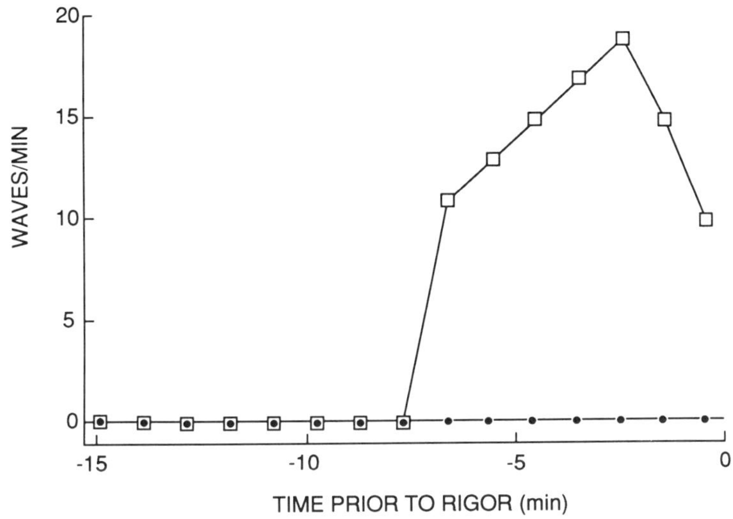

Figure 21 Representative examples of mean wave frequency are plotted as a function of time before rigor contracture for a myocyte exposed to anoxia ($Po_2 < 0.02$ torr; ●) and another cell exposed to hypoxia ($Po_2 = 1$ torr; □) Rigor occurs after a prolonged time period that varies among cells, so the data points are plotted relative to the onset of rigor.

tion between anoxia and hypoxia, which are quite unexpected, has not yet been explained. The simplest explanation would be that cells undergoing ATP depletion might be subject to conflicting processes, one of which suppresses the oscillations and the other, which is time-dependent, exaggerates them. In the hypoxic (as opposed to anoxic) cell, there is a long period of time before rigor during which ATP is probably quite low, and the calcium overloading process would have time to develop. These explanations remain entirely speculative at present. It is equally possible that small concentrations of oxygen might have a direct, deleterious effect on the cell, perhaps by stimulating the formation of oxygen-derived free radicals.

In recent years it has become possible to measure intracellular calcium directly in single myocytes, using either the photoprotein aequorin or the fluorescent probes indo-1 and fura-2. Measurements of intracellular calcium during prolonged hypoxia and reoxygenation display a complex pattern (47). About 5 min before the rigor contracture, the normal intracellular calcium transient provoked by electrical stimulation is abolished. The mechanisms of this change are beyond the scope of this chapter, but are probably principally electrophysiological in nature (46). After this, calcium may rise slowly before rigor but this issue remains controversial. After the development of rigor, intracellular calcium rises continually until the time of reoxygenation. When the cell is reoxygenated, there may be a transient fall in calcium (in cells destined to remain rectangular), after which there is a burst of calcium oscillations (Fig. 22). In cells that round up the calcium signal continues to be high and to show rapid oscillations, while cells which remain rectangular show a gradual decline in the frequency of oscillations and in the level of calcium, and generally return to control condition after about 30–45 min. Cells that have been through the rigor state never regain their original rest length, even when their

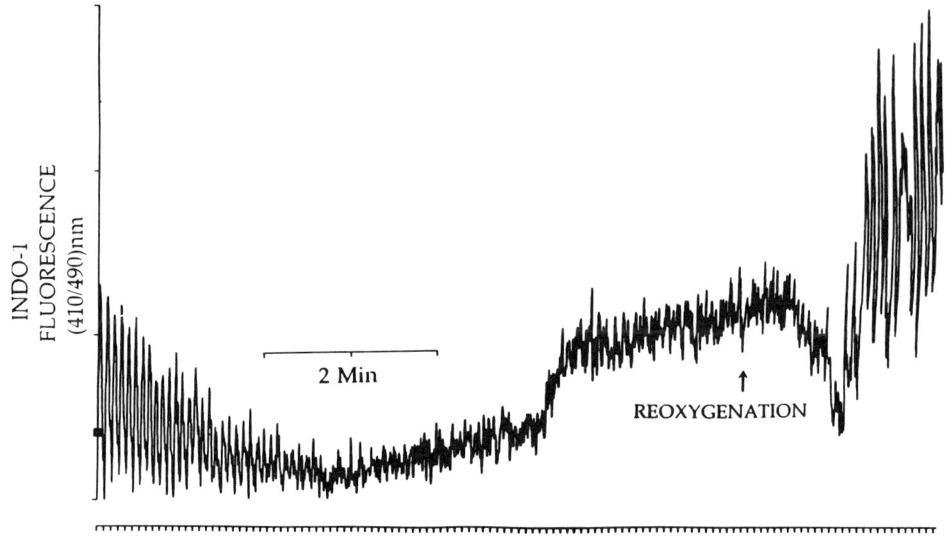

Figure 22 Intracellular calcium (indo-1 fluorescence ratio) in a single rat cardiac myocyte field stimulated at 0.2 Hz is displayed during exposure to anoxia and at reoxygenation. Resting levels of calcium begin to rise after the failure of the calcium transient. Rigor occurs just before the abrupt rise in the fluorescence ratio. Reoxygenation is indicated by the arrow.

calcium homeostasis appears to have returned to normal. This may be because of irreversible changes in myofilament architecture due to the unconstrained shortening that can occur in an isolated cell upon rigor bond formation.

IV. CONCLUSIONS

In summary, spontaneous SR Ca^{2+} release can significantly affect the function of the heart and may be encountered under a variety of pathologic conditions. While there is evidence that the likelihood for spontaneous SR Ca^{2+} release is enhanced by an increase in cell Ca^{2+} loading (e.g., positive inotropic agents, acidosis, hypoxia, and reflow following ischemia), this list is probably still incomplete. Thus, future studies may aim at determining whether spontaneous SR Ca^{2+} release occurs in other pathologic states and whether it has clinical significance.

REFERENCES

1. Olivo O. Sulle modificazioni dell'attivitá contrattile del cuore di embrioni di pollo determinate dall'azione di sali di calcio e di potassio. Arch Fisiol 1924;22:3–36.
2. Fabiato A, Fabiato F. Excitation–contraction coupling of isolated cardiac fibers with disrupted or closed sarcolemma. Calcium dependent cyclic and tonic contractions. Circ Res 1972;31:293–307.
3. Fabiato A, Fabiato F. Activation of skinned cardiac cells. Subcellular effects of cardiac vascular drugs. Europ J Cardiol 1973;1/2:143–55.
4. Fabiato A, Fabiato F. Contractions induced by a calcium-triggered release of calcium from the sarcoplasmic reticulum of single skinned cardiac cells. J Physiol 1975;249:469–95.

5. Dani AM, Cittadini A, Inesi G. Calcium transport and contractile activity in dissociated mammalian heart cells. Am J Physiol 1979;237:C147–55.
6. Chiesi M, Ho MM, Inesi G, Somlyo AV, Somlyo AP. Primary role of sarcoplasmic reticulum in phasic contractile activation of cardiac myocytes with shunted myolemma. J Cell Biol 1981;91:728–42.
7. Bloom S. Spontaneous rhythmic contraction of separated heart muscle cells. Science 1970;167:1727–9.
8. Krueger JW, Pollack GH. Myocardial sarcomere dynamics during isometric contraction. J Physiol 1975;251:627–43.
9. Lappé DL, Lakatta EG. Intensity fluctuation spectroscopy monitors contractile activation in "resting" cardiac muscle. Science NY 1980;207:1369–71.
10. Lakatta EG, Lappe DL. Diastolic scattered light fluctuation, resting force and twitch force in mammalian cardiac muscle. J Physiol 1981;315:369–94.
11. Capogrossi MC, Lakatta EG. Frequency modulation and synchronization of spontaneous oscillations in cardiac cells. Am J Physiol 1985;248:H412–8.
12. Capogrossi MC, Kort AA, Spurgeon HA, Lakatta EG. Single adult rabbit and rat cardiac myocytes retain the Ca^{2+}- and species-dependent systolic and diastolic contractile properties of intact muscle. J Gen Physiol 1986;88:589–613.
13. Capogrossi MC, Suarez-Isla BA, Lakatta EG. The interaction of electrically stimulated twitches and spontaneous contractile waves in single cardiac myocytes. J Gen Physiol 1986;88:615–33.
14. Cobbold PH, Bourne PK. Aequorin measurements of free calcium in single heart cells. Nature 1984;312:444–6.
15. Wier WG, Cannell MB, Berlin JR, Marban E, Lederer WJ. Fura-2 fluorescence imaging reveals cellular and subcellular heterogeneity of $[Ca^{2+}]_i$ in single heart cells. Science 1987;235;325–8.
16. Spurgeon HA, Stern M, Baartz G, Raffaeli S, Hansford RG, Talo A, Lakatta EG, Capogrossi MC. Simultaneous measurement of Ca^{2+}, contraction and potential in cardiac myocytes. Am J Physiol 1990;258:H574–86.
17. Kort AA, Lakatta EG. Calcium-dependent mechanical oscillations occur spontaneously in unstimulated mammalian cardiac tissues. Circ Res 1984;54:396–404.
18. Stern MD, Kort AA, Bhatnagar GM, Lakatta EG. Scattered-light intensity fluctuations in diastolic rat cardiac muscle caused by spontaneous Ca^{2+}-dependent cellular mechanical oscillations. J Gen Physiol 1983;82:119–53.
19. Kort AA, Capogrossi MC, Lakatta EG. Frequency, amplitude, and propagation velocity of spontaneous Ca^{2+}-dependent contractile waves in intact adult rat cardiac muscle and isolated myocytes. Circ Res 1985a;57:844–55.
20. Lakatta EG, Capogrossi MC, Kort AA, Stern MD. Spontaneous myocardial Ca oscillations: overview with emphasis on ryanodine and caffeine. Fed Proc 1985;44:2977–83.
21. Stern MD, Capogrossi MC, Lakatta EG. Spontaneous calcium release from the sarcoplasmic reticulum in myocardial cells: mechanisms and consequences. Cell Calcium 1988;9:247–56.
22. Fabiato A. Time and calcium dependence of activation and inactivation of calcium-induced release of calcium from the sarcoplasmic reticulum of a skinned canine cardiac purkinje cell. J Gen Physiol 1985;85:247–89.
23. Capogrossi MC, Houser S, Bahinski A, Lakatta EG. Synchronous occurrence of spontaneous localized calcium release from the sarcoplasmic reticulum generates action potentials in rat cardiac ventricular myocytes at normal resting membrane potential. Circ Res 1987;61:498–503.
24. Colquhoun D, Neher E, Reuter H, Stevens CF. Inward current channels activated by intracellular Ca in cultured cardiac cells. Nature 1981;294:752–4.
25. Kimura J, Noma A, Irisawa H. Na–Ca exchange current in mammalian heart cells. Nature 1986;319:596–7.

26. Mechmann S, Pott L. Identification of Na–Ca exchange current in single cardiac myocytes. Nature 1986;319:597–9.
27. Clusin WT, Fischmeister R, DeHaan RI. Caffeine-induced current in embryonic heart cells: time course and voltage dependence: Am J Physiol 1983;245:H528–32.
28. Capogrossi MC, Stern MD, Spurgeon HA, Lakatta EG. Spontaneous Ca^{2++} release from the sarcoplasmic reticulum limits Ca^{2+}-dependent twitch potentiation in individual cardiac myocytes: a mechanism for maximum inotropy in the myocardium. J Gen Physiol 1988;91:133–55.
29. Kort AA, Lakatta EG. Biomodel effect of stimulation on light fluctuation transients monitoring spontaneous sarcoplasmic reticulum calcium release in rat cardiac muscle. Circ Res 1988;63:960–8.
30. Kort AA, Lakatta EG. Spontaneous sarcoplasmic reticulum calcium release in rat and rabbit cardiac muscle: relation to transient and rested-state twitch tension. Circ Res 1988;63:969–79.
31. Fabiato A, Fabiato F. Effects of pH on the myofilaments and the sarcoplasmic reticulum of skinned cells from cardiac and skeletal muscles. J Physiol (Lond) 1978;276:233–55.
32. Donaldson SKB, Hermansen L. Differential, direct effects of H^+ on Ca^{2+}-activated force of skinned fibers from the soleus, cardiac and adductor magnus muscles of rabbits. Pflugers Arch 1978;376:55–65.
33. Allen DG, Orchard CH. The effects of changes of pH on intracellular calcium transients in mammalian cardiac muscle. J Physiol (Lond) 1983;335:555–67.
34. Orchard CH. The role of the sarcoplasmic reticulum in the response of ferret and rat heart muscle to acidosis. J Physiol (Lond) 1987;384:431–49.
35. Orchard CH, Houser SR, Kort AA, Bahinski A, Capogrossi MC, Lakatta EG. Acidosis facilitates spontaneous sarcoplasmic reticulum Ca^{2+} release in rat myocardium. J Gen Physiol 1987;90:145–65.
36. Bountra C, Vaughan-Jones RD. Effect of intracellular and extracellular pH on contraction in isolated mammalian cardiac muscle. J Physiol 1989;418:163–87.
37. Lazdunski M, Frelin C, Vigne P. The sodium hydrogen exchange system in cardiac cells: its biochemical and pharmacological properties and its role in regulating internal concentrations of sodium and internal pH. J Mol Cell Cardiol 1985;17:1029–42.
38. Shen AC, Jennings RB. Myocardial calcium and magnesium in acute ischemic injury. Am J Pathol 1972;67:417–40.
39. Carbonin P, di Gennaro M, Valle R, Weisz AM. Inhibitory effect of anoxia on reperfusion- and digitalis-induced ventricular tachyarrhythmias. Am J Physiol 1981;240 (Heart Circ Physiol 9):H730–7.
40. di Gennaro M, Vassalle M, Iacono G, Pahor M, Bernabei R, Carbonin PU. On the mechanisms by which hypoxia eliminates digitalis-induced tachyarrhythmias. Eur Heart J 1986;7:341–52.
41. Stern MD, Weisman HF, Renlund DG, Gerstenblith G, Hano O, Blank PS, Lakatta EG. Laser backscatter studies of intracellular Ca^{2+} oscillations in isolated hearts. Am J Physiol 1989;257(Heart Circ Physiol 26):H665–73.
42. Weiss RG, Gerstenblith G, Lakatta EG. Calcium oscillations index the extent of calcium loading and predict functional recovery during reperfusion in rat myocardium. J Clin Invest 1990;85:757–65.
43. Haworth RA, Hunter DC, Berkoff HA. Contracture in isolated adult rat heart cells: role of Ca^{2+}, ATP and compartmentation. Circ Res 1981;49:1119–28.
44. Hohl C, Ansel A, Altschuldt R, Brierly GP. Contracture of isolated rat heart cells on anaerobic to aerobic transition. Am J Physiol 1982;242:A1022–30.
45. Stern MD, Chien AM, Capogrossi MC, Pelto DJ, Lakatta EG. Direct observation of the "oxygen paradox" in single rat ventricular myocytes. Circ Res 1985;56:899–903.

46. Stern MD, Silverman HS, Houser SR, Josephson RA, Capogrossi MC, Nichols CG, Lederer WJ, Lakatta EG. Anoxic contractile failure in rat heart myocytes is caused by failure of intracellular calcium release due to alteration of the action potential. Proc Natl Acad Sci USA 1988;855:6954–8.
47. Allshire A, Piper HN, Cuthbertson KJR, Cobbold PH. Cytosolic free calcium in single rat heart cells during anoxia and reoxygenation. Biochem J 1987;244:381–5.

4

Effect of Cross-Bridge Kinetics on Force Development and Velocity of Shortening: Implications for Regulation

PIETER P. de TOMBE

The Bowman Gray School of Medicine, Wake Forest University
Winston-Salem, North Carolina

HENK E. D. J. ter KEURS

University of Calgary
Calgary, Alberta, Canada

It is well known that an increase in the contractile state of the heart is usually accompanied by an increase in intracellular calcium in the cardiac myocyte (1,2). Studies by the group of Sonnenblick on isolated papillary muscle have shown that not only developed force but also maximum velocity of muscle shortening (V_{max}) is increased by positive inotropic agents (3,4). The increase in developed force can be explained by an increase in the number of active cross-bridges. The increase in maximum shortening velocity, on the other hand, could indicate an increase in the cycling rate of attached cross-bridges. These results are of interest because they are not predicted by the cross-bridge theory of muscle contraction proposed by A.F. Huxley (5). In this theory, the transition rate of the actomyosin cycle is affected by the relative strain in each attached cross-bridge only, and not by the relative number of cross-bridges actively cycling. Alteration of cross-bridge cycle kinetics by inotropic agents could have important consequences for our understanding of the processes that regulate force development and shortening in cardiac muscle.

Consistent with the results of Sonnenblick's group on intact cardiac muscle (3,4), some investigators have found an effect of free ionized calcium concentration on the unloaded velocity of shortening in skinned skeletal muscle, but conflicting results have been obtained by others, and the subject is still a matter of considerable debate (6–11, for a review see 12). Phosphorylation of specific sites at the myofibrillar proteins by cyclic AMP-dependent kinases could potentially be another site of regulation of cross-bridge kinetics. Indeed, positive inotropic agents operating via the β-receptor in the heart have been shown to alter the biochemical properties of the actomyosin complex (for a review see 13). Recent studies of stiffness of intact (14–17) and chemically skinned (17,18) cardiac papillary muscle preparations by stepwise and sinusoidal length perturbations have likewise suggested that β-adrenergic stimulation increases the cycling rate of cross-bridges during force generation at constant muscle length.

Thus, direct modulation of the actomyosin interaction in the heart might play an important role in the regulation of cardiac muscle. In the intact heart, cycling of cross-bridges results in both pressure development and, via shortening of the muscle fibers in the wall of the heart, propulsion of blood into the circulation. In our studies on isolated cardiac muscle preparations, therefore, we have focused on the factors that determine development of force and velocity of muscle shortening. In this chapter we will review the effects of extracellular calcium concentration, isomyosin composition, and isoproterenol on twitch force and velocity of shortening. For these studies we have used isolated cardiac trabeculae from the right ventricles of rat and cat myocardium.

I. CHOICE OF ISOLATED MUSCLE PREPARATION

One of the major problems in the study of cardiac muscle mechanics is the isolation procedure and the subsequent mounting of the preparation in the experimental apparatus. In the 1970s it was recognized that papillary muscle preparations are grossly nonuniform (19–22). The nonuniformity is a result of the damage inevitably inflicted upon the ends of the muscle preparation during the dissection procedure. This damage will render cardiac muscle preparations more compliant than isolated skeletal muscle. An example of the effect of damaged end compliance in rat cardiac muscle is shown in Figure 1. In this experiment, muscle length, developed force, and sarcomere length were measured in an isolated rat cardiac trabecula. Sarcomere length was measured in the central, presumably undamaged, region of the muscle by a laser diffraction technique, which we will describe in greater detail in a later section. The trabecula was slowly stretched and subsequently released in the experiment shown in Figure 1. Several observations are immediately evident from this experiment. First, even though muscle length was relatively constant during the twitch, the central sarcomeres shortened considerably during the contraction. It is striking that the extent of shortening depended on overall muscle length, and decreased with increasing muscle length, even though force development markedly increased in proportion to muscle length. Second, the central sarcomeres became extremely stiff at sarcomere lengths above 2.3 μm. That is, upon further stretch of the muscle, a large passive force was generated while the length of the central sarcomeres did not increase noticeably. Note, however, that overall muscle length could still be increased by stretching the muscle. Microscopic observation revealed that the additional stretch of the muscle at this sarcomere length was taken up almost completely by the end region that was damaged (23). This result is not a peculiar property of rat cardiac muscle; we have recently shown identical behavior in cat cardiac trabeculae (24). It is clear that the conclusion of this experiment must be that the use of overall muscle length instead of sarcomere length causes one to construct a distorted impression of the mechanical behavior of the cardiac contractile apparatus. For example, cardiac force–length relations determined on the basis of muscle length show a maximum, commonly referred to as L_{max}, and sometimes even a descending limb (Fig. 1; for reviews see 25,26). This result is due solely to the compliance of the damaged ends and can never be observed at the level of the cardiac sarcomere. Shortening of the undamaged sarcomeres during the twitch will invariably lead to *underestimation* of developed force at any particular muscle length. This can best be illustrated as shown in Figure 2. In this experiment, peak twitch force development in a rat trabecula was studied under muscle length isomet-

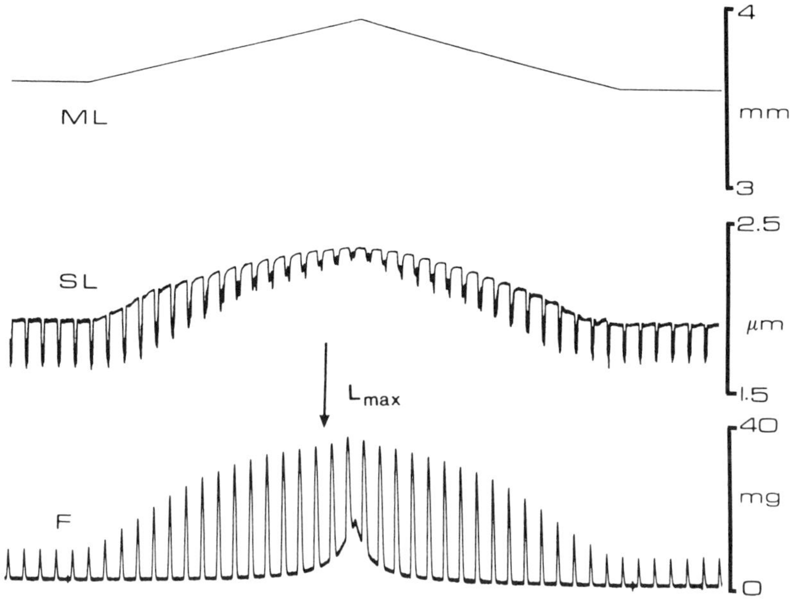

Figure 1 Shortening of central segment sarcomeres in a rat cardiac trabecula during the twitch. Tracings showing the relation between force (F; bottom tracing) muscle length (ML; top tracing), and sarcomere length (SL; middle tracing) in the central region of a representative rat trabecula. Muscle length was varied between 3.5 (slack length) and 4.0 mm. Sarcomere length at rest increased approximately linear in relation to muscle length up to SL=2.3 μm. Sarcomere length increased much less at higher muscle lengths, concomitant with a substantial increase in passive force. Stretch of the damaged ends of the preparation accounted for the difference between stretch of the muscle and stretch of the sarcomeres. The muscle was stimulated every 2 secs. Peak active force development increased with increasing muscle length up to L_{max} (indicated by the arrow). The apparent decrease of actively developed force beyond L_{max} occurred while the sarcomeres in the center of the muscle shortened to a length at which the passive muscle bears no elastic force. Hence, in our studies, peak active developed force is expressed as total peak force minus the passive force that would exist at the same sarcomere length as that existing at peak force. Ca^{2+} concentration in the bathing solution was 1.5 mM at 25.0 C.

ric conditions (left hand panel), and sarcomere isometric conditions (right hand panel). The latter condition was achieved by stretching the muscle from one end during most of the duration of the twitch to such an extent that sarcomere length remained constant well beyond the time of peak twitch force. It is clear that peak force under sarcomere length isometric conditions far exceeded peak force under muscle length isometric conditions. In addition, as we have shown elsewhere (23), relaxation of twitch force is also markedly affected by the shortening of the central sarcomeres during the twitch. We will show below that the unloaded velocity of sarcomere shortening (V_o) is a function of sarcomere length, particularly at lengths below slack length. Hence, shortening of the central sarcomeres during a muscle length isometric twitch in the isolated papillary muscle preparation can severely affect the measurement of the maximum velocity of muscle shortening (V_{max}) since the sarcomere length at which this measurement is made is uncontrolled and *a*

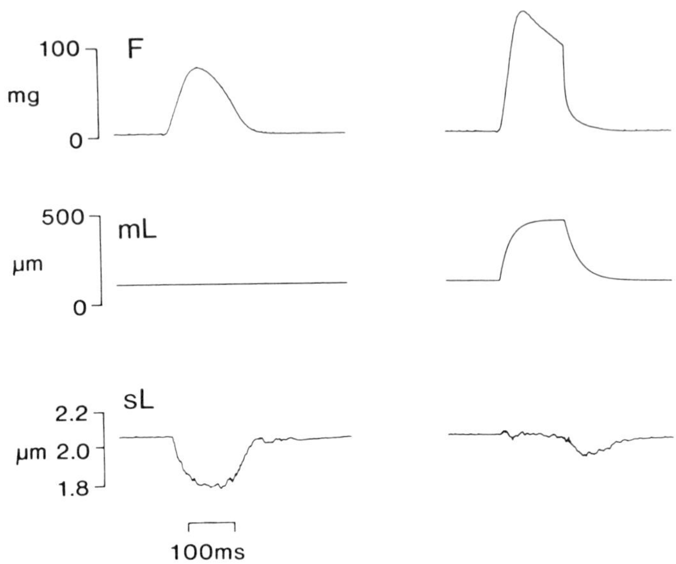

Figure 2 Clamp of sarcomere length during the twitch. Twitch force (F), muscle length (mL), and sarcomere length (sL) were measured in a rat cardiac trabecula. Muscle length was held constant in the left panel. Damaged ends of the preparation allowed substantial sarcomere shortening in the area of measurement during the twitch. In the right panel, internal shortening was prevented during the first two-thirds of the twitch by stretching the muscle by a servo-motor attached to the valvular end of the muscle. This procedure allowed for the measurement of peak twitch force at constant sarcomere length (at about 2.05 μm). $[Ca^{2+}]_o$ = 1.5 mM at 25.0 C. (Modified from Ref. 78 with permission.)

priori unknown. We will describe in a later section the methods we have adopted to circumvent the problems associated with uncontrolled sarcomere shortening in the central segment of the muscle preparation.

II. METHODOLOGIC CONSIDERATIONS

A. Muscle Preparation

The methods we have used to dissect and mount a cardiac trabecula have been described in detail elsewhere (23,27,28). Two 4-month-old Sprague-Dawley rats of either sex, fed ad libitum, were anesthetized with diethyl-ether; kittens, 6–12 weeks of age were anesthetized with 100 mg ketamine. The heart was rapidly excised from the chest and perfused retrogradely via the proximal aortic stump with a modified Krebs–Henseleit solution and placed in a dissection dish beneath a binocular microscope. Thin, unbranched, and uniform trabeculae, running between the free wall of the right ventricle and the atrioventricular ring, were selected. The trabeculae used in our studies were selected for uniformity to prevent potential artifacts associated with the measurement of sarcomere length; they measured 50–200 μm in width, 40–80 μm in thickness for rat trabeculae and 70–150 μm in thickness for cat trabeculae, and 2–5 mm in length. The average success rate in obtaining a suitable preparation was about 25%.

B. Solutions

The standard solution used was a modified Krebs–Henseleit solution with the following composition (mM): Na^+ 140.5, K^+ 5.0, Cl^- 127.5, Mg^{2+} 1.2, $H_2PO_4^-$ 2.0, SO_4^{2-} 1.2, HCO_3^- 19, d-glucose 10.0, and $[Ca^{2+}]_o$ as indicated. The solutions were in equilibrium with a 95% O_2/5% CO_2 gas mixture, resulting in a pH of 7.4 at 25°C. Isoproterenol was infused at the inflow of the muscle bath, to avoid oxidation of the drug. This procedure resulted in a steady-state level of increased twitch force in about 10 minutes (see also Fig. 13).

C. Muscle Bath

The muscles were positioned, under microscopic control, horizontally in an experimental chamber milled from plastic, positioned on the stage of an inverted microscope (cf Fig. 3). Electrical stimulation of the preparation was achieved via platinun electrodes positioned in the wall of the muscle bath along either side of the muscle preparation. Rectangular stimulating pulses were delivered by an isolated pulse generator. Pulse duration was 2 msec, the stimulation frequency was 0.5 Hz at all times. Stimulus strength was adjusted to 50% above the stimulus threshold of the preparation. The stimulator was triggered by a timing device that also controlled the timing of the stretch and release ramps applied to the muscle.

D. Force and Muscle Length

Twitch force was measured with a modified silicon strain gauge (SenSonor; resonance frequency $>$ 10 kHz; cf Fig. 3), attached to a micromanipulator. A lightweight platinum basket glued to the beam of the force transducer provided a stable mounting cradle in which the ventricular end of the trabecula was positioned (cf Fig. 3B). The remnant of the tricuspid valve served as an attachment point to a servo-controlled motor (Cambridge Technology; 90% step response in 300 μsec) via a stainless steel hook (100 μm diameter). The hook was glued onto a lightweight titanium motor arm. During the experiment, muscle length was controlled by three function generators, the output of which were fed into the position command of the servo-control system. The function generators were activated by the timing device. Thus, we were able to construct a complex stretch and release ramp function that we synchronized with the stimulus pulses and applied to the muscle preparation.

E. Sarcomere Length

Sarcomere length was measured in all preparations in a region of the muscle close to the stationary ventricular end mounted in the platinum cradle of the force transducer (cf Fig. 3). Sarcomere length was measured by laser diffraction techniques described in detail elsewhere (19,20,23,29,30). In short, the striations of cardiac muscle act as an optical grating to incident light, in this case the output of a 15 mW He–Ne laser. The trabecula diffract the laser beam into a zero-order band and multiple, spatially symmetrical, higher-order band pairs (19,20) (cf Fig. 3D). The angle between the zero-order band and the first-order diffraction band is proportional to sarcomere length and the wavelength of the laser light (632.8 nm). To measure this angle, the left first-order diffraction band was projected onto a

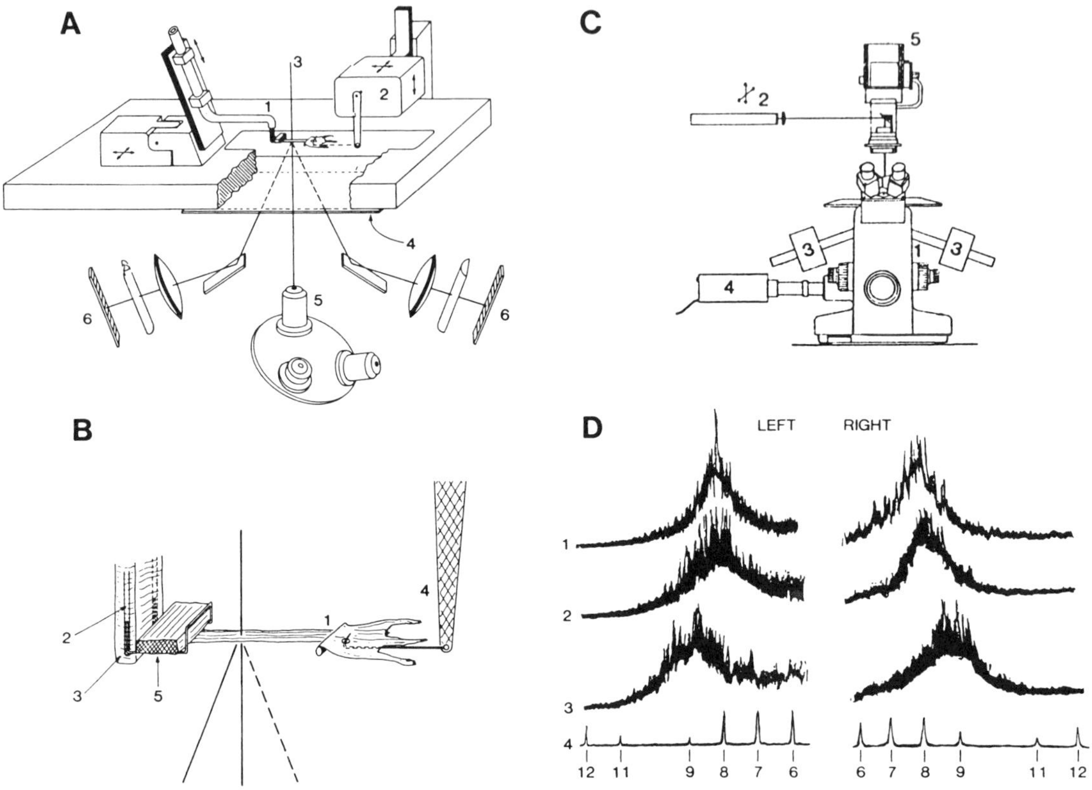

Figure 3 Experimental setup to measure contraction kinetics in cardiac trabeculae. A. Experimental chamber: (1) force transducer; (2) servo-controlled motor, displaced to the right for clarity; (3) He–Ne laser beam; (4) coverslip used as bottom; (5) microscope objective; (6) photodiode array. B. Detailed sketch of the muscle preparation (1) positioned between the force transducer (2), which is insulated with silicon rubber (3), and a servo-controlled motor (4). The remnant of the right ventricular wall (5) rests in the platinum basket. An incident laser beam is diffracted into two symmetrical first-order bands. (Note that the muscle is mounted perpendicular to the incident laser beam). C. The experimental chamber is positioned on the stage of a modified inverted microscope: (1) microscope; (2) He–Ne laser; (3) photodiode array; (4) TV cameras; (5) microscope light source. D. First-order diffraction band distribution of the left and right diffraction band as measured with the photodiode array. The signals were directly derived from the diode array, without zero order compensation. (1) Resting muscle; (2) 70 msec into a twitch in which sarcomere length was kept constant (cf Fig. 2 and text); (3) 14 msec following release at V_o (panels 2 and 3 were slightly retouched); 4) a calibration grating (17.22 μm) was positioned at the level of the muscle. The photodiode array spanned the sixth- through the twelfth-order diffraction lines as indicated. Temperature 24.5 C, $[Ca^{2+}]_o$ = 1.5 mM. (Reproduced from Ref. 28 with permission.)

scanning, 512 element photodiode array (Reticon). In addition, in some muscles the left and right first-order diffraction bands were monitored simultaneously. The photodiode arrays were scanned every 0.5 msec. The median position of the first-order intensity distribution (determined by analog circuitry after correction for the contribution of the zero-order diffraction band and scatter [20,23,30]) was converted into a voltage proportional to sarcomere length by means of a nonlinear amplifier. The transfer function of this amplifier was adjusted by placing standard glass calibration gratings in the same position as the muscle (see Fig. 3D).

III. MEASUREMENT OF SARCOMERE SHORTENING VELOCITY

Velocity of sarcomere shortening as a function of force during shortening was measured by means of the isovelocity release technique (31). The method is illustrated in Figure 4, and several of the factors that affect the measurements used to obtain V_o are illustrated in Figure 5. Sarcomere length was kept constant at 2.1 μm by stretching the muscle from the valvular end (cf Fig. 4). This sarcomere length is chosen because passive force development at this sarcomere length is negligible (see below). When about 70% of isometric twitch force, denoted here as F_o, was

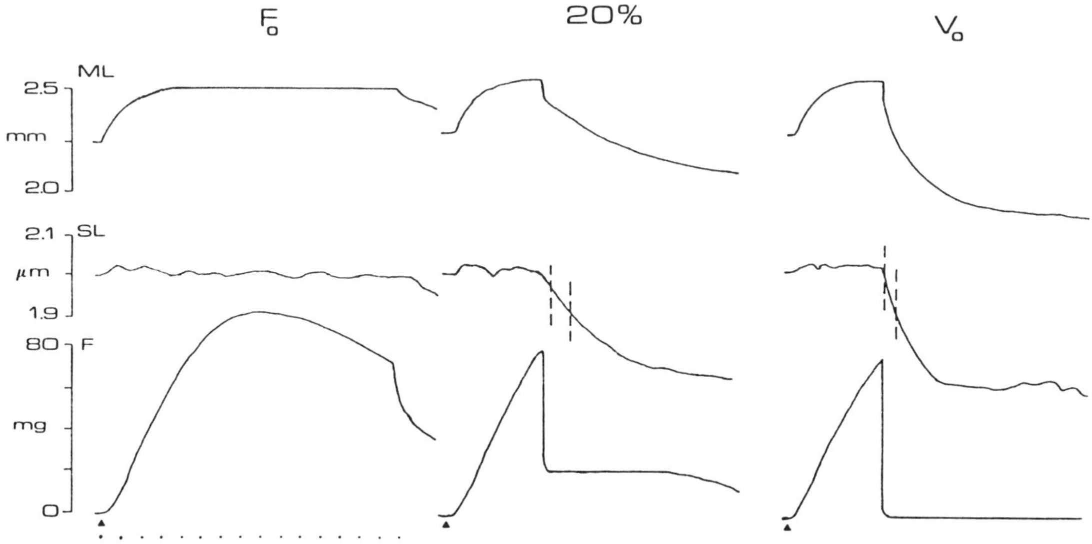

Figure 4 Method to measure force–sarcomere velocity relation. Sarcomere length (middle row) was kept constant by stretching the valvular end of the trabecula (cf muscle length; top row). Peak twitch force (bottom row) was measured at a sarcomere length of 2.0 μm (F_o, left panel) when no shortening step was imposed. The middle panel shows a release to 20% of peak twitch force. Velocity of sarcomere shortening was calculated by linear regression of the digitized sarcomere length values during the initial phase of shortening, when the force was stable, as indicated by the dashed vertical lines. In addition, mean sarcomere length was calculated from the sarcomere lengths during the latter period. A release to zero force is shown in the right panel, which allows *direct* determination of maximum, unloaded velocity of sarcomere shortening (V_o). $[Ca^{2+}]_o$ 1.5 mM; 20 C; time calibration (dots) 20 msec, other calibrations as shown in the left panel. Arrow points indicate the time at which the muscle was stimulated. (From Ref. 28 with permission.)

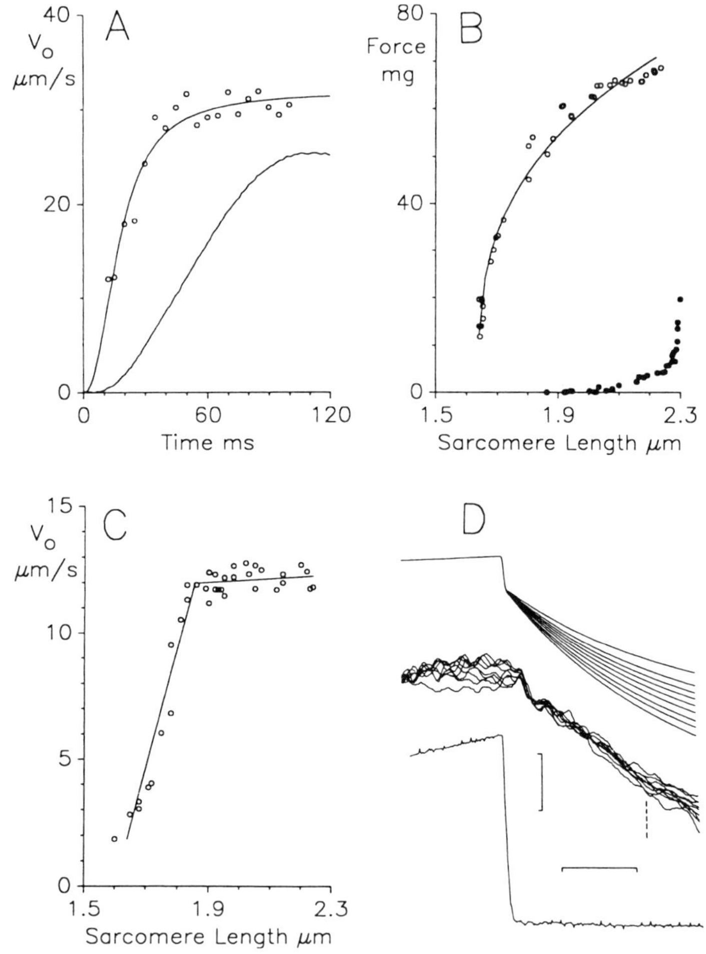
A
40
V_o
μm/s
20
0
0
60
120
Time ms
B
80
Force
mg
40
0
1.5
1.9
2.3
Sarcomere Length μm
C
15
V_o
μm/s
10
5
0
1.5
1.9
2.3
Sarcomere Length μm
D

obtained, the muscle was quickly released to a new load level. This time was chosen because the maximum velocity of sarcomere shortening is stable and maximal during a substantial period after this moment (24,27,28,31) (cf Fig. 5A). Next, a controlled-release ramp was imposed. The speed and amplitude of this release ramp were adjusted so that force was maintained at a constant level. During the first 10–50 msec, average force and the velocity of sarcomere shortening were calculated by linear regression of digitized force and sarcomere values; the window during which the velocity was calculated was inversely proportional to the velocity. The latter calculation also yielded mean sarcomere length during the period of shortening. Care was taken to ensure that minimum sarcomere length was 1.9 μm and that sarcomere shortening during the measurement was limited to 0.2 μm. This procedure removes velocity artifacts that might have been produced by the contribution of passive elastic elements in the muscle preparation (see below). Figure 8 shows examples of shortening velocity plotted as a function of force during shortening, which yields the familiar force–velocity relation. The solid line is a fit of the data to Hill's classic rectangular hyperbola (32):

$$(P+a) \cdot V = (P_o-P) \cdot b$$

In this equation, P stands for the load (i.e., force) during shortening, P_o for isometric load (i.e. F_o), V for velocity, and a and b are constants.

Figure 5 Factors affecting the measurement V_o. A. The effect of time of release on measured V_o in a trabecula. V_o (open circles) was measured as illustrated in Figure 4. Sarcomere length was 1.9–2.0 μm. Twitch force (F; constant sarcomere length) is indicated by the solid line (right and below). Temperature 30 C; $[Ca^{2+}]_o$ = 3.0 mM. Note that V_o is independent of time of release from the time of about 70% F up to peak twitch force development. The relation between V_o and time was fitted to a sigmoidal function; maximum V_o was 32 μm/sec; time at 50% V_o was 21 msec. B. Active (open symbols) and passive (closed symbols) force–sarcomere length relation in a trabecula. Slack sarcomere length was 1.85 μm. The active force–sarcomere length relation was fitted to power function $F=a\cdot(SL - SL_o)^c$, in which SL_o and c are constants. Note that passive force rises steeply at lengths above 2.2 μm. Temperature 25 C, $[Ca^{2+}]_o$ = 1.5 mM. C. The effect of sarcomere length on V_o. V_o was measured at a range of sarcomere lengths (0.1 μm release, average sarcomere length). The data were fitted by linear regression at sarcomere lengths above and below 1.85 μm. The slope of the regression line of V_o vs. sarcomere length above slack length is not significantly different from zero ($p>0.05$). Temperature 25 C, $[Ca^{2+}]_o$ = 1.5 mM. D. The effect of varied release velocity of the muscle on measured V_o. Top panel shows muscle length, middle panel sarcomere length, and bottom panel force development. Releases of the muscle, which resulted in zero force development, are shown. Note that doubling of the velocity of muscle shortening (6–12 muscle lengths/sec) did not affect the velocity of sarcomere shortening, measured close to the ventricular end of the trabecula that rests in the cradle of the force transducer. Extra shortening of the muscle, at velocities of the motor arm larger than required to attain V_o, was completely taken up by buckling of the compliant valve, attached to the motor arm. Temperature 24.3 °C, $[Ca^{2+}]_o$ = 1.5 mM. V_o, measured between the two vertical lines was 11.3 ± 0.25 μm/sec (SD). Calibrations: time 10 msec; sarcomere length 0.1 μm; muscle length 0.2 mm; force 25 mg; resting sarcomere length 2.1 μm. Muscle length was 3.5 mm. Noise on the force tracing was caused by electrical interference from a roller pump. (From Ref. 28 with permission.)

Figure 5D illustrates the method have adopted to ensure that the measurement of V_o occurs at zero external load (28,31). This precaution is necessary because no matter how sensitive the force transducer is, noise and drift will always limit one's ability to measure absolute zero force with sufficient certainty. The method entails imposing a release ramp onto the muscle so that force is zero. Next, starting at the lowest velocity at which force was zero, the velocity of the ramp was gradually increased until the preparation visibly buckled, at which time the diffraction pattern disappeared. At velocities of the ramp between the latter two values, several observations were striking: the velocity of sarcomere shortening in the area of observation was constant; the muscle itself did not buckle; excess shortening was completely taken up by buckling of the valve. Measurements were then performed at a velocity of the motor arm halfway between the value at which force was just zero and the velocity at which buckling of the muscle started to occur.

To examine the effects of inotropic agents on V_o it is essential to eliminate any load on the actomyosin complex during shortening. The total load of the muscle evidently depends on the sum of the external load and the internal load. The internal load, during shortening, depends on inertia, elasticity, and viscosity of the muscle. The inertial term is probably small during shortening at constant velocity. The elastic force, exerted on the sarcomeres, depends on sarcomere length as illustrated by Figures 1 and 5B. If no force on the unstimulated trabeculae is exerted, the sarcomeres are slack at a length of 1.85–1.9 μm. It is evident that stretch induces a small "parallel elastic" force (less than 2% of $F_{o\text{-}max}$), provided that sarcomere length is less than 2.1 μm. After a twitch, sarcomeres elongate spontaneously to slack length, which suggests the presence of "restoring" forces within the trabecula at lengths shorter than 1.9 μm. Apparently the restoring force and the parallel elastic forces balance at slack length. This implies that the sarcomeres in the unstimulated muscle are completely unloaded at that sarcomere length. Hence, to minimize the elastic term we measure V_o at a sarcomere length at or slightly above slack length (i.e., under conditions in which elastic forces are negligible). Figure 5C illustrates V_o measured in a trabecula plotted as function of sarcomere length. It is clear that V_o was nearly independent of sarcomere length in the range 1.9–2.2 μm, as expected from the small passive forces present at these sarcomere lengths. We have recently shown that the viscous component in cardiac trabeculae is small (about 1% of F_o; [27,33]); this force component therefore cannot play an important role at high levels of contractile activation. At lower levels of contractile activation, however, the impact of viscosity can become quite noticeable, as we discuss later.

IV. ARTIFACTS AFFECTING MEASUREMENT OF V_o

We have recently evaluated the impact of several factors that might affect the accuracy of the measurement of sarcomere length and unloaded velocity of sarcomere shortening in cardiac trabeculae (28). Potential sources of error in the use of the laser diffraction technique to measure sarcomere length are Bragg angle reflection, muscle inhomogeneity, and translation of the specimen during shortening.

A population of sarcomeres that are oriented under an angle with respect to the longitudinal axis of a muscle will generate a diffraction pattern with asymmetrical first orders. The asymmetry will manifest itself as differences in intensity and position of the first orders if the population is tilted in the plane of the incident laser beam. These so-called Bragg angle reflections will cause preferential sampling of the tilted population by the corresponding diffractometer (34). The sampled population could potentially change during the twitch, which would give rise to erroneous sarcomere-length readings. Inhomogeneity of the muscle preparation will also result in a change of the sampled population, in this case due to translation of the muscle with respect to a stationary laser beam. We have examined the contribution of asymmetry of the diffraction pattern, due to "Bragg angle" reflections, to errors in the measured median of the sarcomere length distribution with the aid of two diffractometers that sampled the opposite first orders of the diffraction pattern. As Figure 3D shows, we observed nearly identical left and right diffraction patterns during rest, just before release during a sarcomere length clamp, and during shortening at zero external load (i.e., V_o, after about 0.15 μm shortening).

We have also monitored both first-order bands of the diffraction pattern and determined sarcomere length and V_o simultaneously. Figure 6 shows the determination of F_o and $V_o$at 20, 25, and 30°C with the dual diffractometer system. A change in temperature was used in this experiment to alter V_o over a wide range (28). It is clear that sarcomere length and V_o obtained from the opposite first orders of the diffraction patterns differed by less than 4% (the maximal difference in four muscles tested).

The effect of inhomogeneity of the trabeculae on the recorded velocity of shortening was examined in the experiment illustrated in Figure 7. The muscle was translated so that the center of the incident laser beam was at the location indicated in the figure, and V_o was subsequently measured. The valvular end is usually more compliant than the right ventricular end of these preparations. Therefore, regions of the muscle closer to the valvular attachment are expected to move more with respect to a stationary point, such as the laser beam, than those close to the force transducer. V_o measured along the muscle was found to be independent of location, except at positions very close to the valve where lateral translation was largest. A location close to the ventricular end of the muscle was chosen in all the experiments we report in this chapter. Apparently, slight lateral translation in a homogeneous muscle brings only a new population of *functionally identical* sarcomeres into the field of observation.

In summary, we have developed a laser diffraction technique by which we can accurately measure sarcomere length in isolated cardiac trabeculae. The method allows us to measure twitch force at constant sarcomere length, measure the velocity of sarcomere shortening as function of force, and measure the velocity of sarcomere shortening when the external load on the contractile proteins is truly zero (i.e., V_o). Adoption of the laser diffraction technique circumvents the problems associated with the inhomogeneity found in isolated cardiac muscle. We have seen that potential artifacts associated with the use of the diffraction method appear not to play an important role in the measurement of sarcomere length and V_o.

In the following sections we will examine the effects of extracellular calcium concentration ($[Ca^{2+}]_o$), isomyosin composition, and isoproterenol on V_o and isometric twitch force in cardiac trabeculae.

V. EFFECTS OF CHANGES IN $[Ca^{2+}]_o$

Figure 8 shows an example of the force–sarcomere velocity relation measured at $[Ca^{2+}]_o$ = 1.5 mM and $[Ca^{2+}]o$ = 0.5 mM in rat cardiac trabeculae. The solid lines

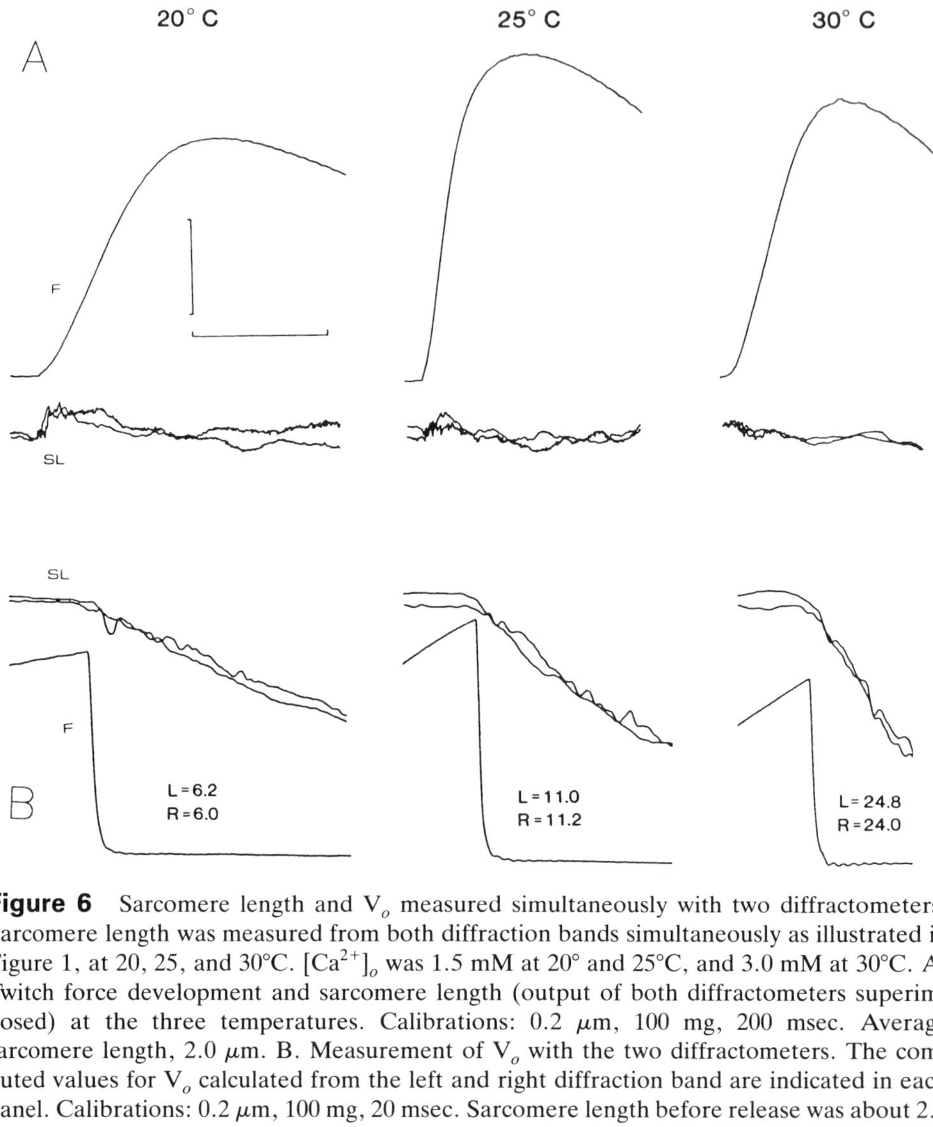

Figure 6 Sarcomere length and V_o measured simultaneously with two diffractometers. Sarcomere length was measured from both diffraction bands simultaneously as illustrated in Figure 1, at 20, 25, and 30°C. $[Ca^{2+}]_o$ was 1.5 mM at 20° and 25°C, and 3.0 mM at 30°C. A. Twitch force development and sarcomere length (output of both diffractometers superimposed) at the three temperatures. Calibrations: 0.2 μm, 100 mg, 200 msec. Average sarcomere length, 2.0 μm. B. Measurement of V_o with the two diffractometers. The computed values for V_o calculated from the left and right diffraction band are indicated in each panel. Calibrations: 0.2 μm, 100 mg, 20 msec. Sarcomere length before release was about 2.1 μm. (From Ref. 28 with permission.)

are fits of the data to Hill's hyperbola (32) for forces below 70% of F_o at each level of $[Ca^{2+}]_o$. The relations deviated from a rectangular hyperbola at forces above 70%. This appears to be a general property of striated muscle; a similar deviation has been observed by us in cat myocardium (24) and by Edman et al. in skeletal muscle (35). Both isometric twitch force and V_o were reduced to about 50% when $[Ca^{2+}]_o$ was lowered from 1.5 mM to 0.5 mM. The shape of the force–velocity relation, however, was not affected by $[Ca^{2+}]_o$, as revealed by the parameters a and b of Hill's hyperbola (see legend). Figure 9 shows the effect of $[Ca^{2+}]_o$ on F_o and V_o in greater detail in both rat (panels A and C) and cat myocardium (panels B and D). It is clear that both F_o and V_o are sigmoidal functions of $[Ca^{2+}]_o$, and that this

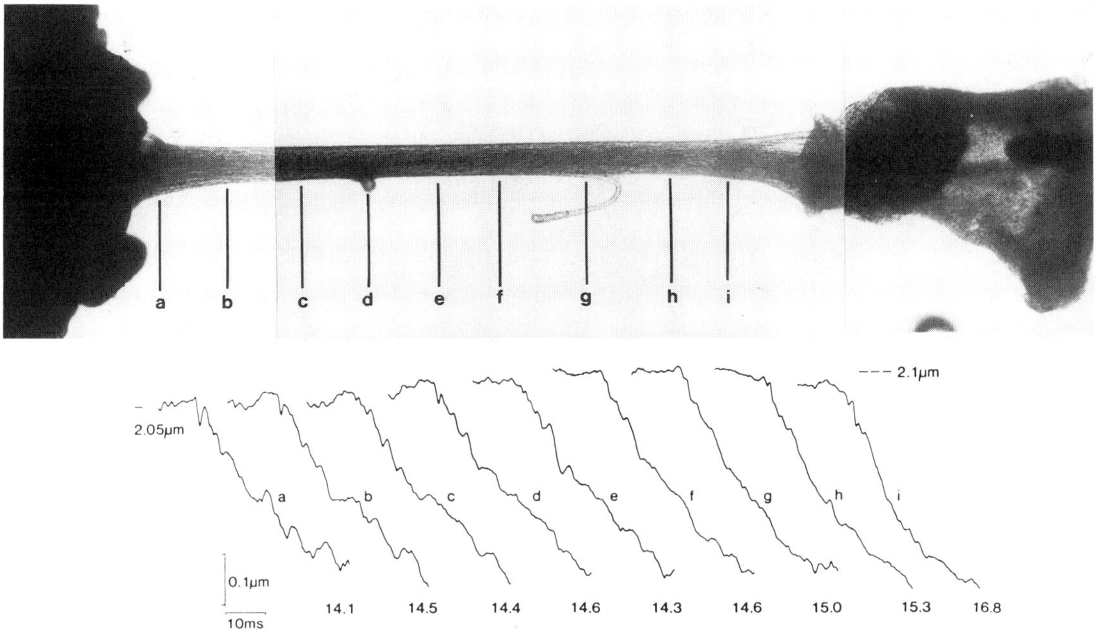

Figure 7 Test of homogeneity of the muscle preparation. Top panel shows a montage of a rat trabecula (3 mm in length, 150 μm in width, 50 μm in thickness). Note the attachment of the valve to the hook on the motor arm on the right. The ventricular end of the preparation is attached to the force transducer on the left. Lines indicate the position (center of the laser beam) at which V_o was measured. Bottom panel shows superimposed (displaced to the right for clarity) sarcomere length recordings during releases at V_o at the positions indicated in the top panel. The values of V_o measured during the first 10 msec of the release are indicated below each trace. Note that lateral translation of the muscle during the shortening ramp was largest at the valvular (right) side of the trabecula, since this end was attached to the motor arm. $[Ca^{2+}]_o$ = 3.0 mM; 0.5 mM procaine; temperature 26.5°C. (From Ref. 28 with permission.)

phenomenon can be observed in both species. The sensitivity of cat myocardium to $[Ca^{2+}]_o$ is substantially less than that in rat myocardium. This difference cannot be ascribed to a difference in the Ca^{2+} sensitivity of the myofilaments; no species difference in the calcium sensitivity for force generation by the myofilaments has been observed in skinned cardiac muscle (36,37). The higher $[Ca^{2+}]_o$ sensitivity of rat myocardium correlates well with the abundance of sarcoplasmic reticulum in this species, which would suggest that rat myocardium depends more on intracellular calcium stores for contractile activation than does myocardium of other mammals (37).

Our results confirm the results of the group of Sonnenblick (3,4) on cat papillary muscle; they showed an increase in the maximum velocity of muscle shortening (V_{max}) upon an increase in $[Ca^{2+}]_o$. However, as we mentioned before, the methods adopted in those studies on isolated papillary muscles probably caused underestimation of V_o. Therefore, comparison between their results and our results is difficult.

The effect of cystolic calcium concentration on V_o has been the subject of considerable debate in the literature (6–12). Our results indicate that V_o depends on extracellular $[Ca^{2+}]_o$ in both rat and cat myocardium. Variation in $[Ca^{2+}]_o$ has been

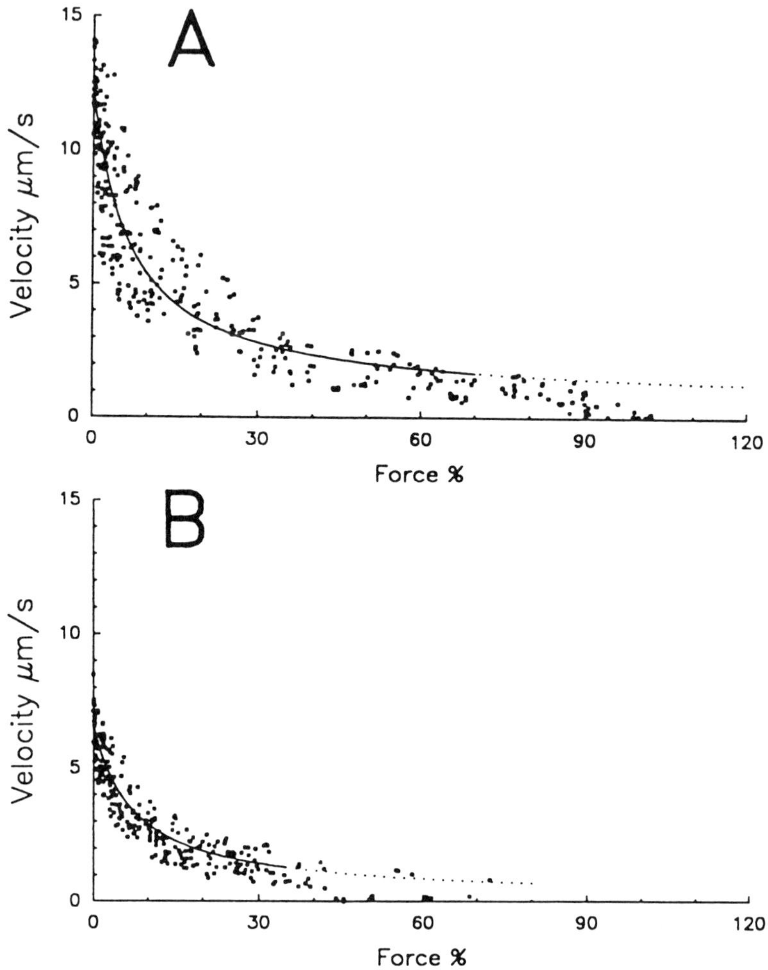

Figure 8 Effect of $[Ca^{2+}]_o$ on force–sarcomere velocity relation. Sarcomere velocity was measured as function of force during shortening in 8 rat trabeculae. Contractile activation was reduced by reducing $[Ca^{2+}]_o$ from 1.5 mM (A) to 0.5 mM (B). The data were fit to the Hill's rectangular hyperbola in each muscle for forces below 70% (solid lines show the average fits). A. $V_o = 12.7 \pm 0.2$ μm/sec; a=9.2 ± 2.7%; b=0.1 ± 0.4 μm/ses; r>0.97. B. $V_o = 6.7 \pm 0.3$ μm/sec; a=13.4 ± 6.4%; b=0.6 ± 0.8 μm/sec; r>0.91. Paired Student's *t*-test revealed p<0.01 for the V_o parameter. Parameters a and b were nonsignificant. Temperature 25°C.

shown to cause proportional variations in cystolic Ca^{2+} (1,2). Hence, one interpretation of our results could be that the concentration of cytosolic Ca^{2+} imposes some form of regulation on the cycling rate of cross-bridges. It is generally assumed that actomyosin interaction is inhibited by low cytosolic calcium concentrations and that this inhibition is relieved by the binding of calcium to troponin-C (for reviews, see 38–41). This theory raises the question of how the overall amount of calcium binding to troponin on the myofilaments can regulate the rate of the actomyosin interaction at the individual cross-bridge sites, and thus regulate V_o. One possible

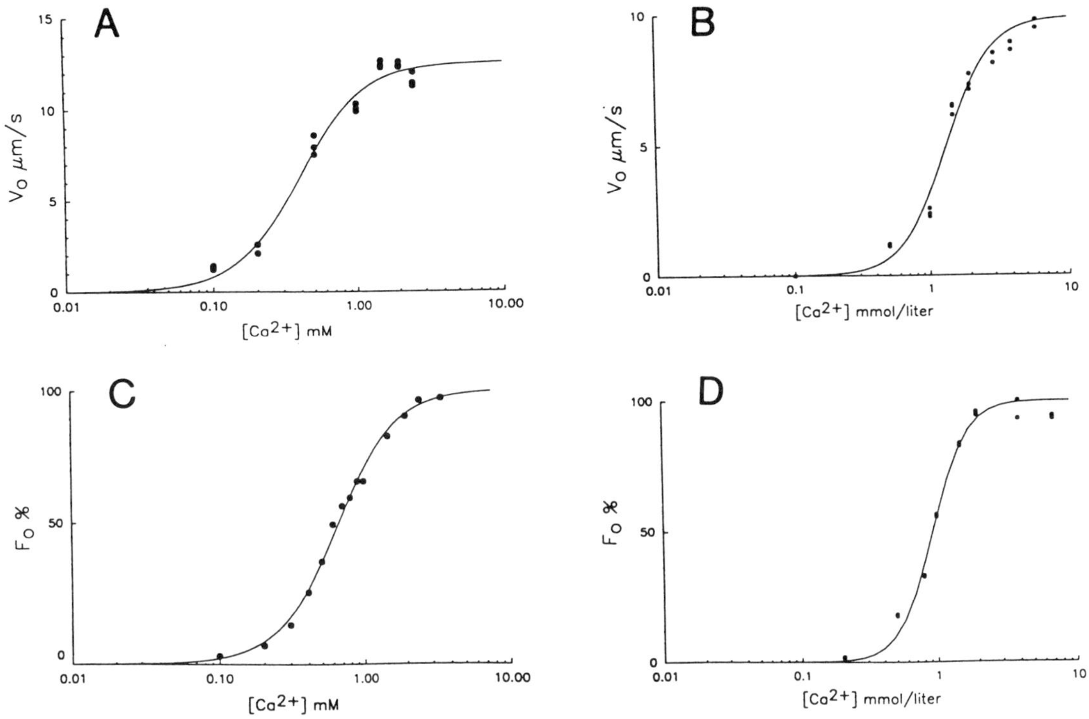

Figure 9 Effect of $[Ca^{2+}]_o$ on F_o and V_o. V_o (top panels) and F_o (bottom panels) shown as function of Ca^{2+} concentration in the bathing solution ($[Ca^{2+}]_o$). The data were measured in a rat trabecula (left hand panels) and a cat trabecula (right hand panels) and were fit to a sigmoidal equation (solid lines). Maximum V_o at saturating $[Ca^{2+}]_o$ was 14.2 ± 0.9 μm/sec in rat trabeculae, and 9.8 ± 0.2 μm/sec in cat trabeculae. The sensitivity of V_o for $[Ca^{2+}]_o$ as expressed by the EC_{50} parameter of the fit to the sigmoidal equation was 0.4 ± 0.04 mM in rat trabeculae and 1.1 ± 0.1 mM in cat trabeculae. EC_{50} values of $[Ca^{2+}]_o$ for F_o were 0.7 ± 0.03 mM and 1.7 ± 0.5 mM in rat and cat trabeculae, respectively. Temperature 25.0°C.

explanation is the presence of an additional calcium regulatory site on myosin, as has been proposed (42–44). Another possible explanation for the effect of $[Ca^{2+}]_o$ on V_o is the existence of an internal elastic (8,45,46) or viscous load (27,33,47,48). Two lines of evidence argue against an elastic, and hence velocity-independent, load. First, we measured V_o at a range of sarcomere lengths at which the passive elastic force must have been negligible. Hence, it is difficult to imagine a structural component of the muscle that would constitute a fixed, internal elastic load at sarcomere lengths slightly above slack length. Second, lowering of $[Ca^{2+}]_o$ from 1.5 mM to 0.5 mM caused a reduction in F_o and V_o, but the shape of the force–sarcomere velocity relation was not affected (cf Fig. 8). A shape change would be expected if sarcomere shortening velocity were limited by a fixed internal load.

We favor the hypothesis that the internal load is formed by the viscous force (F_n), set up during sliding of the filaments. In unstimulated rat cardiac trabeculae we have found that F_n is roughly proportional to the sliding velocity of the sarcomeres; it increases with 0.1% $F_{o\text{-}max}$/μm/sec, where $F_{o\text{-}max}$ is twitch force at 2.0 μm sarcomere length and at $[Ca^{2+}]_o$ = 1.5 mM (27,33). Hence, this viscosity predicts a viscous load of about 1.5% of $F_{o\text{-}max}$ at the maximal active shortening velocity of about 15 μm/sec, which is a typical value for rat cardiac trabeculae, as we have seen earlier.

Introduction of a velocity-dependent load (i.e. $P\eta = \eta \cdot V$) in Hill's rectangular hyperbola (32) relating force and velocity yields:

$$(P + P\eta + a) \cdot V = (P_o - P - P\eta) \cdot b \tag{1}$$

in which P is the load and V is the corresponding velocity; a and b are the asymptotes of the rectangular hyperbola. This predicts for the velocity at zero external load:

$$\eta \cdot V_o^2 + (P_o \cdot b/V_{intr} + \eta \cdot b) \cdot V_o - P_o \cdot b = 0 \tag{2}$$

in which V_{intr} would be truly the unloaded velocity of shortening in the absence of viscous loading (note that the asymptote parameter a has been substituted by $P_o \cdot bV_{intr}$). The positive root of Equation (2) was fit to data such as those shown in Figure 9 in which V_o and F_o were measured at varied $[Ca^{2+}]_o$ in rat trabeculae. As Figure 10 shows, a good fit to the data was obtained for V_{intr} = 15 μm/sec, η=0.14% $F_{o\text{-}max}$/μm/sec, and b=−1.5 μm/sec. These results suggest, to a first approximation, that the relation between the velocity without an external load and activation (or $F_{o\text{-}max}$) can be explained by the presence of a small viscous load, comparable to that generated by the unstimulated muscle on the contractile filaments. This hypothesis is attractive because of its simplicity; no additional calcium regulatory sites that affect the cycling rate of attached cross-bridges need to be invoked in this theory. A more complete and detailed analysis of this hypothesis can be found in references 27 and 33. Note again that restoring forces will reduce V_o further at sarcomere lengths below slack length (SL) (that is, SL<1.9 μm).

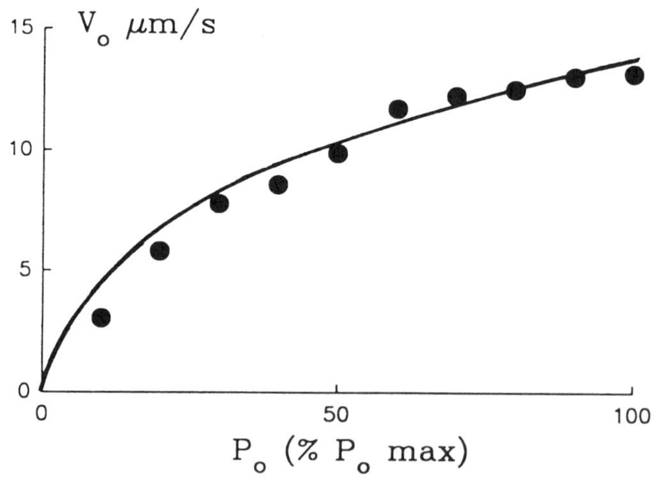

Figure 10 Interrelationship between F_o and V_o. V_o is plotted as function of F_o. The parameters were measured at 1.9 μm sarcomere length in a rat trabeculae under conditions of varied $[Ca^{2+}]_o$ (cf Fig. 9). Solid line shows the correspondence between measured V_o and V_o predicted at varied P_o on the basis of a model in which it was assumed that the contractile system was exposed to an internal load as a result of shortening against a viscous load. See text for details.

VI. EFFECTS OF CATECHOLAMINES AND THYROID STATUS

Recent studies of the stiffness of intact (14–17) and chemically skinned (17,18) cardiac papillary muscle preparations by stepwise and sinusoidal length perturbations have suggested that β-adrenergic stimulation increases the cycling rate of cross-bridges during force generation at constant muscle length, independent of changes in the level of contractile activation. A similar result has also been reported by the group of Winegrad, using ethylene-glycol-tetra acetic-acid (EGTA)-treated muscle (13,49). With this preparation, an increase in maximum calcium-activated force development and myosin ATPase activity has been found upon β-adrenergic stimulation. It seems logical to conclude from these observations that the unloaded shortening velocity of the muscle should also be increased by β-adrenergic stimulation.

Studies by the group of Winegrad have indicated that myocardium that contains predominantly V_1 isomyosin responds to β-adrenergic stimulation, even at saturating concentrations of calcium (13,49). On the other hand, myocardium that contains predominantly V_3 isomyosin does not respond to β-adrenergic stimulation at a saturating calcium concentration (13,49). These results indicate a possible complication in the interpretation of the effect of catecholamines on V_o. In particular, comparison to the results obtained in other species than the rat might be difficult because myosin in the myocardium of larger mammalia is composed mainly of V_3 isomyosin, while myocardium of young adult rats (like most other small rodents) contains predominantly V_1 isomyosin (for a review see reference 50). We therefore induced hypothyroidism in rats by treatment with propylthiouracil (PTU) to induce the synthesis of V_3 isomyosin in the hearts of these animals (50,51).

A. Effects of Hypothyroidism on General Properties of Cardiac Trabeculae

Treatment with PTU lasted 6 weeks and electrophoretic analysis (52) showed that the hearts of hypothyroid animals were composed only of V_3 isomyosin, while the hearts of euthyroid animals were composed predominantly of V_1 isomyosin.

PTU treatment resulted in a significant decline in the serum thyroxine (T4) level at the time of sacrifice of the animal (i.e., from 53 $\pm$ 3.5 nM in euthyroid animals to a nondetectable level in PTU-treated animals; $<$7 nM). Concomitantly, body weight and heart weight were significantly lower in the PTU-treated animals (Fig. 11A, top graphs). Both time to peak twitch force and relaxation were significantly prolonged in the muscle preparations dissected from the hypothyroid animals (Fig. 11A, bottom graphs). These effects have been reported before and are consistent with the complete conversion of the expression of myosin isoenzyme to the V_3 form by PTU treatment (15,16,51).

The effect of hypothyroidism on peak isometric twitch force at saturating concentrations of calcium in the bathing medium (i.e. $>$ 2.5 mM; $F_{o\text{-}max}$) is shown in the bottom right graphs of Figure 11A. $F_{o\text{-}max}$, corrected for cross-sectional area of the muscle, was significantly lower (40%) in hypothyroidism, an observation also made by others (53,54). This observation needs further analysis to ascertain whether the difference is due to an altered fraction of attached cross-bridges at the moment of peak force, an alteration in the level of activation of the contractile filaments by Ca^{2+}, reduced number of myofilaments per cross-sectional area, or all of these possibilities. There is, however, some uncertainty in the measurement of cross-sectional area in our muscle preparations. Hence, in order to investigate the effects

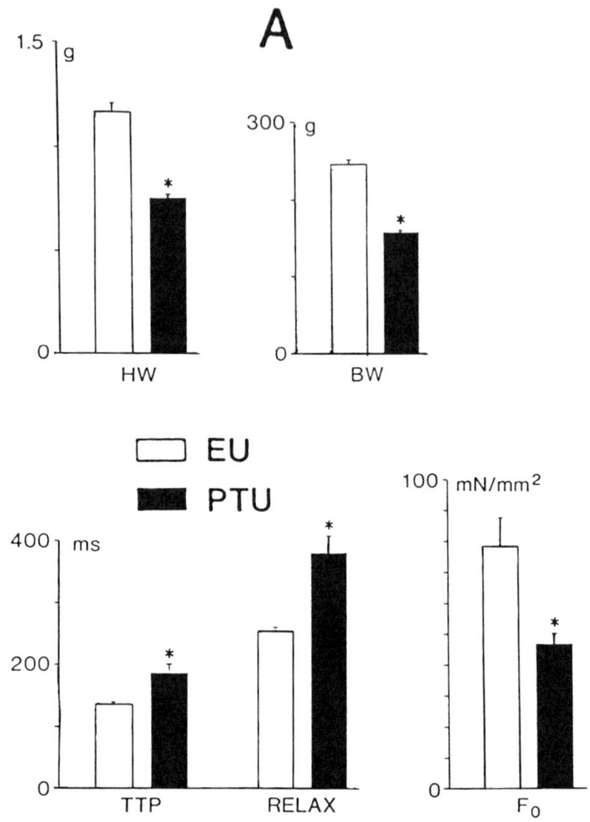

Figure 11 A. Effects of hypothyroidism in rats on body weight (BW), heart weight (HW), time to peak force (TTP), time from peak force to 10% force during relaxation (RELAX) of the twitch at $[Ca^{2+}]_o$ of 1.0 mM, and peak isometric twitch force (F_o) at 2.0 μm sarcomere length and at saturating concentrations of $[Ca^{2+}]_o$ (>2.5 mM). EU, euthyroid animal; PTU, propylthiouracil-treated animal. B. Examples of the measurement of unloaded velocity of sarcomere shortening (V_o) in a euthyroid trabecula (top) and hypothyroid trabecula (bottom). Recordings show tracings of sarcomere length (SL) and force (F) during 30 msec of a release of SL at controlled velocity just before peak force of the twitch. Top tracings show a V_o of 13.2 μm/sec in a trabecula from a euthyroid animal; bottom tracings show that V_o is substantially lower (7.3 μm/sec) in a trabecula from a hypothyroid animal. $[Ca^{2+}]_o$ = 1.5 mM; temperature 25.0°C. Calibrations as indicated. (From Ref. 78 with permission.)

of varied concentrations of external calcium and isoproterenol more precisely, we normalized twitch force to maximum F_o, at saturating $[Ca^{2+}]_o$, in each individual experiment.

The unloaded velocity of sarcomere shortening was reduced in the muscles from hypothyroid animals, as is shown in Figure 11B. This observation has been made previously in myocardium of rat (55), cat (53,56), and rabbit (54,57). In a classic study, Barany (58) showed a close correlation between actomyosin ATPase activity of muscle and maximum shortening velocity. The ATPase activity of V_3 isomyosin is known to be lower than that of V_1 isomyosin (59). The lower value for V_o that we have found in hypothyroidism is thus consistent with Barany's report, and lends

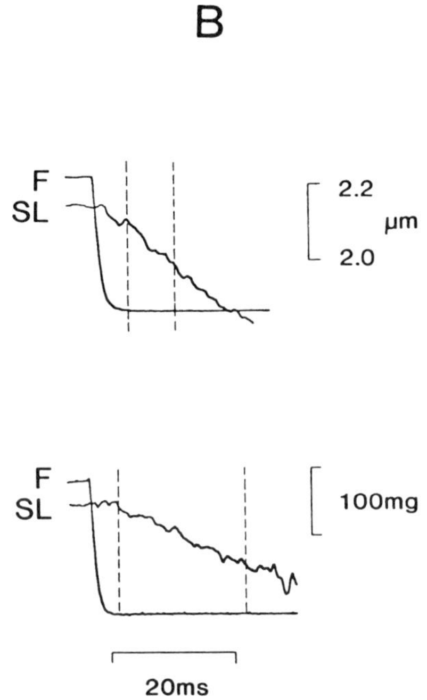

Figure 11 Continued

support to the hypothesis that V_o is controlled by the cycling rate of the cross-bridges.

B. Effects of Isoproterenol on V_o

Catecholamines have been shown to increase intracellular calcium (1,60). This factor complicates efforts to study the effect of β-adrenergic stimulation on V_o *per se,* since V_o is also a function of contractile activation, as we have seen earlier. We therefore varied $[Ca^{2+}]_o$ both in the presence and absence of β-adrenergic stimulation, and thus allow for the effect of changes in the cytosolic calcium concentration on V_o.

In the absence of isoproterenol, V_o and F_o were sigmoidal functions of $[Ca^{2+}]_o$, as we have seen earlier in cardiac trabeculae dissected from euthyroid animals (cf Fig. 9). As Figure 12 shows, this property is not unique to myocardium in which the V_1 form of myosin predominates; a similar interrelationship was also observed in muscles from hypothyroid animals. On average, V_o at saturating $[Ca^{2+}]_o$ was 40% lower in trabeculae dissected from hypothyroid animals: 13.3 ± 0.33 μm/sec and 7.0 ± 0.22 μm/sec in euthyroidism and hypothyroidism, respectively. Note that this difference between the groups can also be appreciated from the measurement of V_o shown in the right-hand panel of Figure 11. The sensitivity for $[Ca^{2+}]_o$, however, judged from the EC_{50} parameters of the sigmoidal fits of F_o and V_o to $[Ca^{2+}]_o$, was not different between the two groups.

We next determined the sensitivity of F_o and V_o to isoproterenol to establish the concentration of isoproterenol at which F_o and V_o were saturated. Isoproterenol

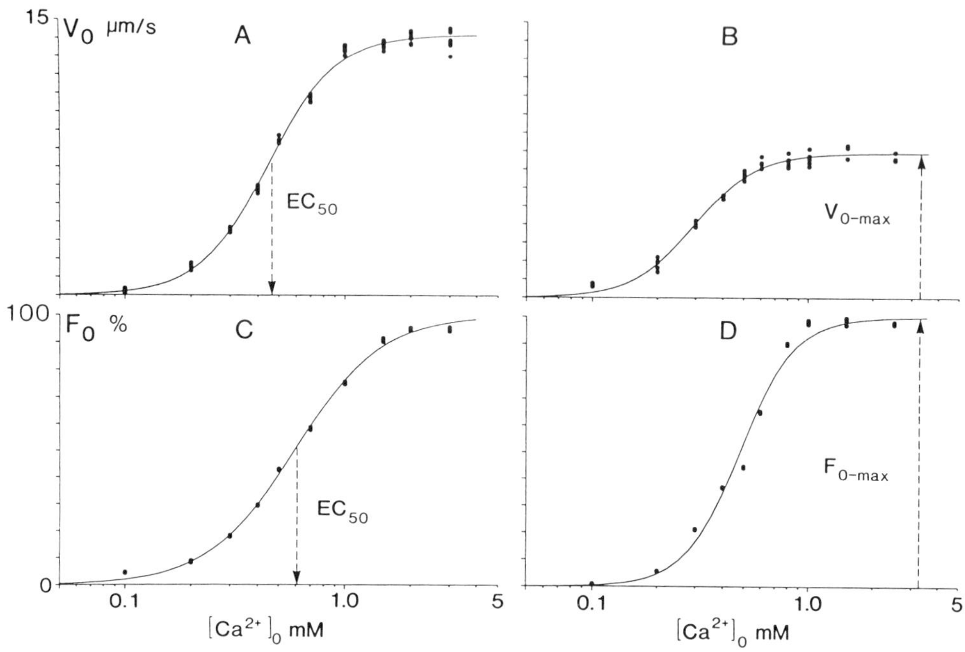

Figure 12 Relations between $[Ca^{2+}]_o$ and unloaded shortening velocity (V_o) or isometric twitch force (F_o) in euthyroidism and hypothyroidism. A and C show results obtained in a trabecula from a euthyroid animal; B and D show the results from a trabecula dissected from a hyperthyroid animal. The data were fit to a sigmoidal equation, which resulted in the parameters EC_{50}, maximal V_o, and maximal F_o as indicated by the dashed arrows. Maximum V_o was 14.2 μm/sec in panel A and 7.9 μm/sec in panel B. EC_{50} of $[Ca^{2+}]_o$ for V_o was 0.41 mM in A and 0.30 mM in B; EC_{50} of $[Ca^{2+}]_o$ for F_o was 0.52 mM in C and 0.48 mM in D. (From Ref. 78 with permission.)

was infused by a mixing pump at the inflow of the muscle bath, which resulted in a steady-state enhancement of contractile state, as shown in Figure 13A. An example of the response of F_o and V_o to increasing concentrations of isoproterenol is shown in Figure 13B. $[Ca^{2+}]_o$ was 0.3 mM in these experiments. As shown before in Figures 9 and 12, at 0.3 mM $[Ca^{2+}]_o$ V_o attains about 50% of maximum V_o at saturating levels of $[Ca^{2+}]_o$ in rat myocardium. The data were fit to the modified Hill sigmoidal equation. On average, isoproterenol reached 50% of its maximum effect on V_o at 7.0 ± 0.6 nM and 12.6 ± 0.52 nM in euthyroidism and hypothyroidism, respectively. Similar values were measured for the F_o parameter. Thus, muscles from euthyroid animals were more sensitive to isoproterenol than muscles from hypothyroid animals, which is consistent with previous reports in the literature (61), and probably due to a reduced number of myocardial β-receptors as a result of hypothyroidism (62).

From the results presented above, it is apparent that both F_o and V_o were a function of the isoproterenol concentration, and saturated at isoproterenol concentrations below 100 nM. Hence, we studied the F_o-$[Ca^{2+}]_o$ and V_o-$[Ca^{2+}]_o$ relations further at a saturated level of β-adrenergic stimulation, that is, 100 nM isoproterenol. Again, both V_o and F_o were sigmoidal functions of $[Ca^{2+}]_o$. Figure 14 shows the

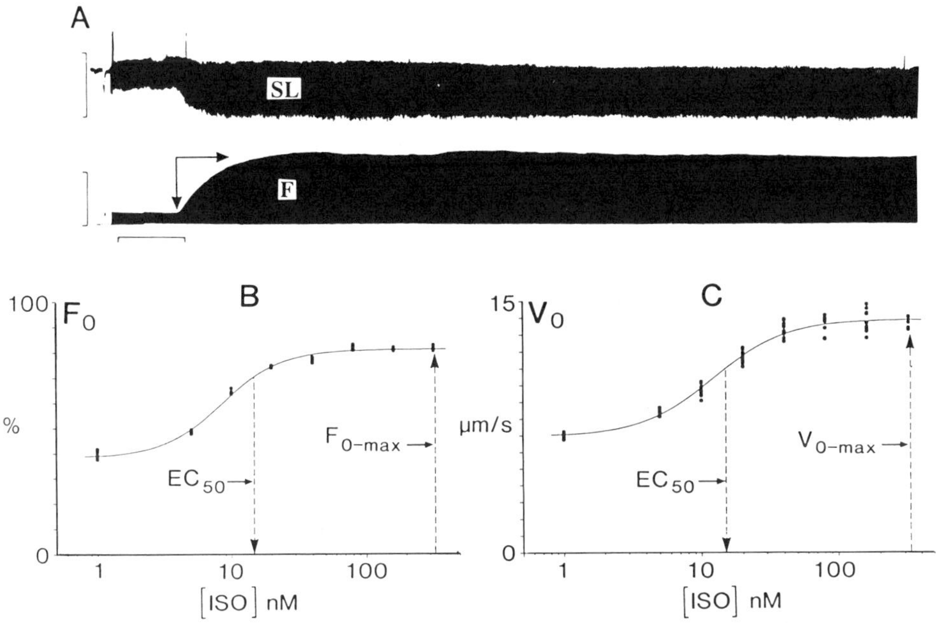

Figure 13 Dependence of twitch force and unloaded shortening velocity on isoproterenol concentration. A. Effect of isoproterenol [ISO] on sarcomere length (SL; top tracing) and twitch force (F; bottom tracing) in a trabecula dissected from a euthyroid animal; $[Ca^{2+}]_o$ was 0.3 mM. Isoproterenol (100 nM) was added at the time indicated by the arrow and subsequently was delivered to the muscle bath via a mixing pump. Calibrations: SL, 0.4 μm. F, 100 mg; time, 5 min. Resting sarcomere length, 2.2 μm. B, C. Examples of the F_o-[ISO] and the V_o-[ISO] relation in euthyroidism. The data were fitted to a sigmoidal equation, which resulted in the parameters EC_{50}, maximal V_o, and maximal F_o as indicated by the dashed arrows. $[Ca^{2+}]_o$ was 0.3 mM. F_o was normalized to the $[Ca^{2+}]_o$ saturated value observed in the absence of isoproterenol (see also Fig. 12). Maximal V_o of this muscle at a saturating $[Ca^{2+}]_o$ and in the absence of isoproterenol was 14.2 μm/sec. Fit parameters (B) EC_{50} = 8.5 nM; maximal F_o = 81.4%; (C) EC_{50} = 12.2 nM; maximal V_o = 13.8 μm/sec. (From Ref. 78 with permission.)

average fit parameters of the sigmoidal relations between F_o and $[Ca^{2+}]_o$ and V_o and $[Ca^{2+}]_o$, both in the presence and absence of isoproterenol. The sensitivity of V_o and F_o to $[Ca^{2+}]_o$ was markedly increased (60–80%) in the presence of isoproterenol, as is evident from the EC_{50} parameters (cf C and D). However, it is clear that regardless of the thyroid state, $V_{o\text{-}max}$ was unaffected by isoproterenol application. $F_{o\text{-}max}$, on the other hand, was significantly reduced (25–32%) in the presence of isoproterenol. β-adrenergic stimulation has been shown to cause phosphorylation of troponin-l, which leads to a reduction of the sensitivity of the myofilaments to calcium ions (13,63,64). The effect of isoproterenol on $F_{o\text{-}max}$ can thus be understood if one realizes that cardiac muscle is never maximally activated. This is probably caused by a limitation of cardiac sarcoplasmic reticulum to store and retain calcium (29,36,37,65,66). We do not think that this reduction in $F_{o\text{-}max}$ by isoproterenol, however, is large enough to explain the lack of effect of isoproterenol on V_o; a significant effect of the level of contractile activation on V_o is only apparent when

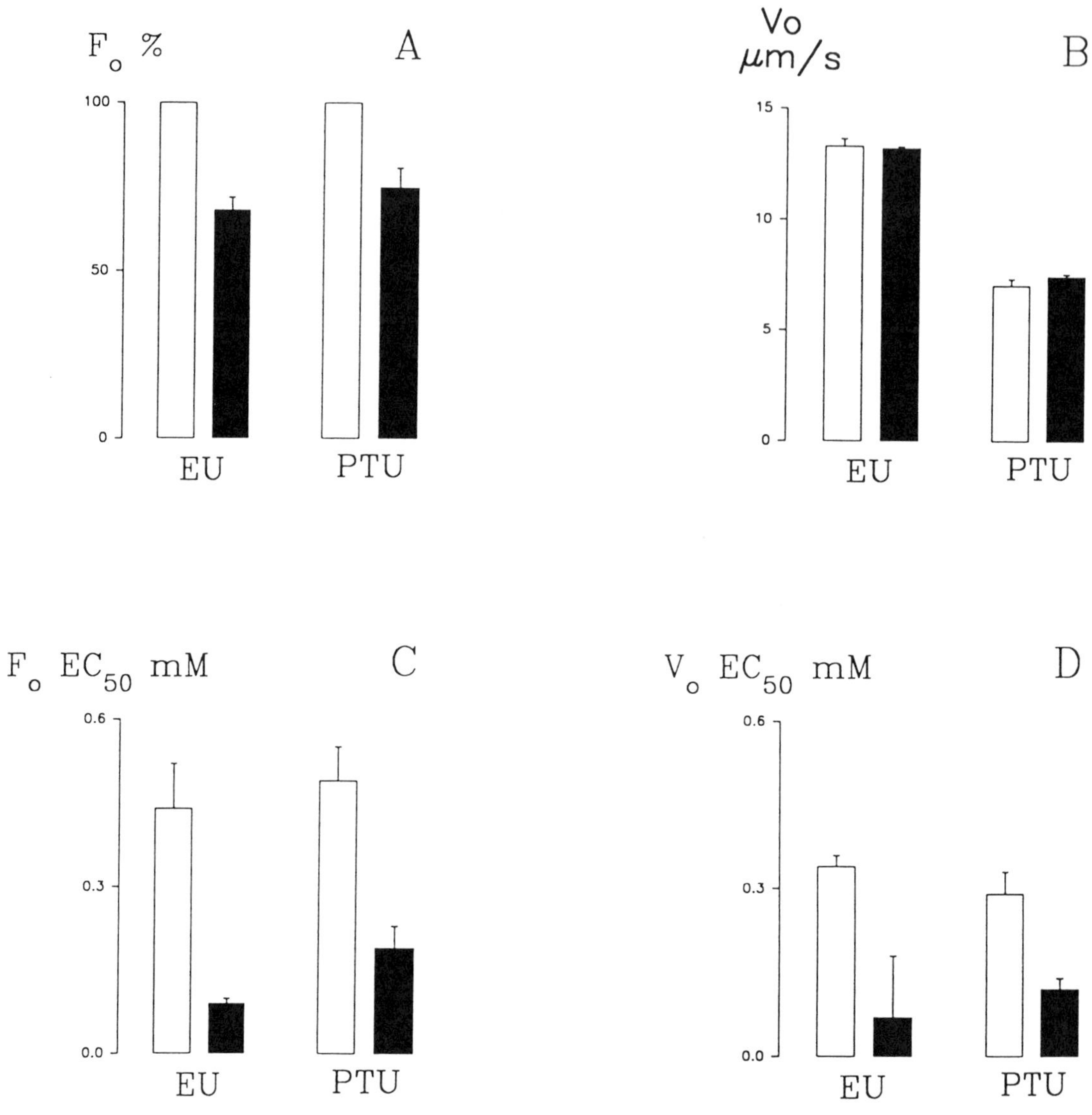

Figure 14 Effect of isoproterenol on maximum F_o, maximum V_o, and on EC_{50} of F_o and V_o for $[Ca^{2+}]_o$. Top panels show the average maximum twitch force (A) and maximum V_o (B) at saturating $[Ca^{2+}]_o$ in the presence (filled bars) and absence (open bars) of 100 nM isoproterenol in euthyroidism and hypothyroidism. Bottom panels show the average EC_{50} for $[Ca^{2+}]_o$ of F_o (C) and V_o (D) in the presence (filled bars) and absence (open bars) of 100 nM isoproterenol in euthyroidism and hypothyroidism.

twitch force is lower than 50% of $F_{o\text{-}max}$, as we have discussed earlier (see also Fig. 10). This conclusion is reinforced by the observation (see, for example, Fig. 13), that when isoproterenol minimally reduced $F_{o\text{-}max}$ (e.g., 10–20%), as it did in several muscles of both groups, maximal V_o was not increased at all above the values measured without isoproterenol.

C. Interpretation of the Results on Isoproterenol

The results on the effects of isoproterenol that we have presented question the appealingly simple prediction that β-adrenergic stimulation should increase the unloaded velocity of sarcomere shortening due to accelerated cross-bridge cycling, as has been shown in studies on dynamic muscle stiffness and kinetics of force development (14–18). The prediction is based on analogy with the correlation between the unloaded velocity of muscle shortening, dynamic muscle stiffness, and the biochemical properties of cardiac myosin isoenzymes (14–16,59). It is well known that the ATPase activity of cardiac muscle depends on the amount of the myosin isoenzyme V_1 relative to the amount of V_3 myosin (59). That this biochemical parameter is reflected in the mechanical properties of cardiac muscle was shown by measurements of the dependence of stiffness on the frequency of small (less than 1%) length perturbations of the muscle during isometric contractures due to constant activation by barium ions (14). The frequency at which stiffness is minimal (approximately 1 Hz) appeared to correlate closely with the isomyosin composition of the muscle (15). Hence, the increase in frequency of minimal stiffness has been attributed to a higher cycling rate of V_1 isomyosin than of V_3 isomyosin (14–16,59). A strong correlation between the unloaded shortening velocity and myocardial isomyosin composition has likewise been demonstrated (54,55,57), which is confirmed by our results. Hence, the assumption that the frequency of minimal stiffness and unloaded shortening velocity is related expressions of the myosin ATPase activity is not unreasonable. β-Adrenergic stimulation of cardiac muscle also has been shown to increase both myosin ATPase activity (13,49) and the frequency of minimal stiffness in papillary muscles during barium contractures (14–16). The hypothesis that β-adrenergic stimulation induces an increase of the cycling rate of cross-bridges was supported by the observation of Saeki et al. (17,18) that catecholamines increased the rate of force redevelopment after small muscle length changes. They also concluded from their observations that an increase of the cross-bridge cycling rate by β-adrenergic stimulation was independent of the level of myofilament activation. In support of this conclusion is the observation in skeletal muscle by Brenner and Eisenberg (67) that the rate of force redevelopment after a quick muscle length change in skeletal muscle is closely correlated with the actomyosin ATPase activity. Hence, by analogy to the correlation between the unloaded shortening velocity and myosin isoenzyme composition, it is possible to predict that β-catecholamines should increase unloaded shortening velocity irrespective of the level of activation of the muscle by calcium ions.

The results of the experiments on rat cardiac trabeculae described here clearly suggest that the latter hypothesis is untenable. This discrepancy raises two intriguing questions. First, which mechanism of operation of the actin–myosin interaction can explain that isoproterenol accelerates the kinetics of isometric force generation but fails to increase the unloaded shortening velocity? Second, is the absence of an effect of β-adrenergic stimulation on unloaded sarcomere shortening velocity a unique property of rat myocardium, or can this phenomenon be expected in cardiac muscle of other species?

The differences of force dynamics and of shortening velocity possibly can be explained by assuming that different steps in the cross-bridge cycle are rate limiting for force generation and for rapid unloaded propulsion of the actin filament.

Siemankowski et al. (68) have likewise proposed that of the different reaction steps of myosin ATPase, one step is rate limiting for unloaded velocity of shortening and another limits the ATPase activity in vitro. Both steps may be affected by modification of the isomyosin composition, but not necessarily by β-adrenergic stimulation. It is likely that the frequency at which stiffness of activated muscle is minimal corresponds to the rate of force redevelopment (14,15), but it is not necessary that this property relates to the unloaded shortening velocity. First, the rate constant of cross-bridge cycling is generally assumed to depend on the strain of the cross-bridges (5), which is evidently high during the test of stiffness. It is also likely that during sinusoidal perturbations, cross-bridges are forced to go through a complete cycle of ATP hydrolysis. On the other hand, the unloaded shortening velocity probably depends on one particular fast-reaction step in the cross-bridge cycle. In fact, a simple calculation shows that the unloaded shortening velocity predicted from the frequency of the stiffness minimum (approximately 1 Hz) and the stroke of the cross-bridges (about 15 nm/half sarcomere) is about two orders of magnitude too slow (0.03 μm/sec vs. 15 μm/sec). Therefore, unloaded shortening velocity and stiffness minimum are not *a priori* expressions of the same molecular reaction processes.

The sensitivity of rat myocardium to $[Ca^{2+}]_o$ is higher than myocardium of other mammals, as we have shown in a previous section of this chapter (cf. Fig. 9). The effects of $[Ca^{2+}]_o$ on the force–sarcomere length and force–sarcomere velocity relation of cat myocardium, however, are in many ways similar to those in rat myocardium (24). The main differences between rat and cat myocardium are slower twitch kinetics and reduced $[Ca^{2+}]_o$ sensitivity in cat myocardium. The similarities between rat and cat cardiac trabeculae suggest that the second question mentioned above can be answered by using cat cardiac trabeculae to test the hypothesis that β-adrenergic stimulation increases the level activation and thereby increases unloaded velocity of shortening velocity in mammalian cardiac muscle.

An increase in force development and ATPase activity upon β-adrenergic stimulation or cyclic AMP application at a saturating calcium concentration that has been reported in EGTA-treated cardiac muscle (13,49). The isomyosin composition appeared to have a major influence on the magnitude of the force response to β-adrenergic stimulation or cyclic AMP at saturating calcium concentrations (13,49). This effect, however, has not been observed in other studies (69,70). In our experiments the response of twitch force to isoproterenol likewise was not affected by the thyroid status. It is not clear what the reason is for these differences. They could be due to the large difference in the techniques used, that is, EGTA-treated fibers vs. intact trabeculae in our experiments.

At first sight, our results would suggest that catecholamines do not increase the unloaded shortening velocity in myocardium. This, however, is not the case under physiological conditions encountered in the intact animal. Under those conditions, the cardiac contractile apparatus is submaximally activated. It is not known at which level of contractile activation the in situ heart operates, but a lower limit estimate can be obtained from our experiments on cat cardiac trabeculae. The free ionized calcium concentration in the blood is about 1 mM. At 25°C and at $[Ca^{2+}]_o$ = 1.0 mM, cat trabeculae develop about 30% of maximum twitch force as at saturating levels of $[Ca^{2+}]_o$ ([24]; cf Fig. 9). Increasing the temperature to 37°C will decrease twitch force about 50% (28). Thus, in the absence of β-adrenergic stimulation and at a physiological temperature, we can assume that the in situ cardiac contractile apparatus is about 15% activated. This value indicates a substantial range over which the contractile state of the in situ heart can be enhanced by catecholamines and other positive inotropic agents. With these considerations in mind it is no surprise that catecholamines increase twitch force and shortening velocity in the in situ heart, a fact well appreciated in the clinical setting. Thus, the unloaded shortening velocity is enhanced by catecholamines only under conditions of submaximal contractile activation, and is due to a greater sensitivity of unloaded shortening velocity to extracellular Ca^{2+}, presumably as a result of enhanced calcium release by intracellular stores, and not due to an intrinsic modification of the rate-limiting step in the actomyosin interaction that determines unloaded shortening velocity of cardiac muscle.

VII. CONCLUSIONS AND FUTURE DIRECTIONS

In this chapter we have presented evidence that showed that isolated cardiac muscle is grossly nonuniform, and that this leads to uncontrolled sarcomere motion in the central region of the muscle preparation during a twitch. We have seen that the laser diffraction technique can be used to overcome the problems associated with this nonuniformity; the technique allows accurate determination of isometric twitch force at constant sarcomere length and velocity of sarcomere shortening.

Unloaded velocity of sarcomere shortening is a function of contractile activation. We have presented evidence that this interrelationship may be due to passive viscous loading of the muscle during shortening, rather than regulation of cross-bridge cycle kinetics by the level of contractile activation. This hypothesis, however, awaits further testing, for example, by experiments with skinned fibers in which it should be possible to manipulate selectively passive viscosity or intrinsic shortening velocity. We have described in this chapter our experiments indicating that catecholamines do not increase the unloaded shortening velocity by a direct effect on the rate-limiting step in the cross-bridges cycle that determines V_o. Rather, these agents appear to enhance greatly the sensitivity of twitch force and V_o to the concentration of extracellular calcium ions. Thus, our results indicate that the kinetics of cross-bridge cycling that pertains to shortening of the cardiac sarcomere is not regulated by phosphorylation of specific sites on the actomyosin complex induced by cyclic AMP-dependent kinases.

We have seen that the level of both activation of the contractile apparatus and catecholamines appears to be without an effect on the fundamental cycling kinetics of the interaction between actin and myosin during shortening at zero load. Hence, one might wonder which, if any, parameters do affect this process. One of the factors we have investigated recently (28) that does have a major effect on unloaded shortening velocity is temperature. Figure 15 shows V_o measured in rat trabeculae plotted as a function of temperature in an Arrhenius plot. Special care was taken in that study (28) to keep the level of contractile activation constant at all temperatures. The Q_{10} for V_o calculated from the slope of this relation was 4.8 (i.e., V_o decreased by a factor of about 5 for each 10°C decrease in temperature). The interpretation of this result is that the activation energy for the rate-limiting step in the cross-bridge cycle that determines V_o is rather high. One could speculate that this fact would cause the reaction associated with the detachment of the cross-

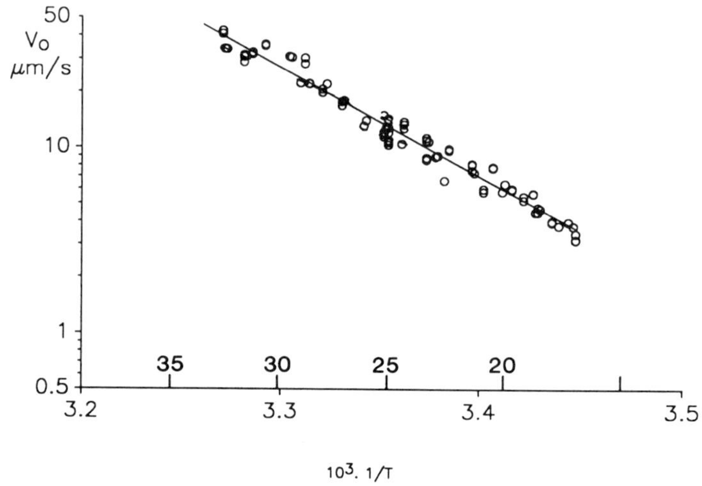

Figure 15 Arrhenius plot of V_o in rat trabeculae. V_o was measured between 17°C and 33°C in rat trabeculae. Contractile activation was kept constant (± 20%) by paired pulse pacing. $[Ca^{2+}]_o$ = 1.5 mM. Regression analysis (solid line) revealed an activation energy of 111.9 ± 2.1 kJ/mol, which corresponds to a Q_{10} of 4.6 (95% confidence limit 4.3–4.8). (Modified from Ref. 28 with permission.)

bridge to proceed virtually undirectionally, thus aiding shortening of the cardiac sarcomere.

Another parameter that affects V_o, albeit on a longer time scale, is the isomyosin composition. V_3 isomyosin was associated with a 40% lower V_o compared to V_1 isomyosin. In rats, not only hypothyroidism but also hypertrophy appears to be associated with the synthesis of the slow V_3 isomyosin (50,71). However, this mechanism is unlikely to play a major role in larger mammals, since the myocardium in those animals (including humans) already contains 100% V_3 isomyosin (50). However, it has been shown that myocardial actomyosin ATPase activity is increased with hyperthyroidism in the dog, despite the fact that the isomyosin composition did not change (i.e., 100% V_3) (72). A similar observation has recently been made in dogs in which heart failure was induced by rapid chronic ventricular pacing (73). In that study, cardiac actomyosin ATPase activity was reduced in the animals with heart failure, while again the isomyosin composition was unaltered from control. These observations suggest that other moietites of the actomyosin complex are important for ATP hydrolysis kinetics and possibly the kinetics of force generation (50,74–76). Whether the unloaded shortening velocity, at the level of the cardiac sarcomere and at saturating levels of contractile activation, is also reduced in these disease states remains to be investigated. We would speculate that this would be the case. For example, we have recently observed a similar disparity between isomyosin composition and unloaded shortening velocity in rats rendered hypothyroid only for a brief period of time; V_o decreased by 35% in cardiac trabeculae from these animals, while the isomyosin composition of the heart was unaltered from control rats (27). This observation lends support to the hypothesis that the isomyosin composition is only one factor of many unknown factors that determine the ATP hydrolysis rate, cross-cycling kinetics, and unloaded velocity of sarcomere shortening in myocardium. Further studies on the effects of disease states on the protein composition of the cardiac myofilaments, and in particular the effects of such changes on force development and sarcomere-shortening velocity of myocardium, are needed to advance the understanding of the mechanisms that cause cardiac disease (77).

ACKNOWLEDGMENTS

This work was supported in part by grants from the Alberta Heritage Foundation for Medical Research (AHFMR) and the Canadian Medical Research council. P.P. de Tombe held a studentship from the AHFMR and HEDJ ter Keurs is a Medical Scientist of the AHFMR.

REFERENCES

1. Allen DG, Kurihara S. Calcium transients in mammalian ventricular muscle. Eur Heart J 1980;1 (Suppl A):5–15.
2. MacKinnon R, Gwathmey JK, Allen PD, Briggs GM, Morgan JP. Modulation by the thyroid state of intracellular calcium and contractility in ferret ventricular muscle. Circ Res 1988;63:1080–9.
3. Sonnenblick EH: Implications of muscle mechanics in the heart. Fed Proc 1962;21:975–93.
4. Brutsaert DL, Parmley WW, Sonnenblick EH. Effects of various inotropic interventions on the dynamic properties of the contractile elements in heart muscle of the cat. Circ Res 1970;27:513–22.
5. Huxley AF. Muscle structure and theories of contraction. Prog Biophys Chem 1957; 7:255–318.
6. Moss RL. Effects on shortening velocity of rabbit skeletal muscle due to variations in the level of thin-filament activation. J Physiol 1986;377:487–505.
7. Julian, FJ, Rome LC, Stephenson DG, Striz S. The influence of free calcium on the maximum speed of shortening in skinned frog muscle fibers. J Physiol 1986;380:257–73.
8. Gulati J, Babu A. Contraction kinetics of intact and skinned frog muscle fibers and degree of activation. J Gen Physiol 1985;86:479–500.
9. Podolsky RJ, Teichholz LE. The relation between calcium and contraction kinetics in skinned muscle fibers. J Physiol 1970;211:19–35.
10. Brenner B. Effect of Ca^{2+} on cross-bridge kinetics in skinned single rabbit psoas fibers: implications for regulation of muscle contraction. Proc Natl Acad Sci (USA) 1988; 85:3265–9.
11. Maughan DW, Low ES, Alpert NA. Isometric force development, isotonic shortening, and elasticity measurements from Ca^{2+}-activated ventricular muscle of the guinea pig. J Gen Physiol 1978;71:431–51.
12. Podolin RA, Ford LE. The influence of calcium on the shortening velocity of skinned frog muscle cells. J Muscle Res Cell Motil 1983;4:263–82.
13. Winegrad S. Regulation of cardiac contractile proteins. Correlation between physiology and biochemistry. Circ Res 1984;55:565–74.
14. Berman MR, Peterson JN, Yue DT, Hunter WC. Effect of isoproterenol on force transient time course and on stiffness spectra in rabbit papillary muscle in barium contracture. J Mol Cell Cardiol 1988;20:415–26.
15. Rossmanith GH, Hoh JFY, Kirman A, Kwan LJ. Influence of V_1 and V_3 isomyosins on the mechanical behaviour of rat papillary muscle as studied by pseudo-random binary noise modulated length perturbations. J Muscle Res Cell Motil 1986;7:307–19.

16. Hoh JFY, Rossmanith GH, Kwan LJ, Hamilton AM. Adrenaline increases the rate of cycling of cross-bridges in rat cardiac muscle as measured by pseudo-random binary noise-modulated perturbation analysis. Circ Res 1988;62:452–61.
17. Saeki Y, Kato C, Yanagisawa K. Catecholamine increases myocardial shortening velocity by an increase in the number and in the cycling rate of cross-bridges. (abstract). J Muscle Res Cell Motil 1989;10:260–61.
18. Saeki Y, Shiozawa K, Shibata T. Adrenaline increases the rate of cross-bridge cycling in rat cardiac-muscle. J Moll Cell Cardiol 1990;22:453–60.
19. Pollack GH, Krueger JW. Sarcomere dynamics in intact cardiac muscle. Eur J Cardiol 1976;4:53–65.
20. Krueger JW, Pollack GH. Myocardial sarcomere dynamics during isometric contraction. J Physiol 1975;251:627–43.
21. Julian FJ, Sollins MR, Moss RL. Absence of a plateau in length-tension relationship of rabbit papillary muscle when internal shortening is prevented. Nature 1976;260:340–2.
22. Julian FJ, Sollins MR. Sarcomere length–tension relation in living rat papillary muscle. Circ Res 1975;37:299–308.
23. ter Keurs HEDJ, Rijnsburger WH, van Heuningen R, Nagelsmit J. Tension development and sarcomere length in rat cardiac trabeculae. Evidence of length-dependent activation. Circ Res 1980;46:703–14.
24. de Tombe PP, ter Keurs HEDJ. Sarcomere dynamics in cat cardiac trabeculae. Circ Res 1991;68:558–596.
25. Physiological basis of Starling's law of the heart. CIBA Foundation Symp 24. Elsevier, Amsterdam, 1974.
26. ter Keurs, HEDJ, Noble MIM. Starling's law of the heart revisited. Dordrecht: Martinus Nijhoff, 1988.
27. de Tombe PP. Determinants of velocity of sarcomere shortening in mammalian myocardium. PhD Thesis, University of Calgary, 1989.
28. de Tombe PP, ter Keurs HEDJ. Force and velocity of sarcomere shortening in trabeculae from rat heart; effects of temperature. Circ Res 1990;66:1239–54.
29. Kentish JC, ter Keurs HEDJ, Ricciardi L, Bucx JJJ, Noble MIM. Comparison between the sarcomere length-force relations of intact and skinned trabeculae from rat right ventricle. Influence of calcium concentrations on these relations. Circ Res 1986;58;755–68.
30. Iwazumi T, Pollack GH. On-line measurement of sarcomere length from diffraction patterns in muscle. IEEE Biomed Eng 1979;26:86–93.
31. Daniels M, Noble MIM, ter Keurs HEDJ, Wohlfart B. Velocity of sarcomere shortening in rat cardiac muscle: relationship to force, sarcomere length, calcium and time. J Physiol 1984;355:367–81.
32. Hill AV. Heat of shortening and the dynamic constants of muscle. Proc Roy Soc 1938;126:136–95.
33. de Tombe PP, ter Keurs HEDJ. An internal viscous element limits unloaded velocity of shortening in rat myocardium. J. Physiol 1992; in press.
34. Rudel R, Zite-Ferenczy F. Interpretation of light diffraction by cross-striated muscle as Bragg reflexion of light by the lattice of contractile proteins. J Physiol 1979;290:317–30.
35. Edman KAP. Double-hyperbolic force-velocity relation in frog muscle fibres. J Physiol 1988;404:301–21.
36. Fabiato A. Myoplasmic free calcium concentration reached during the twitch of an intact isolated cardiac cell and during calcium-induced release of calcium from the sarcoplasmic reticulum of a skinned cardiac cell from the adult rat or rabbit. J Gen Physiol 1981;78:457–97.
37. Fabiato A. Calcium release in skinned cardiac cells: variation with species, tissues, and development. Fed Proc 1982;41:2238–44.

38. Weber A, Murray JM. Molecular control mechanisms in muscle contraction. Physiol Rev 1973;53:612–73.
39. Adelstein RS, Eisenberg E. Regulation and kinetics of the actin-myosin-ATP interaction. Annu Rev Biochem 1980;49:921–56.
40. Woledge RC, Curtin NA, Homsher E. Energetic aspects of muscle contraction. London: Academic Press, 1985.
41. Ruegg JC. Calcium in muscle activation: a comparative approach. Berlin: Springer Verlag, 1986.
42. Morimoto K, Harrington WF. Evidence for structural changes in vertebrate thick filaments induced by calcium. J Mol Biol 1974;88:693–709.
43. Hasselgrove JC. X-ray evidence for conformational changes in the myosin filaments of vertebrate striated muscle. J Mol Biol 1975;92:113–43.
44. Lehman W. Thick-filament-linked calcium regulation in vertebrate striated muscle. Nature 1978;274:80–1.
45. Chiu YL, Ballou EW, LE Ford. Force, velocity and power changes during normal and potentiated contractions of cat papillary muscle. Circ Res 1987;60:446–58.
46. Tsuchiya T. Passive interaction between sliding filaments in the osmotically compressed skinned muscle fibers of the frog. Biophys J 1988;53:415–23.
47. Chiu YL, Ballou EW, Ford LE. Internal viscoelastic loading in cat papillary muscle. Biophys J 1982;40:109–20.
48. Chiu YL, Ballou EW, Ford LE. Velocity transients and viscoelastic resistance to active shortening in cat papillary muscle. Biophys J 1982;40:121–8.
49. Winegrad S, Weisberg A. Isozyme specific modification of myosin ATPase by cAMP in rat heart. Circ Res 1987;60:384–92.
50. Swynghedauw B. Developmental and functional adaptation of contractile proteins in cardiac and skeletal muscles. Physiol Rev 1986;66:710–71.
51. Holubarsch C, Goulette RP, Litten RZ, Martin BJ, Mulieri LA, Alpert NR. The economy of isometric force development, myosin isoenzyme pattern and myofibrillar ATPase activity in normal and hypothyroid rat myocardium. Circ Res 1985;56:78–86.
52. Hoh JFY, McGrath PA, Hale PT. Electrophoretic analysis of multiple forms of rat cardiac myosin: Effects of hypophysectomy and thyroxine replacement. J Mol Cell Cardiol 1977;10:1053–76.
53. Strauer BE, Schulze W. Experimental hypothyroidism: depression of myocardial contractile function and hemodynamics and their reversibility by substitution with thyroid hormones. Basic Res Cardiol 1976;71:624–44.
54. Schwartz K, Lecarpentier Y, Martin JL, Lompre AM, Mercadier JJ, Swynghedauw B. Myosin isoenzymic distribution correlates with speed of myocardial contraction. J Mol Cell Cardiol 1981;13:1071–5.
55. Capelli V, Bottinelli R, Pogessi C, Moggio R, Reggiani C. Shortening velocity and myosin and myofibrillar ATPase activity related to myosin isoenzyme composition during postnatal development in rat myocardium. Circ Res 1989;65:446–57.
56. Buccino RA, Spann JF, Pool PE, Sonnenblick EH, Braunwald E. Influence of the thyroid state on the intrinsic contractile properties and energy stores of the myocardium. J Clin Invest 1967;46:1669–82.
57. Pagani ED, Julian FJ. Rabbit papillary muscle isozymes and the velocity of muscle shortening. Circ Res 1984;54:586–94.
58. Barany M. ATPase activity of myosin correlated with speed of muscle shortening. J Gen Physiol 1967;50:197–216.
59. Pope B, Hoh JFY, Weeds A. The ATPase activities of rat cardiac myosin isoenzymes. FEBS Letts 1980;118:205–8.
60. Kurihara S, Konishi M. Effects of β-adrenoceptor stimulation on intracellular Ca transients and tension in rat ventricular muscle. Pflugers Arch 1987;409:427–37.

61. Scott-Hayes J, Wyss VL, Schenck KS, Cohen ML. Effects of prolonged isoproterenol infusion on cardiac and vascular responses to adrenoceptor agonists. J Pharmacol Exp Ther 1986;237:757–63.
62. McConnaughey MM, Jones, LR, Watenabe AM, Besch HR, Williams LT, Lefkowitz RJ. Thyroxine and propylthiouracil effects on alpha- end beta-adrenergic receptor number, ATPase activities, and sialic acid content of rat cardiac membrane vesicles. J Cardiovasc Pharmacol 1979;1:609–23.
63. Solaro RJ, Rapundalo ST, Garvey JL, Kranias EG. Mechanics of cardiac contraction and the phosphorylation of sarcotubular and myofilament proteins. In ter Keurs HEDJ, Tyberg JV, eds. Mechanics of the circulation. Dordrecht: Martinus Nijhoff, 1987.
64. Rapundalo ST, Solaro RJ, Kranias EG. Inotropic responses to isoproterenol and phosphodiesterase inhibitors in intact guinea pig hearts: comparison of c-AMP levels and phosphorylation of sarcoplasmic reticulum and myofibrillar proteins. Circ Res 1988;64:104–11.
65. Mulder, BM, de Tombe PP, ter Keurs HEDJ. Spontaneous and propagated contraction in rat cardiac muscle. J Gen Physiol 1989;93:943–61.
66. Schouten VJA, Bucx JJJ, de Tombe PP, ter Keurs HEDJ. Sarcolemma, sarcoplasmic reticulum, and sarcomeres as limiting factors in force production in heart. Circ Res 1990;67:913–22.
67. Brenner B, Eisenberg E. Rate of force generation in muscle: correlation with actomyosin ATPase activity in solution. Proc Natl Acad Sci 1986;83:3542–6.
68. Siemankowski RF, Wiseman MO, White HD. ADP dissociation from actomyosin subfragment 1 is sufficiently slow to limit the unloaded shortening velocity in vertebrate muscle. Proc Natl Acad Sci 1985;82:658–62.
69. Miller DJ, Smith GL. The contractile behaviour of EGTA- and detergent-treated muscle. J Muscle Res Cell Motil 1985;6:541–67.
70. Kentish JC, Jewell BR. Some characteristics of Ca^{2+}-regulated force production in EGTA treated muscles from rat heart. J Gen Physiol 1984;84:83–99.
71. Holubarsch C, Litten RZ, Mulieri LA, Alpert NR. Energetic changes of myocardium as an adaption to chronic hemodynamic overload and thyroid gland activity. Basic Res Cardiol 1985;80:582–93.
72. Suga H, Tanaka N, Ohgoshi Y, Futaki S, Yasumura T, Goto Y, Saeki Y, Nakanishi T. Hyperthyroidism like acute inotropic interventions does not affect efficiency of contractile machinery from O_2 consumption to total mechanism energy in canine left ventricle. Proceedings of the 9th international conference of the Cardiovascular Systems Dynamics Society, 1988, Halifax, Canada, pp. 285–288.
73. O'Brien PJ, Ianuzzo CD, Moe GW, Stopps TP, Armstrong PW. Rapid ventricular pacing of dogs to heart failure: biochemical and physiological studies. Can J Physiol Pharmacol 1990;68:34–9.
74. Lauer B, Van Thiem N, Swybghedauw B. ATPase activity of the cross-linked complex between cardiac myosin subfragment 1 and actin in several models of chronic overloading. Circ Res 1989;64:1106–15.
75. Baudet S, Ventura-Clapier R. Differential effects of caffeine on skinned fibers from control and hypertrophied ferrets. Am J Physiol 1990;259:H1803–8.
76. Wankler M, Bohm M, Morano I, Ruegg JC, Eichhorn M, Erdmann E. Calcium sensitivity and myosin light chain pattern of atrial and ventricular skinned cardiac fibers from patients with various kinds of cardiac disease. J Mol Cell Cardiol 1990;22:1425–38.
77. Katz AM. Cardiomyopathy of overload: a major determinant of prognosis in congestive heart failure. N Eng J Med 1990;322:100–10.
78. de Tombe PP, ter Keurs HEDJ. Lack of effect of isoproterenol on unloaded velocity of sarcomere shortening in rat cardiac trabeculae. Circ Res 1991;68:382–391.

5

Calcium Uptake and Release by Cardiac Sarcoplasmic Reticulum

MATTHEW A. MOVSESIAN

University of Utah Medical Center
Salt Lake City, Utah

I. INTRODUCTION

Contraction and relaxation in cardiac myocytes result from the sequential activation and inactivation of the contractile elements by the alternating rise and fall of the cytosolic Ca^{2+} concentration. The sarcoplasmic reticulum is the intracellular membrane system of myocytes that releases and sequesters Ca^{2+} to and from the cytoplasm. Ca^{2+} is also transported across the sarcolemma and mitochondrial membranes, but these systems lack the high Ca^{2+} affinity and capacity of the transport mechanisms of sarcoplasmic reticulum. It is therefore likely that the sarcoplasmic reticulum is the principal organelle through which phasic changes in the cytosolic Ca^{2+} concentration are controlled.

Uptake and release of Ca^{2+} by cardiac sarcoplasmic reticulum occur through separate molecular mechanisms. Alterations in Ca^{2+} uptake might therefore be predicted to have discrete effects on myocardial relaxation, while alterations in Ca^{2+} release would be expected to have discrete effects on contraction. The simplicity of this conceptualization is appealing, but it obscures the possible interdependence of the two processes. Stimulation of Ca^{2+} uptake, for example, might result in a greater accumulation of Ca^{2+} within the sarcoplasmic reticulum, a greater magnitude of subsequent Ca^{2+} release into the cytosol, and a faster rate of contraction. Furthermore, Ca^{2+} storage and release may be linked directly via protein–protein interactions. The complexity of such considerations is becoming more apparent as more is being learned.

In this chapter, aspects of cardiac sarcoplasmic reticulum biochemistry pertinent to Ca^{2+} uptake, storage, and release are reviewed. Special attention is paid to pathophysiological and therapeutic considerations.

II. MORPHOLOGY OF SARCOPLASMIC RETICULUM

With respect to ultrastructure, the sarcoplasmic reticulum can be regarded as comprised of contiguous junctional, corbular, and longitudinal components (1–4). The longitudinal sarcoplasmic reticulum consists of the anastomosing membrane network surrounding the actin and myosin filaments. The junctional sarcoplasmic reticulum consists of portions of the membrane system adjacent to the sarcolemma and transverse tubules (5,6). The corbular sarcoplasmic reticulum consists of globular extensions of the longitudinal sarcoplasmic reticulum that are not immediately adjacent to the sarcolemma and transverse tubules.

Two proteins involved in Ca^{2+} uptake, phospholamban and a Ca^{2+}-transporting ATPase, are primarily localized to the longitudinal and corbular portions of the sarcoplasmic reticulum (7,8). Also localized to these regions are two glycoproteins, alternate-splice products of the same gene, that may be involved in the uptake of Ca^{2+} and its binding within the sarcoplasmic reticulum lumen (9,10). Calsequestrin, another Ca^{2+}-binding protein located within the lumen of the sarcoplasmic reticulum, is found primarily in the corbular and junctional areas, along with a 26,000–32,000 Da calsequestrin-binding protein (11–13). The Ca^{2+}-releasing channels are contained within the high-molecular weight "foot" protein complexes localized to the junctional sarcoplasmic reticulum and spanning the gaps to the sarcolemma and transverse tubule membranes (5,6,14). On the basis of these observations, it appears that Ca^{2+} is taken up principally by the longitudinal and corbular sarcoplasmic reticulum, stored within the lumen of the corbular and junctional sarcoplasmic reticulum, and released via Ca^{2+} channels localized to the latter (see Fig. 1).

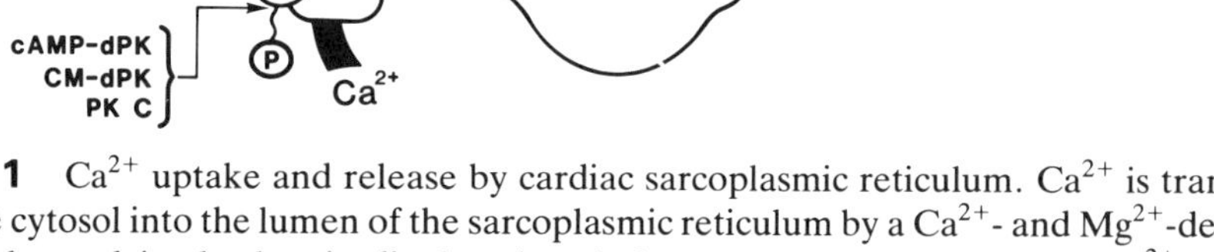

Figure 1 Ca^{2+} uptake and release by cardiac sarcoplasmic reticulum. Ca^{2+} is transported from the cytosol into the lumen of the sarcoplasmic reticulum by a Ca^{2+}- and Mg^{2+}-dependent ATPase located in the longitudinal and corbular sarcoplasmic reticulum. Ca^{2+} uptake is stimulated by phosphorylation of phospholamban (PL) by cAMP-dependent protein kinase (cAMP-dPK), a calmodulin-dependent protein kinase (CM-dPK) and protein kinase C (PK-C). A 53,000-Da glycoprotein (GP_L) may also be involved in regulation.

Within the lumen of the sarcoplasmic reticulum, Ca^{2+} is bound by a 160,000-Da glycoprotein (GP_H) and by calsequestrin (CS). Ca^{2+} is released via the ryanodine-sensitive Ca^{2+} channel (RR) located in the junctional sarcoplasmic reticulum adjacent to the dihydropyridine-sensitive Ca^{2+} channel (DR) of the transverse tubules. Release appears to involve interactions among the ryanodine-sensitive Ca^{2+} channel, calsequestrin, and 26,000–32,000 Da calsequestrin binding protein (CBP).

III. Ca^{2+} UPTAKE

A. Mechanism

Ca^{2+} uptake by cardiac sarcoplasmic reticulum occurs through the activity of a Ca^{2+}- and Mg^{2+}-dependent ATPase. This enzyme transports Ca^{2+} against a high concentration gradient from the cytosol to the lumen of the sarcoplasmic reticulum while hydrolysing ATP to ADP and inorganic phosphate. The cardiac and slow twitch skeletal muscle enzymes are products of the same gene, while the Ca^{2+}- and Mg^{2+}-dependent ATPase of fast twitch skeletal muscle sarcoplasmic reticulum is the product of a separate gene (15). For this reason, molecular mechanisms relating to the Ca^{2+}- and Mg^{2+}-dependent ATPase of fast twitch skeletal muscle, which have been studied in considerable detail, cannot be presumed to apply to the Ca^{2+}- and Mg^{2+}-dependent ATPase of cardiac muscle. The cardiac enzyme has recently been identified in humans, where its molecular weight is 105,000 Da (16).

Ca^{2+} uptake and ATPase activity of sarcoplasmic reticulum are most often studied in microsomes prepared from myocardial homogenates by differential sedimentation. Ca^{2+} uptake (accummulation is a preferable term, since assays measure the net difference between influx and concurrent efflux, but uptake is ubiquitous in the literature) is measured using either radiolabeled Ca^{2+} or Ca^{2+}-sensitive dyes whose fluorescence or absorbance can be measured. Assays of ATPase activity rely upon detection of liberated inorganic phosphate. It is customary in both cases to include oxalate at concentrations of 2.5–10.0 mM in the reaction mixtures. Oxalate, like other dicarboxylic acids, is taken up by the sarcoplasmic reticulum and binds Ca^{2+} within the lumen (17,18). This increases the Ca^{2+} capacity of isolated vesicles markedly, probably by lowering the free Ca^{2+} concentration within the lumen of the sarcoplasmic reticulum and preventing product inhibition of uptake. Ca^{2+} uptake measured under these conditions proceeds linearly over several minutes, and Ca^{2+} uptake rates measured using this method correspond reasonably well to initial Ca^{2+} uptake rates measured in the absence of oxalate (19). It should be noted, however, that the fact that Ca^{2+} uptake is stimulated by oxalate and other Ca^{2+}-binding anions raises the possibility that the Ca^{2+} capacity of sarcoplasmic reticulum may be the factor that limits Ca^{2+} uptake in vivo. The use of such agents may therefore obscure in vivo effects that depend upon changes in Ca^{2+} capacity. In addition, microsomal preparations necessarily entail disruption of the structure of sarcoplasmic reticulum as it exists in vivo, and this may limit the relevance of experiments that rely on their use. The Ca^{2+} capacity of sarcoplasmic reticulum vesicles might depend upon their surface to volume ratio, for example, and this could be affected by methods of preparation.

Ca^{2+} transport and ATPase activity can be characterized in terms of the standard parameters of enzyme kinetics. These include V_{max}, the rate of enzyme activity at saturating substrate concentrations; K_{app}, the apparent dissociation constant of the enzyme–substrate complex (for practical purposes, the substrate concentration at which enzyme activity is half-maximal); and n_{Hill} (Hill coefficient), an index of cooperativity that can be used as a reflection of the number of substrate binding sites. A Hill coefficient between 1.0 and 2.0 is evidence of the existence of at least two substrate binding sites per enzyme molecule; a number between 2.0 and 3.0 is evidence of the existence of at least three sites, and so on. The concentration range over which enzyme activity is a function of substrate concentration can be predicted from the K_{app}. The Hill coefficient is an index of the steepness of the activity vs. substrate concentration curve and hence the sensitivity of enzyme activity to changes in substrate concentration within that range. Specific values for the parameters mentioned above depend upon the conditions under which enzyme activity is assayed.

The two substrates of the Ca^{2+}-transporting ATPase are Ca^{2+} and ATP. With regard to Ca^{2+}, K_{app}s in nonhuman preparations measured under optimal (not necessarily physiological) conditions range from 0.3 to 4.8 μM, with n_{Hill}s ≤ 2.0 (20–22). More recently, Ca^{2+} uptake has been assayed in cardiac sarcoplasmic reticulum isolated from human left ventricular myocardial tissue under conditions designed to approximate the intracellular ionic environment (23). The K_{app} for Ca^{2+} in these preparations was 0.63–0.68 μM, a value that falls within the range of free Ca^{2+} concentrations seen in intact cultured cardiac myocytes during contraction (0.9 μM) and relaxation (0.3 μM) (24). The Hill coefficient in human preparations was 1.6–1.7, implying the existence of at least two cooperatively interacting Ca^{2+} binding sites per ATPase molecule. These data indicate that Ca^{2+} uptake activity is sensitive to small changes in cytosolic Ca^{2+} concentrations within the physiological range. This sensitivity provides an intrinsic mechanism for the regulation of cytosolic Ca^{2+} concentrations during contraction and relaxation. The increase in cytosolic Ca^{2+} concentration following Ca^{2+} release causes an increase in the Ca^{2+} uptake rate of sarcoplasmic reticulum. The resulting reduction in the cytosolic Ca^{2+} concentration leads to relaxation. The reduced cytosolic Ca^{2+} concentration in turn lowers the Ca^{2+} uptake rate to baseline levels, permitting a rapid increase in the cytosolic Ca^{2+} concentration on subsequent release.

With regard to ATP, values for K_{app} ranging from 1.1 μM to 0.18 mM (depending upon assay conditions) have been determined, and no co-operativity has been observed (25–27). These values are very much lower than presently accepted estimates of cytosolic ATP concentrations, which are in the millimolar range even during ischemia (28). It can be concluded that Ca^{2+} uptake rates should not be affected by physiological or pathologic changes in ATP concentrations in intact cells (but see below).

B. Regulation

Ca^{2+} uptake may be regulated through phosphorylation of phospholamban, a 27,000 M_r pentamer that colocalizes with the Ca^{2+} transporting ATPase (8). In vitro, phospholamban can be phosphorylated at separate sites by cAMP-dependent protein kinase, a sarcoplasmic reticulum-associated calmodulin-dependent protein kinase, and protein kinase C. In each case, phosphorylation is accompanied by stimulation of Ca^{2+} uptake rates (29–43). This stimulation results for the most part from an increased affinity for Ca^{2+} (decreased K_{app}) (29,30,35,42,43). Similar stimulation of Ca^{2+} uptake rates can be achieved by selective removal of phospholamban with detergents, proteolysis of its cytoplasmic amino acid side chains with trypsin, or neutralization of the positive charges on these side chains (44–46). It was concluded that the interaction between the positively charged side chains of phospholamban and the Ca^{2+}-transporting ATPase inhibits Ca^{2+} uptake, and that phosphorylation relieves this inhibition by reducing the charge on these side chains. The mechanism has been more recently clarified by experiments demonstrating that cross-linking of the hydrophilic side chain of phospholamban and the Ca^{2+}-transporting ATPase is prevented by phosphorylation of the former (47). In addition, cross-linking is completely inhibited by the presence of 100 μM Ca^{2+}. These observations indicate that the hydrophilic side chains of phospholamban, when unphosphorylated, bind to the Ca^{2+}-transporting ATPase and stabilize it in its Ca^{2+}-free conformation. The lowering of the enzyme's K_{app} for Ca^{2+} can be explained on this basis. There is also evidence that phospholamban can function as a Ca^{2+} channel (48), but the importance of this in the regulation of Ca^{2+} uptake has not been demonstrated. A sarcoplasmic reticulum-associated phosphatase that dephosphorylates the sites phosphorylated by cAMP-dependent and calmodulin-dependent protein kinases has been partially characterized (49, 50).

The effects of hormones on intracellular Ca^{2+} concentrations in cardiac myocytes may occur via phospholamban phosphorylation. Studies with beta-adrenergic agonists provide the strongest evidence for this. Phospholamban is phosphorylated following exposure of isolated rat heart cells to isoproterenol, and is dephosphorylated upon subsequent exposure to propranolol (51). Also, exposure of guinea pig and rabbit heart preparations to isoproterenol in situ is accompanied by phosphorylation of phospholamban and stimulation of Ca^{2+} uptake and ATPase activities in sarcoplasmic reticulum vesicles isolated subsequently (52–54). Finally, muscarinic agonists and adenosine analogs, which oppose the inotropic and chronotropic effects of beta-adrenergic agonists, inhibit beta-adrenergic stimulation of phospholamban phosphorylation (55–57). Calmodulin-dependent phosphorylation might be expected to augment the sensitivity of Ca^{2+} uptake to increases in the cytosolic Ca^{2+} concentrations. Calmodulin-dependent phosphorylation has not been seen in human preparations, however, calling into question the clinical relevance of this hypothesis (58). Protein kinase C, which is activated at cytosolic Ca^{2+} concentrations in the physiological range by diacylglycerol second messengers, is probably responsible for many of the intracellular effects of alpha-adrenergic, muscarinic, and histaminergic agents in diverse cell types (59–61), but whether it phosphorylates phospholamban in cardiac myoctyes in vivo is unclear (41,62,63). It seems unlikely that protein kinase C-catalyzed phosphorylation of sarcoplasmic reticulum proteins would result from phosphatidylinositol hydrolysis occurring within the plasma membrane, since diacylglycerols are not water soluble and should not diffuse through the cytosol to the sarcoplasmic reticulum. It is possible, however, that protein kinase C is activated by phospholipids, and diacylglycerols directly within the sarcoplasmic reticulum membrane.

Ca^{2+} uptake may be regulated via the 53,000 Da glycoprotein present in longitudinal sarcoplasmic reticulum (64). The evidence for this is sparse, however, and the function of this glycoprotein must at present be regarded as unknown. Cytoplasmic factors may also be involved in the regulation of Ca^{2+} uptake. A soluble protein inhibitor of sarcoplasmic reticulum Ca^{2+} uptake was found to be present in ammonium sulfate fractions of cardiac and slow skeletal muscle cytoplasm (65). Subsequent studies identified fractions enriched in actin as having inhibitory activity (66). This inhibition could be antagonized by muscle albumin (67). The potential importance of this form of regulation has not been determined.

C. Pathophysiology

Relaxation has been shown to be abnormal in congestive cardiomyopathy in humans, and the rate of decline of the intracellular Ca^{2+} concentration during diastole is diminished in muscle from failing heart (68,69). These abnormalities might be associated with alterations of Ca^{2+} uptake by sarcoplasmic reticulum and its regulation. In animal models of cardiac hypertrophy and failure, Ca^{2+} uptake rates and capacities of cardiac sarcoplasmic reticulum vesicles are generally diminished, although in milder stages Ca^{2+} uptake rates and capacities are sometimes increased (70–82). Most of these models are simulations of hypertrophic cardiomyopathy, but one study (82) involved a genetically linked dilated cardiomyopathy. In pressure load hypertrophy, steady-state levels of Ca^{2+} ATPase and phospholamban mRNAs are reduced (83,84). A problem in interpreting all these observations is that the extent to which sarcoplasmic reticulum dysfunction is the cause rather than result of the pathologic process is unclear. In animal models of cardiomyopathy associated with doxorubicin toxicity, however, there is in vitro evidence that altered Ca^{2+} uptake by sarcoplasmic reticulum may be pathogenic (85). Stimulation of oxygen free radical formation appears to be involved (86).

Direct evidence for impaired sarcoplasmic reticulum function in human cardiomyopathies has emerged from studies involving tissue homogenates prepared from biopsy specimens of failing and transplanted human hearts, in which decreased Ca^{2+} uptake has been reported (87,88). Whether this impairment reflected with a decrease in Ca^{2+} uptake intrinsic to the sarcoplasmic reticulum was unclear. A comparison of Ca^{2+}-transporting ATPase mRNA levels in myocardium from normal and failing human hearts showed a decrease in the latter relative to the former (89). In contrast, when sarcoplasmic reticulum was isolated from the left ventricular myocardium of normal and failing human hearts (from patients with idiopathic dilated cardiomyopathy), no differences were discovered between the two groups with respect to the V_{max}, K_{app}, or n_{Hill} of unstimulated Ca^{2+} uptake (23). Moreover, the effects of phospholamban phosphorylation on Ca^{2+} uptake in isolated human cardiac sarcoplasmic reticulum were similar to those observed in animal models, and these effects were found to be identical in preparations from normal and failing hearts (90). Yields of sarcoplasmic reticulum from normal and failing human left ventricular myocardium in these studies were comparable. These observations indicate that the decreased Ca^{2+} uptake observed in tissue homogenates does not result from alterations in Ca^{2+} uptake intrinsic to the sarcoplasmic reticulum. Changes involving the intracellular regulation of Ca^{2+} uptake may nevertheless be involved. Decreased Ca^{2+} uptake might reflect the decreased beta-adrenergic receptor density and responsiveness characteristic of heart failure in humans (91), resulting hypothetically in decreased stimulation via cAMP-dependent phosphorylation of phospholamban. It may also reflect the involvement of some of the cytoplasmic factors mentioned earlier (65–67).

Relaxation is abnormal in ischemic myocardium, and impaired Ca^{2+} uptake by sarcoplasmic reticulum may be contributory. Ca^{2+} uptake and ATPase activities are decreased in sarcoplasmic reticulum isolated from ischemic myocardium, suggesting that intrinsic alterations of sarcoplasmic reticulum functions are occurring (92, 93). Other effects may be related to alterations in the cytosolic environment during ischemia. One such effect may involve changes in cytosolic adenine nucleotide concentrations. As noted earlier, Ca^{2+} uptake rates should not be affected significantly by the fall in cytosolic ATP concentrations seen during ischemia. In vivo, however, decreases in cytosolic ATP concentrations result from ATP hydrolysis, and must therefore be accompanied by corresponding increases in cytosolic ADP concentrations. ADP *does* inhibit Ca^{2+}- and Mg^{2+}-dependent ATPase activity at concentrations that would be expected to occur during ischemia (20,28), and this inhibition could explain the abnormal relaxation seen in ischemic hearts.

Impaired Ca^{2+} uptake may also reflect the decrease in cytosolic pH seen during ischemia. As pH falls, so does the apparent affinity of the transport ATPase for Ca^{2+}, suggesting that H^+ and Ca^{2+} compete for the active site of the enzyme (94). Other reports document more complex pH effects, however. The pH optimum for Ca^{2+}- and Mg^{2+}-dependent ATPase activity in isolated sarcoplasmic reticulum is 7.4–8.1, while the pH optimum for Ca^{2+} uptake is 6.6–6.8 (26,31–33). Intracellular acidosis might therefore increase the rate of Ca^{2+} uptake and the number of Ca^{2+} molecules transported per ATP molecule hydrolyzed, an adaptation whose usefulness during energy deprivation is obvious. In contrast, reductions in pH led to reductions in Ca^{2+} uptake and release in mechanically permeablized myofibrils (95). The reason for the differences between in vitro and in situ results is not obvious. Oxygen free radicals, which accumulate in ischemic tissues, may also be pathogenic. Oxygen free radicals decrease Ca^{2+} uptake rates in isolated sarcoplasmic reticulum by increasing the permeability of the vesicles without affecting ATPase activity (96). These effects are Ca^{2+}-calmodulin dependent (97), but the mechanism is unknown.

Finally, changes in Ca^{2+} uptake by sarcoplasmic reticulum may explain some of the abnormalities of cardiac function seen in thyroid disease. Ca^{2+} uptake rates and Ca^{2+} ATPase activity are increased in cardiac sarcoplasmic reticulum isolated from hyperthryoid animals and decreased in cardiac sarcoplasmic reticulum isolated from hypothyroid animals (98–101). These alterations correlate well with changes in cardiac relaxation rates (101). It is interesting that while increases in basal Ca^{2+} uptake were observed in hyperthyroidism, cAMP-dependent stimulation of uptake was found to be diminished (102). Subsequently, hyperthyroidism was shown to increase the level of the Ca^{2+} ATPase and to decrease the level of phospholamban in cardiac sarcoplasmic reticulum (103), and parallel changes were observed in steady-state mRNA levels for the two proteins (84,104). This decrease in the ratio of phospholamban to Ca^{2+} ATPase would explain both the increase in basal Ca^{2+} uptake (relief of inhibition, as discussed above) and the decrease in cAMP-dependent stimulation of Ca^{2+} uptake. Increased Ca^{2+} uptake in hyperthyroidism may also be related to decreased levels of long chain acylcarnitines in sarcoplasmic reticulum membranes (105). Very recently, a thyroid hormone binding protein has been identified as a constituent of cardiac sarcoplasmic reticulum (106).

D. Implications for Therapy

Ca^{2+} uptake by sarcoplasmic reticulum may prove important in the future therapy of heart failure. While some drugs affect Ca^{2+} uptake by cardiac sarcoplasmic reticulum in vitro (107), this occurs only at concentrations several orders of magnitude higher than therapeutic, and no drugs currently used to treat heart failure are believed to work via direct actions on sarcoplasmic reticulum. Recently, however, gingerol, a phenol extract of the rhizome of *Zingiber officinale* Roscoe, was shown to stimulate Ca^{2+} ATPase activity specifically in isolated canine cardiac sarcoplasmic reticulum. The EC_{50} for this effect was 3.8 μM, virtually identical to the value of 4 μM reported for its inotropic and chronotropic effects on guinea pig myocardium (108,109). These reports suggest that the inotropic and chronotropic effects of gingerol derive from its actions on Ca^{2+} uptake by cardiac sarcoplasmic reticulum. In canine cardiac sarcoplasmic reticulum, activation of Ca^{2+} ATPase activity by gingerol is competitive with respect to ATP, suggesting that the drug interacts with the ATP binding site of the enzyme. Activation is mixed with respect to Ca^{2+}, with increases in both V_{max} and K_{app} and no effects on n_{Hill}. This suggests that activation results principally from an increase in the rate constant for enzyme–product dissociation, and that interactions between Ca^{2+} binding sites are not affected. Ca^{2+} ATPase activity is stimulated at Ca^{2+} concentrations greater than 0.24 μM, indicating that physiologically relevant effects are stimulatory. Such effects might be predicted to be synergistic with those of other inotropic agents, which work through different subcellular mechanisms. The development of clinically suitable drugs that stimulate Ca^{2+} uptake by cardiac sarcoplasmic reticulum could therefore provide a major advance in the treatment of heart failure.

Beta-adrenergic agonists and phosphodiesterase inhibitors may stimulate Ca^{2+} uptake by sarcoplasmic reticulum by raising intracellular cAMP concentrations, resulting in activation of cAMP-dependent protein kinase and phosphorylation of phospholamban. This would be expected to speed relaxation and lower end-diastolic Ca^{2+} concentrations, and might contribute to the effects of these drugs on relaxation and (indirectly) on contraction. Beta-adrenergic antagonists, acting via the same pathway, would be predicted to raise end-diastolic Ca^{2+} concentrations and prolong relaxation. Phosphorylation by cAMP-dependent protein kinase can also affect Ca^{2+} influx through the sarcolemma (110,111) and Ca^{2+}-troponin-I binding (112), so that the effects of beta-adrenergic agonists and antagonists and phosphodiesterase inhibitors may be explained through multiple mechanisms. The specific phosphodiesterase inhibited by milrinone, enoximone, and amrinone appears to be associated with the sarcoplasmic reticulum, however, making it possible that the inotropic effects of these drugs result from a selective increase in the phosphorylation of phospholamban (113–118).

IV. Ca^{2+} STORAGE

As noted, Ca^{2+} transport occurs principally in the longitudinal sarcoplasmic reticulum. A 165,000 Da glycoprotein localized to the luminal surface of this region has a high content of acidic amino acid side chains that could allow for Ca^{2+}-binding (10,16). The Ca^{2+} concentration within the longitudinal sarcoplasmic reticulum is several times lower than that of the corbular and junctional sarcoplasmic reticulum, however, suggesting that the latter regions are the principal sites of Ca^{2+} storage (119).

Ca^{2+} is bound within the corbular and junctional sarcoplasmic reticulum by calsequestrin, a highly acidic protein whose apparent molecular weight in humans is 52,000 Da (16). Calsequestrin is also present in the sarcoplasmic reticulum of skeletal muscle, but the cardiac and skeletal forms are products of separate genes and their sequence homology is only 65% (120,121). They differ further in that the cardiac form has an attached high-mannose side chain apparently absent from the skeletal muscle protein. Half-maximal binding occurs at 500 μM Ca^{2+} at high KCl concentrations and at 100 μM Ca^{2+} at low KCl concentrations (122). The binding affinity of calsequestrin for Ca^{2+} is thus quite low, but the binding capacity in these preparations (35 moles of Ca^{2+} per mole calsequestrin) is high, consistent with the notion that calsequestrin serves as an intraluminal Ca^{2+} sponge. There is evidence, however, that calsequestrin's function is more complex: Ca^{2+} binding causes changes in the conformation of calsequestrin that affect its interaction with other proteins located in the junctional sarcoplasmic reticulum (including the ryanodine-sensitive Ca^{2+} channel and an unnamed 26,000–32,000 Da protein), and these effects correlate with changes in the rate of Ca^{2+} release (123). The binding of Ca^{2+} to calsequestrin may therefore be involved in the regulation of the Ca^{2+} release mechanism.

No specific pathologic change associated with calsequestrin has yet been identified. Abnormalities of calsequestrin structure might be expected to affect Ca^{2+} release through the mechanism referred to above. A decrease in the amount of calsequestrin might also be expected to reduce the Ca^{2+} storage capacity of the sarcoplasmic reticulum, and this could result in diminished Ca^{2+} uptake as discussed earlier.

V. Ca^{2+} RELEASE

A. Mechanisms

Ca^{2+} uptake is the result of active transport, through which Ca^{2+} is sequestered against its concentration gradient into a relatively impermeable membrane system. Ca^{2+} release occurs when channels in this membrane system are transiently opened, allowing a passive (thermodynamically favorable) flux of Ca^{2+} from the lumen of the sarcoplasmic reticulum to the cytoplasm.

Most of the initial progress in studying Ca^{2+} release from sarcoplasmic reticulum resulted from experiments involving muscle fibers from which plasma membranes had been removed (124–126). These experiments demonstrated that Ca^{2+} release from sarcoplasmic reticulum could be triggered by rapid increases of the cytosolic Ca^{2+} concentration. Ca^{2+} release was dependent not simply upon the cytosolic Ca^{2+} concentration but also upon the rate of its increase. This Ca^{2+}-induced Ca^{2+} release has been proposed as a mechanism through which excitation and contraction are coupled. According to this hypothesis, depolarization of the plasma membrane results in the opening of dihydropyridine-sensitive Ca^{2+} channels. The resulting influx of Ca^{2+} across the plasma membrane is of a magnitude insufficient to activate the contractile proteins directly, but it brings about a rapid increase in the Ca^{2+} concentration adjacent to the junctional sarcoplasmic reticulum that opens the Ca^{2+} channels of the sarcoplasmic reticulum and releases Ca^{2+} stored within. It is possible that the dihydropyridine-sensitive Ca^{2+} channels of the sarcolemma and transverse tubules also interact directly with the adjacent Ca^{2+} channels of the junctional sarcoplasmic reticulum (127), and sarcolemmal depolarization may open sarcoplasmic reticulum Ca^{2+} channels through such interactions.

Initial attempts to study the mechanism of Ca^{2+}-induced Ca^{2+} release in isolated sarcoplasmic reticulum were frustrated by the fact that release rates measured in vesicle preparations were several orders of magnitude lower than those observed in skinned fibers (128,129). An isolated sarcoplasmic reticulum preparation in which the magnitude of Ca^{2+} release is sufficient to contribute to excitation–contraction coupling has subsequently been described (130). Ca^{2+} release in this preparation is activated by Ca^{2+}, adenine nucleotides, and caffeine and inhibited by Mg^{2+}, H^+, and calmodulin (there is no evidence for involvement of a calmodulin-dependent protein kinase). Ca^{2+}, Mg^{2+}, and adenine nucleotides appear to bind to the Ca^{2+} channel at noninteracting sites. The observation that optimal activation of Ca^{2+} release in the presence of Mg^{2+} and ATP requires Ca^{2+} concentrations several orders of magnitude greater than those seen in intact muscle calls into question the physiological relevance of this mechanism, but it is possible that such Ca^{2+} concentrations exist during contraction in the cytosol immediately adjacent to the junctional sarcoplasmic reticulum. In contrast to results in skinned fibers, Ca^{2+} release in sarcoplasmic reticulum vesicles appears to be sensitive to the extravesicular Ca^{2+} concentration itself rather than to the rate of its increase.

Ca^{2+} release from isolated sarcoplasmic reticulum vesicles can be modulated by the plant alkaloid ryanodine (131–134). The effects are biphasic: Ca^{2+} release is increased when ryanodine is present in the nanomolar range, but is decreased when ryanodine is present at greater than micromolar concentrations. These effects correlate with binding of ryanodine to high- and low-affinity sites in junctional sarcoplasmic reticulum (133–135). Efforts directed at identification of the ryanodine receptor resulted in the purification of a 340,000–450,000 Da protein (14,136,137). When examined under electron microscopy, the purified ryanodine receptor was seen to form complexes having the ultrastructural appearance of the feet structures bridging the junctional sarcoplasmic reticulum and transverse tubules (14, 137). Furthermore, when incorporated into planar bilayers, the ryanodine receptor has Ca^{2+} conductance properties similar to those observed in sarcoplasmic reticulum vesicles (137,138). The most recent studies indicate that the feet structures are oligomers containing four 340,000–450,000 Da polypeptides arranged around a central core (139). This central core may be the actual Ca^{2+} channel.

While the properties of the cardiac and skeletal muscle ryanodine-sensitive Ca^{2+} channels are similar, the two forms differ slightly in their molecular weights and ryanodine-binding properties, and Ca^{2+} release mechanisms in the cardiac and skeletal muscle sarcoplasmic reticulum have different sensitivities to ryanodine and ruthenium red (14,140,141). The cDNA clones of the ryanodine-sensitive Ca^{2+} channels of cardiac and skeletal muscle have been isolated, and it is clear that the cardiac and skeletal muscle proteins are the products of separate genes (142–144). The amino acid sequences of the skeletal and cardiac muscle proteins are only 66% homologous, but the predicted secondary structures are indistinguishable. The C-terminal region of the protein appears to contain the Ca^{2+} channel and modulator-binding moieties localized to the sarcoplasmic reticulum membrane, while the N-terminal region contains the hydrophilic moieties that form the foot structures in the adjacent cytoplasm.

B. Regulation

Ca^{2+} release may be subject to regulation by intracellular messengers. Inositol triphosphate, a product of phosphatidylinositol hydrolysis, has been shown to release Ca^{2+} from the endoplasmic reticulum of a variety of cell types in response to such extracellular agents as alpha-adrenergic agonists, histamine, and muscarinic cholinergic agonists. It has been proposed that this mechanism, through which Ca^{2+}-mediated Ca^{2+} release would be potentiated, operates in cardiac sarcoplasmic reticulum. So far, however, this has been demonstrated only under nonphysiological conditions, and its significance in vivo is controversial (145–156). Guanosine triphosphate has been shown to release Ca^{2+} from the endoplasmic reticulum of neuroblastoma cells, pancreatic islet cells, and macrophages through a mechanism that appears to be separate from that of inositol trisphosphate-induced release (157–160). Whether G proteins similar to those that regulate beta-adrenergic events at the plasma membrane are involved is unknown. If operative in cardiac sarcoplasmic reticulum, guanosine triphosphate-induced release would provide an alternative second messenger system by which agents that increase intracellular guanosine triphosphate concentrations could increase myocardial contractility. To date, however, studies in cardiac sarcoplasmic reticulum have not been reported, and release Ca^{2+} from skeletal muscle sarcoplasmic reticulum by guanosine triphosphate could not be demonstrated (159).

C. Pathophysiology

Presently very little information on the possible involvement of abnormalities of Ca^{2+} release in human pathologic states is available. Decreasing pH has an inhibitory effect on Ca^{2+} release, increasing the optimal free $[Ca^{2+}]$ for triggering release, and this might be important during myocardial ischemia (125,161). Accumulated spontaneous Ca^{2+} release from sarcoplasmic reticulum is capable under some conditions of generating action potentials in rat cardiac myocytes, raising the possibility that this is a potential cause of abnormal automaticity (162). Recent studies of sarcoplasmic reticulum prepared from ischemic canine hearts showed that the decrease in Ca^{2+} uptake rates observed during ischemia was abolished by the addition of ryanodine to the reaction mixtures (163). This suggests that ryanodine-sensitive Ca^{2+} release channels are damaged during ischemia, causing an obligatory leakage of Ca^{2+}. This leakage could lower the Ca^{2+} capacity of the sarcoplasmic reticulum, resulting in higher free cytoplasmic Ca^{2+} concentrations during relaxation and diminished release during activation. Both contraction and relaxation might thereby be impaired.

REFERENCES

1. Forbes MS, Sperelakis N. The membrane systems and cytoskeletal elements of mammalian myocardial cells. In: Dowben RM, Shay JW, eds. Cell and muscle motility, volume 3. New York: Plenum, 1983.
2. Sommer JR, Jennings RB. Ultrastructure of cardiac muscle. In: Fozzard HA, Haber E, Jennings RB, Katz AM, Morgan HE, eds. The heart and cardiovascular system, Volume 1. New York: Raven Press, 1986.
3. Segretain D, Rambourg A, Clermont Y. Three dimensional arrangement of mito-

chondria and endoplasmic reticulum in the heart muscle fiber of the rat. Anat Rec 1981; 200:139–51.
4. Yoshikane H, Niehi T, Moriyama K. Three-dimensional observation of intracellular membranous structure in dog heart muscle cells by scanning electron microscopy. J Submicrosc Cytol 1986; 18:629–36.
5. Somlyo AV. Bridging structures spanning the junctional gap at the triad of skeletal muscle. J Cell Biol 1979; 80:743–50.
6. Franzini-Armstrong C. Structure of sarcoplasmic reticulum. Fed Proc 1980; 39:2403–9.
7. Jorgensen AO, Shen AC-Y, Daly P, MacLennan DH. Localization of Ca^{2+} + Mg^{2+}-ATPase of the sarcoplasmic reticulum in adult rat papillary muscle. J Cell Biol 1982; 93:883–92.
8. Jorgensen AO, Jones LR. Immunoelectron microscopical localization of phospholamban in adult canine ventricular muscle. J Cell Biol 1987; 104:1343–52.
9. Michalak M, Campbell KP, MacLennan DH. Localization of the high affinity calcium binding protein and an intrinsic glycoprotein in sarcoplasmic reticulum membranes. J Biol Chem 1980; 255:1317–26.
10. Leberer E, Charuk JHM, Green NM, MacLennan DH. Molecular cloning and expression of cDNA encoding a lumenal calcium binding glycoprotein from sarcoplasmic reticulum. Proc Natl Acad Sci 1989; 86:6047–51.
11. Jorgensen AO, Campbell KP. Evidence for the presence of calsequestrin in two structurally different regions of myocardial sarcoplasmic reticulum. J Cell Biol 1984; 98:1597–602.
12. Jorgensen AO, Shen AC-Y, Campbell KP. Ultrastructural localization of calsequestrin in adult rat atrial and ventricular muscle cells. J Cell Biol 1985; 101:257–68.
13. Jorgensen AO, McGuffee LJ. Immunoelectron microscopic localization of sarcoplasmic reticulum proteins in cryofixed, freeze-dried, and low temperature-embedded tissue. J Histochem Cytochem 1987; 35:723–32.
14. Inui M, Saito A, Fleischer S. Isolation of the ryanodine receptor from cardiac sarcoplasmic reticulum and identity with the feet structures. J Cell Biol 1987; 262: 15637–42.
15. Brandl CJ, deLeon S, Martin DR, MacLennan DH. Adult forms of the Ca^{2+} ATPase of sarcoplasmic reticulum. J Cell Biol 1987; 262:3768–74.
16. Movsesian MA, Leveille C, Krall J, Colyer J, Wang JH, Campbell KP. Identification and characterization of proteins in human cardiac sarcoplasmic reticulum. J Mol Cell Cardiol 1990; 22:1477–85.
17. Chu A, Bick RJ, Tate CA, Van Winkle WB, Entman ML. Anion effects on in vitro sarcoplasmic reticulum function. J Biol Chem 1983; 258(17):10543–50.
18. Chu A, Tate CA, Bick RJ, Van Winkle WB, Entman ML. Anion effects on in vitro sarcoplasmic reticulum function. J Biol Chem 1983; 258(3):1656–64.
19. Feher JJ, Stephens MJ, Alderson BH, Poland JL. Contribution of the ryanodine-sensitive fraction to capabilities of cardiac SR. J Mol Cell Cardiol 1988; 20:1107–18.
20. Suko J, Hasselbach W. Characterization of cardiac sarcoplasmic reticulum ATP-ADP phosphate exchange and phosphorylation of the calcium transport adenosine triphosphatase. Eur J Biochem 1976; 64:123–30.
21. Sumida M, Wang T, Mandel F, Froehlich JP, Schwartz A. Transient kinetics of Ca^{2+} transport of sarcoplasmic reticulum. J Biol Chem 1978; 253(24):8772–7.
22. Davis BA, Schwartz A, Samaha FJ, Kranias EG. Regulation of cardiac sarcoplasmic reticulum calcium transport by calcium-calmodulin-dependent phosphorylation. J Biol Chem 1983; 258:13587–91.
23. Movsesian MA, Bristow MB, Krall J. Calcium uptake by sarcoplasmic reticulum from patients with idiopathic dilated cardiomyopathy. Circ Res 1989; 65:1141–44.

24. Peeters GA, Hlady V, Bridge JHB, Barry WH. Simultaneous measurement of calcium transients and motion in cultured ventricular cells. Am J Physiol 1987; 253:H1400–8.
25. Tada M, Ohmori F, Yamada M, Abe H. Mechanism of the stimulation of Ca^{2+}-dependent ATPase of cardiac sarcoplasmic reticulum by adenosine 3′:5′-monophosphate-dependent protein kinase. J Biol Chem 1979; 254:319–26.
26. Shigekawa M, Finegan JM, Katz AM. Calcium transport ATPase of canine cardiac sarcoplasmic reticulum. J Biol Chem 1976; 251:6894–900.
27. Altschuld RA, Wenger WC, Lamka KG, Kindig OR, Capen CC, Mizuhira V, VanderHeide RS, Brierley GP. Structural and functional properties of adult rat heart myocytes lysed with digitonin. J Biol Chem 1985; 260:14325–34.
28. Allen DG, Orchard CH. Myocardial contractile function during ischemia and hypoxia. 1987; Circ Res 60:153–68.
29. Davis BA, Schwartz A, Samaha FJ, Kranias EG. Regulation of cardiac sarcoplasmic reticulum calcium transport by calcium-calmodulin-dependent phosphorylation. J Biol Chem 1983; 258:13587–91.
30. Tada M, Ohmori F, Yamada M, Abe H. Mechanism of the stimulation of Ca^{2+}-dependent ATPase of cardiac sarcoplasmic reticulum by adenosine 3′:5′-monophosphate-dependent protein kinase. J Biol Chem 1979; 254:319–26.
31. Simmerman HKB, Collins JH, Thiebert JL, Wegener AD, Jones LR. Sequence analysis of phospholamban. J Biol Chem 1986; 261:13333–41.
32. Iwasa T, Inoue M, Fukunaga K, Isobe T, Okuyama T, Miyamoto E. Purification and characterization of a multifunctional calmodulin-dependent protein kinase from canine myocardial cytosol. Arch Biochem Biophys 1986; 248:21–9.
33. Molla A, Demaille JH. Characterization and partial purification of cardiac sarcoplasmic reticulum phospholamban kinase. Biochemistry 1986; 25:3415–24.
34. Le Peuch CJ, Haiech J, Demaille JH. Concerted regulation of cardiac sarcoplasmic reticulum transport by cyclic adenosine monophosphate dependent and calcium-calmodulin-dependent phosphorylations. Biochemistry 1979; 18:5150–57.
35. Lopaschuk G, Richter B, Katz S. Characterization of calmodulin effects on calcium transport in cardiac microsomes enriched in sarcoplasmic reticulum. Biochemistry 1980; 19:5603–7.
36. Kirchberger MA, Antonetz T. Calmodulin-mediated regulation of calcium transport and (Ca^{2+} + Mg^{2+})-activated ATPase activity in isolated cardiac sarcoplasmic reticulum. J Biol Chem 1982; 257:5685–91.
37. Limas CJ. Phosphorylation of cardiac sarcoplasmic reticulum by a calcium-activated, phospholipid-dependent protein kinase. Biochem Biophys Res Commun 1980; 96: 1378–83.
38. Iwasa Y, Hosey MM. Phosphorylation of cardiac sarcolemma proteins by the calcium-activated phospholipid-dependent protein kinase. J Biol Chem 1984; 259:534–40.
39. Movsesian MA, Nishikawa M, Adelstein RS. Phosphorylation of phospholamban by calcium-activated, phospholipid-dependent protein kinase. J Biol Chem 1984; 259: 8029–32.
40. Imagawa T, Watanabe T, Nakamura T. Subunit structure and multiple phosphorylation sites of phospholamban. J Biochem 1986; 99:41–53.
41. Wegener AD, Simmerman HKB, Liepnieks J, Jones LR. Proteolytic cleavage of phospholamban purified from canine cardiac sarcoplasmic reticulum vesicles. J Biol Chem 1986; 261:5154–9.
42. Tada M, Inui M, Yamada M, Kadoma M, Kuzuya T, Abe H, Kakiuchi S. Effects of phospholamban phosphorylation catalyzed by adenosine 3′:5′-monophosphate-and calmodulin-dependent protein kinases on calcium transport ATPase of cardiac sarcoplasmic reticulum. J Mol Cell Cardiol 1983; 15:335–46.
43. Plank B, Pifl C, Hellmann G, Wyskovsky W, Hoffmann R, Suko J. Correlation be-

tween calmodulin-dependent increase in the rate of calcium transport and calmodulin-dependent phosphorylation of cardiac sarcoplasmic reticulum. Eur J Biochem 1983; 136:215–21.
44. Inui M, Chamberlain BK, Saito A, Fleischer S. The nature of the modulation of Ca^{2+} transport as studied by reconstitution of cardiac sarcoplasmic reticulum. J Biol Chem 1986; 261:1794–1800.
45. Kirchberger MA, Borchman D, Kasinathan C. Proteolytic activation of the canine sarcoplasmic reticulum calcium pump. Biochemistry 1986; 25:5484–92.
46. Xu ZC, Kirchberger MA. Modulation by polyelectrolytes of canine cardiac microsomal calcium uptake and the possible relationship to phospholamban. J Biol Chem 1989; 264:16644–51.
47. James P, Inui M, Tada M, Chiesi M, Carafoli E. Nature and site of phospholamban regulation of the Ca^{2+} pump of the sarcoplasmic reticulum. Nature 1989; 342:90–2.
48. Kovacs RJ, Nelson MT, Simmerman HKB, Jones LR. Phospholamban forms Ca^{2+}-selective channels in lipid bilayers. J Biol Chem 1988; 263:18364–8.
49. Kranias EG. Regulation of calcium transport by protein phosphatase activity associated with cardiac sarcoplasmic reticulum. J Biol Chem 1985; 260:11006–10.
50. Kranias EG, DiSalvo J. A phospholamban protein phosphatase activity associated with cardiac sarcoplasmic reticulum. J Biol Chem 1986; 261:10029–32.
51. Blackshear PJ, Nemenoff RA, Bonventre JV, Cheung JY, Avruch J. Hormonal regulation of protein phosphorylation in isolated rat heart cells. Am J Physiol 1984; 246:C439–49.
52. Kranias EG, Solaro RJ. Phosphorylation of troponin I and phospholamban during catecholamine stimulation of rabbit heart. Nature 1982; 298:182–4.
53. Kranias EG, Garvey JL, Srivastava RD, Solaro RJ. Phosphorylation and functional modifications of sarcoplasmic reticulum and myofibrils in isolated rabbit hearts stimulated with isoprenaline. Biochem J 1985; 226:113–21.
54. Lindemann JP, Jones LR, Hathaway DR, Henry BG, Watanabe AM. Beta-adrenergic stimulation of phospholamban phosphorylation and Ca^{2+}-ATPase activity in guinea pig ventricles. J Biol Chem 1983; 258:464–71.
55. Iwasa Y, Hosey MM. Cholinergic antagonism of beta-adrenergic stimulation of cardiac membrane protein phosphorylation in situ. J Biol Chem 1983; 258:4571–5.
56. Hosey MM, McMahon KK, Green RD. Inhibitory adenosine receptors in the heart: characterization by ligand binding studies and effects on beta-adrenergic receptor stimulated adenylate cyclase and membrane protein phosphorylation. J Mol Cell Cardiol 1984; 16:931–42.
57. Lindemann JP, Watanabe AM. Muscarinic cholinergic inhibition of beta-adrenergic stimulation of phospholamban phosphorylation and Ca^{2+} transport in guinea pig ventricles. J Biol Chem 1985; 260:13122–9.
58. Will H, Kuttner I, Kemsies C, Vetter R, Schubert E. Comparative analysis of phospholamban phosphorylation in crude membranes of vertebrate hearts. Experientia 1985; 41:1052–4.
59. Berridge MJ. Inositol trisphosphate and diacylglycerol as second messengers. Biochem J 1984; 220:345–60.
60. Nishizuka Y. Phospholipid degradation and signal translation for protein phosphorylation. Trends Biochem Sci 1983; 8:13–6.
61. Michell B. Hormone action at membranes. Trends Biochem Sci 1984; 9:3–4.
62. Presti CF, Scott BY, Jones LR. Identification of an endogenous protein kinase C activity and its intrinsic 15-kilodalton substrate in purified canine cardiac sarcolemmal vesicles. J Biol Chem 1985; 260:13879–89.
63. Yuan S, Sen AK. Characterization of the membrane-bound protein kinase C and its substrate proteins in canine cardiac sarcolemma. Biochim Biophys Acta 1986; 886:152–61.

64. Leonards KS, Kutchai H. Coupling of Ca^{2+} transport to ATP hydrolysis by the Ca^{2+}-ATPase of sarcoplasmic reticulum: potential role of the 53-kilodalton glycoprotein. Biochemistry 1985; 24:4876–84.
65. Narayanan N, Newland M, Neudorf D. Inhibition of sarcoplasmic reticulum Ca^{2+} pump by cytosolic protein(s) endogenous to heart and slow skeletal muscle but not fast skeletal muscle. Biochim Biophys Acta 1983; 735:53–66.
66. Chiesi M, Schwaller R. Characterization of heart cytosolic proteins capable of modulating calcium uptake by the sarcoplasmic reticulum. 2. Identification of actin isoforms with inhibitory activity. Eur J Biochem 1987; 162:371–7.
67. Chiesi M, Guerini D. Characterization of heart cytosolic proteins capable of modulating calcium uptake by the sarcoplasmic reticulum. 1. Isolation of a protein with protective activity and its identification as muscle albumin. Eur J Biochem 1987; 162:365–70.
68. Gwathmey JK, Copelas L, MacKinnon R, Schoen FJ, Feldman MD, Grossman W, Morgan JP. Abnormal intracellular calcium handling in myocardium from patients with end-stage heart failure. Circ Res 1987; 61:70–6.
69. Grossman W, McLaurin LP, Rolett EL. Alterations in left ventricular relaxation and diastolic compliance in congestive cardiomyopathy. Cardiovasc Res 1979; 13:514–22.
70. Sordahl LA, McCollum WB, Wood WG, Schwartz A. Mitochondria and sarcoplasmic reticulum function in cardiac hypertrophy and failure. J Physiol 1973; 224:497–502.
71. Ito Y, Suko J, Chidsey CA. Intracellular calcium and myocardial contractility. V. Calcium uptake of sarcoplasmic reticulum fractions in hypertrophied and failing rabbit hearts. J Mol Cell Cardiol 1974; 6:237–47.
72. Lamers JMJ, Stinis JT. Defective calcium pump in the sarcoplasmic reticulum of the hypertrophied rabbit heart. Life Sci 1979; 24:2313–20.
73. Dhalla NJ, Das P, Sharma GP. Subcellular basis of cardiac contractile failure. J Mol Cell Cardiol 1978; 10:363–85.
74. Staley NA, Noren GR, Einzig S. Early alterations in the function of sarcoplasmic reticulum in a naturally occurring model of congestive cardiomyopathy. Cardiovasc Res 1981; 15:276–81.
75. Limas CJ, Spier SS, Kahlon J. Enhanced calcium transport by sarcoplasmic reticulum in mild cardiac hypertrophy. J Mol Cell Cardiol 1980; 12:1103–16.
76. Staley NA, Noren GR, Einzig S, Rublein TG. Effect of early propranolol treatment in an animal model of congestive cardiomyopathy: I. Mortality and Ca^{2+} transport in sarcoplasmic reticulum. Cardiovasc Res 1984; 18:371–6.
77. Dhalla NS, Alto LE, Heyliger CE, Pierce GN, Panagia V, Singal PK. Sarcoplasmic reticular Ca^{2+}-pump adaptation in cardiac hypertrophy due to pressure overload in pigs. Eur Heart J 1984; 5(supplement F):323–8.
78. Malhotra A, Penpargkul S, Schaible T, Scheuer J. Contractile proteins and sarcoplasmic reticulum function in physiologic cardiac hypertrophy. Am J Physiol 1981; 241:H263–7.
79. Fizel A, Turcani M, Fizeliova A, Maasova D, Simko F. Calcium transport by intracellular membrane structures in the myocardium of hypertrophied and failing hearts. Cor Vasa 1986; 28:373–83.
80. Tomlinson CW, Lee SL, Dhalla NS. Abnormalities in heart membranes and myofibrils during bacterial infective cardiomyopathy in the rabbit. Circ Res 1976; 39:82–92.
81. Tahiliani AG, McNeill JH. Diabetes-induced abnormalities in the myocardium. Life Sci 1986; 38:959–74.
82. Whitmer JT, Kuman P, Solaro RJ. Calcium transport properties of cardiac sarcoplasmic reticulum from cardiomyopathic Syrian hamsters (BIO 53.58 and 14.6): evidence for a quantitative defect in dilated myopathic hearts not evident in hypertrophic hearts. Circ Res 1988; 62:81–5.
83. Komuro I, Kurabayashi M, Shibazaki Y, Takaku F, Yazaki Y. Molecular cloning and

characterization of a Ca^{2+} + Mg^{2+}-dependent adenoxine triphosphatase from rat cardiac sarcoplasmic reticulum. J Clin Invest 1989; 83:1102–8.
84. Nayler WG, Merrillees NCR, Chipperfield D, Kurtz JB. Influence of hyperthyroidism on the uptake and binding of calcium by cardiac microsomal fractions and on mitochondrial structure. Cardiovasc Res 1971; 5:469–82.
85. Boucek Jr RJ, Olson RD, Brenner DE, Ogunbunmi EM, Inui M, Fleischer S. The major metabolite of doxorubicin is a potent inhibitor of membrane-associated ion pumps. J Biol Chem 1987; 262:15851–6.
86. Harris RN, Doroshow JH. Effect of doxorubicin enhanced hydrogen peroxide and hydroxyl radical formation on calcium sequestration by cardiac sarcoplasmic reticulum. Biochem Biophys Res Commun 1985; 130:739–45.
87. Limas CJ, Olivari M-T, Goldenberg IF, Levine TB, Benditt DG, Simon A. Calcium uptake by cardiac sarcoplasmic reticulum in human dilated cardiomyopathy. Cardiovasc Res 1987; 21:601–5.
88. Limas CJ, Olivari MT, Benditt DG, Almquist A. Altered calcium uptake by the sarcoplasmic reticulum following cardiac transplantation in humans. Can J Cardiol 1987; 3:215–9.
89. Mercadier JJ, Lompre AM, Duc P, Boheler KR, Fraysse JB, Wisnewsky C, Allen PD, Komajda M, Schwartz K. Altered sarcoplasmic reticulum Ca^{2+}-ATPase gene expression in the human ventricle during end-stage heart failure. J Clin Invest 1990; 85:305–9.
90. Movsesian MA, Colyer J, Wang JH, Krall J. Phospholamban-mediated stimulation of Ca^{2+} uptake in sarcoplasmic reticulum from normal and failing hearts. J Clin Invest 1990; 85:1698–702.
91. Bristow MR, Ginsburg R, Minobe W, Cubicciotti RS, Sageman WS, Lurie K, Billingham ME, Harrison DC, Stinson EB. Decreased catecholamine sensitivity and beta-adrenergic receptor density in failing human hearts. N Engl J Med 1982; 307:205–11.
92. Rapundale ST, Briggs FN, Feher JJ. Effects of ischemia on the isolation and function of canine cardiac sarcoplasmic reticulum. J Mol Cell Cardiol 1986; 18:837–51.
93. Singal PK, Lee SL, Ganguly PK, Panagia V, Dhalla NS. Reversibility of ultrastructural, contractile function and Ca^{2+} transport function changes in guinea pig hearts after global ischemia. Can J Physiol Pharmacol 1986; 64:1368–75.
94. Levitsky DO, Benevolensky DS. Effects of changing Ca^{2+}-to-H^{+} ratio on Ca^{2+} uptake by cardiac sarcoplasmic reticulum. Am J Physiol 1986; 250:H360–5.
95. Fabiato A. Use of aequorin for the appraisal of the hypothesis of the release of calcium from the sarcoplasmic reticulum induced by a change of pH in skinned cardiac cells. Call Calcium 1985; 6:95–108.
96. Okabe E, Odajma C, Taga R, Kukreja RC, Hess ML, Ito H. The effect of oxygen free radicals on calcium permeability and calcium loading at steady state in cardiac sarcoplasmic reticulum. Mol Pharmacol 1988; 34:388–94.
97. Okabe E, Kato Y, Sasaki H, Saito G, Hess ML, Ito H. Calmodulin participation in oxygen radical-induced cardiac sarcoplasmic reticulum calcium uptake reduction. Arch Biochem Biophys 1987; 255:464–8.
98. Suko J. Alterations of Ca^{2+} uptake and Ca^{2+}-activated ATPase of cardiac sarcoplasmic reticulum in hyper- and hypothyroidism. Biochim Biophys Acta 1971; 252:324–7.
99. Nayler WG, Merrillees NCR, Chipperfield D, Kurtz JB. Influence of hyperthyroidism on the uptake and binding of calcium by cardiac microsomal fractions and mitochondrial structure. Cardiovasc Res 1971; 5:469–82.
100. Limas JL. Calcium transport ATPase of cardiac sarcoplasmic reticulum in experimental hyperthyroidism. Am J Physiol 1978; 235(6):H745–51.
101. Rodgers RL, Black S, Katz S, McNeill JH. Thyroidectomy of SHR: effects on ventricular relaxation and on SR calcium uptake activity. Am J Physiol 1986; 250:H861–5.
102. Guarnieri T, Filburn CR, Beard ES, Lakatta EG. Enhanced contractile response and

protein kinase activation to threshold levels of β-adrenergic stimulation of hyperthyroid rat heart. J Clin Invest 1980; 65:861–8.
103. Beekman RE, van Hardeveld C, Simonides WS. On the mechanism of the reduction by thyroid hormone of β-adrenergic relaxation rate stimulation in rat heart. Biochem J 1989; 259:229–36.
104. Rohrer D, Dillmann WH. Thyroid hormone markedly increases the mRNA coding for sarcoplasmic reticulum Ca^{2+}-ATPase in the rat heart. J Biol Chem 1988; 263: 6941–4.
105. Black SC, McNeill JH, Katz S. Sarcoplasmic reticulum Ca^{2+} transport and long chain acylcarnitines in hyperthyroidism. Can J Physiol Pharmacol 1988; 66:159–65.
106. Fliegel L, Burns K, Wlasichuk K, Michalak M. The thyroid hormone receptor of muscle sarcoplasmic reticulum. Biophys J 1989; 55:482a.
107. Movsesian MA, Ambudkar IS, Adelstein RS, Shamoo AE. Stimulation of canine cardiac sarcoplasmic reticulum calcium uptake by dihydropyridine calcium antagonists. Biochem Pharmacol 1985; 34:195–201.
108. Kobayashi M, Shoji N, Ohizumi Y. Gingerol, a novel cardiotonic agent, activates the Ca^{2+}-pumping ATPase in skeletal and cardiac sarcoplasmic reticulum. Biochim Biophys Acta 1987; 903:96–102.
109. Kobayashi M, Ishida Y, Shoji N, Ohizumi Y. Cardiotonic action of [8]-gingerol, an activator of the Ca^{2+}-pumping adenosine triphosphatase of sarcoplasmic reticulum, in guinea pig atrial muscle. J Pharmacol Exp Ther 1988; 246:667–73.
110. Sperelakis N, Schneider JA. A metabolic control mechanism for calcium ion influx that may protect the ventricular myocardial cell. Am J Cardiol 1976; 37:1079–85.
111. Reuter H. Calcium channel modulation by neurotransmitters, enzymes and drugs. Nature 1983; 322:80–3.
112. Buss JE, Stull JT. Calcium binding to cardiac troponin and the effect of cyclic AMP dependent protein kinase. FEBS Lett 1977; 73:101–4.
113. Harrison SA, Reifsnyder DH, Gallis B, Cadd GG, Beavo JA. Isolation and characterization of bovine cardiac muscle cGMP-inhibited phosphodiesterase: a receptor for new cardiotonic drugs. Mol Pharm 1986; 29:506–14.
114. Artman M, Robertson DW, Mahony L, Thompson WJ. Analysis of the binding sites for the cardiotonic phosphodiesterase inhibitor [^{3}H]LY186126 in ventricular myocardium. Mol Pharm 1989; 36:302–11.
115. Kauffman RF, Crowe VG, Utterback BG, Robertson DW. LY195115: A potent, selective inhibitor of cyclic nucleotide phosphodiesterase located in the sarcoplasmic reticulum. Mol Pharm 1986; 30:609–16.
116. Kauffman RF, Utterback BG, Robertson DW. Characterization and pharmacological relevance of high affinity binding sites for [^{3}H]LY186126, a cardiotonic phosphodiesterase inhibitor, in canine cardiac membranes. Circ Res 1989; 65:154–63.
117. Masuoka H, Ito M, Nakano T, Naka M, Tanaka T. Effects of amrinone and enoximone on the subclasses of cyclic AMP phosphodiesterase from human heart and kidney. J Cardiovasc Pharmacol 1990; 15:302–7.
118. Movsesian MA, Smith CJ, Krall J, Bristow MR, Manganiello VC. Sarcoplasmic reticulum-associated cyclic adenosine 5'-monophosphate phosphodiesterase activity in normal and failing human hearts. J Clin Invest 1991; 88:15–19.
119. Jorgensen AO, Broderick R, Somlyo AP, Somlyo AV. Two structurally distinct calcium storage sites in rat cardiac sarcoplasmic reticulum: an electron microprobe analysis study. Circ Res 1988; 63:1060–9.
120. Fliegel L, Ohnishi M, Carpenter MR, Khanna VK, Reithmeier RAF, MacLennan DH. Amino acid sequence of rabbit fast-twitch skeletal muscle calsequestrin deduced from cDNA and peptide sequencing. Proc Natl Acad Sci USA 1987; 84:1167–71.
121. Scott BT, Simmerman HKB, Collins JH, Nadal-Ginard B, Jones LR. Complete amino

acid sequence of canine cardiac calsequestrin deduced by cDNA cloning. J Biol Chem 1988; 263:8958–64.
122. Mitchell RD, Simmerman HKB, Jones LR. Ca^{2+} binding effects on protein conformation and protein interactions of canine cardiac calsequestrin. J Biol Chem 1988; 263:1376–81.
123. Ikemoto N, Ronjat M, Meszaros LG, Koshita M. Postulated role of calsequestrin in the regulation of calcium release from sarcoplasmic reticulum. Biochemistry 1989; 28:6764–71.
124. Fabiato A. Calcium-induced release of calcium from the cardiac sarcoplasmic reticulum. Am J Physiol 1983; 245:C1–C14.
125. Fabiato A. Time and calcium dependence of activation and inactivation of calcium-induced release of calcium from the sarcoplasmic reticulum of a skinned canine cardiac Purkinje cell. J Gen Physiol 1985; 85:247–89.
126. Fabiato A. Simulated calcium current can both cause calcium loading in and trigger calcium release from the sarcoplasmic reticulum of a skinned canine cardiac Purkinje cell. J Gen Physiol 1985; 85:291–320.
127. Block B, Imagawa T, Campbell KP, Franzini-Armstrong. Structural evidence for direct interaction between the molecular components of the traverse tubule/sarcoplasmic reticulum junction in skeletal muscle. J Cell Biol 1988; 107:2587–600.
128. Chamberlain BK, Volpe P, Fleischer S. Calcium-induced calcium release from purified cardiac sarcoplasmic reticulum vesicles. J Biol Chem 1984; 259:7540–6.
129. Chamberlain BK, Volpe P, Fleischer S. Inhibition of calcium-induced calcium release from purified cardiac sarcoplasmic reticulum vesicles. J Biol Chem 1984; 259:7547–53.
130. Meissner G, Henderson JS. Rapid Ca^{2+} release from cardiac sarcoplasmic reticulum vesicles is dependent on Ca^{2+} and is modulated by Mg^{2+}, adenine nucleotide and calmodulin. J Biol Chem 1987; 262:3065–73.
131. Jones LR, Cala SE. Biochemical evidence for functional heterogeneity of cardiac sarcoplasmic reticulum vesicles. J Biol Chem 1981; 256:11809–18.
132. Feher JJ, Lipford GB. Mechanism of action of ryanodine on cardiac sarcoplasmic reticulum. Biochim Biophys Acta 1985; 813:77–86.
133. Fleischer S, Ogunbunmi EM, Dixon MC, Fleer EAM. Localization of Ca^{2+} release channels with ryanodine in junctional terminal cisternae of sarcoplasmic reticulum of fast skeletal muscle. Proc Natl Acad Sci USA 1985; 82:7256–9.
134. Lattanzio FA Jr, Schlatterer RG, Nicar M, Campbell KP, Sutko JL. The effects of ryanodine on passive calcium fluxes across sarcoplasmic reticulum membranes. J Biol Chem 1987; 262:2711–8.
135. McGrew SG, Wolleben C, Siegl P, Inui M, Fleischer S. Positive cooperativity of ryanodine binding to the calcium release channel of sarcoplasmic reticulum from heart and skeletal muscle. Biochemistry 1989; 28:1686–91.
136. Campbell KP, Knudson CM, Imagawa T, Leung AT, Sutko JL, Kahl SD, Raab CR, Madson L. Identification and characterization of the high affinity [^{3}H]Ryanodine receptor of the junctional sarcoplasmic reticulum Ca^{2+} release channel. J Biol Chem 1987; 262:6460–3.
137. Anderson K, Lai FA, Liu QY, Rousseau E, Erickson HP, Meissner G. Structural and functional characterization of the purified cardiac ryanodine receptor-Ca^{2+} release channel complex. J Biol Chem 1989; 264:1329–35.
138. Smith JS, Imagawa T, Ma J, Fill M, Campbell KP, Coronado R. Purified ryanodine receptor from rabbit skeletal muscle is the calcium release channel of sarcoplasmic reticulum. J Gen Physiol 1988; 92:1–26.
139. Wagenknecht T, Grassucci R, Frank J, Saito A, Inui M, Fleischer S. Three-dimensional architecture of the calcium release channel from skeletal muscle. Nature 1989; 338:167–70.

140. Chiesi M, Schwaller R, Calviello G. Inhibition of rapid Ca-release from isolated skeletal and cardiac sarcoplasmic reticulum (SR) membranes. Biochem Biophys Res Commun 1988; 154:1–8.
141. Michalak M, Dupraz P, Shoshan-Barmatz V. Ryanodine binding to sarcoplasmic reticulum membrane; comparison between cardiac and skeletal muscle. Biochim Biophys Acta 1988; 939:587–94.
142. Takeshima H, Nishimura S, Matsumoto T, Isida H, Kangawa K, Minamino N, Matsuo H, Ueda M, Hanaoka M, Hirose T, Numa S. Primary structure and expression from complementary DNA of skeletal muscle ryanodine receptor. Nature 1989; 339:439–45.
143. Zorzato F, Fujii J, Otsu K, Phillips M, Green NM, Lai FA, Meissner G, MacLennan DH. Molecular cloning of cDNA encoding human and rabbit forms of the Ca^{2+} release channel (ryanodine receptor) of skeletal muscle sarcoplasmic reticulum. J Biol Chem 1990; 265:2244–56.
144. Otsu K, Willard HF, Khanna VK, Zorzato F, Green NM, MacLennan DH. Molecular cloning of cDNA and coding the CA^{2+} release channel (ryanodine receptor) of rabbit cardiac muscle sarcoplasmic reticulum. J Biol Chem 1990; 265:13472–83.
145. Streb H, Irvine RF, Berridge MJ, Schulz I. Release of Ca^{2+} from a nonmitochondrial intracellular store in pancreatic acinar cells by inositol-1, 4, 5-triphosphate. Nature 1983; 306:67–9.
146. Prentki M, Biden TJ, Janjic D, Irvine RF, Berridge MJ, Wollheim CB. Rapid mobilization of Ca^{2+} from rat insulinoma microsomes by inositol-1, 4, 5-triphosphate. Nature 1984; 309:562–4.
147. Joseph SK, Thomas AP, Williams RJ, Irvine RF, Williamson JR. Myoinositol-1, 4, 5-trisphosphate. J Biol Chem 1984; 259:3077–81.
148. Volpe P, Salviati G, DiVirgilio F, Pozzan T. Inositol 1, 4, 5-triphosphate induces calcium release from sarcoplasmic reticulum of skeletal muscle. Nature 1985; 316:347–9.
149. Vergara J, Tsien RY, Delay M. Inositol 1, 4, 5-trisphosphate: a possible chemical link in excitation–contraction coupling in muscle. Proc Natl Acad Sci 1985; 82:6352–6.
150. Hirata M, Suematsu E, Hashimoto T, Hamachi T, Koga T. Release of Ca^{2+} from a non-mitochondrial store site in peritoneal macrophages treated with saponin by inositol 1, 4, 5-trisphosphate. Biochem J 1984; 223:229–36.
151. Movsesian MA, Thomas AP, Selak M, Williamson JR. Inositol trisphosphate does not release Ca^{2+} from permeablized cardiac myocytes and sarcoplasmic reticulum. FEBS Lett 1985; 185:328–32.
152. Nosek TM, Williams MF, Ziegler ST, Godt RE. Inositol trisphosphate enhances calcium release in skinned cardiac and skeletal muscle. Am J Physiol 1986; 250:C807–C11.
153. Fabiato A. Inositol 1, 4, 5-trisphosphate-induced release of Ca^{2+} from the sarcoplasmic reticulum of skinned cardiac cells. Biophys J 1986; 49:190A.
154. Scherer NM, Ferguson JE. Inositol 1, 4, 5-trisphosphate is not effective in releasing calcium from skeletal sarcoplasmic reticulum microsomes. Biochem Biophys Res Commun 1985; 128:1064–70.
155. Mikos GJ, Snow TR. Failure of inositol 1, 4, 5-trisphosphate to elicit or potentiate Ca^{2+} release from isolated skeletal muscle sarcoplasmic reticulum. Biochim Biophys Acta 1987; 927:256–60.
156. Lea TJ, Griffiths PJ, Tregear RT, Ashley CC. An examination of the ability of inositol 1, 4, 5-trisphosphate to induce calcium release and tension development in skinned skeletal muscle fibres of frog and crustacea. FEBS Lett 1986; 207:153–61.
157. Gill DL, Ueda T, Chueh SH, Noel MW. Ca^{2+} release from endoplasmic reticulum is mediated by a guanine nucleotide regulatory mechanism. Nature 1986; 320:461–4.

158. Hamachi T, Hirata M, Kimura Y, Ikebe T, Ishimatsu T, Yamaguchi K, Koga T. Effect of guanosine triphosphate on the release and uptake of Ca^{2+} in saponin-permeabilized macrophages and the skeletal-muscle sarcoplasmic reticulum. Biochem J 1987; 242: 253–60.
159. Wolf BA, Florholmen J, Colca JR, McDaniel ML. GTP mobilization of Ca^{2+} from the endoplasmic reticulum of islets. Biochem J 1987; 242:137–41.
160. Ueda T, Chueh SH, Noel MW, Gill DL. Influence of inositol 1, 4, 5-trisphosphate and guanine nucleotides on intracellular calcium release within the N1E-115 neuronal cell line. J Biol Chem 1986; 261:3184–92.
161. Fabiato A. Use of aequorin for the appraisal of the hypothesis of the release of calcium from the sarcoplasmic reticulum induced by a change of pH in skinned cardiac cells. Cell Calcium 1985; 6:95–108.
192. Capogrossi MC, Houser SR, Bahinski A, Lakatta EG. Synchronous occurrence of spontaneous localized calcium release from the sarcoplasmic reticulum generated action potentials in rat cardiac ventricular myocytes at normal resting membrane potential. Circ Res 1987; 61:498–503.
163. Feher JJ, LeBolt WR, Manson NH. Differential effect of global ischemia on the ryanodine-sensitive and ryanodine-insensitive calcium uptake of cardiac sarcoplasmic reticulum. Circ Res 1989; 65:1400–8.

6

Excitation–Contraction Coupling in Human Ventricular Myocardium: Relationship to the Pathophysiology of Heart Failure

JUDITH K. GWATHMEY and PAUL D. ALLEN

Harvard Medical School
Boston, Massachusetts

ROGER J. HAJJAR

Massachusetts General Hospital
Boston, Massachusetts

Congestive heart failure is characterized by two prominent cardiac defects: the inability of the heart muscle to generate ventricular pressure to propel blood adequately through the cardiovascular system and/or the inability of the heart to relax completely and allow sufficient filling during diastole. These defects either independently or together lead to a reduction in cardiac output.

Despite insights into altered excitation–contraction coupling (E-C coupling) in animal models of cardiac disease the question remains: What are the subcellular defects seen in human cardiomyopathy and, more important, what is their functional significance? Through a better understanding of these defects one might possibly better direct the development of cardioprotective as well as therapeutic agents.

Advances in the understanding of disease processes in human myocardium have been limited by investigators' inability to obtain cardiac tissue for detailed study. To gain insight into possible myocardial defects associated with congestive heart failure in humans, we have studied ventricular tissue from normal human hearts received from organ donors without known cardiac disease and hearts of patients with end-stage heart failure undergoing cardiac transplantation due to ischemic, valvular, hypertrophic, viral, and idiopathic cardiomyopathy. We have studied over 40 hearts from patients with end-stage heart failure.

We previously reported some of our findings in normal and diseased human myocardium (1–14). Because the study of human myocardium is relatively new, the related literature is not extensive. Findings in human tissue as well as animal studies in relation to normal and diseased states are covered in other chapters. It is not our intention to cover exhaustively material readily available in the literature, but to emphasize new information that has emerged from our studies.

I. INTRACELLULAR CALCIUM HANDLING IN HUMAN VENTRICULAR MYOCARDIUM

Abnormal intracellular calcium handling has been implicated as pivotal to the contractile abnormalities seen with congestive heart failure and hypertrophy. We have identified abnormalities in the calcium transient that correlate with a prolonged contractile response in congestive heart failure at both 30°C and 37°C, a more physiological temperature (14). In myopathic human ventricular myocardium, the calcium transient consists of a fast component L_1, and a second slower component, L_2 (Fig. 1). The early fast component is similar to that seen in normal human myocardium and in other animal species (15). The early component, L_1, predominantly reflects release and reuptake of calcium by the sarcoplasmic reticulum (SR). The second slower component in the calcium transient (L_2) could be due to a defect at the level of the sarcolemma (i.e., calcium channels, Na^+/Ca^{2+} exchange, Ca^{2+} ATPase), the sarcoplasmic reticulum (i.e., reduced reuptake rate and/or rerelease), mitochondrial calcium buffering, or the result of calcium being released from the myofilaments (i.e., altered affinity of troponin C for Ca^{2+}).

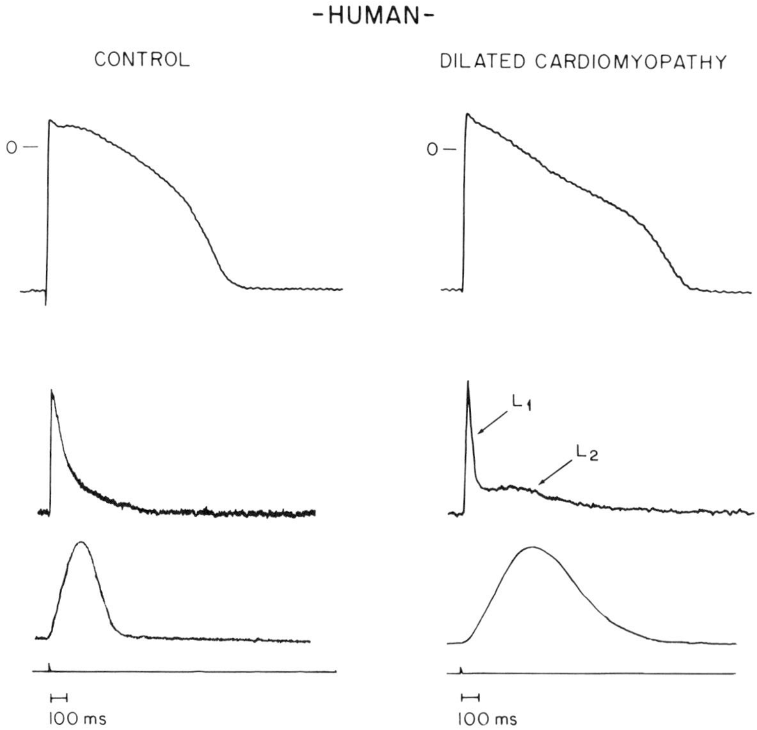

Figure 1 Top panels: Action potentials from control and myopathic myocardium. Middle panels: Calcium transients and associated isometric twitches (lower panels) in a trabeculae carneae from an organ donor without known cardiac disease and from a patient with end-stage heart failure. L_1 is the early fast component typical of normal tissue and calcium transients from other mammalian species. L_2 is the second slower component seen in myopathic human myocardium.

A. Sarcolemma, Calcium Influx, and Sodium–Calcium Exchange

The hypothesis that a defect in sarcolemmal calcium transport is a partial explanation for the qualitatively different calcium transients seen in trabeculae carneae from patients with cardiomyopathy (CMY) is supported by evidence that increasing $[Ca^{2+}]_o$ results in an increase in end-diastolic intracellular calcium concentration ($[Ca^{2+}]_i$) and diastolic tone in CMY muscles (2,6). However, the appearance of L_2 cannot be explained fully by an increase in voltage-dependent slow Ca^{2+} flux demonstrated by addition of verapamil, a calcium channel antagonist. In the presence of verapamil there was equal diminution in amplitude of both components (Fig. 2). If L_2 was due solely to transsarcolemmal calcium influx through the slow voltage-dependent channel, one would expect a much greater effect on its amplitude than L_1. The fact that both components were affected equally suggested that SR loading might play a role. One likewise cannot explain the increase in amplitude of L_2 far out of proportion to L_1 at varying $[Ca^{2+}]_o$ solely on the basis of a defect of the sarcolemma. In atrial myocardium from patients with hypertrophic cardiomyopathy it has been reported that there are a greater number of nitrendipine-binding sites, suggesting that there is increased calcium conductance across the sarcolemma as previously demonstrated in the Syrian hamster (16–18). This finding supports our findings that verapamil abolished the remaining calcium transient after addition of ryanodine, an alkaloid that inhibits sarcoplasmic reticulum calcium release and induces SR calcium "leak" (2). Figure 3 demonstrates a similar effect of caffeine on the amplitude of L_1 and L_2. Caffeine induces SR calcium release and impairs SR calcium reuptake. The addition of 20 mM caffeine completely abolished L_1. L_2 was diminished in amplitude, as was previously reported with ryanodine (2). The fact that in the presence of caffeine L_2 was diminished in amplitude, but was not com-

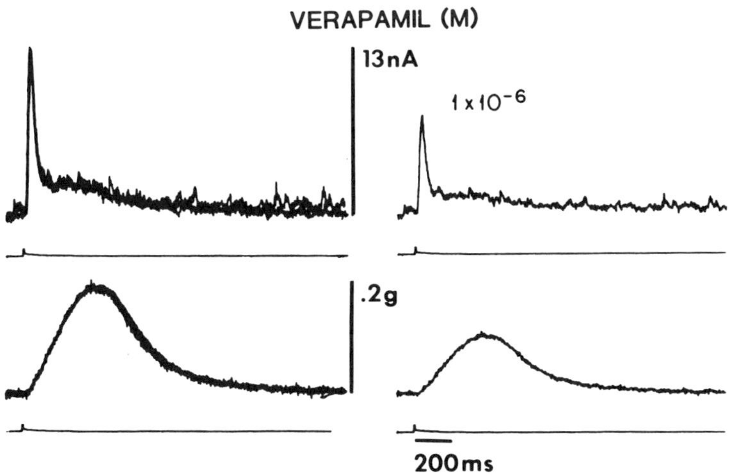

Figure 2 Effect of 1×10^{-6} M verapamil on the amplitude of L_1 and L_2. Notice the suggestion of a greater effect on L_2. Left panel demonstrates that once the calcium transients are electrically amplified to the same height as L_1 before addition of verapamil, there is superimposition of the traces.

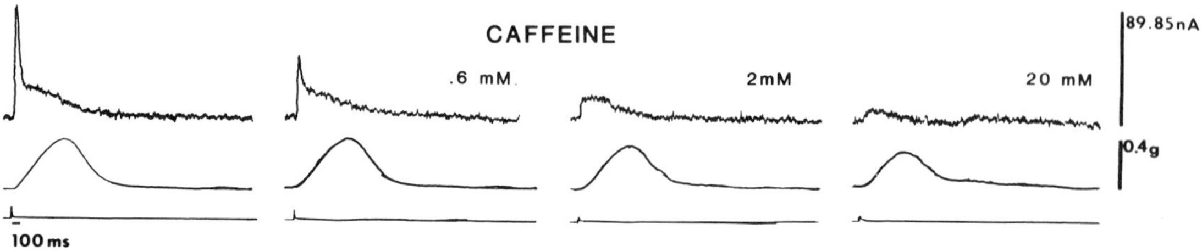

Figure 3 Concentration effect of addition of caffeine. Notice that L_1 is abolished. L_2 is not abolished but is diminished in amplitude. Subsequent addition of verapamil abolished the remaining component.

pletely abolished as was the case with ryanodine, indicates that L_2 arises in part from the sarcoplasmic reticulum. The second component of the calcium transient therefore most likely reflects rerelease of calcium from the SR as opposed to a greatly impaired reuptake of calcium. This conclusion fits well with the observation by Movsesian et al. that in patients with idiopathic dilated cardiomyopathy there is no intrinsic alteration of Ca^{2+} uptake by sarcoplasmic reticulum vesicles (19). They reported that Ca^{2+} uptake by the sarcoplasmic reticulum had a V_{max} of 107.1±15.5 nmol/m min, in nonfailing hearts. The corresponding value in failing hearts was 126.7±14.0 nmol/m min. They also reported that with antiphospholamban stimulation (e.g., similar to cyclic AMP stimulation) there was a 1.93-fold increase in the sarcoplasmic reticulum Ca^{2+} transport from normal human left ventricular myocardium and 1.94-fold increase in sarcoplasmic reticulum prepared from the left ventricle of patients with idiopathic dilated cardiomyopathy (20). Our observation that the rate of rise and decline of the early fast component in myopathic tissue approximates that in normal tissues support this conclusion. We have further demonstrated that the amount of intracellular calcium released by the sarcoplasmic reticulum is not different in the presence of varying frequencies of stimulation or $[Ca^{2+}]_o$ for control or myopathic tissue (6). Recently, in failing human myocardium, Ca^{2+} ATPase messenger RNA has been reported reduced by as much as 50% (13).

There is strong evidence that inositol 1, 4, 5-trisphosphate (IP_3) stimulates Ca^{2+} release from intracellular stores. Recently a ryanodine-like IP_3 receptor was isolated from cardiac sarcoplasmic reticulum (21). Although the mechanism of IP_3-induced Ca^{2+} mobilization is poorly understood, it has been proposed that IP_3 secondarily elicits Ca^{2+} entry by emptying the SR Ca^{2+} pool (22). IP_3-induced Ca^{2+} could explain the appearance of the second slower component. Changes in IP_3 turnover have been reported to result in slow release and reuptake of calcium by the SR (23,24). Further investigation is needed to elucidate the effects of the phosphatidylinositol systems on the SR, and whether there are differences in the response of the SR to IP_3 between control and myopathic hearts.

Calcium release from the sarcoplasmic reticulum is stimulated by a rise in intracellular calcium from the nanomolar to micromolar range (25,26). During the increase in Ca^{2+} around the SR the probability that Ca^{2+} channels are open increases. This is due to an increase in the total number of open events and not to an increase in the open state lifetimes. Open times are not affected over a range of 2–250 μM. Maximum net release occurs when $[Ca^{2+}]_i$ is 1.5–2 μM. Ca^{2+} release declines at both lower and higher [Ca^{2+}]. The release mechanism is then turned off when calcium reaches micromolar concentrations and reuptake is switched on. The K_m for calcium pumping has been reported to be about 2.6 μM while net calcium release is half-maximal at 0.8 μM (26). Calcium affects the duration of the longer closed state in a concentration-dependent manner (faster time constant at higher [Ca^{2+}]) whereas the short closed time is unaffected (25). As the intracellular calcium concentration declines, channels are reset for opening again (open probability decreases). If in myopathic myocardium the kinetics of calcium extrusion is delayed, it is possible to envision how the decline of intracellular calcium in the presence of an elevated resting calcium level might induce a rerelease of a smaller amount of calcium with a slower time course of release and reuptake. Sarcoplasmic reticulum calcium channel activation can be detected at 10^{-7} M calcium concentration. L_2 can range from 400 to 1000 nM, which is well above the [Ca^{2+}] level demonstrated to activate calcium release. The resting [Ca^{2+}] in myopathic tissue is 361±68 μM, compared to 225±52 μM in control tissue (6,27). One must also keep in mind that both Ca^{2+} and ATP are required to activate fully the sarcoplasmic reticulum calcium channels. In diseased myocardium it has been suggested that cAMP is diminished (1). Although this may affect gating kinetics in the intact preparation, it is unlikely to play a significant role because ATP concentrations in myocardium have been reported to be in the millimolar range. High-energy phosphate concentrations have been reported to be low in myopathic myocardium (28,29) and creatine kinase activity lower (3). A combination of rerelease of calcium from the sarcoplasmic reticulum with a lower creatine kinase activity might therefore explain a significant proportion of the diastolic relaxation abnormalities seen in diseased myocardium as well as the negative force–frequency relationship (6).

There is also evidence in human myocardium that transsarcolemmal calcium flux may result in direct activation of the myofilaments (6). This then suggests a potential significant role of SR calcium release and the amplitude of the second component, L_2, in force production and maintenance. Yue (30) reported that when [Ca^{2+}]$_i$ was 0.2μM (0.15–0.3 μM larger than resting [Ca^{2+}]) maximum negative dF/dt was no longer a simple instantaneous function of [Ca^{2+}]$_i$. This value of [Ca^{2+}]$_i$, which he termed the "[Ca^{2+}] 'offset,' " was the same for both physiological and slowed contractions. Yue postulated that the linear relationship of dF/dt to [Ca^{2+}]$_i$ during early phases of tension rise in slowed contractions was due to more spatial uniformity of the slower Ca^{2+} transient during the upstoke. Gwathmey et al. (6) reported that in myopathic tissue L_2 maintains an elevation of intracellular calcium between 0.4 and 1 μM (0.1–0.7 μM larger than resting [Ca^{2+}]$_i$) and occurs at the time of expected maximum negative dF/dt. They proposed that the diastolic dysfunction seen in myopathic tissue could result from an increase in resting intracellular calcium and/or an altered [Ca^{2+}] offset. They further proposed that in myopathic tissue initial negative dF/dt (i.e., initial relaxation) bears a linear relationship to L_2 and that this relationship becomes nonlinear at an altered [Ca^{2+}] offset. These proposals were supported by findings of Movsesian et al. (20). Their findings suggested that stimulation of Ca^{2+} uptake by phospholamban phosphorylation has little effect on the initial phase of relaxation, during which free cytosolic [Ca^{2+}] is 0.8–0.9 μM. They proposed that the principal effects of phosphorylation would instead be reflected in lowering of the free cytosolic [Ca^{2+}] during later stages of relaxation and an increase in the amount of calcium stored in the sarcoplasmic reticulum (and available for subsequent release).

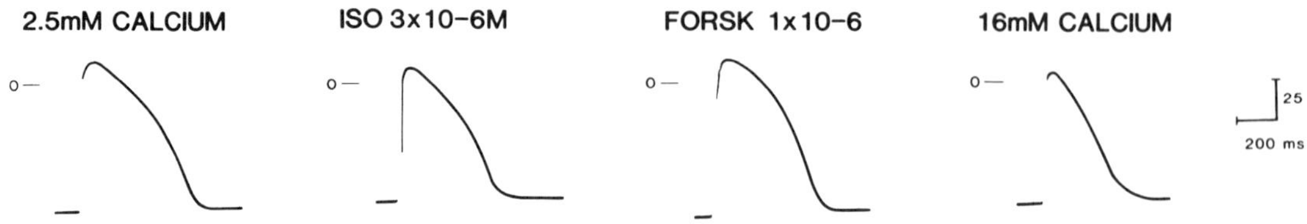

Figure 4 Action potentials obtained in a myopathic muscle after addition of isoproterenol (ISO), a beta-receptor agonist; forskolin (FORSK), an adenylate cyclase activator; and high extracellular calcium. Notice that action potential duration is significantly abbreviated only in the presence of high $[Ca^{2+}]_o$, suggesting inhibition of the I_{Ca}. The observation that isoproterenol did not abbreviate action potential duration as reported in other species suggests that receptor stimulation is altered in the myopathic state.

In diseased human myocardium the action potential duration in multicellular preparations is prolonged (2,4,6) (Figs. 1, 4). The observed prolongation of the action potential might reflect a prolonged inward current (I_{Ca}), delayed inactivation of an outward or rectifying potassium current, or enhanced sodium conductance. Prolongation of the plateau phase of the action potential, suggesting enhanced transsarcolemmal calcium flux, may explain in part the appearance of the slower second component in the calcium transient seen in myopathic human myocardium. The mechanism of action potential prolongation has not been established and awaits voltage clamp studies in isolated myocytes in which the membrane currents can be controlled (31). Action potentials recorded from isolated human myocytes have a resting membrane potential of -75 ± 35 mV in the presence of 6.0 mM K^+ (32). Peak amplitudes average 94 ± 3.6 mV (32). Li et al. reported that isoproterenol resulted in an increase in peak depolarization (104 ± 3.2 mV) and a prolongation of the action potential (33). Similar to action potentials in multicellular preparations (2,4,6), they found that the action potentials from failing human myocytes were abnormally prolonged (33). Li reported that extremely prolonged action potentials were unique to a subset of failing human myocytes (33). One could hypothesize that enhanced calcium flux would augment SR calcium loading and preserve contractility. However, one must keep in mind in the presence of impaired sarcoplasmic reticulum function that the influx of calcium across the sarcolemma may effectively increase free ionized calcium and result in activation of the myofilaments (6). This could potentially lead to diastolic relaxation abnormalities that have been reported in patients with end-stage heart failure. Calcium overload can result not only in diastolic abnormalities with an increase in passive stiffness, but also diminished peak contractile force (2,4,6). Figure 5 demonstrates the effect of stopping the electrical stimulus in the presence of acetylstrophanthidin-induced calcium overload. There is a decrease in resting calcium and tension. Upon restarting the stimulation, the first few contractions are of larger amplitude and have lower end-diastolic tone.

The role played by the sodium–calcium exchange mechanism under normal physiological conditions remains controversial. The sodium–calcium exchanger operating under control electrochemical gradients for sodium and calcium primarily removes calcium from the cytosol. However, when there is a reduction in the sodium electrochemical gradient and/or an increase in the calcium electrochemical

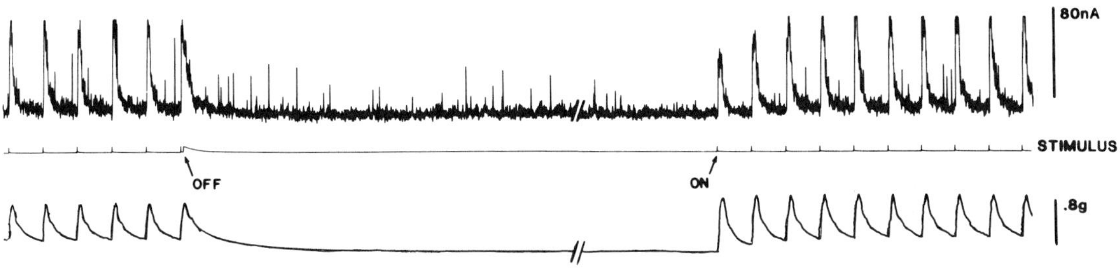

Figure 5 Effect of acetylstrophanthidin toxicity in a myopathic muscle. There is an increase in diastolic calcium and tone. When the stimulus is turned off there is a decrease in diastolic calcium and tone. Note that upon restarting the stimulus the contraction is larger in the absence of a similar increase in the peak amplitude of the calcium transient.

gradient, it is possible for the exchanger to move calcium into the cell (4,34,35). Therefore, sodium–calcium exchange can transport calcium in either direction across the sarcolemma but is involved mainly in the uphill transport of calcium out of the cell in a nonelectrogenic exchange for Na^+, which moves down a concentration gradient. The sodium gradient causes the carrier system that is not energy dependent to establish a gradient for calcium according to the equation

$$[Ca^{2+}]_i/[Ca^{2+}]_o = [Na^+]_i/[Na^+]_o. \quad (1)$$

The coupling ratio for the number of sodium ions transported in relation to the number of calcium ions has been reported to be 3:1 (36). Na^+ and Ca^{2+} appear to bind equally well at both sides of the membrane (i.e., the affinities of the receptor for Na^+ and Ca^{2+} are the same at both sides of the membrane). Sodium–calcium exchange and the effects of intracellular sodium are covered in detail in another chapter.

Sodium–calcium exchange has recently been shown to be capable of not only pumping calcium from the cytosol and causing relaxation but also transporting calcium into the cytosol and producing contraction (4,32,33,37). Under certain conditions, such as intracellular sodium loading in the presence of impaired sarcoplasmic reticulum calcium handling after addition of ryanodine, sodium–calcium exchange (a low-affinity but high-capacity transporter) has been shown to be capable of transporting significant amounts of calcium ($\approx 1\mu M$) into the cytosol, resulting in significant force production (4). Calcium efflux from the cell is attained by sodium–calcium exhange and a sarcolemmal-bound Ca^{2+}–ATPase driven Ca^{2+} pump. A defect in Na^+/Ca^{2+} exchange or Ca^{2+}–ATPase could therefore explain the appearance of the second slow component, L_2. Sarcolemmal Ca^{2+} ATPase activity to date has not been directly investigated in human myocardium.

The fact that with each beat small amounts of calcium enter the cardiac cell without a long-term rise in total cellular calcium indicates that there are functional extrusion mechanisms for calcium from the cell. Acetylstrophanthidin (NASA), a Na^+-K^+ ATPase inhibitor, is reported to exert its positive inotropic effect by blocking Na^+ extrusion from the cell, thereby increasing $[Na^+{}_i]$ and causing an increase in the $[Na^+]_i/[Na^+]_o$ ratio. According to Equation 1 the Ca^{2+} ratio increases so that at a constant level of $[Ca^{2+}]_o$ the sodium pump inhibition causes a net gain in $[Ca^{2+}]_i$ due

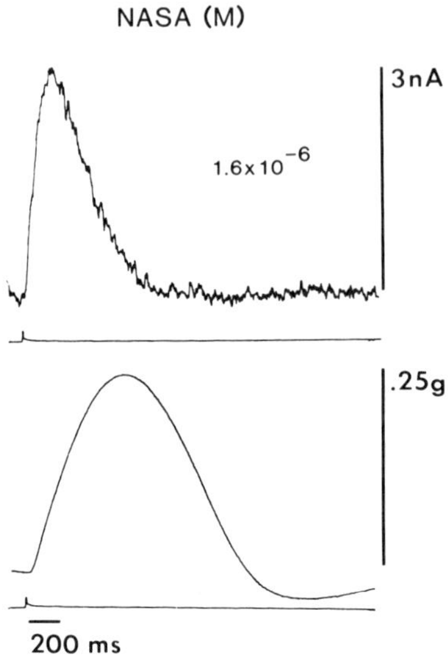

Figure 6 Addition of acetylstrophanthidin (NASA) results in fusion of L_1 and L_2.

to a reduced efflux from the cell. When CMY muscles were exposed to a concentration from 4×10^{-7} M to 1.6×10^{-6} M acetylstrophanthidin, L_2 increased in amplitude and became fused to L_1, as demonstrated in Figure 6.

To address further the question of whether Na^+–Ca^{2+} exchange is altered and whether L_2 is due to Na^+–Ca^{2+}, muscles were exposed to a low extracellular sodium concentration (46 mM) in a choline-chloride-substituted Hepes solution. Reduction of extracellular sodium causes the equilbrium described in Equation 1 to shift so that the ratio $[Ca^{2+}]_i/[Ca^{2+}]_o$ increases. When $[Ca^{2+}]_o$ is held constant, a decrease in $[Na^+]_o$ causes an increase in $[Ca^{2+}]_i$. The initial effect of a reduction in $[Na^+]_o$ is a decrease in the inward movement of sodium and a corresponding increase in calcium influx. The increase in calcium influx causes $[Ca^{2+}]_i$ to rise until the relative rates of sodium and calcium efflux match the newly established relationship between sodium and calcium influx. This new equilibrium is reached, therefore, by an increase in intracellular calcium. When muscles were exposed to a low-sodium bathing medium there was an increase in resting intracellular calcium and the amplitude of L_2, as demonstrated in Figure 7. This suggests that not only is the exchange mechanism intact, but that L_2 also is not due solely to voltage-dependent sarcolemmal flux of Ca^{2+} since the duration of the action potential is not altered under such circumstances. Furthermore, evidence that L_2 is not due to increased intracellular sodium and resultant sodium–calcium exhange is demonstrated in Figure 8. Addition of tetrodotoxin, a sodium channel antagonist, in the presence of the remaining component of L_2 after addition of ryanodine did not affect its amplitude or time course as opposed to verapamil, which abolished it. This indicates that L_2 is not due to a sodium-overloaded state and sodium–calcium exchange, but instead reflects in part another sarcolemmal event (4). Recently, it has been reported that there is no alteration in saxitoxin-binding sites in cardiac tissue from patients with hypertrophic cardiomyopathy (18). These data suggest that sodium overload from Na^{2+} channels cannot explain the abnormal intracellular calcium concentration seen in the myopathic state.

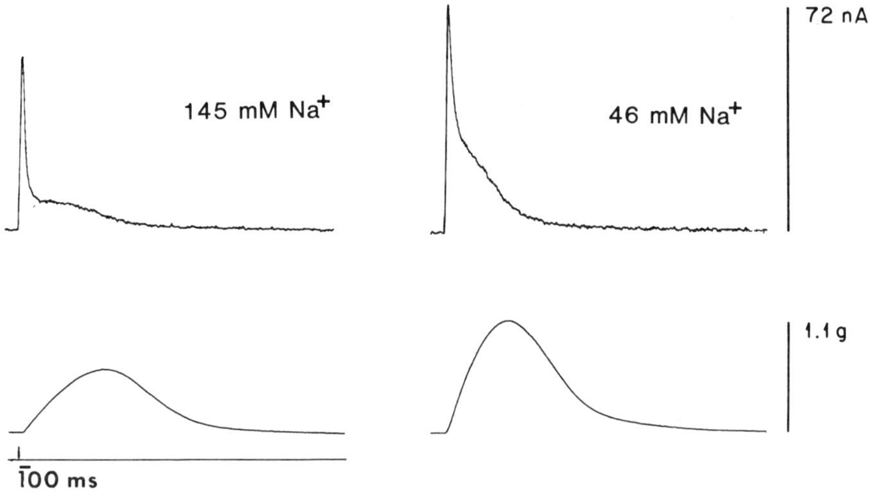

Figure 7 Effect of low extracellular sodium with time on force and intracellular calcium in a myopathic muscle.

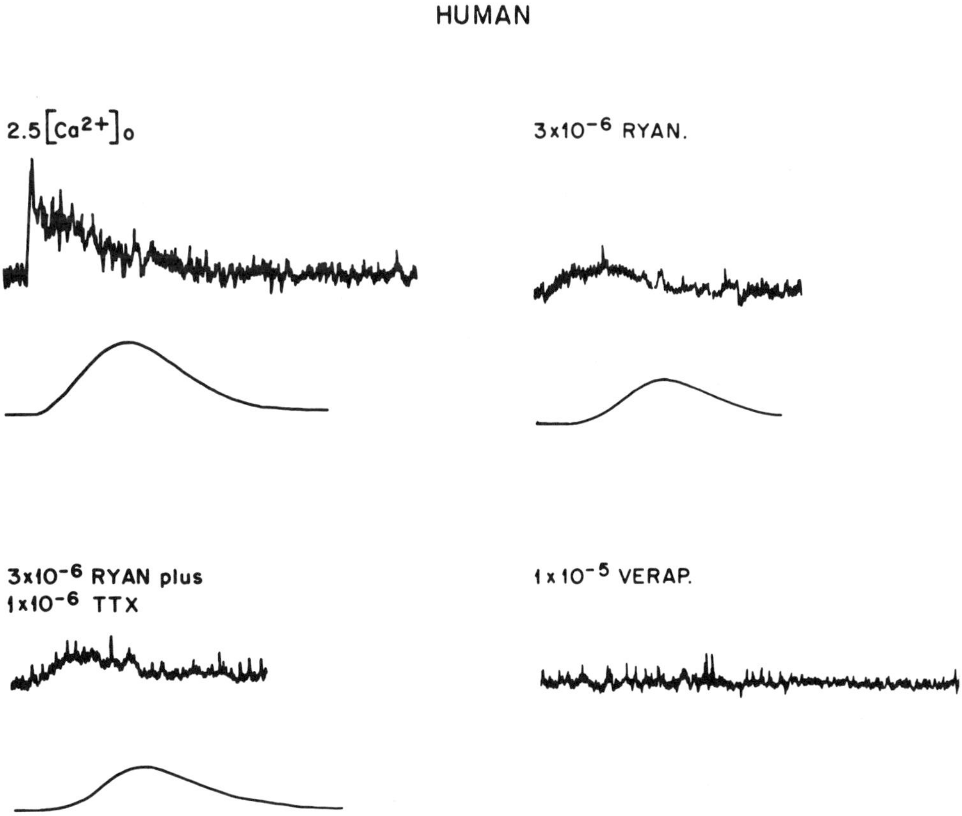

Figure 8 Addition of ryanodine abolished L_1 and diminished the amplitude of L_2. Addition of tetrodotoxin (TTX) did not affect the amplitude or time course of the remaining calcium transient (L_2).

B. Mitochondria, Ca^{2+} ATPase, and Calcium Mobilization

Mitochondrial calcium accumulation is mediated via electron transport, utilizing a proton gradient or via ATP-dependent processes. Previous experiments on isolated mitochondria have established that under physiological loading conditions calcium uptake requires electron transport from any of a series of respiratory substrates and that either Mg^{2+} or phosphate must be present. In addition, calcium uptake under these conditions is inhibited by respiratory uncouplers such as 2,4-dinitrophenol, but not by oligomycin. Addition of oligomycin B during hypoxia has been shown to prevent prolongation of the time course of relaxation seen upon reoxygenation due to calcium release by mitochondria (38). If L_2 reflects abnormal calcium handling by mitochondria, it should be affected by addition of a mitochondrial inhibitor. The addition of oligomycin B, a mitchondrial ATPase inhibitor, should result in an increase in the amplitude of L_2 if the extrusion of calcium from the cell by ATP-dependent Ca^{2+}–ATPase is affected and/or L_2 arises as a result of a buffering effect by mitochondria resulting from mitochondrial calcium extrusion. Addition of oligomycin resulted in a slight decrease in amplitude of the peak calcium transient and second slow component without affecting the time course. These data suggest that mitochondrial calcium handling cannot fully explain the occurrence of the second slow component.

Recently, in isolated myocytes loaded with the fluorescent indicator Fura-2, the calcium transient was found to have two temporally distinct components (39). The first component was identified as being of sarcoplasmic reticulum origin, confirming our findings with aequorin. This suggests that inhomogeneties in conduction are not responsible for the appearance of two components as detected with aequorin. All other animal species studied with aequorin have a monophasic calcium transient. Canine Purkinje fibers, however, have been reported to have two components (40–42). In a porcine model of virally induced myocarditis/cardiomyopathy developed by Gwathmey and Abelmann (43), there is prolongation of the action potential and associated isometric contraction. There are likewise two temporally distinct components to the calcium transient (44). As previously reported in humans, the two components appear to reflect abnormal calcium handling by the sarcoplasmic reticulum and sarcolemma. This finding suggests that cardiomyopathies that result from potentially multiple and differenting causes may reflect similar subcellular defects in electrical and calcium handling events.

C. Sarcoplasmic Reticulum and Calcium Handling

Studies using aequorin have demonstrated that the resting intracellular calcium level is higher in myopathic tissue than in normal myocardium (6). Furthermore, there was no significant difference in the amount of calcium released by the sarcoplasmic reticulum (Fig. 9) (6). These data suggest that contractile failure seen in heart failure is *not* due to diminished availability of intracellular calcium. It should be pointed out that in some muscles from patients with ischemic cardiomyopathy the calcium transient consisted of a single component. The time course of this calcium transient was, however, prolonged compared to the time course of the transient in normal myocardium.

In summary, the occurrence of L_2 and proposed explanations of the effect of various interventions on its amplitude are illustrated in Figure 10. In the presence of

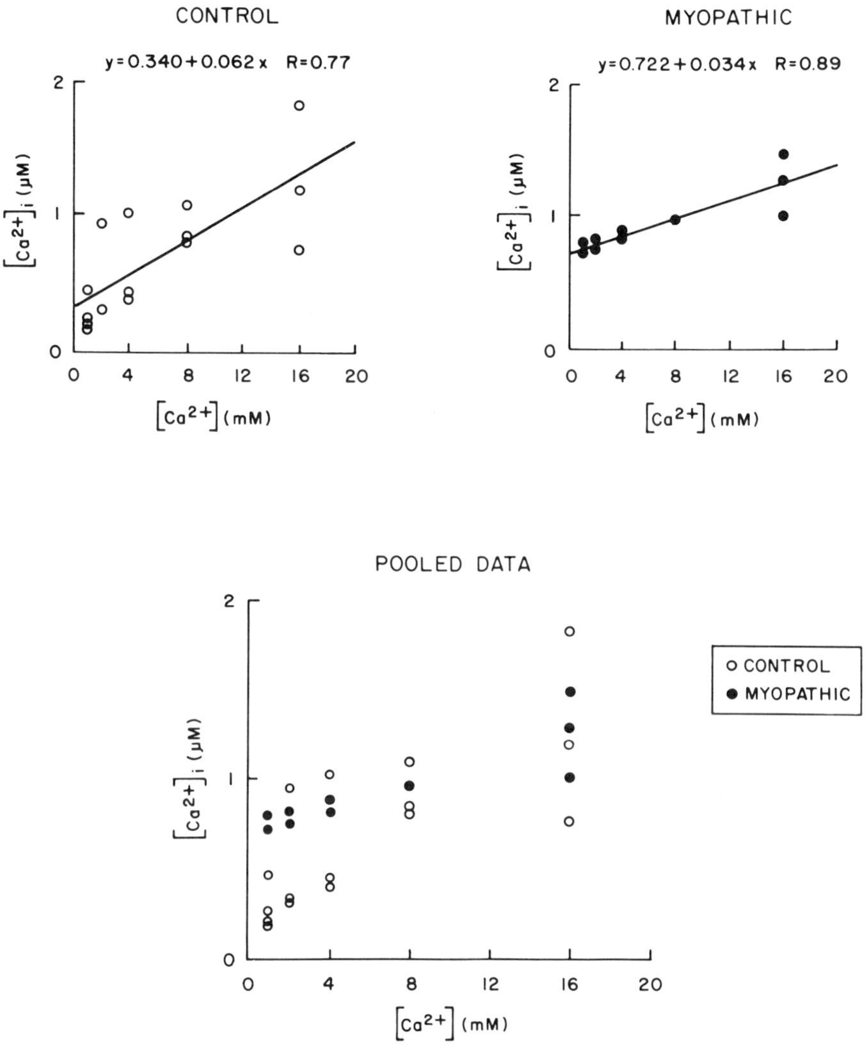

Figure 9 Peak intracellular calcium released in normal and myopathic myocardium exposed to varying extracellular calcium concentrations. A linear regression using a least-squared algorithm was used. Y intercepts and r values are given.

diminished intracellular cyclic AMP, as has been suggested by Feldman et al. (1), there would be the occurrence of L_1 and L_2 (panel A). If the predominant effect of increasing intracellular cyclic AMP is upon phosphorylation of phospholamban, as has been suggested by Garvey et al. (45), the amplitude of L_1 would be increased, and the time course shortened, and there would be a diminished amplitude of L_2 due to increased uptake by the sarcoplasmic reticulum (panel B). This is suggested in Figure 11, in which addition of isoproterenol and forskolin, both of which increase intracellular cyclic AMP and thereby enhance transsarcolemmal calcium influx, are shown to result in abbreviation of the time course of the calcium transient. If, however, there is no change in action potential duration with enhanced

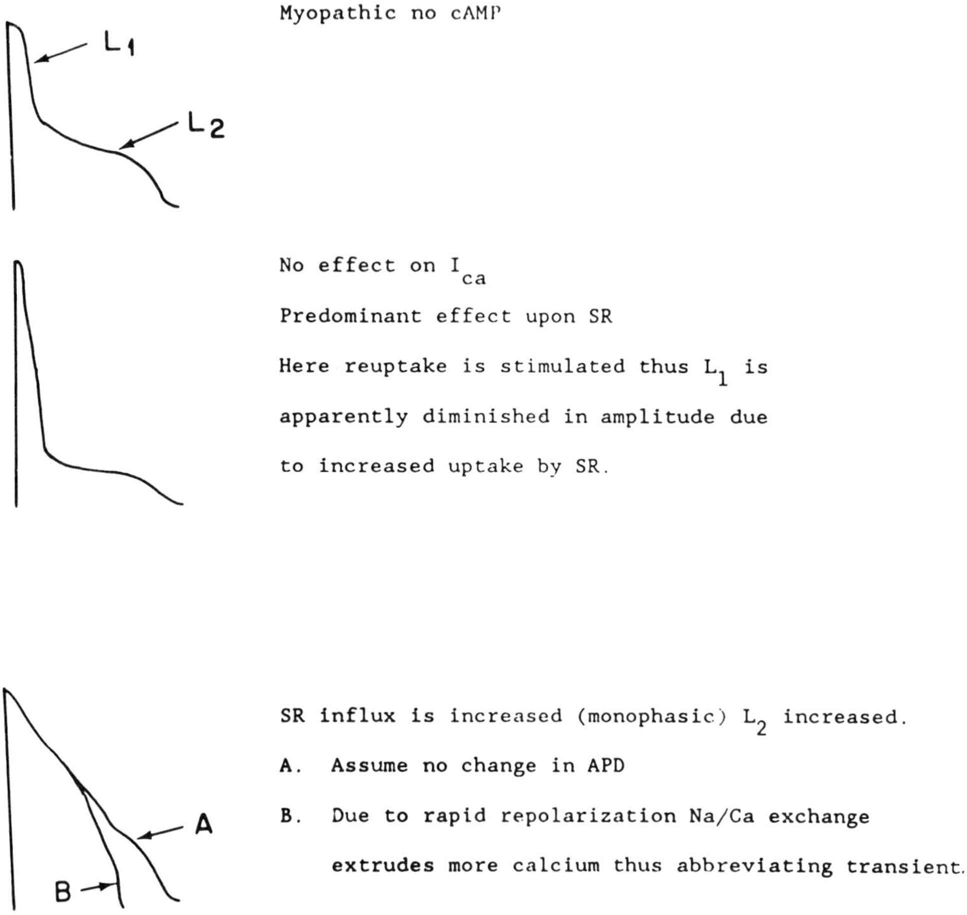

Figure 10 Effect of cyclic AMP and action potential duration on the amplitude of L_2. Proposed mechanisms for changes in the amplitude of L_2 with resultant fusion with L_1.

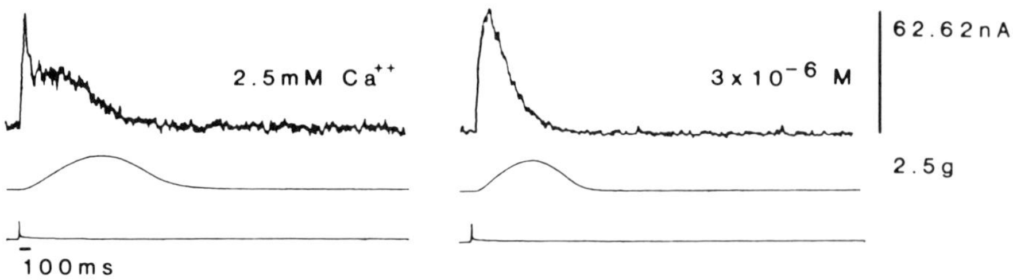

Figure 11 Addition of forskolin to a myopathic muscle. Notice that L_2 is diminished in amplitude. Also notice the lack of inotropic effect of forskolin in this muscle. There is associated abbreviation of the time course of the isometric twitches in the presence of both agents. The abbreviation in the time course of the twitch may reflect phosphorylation of troponin I and/or enhanced uptake by the SR.

calcium and/or sodium loading, the sodium–calcium exchanger would result in a hyperpolarizing current with resulting abbreviation of the duration of L_2. Rapid repolarization would result and Na/Ca exchange would extrude more calcium, thus abbreviating the calcium transient (panel C). Higher frequencies of stimulation and higher $[Ca^{2+}]_o$ could therefore result in a shortened duration of L_2 (or fusion) due to enhanced sodium–calcium exchange, and/or activation of ATP and calcium-dependent potassium channels. The amplitude and time course of L_2 react in a predictable manner to both pharmacologic and physiological perturbations, further substantiating it as a pathophysiological phenomenon.

II. MYOFIBRILLAR CONTENT, Mg^{2+}-ATPASE ACTIVITY, AND MYOFILAMENT RESPONSIVENESS TO CALCIUM

Modulation of contractility is not due solely to variation in the rise in cytoplasmic Ca^{2+} initiated by the action potential. Abnormalities in contracile performance have been associated with alterations in the structure and function of the contractile proteins. It is now clear that properties of the contractile proteins themselves change during physiological regulation of contraction. In intact muscle preparations, a change in contractility may result from changes in contractile proteins, or from changes in other elements of the electromechanical coupling process (e.g., transsarcolemmal Ca^{2+} current and $[Ca^{2+}]_i$ release). Understanding mechanisms that alter the properties of the contractile proteins therefore requires the integration of several different types of information.

We have determined that the enzymatic properties of the myofibrillar proteins are depressed in human heart failure (12). Mg^{2+} ATPase activity was reduced at higher pCa, although not always statistically significant (Table 1). Total protein content per gram wet weight of tissue was not significantly different between the normal group and groups with coronary artery disease, mitral valve insufficiency, and cardiomyopathy. Compared to the normal group, the total recovery of myofibrillar proteins expressed as milligrams protein per gram wet tissue was significantly lower for patients with end-stage failure due to coronary artery disease and cardiomyopathy. Expressing myofibrillar protein recovery as milligrams myofibrillar protein per 100 mg ventricular protein revealed a significantly lower myofibrillar protein content in patients with cardiomyopathy (Table 2). Ca^{2+}–ATPase and actin-activated Mg^{2+}–ATPase of purified myosin isolated from hypertrophied human ventricular muscle has been reported not to be significantly different from normal human myocardium (12). We have found that the Ca^{2+}–ATPase of myosin isolated from hearts with end-stage failure due to cardiomyopathy or coronary artery disease is also not different compared to normal myocardium or patients with

Table 1 Calcium-Dependent Mg^{2+} ATPase (n Mole P_i/mg protein/min)

pCa	6.75	6.25	6.15	6.0	5.85	5.75	5.50	5.0
Normal	8.7	30	23	28	30	35	40	41
Mitral valve insufficiency (class III)	7.8	11	16	19	19.5	20	24	26
Idiopathic myopathy (class IV)	7.5	12	15	18	19	22	25	27
Ischemic myopathy (class IV)	7.6	11	15	18	19	21	25	26

Table 2 Myofibrillar Protein Content (mg/wet weight; Mean±SEM)

Normal	Mitral Valve (Class III)	Idiopathic Myopathy	Ischemic Myopathy (Class IV)
41±1	38±4	25±4*	28±2*

*Significant difference from control $p<0.05$

valve insufficiency. Curves describing the relationship between ionized calcium and normalized Mg^{2+}–ATPase activity were similar, suggesting no change in myofilament sensitivity.

Myofibrillar Ca^{2+} responsiveness has traditionally been studied using the skinned fiber technique in which the sarcolemma and sarcoplasmic reticulum have been destroyed. The skinned fiber technique offers the advantage that intracellular [Ca^{2+}] can be directly controlled at the level of the myofilaments, allowing force–pCa relationships to be studied. We have compared force–pCa relationships in saponin-skinned trabeculae carneae from normal and diseased human myocardium (5). We used a concentration of saponin (250 μg/ml) that has been reported to remove the SR. On a teleologic basis one might expect in failing myocardium a shift to lower pCa to compensate for reduced contractility in the setting of heart failure. As has been reported for animal models of hypertrophy and failure, there was no significant difference in the myofilament force–pCa relationships. These data suggest that the contractile failure seen in heart failure is *not* due to diminished responsiveness of the myofilaments to calcium.

Other studies have suggested that there may be an altered response of receptor expression in hearts from patients with ischemic cardiomyopathy than with idiopathic dilated cardiomyopathy (46). In some patients with coronary artery disease the force–pCa relationship is shifted to the right, suggesting a decreased sensitivity of the myofilaments (Fig. 12). This may reflect an effect of chronic ischemia on myofilament isoforms. Recently, Anderson et al. reported differences in troponin T expression between control and myopathic hearts (47). We have previously proposed that changes in troponin T isoforms may explain the differential effects seen in myopathic myocardium in response to the inotropic agent DPI 201–106 (5). In myopathic tissue the force–pCa relationship was shifted to the left in the presence of 1 μM DPI, suggesting an increase in myofilament sensitivity, whereas in control tissue no change was noted in the force–pCa relationship in the presence of 1 μM DPI.

III. MORPHOLOGIC CORRELATES

Myocardium is limited in its response to insult. The heart can either hypertrophy and/or undergo necrosis with replacement fibrosis (hyperplasia has not been demonstrated in adult myocardium). Of course this is a simplified view, not taking into account dilatation, fiber reorientation, fibrin deposition, vascular changes, and hyperplasia of other cellular components. One marker of idiopathic dilated cardiomyopathy is enlarged, bizarre nuclei and myocyte hypertrophy. We have reported enlargement of nuclear area and fiber diameter in myocardium from patients with end-stage heart failure (2). Therefore, our findings of abnormal calcium

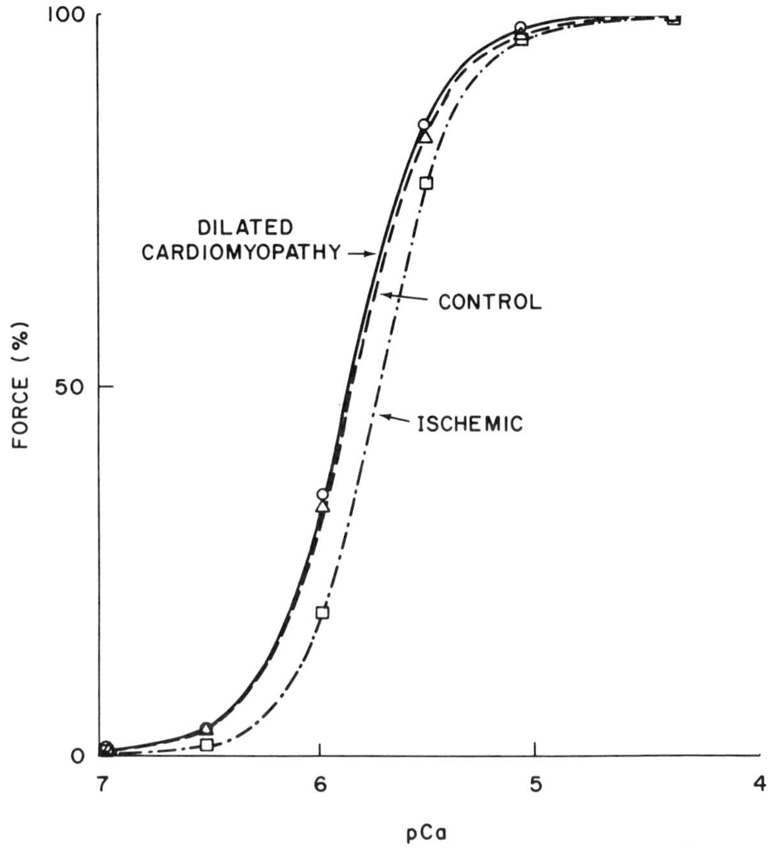

Figure 12 Force–pCa in trabeculae carneae from a normal heart, a patient with ischemic heart disease due to coronary artery disease, and a patient with dilated idiopathic cardiomyopathy.

handling and prolongation of the action potential duration without alteration in myofilament responsiveness may reflect the hypertrophied state in the setting of heart failure.

The effects of fibrous connective tissue on contractility have not been fully assessed. Fibrous connective tissue is increased in animal models of pressure overload hypertrophy and in patients with end-stage heart failure. This is particularly evident in end-stage heart failure patients with coronary artery disease. Using a point-counting technique, we have found the fibrous connective tissue content to be 12±1% in normal human myocardium and 25±10% in diseased myocardium. One can imagine that if the placement of fibrous connective tissue is such that hypertrophied fibers contract against a relatively noncompliant region, that force would be transduced throughout the system, resulting in preserved if not enhanced contractile force (similar to a large spring moving a noncompliant target). Likewise, if the myoctyes are restricted in their contraction due to the presence of fibrous connective tissue, force production would be reduced (48). The relative contribution of fibrous tissue replacement to myocardial failure will have to await further study.

Table 3 Force Potentiation with Increased Stimulation Rate from 0.33 to 1 Hz

Clinical Diagnosis		N
Idiopathic cardiomyopathy	4	9
Coronary artery disease	2	6
Control	2	8
Passive tension ↑	27%	0%
Active tension ↓	60%	0%
Active tension ↑	13%	100%

The similarity in peak contracile force between control and myopathic tissue we have reported (1,2) might therefore be due to selection of muscles relatively free of fibrous connective tissue and scarring, the relatively hypothermic conditions (30°C) under which the muscles were studied, and/or the relatively slow stimulation rates (0.33 Hz) used. In normal human ventricular myocardium there is a positive treppe effect. As demonstrated in Table 3, there is diminished force augmentation at higher frequencies of stimulation in myopathic human myocardium. This is often associated with an increase in end-diastolic tone and resting calcium. The associated Ca^{2+} transient amplitude is unchanged from normal myocardium in myopathic muscles even when a negative treppe effect is observed.

To address the question of whether this might reflect changes in myofilament calcium responsiveness, we used tetanized myocardium from myopathic hearts to obtain steady-state force–calcium relationships. Muscles were tetanized by increasing the stimulation rate to 15–20 Hz with a pulse duration of 50 msec at varying $[Ca^{2+}]_o$. This allowed us to relate tetanus force and $[Ca^{2+}]$. This relationship was described by the modified Hill equation:

$$\frac{F = [Ca^{2+}]^n}{F_{max}[Ca^{2+}]_{50}+[Ca^{2+}]^n}$$

where F is the force developed, F_{max} maximal Ca^{2+} activated force, $[Ca^{2+}]_{50\%}$ the concentration required for 50% activation, and n is the Hill coefficient. We have used this technique to derive information about the sensitivity of the myofilaments to Ca^{2+} in intact preparations. In concordance with our findings in skinned fibers, there was no difference in myofilament calcium responsiveness between control and myopathic tissue when stimulated at a basal frequency of 0.33 Hz followed by immediate tetanization (Fig. 13). The $Ca_{50\%}$ (μM) for normal and myopathic myocardium was 0.56±0.05 vs. 0.54±0.09, respectively; the Hill coefficient was 5.21±0.2 vs 5.61±0.6, respectively (27). To investigate the potential effect of higher frequencies of stimulation in myopathic tissue on force–calcium relationships, tetani were derived after a basal frequency of 1 Hz with and without periods of delay and compared to force–calcium relationships derived in the presence of varying extracellular calcium derived at a basal frequency of 0.33 Hz. As demonstrated in Figure 14, there was no potentiation of force with immediate tetanization after stimulating the muscle at a basal frequency of 1 Hz. However, with varying delays there was potentiation of peak tetanus force. The fact that the intracellular calcium concentrations attained after 1 Hz stimulation with no delay in 2.5 mM $[Ca^{2+}]_o$ were

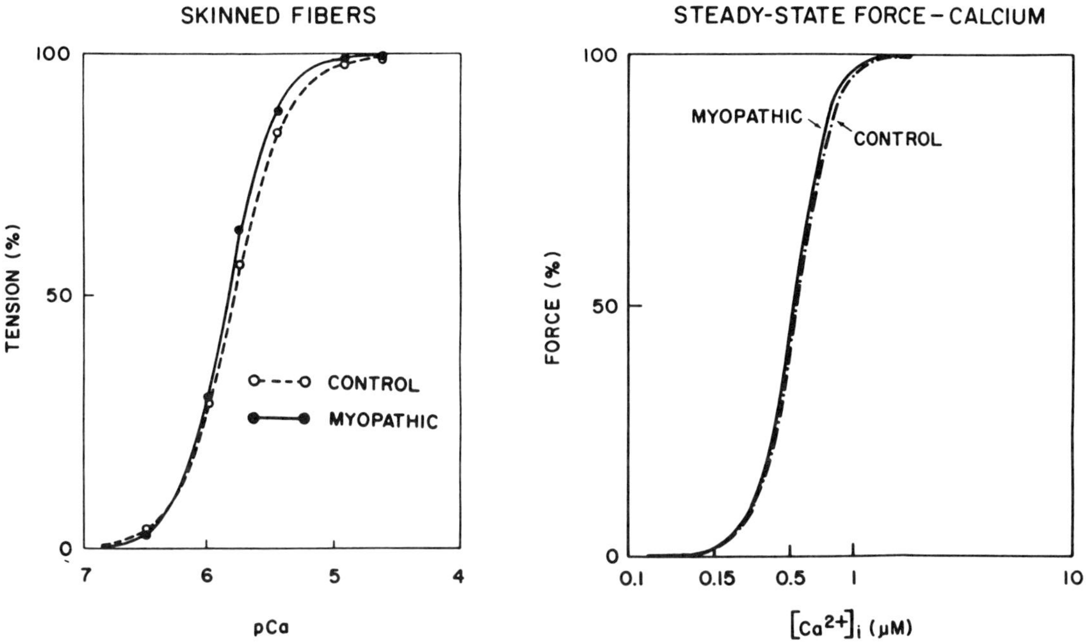

Figure 13 Force–pCa and steady-state force–$[Ca^{2+}]_i$ relationships in control and myopathic myocardium.

similar to that attained at 0.33 Hz in the presence of 8 mM extracellular calcium, yet the force was similar to that attained at 2 mM extracellular calcium, demonstrates a clear decrease in myofilament calcium sensitivity. This is most likely due to accumulation of inorganic phosphate and other metabolites due to high-energy phosphate utilization. Inorganic phosphate has been shown to decrease myofilament calcium sensitivity and to reduce maximal calcium activated force (49). Further, Ingwall et al. have shown that total creatine kinase activity is reduced in hypertrophied and failing human myocardium (3,50).

It has recently been demonstrated in Indo-1-loaded myocytes from the hearts of patients with ischemic cardiomyopathy undergoing cardiac transplantation that there is a progressive rise in resting $[Ca^{2+}]_i$ as well as a decrease in diastolic cell length (31). Resting calcium was ≈ 375 nM after depolarization from −75 mV to −15 mV or −55 mV to +5 mV. This is similar to findings in aequorin-loaded trabeculae carneae (resting calcium 370±10 nM) at 0.33 Hz (6) from patients with ischemic cardiomyopathy undergoing cardiac transplantation. Furthermore, in isolated myoctyes the contractions were found to be more dramatic than the increase in the amplitude of $[Ca^{2+}]_i$ transients superimposed on the rising diastolic $[Ca^{2+}]_i$. The peak I_{Ca} decreased as the contractions increased (31). The effect of $[Ca^{2+}]_i$ on I_{Ca} was proposed as a mechanism in the pathophysiology seen in myopathic myocardium by Gwathmey et al. (6) and is supported by these findings. As demonstrated in Figure 15, there is a progressive abbreviation of the action potential duration by increasing the stimulation rates from 0.33 to 1 Hz in myopathic tissue. In control tissue the action potential abbreviates and stabilizes within a few contrac-

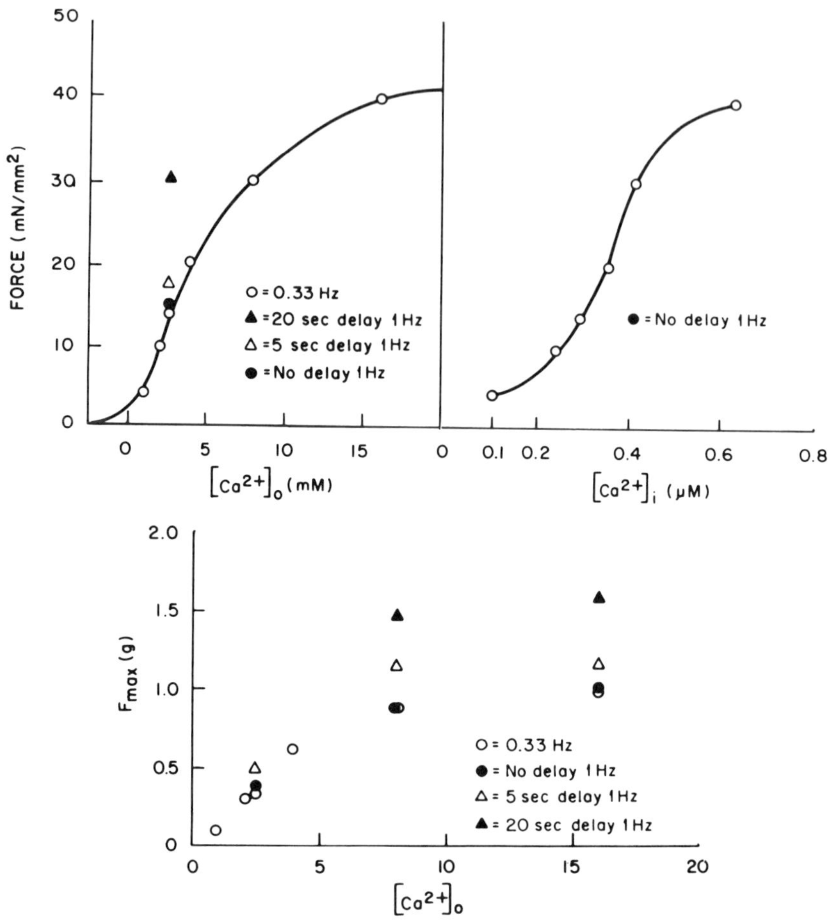

Figure 14 Steady-state force–calcium relationships: effect of tetanizations at 1 Hz basal stimulation rate with and without delays.

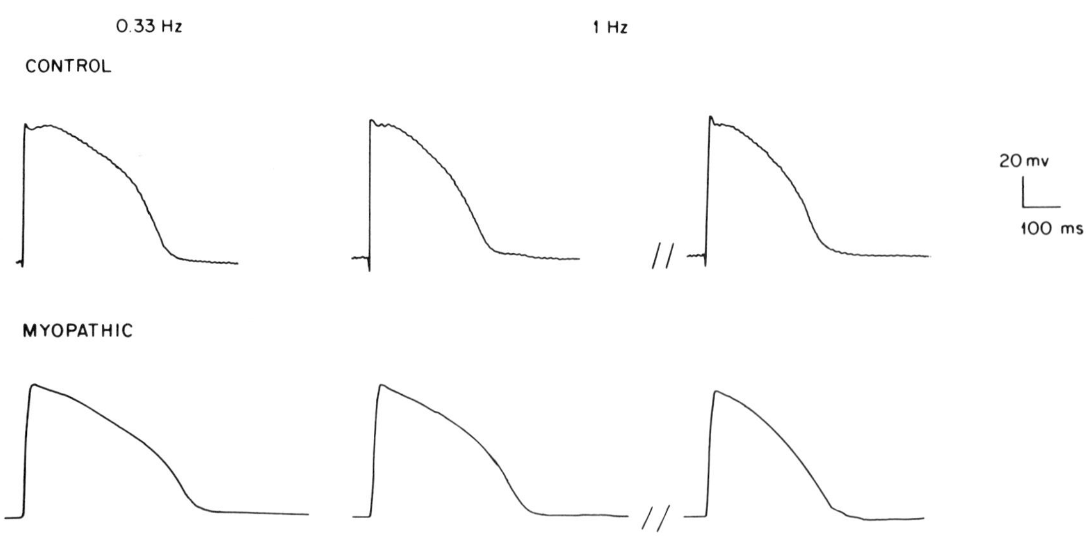

Figure 15 Effect of increasing the stimulation rate in control and myopathic trabeculae on action potential duration.

tions. Lederer et al. (31) arrived at similar conclusions to Gwathmey et al. (6), that even though there may be a progressive loading of the sarcoplasmic reticulum it appears clear that the rising diastolic $[Ca^{2+}]_i$ plays a major role in the contraction staircase. Furthermore, Lederer et al. found that $[Ca^{2+}]$ during rest was about 240 nM at a holding potential of −75 mV. Depolarization to −55 mV led to an increase in $[Ca^{2+}]_i$ to about 290 nM. Thus resting $[Ca^{2+}]_i$ was found to be sensitive to membrane potential as proposed and demonstrated by Gwathmey et al. (4,6). They also found that peak $[Ca^{2+}]_i$ attained during a 60 mV depolarization holding potential was about 1 μM. This is similar to 1.26±0.29 μM reported by Gwathmey et al. (6,27).

These experiments emphasize the importance of physiological perturbations in intact preparations in bringing out functional abnormalities. We have reported no difference in peak developed isometric twitch force between control and myopathic tissues (1,2). One now has to re-evaluate these findings. There is a differential effect between varying the rate and/or pattern of stimulation. The inotropic response to postextrasystolic potentiation was preserved in diseased myocardium. Normal and myopathic tissues attained similar peak twitch force and peak intracellular calcium (2,6). Demonstrated in Figure 16 is the effect of interpolated beats (paired stimulation) on force and calcium in normal and diseased myocardium. These data suggest that if allowed sufficient time to complete restitution processes, myopathic tissue has the potential of attaining similar force as normal myocardium.

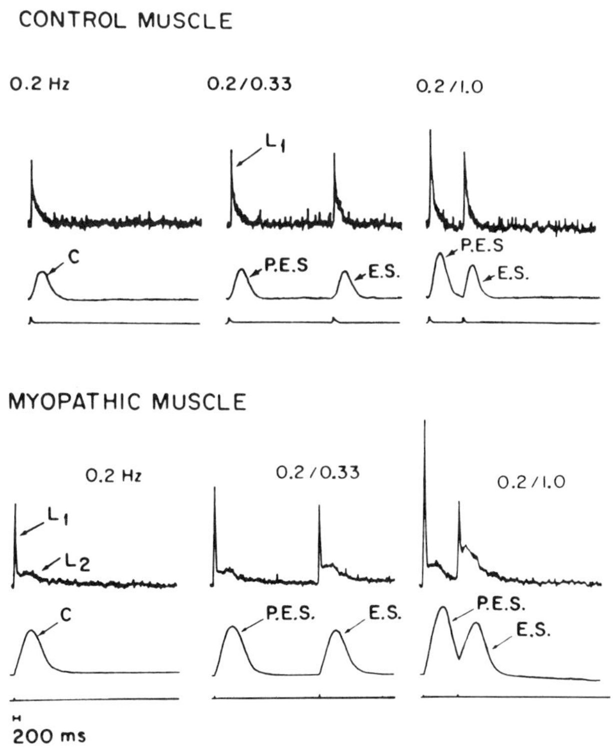

Figure 16 Effect of using the protocol of paired stimulation on force and calcium. P.E.S., postextrasystole; E.S., extrasystole.

Table 4 Time Constants (*T*) and Y Intercepts (Y°) for Postextrasystolic Potentiation in Control and Myopathic Myocardium as a Function of Extrasystolic Interval

	Peak Developed Force		Peak Intracellular Calcium	
	T	Y°	*T*	Y°
Control	5400	216	4900	186
Myopathic	5170	196	4300	204

Postextrasystolic potentiation force curves and restitution curves for extrasystoles both fit a monoexponential using a nonlinear least-squared error algorithm with similar time constants and Y intercepts (Table 4). This suggests a single common underlying mechanism, most likely the sarcoplasmic reticulum. The calcium transients as detected with aequorin for postextrasystole curves similarly fit a monoexponential with similar time constants and Y intercepts for control and myopathic tissue. The extrasystole was potentiated in both control and myopathic myocardium. However, in myopathic tissue L_2 similarly fit a monoexponential for restitution curves. The peak calcium transient associated with the extrasystole was not potentiated. These data suggest that calcium fluxing across the sarcolemma can directly activate the myofilaments in human myocardium. This idea is supported by the observation that the force–frequency relationship fit a double exponential, suggesting at least two underlying factors: sarcolemmal calcium flux and sarcoplasmic reticulum calcium release.

IV. PATHOPHYSIOLOGY OF CARDIOMYOPATHY IN HUMANS

We have demonstrated that excitation–contraction coupling is abnormal in hearts from patients with end-stage heart failure. We have shown that patients with heart failure are not in failure due to a diminished intracellular calcium availability. There is, however, diminished myofibrillar protein content and increased fibrous connective tissue that might explain in part the occurrence of heart failure. The myofilaments' responsiveness to calcium is similarly not altered and cannot explain the reduced contractile performance seen in these hearts. So we are left with the question of why these hearts are in failure. One possible explanation is that failure is related to energy metabolism as well as abnormal calcium mobilization and utilization. A relative "calcium overload" state with resultant additional electrolyte imbalances results in decreased systolic function and decreased diastolic compliance. If this is true, it would explain why tachycardia is so poorly tolerated in patients with significant hypertrophy and failure.

V. THERAPEUTIC IMPLICATIONS

In myopathic myocardium there is not a diminished availability of intracellular calcium. On the contrary, there is elevated resting calcium in the diseased state. Peak intracellular calcium release from the sarcoplasmic reticulum is similar if not greater than that seen in normal myocardium. There is, however, abnormal calcium mobilization in myopathic human myocardium. This may result in a drain on already compromised energy stores in an effort to extrude and reuptake this intracellular calcium. Furthermore, depletion of high-energy phosphates and/or altered utilization and *flux* would result in the accumulation of inorganic phosphate and other metabolites which affect contractile protein activation.

If the contractile failure is due to a "calcium overload" and "energy imbalance," inotropic agents that work solely by increasing intracellular calcium and/or increasing the sensitivity of the myofilaments to calcium would be expected to have little beneficial effect in the treatment of heart failure, and may actually worsen the condition. Agents targeted at improving intracellular calcium mobilization would appear warranted. Agents that specifically improve sarcoplasmic reticulum calcium handling and energetics should prove of benefit. Such agents could then be used in combination with agents such as digitalis that increase intracellular calcium, thereby producing further inotropy. In this scheme it is important to keep in mind the pivotal role played by diastolic function and its interrelationship with systolic performance.

Heart failure is defined as dysfunction of myocardial contractility. Evidence that contractility is depressed in the failing heart has led to the logical corollary that an increase in myocardial contractility should benefit patients with heart failure. The area of cardiovascular treatment and research has focused primarily on the use and development of inotropic agents that increase intracellular calcium concentration. Nevertheless, current treatment modalities have only affected the long-range outcome of congestive heart failure in a palliative way. Therefore, the use of drugs that increase myocardial $[Ca^{2+}]_i$ to alleviate depressed myocardial contractility has been unsuccessful. This lack of success necessitates the investigation of agents that work via mechanisms other than an increase in intracellular calcium availability. Our data suggest that agents that increase intracellular calcium may not only not be curative, but may also in actuality be culprits in the progression of cardiomyopathy.

ACKNOWLEDGMENTS

This work has been supported in part by a Biomedical Research Support Grant, Massachusetts Heart Association Affiliate Grant-in-Aid, CVD Institute, and National Institutes of Health (HL-39091 and HL-36797) to JKG.

Special gratitude is extended to transplant recipients and the families of organ donors. The authors wish to thank the New England Organ bank, for without their cooperation these experiments could not have been performed. Drs. James Marsh and Frederick Schoen are thanked for procurement of diseased tissue. Ms. Joan Burke is thanked for secretarial support.

REFERENCES

1. Feldman MD, Copelas L, Gwathmey JK, Phillips P, Schoen F, Grossman W, Morgan JP. Deficient production of cyclic AMP: pharmacologic evidence of an important cause of contractile dysfunction in patients with end-stage heart failure. Circulation 1987; 75:331–9.
2. Gwathmey JK, Copelas L, MacKinnon R, Schoen FJ, Feldman MD, Grossman W, Morgan JP. Abnormal intracellular calcium handling in myocardium from patients with end-stage heart failure. Circ Res 1987;61:70–6.

3. Ingwall JS, Kramer MF, Fifer MA, Lorell BH, Shemin R, Grossman W, Allen PD. The creatine kinase system in normal and diseased human myocardium. N Engl J Med 1985;313:1050–4.
4. Gwathmey JK, Slawsky MT, Briggs GM, Morgan JP. The role of intracellular sodium in the regulation of intracellular calcium and contractility: the effects of DPI 201-106 on excitation–contraction coupling in human ventricular myocardium. J Clin Invest 1988;82(5):1592–605.
5. Hajjar RJ, Gwathmey JK, Briggs MG, Morgan JP. Differential effects of DPI 201-106 on the sensitivity of the myofilaments to Ca^{2+} in intact and skinned trabeculae from control and myopathic human hearts. J Clin Invest 1988;82(5):1578–84.
6. Gwathmey JK, Slawsky MT, Hajjar RJ, Briggs GM, Morgan JP. Role of intracellular calcium handling in force interval relationships of human ventricular myocardium. J Clin Invest 1990;85:1599–613.
7. Feldman MD, Gwathmey JK, Phillips P, Schoen F, Grossman W, Morgan JP. Reversal of the force–frequency relationship in working myocardium from patients with end-stage heart failure. J Appl Cardiol 1988;3:273–83.
8. Warren SE, Gwathmey JK, Feldman MD, Phillips P, Grossman W, Morgan JP. Inotropic and lusitropic effects of DPI 201-106 on human myocardium. J Appl Cardiol 1989;4:177–88.
9. Warren SE, Kihara Y, Pesaturo J, Gwathmey JK, Phillips P, Morgan JP. Inotropic and lusitropic effects of MCI-154(6-[4-(4-pyridyl)aminophenyl]4,5-dihydro-3)(2H)-pyridazinone) on human myocardium. J Mol Cell Cardiol 1989;21:1037–45.
10. Phillips PJ, Gwathmey JK, Feldman MD, Schoen FJ, Grossman W, Morgan JP. Postextrasystolic potentiation and force frequency relationship: differential augmentation of myocardial contractility in working myocardium from patients with end-stage heart failure J Mol Cell Cardiol 1990;22:99–110.
11. Denniss AR, Colucci WS, Allen PD, Marsh JD. Distribution and function of human ventricular beta adrenergic receptors in congestive heart failure. J Mol Cell Cardiol 1989;21(7):651–60.
12. Pagani ED, Alousi AA, Grant AM, Older TM, Dziuban SW Jr, Allen PD. Changes in myofibrillar content and Mg-ATPase activity in ventricular tissues from patients with heart failure caused by coronary artery disease, cardiomyopathy, or mitral valve insufficiency. Circ Res 1988;63(2):380–5.
13. Mercadier J, Lompre A, Duc P, Boheler KR, Fraysee J, Wisnewsky C, Allen PD, Komajda M, Schwartz K. Altered sarcoplasmic reticulum Ca^{2+}–ATPase gene expression in the human ventricle during end-stage heart failure. J Clin Invest 1990, 85:305–9.
14. Gwathmey JK, Warren S, Briggs GM, Copelas L, Feldman MD, Phillips PJ, Callahan M, Schoen FJ, Grossman W, Morgan JP: Diastolic dysfunction in hypertrophic cardiomyopathy: effect on active force generation during systole. J Clin Invest 1991;87:1023–31.
15. Morgan JP, Morgan KG. Calcium and cardiovascular function: intracellular calcium levels during contraction and relaxation of mammalian cardiac and vascular smooth muscles as detected with aequorin. Am J Med 1984; 77 (Suppl 5A):33–46.
16. Wagner JA, Reynolds IJ, Weisman HF, Dudeck P, Weisfeldt ML, Snyder SH. Calcium antagonist receptors in cardiomyopathic hamster: selective increases in heart, muscle, brain. Science 1986;232:515–8.
17. Finkel MS, Marks ES, Patterson RE, Spier EH, Steadman K, Keiser HR. Increased cardiac calcium channels in hamster cardiomyopathy. Am J Cardiol 1986;57:1205–6.
18. Wagner JA, Sax FL, Weisman HF, Porterfield J, McIntosh C, Weisfeldt ML, Synder SH, Epstein SE. Calcium antagonist receptors in the atrial tissue of patients with hypertrophic cardiomyopathy. N Engl J Med 1989;320:755–61.
19. Movsesian MA, Bristow MR, Krall J. Ca^{2+} uptake by cardiac sarcoplasmic reticulum from patients with dilated cardiomyopathy. Circ Res 1989;65:1141–4.

20. Movsesian M, Colyer J, Wang JH, Krall J. Phospholamban mediated stimulation of Ca^{2+} uptake in sarcoplasmic reticulum from normal and failing hearts. J Clin Invest 1990;85:1698–702.
21. Mignery GA, Sudhof TC, Takei K, De Camilli P. Putative receptor for inositol 1, 4, 5-trisphosphate similar to ryanodine receptor. Nature 1989;342:192–5.
22. Putney JW, Takemura H, Hughes AR, Horstman DA, Thastrup O. How do inositol phosphates regulate calcium signaling? FASEB J 1989;3:1899–905.
23. Vites AM, Pappano AJ. Ryanodine and ruthenium red prevent inositol 1, 4, 5-trisphosphate-induced contractures in atrial muscle. Circulation 1989;80(4):II–445.
24. Kawaguchi H, Shouki M, Yasuda Y. Calcium release from microsomes was stimulated by inositol triphoshate in rat heart Circulation 1989;80(4):II–443.
25. Smith JS, Coronado R, Meissner G. Single channel measurements of the calcium release channel from skeletal muscle sarcoplasmic reticulum. J Gen Physiol 1986; 88:573–88.
26. Chamberlain BK, Volpe P, Fleischer S. Calcium-induced calcium release from purified cardiac sarcoplasmic reticulum vesicles. J of Biological Chemistry 1984;259(12):7540–6.
27. Gwathmey JK, Hajjar RJ. Force–calcium relationships in human myocardium. J Mol Cell Cardiol 1989;21(suppl III):s.10.
28. Swain JL, Sabina RL, Peyton RB, Jones RN, Wechsler AS, Holmes EW. Derangements in myocardial purine and pyrimidine nucleotide metabolism in patients with coronary artery disease and left ventricular hypertrophy. Proc Natl Acad Sci USA 1982;79:655–9.
29. Bashore TM, Magorien DJ, Letterio J, Shaffer P, Unverferth DV. Histologic and biochemical correlates of left ventricular chamber dynamics in man. J Am Coll Cardiol 1987;9:734–42.
30. Yue DT. Intracellular $[Ca^{2+}]$ related to rate of force development in twitch contraction of heart. Am J Physiol 1987;252:H760–70.
31. Lederer WJ, Berlin JR, Cohen NM, Hadley RW, Bers DM, Cannell MB. Excitation–contraction coupling in heart cells. Roles of the sodium–calcium exchange, the calcium current, and the sarcoplasmic reticulum. Ann NY Acad Sci 1990;588:190–206.
32. Hohl CM, Hu B, Wimsatt, Fertel RH, Starling RC, Brierley GP, Altschuld RA. Isolated myocytes from a normal human heart. In: N. Sperelakis, ed. Frontiers in smooth muscle research. New York: Alan R. Liss, 1990.
33. Li Q, Biagi B, Hohl C, Starling R, Stokes B, Altschuld R. Effects of isoproterenol and caffeine on calcium transients and action potentials in human ventricular cardiomyocytes. In: N. Sperelakis, ed. Frontiers in smooth muscle research. New York: Alan R. Liss, 1990.
34. Barcenas-Ruiz L, Beucklemann, Wier WG. Sodium–calcium exchange in heart: membrane currents and changes in $[Ca^{2+}]_i$. Science 1987;238:1720–2.
35. Barcenas-Ruiz L, Wier WG. Voltage dependence of intracellular $[Ca^{2+}]_i$ transients in quinea pig ventricular myocytes. Circ Res 1987;61:148–54.
36. Bridge JHB, Smolley JR, Spitzer KW. The relationship between charge movements associated with I_{ca} and $I_{Na\text{-}Ca}$ in cardiac myocytes. Science 1990;248;376–8.
37. Bridge JHB, Spitzer KW, Ershler PR. Relaxation of isolated ventricular cardiomyocytes by a voltage-dependent process. Science 1988;214:823–5.
38. Pesaturo J, Gwathmey JK. The role of mitochondria and sarcoplasmic reticulum calcium handling upon reoxygenation of hypoxic myocardium. Circ Res 1990;66:696–709.
39. Li Q, Biagi B, Starling R, Hohl C, Altschuld R, Stokes B. Characteristics of calcium transients and electrophysiology in human ventricular myocytes. Biophys J 1989; 55:488a (abstr).
40. Wier WG. Calcium transients during excitation–contraction coupling in mammalian heart: aequorin signals of canine Purkinje fibers. Science 1980;207:1085–7.

41. Wier WG, Isenberg G. Intracellular [Ca^{2+}] transients in voltage clamped cardiac Purkinge fibers. Pflugers Arch 1982;392:284–90.
42. Hess P, Wier WG. Excitation–contraction coupling in cardiac Purkinje fibers: effects of caffeine on the intracellular [Ca^{2+}] transient, membrane currents, and contraction. J Gen Physiol 1984;83:417–33.
43. Gwathmey JK, Nakao S, Come PC, Goad MEP, Serur JR, Als AV, Abelmann WH. An experimental model of acute and subacute viral myocarditis in the pig. JACC 1992;19:864–869.
44. Gwathmey JK, Morgan JP. Calcium handling in myocardium from amphibian, avian, and mammalian species: the search for two components. J Comp Physiol B 1991; 161:19–25.
45. Garvey JL, Kranicis EG, Solaro RJ. Phosphorylation of C-protein, troponin I, and phospholamban in isolated rabbit hearts. Biochem J 1988;249:709–14.
46. Port JD, Larrabee P, Wiederin J, Durham DW, Rasmussen R, Bristow MR. Differences in ventricular myocardial β receptor expression in ischemic vs. idiopathic dilated cardiomyopathy. Circulation 1989:80(4):II–8.
47. Anderson PAW, Malouf NN, Oakeley AE, Pagani ED, Allen PD. Tropmin T isoform expression in humans. A comparison among normal and failing adult heart, fetal heart, and adult and fetal skeletal muscle. Circ Res 1991;69:1226–1233.
48. Doering CW, Janicki JS, Pick R, Shroff SG, Weber KT. Fibrillar collagen and myocardial stiffeners in intact hypertrophied rat left ventricle. Cir Res 1989;64:1041–50.
49. Herzig JW, Peterson JW, Ruegg JC, Solaro RJ. Vanadate and phosphate ions reduce tension and increase cross-bridge kinetics in chemically skinned heart muscle. Biochim Biophys Acta 1981;672:191–6.
50. Nascimben L, Pauletto P, Pessina AC, Reis I, Ingwall JS. Decreased energy reserve may cause pump failure in human dilated cardiomyopathy. Circulation 1991;84:II–563.

7

Cellular Regulation of Smooth Muscle Contraction

R. ANN WORD and JAMES T. STULL

University of Texas Southwestern Medical Center at Dallas
Dallas, Texas

I. INTRODUCTION

It is well established that a number of hormones and neurotransmitters affect cellular functions by regulating cytoplasmic Ca^{2+} concentration ($Ca^{2+}{}_i$). An increase in the concentration of $Ca^{2+}{}_i$, as a primary second messenger, and binding of Ca^{2+} to calmodulin, results in activation of a number of Ca^{2+}-dependent cellular processes, including smooth muscle contraction (1). The regulation of actin–myosin interactions in smooth muscle by Ca^{2+} is more complex than that in skeletal or cardiac muscle, where contraction is effected by Ca^{2+} binding to troponin on thin filaments. The preponderance of biochemical evidence indicates that Ca^{2+}-dependent myosin phosphorylation serves an obligatory role in the regulation of smooth muscle contraction, although additional mechanisms for regulation are not entirely excluded. For example, contractions effected by excitatory agonists result in a greater increase in myosin light-chain phosphorylation relative to the $Ca^{2+}{}_i$ concentration than those obtained with K^+ depolarization (2–4). This alteration in the Ca^{2+}-sensitivity of smooth muscle contractile elements with different modes of cellular stimulation may be related to changes in the extent of activation of protein kinases or phosphatases. In addition, secondary mechanisms of regulation by other cytoplasmic proteins may exist. Thus, contractile elements in smooth muscle cells are not dependent solely on $Ca^{2+}{}_i$, but may employ additional regulatory mechanisms. The focus of this chapter is on the primary and secondary mechanisms involved in the regulation of contractile elements and their contribution to physiological functions of smooth muscle. Other chapters will emphasize cellular processes involved in the regulation of $Ca^{2+}{}_i$ by way of Ca^{2+} channels and pumps.

II. CONTRACTILE PROTEINS

A. Thick Filament System

1. Myosin

Myosin is the primary protein of smooth muscle thick filaments and is composed of two heavy chain subunits (approximately 200 kDa each) and two each of two types of light chain subunits (20 and 17 kDa, respectively) (5). The native hexameric form of myosin is configured as an α-helical coiled tail region embedded in thick filaments and two globular head regions that protrude from the thick filaments at regular intervals to form cross-bridges (Fig. 1). These head regions contain distinct sites for binding to actin, ATP hydrolysis, and association of light-chain subunits.

Two groups of basic amino acid residues located amino terminal to the phosphorylatable serine in either the smooth or skeletal muscle light chains confer substrate specificity for myosin light-chain kinase (6,7). The smooth muscle myosin light-chain kinase requires an arginine that is three residues amino-terminal to the phosphorylatable serine 19, in addition to three basic residues that are six to eight residues amino-terminal to the phosphorylatable serine. Thus, the serine phosphorylation of myosin light chain by myosin light-chain kinase requires a complex arrangement of substrate determinants, resulting in a high degree of substrate specificity (Fig. 1).

Phosphorylation of both light chains in a myosin molecule is required for an increase in the actin-activated MgATPase activity (8–10). Thus, high levels of myosin light-chain phosphorylation are required for significant increases in MgATPase activity, and the relationship between the amount of myosin light chain phosphorylated and MgATPase activity is nonlinear. The actin-binding site and the junction between the head and neck portion of the myosin molecule are the two sites on myosin influenced by light-chain phosphorylation. It has been proposed

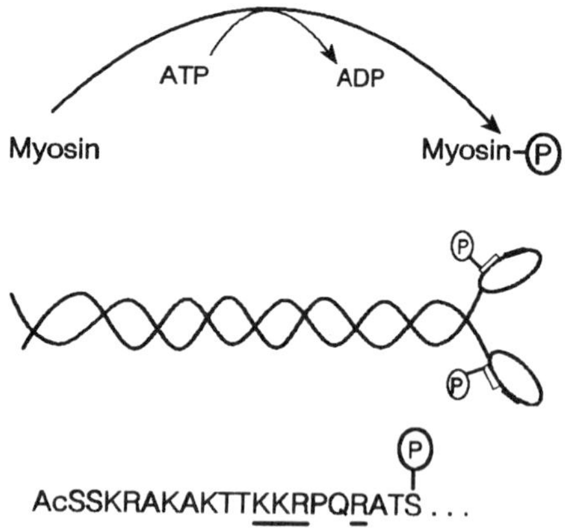

Figure 1 Schematic representation of myosin and its phosphorylation. Two heavy-chain subunits with their respective intertwined tail regions and globular head regions are associated with one each of two types of light chains, the 20 kDa regulatory (or phosphorylatable) light chain and the 17 kDa light chain. The amino acid sequence of the regulatory light chain is provided. The basic residues that confer substrate specificity for Ca^{2+}/calmodulin-dependent myosin light chain kinase are underlined.

that phosphorylation of myosin light chains results in an increased flexibility at the head/neck junction, thereby facilitating actin-activated MgATPase activity (11). Future biochemical investigations will focus on the mechanisms by which this conformational change increases actin-activated MgATPase activity.

In general, there is a linear relationship between myosin light chain phosphorylation and steady state force from 0 to about 50% phosphorylation in intact and skinned smooth muscle fibers (12). Although these physiological results would appear to contradict biochemical reports on the relationship between light-chain phosphorylation and MgATPase activity, the true relationship is obscured by the complexity of the cellular milieu. It is conceivable that under steady-state conditions both regulatory light chains are phosphorylated within a myosin molecule, that is, all of the phosphorylated myosin exists as the diphosphorylated moiety (even at low extents of phosphorylation). Hence, each myosin molecule that had both light chains phosphorylated would express increased actin-activated MgATPase activity. There are no published reports on the kinetic properties of myosin dephosphorylation in respect to monophosphorylated and dephosphorylated myosin nor on the phosphate distribution in myosin under steady-state conditions. Additional investigations are needed to provide insights into this apparent discrepancy between biochemical and physiological results.

2. *Calmodulin*

Calmodulin (CaM) is a regulatory protein involved in a variety of cellular Ca^{2+}-dependent signaling pathways. CaM displays a large number of functions, particularly for a protein of 148 residues (17 kDa). The binding of 4 Ca^{2+} ions results in conformational changes that allow it to modulate the activities and functions of a large number of enzymes and proteins, including myosin light-chain kinase. CaM binds to many target proteins with high affinity, for example, the dissociation constant for myosin light-chain kinase is approximately 1 nM (5). In contrast to CaM, which is highly conserved from *Paramecium* to humans, the CaM-binding domains of its target proteins (including myosin light-chain kinase) are variable in amino acid sequence. However, CaM binds with high affinity and broad specificity to basic amphiphilic α-helical peptides which has allowed development of a molecular model (13).

Smooth muscle cells contain large amounts of CaM (10–40 μM), and CaM is present in excess of myosin light-chain kinase (1 μM) (5). The concentrations of CaM and kinase are 10,000- and 1,000-fold greater, respectively, than the dissociation constant of Ca^{2+}/calmodulin for myosin light-chain kinase. Furthermore, the dissociation constants of CaM for Ca^{2+} are decreased 10–50-fold when CaM binds to target proteins such as myosin light-chain kinase (14). These cellular and biochemical properties dictate positively cooperative activation of myosin light-chain kinase at Ca^{2+} concentrations less than 1 μM, which is the range associated with myosin light-chain phosphorylation in smooth muscle cells.

3. *Myosin Light-Chain Kinase*

Myosin light-chain kinase provides a simple model for the study of Ca^{2+}-calmodulin-regulated enzymes. The inactive enzyme exists as a monomer with an apparent molecular mass ranging from 130,000 to 150,000 in smooth muscle cells from various animal species (5). When Ca^{2+} binds to calmodulin, myosin light-chain kinase is activated by the binding of 1 mol calmodulin mol kinase. The precise biochemical mechanism by which Ca^{2+}/calmodulin activates myosin light-chain kinase is not clear. Limited tryptic cleavage of smooth muscle myosin light-chain kinase results in the generation of an active 61 kDA Ca^{2+}/calmodulin-*independent* myosin light-chain kinase (15–17). The calmodulin-binding domain of myosin light-chain kinase is located between residues 796 and 813 of the chicken smooth muscle myosin light-chain kinase (18,19). Thus, myosin light-chain kinase contains an inhibitory region and a calmodulin-binding domain (19). The inhibitory region has been defined by site-directed mutagenesis to be contained within residues 794–800 and includes the amino acid sequence Tyr-Met-Ala-Arg-Arg-Lys-Trp (20). Synthetic peptides modeled after this region inhibit the kinase activity of the constitutively active 61 kDa myosin light-chain kinase fragment (17). One of these peptides (783–804) is a competitive inhibitor with myosin light chain as substrate, probably due to similarity in structure with the three basic residues. Thus, it has been postulated that the inhibitory region mimics the light-chain substrate, and is a pseudosubstrate prototope that binds to the active site of the kinase in the absence of calmodulin (21). Pseudosubstrates have been proposed as a mechanism of regulating the activity of other allosterically regulated enzymes (15). This mechanism of regulation, however, has not been directly proven for myosin light-chain kinase. Recent kinetic experiments indicate that a more complex model may be required (22). In addition, substitution of these same basic residues to acidic residues in skeletal muscle myosin light chain kinase did not result in a constitutively active kinase (23). However, the affinity of the mutated kinase for CaM was decreased.

A central catalytic core region of the smooth muscle myosin light-chain kinase contains many residues that are highly conserved among protein kinases (24,25). It has recently been suggested that a region immediately amino-terminal to the catalytic core of the rabbit skeletal muscle myosin light-chain kinase is involved in protein substrate binding (25,26). Alteration of one group of acidic residues in this region results in a 10-fold increase in the K_m value for myosin light chain. These acidic residues may bind directly to basic residues in the myosin light-chain substrate. Acidic residues occupy a similar position in the smooth muscle myosin light-chain kinase. Thus, protein kinases may have a common catalytic core with residues involved in the phosphotransferase reaction and an additional distinct region that confers protein substrate specificity.

4. *Protein Phosphatases*

Dephosphorylation of myosin light chain by myosin light-chain phosphatase is also important in the regulation of smooth muscle contractility. Whereas the structure, function, and mechanism of regulation of myosin light-chain kinase have been defined, the structure, function, and regulation of myosin light-chain phosphatase are uncertain. Smooth muscle, like many tissues, contains a number of protein phosphatases most of which have broad and overlapping substrate specificities. The protein phosphatase, responsible for the rapid dephosphorylation of myosin light chain in smooth muscle, has not been clearly established. There are four general classes of serine/threonine protein phosphatases, referred to as types 1, 2A, 2B, and 2C (27). Type 1 protein phosphatase binds to contractile proteins in skeletal and cardiac muscles and catalyzes the dephosphorylation of myosin light chain in vitro (28,29). The catalytic subunit of type 1 phosphatase binds via an unidentified protein (the M subunit) in myofibrils and a different protein (G subunit) in glycogen. Multisite phosphorylation of the glycogen-binding subunit by glycogen synthase kinase 3 and cAMP-dependent protein kinase is associated with release of the catalytic subunit (30). Type 2A protein phosphatase represents the major soluble phosphatase activity toward myosin in cardiac muscle (31).

Bovine aortic smooth muscle myosin light-chain kinase phosphatases have been identified as soluble enzymes with biochemical characteristics of a type 2A phosphatase (32). A multisubunit form of the isolated catalytic subunit of aortic phosphatase 2A dephosphorylates myosin and causes relaxation of skinned fibers from porcine carotid artery (33) and uterine smooth muscle (34). Four protein phosphatases have been purified from gizzard smooth muscle. Smooth muscle myosin phosphatase (SMP IV), which is relatively specific for dephosphorylation of myosin (34), dephosphorylates myosin light chain in skinned muscle fibers (35). A phosphatase with biochemical properties similar to SMP IV is present in rabbit uterine smooth muscle (36). These enzymes are similar but not identical to the more general type 1 protein phosphatase (36). Myosin purified from gizzard smooth muscle also contains type 1-like protein phosphatase activity (36). The mechanism by which it binds to smooth muscle contractile elements has not been defined. In addition, a type 2A-like protein phosphatase also binds to contractile elements in skinned smooth muscle fibers of the ileum (37). By use of the protein phosphatase inhibitors in intact smooth muscle, okadaic acid (more specific for type 2A) (37) and calyculin A (more specific for type I) (38), it appears that type 1 protein phosphatase is the dominant phosphatase that catalyzes the dephosphorylation of myosin light chains. The possibility exists, however, that both protein phosphatases types 1 and 2A may be involved, additional experiments are needed to clarify this problem.

B. Thin Filament System

1. Actin

Although there is general agreement that myosin light-chain kinase phosphorylation plays a major role in the regulation of smooth muscle contraction, there has been considerable effort to investigate other potential regulatory mechanisms, including the identification of proteins associated with actin thin filaments that may alter interactions between myosin cross-bridges and actin. The backbone of the thin filament is organized in a two-stranded helical array of F-actin. The thin filaments in smooth muscle are numerous and appear similar to those of skeletal muscle (39). Of the three major proteins of the contractile apparatus, actin demonstrates the least variation in terms of molecular mass (42 kDa) and ability of G-actin to polymerize to F-actin. Slight differences, however, have been demonstrated by isoelectric focusing. The most acidic form (based on isoelectric points) is α, followed by β and γ (40,41). Within these three classes there are at least six distinct but closely related actin isoforms. In general, the properties of these actins are similar, and most smooth muscles contain a mixture of actin isoforms (39–41). There have been numerous reports on proteins that bind to actin that may either modify polymerization or induce severing of actin filaments (42–44). Although these proteins may influence the assembly and disassembly of thin filaments, their role in the modification of actin isoforms that are more specific to smooth muscle and thus to contractile function is not known.

2. Tropomyosin

Whereas proteins equivalent to the Ca^{2+} regulatory complex troponin (found in cardiac and skeletal muscle) are not present in smooth muscle, tropomyosin is associated with the thin filaments of both skeletal and smooth muscle at a stoichiometry of approximately 1 tropomyosin molecule for each 7 actin molecules. The structure of tropomyosin is conserved among smooth and skeletal types, and despite the absence of troponin in smooth muscle, tropomyosin retains its troponin- and actin-binding sites in smooth muscle (45,46). It is has been shown that smooth muscle tropomyosin modifies actomyosin ATPase activity (in general, a tendency for activation) (39). The position of tropomyosin on smooth muscle thin filaments (as studied by x-ray diffraction) is altered upon activation of smooth muscle (46,47). Thus, it is postulated that tropomyosin may play a role in the regulation of the formation of actomyosin cross-bridges; however, the biochemical mechanism (in the absence of troponin) is incompletely understood in smooth muscle.

3. Caldesmon

Caldesmon is a long, flexible, basic 93 kDa protein associated with actin filaments in smooth muscle and many nonmuscle motile cells (*e.g.*, platelets) (48). On SDS-gels, caldesmon runs as two bands corresponding to 120–140 kDa (caldesmon-*h*) and a smaller isoform (caldesmon-*l*) as an apparent mass of 76–80 kDa. The cDNA clone for the *h*- form has 576 amino acids and a predicted molecular mass of 87 kDa. The predicted molecular mass from cDNA clones of the *l*- form is 58–60 kDa. The anomalous migration on SDS gels is a result of a high content of glutamic and aspartic residues (49). In smooth muscle cells, caldesmon has a concentration of around 10 μM, and contains distinct binding sites for myosin, actin, tropomyosin, and Ca^{2+}/calmodulin (50,51). In vitro, under physiological conditions of temperature and ionic strength, caldesmon inhibits the actin-activated MgATPase activity of phosphorylated myosin (52,53). Its inhibitory activity is reversed by Ca^{2+}/calmodulin (53–55). Phosphorylation of purified caldesmon by protein kinase C (56,57) and Ca^{2+}/calmodulin dependent protein kinase II (58,59) in vitro, likewise acts to relieve the caldesmon inhibition of actin-activated MgATPase activity of myosin. The phosphorylation of caldesmon at two phosphorylation sites (separate from the actin binding site) in intact smooth muscle has been demonstrated (60). The phosphorylation sites, however, are not those obtained with purified caldesmon phosphorylated by protein kinase C or Ca^{2+}/calmodulin-dependent protein kinase II (60). In intact smooth muscle cells, the nonmuscle isoform (caldesmon -l) is phosphorylated by cdc 2 kinase, the catalytic subunit of mitosis promoting factor (MPF,61). Cdc 2 kinase-induced phosphorylation results in dissociation of caldesmon from the microfilaments, an event associated with cell-rounding during mitosis (61). The physiologic role for cdc 2 kinase-induced phosphorylation in smooth muscle cells or for other phosphorylated forms of caldesmon in the regulation of contraction is not completely established. As outlined in the last section of this chapter, experimental approaches that determine unequivocally that Ca^{2+}/calmodulin regulation of caldesmon controls smooth muscle contractility are complex and difficult to accomplish.

4. Calponin

Calponin, a recently discovered heat-stable, basic, 34 kDa actin-binding protein in smooth muscle, has also been proposed as a candidate for thin filament regulation of actin–myosin interactions (62). Calponin is clearly a distinct protein from caldesmon and myosin light chain kinase, and is antigenically related to the C-terminal half of rabbit skeletal and bovine cardiac troponin T (62,63). Like caldesmon, it binds to tropomyosin and actin, and it inhibits the actin-activated MgATPase activity of myosin (63). Phosphorylation of purified calponin relieves this inhibition, primarily by the loss of actin binding upon phosphorylation (63). However, it has been recently reported that calponin is not phosphorylated in resting or contracted arterial smooth muscle (64). The tissue content of calponin (150 μM) is significantly higher than that of caldesmon (10 μM) but otherwise the two proteins exhibit many similarities. Additional physiological and biochemical investigations are needed to establish a role for calponin in the regulation of actin–myosin interactions in smooth muscle.

III. GENERALIZED SCHEME FOR SMOOTH MUSCLE CONTRACTION

A Calcium and Myosin Light-Chain Phosphorylation

Cytoplasmic Ca^{2+} is believed to be a primary determinant of smooth muscle contraction. The increase in $Ca^{2+}{}_i$ via influx of extracellular Ca^{2+} or through mobilization of intracellular Ca^{2+} stores can be induced by two distinct mechanisms of excitation–contraction coupling: electromechanical coupling, mediated through depolarization of the surface membrane by action potentials, and pharmacomechanical coupling, a mechanism by which agents mediate an increase in $Ca^{2+}{}_i$ independent of cell surface membrane potentials. Pharmacomechanical coupling may involve Ca^{2+} influx via receptor-operated Ca^{2+} channels or by receptor-mediated inositol trisphosphate formation and release of Ca^{2+} from intracellular stores in the sarcoplasmic reticulum. Other chapters may be consulted for details regarding these processes.

The scheme generally accepted to be necessary and sufficient for the biochemical activation of smooth muscle contraction is phosphorylation of the 20 kDa regulatory light chain of myosin (Fig. 2). Under relaxed conditions, the free cytoplasmic Ca^{2+} concentration is low (110–150 nM). Myosin light-chain kinase is minimally active resulting in low amounts of phosphorylated myosin light chain ($<10\%$). Initially, smooth muscle cells are stimulated to contract by an agonist binding to its cell surface receptor or by membrane depolarization, both of which result in an increase in the cytoplasmic Ca^{2+} concentration. Ca^{2+} binds to calmodulin, forming a Ca^{2+}/calmodulin complex (65). The second step of the Ca^{2+}-dependent activation involves Ca^{2+}/calmodulin binding to myosin light-chain kinase and activation of the enzyme. Myosin light-chain kinase catalyzes the phosphorylation of a specific amino acid (serine 19) on the 20 kDa light chain subunit of myosin, which results in activation of actomyosin MgATPase, cross-bridge cycling, and mechanical output, that is, force generation and muscle shortening (12,66–68) (Fig. 2). Sequestration or extrusion of Ca^{2+} from the cell results in inactivation of myosin light-chain kinase followed by dephosphorylation of myosin light chain by myosin light-chain phosphatase, inactivation of myosin MgATPase, and smooth muscle relaxation.

B. Biophysical Properties of Smooth Muscle Contraction

The general scheme described above does not adequately describe all of the physiological and cellular processes involved in smooth muscle contraction (12,68,69).

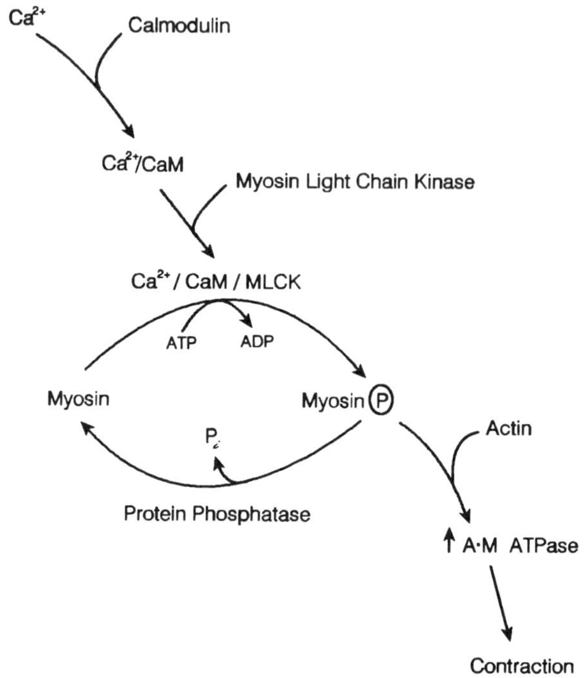

Figure 2 Scheme for regulation of smooth muscle contraction via the myosin light-chain phosphorylation cascade. An increase in cytoplasmic Ca^{2+} ($Ca^{2+}{}_i$) is the primary event that initiates the activation of smooth muscle contractile elements.

Stimulation of many smooth muscles with agonists elicits a transient increase in $Ca^{2+}{}_i$ and myosin light-chain phosphorylation that subsequently declines to low levels while developed force is maintained. The decline in myosin light-chain phosphorylation has also been correlated with a decrease in maximal velocity of shortening, an estimate of cross-bridge cycling rates. Force maintenance with reduced myosin light-chain phosphorylation and maximal shortening velocity has been referred to as a latch state by Murphy and his colleagues (70). These observations have been extended with the development of a quantitative model by which a phosphorylated, myosin cross-bridge may become dephosphorylated while attached to actin. It is proposed that the dephosphorylated cross-bridge (latch bridge) detaches more slowly than the phosphorylated cross-bridge and thus may be responsible for force maintenance at low levels of myosin light-chain phosphorylation (12). Central to this model is the assumption that free and attached cross-bridges are substrates for myosin light-chain kinase and phosphatase, and that the turnover of phosphate in myosin light chain occurs at a relatively high rate. Estimated maximal rates of phosphorylation (1 sec) and dephosphorylation (0.25 sec) are consistent with the model (66,67). The latch bridge model is proposed from physiological experiments and, to date, there have been no biochemical studies that directly demonstrate this unique form of the myosin cross-bridge. Many reports on the correlations between $Ca^{2+}{}_i$, myosin light-chain phosphorylation, maximal shortening velocity, and force in the hog carotid artery are consistent with the latch bridge model as being the primary cellular mechanism regulating contractile properties (12). The latch bridge hypothesis does not, however, exclude secondary mechanisms of regulation.

An alternative explanation for force maintenance in the presence of low levels of myosin light-chain phosphorylation is that there is a single population of force-bearing myosin cross bridges rather than two populations (70). This model requires additional Ca^{2+}-dependent mechanisms to regulate cross-bridge turnover rates and maintenance of force. One possibility proposed is that phosphorylation of myosin heavy light chains by protein kinases (such as protein kinase C) may represent a secondary mechanism of regulation. Purified myosin is phosphorylated at three sites (distinct from the myosin light chain kinase site) by protein kinase C. These sites are not phosphorylated in smooth muscle tissues. In intact smooth muscle, contractions elicited by agonists (carbachol, 5-hydroxytryptamine) and depolarization (KCl) are associated with phosphorylation of myosin light chain at serine 19 (the preferred phosphorylation site of myosin light-chain kinase) with no appreciable phosphate incorporation into protein kinase C sites (71–73). Phosphorylation of purified myosin heavy chain affects the interaction of myosin with actin as well as the assembly of myosin into filaments (74,75). Myosin heavy chain is phosphorylated by protein kinase C and the multifunctional Ca^{2+}/calmodulin-dependent protein kinase II in vitro (75,76). Significant levels of phosphorylation of myosin heavy chain (0.7 mol of phosphate/mol 204 kDa smooth muscle and 0.8 mol phosphate/mol 196 kDa nonmuscle heavy chain) occur in postconfluent smooth muscle cells in culture (77). There is, however, no appreciable myosin heavy-chain phosphorylation in *intact* smooth muscle during relaxation or contraction (71). Thus, under physiological conditions, heavy-chain and light-chain phosphorylation in sites other than serine 19 in the light chain are probably not important in the regulation of smooth muscle contraction.

Although myosin light-chain phosphorylation plays an important role in the initiation of smooth muscle contraction, it is not clear what cellular mechanisms are involved in force maintenance with low levels of myosin light-chain phosphorylation and maximal shortening velocity. Based upon published reports from many laboratories, it appears that the latch bridge hypothesis does not describe all mechansisms regulating smooth muscle contractile elements and that other Ca^{2+}-dependent or perhaps Ca^{2+}-independent processes act in concert with the myosin light chain phosphorylation system (Fig. 3). As mentioned previously, contractions affected by agonists (i.e., carbachol, phenylephrine, $PGF_{2\alpha}$, endothelin) result in greater increases in myosin light-chain phosphorylation relative to $Ca^{2+}{}_i$ than those obtained with K^+ depolarization (2–4), and dissociations between the extent of myosin light-chain phosphorylation and maximal shortening velocity have been observed (78,79). In addition, treatment of bovine tracheal smooth muscle with okadaic acid (a protein phosphatase inhibitor isolated from the marine sponge *Halichondria*) results in a decrease in $Ca^{2+}{}_i$ and relaxation of carbachol-induced contractions despite the maintenance of high levels of myosin light-chain phosphorylation (80). It is clear, then, that other processes may regulate smooth muscle function. This will be discussed in the following section.

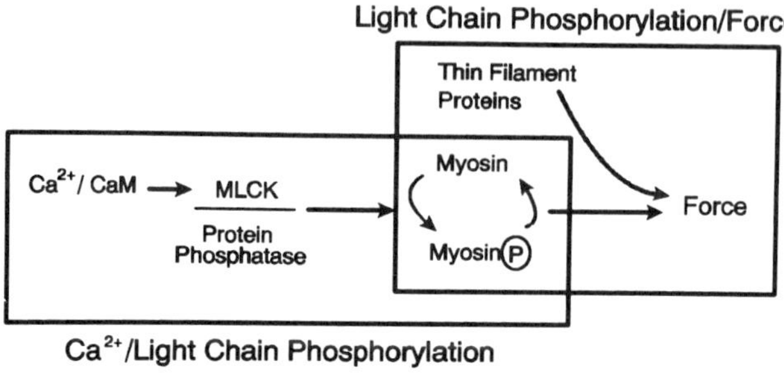

Figure 3 Relationships of different processes in smooth muscle contractile elements. The primary pathway for regulation involves Ca^{2+}-dependent modulation of myosin light-chain kinase activity; however, the relation between Ca^{2+} and light-chain phosphorylation may be modified by additional elements that affect the relative activities of myosin light-chain kinase and phosphatase. It is further hypothesized that the relation between light-chain phosphorylation and force may be affected by other proteins, perhaps residing in the thin filaments.

IV. REGULATION OF THE Ca^{2+} SENSITIVITY OF SMOOTH MUSCLE CONTRACTILE ELEMENTS

In all muscle cells, the cytoplasmic free calcium concentration exerts primary control over the initiation, time course, and force of contraction. Coupling of cell surface signals to intracellular calcium release proceeds by different mechanisms in smooth, cardiac, and skeletal muscle cells. Both voltage-gated calcium channels in the cell surface membranes and intracellular calcium-release channels in the sarcoplasmic reticulum play key roles in smooth muscle contraction.

During force maintenance in the ferret portal vein, phenylephrine-induced contractions are of similar force amplitude to those induced by K^+ depolarization; but the phenylephrine-induced increase in $Ca^{2+}{}_i$ is much less than that obtained with K^+ (2). Thus, the contractile elements are more sensitive to the effects of $Ca^{2+}{}_i$ with phenylephrine stimulation. A number of other investigations have confirmed that the sensitivity of the contractile response (force) to $Ca^{2+}{}_i$ is variable (2–4,81,82). This "sensitization" of the contractile elements to $Ca^{2+}{}_i$ may be a result of changes in two fundamental relationships (Fig. 3): alterations in the $Ca^{2+}{}_i$ dependence of myosin light chain phosphorylation, and changes in the myosin light-chain phosphorylation/force relationship. The $Ca^{2+}{}_i$/myosin light-chain phosphorylation relationship is dependent upon the relative activities of myosin light-chain kinase and phosphatase. The myosin light-chain phosphorylation/force relationship is dependent upon complex interactions within the contractile element system. Both components may be involved in the contracile process.

A. $Ca^{2+}{}_i$/Myosin Light-Chain Phosphorylation

In smooth muscle cells in culture, the cytoplasmic resting Ca^{2+} concentration is low (120–150 nM). Stimulation by agonists (e.g., carbachol, histamine, phenylephrine) or by the Ca^{2+} ionophore, ionomycin, results in an increase in $Ca^{2+}{}_i$ and extent of myosin light-chain phosphorylation. The quantitative relationship between $Ca^{2+}{}_i$ and myosin light-chain phosphorylation is similiar with different agonists (i.e., small increases in $Ca^{2+}{}_i$ lead to increases in myosin light-chain phosphorylation) (83,84). In arterial smooth muscle, there is likewise a single relationship between $Ca^{2+}{}_i$ and the extent of myosin light-chain phosphorylation upon stimulation with various agonists. However, agonist treatment results in greater extents of myosin light-chain phosphorylation at a given $Ca^{2+}{}_i$ compared with the responses obtained with K^+ (4). Thus, there is a decrease in the $Ca^{2+}{}_i$ sensitivity of myosin light-chain phosphorylation with depolarization compared with responses obtained with agonists.

$Ca^{2+}{}_i$-dependent myosin light-chain phosphorylation in smooth muscle is a function of the relative activities of myosin light-chain kinase and myosin light-chain phosphatase. The extent of myosin light-chain phosphorylation may be increased at a specific $Ca^{2+}{}_i$ value due to an increase in myosin light chain kinase activity, a decrease in phosphatase activity, or both (Fig. 4). In addition, a shift in the $Ca^{2+}{}_i$/light-chain phosphorylation curve to the right may result from decreased kinase activity or increased phosphatase activity. Secondary mechanisms of regulation of kinase and phosphatase activities may be important in determining the extent of myosin light-chain phosphorylation, and, ultimately, force development of the muscle.

1. Myosin Light-Chain Kinase Regulation

Purified myosin light-chain kinase from smooth muscle is phosphorylated by a number of different protein kinases in vitro (85–91). The sites of phosphorylation have been identified and mapped to specific regions of myosin light chain kinase (Fig. 5). The phosphorylation of myosin light-chain kinase at a specific regulatory site (site A) adjacent to the calmodulin-binding domain decreases the affinity of the enzyme for Ca^{2+}/calmodulin. Thus, site A phosphorylation will *desensitize* myosin light-chain kinase to activation by Ca^{2+} because higher Ca^{2+} concentrations will be necessary to form more Ca^{2+}/calmodulin required for activation. In vitro, at least three protein kinases catalyze the phosphorylation of myosin light-chain kinase at

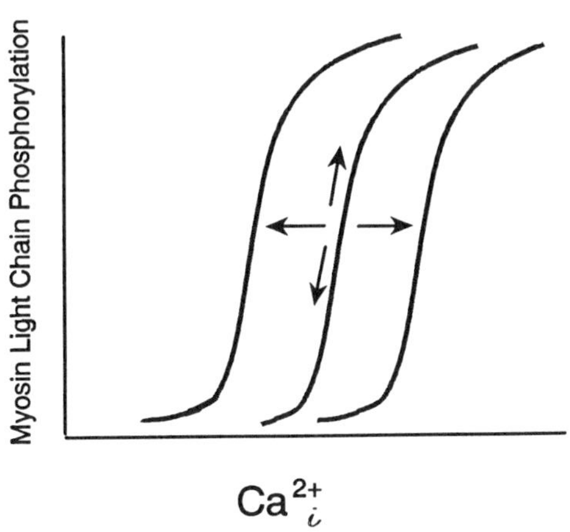

Figure 4 Relationship between free cytosolic Ca^{2+} and extent of myosin light-chain phosphorylation in smooth muscle. Second messenger systems affect myosin light-chain phosphorylation by increasing or decreasing Ca^{2+} concentrations. In addition, the Ca^{2+} dependence of myosin light-chain phosphorylation may change (*i.e.*, shifts in the $Ca^{2+}{}_i$-light chain phosphorylation relationship). These processes have been referred to as sensitization and desensitization when the response curves shift to the left or right, respectively.

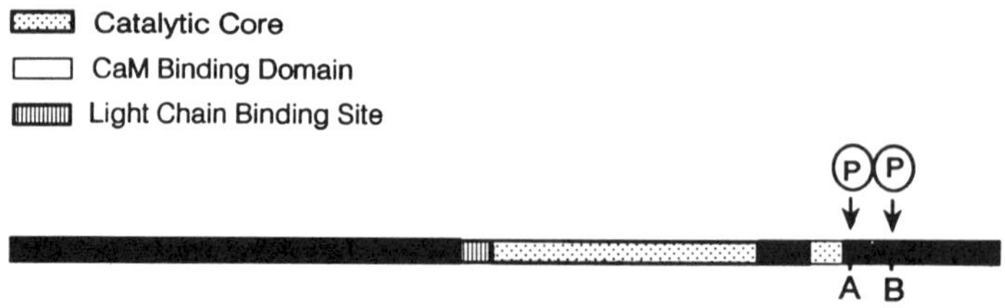

	Phosphorylation Site A	Phosphorylation Site B	Phosphorylation Site Other
cAMP-Dependent Protein Kinase	1	1	
cGMP-Dependent Protein Kinase		1	
Protein Kinase C	1		x
Ca^{2+}/CaM-Dependent Protein Kinase II	1		x

Figure 5 Phosphorylation of smooth muscle myosin light-chain kinase by other protein kinases. A linear schematic of myosin light chain kinase is provided. The phosphorylation of site A results in a 10-fold increase in the concentration of Ca^{2+}/calmodulin required for half-maximal activation of myosin light-chain kinase.

site A by way of cAMP, diacylglycerol, or Ca^{2+}(cAMP-dependent protein kinase, protein kinase C, and Ca^{2+}/calmodulin-dependent protein kinase II).

Myosin light-chain kinase phosphorylation has recently been examined in intact smooth muscle (92). Myosin light-chain kinase contains approximately 0.9 mol of phosphate per mol of kinase in control, relaxed conditions (92). Treatment of tracheal smooth muscle with carbachol, KCl, isoproterenol, or phorbol 12,13-dibutyrate resulted in an increase in the extent of phosphorylation into six primary phosphopeptides (A–F) of myosin light chain kinase (identified by two-dimensional phosphopeptide maps). Site A was phosphorylated to an appreciable extent (up to 0.8 mol ^{32}P incorporated per mol of site A) only with carbachol or KCl, agents that increase $Ca^{2+}{}_i$ and result in contraction of smooth muscle. Cyclic AMP-dependent protein kinase and protein kinase C, therefore, do not affect smooth muscle contractility by phosphorylation of myosin light-chain kinase at site A in vivo. Under steady-state conditions of contraction, site A was phosphorylated to a greater extent with K^+ depolarization than with agonist stimulation (92). Thus, it is possible that the differences in the Ca^{2+} dependencies of myosin light-chain phosphorylation with K^+ and agonists treatments are related to myosin light-chain kinase phosphorylation.

Ionomycin stimulates increases in $Ca^{2+}{}_i$ and a rapid increase in K_{CaM} of myosin light-chain kinase in tracheal smooth muscle cells in culture. Pretreatment with KN-62, an inhibitor of Ca^{2+}/calmodulin-dependent protein kinase II, did not affect the ionomycin stimulated increase in $Ca^{2+}{}_i$ but completely inhibited the associated decrease in the activation properties of myosin light-chain kinase in ionomycin-treated cells (93). Moreover, KN-62 pretreatment was associated with a greater rate and extent of myosin light-chain phosphorylation (93). Thus, Ca^{2+}-dependent phosphorylation of myosin light-chain kinase by Ca^{2+}/calmodulin-dependent protein kinase II may result in desensitization of the contractile elements to $Ca^{2+}{}_i$. Recent experiments conducted in intact tracheal smooth muscle indicate that treatment with KCl results in increases in K_{CaM} that are proportional to increases in $[Ca^{2+}]_i$ (94). Thus, Ca^{2+} desensitization of myosin light chain phosphorylation and force development in KCl-contracted smooth muscle is not mediated by way of a decrease in the calmodulin activation properties of myosin light chain kinase by site A phosphorylation.

Ca^{2+}-dependent myosin light-chain phosphorylation (and tension) is potentially diminished by the Ca^{2+}-dependent phosphorylation of myosin light-chain kinase. Modulation of the affinity of myosin light-chain kinase for Ca^{2+}_i by phosphorylation and dephosphorylation may provide additional fine-tuning mechanisms for light-chain phosphorylation. This process may serve to limit phosphorylation of myosin light chain by way of a negative feedback mechanism, particularly at high levels of Ca^{2+}_i. The affinity of nonphosphorylated CaM-kinase II for calmodulin is much less than myosin light chain kinase. After autophosphorylation of threonine-286, however, there is a marked increase in the affinity of the enzyme for calmodulin (from 45 to 0.06 nM) (95). Thus, greater concentrations of Ca^{2+} may be necessary for activation of Ca^{2+}/calmodulin-dependent protein kinase II, but once activated, calmodulin is slowly released from the enzyme, resulting in prolonged activation. More information is needed regarding the kinetic properties of myosin light chain kinase phosphorylation by this kinase and its role in the regulation of myosin light chain phosphorylation and force development in smooth muscle.

2. *Myosin Light-Chain Phosphatase Regulation*

Another potential mechanism for alteration of the Ca^{2+} sensitivity of myosin light-chain phosphorylation involves regulation of protein phosphatase activity. Evidence has been presented that protein phosphatase types 1 and 2A dephosphorylate smooth muscle myosin (28–38). The activities of these protein phosphatases are regulated in other tissues by inhibitory proteins and phosphorylation of inhibitory proteins and regulatory subunits (27). Types 1 and 2A enzymes are classified into two groups based on whether the enzyme catalyzes the dephosphorylation of the β subunit of phosphorylase kinase (specific for type 1) and on whether it is inhibited by two small heat- and acid-stable proteins, inhibitor-1 and inhibitor-2, in nanomolar concentrations (also type 1). Protein phosphatase type 2 is characteristically *insensitive* to inhibitors 1 and 2 and preferentially dephosphorylates the α subunit of phosphorylase kinase. To add to these complexities, phosphatase subunits and their inhibitor proteins are also regulated by phosphorylation. For example, the phosphorylation of the glycogen-binding subunit of protein phosphatase 1 by cAMP-dependent protein kinase results in dissociation of the catalytic subunit from glycogen and inactivation of the enzyme. Phosphorylation of inhibitor-1 by cAMP-dependent protein kinase results in activation of the inhibitor (thus *inactivation* of protein phosphatase type 1). The complexities of the regulation of protein phosphatase activity within smooth muscle contractile elements are not understood at this time.

A guanine nucleotide-binding protein (G-protein) may be involved in the regulation of myosin light chain phosphatase activity. Treatment of permeabilized smooth muscle with GTPγS increases the sensitivity of the contractile response to activation by Ca^{2+}, and results in a leftward shift of the Ca^{2+}/myosin light chain phosphorylation relationship (96–98). In the presence of GTP, vascular smooth muscle (permeabilized with α-toxin) exhibits an increase in Ca^{2+} sensitivity to agonist treatment and these effects are inhibited by GDPβS (99). Treatment of smooth muscle from the portal vein (also permeabilized with α-toxin) with GTPγS results in increased myosin light-chain phosphorylation (99). These results are supportive of the hypothesis that G-protein Ca^{2+}-sensitizing effects are secondary to increases in myosin light-chain phosphorylation. In skinned bovine tracheal smooth muscle, GTPγS likewise induces myosin light-chain phosphorylation only at the myosin light chain kinase sites, indicating that protein kinase C or other kinases are not responsible for the increase in myosin light-chain phosphorylation (100). Moreover, GTPγS does not enhance okadaic acid-induced contractions. Taken together, these results are consistent with GTPγS-mediated inhibition of myosin light-chain phosphatase, with the resultant increase in myosin light-chain phosphorylation and tension.

The potential regulation of myosin light-chain phosphatase broadens the scope of mechanisms for affecting smooth muscle contractility. This new area of investigation should provide important information since myosin is most likely dephosphorylated by protein phosphatases with broad substrate specificities. Results from these studies could therefore provide insights into regulation of dephosphorylation of many proteins, including proteins present in tissues other than smooth muscle, in addition to providing fundamental information on the smooth muscle contractile element system.

B. Myosin Light-Chain Phosphorylation/Force Relationship

A number of observations in smooth muscles, including various types of vascular tissues, indicate that there may be other important regulatory processes in addition to myosin light-chain phosphorylation. There are at least three examples of dissociation of force development and myosin light chain phosphorylation, other than the latch-state described above. First, in ferret portal vein, 12-deoxyphorbol, 13-isobutyrate 20-acetate, an activator of protein kinase C, acts to cause a slow contraction of similar magnitude to that of K^+ but light chain phosphorylation is not increased (101). It has recently been reported that treatment of the ferret aorta with $PGF_{2\alpha}$ results in not only increased levels of light-chain phosphorylation relative to $Ca^{2+}{}_i$, but also more force development for a given level of light-chain phosphorylation than that obtained with KCl (102). In this unique example, both the $Ca^{2+}{}_i$/light-chain phosphorylation and the light-chain phosphorylation/force curves were shifted to the left by agonist treatment compared with KCl. Experiments conducted in other vascular smooth muscle tissues have demonstrated a single light-chain phosphorylation/force relationship with various agonists (4). Second, in canine tracheal smooth muscle, myosin light-chain phosphorylation is completely dissociated from force development when muscles are stimulated with carbachol in Ca^{2+}-free physiological salt solution and contracted by readmission of $CaCl_2$ (3). In the absence of extracellular Ca^{2+}, carbachol induces an increase in myosin light-chain phosphorylation, yet the muscle remains relaxed. The addition of Ca^{2+} to the bathing medium results in an increase in force and the light chain remains phosphorylated. Lastly, the addition of okadaic acid (a protein phosphatase inhibitor isolated from the marine sponge *Halichondria*) to bovine tracheal smooth muscle contracted with carbachol results in a decrease in Ca_i and relaxation in spite of maintenance of high levels of myosin light chain phosphorylation (80). In this example, ^{32}P was incorporated into serine-19, the site normally phosphorylated by myosin light-chain kinase. This observation is important since phosphorylation of myosin light chain at distinct sites by protein kinase C does not activate myosin MgATPase activity.

It has been proposed that complex interactions of the contractile proteins with thin filament regulatory proteins may alter the myosin light-chain phosphorylation/force relationship. There are two primary problems in the understanding of the physiological role of caldesmon and calponin in the regulation of force development. First, the affinity of myosin light-chain kinase for Ca^{2+}/calmodulin is 2–3 orders of magnitude greater than caldesmon for Ca^{2+}/calmodulin. Thus, it is unlikely that calmodulin will bind to these proteins at low $Ca^{2+}{}_i$, insufficient for full activation of myosin light-chain kinase. Second, in the absence of $Ca^{2+}{}_i$, addition of a partially proteolyzed, calmodulin-*independent* myosin light-chain kinase to skinned fibers results in contraction (103). Similar results have been obtained with microinjection of calmodulin-*independent* myosin light-chain kinase into single smooth muscle cells (104). The binding of calponin or caldesmon to the thin filaments (in the presence of low Ca^{2+} concentrations) acts to inhibit contractions induced by phosphorylated myosin, yet the muscle contracts. Although additional physiological investigations are needed to establish a role for thin-filament proteins in the regulation of smooth muscle function, the possiblity that there are other unidentified proteins that play important regulatory roles in the contractile elements must be considered.

V. SUMMARY

For many years the simple view was held that contractile force in smooth muscle was proportionate to cytoplasmic Ca^{2+} concentrations ($Ca^{2+}{}_i$). With the discovery that phosphorylation of myosin light chain by Ca^{2+}/calmodulin-dependent myosin light-chain kinase initiated contraction, some insight into mechanisms of regulation of the contractile elements was provided. However, it is now clear that this scheme is too simple and that more complex properties of myosin phosphorylation and contraction are evident in smooth muscle cells. Myosin light-chain kinase can be phosphorylated, which desensitizes its activation by Ca^{2+}/calmodulin. Protein phosphatase activity towards myosin may also be negatively regulated, but examples in smooth muscle tissue are sparse. These different mechanisms may be uniquely regulated in smooth muscle cells to affect the Ca^{2+} sensitivity of myosin light chain phosphorylation and contraction (Fig. 6).

The proposal of an attached, dephosphorylated myosin cross-bridge (latch bridge) that can maintain force has evoked considerable controversy about the detailed functions of the myosin phosphorylation system. The latch bridge has been defined by a model based upon physiological properties but has not been identified biochemically. Thin-filament proteins have been proposed as secondary sites of regulation of contractile elements, but additional studies are needed to establish physiological roles. It is apparent that contractile elements in smooth muscle cells are not dependent solely on $Ca^{2+}{}_i$, but employ additional regulatory mechanisms that perhaps involve unidentified proteins. Much research is needed to define further the cellular, biochemical, and molecular basis for these physiological processes involved in the regulation of smooth muscle contraction.

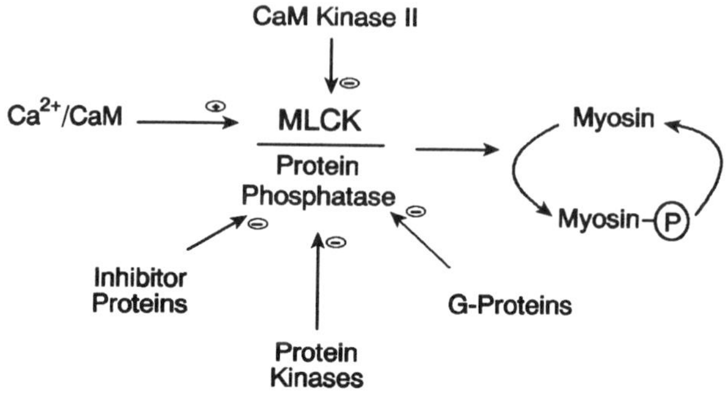

Figure 6 Regulation of the ratio of activities of myosin light-chain kinase and protein phosphatase activities. Ca^{2+} activates myosin light-chain kinase via calmodulin and thereby increases myosin light-chain phosphorylation. Phosphorylation of myosin light-chain kinase by a Ca^{2+}-dependent protein kinase (probably Ca^{2+}/calmodulin-dependent protein kinase II) desensitizes myosin light chain kinase to activation by Ca^{2+}. Although much less is known about the regulation of myosin light-chain phosphatase activity, various mechanisms that potentially involve phosphorylation by protein kinases, inhibitor proteins, and guanine nucleotide-binding proteins result in inhibition of protein phosphatase activity.

REFERENCES

1. Stull JT, Gallagher PJ, Herring, BP, Kamm KE. Vascular smooth muscle contractile elements: cellular regulation. Hypertension 1991;17:723–32.
2. Morgan JP, Morgan KG. Stimulus-specific patterns of intracellular calcium levels in smooth muscle of ferret portal vein. J Physiol 1984;351:155–67.
3. Gerthoffer WT. Calcium dependence of myosin phosphorylation and airway smooth muscle contraction and relaxation. Am J Physiol 1986;250:C597–C604.
4. Rembold CM, Murphy RA. Myoplasmic [Ca^{2+}] determines myosin phosphorylation in agonist-stimulated swine arterial smooth muscle. Circ Res 1988;63:593–603.
5. Kamm KE, Stull JT. The function of myosin and myosin light chain kinase phosphorylation in smooth muscle. Annu Rev Pharmacol Toxicol 1985;25:593–620.
6. Michnoff CH, Kemp BE, Stull JT. Phosphorylation of synthetic peptides by skeletal muscle myosin light chain kinases. J Biol Chem 1986;261:8320–6.
7. Kemp BE, Pearson RB. Spatial requirements for location of basic residues in peptide substrates for smooth muscle myosin light chain kinase. J Biol Chem 1985;260:3355–9.
8. Persechini A, Hartshorne DJ. Evidence for cooperativity between the myosin heads. Science 1981;213:1383–5.
9. Persechini A, Hartshorne DJ. Ordered phosphorylation of the two 20,000 molecular weight light chains of smooth muscle myosin. Biochemistry 1983;22:470–6.
10. Sellers JR, Chock PB, Adelstein RS. The apparently negatively cooperative phosphorylation of smooth muscle myosin at low ionic strength is related to its filamentous state. J Biol Chem 1983;258:14181–8.
11. Ito M, Hartshorne DJ. Phosphorylation of myosin as a regulatory mechanism in smooth muscle. Prog Clin Biol Res 1990;327:57–72.
12. Hai C-M, Murphy RA. Ca^{2+}, cross bridge phosphorylation, and contraction. Annu Rev Physiol 1989;51:285–98.
13. O'Neil, KT, DeGrado, WF. How calmodulin binds its targets: sequence independent recognition of amphiphilic α-helices. TIBS 1990;15:59–64.

14. Olwrin BB, Edelman AM, Krebs EG, Storm DR. Quantitation of energy coupling between Ca^{2+}, calmodulin, skeletal muscle myosin light chain kinase and kinase substrates. J Biol Chem 1984;259:10949–55.
15. Pearson RB, Wettenhall REH, Means AR, Hartshorne DJ, Kemp BE. Autoregulation of enzymes by pseudosubstrate prototopes: myosin light chain kinase. Science 1988; 241:970–3.
16. Ikebe M, Maruta S, Reardon S. Location of the inhibitory region of smooth muscle myosin light chain kinase. J Biol Chem 1989;264:6967–71.
17. Ikebe M, Stephinska M, Kemp BE, Means AR, Hartshorne DJ. Proteolysis of smooth muscle myosin light chain kinase. Formation of inactive and calmodulin-independent fragments. J Biol Chem 1987;260:13828–34.
18. Guerriero V Jr, Russo MA, Olson NJ, Putkey JA, Means AR. Domain organization of chicken gizzard myosin light chain kinase deduced from a cloned cDNA. Biochemistry 1986;25:8372–81.
19. Olson NJ, Pearson RB, Needleman DS, Hurwitz MY, Kemp BE, Means AR. Regulatory and structural motifs of chicken gizzard myosin light chain kinase. Proc Natl Acad Sci USA 1990;87:2284–8.
20. Ito M, Guerriero V, Chen X, Hartshorne DJ. Definition of the inhibitory domain of smooth muscle myosin light chain kinase by site-directed mutagenesis. Biochemistry 1991;30:3498–503.
21. Kemp BE, Pearson RB, Guerriero V Jr, Bagchi IC, Means AR. The calmodulin binding domain of chicken smooth muscle myosin light chain kinase contains a pseudosubstrate sequence. J Biol Chem 1987;262:2542–8.
22. Ikebe M. Mode of inhibition of smooth muscle myosin light chain kinase by synthetic peptide analogs of the regulatory site. Biochem Biophys Res Commun 1990;168:714–20.
23. Herring BP. Basic residues are important for Ca^{2+}/calmodulin binding and activation but not autoinhibition of rabbit skeletal muscle myosin light chain kinase. J Biol Chem 1991;266:11838–41.
24. Hanks SK, Quinn AM, Hunter T. The protein kinase family: conserved features and deduced phylogeny of the catalytic domains. Science 1988;241:42–52.
25. Herring BP, Stull JT, Gallagher PJ. Domain chracterization of rabbit skeletal muscle myosin light chain kinase. J Biol Chem 1990;265:1724–30.
26. Herring BP, Fitzsimons DP, Stull JT, Gallagher PJ. Acidic residues comprise part of the myosin light chain binding site on skeletal muscle myosin light chain kinase. J Biol Chem 1990;265:1724–30.
27. Cohen P. The structure and regulation of protein phosphatases. Annu Rev Biochem 1989;58:453–508.
28. Chisholm AAK, Cohen P. The myosin-bound form of protein phosphatase 1 ($PP\text{-}1_M$) is the enzyme that dephosphorylates native myosin in skeletal and cardiac muscles. Biochim Biophys Acta 1988;971:163–9.
29. Schlender KK, Wang W, Wilson SE. Evidence for a latent form of protein phosphatase 1 associated with cardiac myofibrils. Biochem Biophys Res Commun 1989; 159:72–8.
30. Dent P, Campbell DG, Hubbard MJ, Cohen P. Multisite phosphorylation of the glycogen-binding subunit of protein phosphatase-1_G by cyclic AMP-dependent protein kinase and glycogen synthase kinase-3. FEBS Lett 1989;284:67–72.
31. Mumby MC, Russell KL, Garrard LJ, Green DD. Cardiac contractile protein phosphatases. Purification of two enzyme forms and their characterization with subunit-specific antibodies. J Biol Chem 1987;262:6257–5.
32. Bialojan C, Ruegg JC, DiSalvo J. Phosphatase-mediated modulation of actin–myosin interaction in bovine aortic actomyosin and skinned porcine carotid artery. Proc Soc Exp Biol Med 1985;178:36–45.

33. Haeberle JR, Hathaway DR, DePaoli-Roach AA. Dephosphorylation of myosin by the catalytic subunit of a type-2 phosphatase produces relaxation of chemically skinned uterine smooth muscle. J Biol Chem 1985;260:9965–8.
34. Pato MD, Kerc E. Purification and characterization of a smooth muscle myosin phosphatase from turkey gizzards. J Biol Chem 1985;260:12359–66.
35. Hoar PE, Pato MD, Kerrick WGL. Myosin light chain phosphatase. Effect on the activation and relaxation of gizzard smooth muscle skinned fibers. J Biol Chem 1985;260:8760–4.
36. Pato MD, Kerc E. Comparison of the properties of the protein phosphatases from avian and mammalian smooth muscles: purification and characterization of rabbit uterine smooth muscle phosphatases. Arch Biochem Biophys 1990;276:116–24.
37. Takai Q, Troschka M, Mieskes G, Somlyo AV. Protein phosphatase composition in the smooth muscle of guinea-pig ileum studied with okadaic acid and inhibitor 2. Biochem J 1989;262:617–23.
38. Ishihara H, Ozaki H, Sato K, Hori M, Karaki H, Watabe S, Kato Y, Fusetani N, Hashimoto K, Uemura D, Hartshorne DJ. Calcium-independent activation of contractile apparatus in smooth muscle by calyculin-A. J Pharmacol Exp Ther 1989; 250:388–96.
39. Hartshorne DJ, and Gorecka A. The biochemistry of the contractile proteins of smooth muscle. In: Bohr DF, Somlyo AP, Sparks HV, eds. Handbook of physiology, section 2. The cardiovascular system, vol. II. Vascular smooth muscle. Bethesda, MD: American Physiology Society, 1980.
40. Rubenstein PA, Spudich JA. Actin microheterogeneity in chick embryo fibroblasts. Proc Natl Acad Sci 1977;74:120–3.
41. Whalen RG, Butler-Browne GS, Gros F. Protein synthesis and actin heterogeneity in calf muscle cells in culture. Proc Natl Acad Sci USA 1976;73:2018–22.
42. Craig SW, Pollard TD. Actin-binding proteins. TIBS 1982;7:88–92.
43. Weeds A. Actin-binding proteins-regulators of cell architecture and motility. Nature 1988;2296:811–6.
44. Korn ED. Actin polymerization and its regulation by proteins from nonmuscle cells. Physiol Rev 1982;62:672–37.
45. Hartshorne DJ, Gorecka A, Aksoy MO. Aspects of the regulatory mechanism in smooth muscle. In: Casteels R, Godfrains T, Ruegg JC, eds. Excitation–contraction coupling in smooth muscle. Amsterdam: Elsevier/North-Holland Biomedical Press, 1977.
46. Parry DAD, Squire JM. Structural role of tropomyosin in muscle regulation: analysis of the x-ray diffraction patterns from relaxed and contracting muscle. J Mol Biol 1973; 75:33–55.
47. Vibert PJ, Haselgrove JC, Lowry, J, Poulsen, FR. Structural changes in actin-containing filaments of muscle. J Mol Biol 1972;71:757–67.
48. Moody C, Lehman W, Craig R. Caldesmon and the structure of smooth muscle thin filaments. Electron microscopy of isolated thin filaments. J Muscle Res Cell Motil 1990;11:176–85.
49. Bryan, J. Smooth muscle thin filaments. Caldesmon, acidic amino acids and molecular weight determinations. J Muscle Res Cell Motil 1989;10:95–6.
50. Sobue K, Kanda K, Tanaka T, Ueki N. Caldesmon. A common actin-linked regulatory protein in the smooth muscle and nonmuscle contractile system. J Cell Biochem 1988;37:317–25.
51. Ikebe M, Reardon S. Binding of caldesmon to smooth muscle myosin. J Biol Chem 1988;263:3055–8.
52. Hemric ME, Chalovich JM. Effect of caldesmon on the ATPase activity and the binding of smooth and skeletal myosin subfragments to actin. J Biol Chem 1988;263:1878–85.

53. Ngai PK, Walsh MP. Inhibition of smooth muscle actin-activated myosin Mg^{2+}–ATPase activity by caldesmon. J Biol Chem 1984;259:13656–9.
54. Sutherland C, Walsh MP. Phosphorylation of caldesmon prevents its interaction with smooth muscle myosin. J Biol Chem 1989;264:578–83.
55. Ngai PK, Walsh MP. The effects of phosphorylation of smooth muscle caldesmon. Biochem J 1987;244:417–25.
56. Umekawa H, Hidaka H. Phosphorylation of caldesmon by protein kinase C. Biochem Biophys Res Commun 1985;132:56–62.
57. Tanaka T, Ohta H, Kanda K, Tanaka T, Hidaka H, Sobue K. Phosphorylation of high-Mr caldesmon by protein kinase C modulates the regulatory function of this protein on the interaction between actin and myosin. Eur J Biochem 1990;188:495–500.
58. Scott-Woo GC, Sutherland C, Walsh MP. Kinase activity associated with caldesmon is Ca^{2+}/calmodulin-dependent protein kinase II. Biochem J 1990;268:367–70.
59. Ikebe M, Reardon S. Phosphorylation of smooth muscle caldesmon by calmodulin-dependent protein kinase II. Identification of the phosphorylation sites. J Biol Chem 1990;265:17607–12.
60. Adam LP, Haeberle JR, Hathaway DR. Phosphorylation of caldesmon in arterial smooth muscle. J Biol Chem 1989;264:7698–703.
61. Yamashiro S, Matsumura F. Mitosis-specific phosphorylation of caldesmon: possible molecular mechanism of cell rounding during mitosis. Bioessays 1991;13:563–8.
62. Takahashi K, Hiwada K, Kokubu T. Vascular smooth muscle calponin. A novel troponin T-like protein. Hypertension 1988;11:620–6.
63. Winder SJ, Walsh MP. Smooth muscle calponin. Inhibition of actomyosin MgATPase and regulation by phosphorylation. J Biol Chem 1990;265:10148–55.
64. Barany M, Rokolya A, Barany K. Absence of calponin phosphorylation in contracting or resting arterial smooth muscle. FEBS Letters 1991;279:65–8.
65. Cox JA. Interactive properties of calmodulin. Biochem J 1988;249:621–9.
66. Kamm KE, Stull JT. Activation of smooth muscle contraction: relation between myosin phosphorylation and stiffness. Science 1986;232:80–2.
67. Kamm KE, Stull JT. Myosin phosphorylation, force and maximal shortening velocity in neurally stimulated tracheal smooth muscle. Am J Physiol 1985;249:C238–47.
68. Hartshorne DJ. Biochemistry of the contractile process in smooth muscle. In: Johnson LR, ed. Physiology of the gastrointestinal tract. New York: Raven Press, 1987.
69. Kamm KE, Stull JT. Regulation of smooth muscle contractile elements by second messengers. Annu Rev Physiol 1989;51:299–313.
70. Murphy RA. Special topic: contraction in smooth muscle cells. Annu Rev Physiol 1989;51:275–83.
71. Colburn JC, Michnoff CH, Hsu L, Slaughter CA, Kamm KE, Stull JT. Sites phosphorylated in myosin light chain in contracting smooth muscle. J Biol Chem 1988; 263:19166–73.
72. Kamm KE, Hsu L-C, Kubota Y, Stull JT. Phosphorylation of smooth muscle myosin heavy and light chains: effects of phorbol dibutyrate and agonists. J Biol Chem 1989;264:21223–9.
73. Singer HA, Oren JW, Benscoter HA. Myosin light chain phosphorylation in ^{32}P-labeled rabbit aorta stimulated by phorbol 12,13-dibutyrate and phenylephrine. J Biol Chem 1989;264:21215–22.
74. Trybus KM. Filamentous smooth muscle myosin is regulated by phosphorylation. J Cell Biol 1989;109:2887–95.
75. Greene LE, Sellers JR. Effect of phosphorylation on the binding of smooth muscle heavy meromyosin-ADP to actin. J Biol Chem 1987;262:4177–81.
76. Sutton TA, Haeberle JR. Phosphorylation by protein kinase C of the 20,000-dalton

light chain of myosin in intact and chemically skinned vascular smooth muscle. J Biol Chem 1990;265:2749–54.
77. Kawamoto S, Adelstein RS. The heavy chain of smooth muscle myosin is phosphorylated in aorta cells. J Biol Chem 1988;263:1099–102.
78. Moreland S, Moreland RS, Singer HA. Apparent dissociation between myosin light chain phosphorylation and maximal velocity of shortening in KCl depolarized swine carotid artery: effect of temperature and KCl concentration. Pflugers Arch 1986; 408:139–45.
79. Merkel L, Gerthoffer WT, Torphy TJ. Dissociation between myosin phosphorylation and shortening velocity in canine trachea. Am J Physiol 1990;258:C524–32.
80. Tansey MG, Hori M, Karaki H, Kamm KE, Stull JT. Okadaic acid uncouples myosin light chain phosphorylation and tension in smooth muscle. FEBS Lett 1990;270:219–21.
81. Karaki H. Ca^{2+} localization and sensitivity in vascular smooth muscle. Trends Pharmacol Sci 1989;10:320–5.
82. Somlyo AP, Himpens B. Cell calcium and its regulation in smooth muscle. FASEB J 1989;3:2266–76.
83. Taylor DA, Stull JT. Calcium dependence of myosin light chain phosphorylation in smooth muscle cells. J Biol Chem 1988;263:14456–62.
84. Taylor DA, Bowman BF, Stull JT. Cytoplasmic Ca^{2+} is a primary determinant for myosin phosphorylation in smooth muscle cells. J Biol Chem 1989;264:6206–13.
85. deLanerolle P, Nishikawa M, Yost DA, Adelstein RS. Increased phosphorylation of myosin light chain kinase after an increase in cyclic AMP in intact smooth muscle. Science 1984;223:1415–7.
86. Adelstein RS, Conti MA, Hathaway DR, Klee CB. Phosphorylation of smooth muscle myosin light chain kinase by the catalytic subunit of adenosine 3′: 5′-monophosphate-dependent protein kinase. J Biol Chem 1978;253:8347–50.
87. Conti MA, Adelstein RS. The relationship between calmodulin binding and phosphorylation of smooth muscle myosin kinase by the catalytic subunit of 3′:5′ cAMP-dependent protein kinase. J Biol Chem 1981;256:3178–81.
88. Ikebe M, Inagaki M, Kanamaru K, Hidaka H. Phosphorylation of smooth muscle myosin light chain kinase by Ca^{2+}-activated, phospholipid-dependent protein kinase. J Biol Chem 1985;260:4547–50.
89. Nishikawa M, Shirakawa S, Adelstein RS. Phosphorylation of smooth muscle myosin light chain kinase by protein kinase C. Comparative study of the phosphorylated sites. J Biol Chem 1985;260:8978–83.
90. Hashimoto Y, Soderling TR. Phosphorylation of smooth muscle myosin light chain kinase by Ca^{2+}/calmodulin-dependent protein kinase-II. Comparative study of the phosphorylation sites. Arch Biochem Biophys 1990;278:41–5.
91. Miller JR, Silver PJ, Stull JT. The role of myosin light chain kinase phosphorylation in β-adrenergic relaxation of tracheal smooth muscle. Mol Pharmacol 1983;24:235–42.
92. Stull JT, Hsu L-C, Tansey MG, Kamm KE. Myosin light chain kinase phosphorylation in tracheal smooth muscle. J Biol Chem 1990;265:16683–90.
93. Tansey MG, Word RA, Hidaka H, Singer HA, Schworer CM, Kamm KE, Stull JT. Phosphorylation of myosin light chain kinase by the multifunctional calmodulin-dependent protein kinase II in smooth muscle cells. J Biol Chem 1992;267:12511–6.
94. Tang D-C, Stull JT, Kubota Y, Kamm KE. Regulation of the Ca^{2+} dependence of smooth muscle contraction. J Biol Chem 1992;267:11839–45.
95. Meyer T, Hanson PI, Stryer L, Schulman H. Calmodulin trapping by calcium-calmodulin-dependent protein kinase. Science 1992;256:1199–202.
96. Fujiwara T, Itoh T, Kubota Y, Kuriyama H. Effects of guanosine nucleotides on

skinned smooth muscle tissue of the rabbit mesenteric artery. J Physiol (Lond) 1989;408:535–47.
97. Kitazawa T, Kobayashi S, Horiuti K, Somlyo AV, Somlyo AP. Receptor-coupled, permeabilized smooth muscle. Role of the phosphatidylinositol cascade, G-proteins, and modulation of the contractile response to Ca^{2+}. J Biol Chem 1989;264:5339–42.
98. Nishimura J, Kolber M, Van Breeman C. Norepinephrine and GTPγS increase myofilaments Ca^{2+} sensitivity in α-toxin permeabilized arterial smooth muscle. Biochem Biophys Res Commun 1988;157:677–83.
99. Kitazawa T, Gaylinn BD, Denney GH, Somlyo AP. G-protein-mediated Ca^{2+} sensitization of smooth muscle contraction through myosin light chain phosphorylation. J Biol Chem 1991;266:1708–15.
100. Kubota Y, Kamm KE, Stull JT. Mechanism of GTPγS-dependent regulation of smooth muscle contraction. Biophys J 1990;57:152a(abstr).
101. Jiang MJ, Morgan KG. Intracellular Ca^{2+} levels in phorbol ester-induced contractions of vascular smooth muscle. Am J Physiol 1987;253:H1365–71.
102. Suematsu E, Resnick M, Morgan KG. Change of Ca^{2+} requirement for myosin phosphorylation by prostaglandin $F_{2\alpha}$ Am J Physiol, in press.
103. Walsh MP, Bridenbaugh R, Kerrick WGL, Hartshorne DJ. Gizzard Ca^{2+}-independent myosin light chain kinase: evidence in favor of the phosphorylation theory. Fed Proc 1983;42:45–50.
104. Itoh T, Ikebe M, Kargacin GJ, Hartshorne DJ, Kemp BE, Fay FS. Effects of modulators of myosin light-chain kinase activity in single smooth muscle cells. Nature 1989;338:164–7.

8

Physiology of Vascular Smooth Muscle: Clinical Aspects of Calcium Channel Antagonists and Direct-Acting Vasodilating Agents

JOHN PAWLOWSKI

Beth Israel Hospital
Boston, Massachusetts

I. INTRODUCTION

Each year, cardiovascular disease leads to the death of 1 million Americans and accounts for one-half of all reported fatalities (1). As many as 20% of all Americans have high blood pressure and of these, 85% have essential hypertension (2). The cost of caring for patients with essential hypertension is measured in billions of dollars and the human toll of illness and death is incalculable. Thus, the understanding of the pathophysiology of essential hypertension and the informed therapy of this disease is of enormous importance.

The pathophysiology of essential hypertension involves several abnormalities in the excitation–contraction coupling mechanism of vascular smooth muscle (VSM) cells. Part of understanding hypertension involves understanding the mechanism by which vascular smooth muscle cells develop tension. In addition, local abnormalities in coronary arteries, cerebral vessels, and renal arteries can lead to organ damage of the heart, brain, and kidneys, respectively (3). The vessels of different organs have characteristic contractile responses to stimulation and to vasodilators. Normal and diseased vascular tissue also differ in their responses to agonists and antagonists (4). An understanding of the mechanisms by which vascular smooth muscle contracts and how this contraction is modulated can guide the rational treatment of certain disease states.

This chapter will describe the contractile properties of VSM as presently understood. Vascular smooth muscle will be compared to skeletal and cardiac muscle. Special attention will be paid to the role of intracellular calcium in vascular contraction and the specific mechanisms by which calcium is imported, exported, sequestered, and released. This chapter will not discuss the important role of the endothelium and such substances as endothelium-derived relaxing factors (EDRF) and endothelin. Also mentioned in another chapter are specific receptor-operated mechanisms such as the alpha and beta agonists and antagonists. The new class of potassium channel activators such as cromakalim (5) will be discussed elsewhere. Agents that block angiotensin-converting enzyme such as captopril and drugs that block serotonin receptors such as ketanserin will be described in other chapters. Certain endogenous substances that also act via specific receptors such as adenosine, serotonin, and atrial natriuretic factors (ANF) will not be addressed in this chapter. Therapeutic agents used to treat hypertension that do not have direct effects on vascular smooth muscle, such as diuretics, will be omitted.

Following a brief review of the relevant basic science of the contraction of vascular smooth muscle, this chapter will concentrate on the clinical use of calcium channel antagonists and other smooth muscle dilators. The effects of these agents on general hemodynamics, local organ perfusion, and laboratory tissue preparations will be contrasted where possible. Examples will be cited to illustrate how the discriminant use of specific calcium channel antagonists can ameliorate certain vascular diseases. In addition to the calcium channel blockers, this chapter will discuss the mechanism of action of direct smooth muscle dilators. Specific care will be taken to differentiate arterial from venous effects of vasodilators and conditions that can be improved with vasodilator therapy will be cited.

This chapter is not meant to be an exhaustive review nor is it meant to be irrefutable. An attempt has been made to mention both the commonly used medicines and the experimentally promising agents that affect vascular smooth muscle. To be clinically applicable, there is some mention of dosage schedules as well as discussion of side effects. Only important or unusual side effects are mentioned, however, that might alter the practitioner's choice of medication. Finally, this chapter deals with the effect of certain agents on the vascular smooth muscle and ignores the extremely important effects on myocardial energy metabolism and cardiac function, as well as on other smooth muscle such as that of the gastrointestinal and urogenital systems.

II. CONTRACTILE PROPERTIES OF SMOOTH MUSCLE

Vascular smooth muscle possesses several unique properties of contraction when compared with skeletal muscle. Although smooth muscle contains one-fourth to one-fifth the amount of myosin found in skeletal muscle, it is able to generate twice as much force per cross-sectional area. In addition, smooth muscle is economical, consuming 300 times less energy to maintain tension than skeletal muscle. On the other hand, smooth muscle shows a frequency of cross-bridge cycling and a velocity of shortening several hundred times slower than that of skeletal and cardiac twitch muscle.

Although the architecture is different, smooth muscle contracts with a sliding actin–myosin filament much like skeletal muscle. In Figure 1, Small and Squire depict the arrangement of the smooth muscle cell with its filaments of actin and myosin (6). The smooth muscle cell is elongated and spindle-shaped, with a length of approximately 100 μm and a width of 5–10 to μm. The arrangement of actin and myosin is less regular than in skeletal muscle, although a series of actin and myosin filaments is linked to perform cell contraction. The intermediate actin filaments are connected by dense bodies, here labeled "Z," that are believed to be analogous to the "Z-bands" of cardiac and skeletal muscle. This particular actin–myosin arrange-

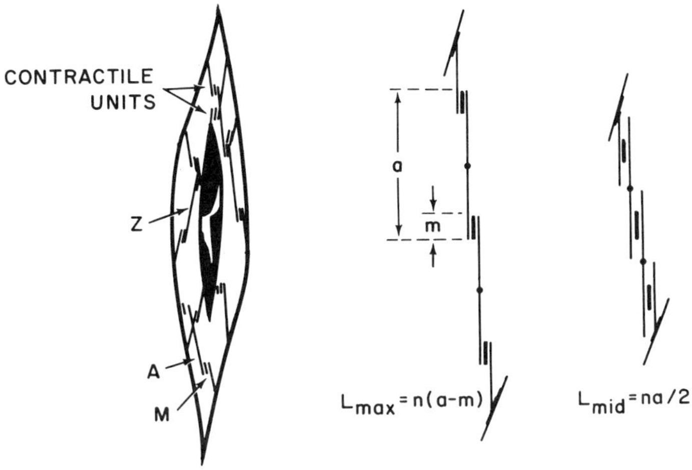

Figure 1 Schematic diagram of a smooth muscle cell showing the general arrangement of the contractile units and a model of a single contractile unit. A, actin; M, myosin. (From Ref. 6 with permission.)

ment allows smooth muscle to contract down to only 20% of its initial length. Smooth muscle myosin differs from skeletal muscle forms because it has two head regions per filament and contains a phosphorylation site on the 20 kDa light chain. The phosphorylation of the myosin light chain is essential for smooth muscle contraction. Troponin is nearly absent in smooth muscle and tropomyosin does not participate in the regulation of contraction, unlike in skeletal and cardiac muscle.

A. Role of Calcium in the Regulation of Contraction

Several experiments have shown a central role for intracellular calcium in the activation of regulatory proteins in smooth muscle cells. The mechanism by which calcium activates the contractile regulating proteins is not fully understood. The theory proposed by Small and Sobieszek (7) remains the most widely accepted: that calcium-activated myosin light-chain kinase (MLCK) causes phosphorylation of the myosin light chain, with calmodulin acting as the receptor for calcium. In the absence of calcium, MLCK becomes inactive, the light chains of myosin are dephosphorylated by a phosphatase, and the actin–myosin cross-bridge detaches with the hydrolysis of ATP. In addition, the affinity of MLCK for calmodulin can be lessened by the phosphorylation of MLCK. Calcium plays central role not only in the initiation of contraction but also in the regulation of the force of contraction through its influences on the sequence of regulatory proteins that modify the actin–myosin crossbridge.

Central to the formation of actin–myosin interactions is the role of MLCK, an enzyme present in high concentrations in smooth muscle cells. Kamm and Stull (1985) have shown the ability of MLCK to phosphorylate the myosin light chain as well as its ability to form an activated complex with calmodulin, an actin-binding protein (8). Calcium is needed for the activation of the 17 kDa protein calmodulin and, presently, there are four distinct calcium-bindings sites on the calmodulin molecule (8). Whether these calcium-binding sites act independently or show coo-

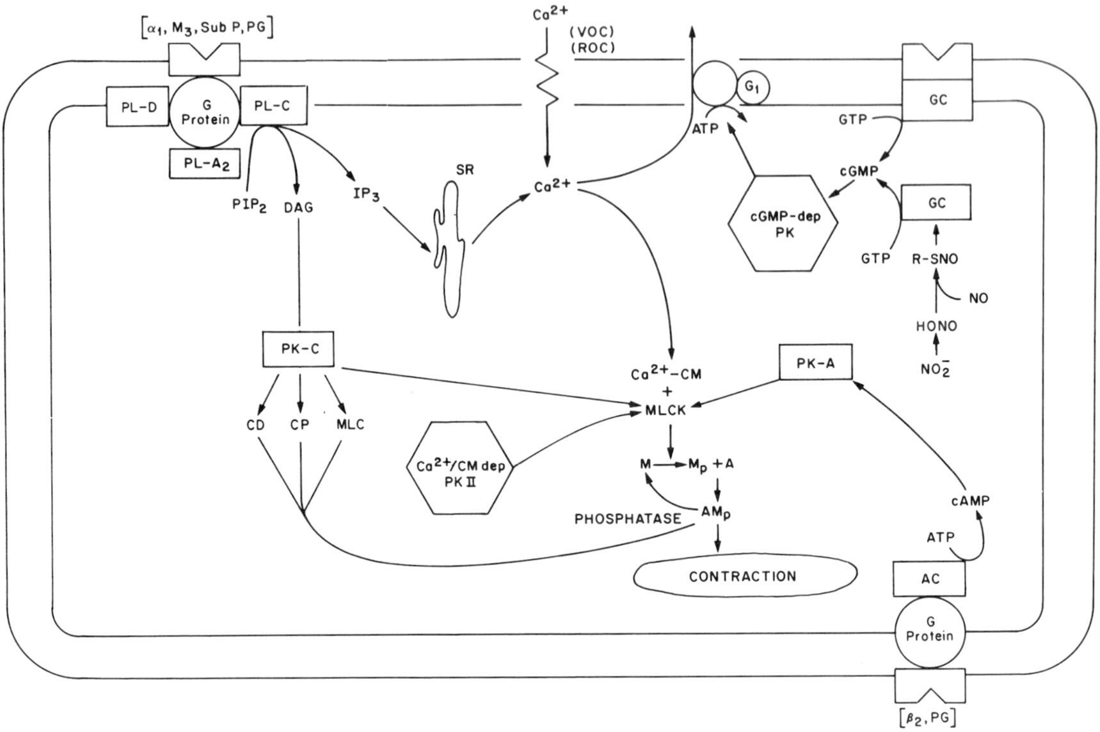

Figure 2 Generalized scheme of the cellular mechanisms regulating contraction and relaxation in vascular smooth muscle. α_1, alpha-adrenergic receptor; M_3, muscarinic receptor; Sub P, substance P receptor; PG, prostaglandin receptor; PL-D, phospholipase D; PL-A_2, phospholipase A_2; PL-C, phospholipase C; PIP_2, phosphatidyl inositol 4,5-bisphosphate; DAG, diacylglycerol; IP_3, inositol 1,4,5 trisphosphate; PK-C, protein kinase C; CD, caldesmon; CP, calponin; MLC, myosin light chain; Ca^{2+}/CM dep PK II, calcium–calmodulin-dependent protein kinase II; M, myosin; Mp, phosphorylated myosin; A, actin; MLCK, myosin light-chain kinase; CM, calmodulin; SR, sarcoplasmic reticulum; VOC, voltage-operated channel; ROC, receptor-operated channel; GC, guanylate cyclase; cGMP-dep PK, cyclic GMP-dependent protein kinase; PK-A, cyclic AMP-dependent protein kinase; AC, Adenylate cyclase; β_2, beta-adrenergic receptor; NO, nitric oxide (e.g., from endothelium). All three phospholipase enzymes are shown bound to the same G-protein for simplicity.

perativity, however, is unresolved. In addition, these calcium-binding sites may be affected by magnesium and hydrogen ions, and the role of secondary ions in the regulation of contraction is poorly understood. Myosin light chain kinase has at least one phosphorylation site, the phosphorylation of which causes much lower specific activity for MLCK.

A number of intracellular molecules exist that can regulate the contractile apparatus of smooth muscle. These regulating molecules include calcium, calmodulin, protein kinase-C, and myosin light chain kinase. In addition, a number of phosphatases exist that can dephosphorylate MLCK and the mysoin light chain itself. Actin-binding proteins caldesmon and calponin appear to play an inhibitory role in the calcium–calmodulin-activated contraction of vascular smooth muscle (10). Both caldesmon and calponin can be phosphorylated in vitro and, thus, the regulation of vascular smooth muscle contraction consists of numerous and complex interactions depicted in the generalized scheme in Figure 2. An understanding of these complexities may lead to more sophisticated clinical control of vascular disease.

A controversial model exists that attempts to explain the sustained development of tension and the economy of energy consumption in smooth muscle (11). In this model, a "Latch" state between actin and myosin would create a rigid cross-bridge that would allow the maintenance of tone without the further expenditure of energy. Evidence for this latch state is demonstrated in the work by Rembolt and Murphy (12); the merit of this theory is discussed in another chapter. Agents that act directly on this latch state are unknown at present, but may prove useful in the future treatment of contractile states such as asthma and vasospasm.

1. Regulation of Calcium

The maintenance of intracellular calcium homeostasis is essential in the development of basal tone. Normal intracellular calcium concentrations range from 120 to 200 nM, which are 10,000 times lower than that of the extracellular fluid (13). The calcium gradient across the cell membrane is maintained by a number of active mechanisms depicted in Figure 3. The plasma membrane contains a calcium–ATPase pump, which causes calcium extrusion. The calcium–extrusion pump is a high-affinity system with a K_m for intracellular calcium of less than 1 μM (14), but with a low capacity. In contrast, the sodium–calcium cotransport (or antiporter) system is a low-affinity, high-capacity system that uses the electrochemical gradient generated from the sodium pump to export calcium. Although recent evidence (15) suggests a significant role in bovine pulmonary artery, other investigators report that the sodium–calcium cotransport system plays a minor role in smooth muscle cells (16). The sodium–calcium cotransport system appears to be important in cardiac muscle, as exemplified by the important actions of cardiac glycosides on failing myocardium.

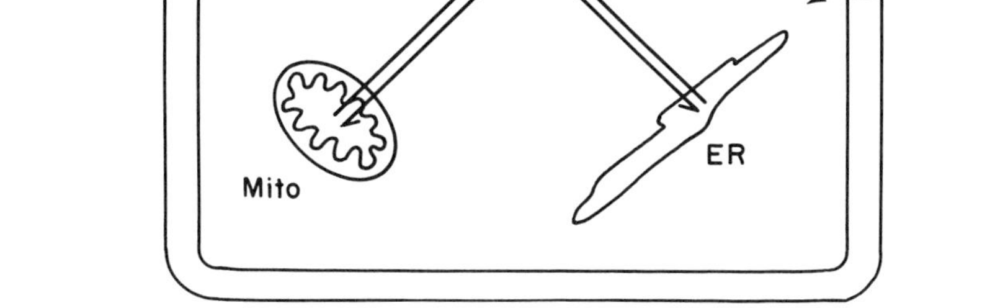

Figure 3 Mechanism controlling cytosolic Ca^{2+} in mammalian cells. Mito, mitochondria; ER, endoplasmic reticulum. (From Ref. 13 with permission.)

In addition to transport systems, a number of calcium channels exist that allow passage of calcium into the cell. In vascular smooth muscle cells, there exist both voltage-sensitive and voltage-insensitive channels. Two different voltage-sensitive channels, designated T and L, allow calcium currents to pass across the cell membrane. The differences between these voltage-sensitive channels will be described in more detail in the section below on calcium channel antagonists. Receptor-operated channels also allow calcium to enter the smooth muscle cells, but these channels and agents that modify them are discussed in another chapter.

In addition to extracellular sources of calcium, several intracellular organelles also contain calcium in relatively high concentrations. Somlyo et al. (17) described the sequestration of calcium by the sarcoplasmic reticulum (SR) as an active process, which requires the hydrolysis of ATP. The calcium uptake into the SR is slow, however, and cannot account for the transient nature of the intracellular calcium peak following certain agonist-induced contractions.

Vascular smooth muscle differs from skeletal muscle and also from certain gut tissues in that depolarization is not essential for contraction. Most agonists that cause vascular smooth muscle contraction cause a transient increase in the concentration of intracellular calcium. The higher calcium triggers the release of additional calcium from the SR, a phenomenon known as "calcium-induced calcium release" that is blocked by specific dihydropyridines. In addition, inositol 1,4,5-triphosphate (IP_3) can cause the release of calcium from intracellular stores. Thus, a common trigger of smooth muscle contraction appears to be an initial rise in intracellular free calcium.

2. *Voltage-Sensitive Calcium Channels*

Of the three known voltage-sensitive calcium channels, two seem to occur frequently in smooth muscle (16). The transient or "T" channel is a short-acting pore that permits the passage of calcium ions but inactivates within 10 msec. In contrast, the long-duration or "L" channel permits sustained calcium currents and inactivates slowly over minutes. The T and L channels are identical to those found in cardiac muscle. The L-type calcium channel is more numerous in smooth muscle, making up about 80% of the voltage-sensitive channels and, therefore, the L-type channel represents the major pathway for calcium entry. The L-type channels are activated by the experimental agent Bay K 8644 and blocked by dihydropyridines. There is also evidence that these channels can be modified by phosphorylation of the channel protein or an associated regulatory protein such as a G protein.

3. *Inositide Metabolism and Calcium*

Recently, the role of inositide metabolism has been elucidated (18) in signal transduction of many cell types. From a number of cell types, Berridge and Irvine (18) provide evidence for inosital 1,4,5-triphosphate causing the release of calcium from intracellular stores. The essential step in the pathway of inositide metabolism is the hydrolysis of phosphatidyl inositol bisphosphate into the soluble components diacylglycerol and inositol triphosphate (IP_3). In the second messenger action of IP_3, there is an amplification by which a single molecule of IP_3 causes the release of 20 calcium ions. The most likely source of the stores of releasable calcium ion is the sarcoplasmic reticulum. Suematsu et al. (19) confirmed the role of IP_3 in vascular smooth muscle using saponin-skinned single muscle cells from porcine coronary artery. In his report, Suematsu shows release of calcium from intracellular stores by IP_3 as well as caffeine. In certain cases of agonist stimulation, the rise in concentration of IP_3 has been shown to precede that of intracellular calcium. Thus, the generation of a calcium trigger to smooth muscle contraction may, under certain circumstances, involve either calcium-induced calcium release (CICR) or IP_3-mediated calcium release.

III. CALCIUM CHANNEL ANTAGONISTS AND CLINICAL USE

Table 1 shows the various agents that block calcium channels. Of these classes, the dihydropyridines, the papaverine derivations, and the benzothiazepines show the most specific action. In the case of the dihydropyridines, for example, van Breeman et al. (19) have shown that these blockers bind to the slow calcium channels more readily in the open state than in the resting or closed state. The dihydropyridines such as nifedipine or nicardipine inhibit calcium influx through voltage-sensitive channels. The effect in VSM from calcium channel blockade is a decrease in force development following stimulation either by action potential depolarization, in the case of visceral muscle, or by potassium depolarization, in the case of arterial smooth muscle (20).

The action of calcium channel blockade has important clinical effects in patients with essential hypertension (21). A hallmark of essential hypertension is an increase in systemic vascular resistance, as shown in studies of forearm blood flow in humans. Calcium channel blockade can decrease systemic vascular resistance with minimal changes in baroreceptor reflex, little reflex tachycardiac or orthostatic hypotension, minimal renal alterations, and no changes in weight. In general, calcium channel blockers work better as therapy for hypertension in the elderly, while beta-blockers work better as initial therapy for hypertension in the young adult. There is some evidence that black patients also show better response to

Table 1 Calcium Channel Antagonists

Dihydropyridine derivatives	*Piperazine derivatives*
Nifedipine	Cinnarizine
Nicardipine	Flunarizine
Niludipine	Lidoflazine
Nisoldipine	
Nitrendipine	*Others*
Nimodipine	Bepredil
Felodipine	Caroverine
FR7534	Fendiline
FR34235	Molsidomine
	Perhexiline
Papaverine derivatives	Prenylamine
Verapamil	PY 106–068
Gallopamil (D600)	Terodiline
Tiapamil	
Benzothiazepine derivatives	
Diltiazem	

calcium channel blockers than to beta-blockers. While monotherapy is the most common initial regimen for hypertension, patients with long-standing or labile hypertension often do better with a combination of a beta-blocker or calcium channel blocker, diuretic, and vasodilator. Later sections will discuss the mechanism of and clinical options in vasodilator therapy.

A. Dihydropyridines

The prototypical and best studied of the dihydropyridines is nifedipine. Nifedipine is a potent vasodilator with an onset time of 10 min when given either orally or sublingually and has an apparent half-life of 4–5 hr. Nifedipine is useful in moderately severe essential hypertension and shows a greater effect in those patients with a higher initial systemic vascular resistance (22). Although there is some myocardial depression when nifedipine is given in combination with beta-blocking agents, nifedipine has been used safely with nitrates, furosemide, anticoagulants, and antidiabetic therapies. Two medicines used in ulcer therapy, ranitidine and cimetidine, tend to raise plasma levels of nifedipine: both antiulcer drugs reduce hepatic blood flow and cimetidine also lowers microsomal enzyme activity, leading to an elevation in plasma nifedipine levels. Plasma levels of nifedipine, however, correlate poorly with the hypotensive effects. One advantage in using nifedipine is that it tends to improve renal function and does not promote renin release. Side effects of nifedipine therapy include tachycardia, a burning sensation of the face, and ankle edema. Oral dosages begin with 10 mg three or four times daily to a maximum daily dose of 120 mg. The usually sublingual dose is 10 mg. Nifedipine has potent antispasmodic action on coronary arteries and is useful in Printzmetal's angina as well as moderate essential hypertension (23).

Of the dihydropyridines other than nifedipine, several show promising therapeutic benefits. Nicardipine is a water-soluble agent that blocks calcium channels as well as inhibits the enzyme phosphodiesterase. Nicardipine has an extensive first-pass clearance and has an apparent half-life of 2 hr: substantially shorter than that of nifedipine. Another agent, nisoldipine, is the most potent of the dihydropyridines and has little effects on heart rate or myocardial contractility. Niludipine is also extremely potent but shows significant depression of AV conduction in clinical studies. An investigational drug, FR-7534, is light stable and, therefore, has a potential advantage over nifedipine. Thus, the dihydropyridines represent a group of agents that antagonize the slow calcium channel currents in smooth muscle and that show varied hemodynamic effects than can be useful clinically.

B. Diphenylalkylamines

Another class of calcium channel blockers is the synthetic papaverine derivatives known as diphenylalkylamines. Of these, verapamil is the best studied. Verapamil is a potent antihypertensive with an apparent half-life of 4 hr that may increase with chronic administration. In contrast to nifedipine, verapamil shows more myocardial depression when used in combination with beta-blockers or with digoxin and in patients with poor left ventricular function. Like nifedipine, plasma levels of verapamil do not correlate with therapeutic hypotensive effects, although better exercise tolerance has been shown in patients whose plasm levels of verapamil were higher than 200 ng/ml. The usual dosage is 80 mg every 8 hr. In addition to the side

Table 2 Specific Action of Common Calcium Channel Antagonists

	Nifedipine	Verapamil	Diltiazem
Afterload	↓↓	↓	↓
Heart rate	↑	–	↓
Coronary blood flow	↑↑	–	↑

effects of headache and dizziness seen with all the calcium blocking agents, verapamil also causes constipation in occasional patients (24).

C. Benzothiazepines

Another separate but specific class of calcium channel antagonists is the benzothiazepines, of which diltiazem is the only agent in current use. Diltiazem blocks the slow calcium channel but there is some evidence that it has a different mechanism of action than the other calcium channel antagonists (25). van Breeman suggests that the action of diltiazem may not be to block calcium entry but rather to interact with the calcium pathway involved in excitation. Diltiazem has an elimination half-life of 4–5 hr and shows extensive hepatic metabolism that can be affected by agents such as cimetidine and barbiturates. In contrast to nifedipine, diltiazem causes slowing of the heart rate and is useful as an antihypertensive in patients who cannot tolerate tachycardia, such as those with ischemic heart disease. The daily dosage is usually 120 mg in three or four divided doses not to exceed 360 mg/day.

In current clinical practice, the three most commonly used calcium channel blockers are nifedipine, verapamil, and diltiazem. Table 2 summarizes the specific hemodynamic effects of these three common therapeutic agents. Of the three, nifedipine is the most potent arterial vasodilator, with its effect both on systemic and coronary vascular resistances. On the other hand, diltiazem produces the most profound bradycardia. All three depress myocardial contractility with minimal venodilatory effects. In choosing a calcium channel blocker, however, one must remember not only the antihypertensive effects but also potential salutary antiarrhythmic effects and detrimental side effects. At present, no single calcium channel blocker is superior in all cases. Until the ideal calcium channel antagonist emerges, the practitioner must choose between a large number of different and imperfect agents.

A number of less-specific calcium channel blocking agents exist that may show clinical benefit under certain conditions. Flunarizine as well as nimodipine appear to be selective cerebral vasodilators. Perhexiline and lidoflazine are long-acting antihypertensives that are efficacious when given once a day but show increased potential toxicity. Cinnarizine has no effect on the inotropic state of the heart, but its complete mechanism of action remains unclear. Although many agents have been shown to be effective monotherapies in mild hypertension, more studies are needed to demonstrate their utility in multidrug therapies for more severe hypertension.

IV. OTHER VASODILATORS

As alluded to previously, multidrug therapy is a common approach to the patient with long-standing or severe hypertension. "Triple" therapy commonly includes a beta-blocker or calcium channel blocker, a diuretic, and a vasodilator. The following section will explore the similarities and varieties of vasodilators in clinical and investigational use.

A. Nitrovasodilators

Recent evidence suggests that a majority of the clinically important vasodilators act in a common manner. Murad suggests the term *nitrovasodilators* to include nitrates, nitrites, nitrosoureas, nitrosamines, azides, hydroxylamine, and hydrazines. All of these agents form a reactive intermediate and cause an increase in cyclic guanosine monophosphate (cGMP) (26). Nitric oxide may also be the transient diffusible substance, endothelium-derived relaxing factor, that mediates endothelium-dependent relaxation (27). Another newly described vasodilator, atrial natriuretic factor, also appears to act by raising cyclic GMP through an endothelium-independent mechanism (28).

In addition to endothelium, a number of vasorelaxants also form nitric oxide. Sodium nitroprusside, for example, spontaneously forms the nitric oxide radical while nitroglycerine forms nitric oxide only in the presence of thiols and under specific conditions and does not stimulate guanylate cyclase in the absence of cysteine. The nitrovasodilators form unstable s-nitrosothiols that are the activators of guanylate cyclase and this instability may explain the short duration of nitric oxide, nitroprusside, and nitroglycerine (25).

Vascular smooth muscle has two isoforms of guanylate cyclase: a particulate and a soluble form that have distinct locations and binding properties. The particulate form is membrane-associated and is activated by atrial natriuretic factor, enterotoxin, and other agents. On the other hand, the soluble isoenzyme is found in the cytosol and is activated by nitric oxide and, therefore, by the nitrovasodilators, and by hydroxyl free radicals. Both forms of guanylate cyclase catalyze the hydrolysis of GTP and the formation of cyclic GMP. Increased cyclic GMP has been associated with the relaxation of tracheal as well as vascular smooth muscle (29–32).

The mechanisms by which increases in cyclic GMP cause relaxation are not understood at present. Cyclic GMP is known to activate cyclic GMP-dependent protein kinase, which phosphorylates a number of smooth muscle proteins (33) and one of these proteins may cause the dephosphorylation of myosin light chain and, thus, reduce its affinity for actin, prevent cross-bridge formation, and lessen smooth muscle contraction (Figure 4). Whether the inhibition of contraction is equal to relaxation is unknown. Although the cyclic GMP-mediated relaxation is calcium-independent, vasorelaxants such as the nitrovasodilators do decrease levels of intracellular calcium, as reported using the fluorescent indicator Quin-2 or aequorin (34). Acting on guanylate cyclase is not the only mechanism of vasodilatation, however, and this section will also mention some vasodilators that act in other ways. The remainder of this section will focus on two of the nitrovasodilators, sodium nitroprusside and nitroglycerin, as well as hydralazine, diazoxide, and flosequinan. The last three agents all have different mechanisms of action that illustrate the complexity of vascular smooth muscle relaxation and also the potential range of options in treating hypertension.

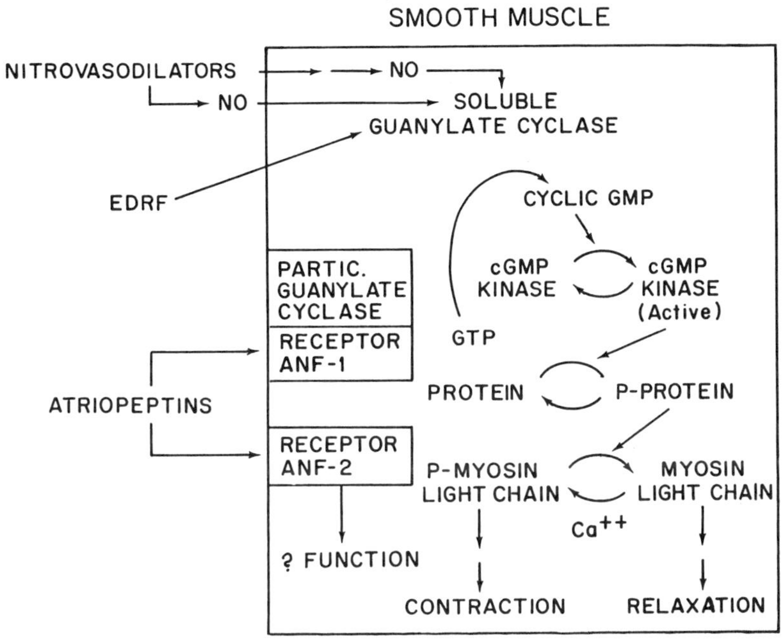

Figure 4 Proposed scheme of a common intracellular mechanism for vasodilation by nitrovasodilators, endothelium-derived relaxing factor (EDRF) and atriopeptins. ANF, atrial natriuretic factor. (From ref. 26 with permission.)

1. Sodium Nitroprusside

Sodium nitroprusside (SNP) or nitroferricyanide consists of a central ferrous atom surrounded by five cyanide moieties and a nitro group. The mechanism of action is similar to all the nitrovasodilators involving the production of nitric oxide and the eventual stimulation of soluble guanylate cyclase (31). SNP relaxes both resistance and capacitance vessels, with a greater effect on arterial smooth muscle, and has no direct central or autonomic activity. Due to a reflex activation of the sympathetic nervous system, the heart rate increases as well as plasma norepinephrine levels with the use of SNP. In normotensive dogs, SNP improves renal perfusion. However, in both hypertensive dogs and patients SNP reduces renal blood flow and fractional sodium excretion and increases plasma renin levels. the metabolism of SNP includes the release of thiocyanate and cyanide ions that have no hemodynamic effects. Cyanide levels can cause toxicity during the prolonged infusion of high doses of SNP, especially in patients with hepatic or renal disease, although the metabolic effects of cyanide toxicity can be reversed using sodium thiosulfate or hydroxocobalamin. The first sign of cyanide toxicity is usually metabolic acidosis. The half-life of SNP is 2–30 min and is excreted mainly in the urine. Sodium nitroprusside is used in hypertensive emergencies and congestive heart failure and is administered intravenously in dosages of 0.5–10 μg/kg/min. Doses higher than 10 μg/kg/min often result in cyanide toxicity and are not recommended. Frequent blood pressure monitoring is essential during the administration of nitroprusside. Rare side effects include hypothyroidism, thrombocytopenia, and methemoglobinuria.

2. Nitroglycerin

Nitroglycerin or trinitroglycerin (TNG) is another member of the nitrovasodilators. Unlike nitroprusside, which acts principally on arterial smooth muscle, TNG acts primarily on venous smooth muscle. The basic mechanism of action for TNG involves the production of nitric oxide and formation of unstable nitrothiol compounds that stimulate guanylate cyclase (31). By reducing venous tone, TNG allows blood to pool in peripheral vessels and leads to a decrease in venous return, lower ventricular volume, and less end-diastolic wall tension (preload). A modest effect on arterial vessels also causes a decline in systemic resistance (afterload). Both effects lead to reduced myocardial oxygen requirements. A third effect of TNG occurs in epicardial coronary arteries, which dilate to improve coronary perfusion further. The specific salutary effect of TNG on coronary arteries makes it useful in ischemic heart disease and in the treatment of variant angina.

Nitrate therapy is available for oral, sublingual, topical, and intravenous routes of administration. The sublingual and intravenous routes show rapid onset of relief from angina. The oral and topical routes provide more gradual onset but more sustained action. Intravenous TNG is used for refractory angina or refractory variant angina and is usually given as a continuous infusion ranging from 0.5 μg/kg/min to 5 μg/kg/min. Nitrate tolerance is well described during chronic or high-dose administration and may be ameliorated using N-acetylcysteine. Side effects include headache, flushing, and methemoglobinemia.

B. Hydralazine

Like nitroprusside, hydralazine also acts primarily as an arterial vasodilator. Hydralazine has forms for both oral and intravenous administration and, therefore, can be used for the treatment of both chronic and acute conditions of hypertension. The precise mechanism of action of hydralazine is unclear but there is some evidence that it lowers intracellular calcium, raises cyclic GMP levels, and decreases myosin light-chain phosphorylation (32). Hydralazine has a number of effects that act to lower blood pressure and raise heart rate and cardiac output. The cardiac effects represent a combination of actions on systemic vascular resistance, the myocardium, and the central nervous system. The sympathetic reflex in response to hydralazine includes tachycardia and activation of the renin–angiotensin–aldosterone system. Thus, hydralazine is usually given with a beta blocker and a diuretic to prevent tachycardia and salt water retention, respectively. The kidney excretes most of the hydralazine after a significant amount of biotransformation in the form of acetylation. Patients who are slow acetylators, therefore, demonstrate higher plasma levels than fast acetylators and are also more prone to develop the side effect of lupus erythematosus syndrome. In addition to the lupus syndrome, hydralazine has rare side effects of peripheral neuropathy, blood dyscrasias, and hepatotoxicity. The adult oral dosage is usually 10–25 mg twice or three times daily. Intravenous doses in adults are usually slow boluses of 5–10 mg to a total of 40 mg. Besides being part of a triple-drug regimen for chronic hypertension, hydralazine is also indicated during hypertensive emergencies, especially acute glomerulonephritis and eclampsia. Two other agents, dihydralazine and minoxidil, have actions similar to those of hydralazine.

C. Diazoxide

Diazoxide is structurally related to the thiazide diuretics, although it has no natriuretic or diuretic effects. Although diazoxide shows a rapid dilating effect on arterioles, it has little effect on veins. Janis et al. (35) have shown that diazoxide can deplete intracellular calcium stores and can depress the vascular reactivity to calcium. Diazoxide does not inhibit carbonic anhydrase and has no direct effects on the heart or autonomic nervous system. Reflex sympathetic activity in response to diazoxide causes an increase in heart rate, plasma catecholamines, renin, angiotensin, and aldosterone, resulting in significant salt and water retention when not used in combination with diuretic. Hyperglycemia and hyperuricemia are two important side effects of diazoxide. Diazoxide appears to have a direct effect on the pancreas to decrease insulin release and results not only in hyperglycemia but also in higher serum levels of free fatty acids. This effect on the pancreas may also result from a mild ability of diazoxide to inhibit phosphodiesterase. Diazoxide also causes rare hypersensitivity reactions and occasional but reversible extrapyramidal symptoms. Excreted in the urine, diazoxide demonstrates a half-life of 20–30 hr, which is much longer than the hypotensive effect. In combination with a beta-blocker and a diuretic, diazoxide is useful in the management of hypertension that is refractory to monotherapy as well as in the management of hypertensive emergencies. The usual dosage schedule for diazoxide is 1–3 mg/kg bolus intravenously to a maximum of 150 mg, followed by an infusion rate of 15–30 mg/min in the adult.

D. Flosequinan

Flosequinan is a recently described quinoline derivative that is an effective arterial and venous dilator (36). In both hypertensive animal and human studies, flosequinan has been shown to lower arterial blood pressure, increase cardiac output, and lower pulmonary arterial occlusion (wedge) pressure that make it a promising drug in the treatment of hypertension and congestive heart failure (37). Sim et al. (38) compared the actions of flosequinan to those of hydralazine and found less tachycardia, lower renin levels, and no change in the renal clearance of creatinine or of para-aminohippurate. Cowley et al. (36) actually report decreases in plasma renin and norepinephrine concentrations in patients given flosequinan. Unlike hydralazine, which causes sodium and water retention, flosequinan actually produces a mild increase in sodium and chloride excretion. In clinical trials, flosequinan has been shown to be effective in the treatment of hypertension both as a monotherapy and in combination with a beta-blocker and diuretic (39). Flosequinan has been shown not to inhibit phosphodiesterase and, therefore, its mechanism of action is unlike the inotrope/vasodilator amrinone. Other investigators are testing the effect of flosequinan on the intracellular calcium pool and initial evidence indicates that flosequinan employs a novel modulation of the contractile apparatus of vascular smooth muscle in addition to a direct depression in the concentration of intracellular calcium (40).

V. CONCLUSION

In the pathophysiology of essential hypertension, the rise in systemic vascular resistance (SVR) plays a central role. One might expect the treatment of hypertension to address the abnormal vascular resistance, but this is not always the case. In fact, beta-blocking agents, when used as a monotherapeutic agent, actually raise SVR. Another class of drugs used to treat hypertension, namely the diuretics, often cause reflex neurohumoral changes, specifically in the renin–angiotensin–aldosterone system that also act to increase systemic vascular resistance.

The focus of this chapter has been the antihypertensive agents that act on calcium channels (41) and that act to stimulate guanylate cyclase. The calcium channel blockers (42,43) and the nitrovasodilators currently constitute the most clinically efficacious of the vasodilators and may be useful in other cardiovascular disorders (44). The contractile apparatus of smooth muscle has a number of regulator proteins that may provide sites of action of antihypertensives. Drugs which affect protein kinase-C, calmodulin, myosin light-chain kinase (45), or the myosin light chains themselves may prove to be useful therapeutic agents. In addition, the phosphatases that inactivate myosin might also be targets for pharmacologic manipulation (46). While several such agents exist in the laboratory, the next decade holds promise for a number of clinical therapeutic agents that act on the central contractile mechanism of vascular smooth muscle tone and, thus, the central pathophysiological cause of essential hypertension.

REFERENCES

1. Braunwald E, ed. Heart disease: a textbook of cardiovascular medicine. Philadelphia: W.B. Saunders, 1980.
2. Laragh JH, Resnick LM. Recognizing and treating two types of long-term vasoconstriction in hypertension. *Kidney Int* 1988; 25:S-162–74.
3. Conway J. Hemodynamic aspects of essential hypertension in human. *Physiol Rev* 1984; 64:617–60.
4. Vanhoutte PM. Aging and vascular responsiveness. *J Cardiovasc Pharmacol* 1988; 12(Suppl 8):S11–8.
5. Longman SD, Clapham JC, Wilson C, Hamilton TC. Cromakalin, a potassium channel activator: a comparison of its cardiovascular haemodynamic profile and tissue specificity with those of pinacidil and nicrorandil. *J Cardiovasc Pharmacol* 1988; 12:535–42.
6. Small JV, Squire JM. Structural basis of contraction in vertebrate smooth muscle. *J Mol Biol* 1972; 67:117–49.
7. Small JV, Sobieszek A. Contractile and structural proteins of smooth muscle. In: Stephens NL *Biochemistry of smooth muscle,* volume 1. Boca Raton, FL: CRC Press, 1986.
8. Kamm KE, Stull JT. The function of myosin and myosin light chain kinase phosphorylation in smooth muscle. *Annu Rev Pharmacol Toxicol* 1985; 25:593–620.
9. Cox JA. Interactive properties of calmodulin. *Biochem J* 1988; 249:621–9.
10. Chalovich JM. Caldesmon and thin-filament regulation of muscle contraction. *Cell Biophysics* 1988; 12:73–85.
11. Naka M, Kureishi Y, Muroga Y, Takahashi K, Ito M, Tanaka T. Modulation of smooth muscle calponin by protein kinase C and calmodulin. *Biochem Biophys Res Commun* 1990; 171:933–7.
12. Rembold CM, Murphy RA. Myoplasmic calcium, myosin phosphorylation and regulation of the crossbridge cycle in swine arterial smooth muscle. *Circ Res* 1986; 58:803–15.
13. Exton JH. Mechanisms of action of calcium-mobilizing agonists: some variations on a young theme. *FASEB J* 1988; 2:2670–6.
14. Eggermont JA, Vrolix M, Raeymaekers L, Wuytack F, Casteels R. Ca^{2+}-transport ATPases of vascular smooth muscle. *Circ Res* 1988; 62:266–78.

15. Birkenhager WH, Reid JL, eds. Handbook of hypertension. Amsterdam: Elsevier, 1984.
16. Bengham CD, Hess P, Tsien RW. Two types of calcium channels in single smooth muscle cells from rabbit ear artery studied with whole-cell and single-channel recordings. *Circ Res* 1987: 61:I10–6.
17. Somlyo AV, Somlyo AP. Electromechanical and pharmacomechanical coupling in vascular smooth muscle. *J Pharmacol Exp Ther* 1968; 159:129–45.
18. Berridge MJ, Irvine RF. Inositol triphosphate, a novel second messenger in cellular single transduction. *Nature* 1984; 312:315–21.
19. Suematsu E, Hirata M, Hashimoto T, Kuriyama H. Inositol 1,4,5-triphosphate releases Ca^{2+} from intracellular store sites in skinned cells of porcine coronary artery. *Biochem Biophys Res Commun* 1984; 120:481–5.
20. van Breeman C, Cauvin C, Yamamoto H, Zschauer A. Vascular smooth muscle channels. *J Cardiovasc Pharmacol* 1987; 10:S10–5.
21. Hermsmeyer K, Sturek M, Rusch NJ. Calcium channel modulation by dihydropyridines in vascular smooth muscle. *Ann NY Acad Sci* 1988; 522:25–31.
22. Bayley S, Dobbs RJ, Robinson BF. Nifedipine in the treatment of hypertension: report of a double-blind controlled trial. *Br J Clin Pharmacol* 1982; 14:509–12.
23. Olivari MT, Bartorelli C, Polese A, Fiorentini C, Moruzzi P, Guazzi MD. Treatment of hypertension with nifedipine, or calcium channel antagonistic agent. *Circulation* 1979; 59:1056–62.
24. Lewis GR. Long-term results with verapamil in essential hypertension and its influence on serum lipids. *Am J Cardiol* 1986; 57:35D–8D.
25. van Breeman C, Hwang OK, Meisheri KD. The mechanism of inhibitory action of diltiazem on vascular smooth muscle contractility. *J Pharmacol Exp Ther* 1981; 218:459–63.
26. Murad F. Cyclic guanosine monophosphate as a mediator of vasodilation. *J Clin Invest* 1986; 78:1–5.
27. Ignarro LJ. Endothelium-derived nitric oxide: actions and properties. *FASEB J* 1989; 3:31–6.
28. Feelisch M, Noack EA. Correlation between nitric oxide formation during degradation of organic nitrates and activation of guanylate cyclase. *Eur J Pharmacol* 1987; 139:19–30.
29. Winquist RJ, Faison EP, Waldman SA, Schwartz K, Murad F, Rapoport RM. Atrial natriuretic factor elicits an endothelium-independent relaxation and activates particulate guanylate cyclase in vascular smooth muscle. *Proc Natl Acad Sci* (*USA*) 1984; 81:7661–4.
30. Murad F, Waldman S, Molina C, Bennett B, Leitman D. Regulation and role of guanylate cyclase-cyclic GMP in vascular relaxation. In: Cabot and McKeehan, eds. *Mechanisms of signal transduction by hormones and growth factors*. New York: Alan R. Liss, 1987.
31. Kreye VA, Hofmann F, Villhauer I. Mode of action of nitrates at the cellular level. *Z Kardiol* 1986; 75(Suppl 3):16–9.
32. Ignarro LJ, Lippton H, Edwards JC, Baricos WH, Hyman AL, Kadowitz PJ, Gruetter CA. Mechanism of vascular smooth muscle relaxation by organic nitrates, nitrites, nitroprusside and nitric oxide: evidence for involvement of s-nitrosothiols as active intermediates. *J Pharmacol Exp Ther* 1981; 219:739–49.
33. Sarcevic B, Brooks V, Martin TJ, Kemp BE, Robinson PJ. Atrial natriuretic peptide-dependent phosphorylation of smooth muscle cell particulate fraction proteins is mediated by cGMP-dependent protein Kinase. *J Biol Chem* 1989; 264(34):20648–54.
34. Jacobs M. Mechanism of action of hydralazine on vascular smooth muscle. *Biochem Pharmacol* 1984; 33:2915–9.

35. Janis RA, Triggle DJ. Effect of diazoxide on aortic reactivity to calcium in spontaneously hypertensive rats. *Can J Physiol Pharmacol* 1973; 51:621.
36. Cowley AJ, Wynn RD, Hampton JR. Flosequinan in heart failure: acute haemodynamic and longer term symptomatic effects. *Eur J Clin Pharmacol* 1987; 33:203–4.
37. Kessler PD, Packer M, Medinea N, Yushak M. Cumulative hemodynamic response to short-term treatment with flosequinan (BTS 49465), a new direct-acting vasodilator drug, in severe chronic congestive heart failure. *J Cardiovasc Pharmacol* 1988; 12:6–11.
38. Sim MF, Yates DB, Parkinson R, Cooling MJ. Cardiovascular effects of the novel arteriovenous dilator agent, flosequinan in conscious dogs and cats. *Br J Pharmacol* 1988; 94:371–80.
39. Cowley AJ, Wynne RD, Stainer K, Fullwood L, Rowley JM, Hampton JR. Flosequinan as a third agent for the treatment of hypertension: a placebo-controlled, double-blind study. *Br Med J* 1988; 297:169–73.
40. Resnick MS, Maitland LA, Morgan KG. Flosequinan, a vasodilator with a novel mechanism of action. *Br J Pharmacol* 1991; 102:974–8.
41. Bohr DF. Actions of calcium on smooth muscle. Historical overview. *Ann NY Acad Sci* 1987; 522:210–5.
42. Laher I, Hwa J, Bevan JA. Calcium and vascular myogenic tone. Ann NY Acad Sci 1987; 522:216–25.
43. Buhler FR. Kiowski W. Calcium antagonists and their potential for antihypertensive therapy. *Ann NY Acad Sci* 1988; 522:584–99.
44. Ferlinz J. Nifedipine in myocardial ischemia, systemic hypertension, and other cardiovascular disorders. *Ann Intern Med* 1986; 105:714–29.
45. Kamm KE, Stull JT. Activation of smooth muscle contraction: relationship between myosin phosphorylation and stiffness. *Science* 1986; 232:80–2.
46. Morgan JP, Morgan KG. Alteration of cytoplasmic ionized calcium levels in smooth muscle by vasodilators in the ferret. *J Physiol* 1984; 357:539–51.

9

The Cardiac Adrenergic Transmembrane Signaling System

WARREN D. ROSENBLUM and ARTHUR M. FELDMAN

Johns Hopkins University School of Medicine
Baltimore, Maryland

I. INTRODUCTION

The heart provides vascular support under resting conditions and allows the body to respond to both abrupt and gradual physiological changes. The physiological responses of cardiac tissue to biological changes are in response to complex neural and hormonal stimuli. Immediate reactions as evidenced by the classic fight or flight response are mediated by neural stimuli. In contrast, slower and more prolonged responses are modulated by hormonal mechanisms. The autonomic nervous system via efferent sympathetic nerve pathways effects rapid and coordinated changes in cardiovascular function. Numerous humoral agents effect similar, albeit slower, physiological changes. Neurohormonal signals are received, processed, and amplified by a complex transmembrane signaling system that is an integral part of myocardial cells. One of the most important and intensively studied transmembrane signaling systems in the heart is the receptor-G protein-adenylyl cyclase (RGC) complex (1; Fig. 1). There are three components of this complex: 1. membrane-bound receptors that are capable of binding either agonists or antagonists, 2. guanine nucleotide-binding regulatory proteins (G proteins) that transduce signals from receptors to effector enzymes and either stimulate (G_s) or inhibit (G_i) the adenylyl cyclase enzyme, and 3. adenylyl cyclase, which catalyzes the conversion of ATP to cyclic AMP (1). Cyclic AMP activates the cyclic AMP-dependent protein kinases resulting in phosphorylation of multiple cardiac proteins. These cardiac proteins include voltage-dependent calcium channels, the sarcoplasmic reticulum protein phospholamban, troponin I, and trans-acting regulatory proteins within the nucleus (2). Steady-state levels of cyclic AMP are also regulated by phosphodiesterases, enzymes that cleave cyclic AMP into an inactive byproduct, 5′AMP.

In the failing heart, the RGC complex plays an important role. As heart failure progresses and the heart must rely on sympathetic stimuli for inotropic support, the

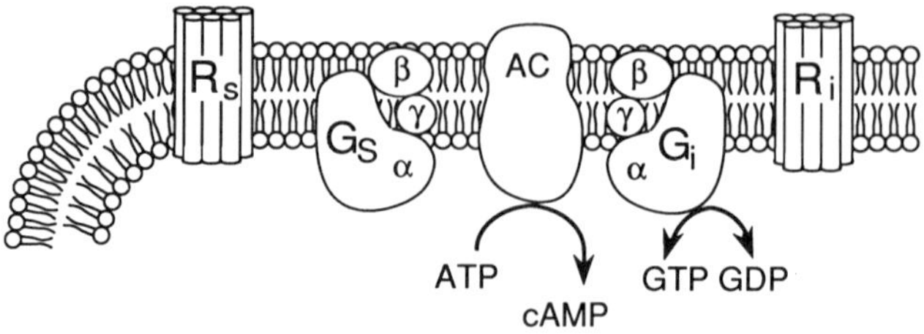

Figure 1 The receptor–adenylyl cyclase complex. R_s, stimulatory receptor; R_i, inhibitory receptor; G_s, stimulatory guanine nucleotide-binding regulatory protein; G_i, inhibitory guanine nucleotide-binding regulatory protein; AC, adenylyl cyclase catalytic unit.

function of the RGC complex paradoxically diminishes. This diminution of the RGC function lessens the effects of adrenergic agonists to improve cardiac contractility. As noted in other chapters, efforts have been directed toward designing pharmacologic agents that could augment cardiac contractility via an interaction with a component of the RGC complex. In this chapter we will discuss the biochemistry, molecular regulation, and pathophysiology of this pathway and address the paradoxic finding that β-adrenergic blockade is beneficial in congestive heart failure.

II. ADRENERGIC RECEPTORS

Over 40 years ago, Ahlquist (3) discovered the existence of two types of receptors that respond to neurohormonal signals and, based on their pharmacologic characteristics, designated them as either α- or β-adrenergic receptors. The α-adrenergic receptors were identified as mediating peripheral vascular constriction while the β-adrenergic receptors mediated peripheral vasodilatation and positive chronotropic and inotropic responses in myocardium. In the ensuing 40 years, this original model has remained virtually unchanged. However, two α-receptors (α_1 and α_2) and two β-adrenergic receptor subtypes (β_1 and β_2) have been identified (see Fig. 2). A third β-receptor has been cloned recently; however, it has not been identified in cardiac tissue (4).

III. α-ADRENERGIC RECEPTORS

Although there are two known subtypes of α-receptors (5), only the α_1-receptors are found in significant biological amounts in cardiac tissue (6,7). α_1-Receptors found postsynaptically are preferentially antagonized by prazosin (8,9) and are coupled by a G protein within the phosphotidylinositol transmembrane signaling system (10; Fig. 3). When an agonist binds the cardiac α_1-receptor, phosphotidylinositol 4,5-biphosphate is hydrolyzed into two intracellular messengers, diacylglycerol and inositol triphosphate (IP3), by the phosphodiesterase phospholipase C (11). Diacylglycerol activates protein kinase C with resultant phosphorylation of multiple cellular proteins. In contrast, IP3 mobilizes intracellular sarcoplasmic reticulum calcium (12,13). Stimulation of the phosphotidylinositol transmembrane pathway can elicit a positive inotropic response in some animals (14,15). However, α_1-receptor density is not altered in failing human myocardium (16), suggesting that α_1-receptors do not provide a compensatory pathway in congestive heart failure. In addition, α_1-recep-

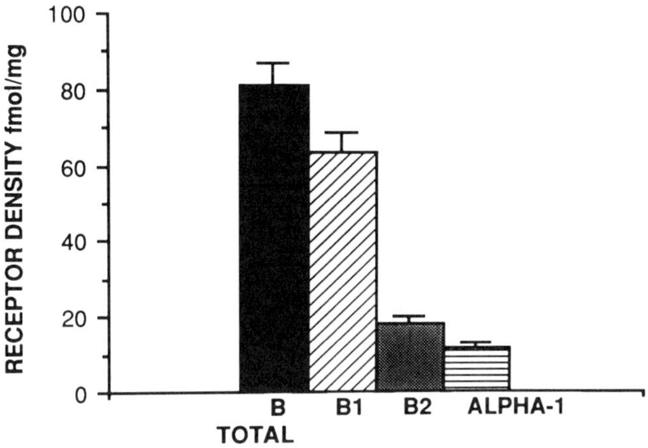

Figure 2 Density measurements of total β, β_1, β_2, and α_1 adrenergic receptors prepared from crude membrane extracts from 18 normal human ventricles. (From Ref. 162.)

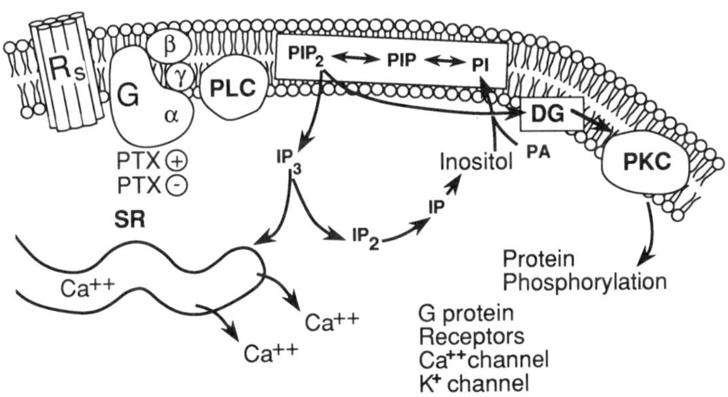

Figure 3 The phosphotidylinositol transmembrane signaling system. R_s, stimulatory receptor; G, stimulatory guanine nucleotide-binding regulatory protein; PLC, phospholipase C; DG, diacylglycerol; IP_3, inositol triphosphate; PIP_2, phosphotidylinositol 4,5,-biphosphate; PIP, phosphotidylinositol 4 phosphate; PI, phosphotidylinositol; IP_2, inositol diphosphate; IP, inositol phosphate; PKC, protein kinase C.

tor density is low, constituting only 14% of the total adrenergic receptor pool (16). In the failing human heart, the proportion of α_1 receptors is increased to 27%; however, this is due to downregulation of the β_1-adrenergic receptors and not to upregulation of the α_1 receptors. Considerable data demonstrates that α_1-receptors are coupled to myocardial growth and hypertrophy (17–19). Stimulation of α-receptors in cultured myocytes enhances the transcriptional expression of structural cardiac proteins, in particular α myosin heavy chain, by stimulating the cyclic AMP-dependent regulatory units of the myosin gene promoter regions.

α_2-Receptor stimulation inhibits adenylyl cyclase via activation of the G inhibitory protein, G_i (20). α_2-Receptors are preferentially antagonized by the yohimbine class of drugs and less so by prazosin (9). Because of their relative absence from human myocardium (7), their relevance to regulation of contractility in the human heart may be insignificant.

IV. β-ADRENERGIC RECEPTORS

Unlike other mammalian species, the human heart has two types of β-receptors (β_1 and β_2), both of which are coupled to adenylyl cyclase and can therefore augment cardiac contractility. These receptors play an important role in the regulation of cardiac contractility and are the most powerful mechanisms by which cardiac contractility can be enhanced physiologically. Although both receptor types are coupled with adenylyl cyclase stimulation, they can be differentiated pharmacologically by their differing affinities for adrenergic agonists. The β_1-receptor binds epinephrine and norepinephrine with equal affinity, while the β_2-receptor preferentially binds norepinephrine approximately 30-fold more than epinephrine (20). In addition, as will be shown subsequently, the two receptors are regulated differently.

V. β-ADRENERGIC RECEPTOR DOWNREGULATION AND MODULATION

It is well known that prolonged exposure to adrenergic agonists eventually results in an attenuated physiological response and that this insensitivity to catecholamines is in part due to desensitization of the β-adrenergic receptors. This decrease in receptor responsiveness with chronic exposure is intuitively rational. The development of the fight or flight response was of major importance in the teleogenesis of higher mammals. Animals with greater adrenergic responses to stressful situations would likely have an increased chance of survival. However, prolonged flight or fight was highly unlikely and the effects of prolonged catecholamine exposure were possibly toxic. Therefore, receptor desensitization may well have developed as a protection against prolonged adrenergic stimulation. The adrenergic receptor is protected from continuous stimulation by two mechanisms. Homologous desensitization enables the receptor to decrease responsiveness to a specific hormone without disrupting receptor sensitivity to other ligands (22,23). In contrast, heterologous desensitization enables the receptor to decrease responsiveness to multiple hormonal stimuli (24). Homologous desensitization can occur quickly, in a matter of minutes (25,26), while heterologous desensitization occurs over a longer period of time and requires the interaction of multiple stimuli (27). Although the exact mechanisms responsible for desensitization are yet to be defined, there is evidence that homologous desensitization occurs at high concentrations of agonist while heterologous desensitization occurs at lower concentrations of agonist (28). Furthermore, heterologous desensitization is mediated in part via a cyclic AMP-dependent protein kinase that phosphorylates the β-adrenergic receptor. Homologous desensitization occurs independent of cyclic AMP-dependent protein kinase (28). Regional sequestration of β-receptors from both the effector enzymes and transduction proteins may be partially responsible for homologous (29) and heterologous (30,31) receptor desensitization. Desensitized receptors can be differentiated from active receptors and selectively quantified utilizing differential sedimentation rates on sucrose density gradients (32). In addition, desensitized (or sequestered) receptors can be identified using binding isotherms with hydrophilic ligands, which bind only surface receptors, and hydrophobic ligands, which bind all receptors including sequestered ones (31). This process of rapid receptor sequestration is reversible, since levels of surface receptors will return to normal without protein synthesis (33,34). Recycling of sequestered receptors occurs when an agonist is removed and has been shown to be an energy-dependent process involving the presence of ATP (34). In contrast, after long-term exposure to agonist, there is loss of β-receptors due to degradation and diminished production as a result of diminished levels of receptor mRNA (M.R. Bristow and A.M. Feldman, unpublished observations). Gradual regeneration of β-receptors after heterologous desensitization may require increased transcription of β-receptor mRNA and subsequent protein synthesis after removal of the agonist (33,35).

Receptor phosphorylation is an important mechanism by which receptors can be downregulated. Both protein kinase A and protein kinase C can facilitate heterologous desensitization by phosphorylating adrenergic receptors (23). In addition, the α_1-receptor and β_2-adrenergic receptor can be phosphorylated in vitro by protein kinase A and protein kinase C. However, when agonist is bound to the receptor, protein kinase C preferentially phosphorylates the α_1-receptor and protein kinase A preferentially phosphorylates the β_2-receptor, allowing for cross-communication between the two agonist signaling systems (36). Phosphorylation of the adrenergic receptor is likewise closely linked to homologous desensitization. Benovic et al. isolated a unique protein kinase for the β-adrenergic receptor (βARK) that can phosphorylate β_2 and α_2-adrenergic receptors in the presence of agonist (37–39). This phosphorylation desensitizes the receptor only to the bound agonist. In addition, investigators have identified a specific cofactor, termed barrestin, that enhances the β-adrenergic receptor kinase's ability to phosphorylate the β-adrenergic receptor (40). An interesting finding is that the β-adrenergic receptor kinases phosphorylate other types of receptors, suggesting that agonist "coupling domains" of different receptors may be highly conserved (41). These findings raise an interesting question: how can an enzyme that is relatively promiscuous in its phosphorylation of receptors mediate homologous desensitization (42)? It may be that βARK can only phosphorylate those receptors that have bound agonist. The agonist may have induced a conformational change in the receptor that allows the sites for phosphorylation to be revealed to the kinase (42). This change in conformation with βARK-dependent phosphorylation may also facilitate receptor coupling with G_s in reconstituted systems (43). It is important to note that sequestration of receptors and phosphorylation-dependent desensitization appear to be independent events (44). This is supported by the fact that the stimulatory guanine nucleotide-binding protein G_s can downregulate receptors without receptor sequestration (44,45). It remains to be elucidated how the mechanisms of downregulation, desensitization, and receptor sequestration are interrelated; however, it is clear that they are complex events.

VI. MOLECULAR BIOLOGY OF THE ADRENERGIC RECEPTORS

The application of molecular biological techniques to the study of receptor function, structure, and biochemistry has provided a wealth of information regarding adrenergic receptors. Purification of the β-adrenergic receptor (46) and deduction of the amino acid sequence (Fig. 4) led directly to the isolation of specific clones from a cDNA library containing the cDNA encoding the β_2-adrenergic receptor

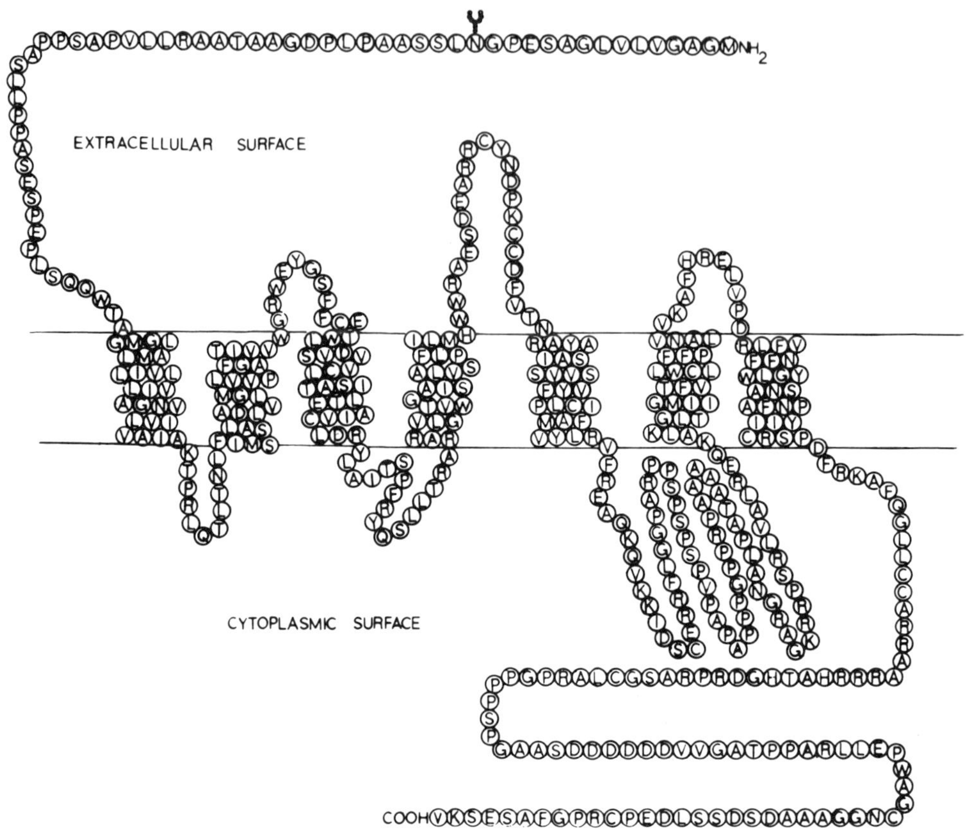

Figure 4 The deduced amino acid sequence of the β_1-adrenergic receptor modified from Frielle et al. (From Ref. 162.)

(47). DNA sequence analysis revealed a gene coding for a 413 amino acid protein (48–50). This gene was notable for the absence of introns (noncoding sequences). Furthermore, hydropathicity studies demonstrated the presence of seven membrane spanning domains (48), a unique structure now known to be present in all known G protein-coupled receptors (51–55). Evidence that this putative β-receptor cDNA did in fact encode the β_2-adrenergic receptor was demonstrated utilizing *Xenopus laevis* oocytes (55). mRNA was transcribed from the cDNA and injected into the *Xenopus* oocytes. This mRNA then encoded receptors in the oocytes that mirrored the pharmacologic characteristics of the β_2-adrenergic receptor (55). These studies produced only a single β-receptor subtype, suggesting that subtype specificity resulted from the presence of homologous yet distinct genes (50). Subsequent somatic cell hybrid analysis studies and in situ hybridization studies localized the β_2-adrenergic receptor to chromosome 5 (48).

Additional studies were carried out to clone and sequence the β_1-adrenergic receptor. Initially, a human genomic clone G-21 was identified that was highly homologous to the β_2-adrenergic receptor and expressed a unique gene product in *Xenopus laevis* oocytes (56). However, this clone proved to represent the gene encoding the serotonin receptor (57) rather than the β_1-adrenergic receptor. Utilizing the serotonin gene as a probe against a human placenta library, investigators were able to isolate and clone the putative β_1-adrenergic receptor cDNA. Expression of this clone in *Xenopus laevis* oocytes confirmed its identity as the β_1-adrenergic receptor gene, since the expressed protein demonstrated pharmacologic characteristics consistent with the β_1-adrenergic receptor. These studies conclusively demonstrated that unique genes encode distinct β_1 and β_2 receptors and that the gene products can be identified by their characteristic pharmacologic properties (50).

The high degree of homology among the different G protein-coupled receptors (58,59) suggests that these various receptors may have evolved from a unique gene (60). By utilizing the *Xenopus laevis* or other expression vectors, investigators have been able to express genes having either mutations or insertions that produce variant gene products (54,61). Chimeric constructs created by splicing sequences from the α_2 and β_2-adrenergic receptor genes were injected into oocytes after being transcribed into mRNA (61). Measurements of adenylyl cyclase activity as well as receptor ligand binding revealed coupling domains within these constructs. G protein coupling was identified between the fifth hydrophobic amino terminus and the sixth hydrophobic carboxyl terminus. Ligand binding domains were found to be within the seven membrane domains while the catecholamine binding site of the β-adrenergic receptor was created by the proximity of the third, fourth, fifth, and seventh domains (62).

α-Adrenergic receptors have also been cloned and sequenced and are highly homologous with other G protein-coupled receptors (54,63,64). α_1-Agonists increase gene transcription in rat myocytes by interacting with *trans*-acting factors in the cell nucleus and possibly by stimulating the expression of early genes such as *c-jun, fos,* and *myc* (65,68).

VII. GUANINE NUCLEOTIDE-BINDING REGULATORY PROTEINS

In 1971, Rodbell and co-workers found that the ability of an adrenergic agonist to promote synthesis of the second messenger cyclic AMP by the enzyme adenylyl cyclase was dependent upon the presence of guanyl nucleotides (69). This landmark finding led to the subsequent discovery of guanine nucleotide-binding regulatory proteins, or G proteins, in the late 1970s (70–72). We now know that these proteins are ubiquitous in eukaryotes and comprise a large family of highly homologous proteins that couple nearly 100 different receptors with effector enzymes (73–76). Furthermore, the receptors and G proteins are intrinsically linked: agonist binding affects G protein conformation while G protein–receptor interactions can modulate receptor affinity. Therefore, the adrenergic receptors cannot be evaluated outside the context of the G proteins.

The G proteins share a heterotrimeric protein structure with subunits designated α, β, and γ. The α-subunits confer specificity upon a G protein and contain GTP-binding sites, intrinsic GTPase activity, and sites that interact with receptors (77), adenylyl cyclase (78), and $\beta\gamma$-subunits (79). The α-subunits of most G proteins also contain a site for bacterial toxin-catalyzed ADP-ribosylation, a finding that led to the initial isolation and characterization of these proteins. Cholera toxin catalyzes a reaction in which NAD^+ is hydrolyzed to ADP-ribose and nicotinamide and the ADP-ribose moiety is covalently bound to specific amino acids on αG_s (80), αG_{olf}

(81), and retinal transducin (82) (which mediates stimulation of cyclic GMP phosphodiesterase by photorhodopsin). The catalytic activity of choleragen can be enhanced by the presence of an ADP ribosylation factor (ARF) (83). ARF is found in both membrane and soluble cell fractions, appears to be ubiquitous in eukaryotic tissues, and its DNA sequence is homologous with the α-subunits of GTP-binding proteins (84,85). Cholera toxin-catalyzed ADP-ribosylation of αG_s stabilizes the GTP-bound conformation of αG_s and decreases its intrinsic GTPase activity, thereby producing continuous stimulation of adenylyl cyclase (86). A paradoxic, finding is that ADP-ribosylation with cholera toxin marks the αG_s protein for accelerated degradation, despite persistence of elevated GTP-dependent adenylyl cyclase activity (87).

Pertussis toxin catalyzes an analogous reaction resulting in attachment of ADP-ribose moieties to different amino acid residues on the α chains of transducin (88), G_i (89), and G_o (90,91), a G protein present in relatively large amounts in brain, but without a known function. In contrast to cholera toxin, pertussis toxin inhibits the functional activity of αG_i (92) and in vivo treatment with pertussis toxin is associated with a decline in G protein β-subunits (93). In addition to ADP-ribosylation, G proteins can also undergo posttranslational modification of myristoylation (94) and phosphorylation (95). Myristoylation affects the binding of the α-subunits to the membrane (96) while phosphorylation may suppress function in hormonal inhibition of adenylyl cyclase (97).

As conceived by Stryer (98), Gilman (99), and their colleagues, the G proteins amplify the effects of receptor activation by a cyclic sequence of steps. When a receptor is occupied by an agonist, GTP binds to αG_s, resulting in the dissociation of the $\beta\gamma$ dimer from αG_s and the activation of the effector by this activated αG_s–GTP complex. In the continued presence of agonist, the activation of the effector enzyme is stopped by the hydrolysis of GTP to GDP by a GTPase located within the αG_s protein. This conversion of GTP to GDP results in a conformational change in αG_s that allows it to reassociate with the $\beta\gamma$ dimer. The associated heterotrimeric form of αG_s results in increased affinity of the β receptor for agonist, whereas dissociation of the heterotrimer (GTP-bound form) decreases receptor affinity. As long as the receptor is occupied by agonist, with GDP–GTP exchange being the rate-limiting step, this cyclic pathway can effect a 100-fold amplification of signal. G_i inhibits adenylyl cyclase by an analogous cycle of dissociation and reassociation; however, in contrast to G_s, the inhibition of adenylyl cyclase may be affected by both the $\beta\gamma$-subunits and αG_i. Free $\beta\gamma$-subunits dissociated from the activated αG_i shift the equilibrium of the G_s heterotrimer toward reassociation by mass action, thereby inactivating G_s (73,100). As an alternative, αG_i (rather than $\beta\gamma$) may mediate inhibition of adenylyl cyclase when G_s is activated by a hormone (101), which would explain the finding that GTP and hormonal stimulation inhibit adenylyl cyclase activity in cells genetically deficient in αG_s (102).

At least four species of αG_s have been recognized having relative molecular weights of 45,000 or 52,000 daltons (103). These various forms are encoded by a single gene and are produced by alternative splicing of the single mRNA precursor (104). It appears that only subtle physiological differences exist between these various forms of αG_s. Three species of αG_i have been identified, each being encoded by a separate gene and having relative molecular weights between 37,000 and 42,000 (105). These distinct αG_i species are differentially regulated in varying tissues; however, it is not known whether they act discretely with selected receptors (106). Therefore, it is not known whether their physiological function differs. The β-subunits of the G heterotrimer have relative molecular weights of either 35,000 or 36,000 daltons and are encoded by at least three distinct genes (107). Multiple genes likewise encode immunologically distinct forms of the 9 kDa γ-subunit (108). It is unclear whether these multiple forms of β and γ-subunits have selective cellular functions (109) or merely represent genetic divergence. The $\beta\gamma$-subunits may function to tether the heterotrimer to the cytoskeleton (110). This hypothesis is supported by the finding that the γ-subunits can be posttranslationally modified by farnesylation (111), isoprenylation (112), and methylation (113), reactions which may regulate binding to $\alpha\beta$-subunits or membranes.

Both the 45,000 and 52,000 dalton forms of αG_s are found in the human heart (114), whereas in canine heart only the 45,000 dalton form is evident (115). The expression of these alternatively spliced gene products is developmentally regulated in rat; neonatal cardiac myocytes contain the M_r 52,000 form whereas adult ventricles have predominantly the M_r 45,000 protein (116).

Identification of the subunits of αG_i is more difficult: αG_{i1} and αG_{i3} are indistinguishable by Western blotting with polyclonal antisera. However, $\alpha G_{i1}/\alpha G_{i3}$ and αG_{i2} have been identified in cultured rat myocytes utilizing immunodetection with selective antisera (116). In the human heart, immunoblotting has identified an M_r 40,000 protein that comigrates with the pertussis toxin substrate as well as an M_r 38,000 protein (117). While the M_r 41,000 peptide is likely to represent $\alpha G_{i1}/\alpha G_{i3}$, the identity of the M_r 38,000 peptide is unclear. The level of αG_i is several times greater than that of αG_s in canine ventricular membranes; however, the $\alpha G_s/\alpha G_i$ ratio appears to be reversed at the mRNA level (118). The deduced amino acid sequence of canine cardiac αG_{i2} differs from that of other species by several amino acids; however, it is unclear whether it differs from αG_{i2} in other canine tissues (118). Like the splice variants of αG_s, the αG_i species are developmentally regulated with an increase in αG_i during embryonic development (119–121). However, culture conditions can substantially alter both the expression (116) and function of G proteins in cultured myocytes (122). The mRNA encoding αG_x (123)/αG_z (124), a bacterial toxin-insensitive αG protein with unique biochemical properties (125,126), has not been found in heart; however, a single report has identified αG_z protein in heart by immunodetection (127). The presence of αG_o is more controversial. Although immunodetectable levels of αG_o are evident in purified sarcolemmal preparations of rat heart (128,129), they cannot be detected in particulate fractions of either rat (130) or human heart (117) using the same antibodies. Furthermore, expression of αG_o mRNA is less in heart than in other tissues (131) and appears to be selective for αG_oA (132). The physiological significance of these levels of αG_o protein in ventricular myocardium remains unclear.

Adrenergic agonists effect an almost instantaneous increase in both heart rate and contractility. Therefore, it was difficult to understand how such a rapid effect could be mediated by the somewhat slow cyclic AMP–protein kinase A-dependent pathway. However, in a series of seminal papers, investigators demonstrated that β-adrenergic agonists effect rapid modulation of cardiac calcium channel currents by a direct effect of G_s independent of cyclic AMP (133–135). This membrane-delimited pathway also affects stimulation (via G_s) and inhibition (via G_i) of the atrial cardiac pacemaker channel (136). Therefore, activation of G_s can effect an increase in cardiac performance within a single beat. αG_i Activates muscarinic-gated K^+ channels in atria (75,137,138) and ATP-blockable channels in ventricle (139). However, the role of the $\beta\gamma$-subunits in regulation of atrial muscarinic K^+ channels remains undefined (140–142). These results in heart and recent studies in noncardiac tissue suggest that the pathways coupling G proteins to ion channels are complex and that multiple mechanisms of action may occur (143,144).

In multiple tissues including the heart, α_1-adrenergic stimulation is coupled to polyphosphoinositide-specific phospholipase C by both pertussis toxin-sensitive and -insensitive G proteins (145–147). Also, arachidonic acid release by phospholipase A_2 is mediated by a G protein-coupled receptor (148). However, the G proteins associated with these pathways have not yet been identified.

Unlike cardiac proteins such as myosin and myoglobin, which have undergone extensive molecular investigation, little is known about the regulation of G protein gene transcription. Many genes of higher eukaryotes have several characteristic elements that regulate basal levels of transcription (core promoter elements) and can be induced by a variety of effector mechanisms and stimuli (inducible promoter elements) to augment or attenuate gene transcription (149). These elements are found in the promoter region of the gene and include "TATA," "CCAAT," and "GC" boxes (150–151). The 5′ flanking region of αG_{i2} contains two typical CCAAT boxes and multiple GC box consensus sequences; however, it lacks a consensus TATA-like sequence (152). In contrast, αG_{i3} has a TATA-like sequence as well as GC boxes in its 5′ flanking region, but lacks a typical CCAAT box. As expected with a highly regulated gene, hormonal stimulation alters gene transcription: αG_i gene transcription is enhanced by both thyroid hormone (153) and adrenergic stimulation (154). However, experiments have not been performed to link definitively a hormone or second messenger with increased transcriptional activity. Such experiments can be performed by coupling a putative promoter region with a reporter gene and assessing reporter gene activity in the presence and absence of hormone (155). In contrast to the αG_is, the putative 5′ flanking region of αG_s contains neither TATA nor CCAAT box sequences (156). This finding led investigators to hypothesize that the αG_s gene may be a "housekeeping" gene that is constitutively regulated. However, experimental evidence does not support this hypothesis: studies in noncardiac tissue suggest that pharmacologic perturbations can alter αG_s gene expression (157). Recently, unexpressed upstream exons have been identified in canine αG_s (158). Therefore, αG_s gene transcription may be regulated "upstream" of an exon that is not expressed as a result of splicing of the initial transcript.

VIII. HEART-FAILURE-ASSOCIATED CHANGES IN THE RGC COMPLEX

It is well known that congestive heart failure in humans is associated with a substantial increase in sympathetic nervous system activity (159). In 1965, Chidsey et al. (159) demonstrated that the decrease in cardiac contractility in the failing human heart was associated with increased norepinephrine secretion. Cardiac norepinephrine levels are not elevated (160–162), probably as a result of impaired uptake (163). This increase in adrenergic drive is maladaptive: there is a positive relationship between levels of circulating catecholamines and mortality in patients with congestive heart failure (164).

One direct effect of high circulating catecholamine levels appears to be down-regulation of the β_1-adrenergic receptor in human ventricular myocardium (165–

168). This loss of β-receptors is selective: the density of the $\beta_1$receptor is altered while that of the β_2-receptor remains unchanged (169) (see Fig. 5). As a result, the proportion of β_1-receptors compared with β_2-receptors shifts from approximately 80:20 in nonfailing heart to 60:40 in failing ventricular myocardium (169). Although the β_2-receptor provides a greater degree of inotropic support in the failing myocardium, studies with selective and nonselective adrenergic agonists have demonstrated that the β_2-adrenergic receptor is partially uncoupled from the effector enzyme adenylyl cyclase (169,170). As discussed below, this uncoupling may be a result of alterations in the activity of the G transduction proteins. Recent studies have also demonstrated that long-term adrenergic stimulation induces in vivo functional changes that occur in a subtype-selective fashion (171).

The selective loss of β_1-receptors has profound functional consequences: it results in a near-total loss of β_1-stimulated muscle contraction and a marked decrease in the ability of β_1-agonists to stimulate adenylyl cyclase activity in failing human heart (170,172). Furthermore, there is a direct relationship between the degree of cardiac dysfunction and downregulation of β_1-adrenergic receptors. Patients with mild congestive heart failure ([ejection fraction] 40–50%) demonstrated only a 38.2% reduction in receptor density compared with a 57.7% decrease in adrenergic receptor density in patients with severe disease (EF < 20%) (173).

Initial studies of adrenergic receptor activity in failing human heart utilized tissue obtained from patients with idiopathic dilated cardiomyopathy. However, studies of experimental ischemia in animal models suggested abnormalities in G protein-mediated signal transduction (174). Furthermore, tissue obtained from a small group of patients with congestive heart failure secondary to ischemic heart disease

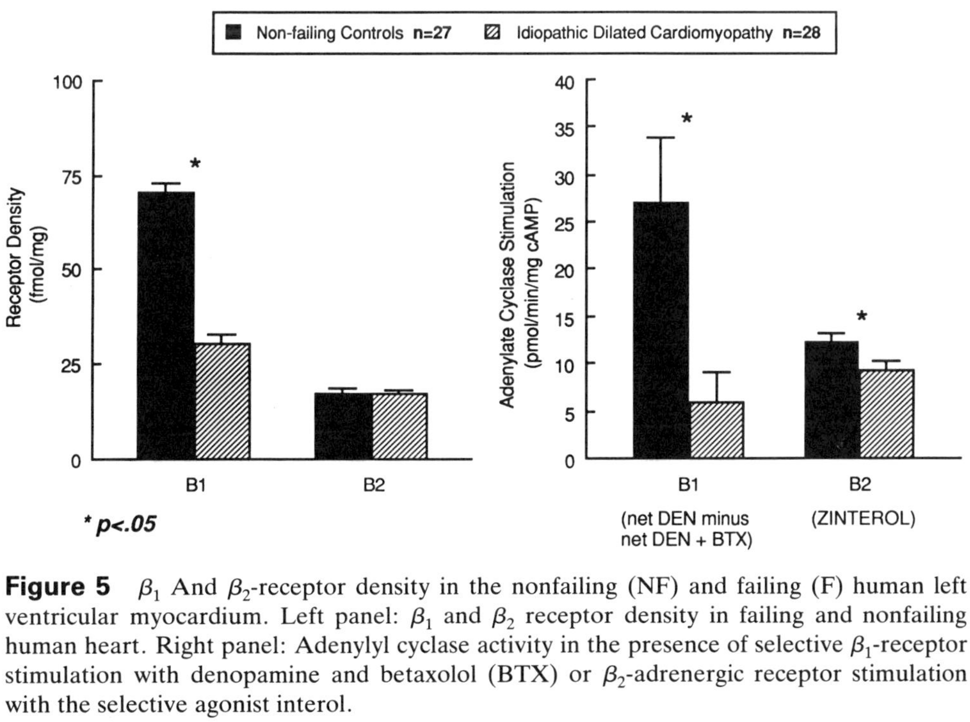

Figure 5 β_1 And β_2-receptor density in the nonfailing (NF) and failing (F) human left ventricular myocardium. Left panel: β_1 and β_2 receptor density in failing and nonfailing human heart. Right panel: Adenylyl cyclase activity in the presence of selective β_1-receptor stimulation with denopamine and betaxolol (BTX) or β_2-adrenergic receptor stimulation with the selective agonist interol.

suggested comparable decreases in receptor density in failing and nonfailing human heart (175). However, a recent study has assessed β-adrenergic neuroeffector mechanisms in a large cohort of patients with either idiopathic dilated cardiomyopathy or ischemic dilated cardiomyopathy (176). This study demonstrated 1. a greater degree of downregulation of total β or β_1-adrenergic receptors in both left and right ventricular myocardium of patients with idiopathic dilated cardiomyopathy; 2. a greater degree of functional uncoupling of the left ventricular β-adrenergic receptors from adenylyl cyclase and a greater uncoupling of right ventricular β-adrenergic receptors from a positive inotropic response in patients with ischemic disease; 3. a selective decrease in adenylyl cyclase activity in the right ventricles of patients with idiopathic dilated cardiomyopathy; and 4. differences in the ability of G protein agonists to augment adenylyl cyclase activity in idiopathic compared with ischemic dilated cardiomyopathies. These studies suggested that potentially important differences exist in the regulatory behavior of components of the RGC complex in idiopathic and ischemic dilated cardiomyopathy, which are presumed to relate to the distinct pathophysiologies of these two types of heart muscle disease.

Little is known about the biology of β-receptor downregulation in failing human heart. Several investigators (170,172,177,178) have recently demonstrated that the levels of β_2-receptor mRNA reflect receptor density in a smooth muscle cell line and that increased lability of the message on exposure to agonist may contribute to the decline in receptor mRNA. Furthermore, exposure of cultured embryonic chick heart cells to norepinephrine results in a rapid decrease in both receptor density and steady-state levels of β_1-receptor mRNA levels (179). Although presently undefined, the molecular mechanisms by which receptors downregulate when exposed to agonist are receiving considerable attention.

It is now well documented that alterations in the functional activity of the G inhibitory protein contribute to the adrenergic insensitivity of the failing human heart. In 1988, we first demonstrated that human hearts with idiopathic dilated cardiomyopathy had diminished adenylyl cyclase activity (see Fig. 6) and that this was associated with an increase in the levels of a pertussis toxin substrate with a relative molecular weight of 40,000 daltons (114; Fig. 7). We were not able to demonstrate an alteration in the activity of αG_s since fluoride-stimulated adenylyl cyclase activity, cholera toxin ADP-ribosylation substrates, and reconstitution studies with cyc- membranes (genetically deficient in αG_s) were not different in failing and nonfailing human hearts. These findings were confirmed by others who demonstrated an increase in pertussis toxin substrate (175,180,181), a lack of change in αG_s, (182), as well as a decrease in guanine nucleotide-stimulated adenylyl cyclase activity (175,183,184) in failing human heart. A functional link between the increase in pertussis toxin substrate and diminished adenylyl cyclase activity was supported by the fact that inhibition of αG_i by pertussis toxin eliminated the differences in effector-stimulated cyclase activity in membranes from failing and nonfailing heart (114). These changes in G_i activity do not appear to be associated with alterations in the absolute amount of protein present in the failing human hearts. Immunochemically detectable levels of αG_i are not altered in failing human heart when compared with nonfailing controls (117; Fig. 7). Steady-state levels of the mRNAs encoding αG_s and αG_i, when measured utilizing quantitative polymerase chain reaction (185), are likewise unaltered in heart failure (186). These latter results differ from those of earlier

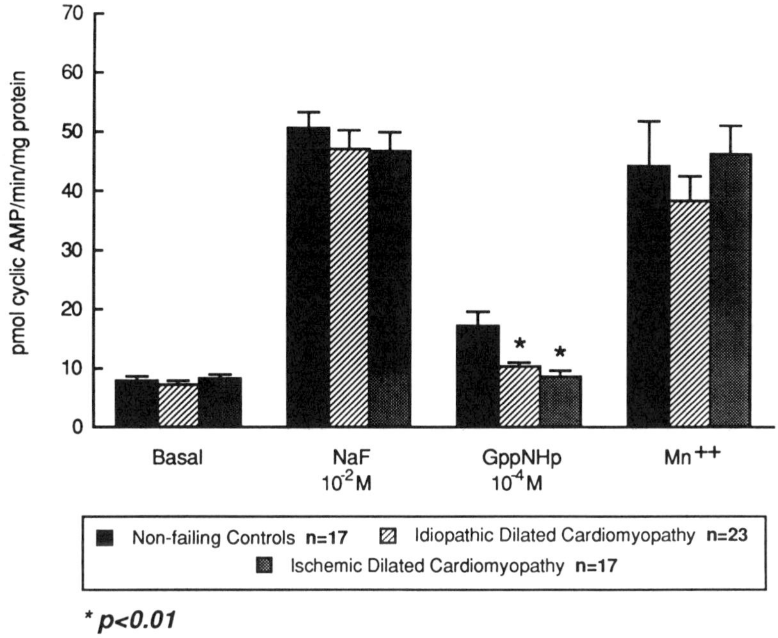

Figure 6 Adenylyl cyclase activity in left ventricular myocardium from failing and nonfailing human hearts. Measurements were obtained under basal conditions and in the presence of the αG_s agonist fluoride, the nonhydrolyzable GTP analog Gpp(NH)p, and the adenylyl cyclase agonist Mn^{++} (see 114, 216).

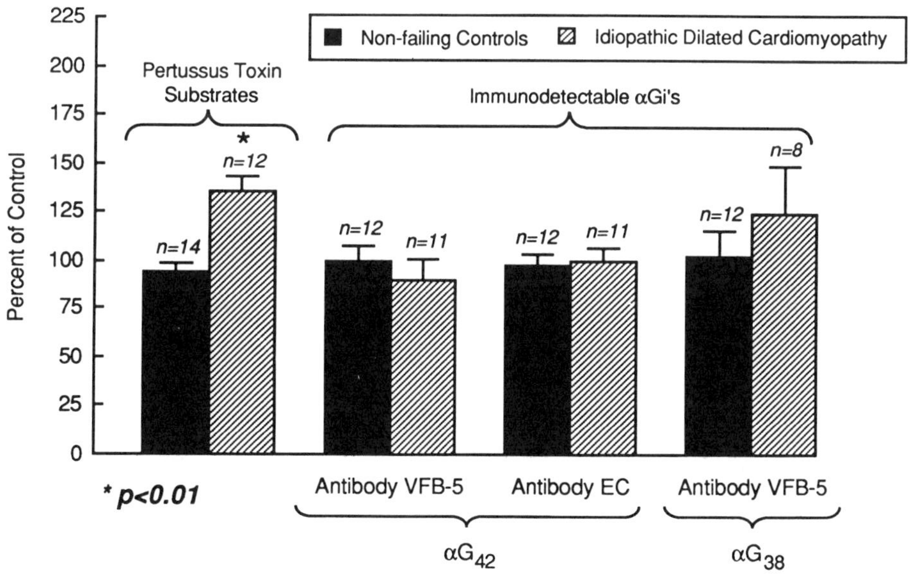

Figure 7 Quantification of αG_i proteins in failing or nonfailing left ventricular myocardium. Levels were assessed by ADP-ribosylation of pertussis toxin substrates (αG_i) or by immunodetection utilizing αG_i specific antibodies. Antibody VFB-5 and EC were raised against amino acid sequences deduced from the nucleotide structures of the cDNAs encoding the 3 αG_i subspecies. These antibodies detected peptides having relative molecular weights of 38,000 and 42,000 daltons, the latter peptide comigrating with the pertussis toxin substrate (see 114 and 117 for details).

studies from our laboratory using standard Northern blot analysis; however, the earlier studies normalized the data to levels of cytoskeletal actin, a quantitative technique that biased the results (187). Therefore, since the functional activity of G_i is increased in the absence of an increase in the actual amounts of αG_i protein, we can assume that the alteration in αG_i activity in failing human heart is a result of posttranslational modification of the αG_i protein.

IX. ANIMAL MODELS OF CONGESTIVE HEART FAILURE

From a teleologic standpoint alterations have occurred not only in the components of the RGC complex but also in the mechanisms that control the activities of adrenergic receptors, G proteins, and effector enzymes. Therefore, it is important to recognize the differences between the human heart and animal models of heart disease in order to interpret accurately experimental results (185). For example, only β_1-adrenergic receptors are found in dog myocardium (188). In contrast, the rat myocardium has an abundance of α_1-receptors, while it appears that histamine receptors play a more prominent role in guinea pig myocardium (189).

In addition, alterations in the functions of the RGC complex are both intervention and species dependent. Congestive failure after aortic banding in the dog (115,190), volume overload hypertrophy in the pig (191), the hereditary myopathy of the Syrian hamster (192), and chronic ischemia (174) are all associated with decreased functional activity (although not necessarily quantity) of αG_s and variable alterations in receptor density. In fact, in the aortic banded dog with congestive heart failure, β-receptor density actually increases (190). In contrast, cardiac denervation (193,194), the myocardial changes associated with hypothyroidism (153), and chronic adrenergic stimulation (154,195) are all associated with increased levels of αG_i and again receptor levels are variable. Although receptor desensitization after chronic exposure to catecholamines was accompanied by an increase in αG_i activity in cultured mammalian cells (154,195), receptor downregulation occurred independent of changes in G protein function in cultured chick myocytes (unpublished observations). Furthermore, two closely related strains of myopathic hamsters demonstrate substantial differences in receptor–effector coupling (192,196). Therefore, to date, data in experimental animals do not reflect the pathophysiology of human disease.

X. THERAPEUTIC USES OF β-ANTAGONISTS

A vast amount of knowledge has been accrued during the past few years regarding the biochemistry, molecular biology, and pathophysiology of receptor–effector coupling in the normal and failing myocardium. However, only recently has this information been brought to the bedside and utilized in the development of approaches to the treatment of heart failure. We would expect intuitively that stimulation of adrenergic drive would improve cardiovascular function in patients with congestive heart failure. However, in practice only the β-selective agonist dobutamine has proved clinically useful in patients with end-stage heart failure (197). Since dobutamine can only be administered intravenously, its use had been limited.

A large amount of interest has, however, been directed at the use of β-adrenergic antagonists in the therapy of congestive heart failure. The potential usefulness of β-

blockers in heart failure is based on several hypotheses. First, β-blocker therapy could effect upregulation of the β-receptors (1,198,199). Under conditions of adrenergic discharge, the endogenous catecholamines would then effectively compete with the β-antagonist for an increased population of adrenergic receptors (200). Second, β-blockers may provide beneficial effects by inhibiting the cardiotoxic effects of chronic adrenergic stimulation (1,199). Support for the first hypothesis comes from studies in which metoprolol had little effect on resting cardiac function, but improved functional performance during exercise (196,199,200). Furthermore, since human myocardium contains few or no spare β-adrenergic receptors, upregulation of receptors would restore the adrenergic pathway to full activity. A 50% decrease in receptor density would likewise be expected to diminish the contractile response by an equal amount. As an alternative, the latter hypothesis is strengthened by the finding that chronic adrenergic stimulation can independently contribute to the development of a dilated cardiomyopathy (203–207).

First proposed as a therapy for congestive heart failure by a group of investigators in Göteborg, Sweden, in 1975 (208), short-term therapy with β-blockers was shown in initial clinical studies to have little clinical usefulness (209,210). However, subsequent investigations demonstrated that long-term therapy with β-blockers improved clinical symptoms in patients with congestive heart failure and improved exercise capacity as well as left ventricular function (198–202). More recently, metoprolol has been shown to improve exercise tolerance, an effect associated with upregulation of β-adrenergic receptors (198; Fig. 8). Although mortality studies have not been performed prospectively in patients with idiopathic dilated cardio-

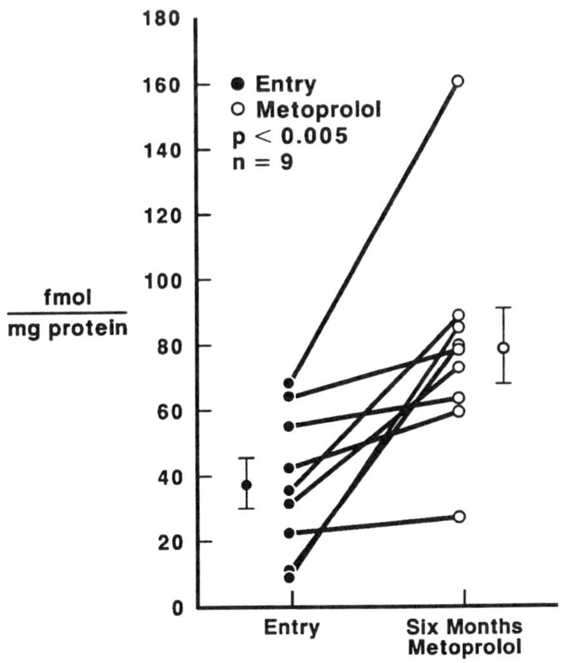

Figure 8 Measurements of β-adrenergic receptor densities (fmole/mg protein) at entry and after 6 months of metoprolol therapy (see 198).

myopathy, it is relevant to note that in several large studies investigating the use of β-blockers after myocardial infarction, the patients who exhibited the best response in terms of improved survival were those with significant left ventricular dysfunction (202,211,212).

Several early studies with β-blockers in patients with congestive heart failure have either failed to show a positive effect or have been detrimental (198,201,207,208). This disparity is likely due to the use of high-dosage β-blockade in several of these studies, and treatment of patients with minimal cardiac dysfunction in the remaining studies. However, it should be noted that as many as 10% of patients will not be able to tolerate β-blocker therapy. Most of the adverse effects are noted early, often with the first dose. In addition, it must be emphasized that β-blocker therapy has only been utilized in the context of clinical trials and requires initiation of therapy at very low dosages with a slow and gradual upward titration over as many as 6 months.

A unique pharmacologic agent, bucindolol, has recently been evaluated. This agent is a potent nonselective β-blocker with weak vasodilator activity (213–215). Short-term administration of bucindolol resulted in a modest, but significant, decrease in heart rate, systemic arterial pressure, and systemic vascular resistance (213,214). The reflex vasoconstriction that accompanies β-blocker-mediated cardiac depression was not seen with bucindolol, presumably because of its vasodilator action. With long-term therapy, bucindolol improved resting cardiac function (213) and left ventricular contractility (214). In addition, maximal exercise performance was improved, although maximal exercise heart rate was decreased. Because bucindolol is a mixed-action drug, it is not clear whether the beneficial effects were a result of β-blockade, vasodilation, or both. However, its positive effects provide a potentially exciting new agent for treating patients with symptomatic heart failure.

REFERENCES

1. Feldman A M, Bristow M R. The β-adrenergic pathway in the failing human heart: implications for inotropic therapy. *Cardiology* 77 1990; (suppl. 1):1–32.
2. Opie L H. Effects on catacholamines on normal myocardium: implications for the failing heart. *Heart Failure 1986;* 2:104–9.
3. Ahlquist R P. A study of the adrenotropic receptors. *Am J Physiol* 1948; 153:586–600.
4. Emorine L J, Marullo S, Briend-Sutren M M, Patey H, Tate K, Delavier-Klutchko C, Strosberg A D. Molecular characterization of the human β_3-adrenergic receptor. *Science* 1989; 1118–21.
5. Starke K, Docherty J R. alpha1- and Alpha2-adrenoceptors: pharmacology and clinical implications. *J. Cardio. Phar.* 3:S14–S23, 1981.
6. Bohm, M., Diet, F., Feiler, G., Kemkes, B., and Erdmann, E. α-adrenoceptors and α-adrenoceptor-mediated positive inotropic effects in failing human myocardium. *J Cardiovasc Pharmacol* 1988; 12:357–64.
7. Braunwald E, Sonnenblick E H, Ross J. Mechanisms of cardiac contraction and relaxation. In: Braunwald E, ed. *Heart disease, a textbook of cardiovascular medicine.* Philadelphia: W B Saunders, 1988; 383–425.
8. Colucci W S. Alpha-adrenergic receptor blockade with prazosin. *Ann Intern Med* 1982; 97:67–77.
9. Hoffman B B, Lefkowitz R J. Alpha-adrenergic receptor subtypes. *N Eng J Med* 1980; 302:1390–6.

10. Berridge M J, Irvine R F. Inositol triphosphate, a novel second messenger in cellular signal transduction. *Nature* 1984; 312:315–21.
11. Brown J H, Jones L G. Phosphoinositides in the heart. In: Perry J W, ed. Phosphoinositide and receptor mechanisms. New York: Alan R. Liss, 1986; 245–70.
12. Hunter T. A thousand and one protein kinases. *Cell* 1987; 50:823–9.
13. Majerus P W, Connolly T M, Bansal V S, Inhorn R C, Ross T S, Lips D L. Inositol phosphates: synthesis and degradation. *J Bio Chem* 1988; 263:3051–4.
14. Endoh M, Blinks J R. Actions of sympathomimetic amines on the Ca^{2+} transients and contractions of rabbit myocardium: reciprocal changes in myofibrillar responsiveness to Ca^{2+} mediated through α- and β-adrenoceptors. *Circ Res* 1988; 62:247–65.
15. Hayes J S, Bowling N. Role of the alpha agonist activity of dobutamine in mediating cardiac output: effects of prolonged isoproterenol infusion. *Pharmacol Exp Ther* 1987; 241:861–9.
16. Bristow M R, Minobe W, Rasmussen R, Hershberger R E, Hoffman B B. Alpha-1 adrenergic receptors in the nonfailing and failing human heart. *J Pharmacol Exp Ther* 1988; 247:1039–45.
17. Simpson P. Norepinephrine-stimulated hypertrophy of cultured rat myocardial cells in an $alpha_1$ adrenergic response. *J Clin Invest* 1983; 72:732–8.
18. Waspe L E, Ordahl C P, Simpson P C. The cardiac beta-myosin heavy chain isogene is induced selectively in alpha 1- adrenergic receptor-stimulated hypertrophy of cultured rat heart myocytes. *J Clin Invest* 1990; 85(4):1206–14.
19. Long C S, Ordahl C P, Simpson P C. Alpha 1-adrenergic receptor stimulation of sarcomeric actin isogene transcription in hypertrophy of cultured rat heart muscle cells. *J Clin Invest* 1989; 83(3):1078–82.
20. Gilman A G. G proteins: transducers of receptor-generated signals. *Annu Rev Biochem* 1987; 56:615–49 (abstr).
21. Bristow M R, Sandoval, A B, Gilbert E M, Deisher T, Minobe W, Rasmussen R. Myocardial α- and β-adrenergic receptors in heart failure: is cardiac derived norepinephrine the regulatory signal? *Eur. Heart J* 1988; 9:35–40.
22. Harden T K. Agonist-induced desensitization of the β-adrenergic receptor-linked adenylate cyclase. *Pharmacol Rev* 1983; 35:5–7.
23. Sibley D R, Benovic J L, Caron M G, Lefkowitz R J. Regulation of transmembrane signaling by receptor phosphorylation. *Cell* 1987; 48:913–22.
24. Clark R B. Desensitization of hormonal stimuli coupled to regulation of cyclic amp levels. *Adv Cyclic Nucleotide Res* 1986; 20:151–3.
25. Su Y F, Johnson G L, Cubeddu L, Leichtling G H, Ortmann R, Perkins J P. Regulation of adenosine 3′:5′-monophosphate content of human astrocytoma cells: mechanisms of agonist-specific desensitization. *J Cyclic Nucleotide Res* 1976; 2:271–85.
26. Su Y F, Cubeddu L, Perkins J P. Regulation of adenosine 3′:5′—monophosphate content of human astrocytoma cells: desensitization to catecholamines and prostaglandins. *J Cyclic Nucleotide Res* 1976; 2:257–70.
27. Livitski A. From epinephrine to cyclic AMP. *Science* 1988; 241:800–6.
28. Clark R B, Kunkel M W, Friedman J, Goka T J, Johnson J A. Activation of cAMP-dependent protein kinase is required for heterologous desensitization of adenylyl cyclase in S49 wild-type lymphoma cells. *Proc Natl Acad Sci USA* 1988; 85:1442–6.
29 Strasser R H, Lefkowitz, R J. Homologous desensitization of β-adrenergic receptor coupled adenylate cyclase. *J Bio Chem* 1985; 260:4561–4.
30. Stadel J M, Strulolvici B, Nambi P, Lavin T N, Briggs M M, Caron M G, Lefkowitz R J. Desensitization of the β-adrenergic receptor of frog erythrocytes: recovery and characterization of the down-regulated receptors in sequestered vesicles. *J Bio Chem* 1983; 258:3032–8.

31. Limas C J, Limas L. Phorbol ester- and diacylglycerol-mediated desensitization of cardiac β-adrenergic receptors. *Circ Res* 1985; 57:443–9.
32. Waldo G L, Northup J K, Perkins J P, Harden T K. Characterization of an altered membrane form of the β-adrenergic receptor produced during agonist-induced desensitization. *J Bio Chem* 1983; 258:13900–8.
33. Doss R C, Perkins J P, Harden T K. Recovery of β-adrenergic receptors following long term exposure of astrocytoma cells to catecholamine: role of protein synthesis. *J Bio Chem* 1981; 256:12281–6.
34. Limas C J, Limas C. Rapid recovery of cardiac β-adrenergic receptors after isoproterenol-induced down-regulation. *Circ Res* 1984; 55:524–31.
35. Hadcock J R, Malbon C C. Down-regulation of β-adrenergic receptors: agonist-induced reduction in mRNA levels. *Proc Natl Acad Sci* 1988; 85:5021–5.
36. Bouvier M, Leeb-Lundberg L M F, Benovic J L, Caron M G, Lefkowitz R J. Regulation of adrenergic receptor function by phosphorylation II. Effects of agonist occupancy on phosphorylation of α_1- and β_2-adrenergic receptors by protein kinase C and the cyclic AMP-dependent protein kinase. *J Bio Chem* 1987; 262:3106–13.
37. Benovic J L, Strasser R H, Caron M G, Lefkowitz R J. β-Adrenergic receptor kinase: identification of a novel protein kinase that phosphorylates the agonist-occupied form of the receptor. *Proc Natl Acad Sci USA* 1986; 83:2797–801.
38. Benovic J L, Mayor F Jr, Staniszewski C, Lefkowitz R J, Caron M G. Purification and characterization of the beta-adrenergic receptor kinase. *J Bio Chem* 1987; 262:9026–32.
39. Benovic J L, Regan J W, Matsui H, Mayor F Jr, Cotecchia S, Leeb-Lundberg L M, Caron M G, Lefkowitz R J. Agonist-dependent phosphorylation of the α_2-adrenergic receptor of the β-adrenergic receptor kinase. *J Bio Chem* 1987; 262:17251–3.
40. Lohse M J, Benovic J L, Codina J, Caron M G, Lefkowitz R J. Barrestin—a novel protein that regulates β-adrenergic receptor function. *Circulation* 1990; 82 (suppl III):III–L.
41. Mayor F Jr, Benovic J L, Caron M G, Lefkowits, R J. Somatostatin induces translocation of the beta-adrenergic receptor kinase and desensitizes somatostatin receptors in S49 lymphoma cells. *J Bio Chem* 1987; 262:6468–71.
42. Lefkowitz R J, Caron M G. Adrenergic receptors: models for the study of receptors coupled to guanine nucleotide regulatory proteins. *J Bio Chem* 1988; 263:4993–6.
43. Benovic J L, Kuhn H, Weyand I, Codina J, Caron M G, Lefkowitz R J. Functional desensitization of the isolated β-adrenergic receptor by the β-adrenergic receptor kinase: potential role of an analog of the retinal protein arrestin (48-kDa protein). *Proc Natl Acad Sci USA* 1987; 84:8879–82.
44. Mahan L C, Koachman A M, Insel, P A. Genetic analysis of β-adrenergic receptor internalization and down-regulation. *Proc Natl Acad Sci USA* 1985; 82:129–33.
45. Kassis S, Olasmaa M, Sullivan M, Fishman P H. Desensitization of the β-adrenergic receptor-coupled adenylate cyclase in cultured mammalian cells. *J Bio Chem* 1986; 261:12233–7.
46. Benovic J L, Shorr R G L, Caron M G, Lefkowitz R J. The mammalian β_2-adrenergic receptor: purification and characterization. *Biochemistry* 1984; 23:4510–8.
47. Dixon R A F, Kobilka B K, Strader D J, Benovic J L, Dohlman H G, Frielle T, Bolanowski M A, Bennett C D, Rands E, Diehl R E, Mumford R A, Slater E E, Sigal I S, Caron M G, Lefkowitz R J, Strader C D. Cloning of the gene and cDNA for mammalian β-adrenergic receptor and homology with rhodopsin. *Nature* 1986; 321:75–9.
48. Kobilka B K, Dixon R A F, Frielle T, Dohlman H G, Bolanowski M A, Sigal I S, Yang-Feng T L, Francke U, Caron M G, Lefkowitz R J. cDNA for the human β_2-adrenergic receptor: a protein with multiple membrane-spanning domains and encoded by a gene whose chromosomal location is shared with that of the receptor for platelet-derived growth factor. *Proc Natl Acad Sci USA* 1987; 84:46–50.

49. Kobilka B K, Freille T, Dohlman H G, Blanowski M A, Dixon R F, Keller P, Caron M G, Lefkowitz R J. Delineation of the intronless nature of the genes for the human and hamster. *J Bio Chem* 1987; 262:7321–7.
50. Bahouth S W, Hadcock J R, Malbon C C. Expression of mRNA of β_1- and β_2-adrenergic receptors in xenopus oocytes results from structurally distinct receptor mRNAs. *J Bio Chem* 1988; 263:8822–6.
51. Masu Y, Nakayama K, Tamaki H, Harada Y, Kuno M, Nakanishi S. cDNA cloning of bovine substance-K receptor through oocyte expression system. *Nature* 1987; 329:836–8.
52. Nathans J, Hogness D S. Isolation and nucleotide sequence of the gene encoding human rhodopsin. *Proc Natl Acad Sci USA* 1984; 81:4851–5.
53. Kubo T, Maeda A, Sugimoto K, Akiba I, Mikami A, Takahashi H, Haga T, Haga K, Ichiyama A, Kangawa K, Matsuo H, Hirose T, Numa S. Primary structure of porcine cardiac muscarinic acetylcholine receptor deduced from the cDNA sequence. *FEBS* 1986; 209:367–72.
54. Kobilka B K, Matsui H, Kobilka T S, Yang-Feng T L, Francke U, Caron M G, Lefkowitz R J, Regan J W. Cloning, sequencing, and expression of the gene coding for the human platelet α_2-adrenergic receptor. *Science* 1987; 238:650–6.
55. Kubo T, Fukuda K, Mikami A, Maeda A, Takahashi H, Mishina M, Haga T, Haga K, Ichiyama A, Kangawa K, Kojima M, Matsuo H, Hirose T, Numa S. Cloning, sequencing and expression of complementary DNA encoding the muscarinic acetylcholine receptor. *Nature* 1986; 323:411–6.
56. Kobilka B K, Frielle T, Collins S, Yang-Feng T, Kobilka T S, Francke U, Lefkowitz R J, Caron M G. An intronless gene encoding a potential member of the family of receptors coupled to guanine nucleotide regulatory proteins. *Nature* 1987; 329:75–9.
57. Fargin A, Raymond J R, Lohse M J, Koblika B K, Caron M G, Lefkowitz R J. The genomic clone G-21 which resembles a β-adrenergic receptor sequence encodes the 5-HT_{1a} receptor. *Nature* 1988; 335:358–60.
58. Dohlman H G, Caron M G, Lefkowitz R J. A family of receptors coupled to guanine nucleotide regulatory proteins. *Biochemistry* 1987; 26:2657–64.
59. Hanley M R, Jackson T. Return of the magnificent seven. *Nature* 1987; 329:766–7.
60. Frielle T, Kobilka B, Lefkowitz R J, Caron M G. Human β_1-and β_2-adrenergic receptors: structurally and functionally related receptors derived from distinct genes. *TINS* 1988; 11:321–4.
61. Kobilka B K, Kobilka T S, Daniel K, Regan J W, Caron M G, Lefkowitz R J. Chimeric α_2-, β_2-adrenergic involved in effector coupling and ligand binding specificity. *Science* 1988; 240:1310–6.
62. Wong S K F, Slaughter C, Ruoho A E, Ross E M. The catecholamine binding site of the β-adrenergic receptor is formed by juxtaposed membrane-spanning domains. *J Bio Chem* 1988; 263:7925–8.
63. Cotecchia S, Schwinn D A, Randall P R, Lefkowitz R J, Caron M G, Koblika T S. Molecular cloning and expression of the cDNA for the hamster α_1-adrenergic receptor. *Proc Natl Acad Sci USA* 1988; 85:7159–63.
64. Insel P A. Structure and function of alpha-adrenergic receptors. *Am J Med* 1989; 87 (suppl. 2A):12–8s.
65. Lee H R, Henderson S A, Reynolds R, Dunnmon D, Yuan D, Chein K R. Alpha_1 adrenergic stimulation of cardiac gene transcription in neonatal rat myocardial cells: effects of myosin light chain-2 gene expression. *J Biol Chem* 1988; 263:7352–8.
66. Simpson P, Bishopric N, Coughlin S, Karliner J, Ordahl C, Starksen N, Tsao T, White N, Williams L. Dual trophic effects of the alpha_1 adrenergic receptor in cultured neonatal rat heart muscle cells. *J Moll Cell Cardiol* 1986; 18(suppl V):V-45–58.
67. Iwaki K, Sukhatme V P, Shubeita H E, Chien H R. Alpha-and beta-adrenergic stimulation induces distinct patterns of immediate early gene expression in neonatal rat myocar-

dial cells. Fos/jun Expression is associated with sarcomere assembly; Egr-1 induction is primarily an alpha 1-mediated response. *J Biol Chem* 1990; 265(23):13809–17.
68. Simpson P C. Role of proto-oncogenes in myocardial hypertrophy. *Am J Cardiol* 1988; 62(11):13–9G.
69. Rodbell M, Birnbaumer L, Pohl S L, Krans H M. The glucagon-sensitive adenyl cyclase system in plasma membranes of rat liver V. An obligatory role of guanyl nucleotides in glucagon action. *J Biol Chem* 1971; 246:1877–82.
70. Pfeuffer T, Helmreich E J M. Activation of pigeon erythrocyte membrane adenylate cyclase by guanyl nucleotide analogs and separation of nucleotide binding protein. *J Biol Chem* 1975; 250:867–76.
71. Ross E M, Gilman A G. Resolution of some components of adenylate cyclase necessary for catalytic activity. *J Biol Chem* 1977; 252:6966–9.
72. Johnson G L, Kaslow H R, Bourne H R. Reconstitution of cholera toxin-activated adenylate cyclase. *Proc Natl Acad Sci* 1978; 75:3113–7.
73. Gilman A G. G proteins: transducers of receptor-generated signals. *Annu Rev Biochem* 1987; 56:615–49.
74. Johnson G L, Dhanasekaran N. The G-protein family and their interaction with receptors. *Endocrine Rev* 1989; 10:317–31.
75. Birnbaumer L, Abramowitz J, Brown A M. Receptor–effector coupling by G proteins. *Biochim Biophys Acta* 1990; 1031:163–224.
76. Ross E M. Signal sorting and amplification through G protein-coupled receptors. *Neuron* 1989; 3:141–52.
77. Masters S B, Sullivan K A, Miller R T, Beiderman B, Lopez N G, Ramachandran J, Bourne H R. Carboxyl terminal domain of $G_{s\alpha}$ specifies coupling of receptors to stimulation of adenylyl cyclase. *Science* 1988; 241:448–51.
78. Bourne H R, Sanders D A, McCormick F. The GTPase superfamily: conserved structure and molecular mechanism. *Nature* 1991; 349:117.
79. Neer E J, Pulsifer L, Wolf L G. The amino terminus of G protein α-subunits is required for interaction with $\beta\gamma$. *J Biol Chem* 1988; 263:8996–9000.
80. Gill D M, Meren R. ADP-ribosylation of membrane proteins catalyzed by cholera toxin: basis of the activation of adenylate cyclase. *Proc Natl Acad Sci* 1978; 75:3050–4.
81. Brown A M, Birnbaumer L. Ionic channels and their regulation by G protein subunits. *Annu Rev Physiol* 1990; 52:197–213.
82. Van Dop C, Tsubokawa M, Bourne H R, Ramachandran J. Amino acid sequence of retinal transducin at the site ADP-ribosylation by cholera toxin. *J Biol Chem* 1984; 259:696–8.
83. Vaughn M, Tsai S C, Noda M, Adamik R, Moss J. Participation of a guanine nucleotide-binding protein cascade in cholera toxin activation of adenylate cyclase. *J Mol Cell Cardiol* 1989; 21(Suppl):97–102.
84. Sewell J L, Kahn R A. Sequences of the bovine and yeast ADP-ribosylation factor and comparison to other GTP-binding sites. *Proc Natl Acad Sci USA* 1988; 86:4620–4.
85. Bobak D A, Nightgale M S, Murtagh J J, Price S R, Moss J, Vaughan M. ADP-ribosylation factors: two guanine nucleotide-dependent activators of cholera toxin. *Proc Natl Acad Sci USA* 1989; 86:6101–5.
86. Cassel D, Selinger Z. Mechanism of adenylate cyclase activation by cholera toxin: inhibition of GTP hydrolysis at the regulatory site. *Proc Natl Acad Sci USA* 1977; 74:3307–11.
87. Chang F H, Bourne H R. Cholera toxin induces cAMP-independent degradation of G_s. *J Biol Chem* 1989; 264:5352–7.
88. Van Dop C, Yamanaka G, Steinberg F, Sekura R D, Manclark C R, Stryer L, Bourne H R. ADP-ribosylation of transducin by pertussis toxin blocks the light-stimulated hydrolysis of GTP and cGMP in retinal photoreceptors. *J Biol Chem* 1984; 259:23–36.

89. Katada T, Ui M. Direct modification of the membrane adenylate cyclase system by islet-activating protein due to ADP-ribosylation of a membrane protein. *Proc Natl Acad Sci USA* 1982; 79:3129–33.
90. Sternweis P C, Robishaw J D. Isolation of two proteins with high affinity for guanine nucleotide from membranes of bovine brain. *J Biol Chem* 1984; 259:13806–13.
91. Neer E J, Lok J M, Wolf L G. Purification and properties of the inhibitory guanine nucleotide regulatory unit of brain adenylate cyclase. *J Biol Chem* 1984; 259:14222–9.
92. Murayama T, Ui M. Loss of the inhibitory function of the guanine nucleotide regulatory component of adenylate cyclase due to its ADP ribosylation by isle-activating protein, pertussis toxin, in adipocyte membranes. *J Biol Chem* 1985; 260:7226–33.
93. Watkins D C, Northup J K, Malbon C C. Pertussis toxin treatment *in vivo* is associated with a decline in G protein β-subunits. *J Biol Chem* 1989; 264:4186–94.
94. Buss J E, Mumby S M, Casey P J, Gilman A G, Sefton B M. Myristoylated α-subunits of guanine-nucleotide-binding regulatory proteins. *Proc Natl Acad Sci USA* 1987; 84:7493–7.
95. Bushfield M, Murphy G J, Lavan B E, Parker P J, Hruby V J, Milligan G, Houslay M D. Hormonal regulation of G_i2 α-subunit phosphorylation in intact hepatocytes. *Biochem J* 1990; 268:449–57.
96. Williams R S. Genetic mechanisms that determine oxidative capacity of striated muscles: control of gene transciption. *Circulation* 1990; 82:319–31.
97. Katada T, Gilman A G, Watanabe Y, Bauer S, Jakobs K H. Protein kinase C phosphorylates the inhibitory guanine–nucleotide-binding regulatory component and apparently suppresses its function in hormonal inhibition of adenylate cyclase. *Eur J Biochem* 1985; 151:431–37.
98. Fung B K K, Hurley J B, Stryer L. Flow of information in the light-triggered cyclic nucleotide cascade of vision. *Proc Natl Acad Sci USA* 1981; 78:152–6.
99. Casey P J, Gilman A C. G protein involvement in receptor–effector coupling. *J Biol Chem* 1988; 263:2577–80.
100. Katada T, Northup J K, Bokoch G M, Ui M, Gilman A G. The inhibitory guanine nucleotide-binding regulatory component of adenylate cyclase. Subunit dissociation and guanine nucleotide-dependent hormonal inhibition. *J Biol Chem* 1984; 259: 3578–85.
101. Katada T, Bokoch G M, Northup J K, Ui M, Gilman A G. The inhibitory guanine nucleotide-binding regulatory component off adenylate cyclase: properties and function of the purified protein. *J Biol Chem* 1984; 259:3568–77.
102. Jakobs K H, Aktories K, Schultz G. A nucleotide regulatory site for somatostatin inhibition of adenylate cyclase in S 49 lymphoma cells. *Nature* (London) 1983; 303:1777–78.
103. Katada T, Bokoch G M, Northup, J K, Ui M, Gilman A G. The inhibitory guanine nucleotide-binding regulatory component off adenylate cyclase: properties and function of the purified protein. *J Biol Chem* 1984; 259:3568–77.
104. Robishaw J D, Smigel M D, Gilman A G. Molecular basis for two forms of the G protein that stimulates adenylate cyclase. *J Biol Chem* 1986; 261:9587–90.
105. Jones D T, Reed R R. Molecular cloning of five GTP-binding protein cDNA species from rat olfactory neuroepithelium: the large and small forms of G_s and the olfactory-specific G-protein, G_{olf}. *J Biol Chem* 1987; 265:4507–14.
106. Senogles S E, Spiegel A M, Padrell E, Iyengar R, Caron M G. Specificity of receptor-G protein interactions: discrimination of G_i subtypes by the D_2 dopamine receptor in a reconstituted system. *J Biol Chem* 1987; 262:14241–9.
107. Levine M A, Smallwood P M, Moen P T, Heleman L J, Ahn T G Molecular cloning of $\beta3$ subunit, a third form of the G protein β-subunit polypeptide. *Proc Natl Acad Sci USA* 1990; 87: 2329–33.

108. Robishaw J D, Kalman V K, Moomaw C R, Slaughter C A. Existence of two γ-subunits of the G proteins in brain. *J Biol Chem* 1989; 264:15758.
109. Gautam N, Northup J, Tamir H, Simon M I. G protein diversity is increased by associations with a variety of γ subunits. *Proc Natl Acad Sci USA* 1990; 87:7973–7.
110. Sternweis P C. The purified alpha subunits of G_o and G_i from bovine brain require beta gamma for association with phospholipid vesicles. *J Biol Chem* 1986; 261:631–7.
111. Fuklada Y, Takao T, Ohguro H, Yoshizawa T, Akino T, Shimonishi Y. Farnesylated γ-subunit of photoreceptor G protein indispensable for GTP-binding. *Nature* 1990; 346:658–60.
112. Mumby S M, Casey P J, Gilman A G, Gutowski S, Sternweis P C. G protein γ subunits contain a 20-carbon isoprenoid. *Proc Natl Acad Sci USA* 1990; 87:5873–7.
113. Backlund P S, Simonds W F, Spiegel A M. Carboxyl methylation and COOH-terminal processing of the brain G-protein V-subunit. *J Biol Chem* 1990; 265:15572–76.
114. Feldman A M, Cates A E, Veazey W B, Hershberger R E, Bristow M R, Baughman K L, Baumgartner W A, Van Dop C. Increase of the 40,000-mol wt pertussis toxin substrate (G protein) in the failing human heart. *J Clin Invest* 1988; 82:189–97.
115. Longabaugh J P, Vatner D E, Vatner S F, Homcy C J. Decreased stimulatory guanosine triphosphate binding protein in dogs with pressure-overload left ventricular failure. *J Clin Invest* 1988; 81:420–4.
116. Foster K A, McDermott P J, Robishaw J D. Expression of G proteins in rat cardiac myocytes: effect of KCl depolarization. *Am J Physiol* 1990; 259:H432–41.
117. Feldman A M, Jackson D G, Bristow M R, Cates A E, Van Dop C. Immunodetectable levels of the inhibitory guanine nucleotide-binding regulatory proteins in failing human heart: discordance with measurements of adenylate cyclase activity and levels of pertussis toxin substrate. *J Mol Cell Cardiol,* 1991; 23:439–452.
118. Holmer S R, Stevens S, Homcy C J. Tissue- and species-specific expression of inhibitory guanine nucleotide-binding proteins: cloning of a full-length complementary DNA from canine heart. *Circ Res* 1989; 65:1136–40.
119. Liang B T, Hellmich M R, Neer E J, Galper J B. Development of muscarinic cholinergic inhibition of adenylate cyclase in embryonic chick heart. *J Biol Chem* 1986:9011–21.
120. Han H M, Robinson R B, Bilezikian J P, Steinberg S F. Developmental changes in guanine nucleotide regulatory proteins in the rat myocardial α_1-adrenergic receptor complex. *Circ Res* 1989:1763–73.
121. Luetje C W, Gierschik P, Milligan G, Unson C, Spiegel A, Nathanson N M. Tissue specific regulation of GTP-binding protein and muscarinic acetylcholine receptor levels during cardiac development. *Biochemistry* 1987; 26:4876–84.
122. Allen I S, Gaa S T, Rogers T B. Changes in expression of a functional G_i protein in cultured rat heart cells. *Am J Physiol* (Cell Physiol 24) 1988; 255:C51–9.
123. Matsuoka M, Itoh H, Kozasa T, Kaziro Y. Sequence analysis of cDNA and genomic DNA for a putative pertussis toxin-insensitive guanine nucleotide-binding regulatory protein α subunit. *Proc Natl Acad Sci USA* 1988; 85:5384–88.
124. Fong H K W, Yoshimoto K K, Eversole-Cire P, Simon M I. Identification of a GTP-binding protein α subunit that lacks an apparent ADP-ribosylation site for pertussis toxin. *Proc Natl Acad Sci USA* 1988; 85:3066–70.
125. Casey P J, Fong H K W, Simon M I, Gilman A G. G_z, a guanine nucleotide-binding protein with unique biochemical properties. *J Biol Chem* 1990; 265:2383–90.
126. Matsuoka M, Itoh H, Kaziro Y. Characterization of the human gene for $G_x\alpha$, a pertussis toxin-insensitive regulatory GTP-binding protein. *J Biol Chem* 1990; 265:13215–20.
127. Spicher K, Hinsch K D, Gausepohl H, Frank R, Rosenthal W, Schultz G. Immunochemical detection of the alpha-subunit of the G protein, G_s in membranes and cytosols of mammalian cells. *Biochem Biophys Res Commun* 1988; 157:883–90.

128. Mumby S M, Kahn R A, Manning D R, Gilman A C. Antisera of designed specificity for subunits of guanine nucleotide-binding regulatory proteins. *Proc Natl Acad Sci USA* 1986; 83:265–9.
129. Scherer N M, Toro M J, Entman M L, Birnbaumer L. G-protein distribution in canine cardiac sarcoplasmic reticulum and sarcolemma: comparison to rabbit skeletal muscle membranes and to brain and erythrocyte G-proteins. *Arch Biochem Biophys* 1987; 259:431–40.
130. Mumby S, Pang I H, Gilman A G, Sternweis P C. Chromatographic resolution and immunologic identification of the α_{40} and α_{41} subunits of guanine nucleotide-binding regulatory proteins from bovine brain. *J Biol Chem* 1988; 263:2020–6.
131. Price S R, Tsai S C, Adamik R, Angus C W, Serventi I M, Tsuchiya M, Moss J, Vaughan M. Expression of $G_{o\alpha}$ mRNA and protein in bovine tissues. *Biochemistry* 1989; 28:3803–7.
132. Strathmann M, Wilkie T M, Simon M I. Alternative splicing produces transcripts encoding two forms of the α subunit of GTP-binding protein G_o. *Proc Natl Acad Sci USA* 1990; 87:6477–81.
133. Yatani A, Codina J, Imoto Y, Reeves J P, Birnbaumer L, Brown A M. A G protein directly regulates mammalian cardiac calcium channels. *Science* 1987; 238:1288–92.
134. Yatani A, Brown A M. Rapid β-adrenergic modulation of cardiac calcium channel currents by a fast G protein pathway. *Science* 1987; 238–1288–92.
135. Pelzer S, Shuba Y M, Asai T, Codina J, Birnbaumer L, McDonald T F, Pelzer D. Membrane-delimited stimulation of heart cell calcium current by β-adrenergic signal-transducing G_s protein. *Am J Physiol* 1990; 259:H264–7.
136. Yatani A, Okabe K, Codina J, Birnbaumer L, Brown A M. Heart rate regulation by G proteins acting on the cardiac pacemaker channel. *Science* 1990; 249:1163–6.
137. Yatani A, Codina J, Brown A M, Birnbaumer L. Direct activation of mammalian atrial muscarinic potassium channels by GTP regulatory protein G_k. *Science* 1987; 235:207–11.
138. Mattera R, Yatani Y, Kirsch G E, Graf R, Okabe K, Olate J, Codinal J, Brown A M, Birnbaumer L. Recombinant α_1-3 subunit of G protein activates G_k-gated K^+ channels. *J Biol Chem* 1989; 264:465–71.
139. Kirsch G E, Codina J, Birnbaumer L, Brown A M. Coupling of ATP-sensitive K^+ channels to A_1 receptors by G proteins in rat ventricular myocytes. *Am J Physiol* 1990; 259:H820–6.
140. Logothetis D E, Kurachi Y, Galper J, Neer E J, Clapham D E. The $\beta\gamma$ subunits of GTP-binding proteins activate the muscarinic K^+ channel in the heart. *Nature* 1987; 325:321–6.
141. Logothetis D E, Kim D, Northup J K, Neer E J, Clapham D E. Specificity of action of guanine nucleotide-binding regulatory protein subunits on the cardiac muscarinic K^+ channel. *Proc Natl Acad Sci USA* 1988; 85:5814–8.
142. Okabe K, Yatani A, Evans T, Ho Y K, Codina J, Birnbaumer L, Brown A M. $\beta\gamma$ dimers of G proteins inhibit atrial muscarinic K^+ channels. *J Biol Chem* 1990; 265:12854–8.
143. Sternweis P C, Pang I H. The G protein-channel connection. *TINS* 1990; 4:122–6.
144. Brown A M, Birnbaumer L. Ionic channels and their regulation by G protein subunits. *Annu Rev Physiol* 1990; 52:197–213.
145. Steinberg S F, Kaplan L M, Inouye T, Zhang J F, Robinson R B. Alpha-1 adrenergic stimulation of 1,4,5-inositol triphosphate formation in ventricular myocytes. *J Pharmacol Exp Ther* 1989; 250:1141–8.
146. Moriarty T M, Sealfon S C, Carty D J, Roberts J L, Iyengar R, Landau E M. Coupling of exogenous receptors to phospholipase C in *Xenopus* oocytes through pertussis toxin-sensitive and -insensitive pathways: cross-talk through heterotrimeric G-proteins. *J Biol Chem* 1989; 264:13524–30.

147. Ashkenazi A, Peralta E G, Winslow J W, Ramachandran J, Capon D J. Functionally distinct G proteins selectively couple different receptors to PI hydrolysis in the sam cell. *Cell* 1989; 56:487–93.
148. Burch R M. Regulation of phospholipase A_2 by G proteins. In: Naccache P, ed. G proteins and calcium signalling. Boca Raton, FL: CRC Press, 1990; 47–58.
149. Williams R S. Genetic mechanisms that determine oxidative capacity of striated muscles: control of gene transcription. *Circulation* 1990; 82:319–31.
150. Cynan W S, Tijan R. Control of eukaryotic messenger RNA synthesis by sequence-specific DNA-binding proteins. *Nature* 1985; 316:774–8.
151. Briggs M R, Kadonaga J T, Bell S P, Tijan R. Purification and biochemical characterization of the promoter-specific transcription factor, Spl. *Science* 1986; 234:47–52.
152. Itoh H, Toyama R, Kozasa T, Tsukamoto T, Matsuoka M, Kaziro Y. Presence of three distinct molecular species of G_i protein α subunit: structure of rat cDNAs and human genomic DNAs. *J Biol Chem* 1988; 263:6656–64.
153. Levine M A, Feldman A M, Robishaw J D, Ladenson P W, Ahn T G, Moroney J F, Smallwood P M. Influence of thyroid hormone status on expression of genes encoding G protein subunits in the rat heart. *J Biol Chem* 1990; 265:3553–60.
154. Reithmann C, Gierschik P, Sidiropoulos D, Werdan K, Jakobs K H. Mechanism of noradrenaline-induced heterologous desensitization of adenylate cyclase stimulation in rat heart muscle cells: increase in the level of inhibitory G-protein α-subunits. *Eur J Pharmacol* 1989; 172:211–21.
155. Williams R S. Genetic mechanisms that determine oxidative capacity of striated muscles: control of gene transcription. *Circulation* 1990; 82:319–31.
156. Kozasa T, Itoh H, Tsukamoto T, Kaziro Y. Isolation and characterization of the human $G_s\alpha$ gene. *Proc Natl Acad Sci USA* 1988; 85:2081–5.
157. Rodan S B, Rodan G A. Dexamethason effects on β-adrenergic receptors and adenylate cyclase regulatory proteins G_s and G_i in ROS 17.2.8 cells. *Endocrinology* 1986; 118:2510–8.
158. Ishaidawa Y, Bianchi C, Nadal-Ginard B, Homcy C J. Alternative promoter and 5′ exon generate a novel $G_{s\alpha}$ mRNA. *J Biol Chem* 1990; 265:8485–62.
159. Chidsey C A, Braunwald E, Morrow A G. Catecholamine excretion and cardiac stores of norepinephrine in congestive heart failure. *Am J Med* 1965; 39:442–51.
160. Petch M C, Nayler W G. Uptake of catecholamines by human cardiac muscle in vitro. *Br Heart J* 1979; 41:336–9.
161. Petch M C, Nayler W G. Concentration of catecholamines in human cardiac muscle. *Br Heart J* 1979; 41:340–4.
162. Bristow M R, Hershberger R E, Port J D, Rasmussen R, Cates A E, Feldman A M. β-Adrenergic pathways in nonfailing and failing human ventricular myocardium. *Circulation* 1990; 82(suppl. I):I12–25.
163. Port J D, Gilbert E M, Larrabee P, Mealey P, Volkman K, Ginsburg R, Hershberger R E, Murray J, Bristow M R. Neurotransmitter depletion compromises the ability of indirect-acting amines to provide inotropic support in the failing human heart. *Circulation* 1990; 81:929–38.
164. Swedburg K, Eneroth P, Kjekshus J, Wilhensen L. Hormones regulating cardiovascular function in patients with severe congestive heart failure and their relation to mortality. *Circulation* 1990; 82:1730–6.
165. Bristow M R, Ginsburg R, Minobe W, Cubicciotti R S, Sageman W S, Lurie K, Billingham M E, Harrison D C, Stinson E B. Decreased catecholamine sensitivity and β-adrenergic-receptor density in failing human hearts. *N Engl J Med* 1982; 307:205–11.
166. Bristow M R, Ginsburg R, Sageman W S, Billingham E, Stinson E B. Analysis of the β-adrenergic receptor pathway in myocardial disease. *Circulation* 1981; 64(suppl IV):IV-286.

167. Bristow M R, Ginsburg R, Minobe W, Harrison D C, Reitz B A, Stinson E B. β-Adrenergic receptor measurements in normal and failing human right and left ventricle. *Circulation* 1982; 66(suppl II):II-207.
168. Ginsburg R, Bristow M R, Billingham M E, Stinson E B, Schroeder J S, Harrison D C. Study of the normal and failing isolated human heart to isoproterenol. *Am Heart J* 1983; 106:535–40.
169. Bristow M R, Ginsburg R, Umans V, Fowler M, Minobe W, Rasmussen R, Zera P, Menlove R, Shah P, Jamieson S, Stinson E B. β_1- and β_2-adrenergic-receptor subpopulations in nonfailing and failing human ventricular myocardium: coupling of both receptor subtypes to muscle contraction and selective β_1-receptor down-regulation in heart failure. *Circ Res* 1986; 59:297–309.
170. Bristow M R, Hershberger R E, Port J D, Minobe W, Rasmussen R. β_1- And β_2-adrenergic receptor-mediated adenylate cyclase stimulation in nonfailing and failing human ventricular myocardium. *Mol Pharmacol* 1988; 35:295–303.
171. Brodde O E, Daul A, Michel-Reher M, Boomsma F, Man in't Veld A J, Schlieper P, Michel M C. Agonist-induced desensitization of β-adrenergic function in humans. *Circulation* 1990; 81:914–20.
172. Bristow M R, Ginsburg R, Umans V, Fowler M, Monobe W, Rasmussen R, Zera P, Menlove R, Shah P, Jamieson S, Stinson E B. β_1- And β_2-adrenergic-receptor subpopulations in nonfailing and failing human ventricular myocardium: coupling of both receptor subtypes to muscle contraction and selective β_1-receptor down-regulation in heart failure. *Circ Res.* 1986; 59:267–309.
173. Fowler M B, Laser J A, Hopkins G L, Minobe W, Bristow M R. Assessment of the β-adrenergic receptor pathway in the intact failing human heart: progressive receptor down-regulation and subsensitivity to agonist response. *Circulation* 1986; 6:1290–302.
174. Karliner J S, Stevens M B, Honbo N, Hoffman J I E. Effects of acute ischemia in the dog on myocardial blood flow, beta receptors, and adenylate cyclase activity with and without chronic beta blockade. *J Clin Invest* 1989; 83:474–81.
175. Bohm M, Gierschik P, Jakobs K H, Pieske B, Schnabel P, Ungerer M, Erdmann E. Increase of $G_{i\alpha}$ in human hearts with dilated but not ischemic cardiomyopathy. *Circulation* 1990; 82:1249–65.
176. Bristow M R, Anderson F L, Port J D, Skerl L, Hershberger R E, Larrabee P, O'Connell J B, Renlund D G, Volkman K, Murray J, Feldman A M. Differences in β-adrenergic neuroeffector mechanisms in ischemic vs idiopathic dilated cardiomyopathy. *Circulation,* 1991; 84:1024–1039.
177. Hadcock J R, Malbon C C. Down-regulation of β-adrenergic receptors: agonist-induced reduction in receptor mRNA levels. *Proc Natl Acad Sci USA* 1988; 85: 5021–5.
178. Hadcock J R, Wang H Y, Malbon C C. Agonist-induced destabilization of β-adrenergic receptor mRNA. *J Biol Chem* 1989; 264:19923–33.
179. Bristow M R, Durham C, Kline J, Rasmussen R, Port J D, Gesteland R R, Barry W H, Feldman A M. Down-regulation of β-adrenergic receptors and receptor RNA in heart cells chronically exposed to norepinephrine. *Clin Res* 1991; 39(2):159A.
180. Neumann J, Scholz H, Doring V, Schmitz W, Meyernick L V, Kalmar P. Increase in myocardial G_i-proteins in heart failure. *Lancet* 1988; 22:936–7.
181. Bohm M, Gierschik P, Jakobs K H, Schnabel P, Kemkes B, Erdmann E. Localization of a postreceptor defect in human dilated cardiomyopathy. *Am J Cardiol* 1989; 64:812–4.
182. Schnabel P, Bohm M, Gierschik P, Jakobs K H, Erdmann E. Improvement of cholera toxin-catalyzed ADP-ribosylation by endogenous ADP-ribosylation factor from bovine brain provides evidence for an unchanged amount of $G_{s\alpha}$ in failing human myocardium. *J Mol Cell Cardiol* 1990; 22:73–82.

183. Karliner J S, Scheinman M. Adenylate cyclase activity coupled to the stimulatory guanine nucleotide binding protein in patients having electrophysiologic studies and either structurally normal hearts or idiopathic myocardial disease. *Am J Cardiol* 1988; 62:1129–39.
184. Denniss A R, Marsh J K, Quigg R J, Gordon J B, Colucci W S. β-Adrenergic receptor number and adenylate cyclase function in denervated transplanted and cardiomyopathic human hearts. *Circulation* 1989; 79:1028–34.
185. Venter JC. Adrenoceptors, adenylate cyclase, and the adrenergic control of cardiac contractility. In: Kunos G, ed. *Adrenoceptors and catecholamine action, Vol. 1.* New York: Wiley, 1981:213–246.
186. Feldman A M, Ray P E, Johns D C, Han R. Molecular regulation of signal transduction proteins in heart failure. *J Mol Cell Cardiol* 1991; 23(suppl III):S24.
187. Feldman A M, Cates A E, Bristow M R, Van Dop C. Altered expression of α-subunits of G proteins in failing human hearts. *J Mol Cell Cardiol* 1989; 21:359–65.
188. Vatner S F. In: Kunos G, ed. *Adrenoceptors and catecholamine action, vol. 1.* New York: Wiley, 1991; 83:1866–1872.
189. Katada T, Gilman A G, Watanabe Y, Bauer S, Jakobs K H. Protein kinase C phosphorylates the inhibitory guanine-nucleotide-binding regulatory component and apparently suppresses its function in hormonal inhibition of adenylate cyclase. *Eur J Biochem* 1985; 151:431–7.
190. Vatner D E, Vatner, S F, Fujii A M, Homcy C J. Loss of high affinity cardiac beta-adrenergic receptors in dogs with heart failure. *J Clin Invest* 1985; 76:2259–64.
191. Hammond, H K, Ransnas L A, White F A, Bloor C M, Insel P. Myocardial β-receptors number, pharmacological responsiveness, and G_s in volume overload hypertrophy in pigs. *Circulation* 1988; 78(suppl II):II-63 (abstr).
192. Kessler P D, Cates A E, Van Dop C, Feldman A M. Decreased bioactivity of the guanine nucleotide-binding protein that stimulates adenylate cyclase in hearts from cardiomyopathic Syrian hamsters. *J Clin Inves* 1989; 84:244–52.
193. Hodges T D, Bailey J C, Fleming J W, Kovacs R J. Selective parasympathectomy increases the quantity of inhibitory guanine nucleotide-binding proteins in canine cardiac ventricle. *Mol Pharmacol* 1989; 36:72–7.
194. Hershberger R E, Feldman A M, Anderson F L, Kimball J A, Wynn J R, Bristow M R. A M_r 40,000 pertussin toxin substrate is increased in surgically denervated dog heart. *J Cardiovasc Pharmacol* 1991; 17:568–75.
195. Reithmann C, Gierrschik P, Muller U, Werdan K, Jakobs K H. *Pseudomonas* exotoxin A prevents β-adrenergic-induced up-regulation of G_i protein α subunits and adenylyl cyclase desensitization in rat heart muscle cells. *Mol Pharmacol* 1990; 37:631–8.
196. Feldman A M, Tena R G, Kessler P D, Weisman H F, Schulman S P, Blumenthal R S, Jackson D G, Van Dop C. Diminished β-adrenergic receptor responsiveness and cardiac dilation in hearts of myopathic Syrian hamsters (BIO 53.58) are associated with a functional abnormality of the G stimulatory protein. *Circulation* 1990; 81: 1341–52.
197. Leier C V, Unverferth V. Drugs five years later. Dobutamine. *Ann Intern Med* 1983; 99:490–6.
198. Heilbrunn S M, Shah P, Bristow M R, Valantine H A, Ginsburg R, Fowler M B. Increased β-receptor density and improved hemodynamic response to catecholamine stimulation during long-term metoprolol therapy in heart failure from dilated cardiomyopathy. *Circulation* 1989; 79:483–90.
199. Imperato-McGinley J, Gautier T, Ehlers K, Zullo M A, Goldstein D S, Vaughan E D, Jr. Reversibility of catecholamine-induced dilated cardiomyopathy in a child with a pheochromocytoma. *N Eng J Med* 1987; 316:793–7.

200. Fowler M B, Bristow M R. Rationale for beta-adrenergic blocking drugs in cardiomyopathy. *Am J Cardiol* 1985; 55:120–4D.
201. Gilbert E M, Anderson J L, Deitchman D, Yanowitz P G, O'Connell J B, Renlund D G, Bartholomew M, Mealey P C, Larrabee P, Bristow M R. Chronic beta-blockade with bucindolol improves resting cardiac function in dilated cardiomyopathy. *Circulation* 1987; 76:1423.
202. Engelmeir R S, O'Connell J B, Walsh R, Rad N, Scanlon P J, Gunnar R M. Improvement in symptoms and exercise tolerance by metoprolol in patients with dilated cardiomyopathy: a double-blind, randomized, placebo-controlled trial. *Circulation* 1985; 72:536–46.
203. Yates J C, Beamish R E, Dhalla N S. Ventricular dysfunction and necrosis produced by adrenochrome metabolite of epinephrine: relation to pathogenesis of catecholamine cardiomyopathy. *Am Heart J* 1981; 102:210–21.
204. Tanaka M, Tsuchihashi Y, Katsumi H, Ijichi H, Ibata Y. Comparison of cardiac lesions induced in rats by isoproterenol and by repeated stress of restraint and water immersion with special reference to etiology of cardiomyopathy. *Jpn Circ J* 1980; 44:971–80.
205. Imperato-McGinley J, Gautier T, Ehlers K, Zullo M A, Goldstein D S, Vaughan E D Jr. Reversibility of catecholamine-induced cardiomyopathy in a child with a pheochromocytoma. *N Eng J Med* 1987; 316:793–7.
206. Rosenbaum J S, Ginsburg R, Billingham M E, Hoffman B B. Effects of adrenergic receptor antagonists on cardiac morphological and functional alterations in rats harboring pheochromocytoma. *J Pharmacol Exp Ther* 1987; 241:354–60.
207. Schaffer M S, Zuberbuhler P, Wilson G, Rose V, Duncan W J, Rowe R D. Catecholamine cardiomyopathy: an unusual presentation of pheochromocytoma in children. *J Pediatr* 1981; 99:276–9.
208. Waagstein I, Hjalmarson Å, Varnauskas E, Wallentin I. Effect of chronic beta-adrenergic receptor blockade in congestive heart failure. *Br Heart J* 1975; 37:1022–36.
209. Currie P J, Kelly M J, McKenzie A, Harper R W, Lim Y L, Federman J, Anderson S T, Pitt A. Oral beta-adrenergic blockade with metoprolol in chronic severe dilated cardiomyopathy. *J Am Coll Cardiol* 1984; 3:203–9.
210. Ikram H, Fitzpatrick D. Double-blind trial of chronic oral beta blockade in congestive cardiomyopathy. *Lancet* 1981; 2:490–3.
211. Chadda K, Goldstein S, Byington R, Curb J D. Effect of propranolol after acute myocardial infarction in patient with congestive heart failure. *Ther Prev* 1986; 73(3):503–10.
212. Swedberg K, Waagstein F, Hjalmarson Å, Wallenton I. Prolongation of survival in congestive cardiomyopathy by beta-receptor blockade. *Lancet* 1979; 1:1374–6.
213. Gilbert E M, Anderson J L, Deitchman D, Yanowitz F G, O'Connell J B, Renlund D G, Bartholomew M, Mealey P C, Lararabee P, Bristow M R. Long-term β-blocker vasodilator therapy improves cardiac function in idiopathic dilated cardiomyopathy: a double-blind, randomized study of bucindolol versus placebo. *Am J Med* 1990; 88:223–9.
214. Eichhorn E J, Bedotto J B, Malloy C R, Hatfield B A, Deitchman D, Brown M, Williard J E, Grayburn P A. Effect of β-adrenergic blockage on myocardial function and energetics in congestive heart failure. *Circulation* 1990; 82:473–83.
215. Pollock S G, Lystash J, Tedesco C, Craddock G, Smucker M L. Usefulness of bucindolol in congestive heart failure. *Am J Cardiol* 1990; 66:603–7.
216. Feldman A M. Experimental issues in the assessment of G protein function in cardiac disease. *Circulation,* 1991; 84:1852–1861.

10

α_1-Adrenergic Receptors and Heart Failure

HOWARD R. LEE

Heart Center of Salt Lake
Salt Lake City, Utah

I. INTRODUCTION

Downregulation of the myocardial β_1-adrenergic receptor (β_1AR) subtype is associated with a corresponding decrease in myocardial function and has been implicated in the pathophysiology of end-stage heart failure in humans (1–3). Treatment with exogenous βAR agonist drugs is also associated with downregulation of the lymphocyte β_2AR, which may account for the phenomenon of tachyphylaxis (4). For these reasons, βAR agonist drugs hold limited promise in the treatment of chronic heart failure. Thus, it is of interest whether drugs that stimulate the α_1-adrenergic receptor (α_1AR) may assume additional importance in heart failure, acting as an "adrenergic reserve." The presence of the α_1AR has been amply demonstrated in mammalian myocardium using pharmacologic as well as direct radioligand receptor binding assays (5,6). Positive inotropic responses result from α_1AR stimulation (5,6). In this chapter, the effects of α_1AR stimulation on myocardial contractile function will be examined, with particular emphasis on the effects in failing and nonfailing human myocardium.

II. RECEPTOR CLASSIFICATION

Adrenergic receptors may be classified into α and β receptors (7). This classification is based, at least in part, on the pharmacologic response of tissues to various agonist drugs, and the pharmacologic blockade by specific receptor antagonists. The βAR demonstrate an agonist rank potency of isoproterenol $>$ epinephrine $\geq$ norepinephrine $>$ phenylephrine. In contrast, α_1AR show a rank potency of epinephrine $\geq$ norepinephrine $>$ phenylephrine $>$ isoproterenol. Propranolol is the prototypic βAR antagonist, while the αAR may be further subclassified based on differential response to antagonists. Thus, α_1AR are selectively blocked by prazosin, while α_2AR are blocked by yohimbine. Of practical consideration in the design of experiments, phenylephrine is often described as an α_1AR agonist, but does have βAR properties at higher concentrations (8). To ensure a pure α_1AR agonist effect, phenylephrine should be studied in the presence of propranolol.

Beta adrenergic receptor stimulation results in a rapid development of muscle contraction as well as shortening of the relaxation time. In contrast, positive inotropic responses by α_1AR agonist drugs are slow in tension development, the action potential is lengthened, and there are no lusitropic effects (8). In muscle bath studies on rat papillary muscle, the α_1AR effects are triphasic, with an initial, transient (peak is at 30 sec) positive inotropic effect that appears immediately after drug stimulation (9). This is followed by a second phase that consists of a negative inotropic effect that reaches a maximal level 80–90 sec after stimulation. Finally, the third phase consists of a sustained, more pronounced positive inotropic effect that reaches a maximum at 5–6 min and continues for up to 20 min (9). In contrast, in human ventricular tissue no transient negative inotropic effect can be demonstrated after αAR stimulation (10).

In the adult rat heart, α_1AR stimulation results in negative chronotropic effects (11). In contrast, isolated neonatal rat myocytes in culture respond with a positive chronotropic effect (11–13). When these neonatal myocytes are cocultured with sympathetic neurons and are innervated, α_1AR stimulation results in a positive chronotropic response. The biochemical mechanism for this phenomenon is unclear, but may involve the appearance of a pertussis-toxin-sensitive G protein associated with innervation (12).

The myocardial mechanical responses to α_1AR stimulation are variable in different mammalian species. This has been documented in studies with direct comparisons in rat, guinea pig, and rabbit heart (14). In contrast, studies in dogs have not demonstrated any effects on left ventricular dP/dt or heart rate (15). Potential reasons for the species variability may include the relative contribution of α_1AR to the total cardiac adrenergic ($\alpha + \beta$) receptor population, receptor coupling mechanisms, as well as experimental conditions.

Studies with human atrial tissue consistently show a positive inotropic effect, which is frequency dependent (16–18). However, conflicting results have been obtained in experimental studies with human ventricular tissue (Table 1) (10,19–24).

In four studies, muscle bath experiments were used in studying isolated papillary muscles obtained at the time of mitral valve surgery. After pretreatment with propranolol, phenylephrine resulted in positive inotropic responses in isolated papillary muscles in 9 of 14 patients (10). The pharmacologic effects were consistent with an α_1AR-mediated event, since prazosin nearly abolished the inotropic effect and propranolol was ineffective (10). Furthermore, prolongation of isometric contraction was consistent with an α_1AR-mediated effect. In the presence of propranolol, phenylephrine increased the force of contraction 235% of control in right ventricular trabeculae carneae obtained from three nonfailing human hearts that could not be used as donor hearts (24). The responses were concentration dependent, with a maximum response at 100–300 μmol phenylephrine. The magnitude of this α_1AR-mediated force of contraction was approximately one-third that of isoproterenol, which suggests that the α_1AR may be of clinical relevance in humans (24).

In contrast, several studies have demonstrated no significant effects of α_1AR agonists in ventricular contractile responses. Methoxamine (10 μM), a pure α_1AR

Table 1 Inotropic Effects on Human Ventricular Myocardium

Drug	PIE	Comments	Reference
Phenylephrine + propranolol	Yes	Mitral valve surgery; LV papillary muscles;	10
Norepinephrine + timolol	Yes	Mitral valve surgery; contraction–relaxation consistent with αAR	19
Methoxamine	No	Cardiac transplantation; RV trabeculae	20
Dobutamine + phentolamine	No	Left main coronary artery infusion; measure LV dP/dt	21
Phenylephrine + propranolol	Yes	Cardiac transplant or mitral valve surgery	22
Phenylephrine + propranolol; norepinephrine or epinephrine	Yes	Mitral valve surgery; αAR response only 8–10% of βAR	23
Phenylephrine + propranolol	Yes	RV trabeculae from nonfailing hearts	24

Studies were performed in muscle bath preparations except for reference 21, which involved hemodynamic measurements during cardiac catheterization.
PIE, positive inotropic effect; LV, left ventricular; RV, right ventricular.

agonist, had no effect in muscle bath studies on isolated right ventricular trabeculae carneae in eight failing hearts and one nonfailing heart (20). In another study, the contribution of α_1AR stimulation was examined indirectly (21). The objective was to determine whether the inotrope, dobutamine, a mixed β- and α_1AR agonist, mediates at least part of its effect through the myocardial α_1AR. Intracoronary infusion of dobutamine was performed in 13 patients with New York Heart Association (NYHA) class III and IV heart failure. This infusion approach was used to minimize peripheral effects of dobutamine. As expected, dobutamine resulted in significant increases in left ventricular dP/dt. Coadministration of phentolamine with dobutamine did not alter the increase in dP/dt, which implied that the positive inotropic effects of dobutamine were predominantly mediated via the βAR (21). However, left ventricular dP/dt may be an insensitive measure of the αAR-mediated response, and is highly dependent on loading conditions.

Another study performed on human papillary muscle samples obtained at the time of mitral valve surgery demonstrated minimal effects ($\approx 10\%$ of βAR stimulation) on inotropy by phenylephrine + propranolol (23). No significant change in the action potential configuration provided additional evidence against a significant α_1AR-mediated effect.

In summary, several studies in human tissue have demonstrated positive inotropic effects due to α_1AR stimulation, which were not blocked by βAR antagonists. In contrast, other studies have demonstrated minimal effects. In any case, along with any direct positive inotropic effects, stimulation of vascular α_1AR increases peripheral vascular resistance and will counteract any positive inotropic effects attributable to myocardial α_1AR stimulation.

III. RECEPTOR PHARMACOLOGY

A single population of high-affinity, saturable α_1AR binding sites is found in mammalian ventricular myocardium using the radioligands [^{3}H]prazosin or [^{125}]IBE 2254 (25–34). These receptor binding sites demonstrate the appropriate stereospecificity and rank potencies of antagonists (prazosin ≈ BE 2254 > phentolamine > yohimbine).

Table 2 lists α_1AR binding characteristics for a number of mammalian species, including humans. Most striking is the obvious difference in total receptor density (B_{max}), ranging from 13 femtomoles/mg protein in cats to 190 femtomoles/mg protein in rabbits. Some of the variability in these values may be attributable to tissue preparation and experimental conditions. For example, a highly purified sarcolemma preparation would be expected to be enriched in cell surface membrane markers, including the α_1- and βAR. Another way to compare the data is to determine the relative percentage of α_1AR in the total adrenergic ($\alpha_1 + \beta$) population (Table 3), since myocardial α_2AR are virtually absent (26). In rats and rabbits, the

Table 2 α_1-Adrenergic Receptor Binding Characteristics in Ventricular Myocardium

Species	K_D (nM)	B_{max} (fmol/mg protein)	G Shift	Reference
Guinea Pig	0.58	70	NR*	25
Adult rat	0.10	36	NR	26
Cat	2.83	12.5	NR	27
Neonatal rat	0.32	60	NR	28
Adult rat	0.09	NR	(−)	29
Adult rat	5.84	167	NR	30
Rabbit	9.5	191	NR	30
Dog	7.0	54.6	NR	30
Adult rat	0.16	111	(+)	31
Adult rat	0.08	70	(+)	32
Human	0.04	14.1	NR	33
Human	0.90	30	(−)	34

NR, not reported

Table 3 Relative α_1- and β-Adrenergic Receptor Density

Species	α/β Ratio	% α_1	Reference
Cat	0.13	11.4	27
Rat	1.10	52.4	30
Rabbit	1.27	56.0	30
Dog	0.18	14.9	30
Human (LV)	0.19	15.9	33
(RV)	0.13	11.9	
Human (NYHA II & III)	0.30	23.3	22
(NYHA IV)	0.62	38.3	
Human (nonfailing)	0.02	2.1	34
(failing)	0.10	8.7	

LV, left ventricle; RV, right ventricle.

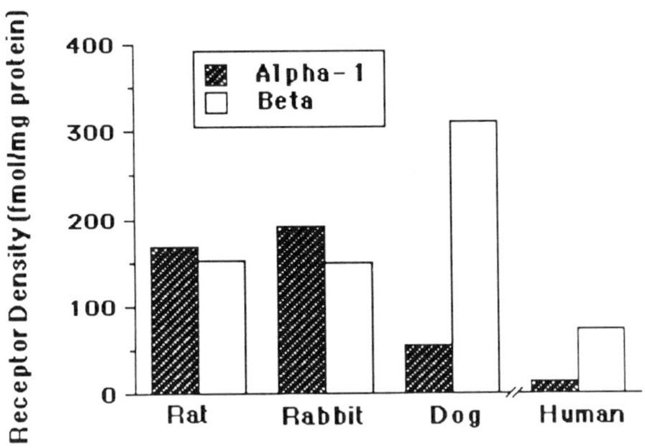

Figure 1 Total myocardial α_1- and β-adrenergic receptor density for various mammalian species. The relative proportion of α_1-adrenergic receptors is high for rat and rabbit. (Data for rat, dog, and rabbit from Ref. 30; human data from Ref. 33.)

proportion of α_1AR is quite high, whereas in cats, dogs, and humans, the proportion is low (Fig. 1). It might be predicted, then, that inotropic effects after α_1AR stimulation might be substantial in rats, since α_1AR account for greater than 50% of the adrenergic population in the heart, while in humans the effect might be a great deal less.

Norepinephrine and epinephrine competition binding curves with [^{3}H]prazosin are shallow (Hill slope $<< 1.0$) or biphasic, suggesting the presence of two affinity states or receptor subtypes (31,32). Addition of guanine nucleotides results in a shift of high-affinity sites to a single population of lower affinity sites. These "GTP" shifts imply the presence and coupling of the cell surface receptor to a guanine nucleotide-binding protein (G protein), analogous to the βAR-G protein–adenyl cyclase system (7). More recently, evidence has been produced for α_1AR subtypes coupled to different second messenger systems (35). This latter issue may be further elucidated by isolating and characterizing the genes involved in coding for the α_1AR (36).

A. Receptor Coupling Mechanisms

It has been well established that βAR stimulation results in activation of adenyl cyclase with the formation of cyclic AMP. Cyclic AMP-dependent protein kinase A then phosphorylates various proteins, including calcium channels (7,37). Until recently, it was unclear what second messenger system was coupled to the α_1AR. Early studies demonstrated no apparent effect on cyclic AMP levels. Furthermore, phosphodiesterase inhibitors did not potentiate the effect of α_1AR agonists, as would be expected for a system derived from cAMP stimulation (5).

Recent data suggest that α_1AR stimulation results in hydrolysis or turnover of polyphosphoinositides in sarcolemmal membranes (9,24,38–40). Two second messengers are formed, inositol 1,4,5-triphosphate (designated IP3 and other inositol phosphates) and diacylglycerol (DAG) (41,42). IP3 triggers release of Ca^{2+} from internal stores, and DAG acts as a cofactor in the activation of protein kinase C (41,42). PI turnover had been amply demonstrated in various animals, but several recent studies also document PI turnover in human myocardium (24,33,40).

There is evidence for involvement by a G protein since pertussis toxin abolishes α_1AR-mediated phosphoinositide hydrolysis in rat neonatal cardiac myocytes (43). Other studies have not been able to demonstrate an effect of pertussis toxin on rat atrial contractions or on inositol phosphate formation (44,45). In addition, there may be pertussis toxin-insensitive mechanisms for α_1AR stimulation of cardiac phosphodiesterase (46).

Several lines of evidence suggest that PI turnover is directly involved in the mechanisms of cardiac contraction (9). This evidence has been developed, in part, from rat heart models: 1. IP3 is rapidly formed upon stimulation by phenylephrine and correlates with the initial phase of contraction; 2. neomycin, a partial inhibitor of PI turnover results in decreased IP3 formation with a resultant decrease in the initial phase of contraction as well as the transient negative inotropic effect; 3. 2,3-diphosphoglyceric acid, a competitive inhibitor of IP3 phosphatase, potentiates the initial contraction phase; 4. active phorbol esters, which mimic the actions of DAG, potentiate the phase 3 effect of α_1AR stimulation. Other studies have demonstrated that phorbol esters may antagonize α_1AR-mediated positive inotropic effects in rabbit papillary muscles (47). Thus, the role of protein kinase C in α_1AR-mediated cardiac contraction is unclear.

B. Receptor Regulation

Chronic catecholamine stimulation of the myocardial βAR is associated with downregulation of the β_1-AR subtype in humans, as well as slight uncoupling of the receptor–adenyl cyclase system (1,2). The behavior of the cardiac α_1AR in response to chronic catecholamine stimulation or various disease states is less characterized.

In one study, chronic infusion of phenylephrine into rats resulted in a 39% decrease in the density of α_1AR (48). However, the inotropic responses of isolated ventricular strips were similar in treated and control rats, despite the apparent downregulation of the α_1AR (48). Others have found no apparent change in α_1AR binding characteristics in rats infused with isoproterenol or norepinephrine (49). Thyroid status appears to regulate α_1AR density, since ventricular receptors are significantly decreased in hyperthyroid rats and increased in hypothyroid rats (50). An interesting finding in this same study was that no changes were observed in the vas deferens, caudal artery, or cerebral cortex of these same animals. This suggests that thyroid hormonal status regulates the α_1AR in a tissue-specific manner (50). Increased receptor density is noted after acute myocardial infarction (27), and after chronic treatment with propranolol (51), whereas decreased receptor density is noted in acute diabetic rats (52).

Limited information is available regarding the α_1AR in heart failure. After aortic banding, guinea pigs develop congestive heart failure. Measurement of the βAR density by (−) [^{3}H]dihydroalprenolol showed a 93% increase in failing hearts (53). Using [^{3}H]prazosin, the cardiac α_1AR density was also increased 79% in the failing hearts (53). Before these data can be extrapolated to human heart failure, it must be pointed out that a *decrease* in βAR density is found in humans, in direct contrast to the pressure-overloaded heart failure in the guinea pig model (1,2).

Two studies have compared the α_1AR binding characteristics in failing and nonfailing human hearts (Table 4) (33,34). In one study, α_1AR were measured in failing hearts obtained at the time of cardiac transplantation, and compared to

Table 4 α_1-Adrenergic Receptors in Nonfailing and Failing Human Hearts

	B_{max} (fmol/mg protein)	Reference
LV		
Nonfailing (n = 9)	14.1	33
Failing (n = 12)	18.2	
RV		
Nonfailing (n = 4)	10.2	
Failing (n = 17)	17.0	
LV		
Nonfailing (n = 3)	30	34
Failing (n = 9)	58*	
Papillary muscles		
NYHA Class II–III (n = 12)	6.7	22
NYHA Class IV (n = 9)	7.4	

B_{max}, total receptor density; LV, left ventricle; RV, right ventricle; NYHA, New York Heart Association.
*$p < 0.01$ vs. respective nonfailing controls.

nonfailing donor hearts that could not be matched with suitable recipients. Using ^{125}IBE 2254, no significant differences in receptor density were noted in failing and nonfailing left or right ventricles, although there was a trend for increased α_1AR in the failing hearts (33). Of particular note is the low α_1AR density (10–18 femtomoles/mg protein) and the low proportion of α_1AR in the total adrenergic receptor population (Table 3). Because of the selective decrease in the β_1AR subtype, the relative proportion of α_1AR is increased in human heart failure. In a second study, α_1AR density was increased in failing hearts compared to one donor heart and two nonfailing hearts obtained at autopsy. The latter hearts were harvested approximately 1 hr after death, and may not reflect the actual α_1AR densities (34). GTP effects on the competition-binding curves were noted only in failing myocardium (34). The issue of alterations in α_1AR density in clinical end stage heart failure is unclear at present due to the limited number of studies, but is certainly worthy of further investigation.

A third study also demonstrated low abundance of α_1AR in NYHA II–IV heart failure patients at the time of mitral valve surgery (22). Because of the decreased βAR density, the relative proportion of α_1AR was increased. Thus, it is possible that the α_1AR may serve a more important role in the inotropic response to catecholamines in failing human ventricles. In addition, it might be speculated that changes in the proportion of α_1AR in the total adrenergic receptor population may be involved in the pathogenesis of ventricular arrhythmias often associated with left ventricular dysfunction (6,54).

IV. α_1-ADRENERGIC RECEPTOR AND CARDIAC HYPERTROPHY

Although the actual stimuli for cardiac hypertrophy are unknown, there has been significant interest in the role that chronic catecholamine stimulation might play (55). Animal studies suggest that “subhypertensive” dosages of catecholamines may induce cardiac hypertrophy (56). Nevertheless, these studies are complicated by a number of factors, including reflex neurohumoral changes and loading conditions.

To circumvent these problems, a rat cell culture model of cardiac hypertrophy has been developed (57). Addition of norepinephrine results in increased cell size, protein incorporation, and myofibrillar protein accumulation (i.e., hypertrophy or growth) (13,57,58). These biochemical effects are blocked by prazosin, but not by propranolol or yohimbine, pointing to an α_1AR-mediated effect. The biochemical mechanisms responsible for this cardiac myocyte hypertrophy may be due, in part, to increased gene transcription (59). Increased beating or contraction does not appear to be the stimulus for hypertrophy in this model, since both α_1- and βAR stimulation are required to increase beating rate (13). The relevance of this neonatal rat model to actual cardiac hypertrophy is unknown. Other investigators have suggested that stretch or load of the myocyte is a more important factor (60–62).

More intriguing is that α_1AR stimulation of neonatal rat cardiac myocytes is associated with a transient increase in the myocyte content of c-myc mRNA (63), and altered gene expression of muscle mRNA isoforms (64). The proto-oncogene c-myc has previously been implicated in various growth processes as well as cell transformation, but c-myc expression must now also be considered a putative early signal for cardiac hypertrophy. The expression of various protooncogenes should be investigated in failing and nonfailing human myocardium, as well as in idiopathic hypertrophic cardiomyopathy.

V. CONCLUSIONS

α_1-Adrenergic receptors have been directly identified in mammalian myocardium, including human. Positive inotropic responses have been noted in many animals and, clearly, in human atria and ventricles. Myocardial α_1AR density is low in humans, but the proportion of α_1AR does increase in heart failure, and thus may subserve a greater importance. However, presently available pharmacologic α_1AR agonists also stimulate vascular α_1AR, resulting in peripheral vasoconstriction, and increased afterload (65). The net result is that left ventricular performance may not be improved or even worsened. Overall, the role of the α_1AR remains unclear in the normal and failing human heart. Future investigation should be focused on the potential interaction of α_1AR stimulation and expression of proto-oncogenes in the control of cardiac hypertrophy or growth.

REFERENCES

1. Bristow MR, Ginsburg R, Minobe WA, et al. Decreased catecholamine sensitivity and β-adrenergic receptor density in failing human hearts. N Engl J Med 1982;307:205–11.
2. Bristow MR, Ginsburg R, Umans V, et al. β_1 and β_2-adrenergic receptor subpopulations in normal and failing human ventricular myocardium: coupling of both receptor subtypes to muscle contraction and selective β_1 receptor down-regulation in heart failure. Circ Res 1986;59:297–309.
3. Bristow MR, Sandoval AB, Gilbert EM, et al. Myocardial α- and β-adrenergic receptors in heart failure: is cardiac-derived norepinephrine the regulatory signal? Eur Heart J 1988;9(Suppl H):35–40.
4. Colucci WS, Alexander RW, Williams GH, et al. Decreased lymphocyte β-adrenergic

receptor density in patients with heart failure and tolerance to the β-adrenergic agonist pirbuterol. N Engl J Med 1981;305:185–90.
5. Bruckner R, Mugge A, Scholz H. Existence and functional role of alpha$_1$-adrenoreceptors in the mammalian heart. J Mol Cell Cardiol 1985;17:639–45.
6. Benfey BG. Function of myocardial α-adrenoceptors. J Appl Cardiol 1987;2:49–70.
7. Lefkowitz RJ, Caron MG, Stile GL. Mechanisms of membrane-receptor regulation. Biochemical, physiological, and clinical insights derived from studies of the adrenergic receptors. N Engl J Med 1984;310:1570–9.
8. Scholz H. Effects of beta- and alpha-adrenoceptor activators and adrenergic transmitter releasing agents on the mechanical activity of the heart. In: Szekeres L, ed. Adrenergic activators and inhibitors (Part I). Handbook of experimental pharmacology. Berlin: Springer-Verlag, 1980;54:651–733.
9. Otani H, Otani H, Das DK. α_1-adrenoceptor-mediated phosphoinositide breakdown and inotropic response in rat left ventricular papillary muscles. Circ Res 1988;62:8–17.
10. Bruckner R, Meyer W, Mugge A, et al. α-adrenoceptor-mediated positive inotropic effect of phenylephrine in isolated human ventricular myocardium. Eur J Pharmacol 1984;99:345–7.
11. Drugge ED, Rosen MR, Robinson RB. Neuronal regulation of the development of the α-adrenergic chronotropic response in the rat heart. Circ Res 1985;57:415–23.
12. Steinberg SF, Drugge ED, Bilezikian JP, Robinson RB. Acquisition by innervated cardiac myocytes of a pertussis toxin-specific regulatory protein linked to the α_1-receptor. Science 1985;230:186–8.
13. Simpson P. Stimulation of hypertrophy of cultured neonatal rat heart cells through an α_1-adrenergic receptor and induction of beating through an α_1- and β_1-adrenergic receptor interaction. Evidence for independent regulation of growth and beating. Circ Res 1985;56:884–94.
14. Shibata S, Seriguchi DG, Iwadare S, et al. The regional and species differences on the activation of myocardial alpha-adrenoceptors by phenylephrine and methoxamine. Gen Pharmacol 1980;11:173–80.
15. Woodman OL, Vatner SF. Cardiovascular responses to the stimulation of alpha-1 and alpha-2 adrenoceptors in the conscious dog. J Pharmacol Exp Ther 1986;237:86–91.
16. Schumann HJ, Wagner J, Knorr A, et al. Demonstration in human atrial preparations of α-adrenoceptors mediating positive inotropic effects. Naunyn-Schmiedebergs Arch Pharmacol 1978;302:333–6.
17. Wagner J, Schumann HJ, Knorr A, et al. Stimulation by adrenaline and dopamine but not by noradrenaline of myocardial α-adrenoceptors mediating positive inotropic effects in human atrial preparations. Naunyn-Schmiedebergs Arch Pharmacol 1980;312: 99–102.
18. Skomedal T, Aass H, Osnes J, et al. Demonstration of an alpha adrenoceptor-mediated inotropic effect of norepinephrine in human atria. J Pharmacol Exp Ther 1985;233: 441–6.
19. Aass H, Skomedal T, Osnes J, et al. Noradrenaline evokes an α-adrenoceptor-mediated inotropic effect in human ventricular myocardium. Acta Pharmacol Toxicol 1986;58: 88–90.
20. Gristwood R, Ginsburg R, Zera P. Are alpha-adrenoceptors coupled to contraction in human heart? Circulation 1986;74(Suppl II):374.
21. Colucci WS, Denniss AR, Quigg R, et al. Lack of positive inotropic effect of alpha-adrenergic receptor stimulation by dobutamine in patients with congestive heart failure. Circulation 1987;75(Suppl IV):71.
22. Bohm M, Diet F, Feiler G, et al. α-Adrenoceptors and α-adrenoceptor-mediated positive inotropic effecfs in failing human myocardium. J Cardiovasc Pharmacol 1988;12: 357–64.

23. Jakob H, Nawrath H, Rupp J. Adrenoceptor-mediated changes of action potential and force of contraction in human isolated ventricular heart muscle. Br J Pharmacol 1988;94:584–90.
24. Kohl C, Schmitz W, Scholz H, et al. Evidence for α_1-adrenoceptor-mediated increase of inositol triphosphate in the human heart. J Cardiovasc Pharmacol 1989;13:324–7.
25. Karliner JS, Barnes P, Hamilton CA, Dollery CT. Alpha$_1$-adrenergic receptors in guinea pig myocardium: identification by binding of a new radioligand, [^{3}H]-prazosin. Biochem Biophys Res Commun 1979;90:142–9.
26. Williams RS, Dukes DF, Lefkowitz RJ. Subtype specificity of α-adrenergic receptors in rat heart. J Cardiovasc Pharmacol 1981;3:522–31.
27. Corr PB, Shayman JA, Kramer JB, Kipnis RJ: Increased α-adrenergic receptors in ischemic cat myocardium. A potential mediator of electrophysiological derangements. J Clin Invest 1981;67:1232–6.
28. Kupfer LE, Robinson RB, Bilezikian JP. Identification of α_1-adrenergic receptors in cultured rat myocardial cells with a new iodinated α_1-adrenergic antagonist, [^{123}I]IBE 2254. Circ Res 1982;51:250–4.
29. Stiles GL, Hoffman BB, Hubbard M, et al. Guanine nucleotides and alpha$_1$ adrenergic receptors in the heart. Biochem Pharmacol 1983;32:69–71.
30. Mukherjee A, Haghani Z, Brady J, et al. Differences in myocardial α- and β-adrenergic receptor numbers in different species. Am J Physiol 1983;245:H957–61.
31. Colucci WS, Gimbrone MA Jr, Alexander RW. Regulation of myocardial and vascular α-adrenergic receptor affinity. Effects of guanine nucleotides, cations, estrogen, and catecholamine depletion. Circ Res 1984;55:78–88.
32. Buxton ILO, Brunton LL. α-Adrenergic receptors on rat ventricular myocytes: characteristics and linkage to cAMP metabolism. Am J Physiol 1986;251:H307–13.
33. Bristow MR, Minobe W, Rasmussen R, et al. Alpha-1 adrenergic receptors in the nonfailing and failing human heart. J Pharmacol Exp Ther 1988;247:1039–45.
34. Vago T, Bevilacqua M, Norbiato G, et al. Identification of α_1-adrenergic receptors on sarcolemma from normal subjects and patients with idiopathic dilated cardiomyopathy: characteristics and linkage to GTP-binding protein. Circ Res 1989;64:474–81.
35. Han C, Abel PW, Minneman KP. Heterogeneity of α_1-adrenergic receptors revealed by chlorethylclonidine. Mol Pharmacol 1987;32:505–10.
36. Cotecchia S, Schwinn DA, Randall RR, et al. Molecular cloning and expression of the cDNA for the hamster α_1-adrenergic receptor. Proc Natl Acad Sci USA 1988;7159–63.
37. Lindemann JP: α-Adrenergic stimulation of sarcolemmal protein phosphorylation and slow responses in intact myocardium. J Biol Chem 1986;261:4860–7.
38. Brown JH, Buxton IL, Brunton LL. α_1-Adrenergic and muscarinic cholinergic stimulation of phosphoinositide hydrolysis in adult rat cardiomyocytes. Circ Res 1985;57: 532–7.
39. Schmitz W, Scholz H, Scholz J, Steinfath M. Increase in IP_3 precedes α-adrenoceptor-induced increase in force of contraction in cardiac muscle. Eur J Pharmacol 1987;140: 109–11.
40. Scholz J, Schaefer B, Schmitz W, et al. Alpha-1 adrenoceptor-mediated positive inotropic effect and inositol triphosphate increase in mammalian heart. J Pharmacol Exp Ther 1988;245:327–35.
41. Berridge MJ, Irvine RF. Inositol triphosphate, a novel second messenger in cellular signal transduction. Nature 1984;312:315–21.
42. Kiukawa U, Nishizuka Y. The role of protein kinase C in transmembrane signalling. Annu Rev Cell Biol 1986;2:149–78.
43. Steinberg Sf, Chow YK, Robinson RB, Bilezikian JP. A pertussis toxin substrate regulates α_1-adrenergic dependent phosphatidylinositol hydrolysis in cultured rat myocytes. Endocrinology 1987; 120:1889–95.

44. Bohm M, Schmitz W, Scholz H. Evidence against a role of a pertussis toxin-sensitive guanine nucleotide-binding protein in the alpha$_1$-adrenoceptor-mediated positive inotropic effect in the heart. Naunyn-Schmiedebergs Arch Pharmacol 1987;335:476–9.
45. Schmitz W, Scholz H, Scholz J, et al. Pertussis toxin does not inhibit the α_1-adrenoceptor-mediated effect on inositol phosphate production in the heart. Eur J Pharmacol 1987;134:377–8.
46. Buxton ILO, Brunton LL. Action of the cardiac α_1-adrenergic receptor. Activation of cyclic AMP degradation. J Biol Chem 1985;26:6733–7.
47. Kushida H, Hiramoto T, Satoh H, Endoh M. Phorbol ester does not mimic, but antagonizes the alpha-adrenoceptor-mediated positive inotropic effect in the rabbit papillary muscle. Naunyn-Schmiedebergs Arch Pharmcol 1988;337:169–76.
48. Gengo PJ, Bowling N, Wyss VL, Hayes JS. Effects of prolonged phenylephrine infusion on cardiac adrenoceptors and calcium channels. J Pharmacol Exp Ther 1988;244: 100–5.
49. Chang HY, Klein RM, Kunos G. Selective desensitization of cardiac beta adrenoceptors by prolonged in vivo infusion of catecholamines in rats. J Pharmacol Exp Ther 1982;221:784–9.
50. Fox AW, Juberg EN, May JM, et al. Thyroid status and adrenergic receptor subtypes in the rat: comparison of receptor density and responsiveness. J Pharmacol Exp Ther 1985;235:715–23.
51. Mugge A, Reupcke, Scholz H. Increased myocardial α_1 adrenoceptor density in rats chronically treated with propranolol. Eur J Pharmacol 1985;112:249–52.
52. Wald M, Borda ES, Sterin-Borda L. α-Adrenergic supersensitivity and decreased number of α-adrenoceptors in heart from acute diabetic rats. Can J Physiol Pharmacol 1988;66:1154–60.
53. Kaliner JS, Barnes P, Brown M, Dollery C. Chronic heart failure in the guinea pig increases cardiac α_1- and β- adrenoceptors. Eur J Pharmacol 1980;67:115–8.
54. Apkon M, Nerbonne JM. α_1-Adrenergic agonists selectively suppress voltage-dependent K^+ currents in rat ventricular myocytes. Proc Natl Acad USA 1988;85:8756–60.
55. Ostman-Smith I. Cardiac sympathetic nerves as the final common pathway in the induction of adaptive cardiac hypertrophy. Clin Sci 1981;61:265–72.
56. Laks MM, Morady F, Swan HJC. Myocardial hypertrophy produced by chronic infusion of subhypertensive doses of norepinephrine in the dog. Chest 1973;64:75–8.
57. Simpson P. Norepinephrine-stimulated hypertrophy of cultured rat myocardial cells is an alpha$_1$ adrenergic response. J Clin Invest 1983;72:732–8.
58. Meidell RS, Sen A, Henderson SA, et al. α_1-Adrenergic stimulation of rat myocardial cells increases protein synthesis. Am J Physiol 1986;251:H1076–84.
59. Lee HR, Henderson SA, Reynolds R, et al. α_1-Adrenergic stimulation of cardiac gene transcription in neonatal rat myocardial cells. J Biol Chem 1988;263:7352–8.
60. Marino TA, Kuseryk L, Lauva IK. Role of contraction in the structure and growth of neonatal rat cardiocytes. Am J Physiol 1987;253:H1391–9.
61. Cooper G IV, Mercer WE, Hoober JK, et al. Load regulation of the properties of adult feline cardiocytes. The role of substrate adhesion. Circ Res 1986;58:692–705.
62. Cooper G IV: Cardiocyte adaptation to chronically altered load. Annu Rev Physiol 1987;49:501–18.
63. Starksen NF, Simpson PC, Bishopric N, et al. Cardiac myocyte hypertrophy is associated with c-myc protooncogene expression. Proc Natl Acad Sci USA 1986;83:8348–50.
64. Bisphopric NH, Simpson PC, Ordahl CP. Induction of the skeletal α-actin gene in α_1-adrenoceptor-mediated hypertrophy of rat cardiac myocytes. J Clin Invest 1987;80:1194–9.
65. Francis GS, Goldsmith SR, Levine TB, et al. The neurohumoral axis in congestive heart failure. Ann Intern Med 1984;101:370–7.

11

β-Adrenergic Agonists, Partial Agonists, and Antagonists

WILSON S. COLUCCI

Brigham and Women's Hospital and Harvard Medical School
Boston, Massachusetts

The effects of the sympathetic nervous system on the myocardium are mediated entirely via α- and β-adrenergic receptors located on the myocardial cell. Although there is evidence that α-adrenergic receptor stimulation can exert a positive inotropic effect in the myocardium, it appears that the major inotropic and chronotropic effects of the sympathetic nervous system are mediated through β-adrenergic receptors. An exogenously administered β-adrenergic agonist or antagonist likewise may affect myocardial function directly through stimulation or inhibition of the myocardial β-adrenergic receptor.

Adrenergic nervous system activity is frequently increased in patients with congestive heart failure (CHF), and is generally believed to play a beneficial role in supporting cardiovascular function in such patients. It is not surprising that there has been substantial effort over the last several years to develop orally active β-adrenergic agonists for the treatment of patients with CHF. More recently, the possibility that excessive sympathetic stimulation may adversely affect the myocardium has led to the evaluation of β-adrenergic antagonists in patients with CHF. Finally, there is at least theoretical reason to believe that a partial β-adrenergic agonist might provide the benefits of both an agonist and an antagonist while avoiding their respective limitations. Thus, an interesting situation exists in which β-adrenergic agonists, antagonists, and partial agonists are all under active investigation as therapeutic modalities in patients with CHF.

I. GOALS OF THERAPY FOR CONGESTIVE HEART FAILURE

Although there are multiple goals in the treatment of patients with CHF, three broad areas of efficacy can be defined. First, an agent may be efficacious in improving the function of the heart, thereby resulting in hemodynamic improvement. Second, an agent may result in an improved functional status of the patient, most commonly assessed as an improvement in exercise capacity. Such improvement may also be associated with improved clinical well-being, as related to less frequent hospitalizations, reduced requirements for other medications, and/or a decrease in morbid events. Finally, a pharmacologic agent may influence the rate of disease progression and/or mortality from the disease process. As experience with various pharmacologic agents is gained, it is apparent that some agents may affect only one of these efficacy parameters. In addition, it is theoretically possible to exert a beneficial effect in one or more areas but a deleterious effect in another.

When β-adrenergic agonists are administered on a short-term basis, as is commonly done in the intensive care unit, efficacy is most often defined simply as an improvement in hemodynamic performance. A beneficial effect may manifest as an increase in stroke volume, stroke work, or cardiac index with little or no increase in heart rate, and may be associated with a decrease in left and/or right heart filling pressures. In this situation, the goal is to improve the hemodynamic stability of the patient, thereby improving perfusion to vital organs. The duration of such therapy is generally limited to several hours to a few days.

In the ambulatory patient with CHF, the goal is most often to improve functional capacity and reduce the reliance on hospitalization. It is interesting that although one would anticipate a clear relationship between the acute hemodynamic actions of an agent and its long-term clinical effects, this is often not the case. An improvement in hemodynamic performance, per se, does not necessarily result in improved functional capacity or clinical well-being. Predicting the long-term clinical effects of an agent is further complicated by the possibility that an agent may exert a beneficial effect on short-term function but an adverse effect on long-term survival. Conversely, it is possible that an agent may exert an adverse effect on short-term hemodynamics but a beneficial effect on long-term survival. Finally, the acute hemodynamic effects of an agent may not be maintained due to the development of pharmacologic tolerance. At the present time, it is difficult to predict the clinical effects of any therapeutic agent in patients with CHF, and therefore, it is important that the precise goals of therapy be defined and carefully evaluated for each agent.

II. DYNAMIC NATURE OF THE β-ADRENERGIC PATHWAY

The β-adrenergic pathway in the myocardium consists of the β-adrenergic receptor, one or more guanine nucleotide-sensitive coupling proteins, and the enzyme adenylate cyclase (1). Stimulation of the receptor causes an increase in the production of cAMP, which in turn has several effects. These include 1. an increase in contractile force due to an increase in inward Ca^{++} conductance via voltage-dependent Ca^{++} channels, 2. an increase in the rate of relaxation due to an increased reuptake of Ca^{++} by the sarcoplasmic reticulum and 3. phosphorylation of the β-adrenergic receptor and activation of β-adrenergic receptor kinase (BARK), actions which play a key role in regulating the subsequent uncoupling and internalization/downregulation of β-adrenergic receptors in response to agonist. There are at least two abnormalities of the β-adrenergic receptor pathway in the myocardium from patients with CHF. First, the density of β-adrenergic receptors is decreased (2–4): The extent of this receptor downregulation appears to be inversely related to the degree of sympathetic nervous system activation and/or the severity of the heart failure state. Second, there is evidence that at least one of the G-proteins (G_i) is altered in some patients with CHF (5). As a consequence of one or both of these abnormalities in the β-adrenergic pathway, the myocardial responsiveness to β-adrenergic receptor stimulation is decreased in patients with CHF. Thus, the β-adrenergic receptor-stimulated increase in contractile force in myocardium is reduced in vitro (2–4) and in situ (6). In patients with New York Heart Association (NYHA) class III–IV CHF, the positive inotropic response to dobutamine, a β-adrenergic agonist, is reduced on the order of 50% (6). In addition, there is evidence that the chronotropic response to β-adrenergic stimulation is decreased in patients with CHF (7), presumably reflecting similar alternations in the β-adrenergic pathway in the sinoatrial node.

The degree of downregulation and/or desensitization of the myocardial β-adrenergic pathway in patients with CHF is dynamic. Thus, it is possible that the administration of a β-adrenergic agonist and/or antagonist may further modify the status of the β-adrenergic pathway, either through direct effects on the receptor, or, secondarily, through indirect reflex effects consequent to the agent's hemodynamic actions. Although it might be anticipated that a β-adrenergic agonist would cause further desensitization of the pathway, whereas a β-adrenergic antagonist might lead to resensitization of the pathway, it is important to note that the secondary effects of β-adrenergic agonists and antagonists on automatic tone might actually play a more important role in determining the eventual effects of the pharmacologic agent. For instance, in patients with severe CHF and markedly increased sympathetic tone, the effect of dobutamine to improve hemodynamic performance can result in a withdrawal of sympathetic tone (6), and there is some evidence that dobutamine administration might lead to upregulation of β-adrenergic receptors in the myocardium of such patients.

In predicting the effect of sympathetic nervous system stimulation on the β-adrenergic receptor pathway in human myocardium, it is important to consider the relationship between receptor number and tissue responsiveness. Although in several species there is evidence of a marked redundancy in the β-adrenergic receptor occupancy/response relationship (i.e., a full physiological response may be achieved with occupancy of only a small fraction of the total receptor number), studies in humans (6) suggest that this relationship is much more linear in humans. An important implication of this finding is the prediction that an alteration in β-adrenergic receptor density will have a direct influence on the maximum physiological response to β-adrenergic stimulation.

III. β-ADRENERGIC AGONISTS

Several catecholamines and sympathomimetics commonly used in clinical practice exert a significant β-adrenergic agonist effect. These agents differ substantially in their pharmacologic specificity for α- and β-adrenergic receptors, as well as for the subtypes of α- and β-adrenergic receptors. For instance, norepinephrine, phenylephrine, and neosynephrine exert substantial agonist activity at α_1-adrenergic receptors, and therefore are potent vasoconstrictors. Although β-adrenergic stimulation may contribute to the overall clinical effect of these agents, particularly in patients with decreased myocardial function, these agents are most often used as vasoconstrictors to increase blood pressure. Isoproterenol nonselectivity stimulates β_1- and β_2-adrenergic receptors, and therefore its positive inotropic effect is generally accompanied by substantial vasodilation (vascular β_2-adrenergic receptors) and tachycardia (sinoatrial β_2-adrenergic receptors). Dobutamine and dopamine are among the most widely used β-adrenergic agonists in clinical practice. As discussed below, the pharmacology of these agents is also relatively complex, but each provides a unique spectrum of activity that is of value in clinical practice. Although some orally active β-adrenergic agonists are currently available for the treatment of bronchoconstriction, no orally active β-adrenergic agonist has been shown to be efficacious for the treatment of CHF. Nevertheless, the development of orally active β-adrenergic agonists continues to be an active area of research, as discussed below.

A. Dobutamine

Dobutamine serves as the prototype β-adrenergic agonist (8). Dobutamine is a synthetic agent that stimulates β_1 and β_2 adrenergic receptors, as well as α-adrenergic receptors in the myocardium and vascular smooth muscle. Unlike dopamine, it has no activity at dopaminergic receptors. In animals there is evidence that the positive inotropic effect of dobutamine is due both to its β-adrenergic and α-adrenergic actions (9). Since a significant percentage of human myocardial β-adrenergic receptors are of the β_2 subtype (3), a portion of dobutamine's positive inotropic effect may also be due to β_2 receptor stimulation. Indeed, since it appears that β_2-adrenergic receptors may be less sensitive to downregulation in patients with CHF (3), the β_2-adrenergic component of dobutamine may be of increased importance in such patients. The peripheral α-adrenergic vasoconstrictor effects of dobutamine are generally not evident, due most likely to the offsetting vasodilating effects of β_2 receptor stimulation. In addition, although the levo-isomer of dobutamine (dobutamine is a racemic mixture of levo and dextro-isomers in equal proportion) is an α-agonist, the dextro-isomer is a weak partial agonist that may therefore inhibit the α-agonist activity of the levo-isomer.

The major use of dobutamine is in the short-term hemodynamic support of patients with left ventricular failure. In patients with CHF secondary to left ventricular dysfunction, dobutamine increases stroke volume and cardiac output, with relatively little effect on heart rate. Systolic, mean, and diastolic blood pressures change very little, although at higher dosages, systolic blood pressure may increase as a result of an increase in cardiac output. Small decreases may occur in systemic vascular resistance and left and right heart filling pressures, probably reflecting a combination of actions, including improvement in systolic and diastolic pump function, direct arterial and venous dilation secondary to β_2-adrenergic receptor stimulation, and reflex withdrawal of sympathetic nervous system tone secondary to improved hemodynamic performance. The hemodynamic effects of dobutamine are dose-related. The usual clinical range is from 2 to 15 μg/kg/min. Higher dosages are occasionally useful, but are more likely to be associated with excessive tachycardia and increased ventricular and/or atrial arrhythmias. The dosage of dobutamine is best established by titrating the infusion rate based on the desired hemodynamic effect, which most often is quantitated by measurement of cardiac output. The dosage of dobutamine may be limited in some patients by tachycardia or the emergence of arrhythmias.

There is evidence that the hemodynamic effect of dobutamine may diminish over a prolonged period of continuous administration, ranging from several hours to days. Unverferth et al. (10) found that when the hemodynamic effect of intravenous dobutamine was normalized for a constant plasma concentration of drug, the increase in cardiac output caused by drug decreased by as much as 45% over 96 hr of continuous infusion. It is presumed, although not proven, that this type of tolerance is the result of agonist-stimulated desensitization and/or downregulation of the β-adrenergic receptor pathway. Theoretically, further desensitization of the β-adrenergic receptor pathway could limit the therapeutic potential of the agent. In clinical practice it is generally possible to overcome this phenomenon by titrating the drug to a higher dose. This ability to retitrate to an effective dose is not surprising since it is likely that the therapeutic concentrations of dobutamine in usual clinical practice are at the low end of the dose–response curve for the β-adrenergic receptor in the myocardium (6).

Dobutamine can be combined with several other positive inotropic and/or vasoactive agents to achieve a more tailored therapeutic effect (11). Low-dosage dopamine ($\leq$4 μg/kg/min) exerts a beneficial effect on renal blood flow and urinary output, and therefore is frequently added to dobutamine. In this case, the positive inotropic effect of dobutamine is titrated, whereas the dosage of dopamine is held low in order to avoid the vasoconstrictor effects associated with higher infusion rates. Higher dosages of dopamine, which exert a vasoconstrictor effect, may be added to dobutamine in patients in whom systemic blood pressure is excessively low. As an alternative, vasodilator agents such as nitroprusside or nitroglycerin may be used concomitantly with dobutamine when it is desirable to reduce arterial and/or venous pressures. Finally, there is good evidence that β-adrenergic agonists such as dobutamine can be combined with phosphodiesterase inhibitors such as amrinone (12) or milrinone (6). By doing so, there is the additional vasodilator action of the phosphodiesterase inhibitor as well as the additive positive inotropic effect that results when positive inotropic agents acting at different sites in the β-adrenergic pathway are combined.

B. Intermittent Dobutamine Infusion

Although dobutamine is not available as an orally active agent, there has been experience with the use of intermittent dobutamine infusions, both in hospital and out of hospital. Unverferth et al. (13) found evidence of clinical improvement for up to 10 weeks following a 3 day infusion of dobutamine to patients with severe CHF. Subsequently, Leier et al. (14) showed that a 4 hr infusion of dobutamine weekly for 24 weeks resulted in significant improvements in left ventricular systolic performance and exercise duration. These objective findings were associated with improvement in functional classification in 12 of 15 dobutamine-treated patients, but in only 2 of 11 control patients. Liang et al. (15) evaluated the long-term effects of a 3 day infusion of dobutamine in 15 patients with NYHA class III and IV CHF randomized to receive either dobutamine or placebo. Patients who received dobutamine showed significant improvements in maximal exercise duration and left ventricular ejection fraction throughout the 4 week period following administration of dobutamine. These objective findings were associated with improvement in functional class in six of eight dobutamine-treated patients, but only two of seven control patients.

The mechanisms by which dobutamine exposure might cause these effects is not known. Liang et al. (16) found that intermittent dobutamine infusion to dogs over a period of 5 weeks elicited many of the characteristic hemodynamic and metabolic changes of exercise conditioning. More recently, Sullivan et al. (17) studied the effect of intermittent dobutamine infusion in normal human volunteers. They found that a daily 2 hr infusion of dobutamine over a 3 week period prevented deconditioning and increased the extraction of oxygen across the exercising limb. This was associated with induction of the oxidative enzymes, citrate synthetase and succinate dehydrogenase. These studies therefore raise the possibility that the effects of intermittent dobutamine exposure may be due, at least in part, to a conditioning effect on the peripheral musculature.

There have been attempts to administer intermittent dobutamine on an outpatient basis. Applefeld et al. (18) have used portable infusion pumps to administer dobutamine to ambulatory patients. Krell et al. (19) evaluated the clinical benefits of *intermittent* dobutamine infusion in 13 ambulatory patients who received dobutamine for *48 hr per week at home.* In this uncontrolled study, although 7 of the patients appeared to improve functionally, only 3 survived for 26 weeks, and 6 of the 13 patients experienced sudden death. A larger, multicenter, controlled trial involving 60 ambulatory patients evaluated the efficacy of a weekly 48 hr dobutamine infusion (20). The dobutamine treatment group showed an increase in exercise performance and a reduction in episodes of clinical deterioration compared to the placebo-treated group. However, of 18 deaths during the study, 13 were in the dobutamine treatment group. Furthermore, sudden death occurred in 10 of the dobutamine-treated patients, but only 4 of the placebo-treated patients. Although the results of this study were inconclusive due to the premature conclusion of the trial, they raised concern that ambulatory dobutamine could be associated with increased mortality, presumably in part related to arrhythmias. Further studies will be needed to evaluate the ultimate clinical role of intermittent dobutamine therapy and the relative safety of in-hospital vs. outpatient infusion.

C. Orally Active β-Adrenergic Agonists

Several orally active sympathomimetic agents with activity at β-adrenergic receptors have been evaluated in patients with CHF. Although these agents show a wide diversity with regard to β_1 vs. β_2 selectivity, in general, they share the property of partial agonism for β-adrenergic receptors. Thus, even at maximal drug concentrations in vitro, the maximal physiological response is, by definition, less than that to a full agonist such as isoproterenol or norepinephrine. The degree of partial agonist activity, frequently referred to as intrinsic sympathomimetic activity (ISA), can range widely. For instance, dobutamine is essentially a full agonist whereas pindolol, an agent with a relatively low ISA of approximately 25%, is primarily a β-adrenergic antagonist. Prenalterol and pirbuterol, two agents that have been evaluated in patients with CHF, are relatively potent agonists with ISAs in the range of 70%, whereas another recently evaluated agent, xamoterol, is intermediate with an ISA in the range of 45%.

The hemodynamic effects of a partial agonist will be critically determined by at least two factors: the ambient level of sympathetic stimulation of β-adrenergic receptors, and the status of the β-adrenergic receptor pathway. Since partial agonists exert both agonistic and antagonistic effects, the response to a partial agonist is, to a large extent, determined by the pretreatment level of receptor stimulation. If there is relatively low ambient sympathetic tone, even a mild partial agonist will exert a stimulatory effect, as evidenced by increases in heart rate and contractility. As an alternative, if sympathetic tone is high, as for instance in patients with severe CHF or during exercise, a partial agonist will act as a weak β antagonist. The level of sympathetic tone at which the agonist and antagonist activities of the agent crossover is roughly proportional to the ISA of the drug. Thus, agents with higher degrees of ISA will exert stimulatory actions, even in patients with some elevation of sympathetic tone. In theory, a partial agonist might be better tolerated than a full antagonist, and yet provide some degree of β-adrenergic blockade at times of increased sympathetic stress.

The stimulatory effects of a partial agonist are particularly sensitive to downregulation and/or desensitization of the β-adrenergic pathway in human myocardium for two reasons. First, a partial agonist, by definition, is one that exerts less than the maximal response that would be obtained with a full agonist. Second, it appears that in human myocardium, as opposed to several other animal species, there are no spare β-adrenergic receptors (6). As a consequence, this pathway exhibits little redundancy and, therefore, a reduction in β-adrenergic receptor density will translate directly into a reduction in maxmial response. In view of these theoretical points, it is perhaps not surprising that long-term oral administration of partial β-adrenergic agonists has so far been relatively unsuccessful, with little evidence of maintenance of the initial hemodynamic response to the agent (21,22).

Xamoterol is a partial β-adrenergic agonist with a modest degree of ISA. This compound is particularly interesting since its level of ISA (approximately 45%) is such that it exerts a mild stimulatory effect in patients with CHF and moderately elevated sympathetic activity, but acts as an antagonist when such patients exercise. It has been proposed that this dual action, with a particularly favorable "crossover point," might be of more clinical value in patients with CHF than agents with either higher or lower levels of ISA (23). Although some data have suggested the clinical utility of xamoterol in patients with CHF (24,25), final conclusions regarding its role in ambulatory heart failure patients cannot be determined at the present time.

D. Dopamine

Dopamine, the endogenous precursor of the catecholamines epinephrine and norepinephrine, acts by stimulating α- and β-adrenergic receptors, as well as dopaminergic receptors (26). The effects on various receptor systems are extremely dose-dependent. At low infusion rates (generally less than 4 μg/kg/min), dopamine stimulates almost exclusively dopaminergic receptors located in renal, splanchnic, cerebrospinal, and coronary vascular beds, to cause vasodilation. Although this is associated with a small decrease in net systemic vascular resistance, the major benefit of this activity is to increase renal blood flow and glomerular filtration rate. At higher infusion rates, dopamine begins to stimulate β-adrenergic receptors, primarily in the myocardium, and α-adrenergic receptors, primarily in the peripheral vasculature. Thus, at higher infusion rates, dopamine exerts both positive inotropic and a vasoconstrictor actions. High vasoconstrictor dosages may attenuate the renal effects of dopamine, and can cause increases in right or left heart filling pressures due to increased venous return as a consequence of venoconstriction (27). It is therefore not surprising that when administered to patients with CHF, dopamine is frequently combined with a vasodilator agent such as nitroprusside or nitroglycerin to mitigate the vasoconstrictor effect. The positive inotropic effects of dopamine are medicated primarily through its β-adrenergic receptor stimulating actions. It is also possible, but unproven, that its α-adrenergic receptor stimulating action could contribute to the positive inotropic effect.

E. Levodopa

One interesting approach to the therapy of ambulatory patients with CHF has been the administration of levodopa, the precursor of dopamine, which is converted to dopamine after oral ingestion (28). In a limited number of studies, patients with CHF have received levodopa in dosages of 6–8 g/day, with resultant improvement in hemodynamic parameters. The actual mechanism of this beneficial effect is not clear, but it appears that the plasma levels of dopamine achieved with these oral dosages are relatively low, in the range associated with "low-dose" dopamine infusions. Thus, the hemodynamic benefits of oral levodopa may be due primarily to its vasodilator effect. Data are not available with which to evaluate the clinical utility of chronic ambulatory therapy with levodopa.

F. Orally Active Dopamine Agonists

A number of orally active dopamine agonists have been developed, and some have been tested in patients with CHF. Ibopamine is an orally active compound that is metabolized to N-methyl dopamine (epinine) after oral ingestion. The hemodynamic and renal effects of ibopamine appear similar to those of dopamine, and this agent is therefore of potential interest in the chronic therapy of CHF (29). Other sympathomimetic agents that exert a dopaminergic effect include propylbutyl dopamine, dopexamine, and feloldapine.

IV. β-ADRENERGIC ANTAGONISTS

Since the sympathetic response to CHF is an important compensatory mechanism that helps to support the hemodynamic function of the failing heart, it is not surprising that the use of β-adrenergic antagonists in patients with CHF was met with skepticism. However, a growing body of data provides evidence that β-adrenergic antagonists may be of benefit in some patients with severe cardiomyopathy and symptomatic CHF (30). Early uncontrolled studies from Sweden suggested that β-adrenergic therapy could improve clinical symptoms and left ventricular performance in patients with dilated cardiomyopathy (31,32). Subsequently, Swedborg et al. (33) also provided uncontrolled evidence to suggest that metoprolol might improve the survival of patients with idiopathic cardiomyopathy since in a study of 24 patients, the 1 and 2 year survivals were substantially higher than might have been anticipated based on historical control populations.

There have been relatively few controlled studies of the use of β-adrenergic antagonists in cardiomyopathy. Currie et al. (34) performed a double-blind crossover trial of metoprolol therapy for 4 weeks in patients with NYHA class III CHF due either to idiopathic cardiomyopathy or coronary artery disease. Metoprolol had no effect on exercise performance, chest x-ray findings, or clinical symptoms. Likewise, a study by Ikram et al. (35), also of short duration, failed to see any evidence of clinical improvement with β antagonist therapy. More recently, Anderson et al. (36) randomized 50 patients with idiopathic dilated cardiomyopathy to therapy with low-dose metoprolol vs. placebo. Metoprolol was tolerated on a long-term basis in 80% of patients, and there was a significant improvement in functional capacity in the metoprolol-treated patients, although exercise performance time was not significantly improved. Engelmeier et al. (37) evaluated metoprolol in 8 patients using a double-blind randomized protocol over a period of 12 months. In this study, NYHA functional classification and exercise performance both improved significantly. Left ventricular ejection fraction and end-diastolic diameter, on the other hand, were unchanged.

Although the currently existing data do not allow strong conclusions to be drawn regarding the clinical efficacy of β antagonist therapy in patients with severe CHF, the data are consistent with the view that the effects of β-antagonists require a relatively prolonged period of time to be manifest since the most encouraging findings have been in patients who have been treated for several months. There is also relatively little information regarding the best agent. Most of the data so far have evaluated metoprolol, a relatively β_1-selective adrenergic antagonist that has the theoretical advantage that it would leave myocardial β_2-adrenergic receptors unopposed, and therefore might be better tolerated hemodynamically.

The mechanism by which β-adrenergic antagonists might be beneficial in patients with severe CHF is not known, and has not been directly addressed so far. Catecholamines in high concentration can have deleterious effects on the myocardium, resulting in necrosis and inflammatory changes, actions that appear to be mediated largely, but not exclusively, through β-adrenergic receptors (38). Therefore, it is possible that β-adrenergic antagonists may help to protect the myocardium from the toxic effects of excess sympathetic stimulation that occurs in response to hemodynamic deterioration in patients with CHF. β-Adrenergic tone might also be an important component in the arrhythmias and/or sudden death of patients with severe CHF. In patients with existing coronary artery disease, β-adrenergic stimulation may provoke further ischemia, particularly if associated with excess tachycardia. β-Adrenergic tone may be involved in the regulation of vascular tone through its indirect effects on renin, angiotensin, aldosterone, vasopressin, and, potentially, other vasoactive hormones. Finally, there is theoretical reason to believe that β-adrenergic antagonists would result in upregulation and/or resensitization of the β-adrenergic pathway in myocardium of patients with severe CHF. One study by Heilbrunn et al. (39) has provided direct evidence that the density of myocardial β-adrenergic receptors increases significantly in patients treated with metoprolol for 6 months. In this study, the increased β-adrenergic density was associated with a significant improvement in the hemodynamic performance and an increase in the responsiveness to β-adrenergic stimulation, suggesting that resensitization of the β-adrenergic pathway might also contribute to the beneficial effects of β-adrenergic antagonists. However, since this study was not controlled, it cannot be concluded with certainty that the improvement in hemodynamics was due to the β antagonist. Nevertheless, these data suggest that there may be potentially important alterations in the end-organ β-adrenergic pathway in response to β-adrenergic antagonist therapy.

A large multicenter trial, the Metoprolol in Idiopathic Dilated Cardiomyopathy Trial (MIDC), is underway and promises to provide important information regarding the clinical utility and safety of β-adrenergic antagonist therapy in patients with idiopathic dilated cardiomyopathy (30).

REFERENCES

1. Stiles GL, Caron MG, Lefkowitz, RJ. β-Adrenergic receptors: biochemical mechanisms of physiological regulation. Physiol Rev 1984; 64:661–743.
2. Bristow MR, Harrison DC, Stinson EB. Decreased catecholamine sensitivity and β-adrenergic receptor density in failing human hearts. N Eng J Med 1982; 307:205–11.
3. Bristow MR, Ginsberg R, Umans V, Fowler M, Minobe W, Rasmussen R, Zera P, Menlove R, Shah P, Jamieson S, Stinson EB. β_1- and β_2-Adrenergic receptor subpopulations in nonfailing and failing human ventricular myocardium. Coupling of both receptor subtypes to muscle contraction and selective β_1 receptor down-regulation in heart failure. Circ Res 1986; 59:297–309.
4. Denniss AR, Colucci WS, Allen PD, Marsh JD. Distribution and function of human ventricular beta-adrenergic receptors in congestive heart failure. J Mol Cell Cardiol 1989; 21:651–60.
5. Feldman AM, Cates AE, Veazey WB, Hershberger RE, Bristow MR, Baughman KL, Baumgartner WA, Van Dop C. Increase of the 40,000–mol wt pertussis toxin substrate (G protein) in the failing human heart. J Clin Invest 1988; 82:189–97.
6. Colucci WS, Denniss AR, Leatherman GF, Quigg RJ, Ludmer PL, Marsh JD, Gauthier DF. Intracoronary infusion of dobutamine to patients with and without severe congestive heart failure. Dose-response relationships, correlation with circulating catecholamines, and effect of phosphodiesterase inhibition. J Clin Invest 1988; 81:1103–10.
7. Colucci WS, Ribeiro JP, Rocco MB, Quigg RJ, Creager MA, Marsh JD, Gauthier DF, Hartley LH. Impaired chronotropic response to exercise in patients with congestive heart failure. Role of postsynaptic β-adrenergic desensitization. Circulation 1989; 80:314–23.
8. Leier CV, Unverferth, DV. Drugs five years later: dobutamine. Ann Intern Med 1983; 99:409–96.
9. Ruffolo RR, Spradlin TA, Pollock GD, Waddell JE, Murphy PJ. Alpha and beta-adrenergic effects of the steroisomers of dobutamine. J Pharmacol Exp Ther 1981; 219:447–52.
10. Unverferth DV, Blanford M, Kates RE, et al. Tolerance to dobutamine after a 72 hour continuous infusion. Am J Med 1980; 69:262–66.
11. Colucci WS. Dobutamine in combination with other positive inotropes. In: Chatterjee K, ed. Dobutamine, a ten-year review. NCM Publishers, New York, 1989: 139–54.
12. Gage J, Rutman H, Lucido D, LeJemtel TH. Additive effects of dobutamine and amrinone on myocardial contractility and ventricular performance in patients with severe heart failure. Circulation 1986; 74:367–73.
13. Unverferth DV, Magorien RD, Lewis RP, Leier CV. Long-term benefit of dobutamine in patients with congestive cardiomyopathy. Am Heart J 1980; 100:622–30.
14. Leier CV, Huss P, Lewis RP, Unverferth DV. Drug-induced conditioning in congestive heart failure. Circulation 1982; 65:1382–7.
15. Liang CS, Sherman LG, Doherty JU, Wellington K, Lee VW, Hood WB, Jr. Sustained improvement of cardiac function in patients with congestive heart failure after short-term infusion of dobutamine. Circulation 1984; 69:113–9.
16. Liang CS, Tuttle RR, Hood WB Jr, Gavras H. Conditioning effects of chronic infusions of dobutamine: comparison with exercise training. J Clin Invest 1979; 64:613–9.

17. Sullivan MJ, Binkley PF, Unverferth DV, Ren J-H, Boudoulas H, Bashore TM, Merola AJ, Leier CV. Prevention of bedrest-induced physical deconditioning by daily dobutamine infusions. Implications for drug-induced physical conditioning. J Clin Invest 1985; 76:1632–42.
18. Applefeld MM, Newman KA, Grove WR, Sutton FJ, Roffman DS, Reed WP, Linberg SE. Intermittent, continuous outpatient dobutamine infusion in the management of congestive heart failure. Am J Cardiol 1983; 51:455–8.
19. Krell MJ, Kline EM, Bates ER, Hodgson J McB, Dilworth LR, Laufer N, Vogel RA, Pitt B. Intermittent, ambulatory dobutamine infusions in patients with severe congestive heart failure. Am Heart J 1986; 112:787–90.
20. Dies F. Intermittent dobutamine in ambulatory patients with chronic cardiac failure. Br J Clin Pract. 1986; 45:37–40.
21. Colucci WS, Alexander RW, Williams GH, et al. Decreased lymphocyte β-adrenergic receptor density in patients with heart failure and tolerance to the β-adrenergic agonist pirbuterol. N Engl J Med 1981; 305:185–90.
22. Colucci WS, Wright RF, Braunwald E. New positive inotropic agents in the treatment of congestive heart failure. N Engl J Med 1986; 314:290–9.
23. Sato H, Inoue M, Matsuyama T, Ozaki H, Shimazu T, Takeda H, Ishida Y, Kamada T. Hemodynamic effects of the β_1-adrenoceptor partial agonist xamoterol in relation to plasma norepinephrine levels during exercise in patients with left ventricular dysfunction. Circulation 1987; 75:213–20.
24. Pouleur H, Rousseau MF, Mengeot P, Veriter C, Vincent MF, Brasseur LA. Improvement in global and regional left ventricular function in patients with previous myocardial infarction by a new β_1-adrenoreceptor partial agonist, ICI 118,586. Eur Heart J 1982; 3:123–7.
25. The German and Austrian Xamoterol Study Group. Double-blind placebo-controlled comparison of digoxin and xamoterol in chronic heart failure Lancet 1988; 1: 489–93.
26. Goldberg LI, Rajfer SI. Dopamine receptors: application in clinical cardiology. Circulation 1985; 72:245–8.
27. Lang RM, Carrol JD, Nakamura S, Itoh H, Rajfer SI. Role of adrenoceptors and dopamine receptors in modulating left ventricular diastolic function. Circ Res 1988; 63:126–34.
28. Rajfer SI, Anton AH, Rossen JD, Goldberg LI. Beneficial hemodynamic effects of oral levodopa in heart failure. N Engl J Med 1984; 310:1357–62.
29. Dei Cas L, Bolognesi R, Cucchini F, Fappani A, Riva S, Visioli O. Hemodynamic effects of ibopamine in patients with idiopathic congestive cardiomyopathy. J Cardiovasc Pharmacol 1983; 5:249–53.
30. Shanes JG. β-Blockade—rational or irrational therapy for congestive heart failure? Circulation 1987; 76:971–3.
31. Swedberg K, Hjalmarson A, Waagstein F, Wallentin I, Saunders R, Fletcher RD, Loeb HS, Hughes VC, Baker B. Beneficial effects of long-term beta-blockade in congestive cardiomyopathy. Br Heart J 1980; 44:117.
32. Waagstein F, Hjalmarson A, Swedberg K, Wallentin I, Saunders R, Fletcher RD, Loeb HS, Hughes VC, Baker B. Beta blockers in dilated cardiomyopathies: they work. Eur Heart J 1983; 4:173.
33. Swedberg K, Hjalmarson A, Waagstein F, Wallentin I, Saunders R, Fletcher RD, Loeb HS, Hughes VC, Baker B. Prolongation of survival in congestive cardiomyopathy by beta receptor blockade. Lancet 1979; 1:1374.
34. Currie, PJ, Kelly MJ, McKenzie A, Harper RW, Lim YL, Federman J, Anderson ST, Pitt A. Oral beta-adrenergic blockade with metoprolol in chronic severe dilated cardiomyopathy. J Am Coll Cardiol 1984; 3:203–9.

35. Ikram H, Fitzpatrick D. Double-blind trial of chronic oral beta blockade in congestive cardiomyopathy. Lancet 1981; 1:490.
36. Anderson JL, Lutz JR, Gilbert EM, Sorensen SG, Yanowitz FG, Menlove RL, Bartholomew M. A randomized trial of low-dose beta-blockade therapy for idiopathic dilated cardiomyopathy. Am J Cardiol, 1985; 55:471–5.

12

Use of Beta-Blockers in the Treatment of Dilated Cardiomyopathy

ÅKE HJALMARSON and FINN WAAGSTEIN

Sahlgren's Hospital
University of Göteborg
Göteborg, Sweden

For more than a century digitalis and diuretic drugs have been used for the treatment of congestive heart failure. During the last 20 years new treatments have been introduced including venodilators, vasodilators, and new inotropic agents. The aim of the treatment has mainly been to reduce symptoms such as dyspnea, fatigue, and edema. Until recently there has been a lack of influence on long-term morbidity and mortality from any of the pharmacologic interventions in patients with congestive heart failure. During the last few years randomized trials of patients with chronic congestive heart failure have demonstrated a significant reduction in mortality (1,2). A combination of nitroglycerin and hydralazine reduced long-term mortality in patients with chronic congestive heart failure as reported by Cohn and co-workers in 1986 (1). The Consensus Trial study group reported a significant reduction in mortality among patients with severe congestive heart failure with the angiotensin-converting enzyme inhibitor enalapril compared to placebo in 1987 (2). Studies on various new inotropic agents, beta-adrenergic agonists, and phosphodiesterase inhibitors on the other hand, have not resulted in long-term improvement of cardiac function, exercise capacity, or survival. During the last few years, it has been clarified that beta-adrenergic agonists cause desensitization and in order to maintain long-term stimulatory effects only partial agonists can be used.

This chapter discusses the controversial use of beta-blockers in the treatment of patients with congestive heart failure due to dilated cardiomyopathy.

I. MILD TO MODERATE CONGESTIVE HEART FAILURE AFTER ACUTE MYOCARDIAL INFARCTION

In the 1960s the use of beta-blockers in the treatment of patients with hypertension, angina pectoris, and supraventricular arrhythmias was well established. It was proposed as early as 1965 that beta-blockers could be of value in improving survival in patients after acute myocardial infarction. However, a large number of randomized placebo-controlled trials failed to show any significant effect on survival after myocardial infarction (3). In addition, several case reports suggested that beta-blockers might cause deleterious effects, especially in patients with congestive heart failure after myocardial infarction. In 1981, three large placebo-controlled trials reported a significant reduction in mortality after myocardial infarction with the use of beta-blocking agents. In two of these trials, the treatment with beta-blockers started about 2 weeks after onset of infarction and continued for about 2 years. The Norwegian Timolol Trial (4) and the American BHAT Trial (5) demonstrated a significant reduction in long-term mortality and morbidity including reduction in nonfatal reinfarctions. The third study report in 1981 was the Göteborg Metoprolol Trial (6) in which beta-blockers were given intravenously shortly after patients' hospital arrival with suspected infarction followed by oral long-term treatment. In this study there was reduction in 3 month mortality and prevention of all types of infarct complications including development of congestive heart failure. Later, two very large trials aimed at early mortality reduction, the MIAMI Trial on metoprolol (7) and the ISIS-1 Trial on atenolol (8) showed favorable effects on 1–2 week mortality after the onset of infarction and hospital complications. A major finding from all early and late intervention trials on beta-blockers in patients after myocardial infarction was a major benefit found in older and/or sicker patients. Thus, favorable results were obtained among patients with slight to moderate congestive heart failure. Furthermore, pooling all studies using beta-blockers after myocardial infarction including about 50 studies in 50,000 patients have clearly demonstrated that the use of beta-blockers did not cause adverse reactions with worsening of heart failure. It should be stated, however, that patients with severe heart failure were excluded from these randomized trials on beta-blockers.

In the early 1970s our group started to use beta-blockers in patients with acute myocardial infarction. A number of favorable effects of beta-blockers were obtained, such as reduction of chest pain, ST segment elevation, lactate release, and supraventricular and ventricular arrhythmias. Patients with moderate to severe heart failure were excluded from these studies. We decided to evaluate whether cardiac dysfunction due to acute myocardial ischemia could be favorably influenced by the use of beta-blockers. In five consecutive patients with acute myocardial infarction complicated by pulmonary edema and with heart rates above 90 beats/min, intravenous injections of practolol were given. It was hypothesized that in patients with marked tachycardia a reduction in heart rate by beta-blockade might improve rather than depress cardiac function. Without the institution of any other therapy for the heart failure, a careful and stepwise increase in the dosage of practolol caused subjective and objective improvement of the patients and disappearance of the pulmonary edema (9). The heart rate among these patients ranged from 110 to 150 beats/min and two of the five patients had atrial fibrillation. Our interpretation of the findings was that the reduction of high heart rates among these patients reduced the severity of myocardial ischemia and thereby improved their myocardial function.

II. IDIOPATHIC DILATED CARDIOMYOPATHY

The first study to suggest that chronic administration of beta-blocking agents could be useful in some forms of severe heart failure due to idiopathic dilated cardiomyopathy was published by our group in 1975 (10). This was a report from our first seven consecutive patients who were given long-term treatment with the beta-blockers practolol and alprenolol. In several of these patients, the first dose of the beta-blocker was given intravenously and there was a careful titration of the dosage because of potential adverse effects. Long-term treatment over 6–12 months caused a more or less marked improvement in various indices of heart function, functional class, and exercise capacity. During the following 15 years several studies from our group and from others have reported favorable effects of long-term beta-blockade in patients with congestive heart failure due to idiopathic dilated cardiomyopathy (Table 1). In nine different studies, including a total of 170 patients with idiopathic dilated cardiomyopathy, mostly in New York Heart Association (NYHA) functional class III–IV, significant improvement of cardiac function has been demonstrated in all studies based upon noninvasive as well as invasive hemodynamic findings (10–18). The median duration of treatment in the studies varies from 2 to 19 months. In most of the patients the $beta_1$-selective blocker metoprolol was used (127 patients) but there were also favorable effects on nonselective blockers such as bucindolol (13 patients), labetalol (12 patients), and alprenolol-propranolol (10 patients). In most of the studies detailed information is given (whether there was an improvement in cardiac function or exercise capacity, no changes, deterioration, or death) in individual patients. Of 144 such patients with detailed information provided in Table 1, 66% of the patients were estimated to be improved, 19% unchanged and 15% deteriorated or died.

In our first report (10), practolol was given to six of the seven patients. It was hypothesized early by our group that a $beta_1$-selective blocking agent would be preferable in patients with depressed cardiac function such as in acute myocardial infarction. $Beta_2$-blocking property would cause unmasking of alpha-receptors in the peripheral arteries with a potential risk of an increase in vascular resistance. It was assumed that the acute administration of a beta-blocker should reduce cardiac work and oxygen consumption due to a reduction in heart rate and rate of pressure development. After the toxic reports for practolol we started to use another $beta_1$-selective blocker, metoprolol. In four studies from 1975 to 1989, our group with Waagstein, Swedberg, Hjalmarson, and others (10–12,17) has reported favorable effects in about two-thirds of the 86 patients with idiopathic dilated cardiomyopathy. Most of the patients were treated with metoprolol and all in an open study design.

Three groups of US investigators in Chicago, Salt Lake City, and at Stanford University were interested in our use of beta-blockers in patients with idiopathic dilated cardiomyopathy (13–15). In all of these studies, metoprolol was used as in our studies, and the median duration of treatment was 6–19 months. All patients had idiopathic dilated cardiomyopathy and in two of the studies, by Engelmeier and co-workers (13) and Anderson and co-workers (14), there was a double-blind design. All three studies (13–15) showed clear improvement in indices of cardiac function and in exercise capacity. Later, the group in Salt Lake City with Anderson, Bristow, O'Connell, and co-workers (16) showed significant and favorable effects of the nonselective beta-blocking agent bucindolol in a double-blind study over 3 months. More recently, Leung and co-workers (18) reported favorable effects also of labetalol on cardiac function and exercise capacity in a double-blind study over 2 months. It can be concluded that treatment with beta-blocking agents over a period of more than 2 months clearly improves cardiac function and exercise capacity in

Table 1 Studies on Beta-Blockers in Idiopathic Dilated Cardiomyopathy

Authors (ref.)	No pts	NYHA FC	Study Design	Duration of treatment (months)	Beta-blocker (number of pts)	Effects in beta-blocker-treated patients: Improvement	Unchanged	Deterior. or death	Significant improvement
Waagstein et al. (10)	7	III–IV	Open	5	Practolol (6) Alprenolol (1)	7	0	0	+
Swedberg et al. (11)	28	III–IV	Open	12	Alprenolol (7) Practolol (2) Propranolol (2) Metoprolol (17)	15	12	1	+
Waagstein et al. (12)	18[a]	III–IV	Open	6	Metoprolol (18[a])	14	1	3	+
Engelmeier et al. (13)	25	II–IV	Open + double-blind	12	Metoprolol (20)	14	4	2	+
Anderson et al. (14)	50	II–IV	Double-blind	19	Metoprolol (25)	13 (?)	6 (?)	6	+
Heilbrunn et al. (15)	14	I–III	Open	6	Metoprolol (14)	10	2	2	+
Gilbert et al. (16)	24	II–III	Double-blind	3	Bucindolol (13)	?	?	?	+
Waagstein et al. (17)	33	II–IV	Open	16	Metoprolol (33)	24	2	7	+
Leung et al. (18)	12	II–IV	Double-blind	2	Labetalol (12)	?	?	?	+
Totals 9 studies	211			2–19 months	170 Metroprolol 127 Bucindolol 13 Labetalol 12 Other 18	97 (66%)	27 (19%)	21 (15%)	Improved in all studies

NYHA FC, New York Heart Association functional class.
[a]patients not included in previous studies.

selected patients with congestive heart failure due to idiopathic dilated cardiomyopathy. The effect has been obtained with various beta-blocking agents (i.e., $beta_1$-selective, nonselective with and without vasodilator properties). About two-thirds of the patients in the studies performed (Table 1) were improved, while one-third were either unchanged, deteriorated, or died.

III. OTHER FORMS OF DILATED CARDIOMYOPATHY

It has been questioned whether similar effects of beta-blockers could be obtained also in other forms of congestive heart failure. During 1986 to 1989, seven studies have addressed this question (Table 2). The first study by Eiswirth and co-workers in 1986 (19) treated 6 patients with adriamycin-induced dilated cardiomyopathy over 3 months and found improvement of cardiac function. This was followed by three studies including patients with ischemic cardiomyopathy due to coronary artery disease and three studies with a mixed group of patients with dilated cardiomyopathy who were not otherwise defined (20–25). These studies included 120 patients treated with bucindolol (38 patients), metoprolol (27 patients), and carvedilol (16 patients) over 2–12 months showed improvement in cardiac function and/or exercise capacity. Of the patients included, 50 were defined as having coronary artery disease due to adriamycin (6 patients), valvular heart disease (2 patients), diabetes (1 patient), or were not specified (61 patients).

In 10 studies (Table 3) including 153 patients (idiopathic in 107 patients, coronary artery disease in 27 patients, and other forms in 19 patients) measurement of ejection fraction from noninvasive or invasive recordings was reported before and after 2–16 months of treatment. These studies showed statistically significant improvement in ejection fraction and the pooled results from all studies showed a 40% increase in ejection fraction from 27% before to 38% after long-term beta-blockade ($p<0.001$).

IV. INCONCLUSIVE SHORT-TERM STUDIES

After the first favorable reports of chronic beta-blockade in patients with idiopathic dilated cardiomyopathy, two studies showed nonconclusive results (Table 4). Ikram and Fitzpatrick reported in 1981 a double-blind study in which acebutolol and placebo were given for 1 month to patients with dilated cardiomyopathy (26). There were no changes in indices of cardiac function or in exercise capacity. In this double-blind crossover trial 17 patients in NYHA functional class II–III were included: 12 with alcohol cardiomyopathy and 5 with idiopathic cardiomyopathy. Acebutolol, a nonselective beta-blocker (selectivity when given intravenously but orally nonselective) with intrinsic stimulatory activity was given in a dosage of 200 mg twice daily. The rather high starting dosage is in contrast with all other studies in which a much lower initial dosage was utilized (see Table 5). However, later Currie and co-workers (27) reported lack of effects of metoprolol also in a double-blind study over 1 month in patients with dilated cardiomyopathy, NYHA functional class III. In this study six patients had idiopathic dilated cardiomyopathy and four coronary artery disease. A smaller dosage of metoprolol was administered: 25 mg twice daily with a stepwise increase over the following week to a maximum dosage of 100 mg twice daily or maximal dose tolerated. The study demonstrated no beneficial effect on

Table 2 Effects of Long-Term Beta-Blockade on Patients with Other Forms of Dilated Cardiomyopathy Excluding Idiopathic Cardiomyopathy

Authors (ref.)	No pts	Type of cardiomyopathy	Beta-blocker	No pts on beta-blockade	Duration (months)	Significant improvement
Eiswirth et al. (19)	6	Adriamycin-induced DC	Metoprolol	6	3	+
Waagstein et al. (20)	13	CAD 10 valvular 2 diabetes 1	Metoprolol	13	12	+
DasGupta et al. (21)	16	CAD	Carvedilol	16	2	+
Eichhorn et al. (22)	11	Other DC	Bucindolol	11	3	+
Polloc et al. (23)	20	Other DC	Bucindolol	13	3	+
Sano et al. (24)	30	Other DC	Metoprolol	8	12	+
Woodley et al. (25[a])	24	CAD 24	Bucindolol	14	3	+
Totals 7 studies	120	CAD 50 Other DC 70	Bucindolol Metoprolol Carvedilol	38 27 16	2–12	Improvement in all 7 studies

[a]pts with IDC (23) included in Gilbert et al. (Table 1).
DC, dilated cardiomyopathy; CAD, coronary artery disease.

Table 3 Effects of Long-Term Beta-Blockade on Ejection Fraction in Patients with Dilated Cardiomyopathy

Authors (ref.)	No. pts	Type of cardiomyopathy	Beta-blocker	Duration (months)	Ejection fraction (%)		p
					Before	After	
Swedberg et al. (11)	15	IDC	Metoprolol	12	33 ± 2	42 ± 4	<0.05
Waagstein et al. (12)	32	IDC	Metoprolol	6	34 ± 5	50 ± 5	<0.001
Engelmeier et al. (13)	8	IDC	Metoprolol	12	13 ± 6	21 ± 10	<0.02
Waagstein et al. (20)	11	CAD	Metoprolol	12	23 ± 6	32 ± 8	<0.01
Heilbrunn et al. (15)	13	IDC	Metoprolol	6	26 ± 3	39 ± 3	<0.05
Gilbert et al. (16)	13	IDC	Bucindolol	13	26 ± 2	35 ± 3	<0.003
Waagstein et al. (17)	26	IDC	Metoprolol	16	25 ± 6	41 ± 13	<0.001
Eichhorn et al. (22)	11	DC	Bucindolol	11	23 ± 11	29 ± 13	<0.05
DasGupta et al. (21)	16	CAD	Carvedilol	2	28 ± 9	33 ± 10	<0.02
Sano et al. (24)	8	CD	Metoprolol	12	24 ± 3	31 ± 2	<0.05
Totals							
10 studies	153	IDC 107 CAD 27 DC 19	Metoprolol 113 Bucindolol 24 Carvedilol 16	2–16 months	27	38	<0.001

IDC, idiopathic dilated cardiomyopathy; CAD, coronary artery disease; DC, dilated cardiomyopathy.

Table 4 Short-Term Studies with Beta-Blockers in Patients with Dilated Cardiomyopathy

Authors (ref.)	No pts	NYHA FC	Type of Cardiomyopathy	Study Design	Duration of Treatment (n)	Beta-Blocker (n)	Overall Effects
Ikram & Fitzpatrick (26)	17	II–III	IDC 5 Alcohol-induced 12	Double-blind	1 month	Acebutolol (15)	No changes
Currie et al. (29)	10	III	IDC 6 CAD 4	Double-blind	1 month	Metoprolol (10)	No changes

Table 5 Types of Beta-Blockers and Daily Doses

	Daily Dose (mg)[a]	
Beta-Blocker	Initially	Maximum final
Acebutolol	400	400
Alprenolol	50	200
Bucindolol	25	200
Labetalol	100	400
Metoprolol	10	200
Practolol	25	800
Propranolol	40	120

[a]In two or three daily divided doses.

symptoms or cardiac function. It seems most likely that the lack of effects in the two studies referred to is due to the short duration of treatment. All other studies listed in Tables 1 and 2 (16 studies in 251 beta-blocker-treated patients) had a median treatment duration of 2–16 months (most above 6 months). Another explanation might be selection of patients, but this argument should only be valid for the study of Ikram and Fitzpatrick (26), which included 12 patients with alcohol as a possible cause of cardiomyopathy among 17 cases. However, in the 2 short-term studies there was no support for favorable effects among the 11 patients with idiopathic dilated cardiomyopathy and the 4 with ischemic cardiomyopathy. This is in contrast with the findings reported in Tables 1 and 2.

V. TYPE OF BETA-BLOCKER AND DAILY DOSE

Table 5 lists the beta-blockers that have been used in most of the studies of patients with dilated cardiomyopathy and in which dosage regimes were given. As can be seen from the table, the initial daily dosage is rather small and there is a stepwise increase over several weeks to the maximal or final dosage listed. The maximal daily dosages for the various beta-blockers are comparable to those used in the treatment of patients with, for example, angina pectoris or hypertension. In most studies, the beta-blockers were given in two to three daily divided doses. In only one study, the short-term double-blind study on acebutolol (26), was the same dosage of acebutolol used from start to end of treatment. It can be concluded that a large range of different beta-blockers has been used in long-term studies with favorable effect on cardiac function and/or exercise capacity in patients with dilated cardiomyopathy. It seems reasonable to assume that the most important property for the favorable effects is the $beta_1$-adrenoreceptor blockade. The importance of $beta_2$-blockade and alpha receptor blockade or other vasodilating properties is, at present, uncertain.

VI. ACUTE VS. LONG-TERM EFFECTS OF BETA-BLOCKERS IN DILATED CARDIOMYOPATHY

Several studies from our group (12,17,29) have demonstrated that acute administration of metoprolol caused a drop in heart rate, cardiac output, and systolic blood

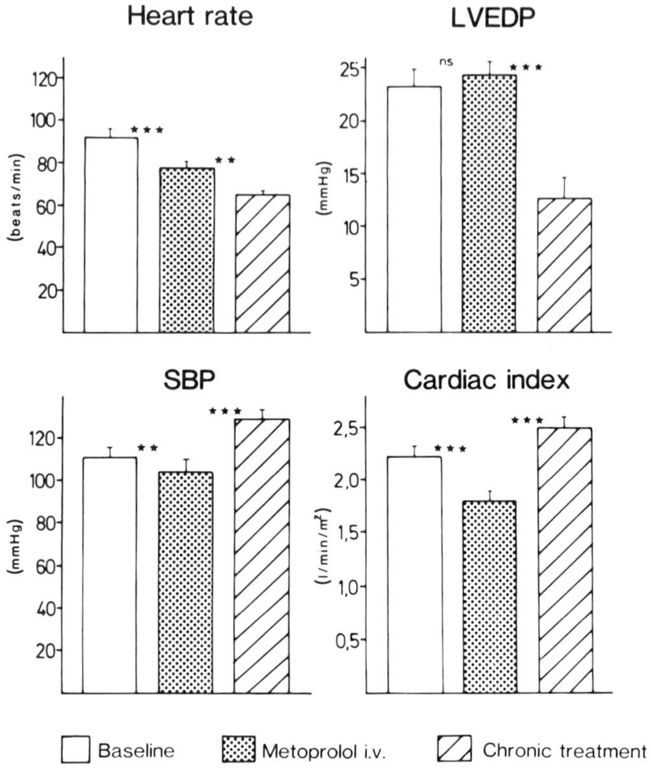

Figure 1 Effects of acute administration and of long-term treatment with metoprolol compared to baseline values in patients with idiopathic dilated cardiomyopathy. LVEDP, left ventricular end-diastolic pressure; SBP, systolic blood pressure; **$p<0.01$; ***$p<0.001$.

pressure, whereas there were no effects on right and left ventricular filling pressures (Fig. 1). Even in patients with markedly depressed cardiac function with low ejection fraction, high filling pressures, and in functional class IV, no changes were seen in filling pressures or in ejection fraction after intravenous injections of 10–15 mg metoprolol. We have therefore suggested that there is a good tolerance for acute intravenous administration of metoprolol in patients with idiopathic dilated cardiomyopathy. Similar acute effects have been reported also by other investigators (30,31), in which acebutolol and pindolol were given intravenously. It has been suggested that the good tolerance for acute intravenous administration of beta-blockers in dilated cardiomyopathy is due to improved compliance and a decreased stiffness constant noted after intravenous administration of acebutolol (30). The short-term studies in which beta-blockers were given only for 1 month show results similar to those after acute administration of beta-blockers intravenously. Acute and short-term administration causes a fall in heart rate and blood pressure, unchanged filling pressures and ejection fraction. The overall acute and short-term effect with a reduction of cardiac work indicates a lowering of myocardial oxygen consumption that may be of value for the long-term benefits. Our own findings when using metoprolol during long-term treatment have shown that there are no effects on cardiac function after 1 month of metoprolol treatment. Clear improvement in cardiac function and in exercise capacity is not demonstrated among responders until 3 months of treatment (12,17; Fig. 1).

VII. EFFECTS OF BETA-BLOCKERS ON MORTALITY IN IDIOPATHIC DILATED CARDIOMYOPATHY

It was first suggested by Swedberg and co-workers that long-term beta receptor blockade in patients with dilated cardiomyopathy might prolong survival (32). In this study 24 patients with idiopathic dilated cardiomyopathy treated with metoprolol in addition to digitalis and diuretics were compared to a control group without beta-blocker treatment. The two groups were very comparable as to age, sex, duration of disease, and cardiac function based upon careful noninvasive measurements. All patients belonged to NYHA functional class III–IV. As can be seen from Figure 2A, all patients in the group without beta-blocker treatment had died after 3 years. At this time the beta-blocker group had a 52% survival ($p<0.01$). In this study beta-blocker treatment caused improvement in myocardial function and in exercise capacity. In the control group, most patients died of progressive congestive heart failure, while the deaths in the beta-blocker-treated group tended to be more sudden without prior worsening of heart failure symptoms. A more recent long-term follow-up of another group of patients with idiopathic dilated cardiomyopathy (Fig. 2B) showed similar results, with long-term survival of about 50% (12). The results of the two studies suggesting improved survival on long-term beta-blocker therapy for patients with idiopathic dilated cardiomyopathy needs to be followed by a large randomized placebo-controlled trial. At present there is only one small randomized study comparing conventional standard therapy alone or with addition of the beta-blocking agent metoprolol (14). However, in this small study there were only 11 deaths and by intention-to-treat there were 5 deaths in the beta-blocker group and 6 in the control group. By actual treatment three patients on long-term treatment with beta-blockers died compared to eight patients without beta-blockade. However, two of the control patients were crossed over from the beta-blocker group since they were intolerant to the initial metoprolol dosages. A large international multicenter trial, the MDC Trial, is in progress to compare long-term metoprolol and placebo treatment in addition to conventional heart failure treatment in patients with idiopathic dilated cardiomyopathy. Very recently a first presentation of the MDC Trial showed that metoprolol compared to placebo reduced the sum of death and need for heart transplantation in 283 patients with idiopathic dilated cardiomyopathy, an estimated risk reduction of 34% ($p=0.0058$) (to be published, personal communication).

VIII. ADVERSE EFFECTS OF BETA-BLOCKER WITHDRAWAL IN IDIOPATHIC DILATED CARDIOMYOPATHY

Two studies have investigated the effects of withdrawal of beta-blockade after long-term administration. In 1980 Swedberg and co-workers (32) demonstrated that chronic treatment with metoprolol for 6–50 months had caused a significant improvement in cardiac function and exercise capacity and that withdrawal of beta-blockade caused a more or less marked deterioration of cardiac function in most of the patients within 3–4 months. Some of the patients had a very dramatic deterioration, with severe tachycardia and pulmonary edema, and there were deaths within

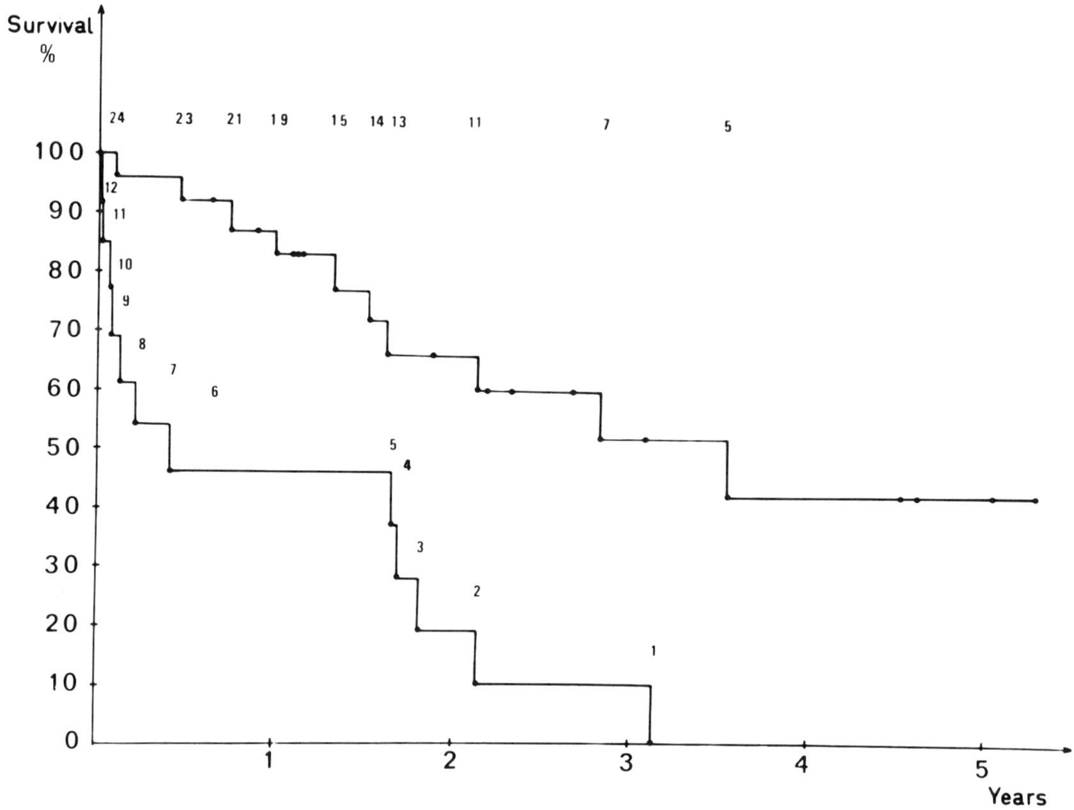

Figure 2 Survival curves for patients with idiopathic dilated cardiomyopathy. (A) Comparison between patients on conventional treatment with digitalis and diuretics with addition of a beta-blocker (upper graph, 24 patients) and without (13 control patients). The difference between the curves is significant ($p<0.01$; data from Ref. 32). (B) Survival among 46 patients all treated with digitalis, diuretics, vasodilators, and beta-blockers up to 9 years with a mortality rate similar to that among beta-blocker-treated patients in A. (From Ref. 12.)

a few weeks. A plan to study withdrawal in a larger number of patients had to be stopped for ethical reasons. In this study myocardial biopsies were not taken routinely and it could be argued whether some of the patients without deterioration could have had myocarditis with spontaneous improvement or improvement due to beta-blocker treatment. In a second study in 1989 by our group (17), all patients had an initial endocardial biopsy and there was no sign of myocarditis among the patients included. As can be seen from Figure 3, patients who improved during chronic treatment with metoprolol had a worsening of their general condition and in NYHA class after withdrawal, but were again improved after readministration of the beta-blocker. All of these changes were significant ($p<0.001$). The major results from the two studies are summarized in Table 6. A total of 39 patients were improved after long-term treatment with beta-blockers and withdrawal caused significant worsening of cardiac function variables such as ejection fraction, left atrial end-ventricular diameter, and rapid filling wave ratio. As discussed by Waagstein and co-workers (17), the deterioration of cardiac function and general condition

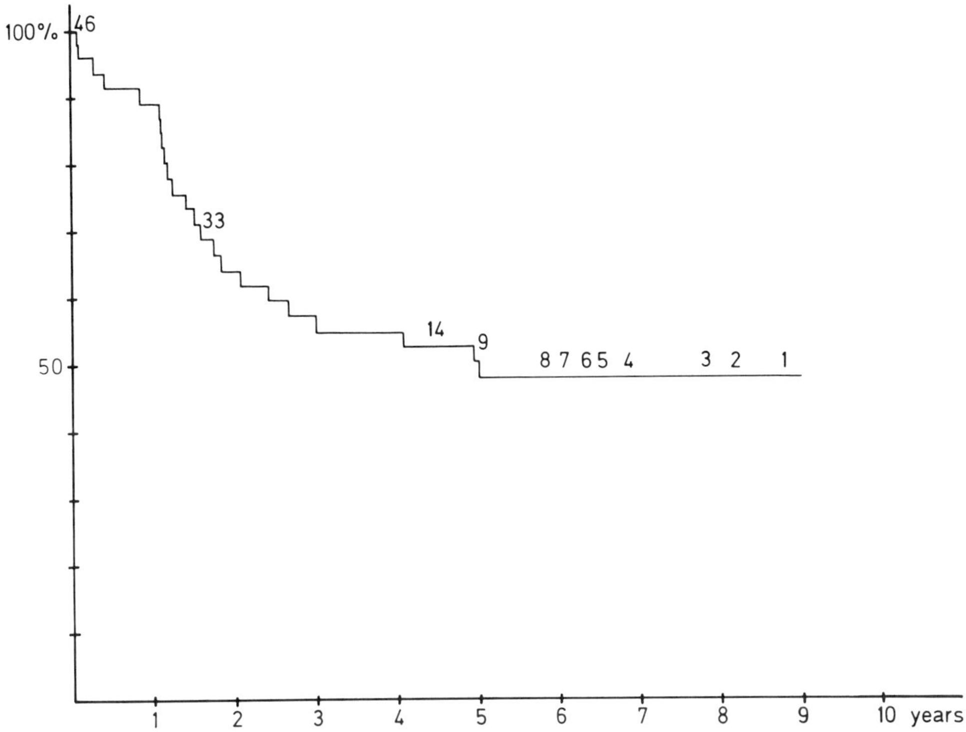

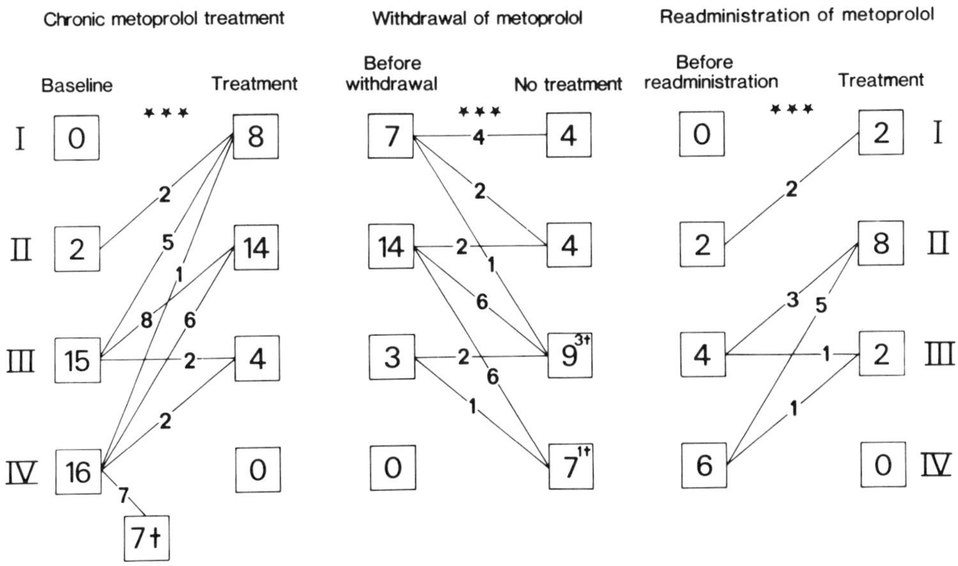

Figure 3 New York Heart Association (NYHA) Functional Class in patients with idiopathic dilated cardiomyopathy before and after chronic treatment with metoprolol, after withdrawal and readministration of metoprolol.

Table 6 Effect of Withdrawal of Beta-Blockade

	Swedberg et al. (1) (n=15).			Waagstein et al. (2) (n=24)		
	C	W	P	C	W	P
Ejection fraction	0.42	0.35	<0.01	0.41	0.32	<0.0001
Left atrial diameter	No change			5.54	4.80	<0.02
Left ventricular end-diastolic diameter	No change			6.44	6.81	<0.001
Rapid filling wave ratio	Increase in 8/23 pts		<0.05	6.20	11.30	=0.067
	Follow-up time: mean 1.3 months			Follow-up time: mean 7.9 months		
Survivors	14/15			20/24		

C, control before withdrawal of chronic beta-blockade; W, withdrawal (when symptoms of dyspnea, decompensation, or sudden death occurred, or the patient had been followed for 4 months or 18 months without any signs of deterioration).

after withdrawal and the improvement after reinstitution of beta-blocker treatment strongly suggest that the favorable effects of beta-blockers represent a true pharmacologic effect and are not due to a spontaneous improvement.

IX. POSSIBLE MECHANISMS FOR FAVORABLE EFFECTS OF BETA-BLOCKERS IN DILATED CARDIOMYOPATHY

It is now well established that long-term administration of beta-blockers to patients with idiopathic dilated cardiomyopathy causes improvement of cardiac function and of exercise capacity in some patients. On the other hand, there are patients who will either not tolerate beta-blocker treatment or will be unchanged or deteriorate during long-term treatment. During the last few years it has become obvious that similar improvement by long-term beta-blockade can be obtained also among other patients with congestive heart failure (e.g., due to coronary artery disease, adriamycin-induced, or secondary to valvular heart disease). It is not yet clear why some patients respond favorably to the treatment while others are nonresponders. It was recently suggested by Woodley and co-workers (25) that patients with idiopathic dilated cardiomyopathy should respond better than the ischemic patients. However, this is not the experience from our studies on patients with idiopathic and ischemic cardiomyopathy (11,12,17,20). In fact, we have not been able to identify any factor that seems to be correlated with a better response to chronic beta-blockade. It was first thought that patients with tachycardia would respond more favorably but it was later found that also patients with atrioventricular (AV) block and pacemakers responded with marked improvement in some cases. Age, duration of disease, or severity of heart failure does not predict if the patient will respond favorably. Recently, Gilbert and co-workers compared patients with idiopathic dilated cardiomyopathy who were responders to the beta-blocking agents metoprolol or bucindolol to nonresponders (34). There was no difference between the groups as regards entry variables such as resting or exercise ejection fraction, heart rate, cardiac index, filling pressure, blood pressure, or exercise capacity. The only difference noted was a trend toward higher venous norepinephrine concentration among patients responding favorably to beta-blocker therapy.

A number of effects of beta-blockers has been suggested to explain the improvement in patients with dilated cardiomyopathy.

1. In patients with congestive heart failure there is a high mechanical workload of the myocardium due to tachycardia and wall stress. Reduction of heart work and cardiac output by acute administration of beta-blockers causes a reduction in oxygen consumption and lactate release (12). These favorable effects might be, to some extent, counteracted by an increase in vascular resistance due to a marked compensatory increase in sympathetic activity (30,31) with an increase in vascular resistance. Long-term treatment might, however, change this due to improved cardiac function and adaptive changes of the peripheral arteries during long-term beta-blocker treatment (35). A reduction in metabolic demand during long-term treatment might reduce any ischemia-like changes with more favorable energy utilization.

2. In ischemic heart disease it has clearly been demonstrated that catecholamines cause a decrease in left ventricular compliance while beta-blockade has the opposite effect. Based upon the information of marked lactate release during exercise and pacing in patients with idiopathic dilated cardiomyopathy (29), beta-blockade may cause favorable effects in congestive heart failure by improving left ventricular compliance. This idea is in agreement with a finding of marked improvement of diastolic function during the early phase of chronic beta-blocker treatment (within the first few months; 12). The reduction in heart rate per se increases the time of filling and emptying of the cardiac ventricles. Chronic treatment causes a marked reduction in left ventricular filling pressures and of the rapid filling wave.

3. An increased sympathetic activity with marked release of catecholamines from sympathetic nerve endings in the myocardium (29) may cause direct toxic effects on the myocytes (36).

4. Gwathmey and co-workers have demonstrated an abnormal intracellular calcium handling in human myocardium that may cause systolic and diastolic dysfunction in heart failure (37). Direct or indirect effects of sympathetic overactivity through receptor desensitization may cause this abnormality. Myocardial ischemia is also known to cause defects in intracellular calcium release and reuptake.

5. Secondary to sympathetic overactivity there is a marked downregulation of beta-receptor density of the failing human myocardium (15,17,38,39). Our group and others have shown that long-term treatment with metoprolol causes a receptor upregulation to the level somewhat below the values seen in normal individuals (15,17). Bristow and co-workers have demonstrated that the downregulation mainly affects the beta$_1$-receptor population of the failing human myocardium (38).

6. Recent data also indicate the role for G-protein changes in cardiovascular disease (40). These are the coupling membrane proteins activated by the receptor—agonist complex causing an activation of second messenger effector systems. It has been found that there is not only a downregulation of the beta-adrenergic receptor but also an uncoupling of the receptor from adenylate cyclase. It has recently been found that there is an impaired activation of the stimulatory G-protein G_s by GTP in heart membranes from failing human hearts (41). Our group (42) reported that membranes from the failing human heart had a more marked depression of adenylate cyclase activity after addition of muscarinic agonists. This indicated a

tight coupling between the muscarinic receptor and adenylate cyclase. It was later proposed that there is an increased content of G_i-proteins in membranes from failing human myocardium (43–45). Such an increase in G_i-proteins might explain a more marked depression of adenylate cyclase activity after addition of muscarinic agonists, but might also indirectly influence the adrenergic receptor-adenylate cyclase coupling. It has recently also been found that the G-proteins influence cardiac calcium channels via two pathways: direct coupling between G_s-protein and calcium channels and indirectly through the cyclic AMP cascade (46,47).

7. As discussed above, it has been thought that the decreased responsiveness to beta-agonists of the failing human heart with a lower number of membrane beta-receptors, uncoupling of receptors to adenylate cyclase, and decreased positive inotropic effects are caused by sympathetic overactivity. However, the mechanisms behind this desensitization have not been fully clarified and there might be other factors involved. Recently Limas and co-workers reported that autoantibodies directed against cardiac beta-adrenoceptors were present in sera from patients with idiopathic dilated cardiomyopathy (48). Independent of their work, our group took a new approach towards detection of receptor autoantibodies versus human beta_1-adrenergic receptors (49). Peptides corresponding to the predicted sequence of the second extracellular loop of the human beta_1- and beta_2-adrenergic receptors were used as antigens in an enzyme immunoassay to screen sera from patients with dilated cardiomyopathy. One-third of the patients with idiopathic dilated cardiomyopathy had antibodies directed exclusively against the beta_1-peptide. None of the patients with congestive heart failure due to ischemic heart disease had such antibodies. Autoimmunity has been claimed as one of the pathologic processes involved in idiopathic dilated cardiomyopathy (50). Further studies are needed to evaluate whether autoantibodies versus the myocardial beta-adrenergic receptors are of etiologic, prognostic, or therapeutic value in patients with idiopathic dilated cardiomyopathy.

It is obvious that there are a number of possible mechanisms behind the favorable effects of beta-blockers in patients with dilated cardiomyopathy. These mechanisms involve mechanical work, energy utilization, membrane receptor modification, changes in G-proteins and the cyclic AMP cascade, and through intracellular calcium handling. Some of the changes described in heart failure have been partly corrected by chronic beta-blocker treatment, which might give support for the mechanisms involved. Much more work is, however, needed before the effects of long-term beta-blocker treatment are fully understood. The positive findings of the MDC Trial with a 34% risk reduction of death or need for cardiac transplantation by metoprolol compared to placebo will add new important information about possible mechanisms."

X. CONCLUSION

A large number of studies have clearly demonstrated that some patients with congestive heart failure due to various causes can be improved by long-term beta-blocker treatment. This was first reported by our group in 1975 for patients with idiopathic dilated cardiomyopathy. It was later found that other forms of dilated cardiomyopathy might respond favorably. Among factors that may predict whether a patient will respond favorably or not has been suggested a marked elevation of venous norepinephrine concentration. This needs to be explored in studies involving larger numbers of patients to allow for careful subgroup analysis. Long-term treatment with beta-blockers seems to improve some patients during maintenance treatment, but withdrawal of treatment causes more or less marked deterioration, suggesting that it is not possible to obtain a healing of the myocardial defect in dilated cardiomyopathy.

ACKNOWLEDGMENT

Our investigations have been supported by the Swedish Medical Research Council and the Swedish National Association Against Heart and Chest Diseases.

REFERENCES

1. Cohn JN, Archibald DG, Ziesche S, Franciosa JA, Harston WE, Tristani FE, Dunkman WB, Jacobs W, Francis GS, Flohr KH, Goldman S, Cobb FR, Shah PM, Saunders R, Fletcher RD, Loeb HS, Hughes VC, Baker B. Effect of vasodilator therapy on mortality in chronic congestive heart failure. Results of a Veterans Administration Cooperative Study. N Engl J Med 1986;314:1547–52.
2. The Consensus Trial Study Group. Effects of enalapril on mortality in severe congestive heart failure. N Engl J Med 1987; 316: 1429–35.
3. Hjalmarson Å. International beta-blocker review in acute and postmyocardial infarction. Am J Cardiol 1988; 61 (3):26–9B.
4. The Norwegian Multicenter Study Group. Timolol-induced reduction in mortality and reinfarction in patients surviving acute myocardial infarction. N Engl J Med 1981; 304: 801–7.
5. Beta-Blocker Heart Attack Study Group. The beta-blocker heart attack trial (BHAT). JAMA 1981; 246: 2073–4.
6. Hjalmarson Å, Elmfeldt D, Herlitz J, Holmberg S, Málek I, Nyberg G, Rydén L, Swedberg K, Vedin A, Waagstein F, Waldenström A, Waldenström J, Wedel H, Wilhelmsen L, Wilhelmsson C. Effect on mortality of metoprolol in acute myocardial infarction. A double-blind randomized trial. Lancet 1981; 2: 823–7.
7. The MIAMI Trial Research Group. Metoprolol in acute myocardial infarction (MIAMI). A randomized placebo-controlled international trial. Eur Heart J 1985; 6: 199–226.
8. ISIS-1 (First International Study of Infarct Survival) Collaborative Group. Randomized trial of intravenous atenolol among 16027 cases of suspected acute myocardial infarction: ISIS-1. Lancet 1986; 2: 57–66.
9. Waagstein F. The use of beta-adrenergic blockade in the critically diseased heart. A study in acute myocardial infarction and congestive cardiomyopathy. Thesis, Faculty of Medicine, University of Göteborg, Sweden, 1976.
10. Waagstein F, Hjalmarson Å, Varnauskas E, Wallentin I. Effect of chronic beta-adrenergic receptor blockade in congestive cardiomyopathy. Br Heart J 1975; 37: 1022–36.
11. Swedberg K, Hjalmarson Å, Waagstein F, Wallentin I. Beneficial effects of long-term beta-blockade in congestive cardiomyopathy. Br Heart J 1980; 44: 117–33.
12. Waagstein F, Hjalmarson Å, Swedberg K, Wallentin I. Beta-blockers in dilated cardiomyopathies: they work. Eur Heart J 1983; 4 (suppl. A): 173–8.
13. Engelmeier RS, O'Connell JB, Walsh R, Rad N, Scanlon PF, Gunnar RM. Improvement in symptoms and exercise tolerance by metoprolol in patients with dilated cardiomyopathy: a double-blind, randomized, placebo-controlled trial. Circulation 1985; 72: 536–46.
14. Anderson JL, Lutz JR, Gilbert EM, Sorenson SG, Yanowitz FG, Menlove RL, Bar-

tholomew M. A randomized trial of low-dose beta-blockade therapy for idiopathic dilated cardiomyopathy. Am J Cardiol 1985; 55: 471–5.
15. Heilbrunn SM, Shah P, Bristow MR, Valantine HA, Ginsburg R, Fowler MB. Increased beta-receptor density and improved hemodynamic response to catecholamine stimulation during long-term metoprolol therapy in heart failure from dilated cardiomyopathy. Circulation 1989; 79: 483–90.
16. Gilbert EM, Anderson JL, Deitchman D, Yanowitz FG, O'Connell JB, Renlund DG, Bartholomew M, Mealey PC, et al. Long-term beta-blocker vasodilator therapy improves cardiac function in idiopathic dilated cardiomyopathy: a double-blind, randomized study of bucindolol versus placebo. Am J Med 1990;88:223–9.
17. Waagstein F, Caidahl K, Wallentin I, Bergh C-H, Hjalmarson Å. Long-term beta-blockade in congestive cardiomyopathy. Effects of acute and chronic metoprolol treatment followed by withdrawal and readministration of metoprolol. 1989; 80: 551–63.
18. Leung W-H, Lau C-P, Wong C-K, Cheng C-H, Tai Y-T, Lim S-P. A double-blind crossover trial of labetalol in patients with idiopathic dilated cardiomyopathy. Circulation 1989; 80 (suppl II): II–118.
19. Eiswirth CC, Bowden RE, Kazamias T, Fowler M, Bristow MR. Treatment of adriamycin cardiomyopathy with metoprolol. Circulation 1986; 74 (suppl II): 310.
20. Waagstein F, Blomström-Lundquist C, Andersson B, Hjalmarson Å, Wallentin I. Long-term effects of metoprolol in severe heart failure due to ischemic cardiomyopathy, primary valve disease and diabetes. Circulation 1987; 76 (suppl IV): IV–358.
21. DasGupta P, Broadhurst PA, Lahiri A. Improvement in congestive heart failure following chronic therapy with a new vasodilating betablocker: carvedilol. Circulation 1989; 80 (4) (suppl. II): II–117.
22. Eichhorn EJ, McGhie AI, Bedotto JB, Corbett JR, Malloy CR, Hatfield BA, Deitchman D, Willard JE, Grayburn PA. Effects of bucindolol on neurohormonal activation in congestive heart failure. Am J Cardiol 1991;67:67–73.
23. Pollock SG, Lystash J, Tedesco C, Craddock G, Smucker ML. Usefulness of bucindolol in congestive heart failure. Am J Cardiol 1990;66:603–7.
24. Sano H, Kawabata N, Yonezawa K, Hirayama H, Sakuma I, Yasuda H. Metoprolol was more effective than captopril for dilated cardiomyopathy in Japanese patients, Circulation 1989; 80 (4) (suppl. II): II–118.
25. Woodley SL, Gilberg EM, Anderson JL, O'Connell JB, Deitchman D, Yanowitz FG, Mealey PC, Volkman K, et al. Beta-blockade with bucindolol in heart failure caused by ischemic versus idiopathic dilated cardiomyopathy. Circulation 1991;84:2426–41.
26. Ikram H, Fitzpatrick D. Double-blind trial of chronic oral beta-blockade in congestive cardiomyopathy. Lancet 1981; 2: 490–2.
27. Currie PJ, Kelly MJ, McKenzie A, Harper RW, Lim YL, Federman J, Anderson ST, Pitt, A. Oral beta-adrenergic blockade with metoprolol in chronic severe dilated cardiomyopathy. J Am Coll Cardiol 1984; 3: 203–9.
28. Shanes JG. Beta-blockade—rational or irrational therapy for congestive heart failure? (Editorial). Circulation 1987; 76: 971–3.
29. Swedberg K, Hjalmarson Å, Holmberg S. Effects of work and acute beta-receptor blockade on myocardial noradrenaline release in congestive cardiomyopathy. Clin Cardiol 1979; 2: 424–30.
30. Ikram H, Chan W, Bennett SI, Bones PJ. Haemodynamic effects of acute beta-adrenergic receptor blockade in congestive cardiomyopathy. Br Heart J 1979; 42: 311–5.
31. Binkley PF, Lewe RF, Lima JL, Al-Awwa A, Unverferth DV, Leier CV. Hemodynamic–inotropic response to beta-blocker with intrinsic sympathomimetic activity in patients with congestive cardiomyopathy. Circulation 1986; 74 (6): 1390–8.

32. Swedberg K, Hjalmarson Å, Waagstein F, Wallentin I. Prolongation of survival in congestive cardiomyopathy during treatment with beta-receptor blockade. Lancet 1979; 1: 1374–6.
33. Swedberg K, Hjalmarson Å, Waagstein F, Wallentin I. Adverse effects of beta-blockade withdrawal in patients with congestive cardiomyopathy. Br Heart J 1980; 44 (2): 134–42.
34. Gilbert EM, Mestroni L, Anderson JL, Woodley SL, Bristow MR. Can response to beta-blocker therapy in idiopathic dilated cardiomyopathy be predicted by baseline parameters? Circulation 1989; 80 (4) (suppl. II): II–428.
35. Wikstrand J, Trimarco B, Buzzetti G, Ricciardelli B, de Luca N, Volpe M, Condorelli M. Increased cardiac output and lowered peripheral resistance during metoprolol treatment. Acta Med Scand 1983; (suppl. 672): 105–10.
36. Reichenbach DD, Benditt EP. Catecholamine and cardiomyopathy: the pathogenesis and potential importance of myofibrillar degeneration. Hum Pathol 1970; 1: 125–50.
37. Gwathmey JK, Copelas L, MacKinnon R, Schoen FJ, Feldman MD, Grossman W, Morgan JP. Abnormal intracellular calcium handling in myocardium from patients with end-stage heart failure. Circ Res 1987; 61: 70–6.
38. Bristow MR, Ginsburg R, Umans V, Fowler M, Minobe W, Rasmussen R, Zera P, Menlove R, Shah P, Jamieson S, Stinson EB. $Beta_1$- and $beta_2$- adrenergic receptor subpopulations in nonfailing and failing human ventricular myocardium: coupling of both receptor subtypes to muscle contraction and selective $beta_1$-receptor down-regulation in heart failure. Circ Res 1986; 59: 297–309.
39. Bristow MR, Ginsburg R, Minobe W, Cubicciotti RS, Sageman WS, Lurie K, Billingham ME, Harrison DC, Stinson EB. Decreased catecholamine sensitivity and beta-adrenergic receptor density in failing human hearts. N Engl J Med 1982; 307: 205–11.
40. Insel PA, Ransnäs LA. G-proteins and cardiovascular disease. Circulation 1988; 78: 1511–13.
41. Ransnäs LA, Hjalmarson Å, Insel PA. Dilated cardiomyopathy is associated with an impaired activation of the stimulatory G protein, G_s, by GTP in heart membranes. Circulation 1988; 78 (suppl II): II–178.
42. Fu XL, Waagstein F, Hjalmarson Å. Abnormalities of adrenergic and muscarinic receptor control of human myocardial membranes in idiopathic dilated cardiomyopathy. (To be published).
43. Feldman AM, Cates AE, Veazey WB, Hershberger RE. Increase of the 40,000 mol wt pertussis toxin substrate (G protein) in failing human heart. J Clin Invest 1988; 82: 189–97.
44. Neumann J, Schmitz W, Scholz H, von Meyerinck L, Döring V, and Kalmár P. Increase in myocardial G_i-proteins in heart failure. Lancet 1988; 2: 936–7.
45. Imoto, Yatani A, Reeves JP, Codina J. Alpha-subunit of G_s directly activates cardiac calcium channels in lipid bilayer. Am J Physiol 1988; 255(4 part 2): H722–8.
46. Brown AM, Birnbauer L. Direct G protein gating of ion channels. Am J Physiol 1988; 254: H401–10.
47. Limas CJ, Goldenberg IF, Limas C. Autoantibodies against beta-adrenoceptors in human idiopathic dilated cardiomyopathy. Circ Res 1989; 64: 97–103.
48. Magnusson Y, Marullo S, Höyer S, Waagstein F, Andersson B, Vahlne A, Guillet JG, Hjalmarson Å, Hoebeke J. Mapping of a functional autoimmune epitope on the $beta_1$-adrenergic receptor in patients with idiopathic dilated cardiomyopathy. J Clin Invest 1990;86:1658–63.
49. Goodwin JF. Mechanisms in cardiomyopathies. J Moll Cell Cardiol 1985; 17: 5–9.

13

Muscarinic Receptors: Basic Science and Experimental Pharmacology

JONAS B. GALPER and JOEY V. BARNETT

Brigham and Women's Hospital and Harvard Medical School
Boston, Massachusetts

I. INTRODUCTION

In this chapter we summarize recent insights gained into the mechanism of muscarinic cholinergic modulation of cardiac function. Vagal stimulation of the heart results in a decrease in the rate and force of contraction. These effects have been related to the ability of muscarinic stimulation to increase K^+ permeability of the heart cell membrane (1) and to antagonize the elevation of cyclic AMP levels mediated by the sympathetic nervous system (2). In addition, the response of the heart to muscarinic stimulation is also associated with a decrease in Ca^{+2} permeability (3), increased levels of cyclic GMP (4), and increased turnover of phosphatidyl inositol with production of diacylglycerol and inositol phosphates (5,6).

Recent studies have demonstrated that transduction of muscarinic and many other receptor-initiated signals across the cell membrane involves at least three components: binding of the hormone or neurotransmitter to a receptor, the coupling of the receptor–agonist complex to a guanine nucleotide-binding protein, and the GTP-dependent activation of an effector within the cell. Molecular biological studies of muscarinic receptors and the guanine nucleotide-binding proteins (G-proteins) that couple the receptor to a physiological response in the cell demonstrate that both muscarinic receptors and G-proteins exist as multiple isoforms in the cell. Furthermore, the effector molecules to which these G-proteins are coupled also appear to exist as multiple isoforms. The specificity of receptors, G-proteins, and effector isoforms for a given tissue and a given physiological response is not well understood. In this chapter we will review classic studies of muscarinic receptor function and mechanisms of parasympathetic modulation of cardiac function as well as more recent findings utilizing molecular biological approaches to help understand the relationship between receptor—effector coupling and parasympathetic responsiveness in the heart.

II. VAGAL EFFECTS OF THE HEART: HISTORICAL PERSPECTIVE

The autonomic nervous system is characterized by a two-neuron chain. Bodies of primary preganglionic neurons are located in the central nervous system and send out axons to synapse with secondary postganglionic neurons whose cell bodies are located in a peripheral autonomic ganglion. The postganglionic axons then pass to their distribution in the innervated organ. The parasympathetic input to the vagus nerve originates in the dorsal motor and salivatory nuclei of the medulla oblongata. The dorsal motor nucleus is the principal source of preganglionic parasympathetic fibers destined to innervate the heart. Fibers in the cardiac plexus synapse with ganglia located primarily in the atria, with a particularly rich collection of ganglia in the region of the sinoatrial and atrioventricular nodes (7,8).

In 1921, Otto Loewi described the release of a chemical substance from the vagus nerve that he termed "*vagusstoff*" or parasympathin (9). Vagusstoff was shown to be released by electrical stimulation of the vagus nerve and to slow the rate of the perfused heart. Feldberg and Krayer later determined that vagusstoff was acetylcholine (10). The postsynaptic site on which acetylcholine exerted its effects was defined by Dale as the muscarinic receptor (11). This receptor site was specifically stimulated by acetylcholine and selectively antagonized by the belladonna alkaloid, atropine. Dale's description of the response of the heart to the mushroom alkaloid muscarine constitutes the classic definition of muscarinic cholinergic receptor still in use today (3). However, drugs such as nicotine and dimethylphenylpiperazinium, which are selective nicotinic agonists, also suppressed sinoatrial pacemaker activity in isolated chick embryo hearts (12). This apparent discrepancy was resolved when it was determined that preganglionic cholinergic receptors are nicotinic while postganglionic receptors in the heart are muscarinic (2). Thus acetylcholine was shown to be a neurotransmitter at both preganglionic and postganglionic parasymathetic fibers (1).

III. CLASSIC PHYSIOLOGICAL RESPONSES OF THE HEART TO MUSCARINIC STIMULATION

Vagal stimulation of the heart or exposure of the heart to acetylcholine produces characteristic changes in both the sinus venosus and atrial muscle that include hyperpolarization of the resting membrane potential and shortening of the action potential duration. These changes are associated with increased K^+ permeability and decreased Ca^{2+} permeability.

A. Effects on K^+ Permeability

Early studies by Hutter and Trautwein documented a hyperpolarization of the heart cell membrane in response to vagal stimulation and also accelerated repolarization of the action potential in atrial tissue and sinoatrial node, resulting in decreased action potential duration (13). These effects were found to be sensitive to extracellular K^+ concentration. Harris and Hutter documented that vagal stimulation of the heart or exposure to acetylcholine resulted in an increase in the rate of $^{42}K^+$ efflux from a sinus venosus preparation loaded with $^{42}K^+$ (14). It is now widely accepted that the negative chronotropic response to muscarinic stimulation involves an increase in K^+ conductance of the heart cell membrane. This has been extensively quantified by Glitsch and Pott using voltage clamp techniques (15).

B. Effects of Muscarinic Stimulation on Calcium Currents

In electrically paced guinea pig atria, acetylcholine decreased contraction amplitude by 80% concomitant with a 40% decrease in $^{45}Ca^{2+}$ uptake over 5 min (16). These and other studies supported the conclusion that muscarinic stimulation decreased calcium flux in atrial preparations (17,18). Modulation of cyclic GMP and cyclic AMP levels by muscarinic agonists appears to be the mechanism by which parasympathetic stimulation decreases Ca^+ uptake and contractile force. Increases in cyclic AMP levels have been shown to correlate with increases in slow inward current (I_{si}) and enhanced contractility. In addition, agents including histamine and phosphodiesterase inhibitors, which increase intracellular cAMP levels independent of the effects of beta-adrenergic stimulation, also increase I_{si} and increase contractility (19,20). Hence cAMP, presumably acting through the stimulation of protein phosphorylation via cyclic AMP-activated protein kinase, is capable of increasing Ca^{2+} influx. It is now well established that the antagonist effects of parasympathetic stimuli on the response to sympathetic stimulation are mediated, at least in part, by the ability of muscarinic agonists to lower intracellular cyclic AMP levels (21,22).

IV. DEVELOPMENT OF PARASYMPATHETIC RESPONSIVENESS IN THE HEART

The ontogenesis of parasympathetic responsiveness of the heart has been most fully described in the chick embryo. Gestation of the chick embryo requires 21 days. In the chick embryo, vagal fibers appear in the region of the truncus arteriosis during the 3rd day in ovo, reach the atria toward the end of the 4th day in ovo, and the interatrial septum on the 5th day in ovo (12,23). Innervation of the sinoatrial node and atrial wall has been demonstrated on days 6 and 7 in ovo, respectively. The atrial ventricular groove is reached by vagal fibers by the 9th day. Far less is known regarding the development of the parasympathetic innervation of the human heart. Nerve cells are known to be present at about 5 weeks of gestation while ganglia appear to develop between the 5th and 12th weeks of gestation (24).

In the chick heart inhibitory transmission between postganglionic neurons and sinoatrial pacemaker cells appears on the 12th day in ovo (25). Evidence indicates that muscarinic receptors are present in the embryonic chick heart for a substantial period prior to ingrowth of the vagus nerve (26–28). However, exogenously added acetylcholine mediates only a very modest decrease in atrial beating rate of chick hearts 2–3 days in ovo; enhanced sensitivity of beating to acetylcholine increases gradually between the 5th and 10th day in ovo, a time well after vagal innervation (29,30). It has been known for some time now that autonomic responsiveness in the embryonic chick heart proceeds noncoordinately. Before days 4 and 5 in ovo, beta-adrenergic stimulation by exogenous norepinephrine results in cardioacceleration (31). Some of the molecular mechanisms responsible for the noncoordinate development are described below.

V. BIOCHEMICAL ASPECTS OF MUSCARINIC RESPONSIVENESS IN THE HEART

The availability of ligands radiolabeled to high specific activity allowed the study of developmental changes in receptors and their coupling to physiological responses in the heart. During embryonic development, chick hearts 2–4 days in ovo decreased beat rate by less than 10% in response to 1 mM carbamylcholine, while beat rates in embryos 5–6 days in ovo decreased by 90% at the same carbamylcholine concentration (26). Embryonic chick heart sensitivity continued to increase rapidly by days 7–12 in ovo, with beating being totally inhibited by 10^{-6} M carbamycholine (26). From days 2-½ to 12 in ovo, the number of muscarinic receptors per mg of cell protein remained unchanged as measured by binding of the labeled muscarinic antagonist [^{3}H]-quinuclidinylbenzilate (QNB) (32). Thus, muscarinic receptors are present before ingrowth of the vagus nerve at a time when these receptors are relatively insensitive to muscarinic agonists. Hence, the development of sensitivity following vagal innervation does not appear to be due to an alteration in receptor number but rather to the absence of coupling of these receptors to effectors.

A. Role of a GTP-Binding Protein in Determining the Affinity State of Muscarinic Receptors

Competition binding between carbamylcholine and 1 mM [^{3}H]QNB to homogenates of cultures of hearts from embryos 10 days in ovo demonstrated at least two agonist binding sites: high-affinity binding sites (R_H) constituting 26% of total sites with an IC_{50} for inhibition of [^{3}H]QNB binding of 3.9×10^{-7} M; and low-affinity sites (R_L) with an IC_{50} of 4.5×10^{-5} M for inhibition of antagonist binding (33).

Using analogous competitive binding methods, Rosenberger and colleagues (34) found that guanine nucleotides and Na^+ decreased the affinity of the muscarinic receptor for agonist. In homogenates of cultures of embryonic chick heart cells, guanine nucleotides had no effect on the total number of receptors, but resulted in the conversion of the subset of 26% of high-affinity receptors to a low-affinity form (33). In intact cells exposed briefly (1–5 min) to muscarinic agonists and washed carefully to remove unbound agonists prior to homogenization, the number of receptors decreased by 26% as judged by [^{3}H]QNB binding (34) and all of the remaining sites were in the low-affinity form. These findings suggested that the loss of receptors following brief exposure to agonist may involve persistent binding of agonist to the high-affinity form of the receptor, leaving these high-affinity receptors unavailable for labeled antagonist binding.

Radiolabeled muscarinic agonist binding has also demonstrated loss of high-affinity sites in response to guanine nucleotides. [^{3}H]Oxotremorine-M and [^{3}H]cis-dimethyldioxalane, both muscarinic agonists, bind to cell homogenates and give high levels of specific binding, to a high-affinity site (K_D, for [^{3}H]cis-methyldioxalane of 16×10^{-9} M) and a low-affinity site (K_D, 4×10^{-7} M). The fraction of [^{3}H]cis-dimethyldioxalane with the more rapid dissociation rate increased in the presence of guanine nucleotides with a half-maximal effect at 10^{-6}M Gpp(NH)p (35). These findings are consistent with the view that muscarinic receptors exist in at least two forms, and that guanine nucleotides mediate the conversion of the high-affinity receptor to a low-affinity form. The data further support the view that agonists persistently bound to the high-affinity receptors are released during guanine nucleotide-mediated conversion to the low-affinity form (36,37).

B. Ternary Complex Model for the Interaction of Muscarinic Agonists, Receptors, and Guanine Nucleotide-Binding Proteins

The data cited above suggest the following model for the interaction of muscarinic agonist, high-affinity receptor, and G-protein. This scheme parallels that presented by DeLean et al. (38) for the β-adrenergic receptor.

$R_HG_i + A$ (Step 1)$\rightarrow R_HG_iA + GTP$ (Step 2)$\rightarrow (AR_HG_i\text{-}GTP)$ (Step 3)$\rightarrow R_L + (G_i - GTP) + A$.

In this scheme R_H is a high-affinity receptor, R_L is a low-affinity receptor, G_i is an inhibitory G-protein, and A is the agonist. Only indirect evidence is available for the species in parentheses. According to this model, in the absence of GTP, agonist binds persistently to R_HG_i to form $R_H\ G_iA$ (step 1) thus causing these R_H sites to be unavailable for binding of labeled antagonists. This explains why brief exposure to agonist results in the loss of 26% of [^{3}H]QNB binding sites (33). According to this scheme, binding of A and formation of R_HG_iA permits interaction of R_HG_iA with GTP, with release of agonist (step 2) and regeneration of the receptor in a low affinity form (step 3). It is obvious that a G-protein must be present in order for the muscarinic receptor to interact with guanine nucleotides. The absence of a significant effect of guanine nucleotides on the affinity of R_L for agonist indicates that G_i may be associated only with the high-affinity state of the receptor. Hence the conversion of R_H to R_L in the presence of GTP is associated with the release of the G-protein (step 3). Furthermore, Florio and Sternweiss (39) demonstrated that reconstitution of phospholipid vesicles containing muscarinic receptors in the low-affinity form with G_i resulted in the appearance of the high-affinity form of the receptor and the development of sensitivity of agonist binding to guanine nucleotides. Hence, regeneration of R_H from R_L is associated with the binding of an inhibitory G-protein to a low-affinity form of the receptor.

C. Role of Changes in Levels of GTP-Binding Proteins in the Ontogenesis of Parasympathetic Responsiveness in the Embryonic Chick Heart

We have demonstrated that early in embryonic development, at a time when muscarinic agonists are incapable of mediating a negative chronotropic response in cultured chick atrial cells, guanine nucleotides have no effect on conversion of muscarinic receptors from the high-affinity to the low-affinity form. One interpretation of these data is that early in embryonic development certain G-proteins are either absent or markedly decreased in these cells (40). Liang et al. (32) demonstrated that during embryonic development of the chick heart (between days 2-½ and 10 in ovo) levels of certain G-proteins increased threefold in parallel with the increased ability of muscarinic agonists to inhibit isoproterenol-stimulated adrenylate cyclase activity. Furthermore, homogenates of hatched chick hearts in which both muscarinic receptors and adenylate cyclase activity had been inactivated, when reconstituted with membranes from embryonic chick hearts 2-½ days in ovo, enhanced the ability of muscarinic agonists to inhibit isoproterenol-stimulated adylate cyclase activity (41). The factor in the hatched chick homogenates responsible for reconstituting enhanced muscarinic inhibition of adenylate cyclase activity was shown to be a G-protein. These data suggested that the embryonic development of a muscarinic response in the chick heart may require the appearance of increased levels of G-proteins or expression of a new G-protein isoform.

VI. ROLE OF GTP-BINDING PROTEINS IN COUPLING OF THE MUSCARINIC RECEPTOR TO A PHYSIOLOGICAL RESPONSE

A. GTP-Binding Proteins: α, β, and γ Subunits

1. Studies with Bacterial Toxins

The physiology and biochemistry of G-proteins have been extensively studied using bacterial toxins that catalyze the transfer of an ADP–ribose moeity from nicotinamide adenine dinucleotide (NAD) to the α subunit of many G-proteins. A protein initially referred to as "islet activating protein" (IAP) isolated from cultures of *Bordetella pertussis* was shown to potentiate the effects of various insulin secretogogues when incubated with pancreatic islet cells (42). This effect was associated with an increase in cyclic AMP levels. Hazeki and Ui demonstrated that levels of cAMP in isoproterenol-stimulated heart cells were significantly higher in cells preincubated with IAP (43). Although muscarinic agonists markedly inhibited cAMP accumulation in isoproterenol-stimulated rat heart myocyte cultures, muscarinic agonists had no effect on isoproterenol-stimulated cAMP levels in cells pretreated with IAP. These data suggested that IAP interfered with the action of agonists that inhibited adenylate cyclase activity.

It is well established that both isoproterenol and GTP stimulate adenylate cyclase activity (44). Katada and Ui (46) demonstrated that IAP (now referred to as pertussis toxin) enhanced the effect of GTP or GTP plus isoproterenol on cAMP production in membranes from cultured neural cells. Nicotinamide adenine dinucleotide and ATP were required for this effect and the reaction was shown to involve the transfer of an ADP ribose moiety from NAD to a 41,000 dalton protein. Katada and Ui further demonstrated that pertussis toxin treatment converted the muscarinic receptor from a high-affinity to a low-affinity form by interfering with the interaction of the receptor and G-protein. Hence not only is hormonal inhibition of adenylate cyclase activity prevented, but basal levels of adenylate cyclase activity are also increased by release of adenylate cyclase from a tonic inhibition by an inhibitory G-protein.

Inhibitory G-proteins have been termed G_i and have been shown to exist as heterotrimers composed of three subunits designated α, β, and γ (46–49). The α subunit has been shown to be a protein that varies in molecular weight from 39 to 41 kD, binds GTP, catalyzes the hydrolysis of GTP to GDP, and is the substrate for pertussis toxin. The β subunit is a 35 kD protein usually found in association with a 9 kD γ subunit (50).

A second toxin derived from *Vibrio cholera* has been shown to enhance the activity of adenylate cyclase by catalyzing the transfer of ADP-ribose from NAD to a 45 kD dalton GTP-binding protein designated α_s. The α_s subunit has been found to associate with a $\beta\gamma$ subunit identical to that associated with α_i and is responsible for coupling stimulatory receptors to adenylate cyclase (51).

2. A Family of GTP-Binding Proteins

Jones and Reed (52) demonstrated the presence of five G-proteins cloned from rat olfactory neuroepithelium. The majority of clones encoded the α subunit of G_s, while the remaining clones encoded G-proteins that were pertussis toxin substrates, $G\alpha_o$, a 39 kD protein found in high levels in the brain, and three other proteins designated $G\alpha_{i-1}$, $G\alpha_{i-2}$, and $G\alpha_{i-3}$. More recently Strathmann et al. (53) cloned five new G-proteins utilizing the polymerase chain reaction (PCR) with a template cDNA prepared from total RNA from adult mouse brain and mouse spermatids and an oligonucleotide primer 95% identical to sequences in G_s, G_o, G_i, and transducin. These data suggest that the family of G-proteins may contain more than 15 members.

B. Receptor–Effector Coupling via G-Proteins

Two forms of the α subunit of the G-protein transducin, a pertussis toxin substrate found in the eye, have been demonstrated. One form is found only in retinal rods and the other only in retinal cones, suggesting that these two α subunits have specific functions within the two different cell types. However, hormone receptor-linked α subunits appear to be less specific in their distribution among different cell types. Thus, α_s is universally present in all cells and many cells have all three major forms of α_i ($G\alpha_i$-1, $G\alpha_i$-2, $G\alpha_i$-3). However, bone marrow cells contain α_{i-2} and α_{i-3}, but lack α_{i-1} (54,55). As noted above, Strathmann et al. (53) recently demonstrated the presence of five new members of the α subunit family. The relationship of these new G-proteins to previously described members of this family is currently being established. Hence, the significance of the complexity of G-proteins, both in terms of their specificity for a given physiological response and their tissue-specific distribution, remains to be established.

1. Inhibition of Adenylate Cyclase Activity

Although the identity of the specific G-protein isoform involved in the muscarinic inhibition of adenylate cyclase activity has not been unequivocally established, data have demonstrated that both the α subunit and $\beta\gamma$ subunit of an inhibitory G-protein are involved in the muscarinic inhibition of hormone-stimulated adenylate cyclase activity. Northrup et al. (51) demonstrated that the $\beta\gamma$ subunit is capable of inactivating GTP or fluoride-stimulated adenylate cyclase activity in the presence of α_s. These authors suggested that hormone–receptor interaction resulted in release of $\beta\gamma$ from α_i and that the association of free $\beta\gamma$ with α_s resulted in inactivation of the GTP or fluoride-dependent α_s activation of adenylate cyclase. Evidence has also been presented suggesting that α_i alone is capable of exerting an inhibitory effect on adenylate cyclase activity (46). The relative contribution of $\beta\gamma$ subunit interaction with α_s and the direct effect of α_i in the regulation of adenylate cyclase activity are unclear (Fig. 1).

2. Muscarinic Stimulation of K^+ Channel Activity: Role of $\beta\gamma$ and α_{i-3}

We have previously outlined the classic studies of the effects of muscarinic stimulation on K^+ permeability and its relationship to changes in the chronotropic state of the heart. More recently, Martin et al. (56) demonstrated that pertussis toxin treatment of cultured embryonic chick heart cells interfered with muscarinic stimulation of $^{42}K^+$ uptake. Pfaffinger et al. (57) demonstrated that coupling of the muscarinic

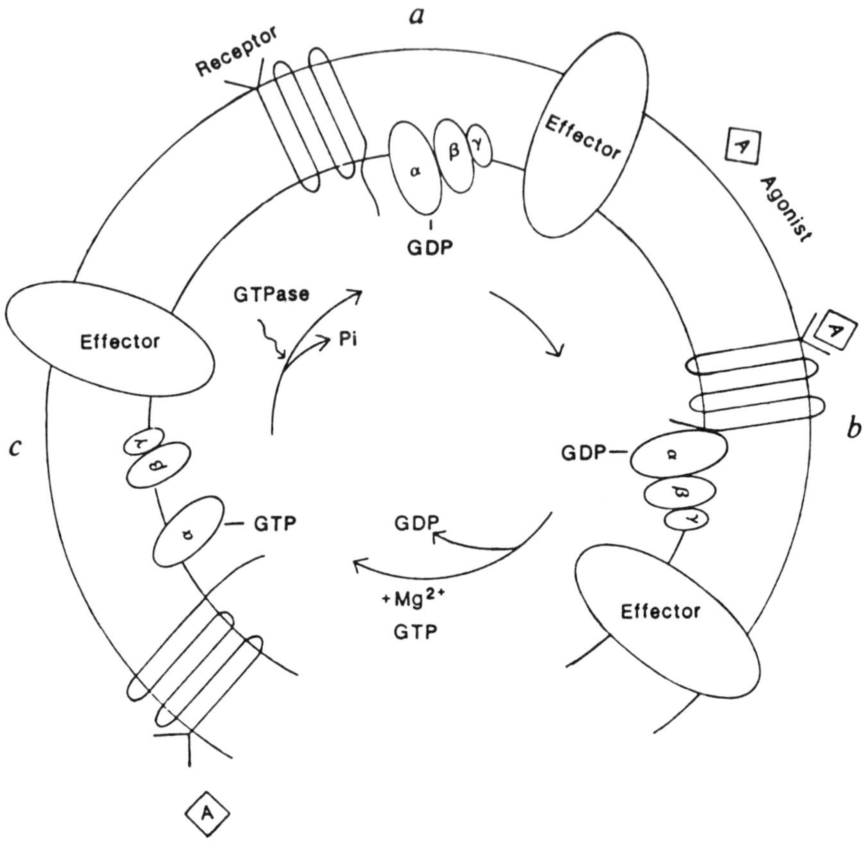

Figure 1 Simple scheme for G protein signal transduction. From the unliganded state (a), receptor binds agonist A (for example, epinephrine, acetylcholine) which produces a change (b) in receptor-G protein interaction, allowing GTP in the presence of Mg^{2+}, to replace GDP on the subunit α. The activated α-GTP subunit and the $\beta\gamma$ subunits dissociate and one or both interacts with effectors (for example, adenylyl cyclase, K^+ channel). Alternatively, free $\beta\gamma$ may bind other α subunits. The intrinsic GTPase activity of the α subunit hydrolyses GTP to GDP, releasing inorganic phosphate (P_i), and α-GDP recombines with $\beta\gamma$ (c), ending the activation cycle. Nonhydrolysable analogues of GTP such as Gpp(NH)p or $GTP_\gamma S$ produce persistent activation of α subunits and persistent dissociation of α from $\beta\gamma$ because activation cannot be reversed by hydrolysis of these nucleotide analogues to GDP. Neer and Clapham, Nature 33,129–134, 1988. With permission from Nature.

receptor in embryonic chick atrial cells to an inward rectifying potassium channel required intracellular GTP. Pretreatment of cells with pertussis toxin eliminated the acetylcholine-induced inward rectification (58). Logothetis et al. (58) demonstrated that addition of the purified $\beta\gamma$ complex reproducibility increased i_{K-Ach} in inside-out patches in which K^+ channels had been uncoupled from the muscarinic receptor by pertussis toxin-catalyzed ADP ribosylation of endogenous α proteins. Neither a GTP-liganded α subunit nor a GTPγS-liganded α subunit was capable of activating this current. However, when the α subunits were added in excess over $\beta\gamma$ they inhibited activation of K channels by $\beta\gamma$, presumably by binding the $\beta\gamma$ and rendering it unavailable for activation of the K channel. Logothetis et al. (59) subsequently demonstrated that at concentrations of 200 pM, $\beta\gamma$ activated K channels in patches from rat and chick atria 97% of the time. Activation was maximal at 10 nM. They further demonstrated that activated α subunits purified from human erythrocytes, α40-GTPγS, or bovine α39-GTPγS at concentrations of 10 pM or greater opened K channels in chick atrial patches (5 of 27) and rat atrial patches (5 of 11). Hence activation of the channel by both $\beta\gamma$ and α subunits appears to be possible. Recently, a product of phospholipase A2 activity has been implicated in the response of chick atrial patches to $\beta\gamma$ subunits via production of a lipoxygenase-derived second messenger (60,61).

Yatani et al. (62) have demonstrated that activation of mammalian atrial muscarinic potassium channels by a human erythrocyte pertussis toxin-sensitive G-protein, Gk, which they have identified as α_i-3 (64), is responsible for coupling muscarinic stimulation to activation of the acetylcholine-sensitive K channel. This effect takes place at pM concentrations of Gk, whereas nM concentrations of human red blood cell Gs were ineffective. In their hands, $\beta\gamma$ dimers at nM concentrations had no effect on these K currents. The lack of effect of $\beta\gamma$ on atrial K channels in their hands is unexplained (64–67).

3. Muscarinic-Stimulated Inositol Phosphate Production

The hydrolysis of membrane-bound phosphotidylinositol (4,5) P_2 has emerged as a major intracellular signaling pathway. Since the initial report of Hokin and Hokin in 1954 (68) describing the release of inositol phosphates from stimulated cells, phospholipase C activation resulting in inositol phosphate release has been demonstrated in many tissues and in response to stimulation by a large number of agonists (for a review, see 69). The hydrolysis of phosphotidylinositol (4,5)P_2 yields both inositol (1,4,5)P_3, which releases Ca^{2+} from intracellular stores (70,71), and 1,2-diacylglycerol, which activates protein kinase C. It has recently been suggested that phosphorylation metabolites of inositol (1,4,5)P_3 may be physiologically active. For example, inositol (1,3,4,5)P_4 (72–74) may modulate calcium levels and inositol P_5 and inositol P_6 may act as extracellular signals (75). Muscarinic-stimulated inositol phosphate production in the heart was demonstrated by Masters et al. (76) using chick ventricular cells 13 days in ovo cultured for 24 hr. The EC_{50} for muscarinic-stimulated inositol phosphate production in the ventricle was reported to be 20–30 μM, which is in agreement with the value subsequently reported in chick atria. This study also demonstrated that total inositol phosphate formation produced in response to muscarinic stimulation was insensitive to pertussis toxin. Jones et al. (77), using chick ventricular cells 13 days in ovo cultured for 24 hr, also demonstrated that inositol phosphate production was stimulated by GTPγS in saponin-permeabilized chick ventricular cells. These data suggested that in ventricular cells a pertussis toxin-insensitive G-protein coupled the muscarinic receptor to phospholipase C activation.

Recent studies by Barnett et al. (78,79) have described the ontogenesis of muscarinic-stimulated inositol phosphate production in cultures of chick heart cells from both atria and ventricle. These studies demonstrated different mechanisms of coupling of muscarinic receptors to phospholipase C in atrium and ventricle. In agreement with the work of Masters et al. (76), ventricular cells cultured from embryos 5, 7, 10, 12, and 14 days in ovo demonstrated a developmental decrease of

50% in the ability of muscarinic-agonists to stimulate inositol phosphate production. Thus, in the ventricle muscarinic stimulation of phospholipase C activity was insensitive to pertussis toxin at all ages studied (79).

In atrial cells muscarinic-stimulated inositol phosphate production also decreased by 50% between 5 and 14 days in ovo. However, pertussis toxin-sensitive muscarinic-stimulated inositol phosphate production in atrial cells increased from undetectable levels at day 5 in ovo to 40% of the total production of inositol phosphates by day 12 in ovo (79). The time course of the development of pertussis toxin-sensitive inositol phosphate production in the atria is coincident with the time course of increase in the levels of pertussis toxin substrates during the development of the chick heart described previously (32).

In cultured chick heart cells from both atria and ventricle from hearts 5 days in ovo permeabilized with saponin GTPγS stimulated pertussis toxin-insensitive inositol phosphate production. In cultures of atria and ventricles 14 days in ovo permeabilized with saponin, pertussis toxin was able to inhibit a fraction of the response stimulated by GTPγS only in the atrium (78,79). These data taken together suggest that, in ventricle, a pertussis-toxin-insensitive G-protein couples the muscarinic receptor to phospholipase C activation. However, in atria, phospholipase C activity is initially coupled to a pertussis-toxin-insensitive G-protein, but during the course of development coupling of phospholipase C to the muscarinic receptor occurs via two separate G-proteins: one a pertussis-toxin-sensitive G-protein, and the other a pertussis-toxin- insensitive G-protein.

Inositol phosphate production in the mammalian heart is less well described. Poggioli et al. (80) demonstrated IP_3 production in intact rat heart in response to α_i-adrenergic, muscarinic cholinergic, and electrical stimulation. Schmitz et al. (81) have reported that both the α_1-adrenergic receptor-mediated inotropic effect and α_1 adrenergic-stimulated IP_3 production are insensitive to pertussis toxin. In this study IP_3 production was found to precede the inotropic effect of α_i-adrenergic receptor stimulation consistent with a role of IP_3 in mediating the inotropic effect of α_1-adrenergic stimulation of the heart. However, total inositol phosphate production in response to α_1-adrenergic stimulation in cultured rat cardiac myocytes has been reported by Steinberg et al. (82) to be partially sensitive to pertussis toxin. Renaud and Poggioli (83) have determined that rat heart homogenates can convert 1,4,5, IP_3 to IP_4, but Woodcock et al. (84) were unable to demonstrate IP_4 in mammalian heart.

The physiological role of inositol phosphate production in the heart and the significance of its differential coupling in the atria and ventricle are unknown. It has been determined that the predominant product formed following muscarinic stimulation of chick atria and ventricle from 5 to 14 days in ovo is inositol(1,3,4,5)P_4 (78,79). Studying the effects of this isomer on the heart may yield the answer to the physiological role of inositol phosphate production in the heart. Although IP_3 has not been demonstrated to release Ca^{+2} from permeabilized rat myocytes (85), it is tempting to speculate that inositol(1,3,4,5)P_4 will play a role in determining the steady-state calcium level in cardiac cells.

4. *Muscarinic Stimulation of Diacylglycerol Formation*

Recent studies (86) have demonstrated that although a fraction of diacylglycerol is produced via direct action of phospholipase C on phosphatidyl inositolbisphosphate to produce IP_3 and diacylglycerol, a large fraction of diacylglycerol is generated via the action of phospholipase D on phosphatidyl inositol. Phospholipase D has been shown to cleave the phosphodiester bond between the phosphate and polar head groups of the phospholipid releasing the polar moiety and phophatidic acid.

Muscarinic stimulation of chick atrial cells whose phospholipids have been labeled with [^{3}H]arachidonic acid results in the initial appearance of phosphatidic acid followed by an increase in diacylglycerol levels and a parallel decrease in phosphatidyl inositol, suggesting a role for phospholipase D in the hydrolysis of phosphotidyl inositol and the production of diacylglycerol. Although in other tissues phosphatidylcholines have been shown to be a substrate for phospholipase D, no evidence for the release of [^{3}H]choline has been obtained following muscarinic stimulation of chick atrial cells labeled overnight with [^{3}H]choline.

Muscarinic stimulation of diacylglycerol production is partially sensitive to pertussis toxin in the atrium, but insensitive to pertussis toxin in the ventricle. Furthermore, the GTPγS-stimulated production of phosphatidic acid and diacylglycerol in the atrium was partially sensitive to pertussis toxin, consistent with the hypothesis that phospholipase D activity in the atrium is coupled to the muscarinic receptor via two separate G proteins.

The ontogenesis of diacylglycerol formation in the chick atrium further supports the hypothesis that the muscarinic receptor is coupled to inositol phosphate metabolism and to diacylglycerol production via separate pathways. Thus, unlike muscarinic-stimulated phospholipase C activity, which decreases by 50% between days 5 and 12 in ovo, levels of muscarinic-stimulated diacylglycerol formation do not change with development (87).

Although Leatherman et al. (47) demonstrated that brief (5 min) exposures of cultured rat ventricular cells to high doses of phobol esters resulted in a significant negative inotropic effect and a decrease in $^{45}Ca^{+2}$ uptake into cultured chick ventricular cells, no clear demonstration of the physiological role of either diacylglycerol or the activation of protein kinase C has been demonstrated.

VII. DOWN REGULATION OF MUSCARINIC RECEPTORS FOLLOWING PROLONGED AGONIST EXPOSURE

Cultured chick heart cells respond to a 3 hr exposure to muscarinic agonist with a decrease of up to 70% in the number of muscarinic receptor sites as judged by [^{3}H]QNB binding to homogenates of heart cell cultures (88). The remaining receptors show an unchanged affinity for [^{3}H]QNB, indicating that the reduced number of receptors reflected a loss of binding sites rather than a change in affinity for the antagonist.

The physiological response to muscarinic stimulation in the heart requires the interaction of agonist with receptors on the cell surface. Thus, the number of receptors measured in homogenates of cells may not reflect receptors on the surface of the intact cell capable of binding agonist. We developed an assay for the binding of the muscarinic antagonist [^{3}H]methylscopolamine ([^{3}H]MS) to intact cultured heart cells (34). Unlike QNB, [^{3}H]MS is a highly charged muscarinic agonist that does not enter the hydrophobic environment of the cell membranes and thus binds only to cell surface receptors. Binding of [^{3}H]MS was saturable, of high affinity, and the relative potency of muscarinic ligands to compete with

[^{3}H]MS for binding to intact cells followed the order expected for binding to a muscarinic receptor.

The cultured heart cell preparation provided a suitable model system for the study of changes in the number of [^{3}H]MS-binding sites in the intact cell after preexposure to agonist for various times. In cells incubated with the muscarinic agonist carbomylcholine, a brief lag phase was followed by a 72% decrease in the number of [^{3}H]MS binding sites over 6 hr with a half-time of 30 min (33). Binding sites recovered over a 12 hr incubation period in the presence of fresh media and recovery was inhibited by the protein synthesis inhibitor cycloheximide. A close correlation existed between the time course of the agonist-mediated decrease in binding of [^{3}H]MS and the time course of the decrease in the ability of agonist to increase K^+ permeability and decrease beating rate. All three of these parameters showed a 15-min lag period followed by decreases that were maximal after 6 hr and half-maximal at about 30 min (34). This close relationship between the number of receptors on the surface of the intact cell and the physiological responsiveness of the cell suggests that agonist modulation of receptor number constitutes a sensitive mechanism for the control of muscarinic responsiveness of the cultured heart cell.

In several well-studied systems, binding of a ligand to a receptor results in a process known as receptor-mediated endocytosis (44,88,89). Agents including colchicine and vinblastine that inhibit microtubule function interfere with the process of endocytosis (90). We found that intact cultured heart cells pre-exposed to muscarinic agonists in the presence of colchicine and vinblastine showed a marked decrease in the loss of receptors compared to cells exposed to agonist alone (88). These findings are consistent with the hypothesis that agonist exposure causes a change in the configuration of the receptor in the cell membrane, or some other alteration in receptor state, which renders the receptor inaccessible to ligand binding and subject to endocytosis.

Although following prolonged agonist exposure the receptor may not be capable of stimulating physiological response to agonist binding, it is possible that a hydrophobic radioligand might continue to bind specifically to such an altered form of the receptor. To test this hypothesis, we compared the binding of [^{3}H]MS and the more hydrophobic antagonist [^{3}H]QNB to cells subjected to prior agonist exposure for various times (34). The results of these experiments show that [^{3}H]QNB continued to bind specifically to muscarinic receptors for 90 min after [^{3}H]MS binding had essentially disappeared. Analysis of these data suggested a sequential conversion of the receptor from a form, A, that gave a physiological response to agonist and bound both [^{3}H]QNB and [^{3}H]MS to a form, B, that bound only [^{3}H]QNB and did not give a physiological response to agonist. B was converted to a form, C, presumably a degraded form of the receptor, that was able to bind neither [^{3}H]MS nor [^{3}H]QNB. Thus, B may constitute an intermediate state of the receptor formed during endocytosis that is more intimately associated with the cell membrane, but is inaccessible to agonist and has not yet progressed to a degraded state.

Kwatra et al. (91,92) demonstrated that prior exposure of chick hearts to muscarinic agonists resulted in the phosphorylation of a 79kD protein that was identified as a muscarinic receptor. They further suggested a parallel between this phosphorylation and the loss of the ability of the receptor to mediate a negative inotropic response to muscarinic agonists. These authors suggested that the phosphorylation of the cardiac muscarinic receptor required agonist occupancy and was related to muscarinic receptor desensitization.

VIII. MULTIPLE SUBTYPES OF THE MUSCARINIC RECEPTOR

One explanation for the absence of a physiological response to muscarinic agonists early in embryonic development (Sec. IV) is that muscarinic receptors exist in several isoforms and that embryonic development of the muscarinic response in the heart involves expression of isoforms not present at early embryonic age. In recent years studies using both specific muscarinic ligands and molecular biological approaches have demonstrated at least five classes of muscarinic receptors.

A. Pharmacologic Evidence for Muscarinic Receptor Heterogeneity

Studies by Barlow et al. (93) in 1976 implied that different muscarinic receptors were present in atria and ilium. The antagonist 4-diphenyl-acetoxy-N-methyl-piperadine methiodide (4-DAMP) showed a 10-fold selectivity for binding to atrial muscarinic receptors over the muscarinic receptors present in the ilium. Rattan and Goyal (94) demonstrated in 1978 that two subpopulations of muscarinic receptors are responsible for eliciting a rise and subsequently a fall in lower esophageal sphincter pressure in the opossum. These investigators determined that muscarinic receptors present on inhibitory neurons in the vagus nerve that innervates the sphincter muscle caused a fall in pressure by relaxing the sphincter muscle. This population of receptors was specifically activated by McN-A343 (4-hydroxy-2-butynyl trimethylammonium chloride-m-chlorocarbinilate) (94), a compound now identified as a selective agonist for activating muscarinic receptors found in ganglia (96–98). The subpopulation of muscarinic receptors that decreased lower esophageal pressure were termed M1 receptors (98). A different subpopulation of muscarinic receptors, which caused a rise in sphincter pressure and were selectively activated by bethanacol and carbachol, were located directly on the sphincter muscle itself and termed M2 receptors (98).

Hammer et al. in 1980 (99)—using pirensepine, a compound which inhibited gastric acid secretion (100,101), antagonized muscarinic agonist-stimulated ilial smooth muscle contraction, elicited tachycardia, and blocked salivation—presented data which suggested the presence of multiple muscarinic receptors. He demonstrated that the dosage of pirenzepine necessary to inhibit these effects varied markedly. For example, very low concentrations of pirenzepine were required to block gastric acid secretion compared to the dosages required to block the effects of cholinergic agonists on smooth muscle and the heart (101). While these physiological studies suggested multiple muscarinic receptor subtypes, the advent of radioligand binding made the examination of these receptor subtypes possible. Patton and Rang in 1965 were the first to use radioligand binding to study the muscarinic receptor (102). Relatively few of the [^{3}H]QNB binding sites in rat heart, ilium, and cerebellum exhibited high-affinity binding for pirenzepine (103,104). Only half of the [^{3}H]QNB-binding sites in cortex, hippocampus, and cerebellum demonstrated high affinity for prizanzepine. Luthin and Wolfe (105) demonstrated that these differences in the binding site densities for these two ligands, [^{3}H]QNB and [^{3}H]pirenzepine, were not due to differences in the rate of interconversion between two forms of the receptor–ligand complex. Therefore, it appears that QNB and pirenzepine are recognizing functionally distinct stable receptor types as opposed to transitory intermediates or conformational states of the same protein. Hence, studies with pirenzepine have confirmed the initial division of the muscarinic receptor into two subtypes. The M1 subtype muscarinic receptor has a high affinity for pirenzepine, kD values from 5 to 20 nM, which are located primarily in cerebral cortex, hippocampus, striatum, and peripheral ganglia, whereas the M2 subtypes have a low affinity for pirenzepine with kD values from 200 to 800 nM and are located in peripheral tissues such as smooth muscle and atria. Since this work by Hammer and others (99), many groups have defined subtypes of muscarinic receptors and have attempted to develop a systematic organization of these subtypes.

One of these groups, Lambrecht et al. (106–109) developed novel cholinergic antagonists to subclassify muscarinic receptors further. In this scheme receptors are initially classified as M1 or M2 based on their affinity for pirenzepine. Within these groups the authors further subclassified the M1 and M2 receptors as M1α, M1β, M2α, and M2β based on relative inhibition by pirenzepine, hexahydro-sila-difenidol (HHSID), and methoctramine. Lambrecht further characterized the four forms of the receptor by site of localization. For example, M1α is found primarily in the hippocampus, M1β is in ganglia and cortex, M2α in smooth muscle, and M2β in exocrine glands. This classification closely parallels data from molecular biological studies outlined below.

In several studies, attempts were made to link specific muscarinic receptor subtypes to specific biochemical responses. Gil and Wolfe (110) compared the ability of pirenzepine and atropine to inhibit muscarinic stimulation of IP_3 production or muscarinic inhibition of adenylate cyclase activity. They demonstrated a 15-fold difference in K_i for pirenzepine inhibition of muscarinic stimulation of adenylate cyclase compared to pirenzepine inhibition of phospholipase C activity. These results lead Gil and Wolfe to conclude that stimulation of phosphoinositide hydrolysis was mediated by an M_1 receptor that exhibits a low K_D value for pirenzepine and inhibition of adenylate cyclase was mediated by an M_2 receptor that exhibits a higher K_D value for pirenzepine.

B. Molecular Biological and Biochemical Approaches to Receptors and Receptor Coupling: Identification and Characterization of Muscarinic Receptor Isoforms

Molecular biological approaches have confirmed the existence of multiple muscarinic receptor subtypes. Cloning of the muscarinic receptors involved initial purification of the receptor from the porcine atrium (111). The 80kD purified protein demonstrated a high affinity for the muscarinic antagonist QNB, with a binding capacity of 12.4 nM/mg of protein. Peralta et al. (112) determined the amino acid sequence of tryptic peptides derived from the receptor. Oligonucleotides corresponding to the sequence of these tryptic peptides were used to screen a cDNA library prepared from porcine atria. Analysis of the longest clone obtained demonstrated an open reading frame of 466 amino acids, giving a protein of molecular weight of 51,700 dalton. The putative M_2 atrial receptor sequence gave a 30% amino acid identity with the beta-adrenergic receptor from the turkey erythrocyte. Hydropathy plots of the amino acid sequence of the M_2 receptor suggested that atrial muscarinic receptors had seven transmembrane-spanning domains of 27 amino acids, as suggested by the sequence homology with the beta-adrenergic receptor. Expression of this cDNA in Chinese hamster ovary cells (CHO) demonstrated high-affinity [^{3}H]QNB binding of 10 pmol/mg protein, compared to less than 5 fmol/mg protein in nontransfected CHO cells. These transfected receptors bound QNB with high affinity and pirenzepine with a low affinity, consistent with the identity of the receptor as the M2 type. The use of this cDNA probe to establish the structure of the atrial muscarinic receptor gene demonstrated that the coding region of this gene existed as a single exon.

Kubo et al. (113), utilizing a partial amino acid sequence from an M_1 muscarinic receptor purified from bovine brain, cloned a muscarinic receptor with 38% homology overall with that reported by Peralta et al. (112) and extensive local identities found in transmembrane domains (50–91%) as well as identity in small connecting loops (40–76%). The porcine cerebral muscarinic receptor contained 460 amino acid residues with a calculated molecular weight of 51,416 daltons. Hydropathy plots of the amino acid sequence demonstrated the presence of seven hydrophobic segments. The gene coding for this cDNA was also demonstrated to be intronless and expression studies of the cDNA in xenopus oocytes demonstrated the appearance of an inward rectifying K^+ current in response to acetylcholine that was abolished by 10 nM atropine. Extracts prepared from oocytes injected with the mRNA coding for this gene exhibited (^{3}H)QNB binding capacity ranging from 3.2 to 6.8 fmol/oocyte, whereas no measurable binding was observed with extracts derived from control oocytes. These binding sites demonstrated a high affinity for pirenzepine, as expected for an M_1 receptor. Hybridization analysis of Poly-A RNA from different porcine tissues with a muscarinic acetylcholine receptor cDNA probe demonstrated high concentrations of the M_1 receptor mRNA in cerebral cortex, a somewhat decreased level in corpus striatum, and the complete absence of this mRNA in the medulla, pons, and atrium (113).

Bonner et al. (114) screened a rat cerebral cortex cDNA library with a portion of cDNA taken from the beginning of the second transmembrane region of the porcine brain cDNA and obtained four different clones. The first clone was identical to the M_1 clone previously isolated by Kubo et al. (115) from the cerebral cortex. The second clone coded for a 586 amino acid protein with 98% identity to porcine M_1. The third clone isolated coded for a 589 amino acid protein that differed from both the M_1 and M_2 clones and was referred to by Bonner as M_3. A fourth clone coding for a protein containing 478 amino acids was designated M_4. Comparison of these sequences with those of the porcine receptor showed a high degree of conservation in the regions corresponding to postulated transmembrane regions 1–5 and 6–7 with much less homology in the amino terminal and carboxyterminal regions (Fig. 2). In addition, a large cytoplasmic loop between transmembrane regions 5 and 6 varying in size from 157 to 203 amino acids showed little similarity among M_1 through M_4, except for a large fraction (17–20%) of basic residues. This loop is much smaller in the beta-adrenergic receptor and rhodopsin than it is in the muscarinic receptor. If one excludes this loop and the amino and carboxyterminal ends from the comparison, the M_3 sequence has 79% identity with the M_1 sequence. The M_4 receptor sequence is 65% identical to M_3 but is more closely related to the porcine M_2 receptor, with 85% identity. The poor homology between the amino acid terminals and the large cytoplasmic loop of the M_2 receptor with the corresponding regions of the M_4 receptor indicates that the M_4 receptor is not the rat

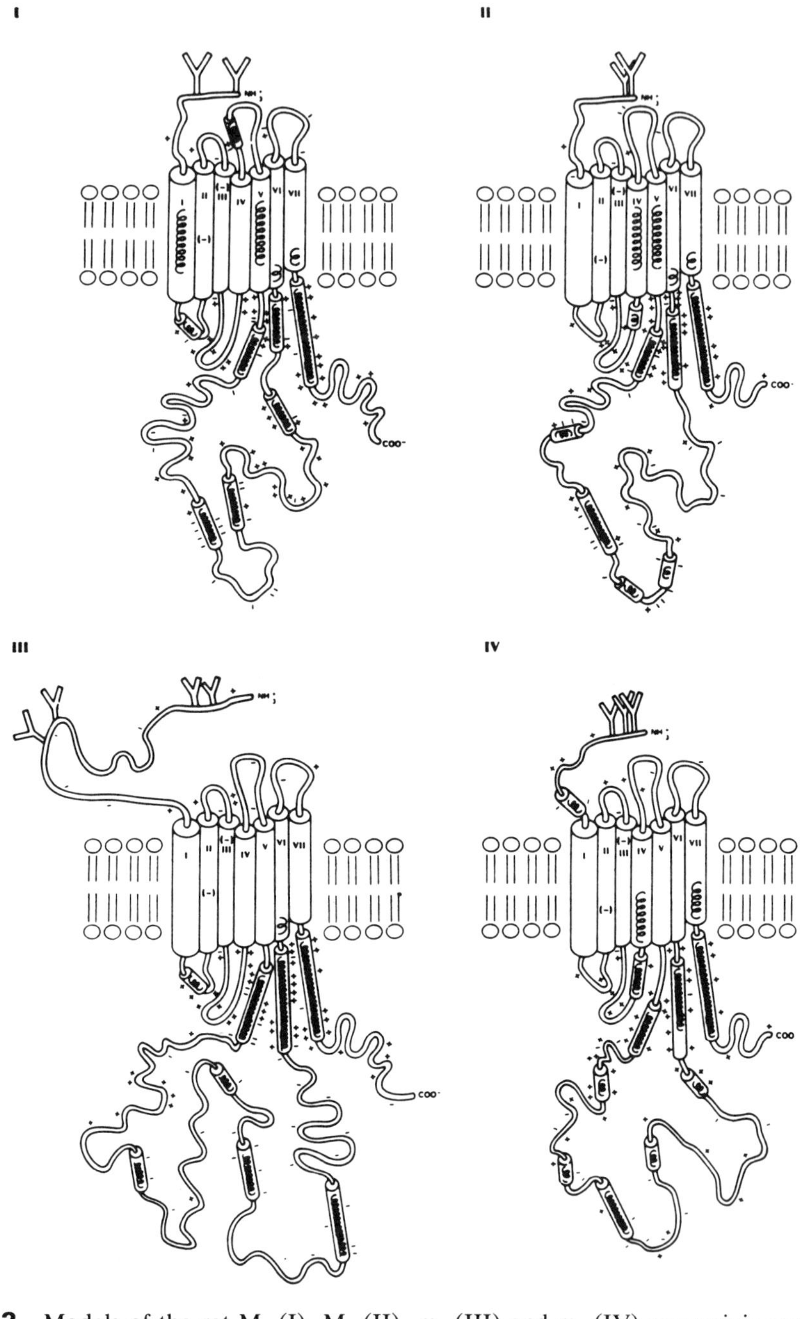

Figure 2 Models of the rat M_1 (I), M_2 (II), m_3 (III) and m_4 (IV) muscarinic receptors. Positively charged (including histidine) and negatively charged side chains are indicated. Coils represent regions predicted to be α-helical. Kerlavage et al. Trends in Pharmacology Sciences 8, 426–431, 1987. With permission from TIPS.

homologue of the porcine M_2 receptor. Each of the four receptors appears to be the product of intronless gases. More recently, a fifth muscarinic receptor has been cloned from human and rat genes and expressed in mammalian cells (116). The mammalian gene coded for a 532 amino acid protein with 89% sequence identity to the 531 amino acid rat protein and was most closely related to the M_3 receptor. Both the rat and human proteins are encoded by a single exon.

1. Binding Properties of Receptor Subtypes

All five muscarinic–cholinergic receptors were stably expressed in CHO-K1 hamster ovary cells (117). Studies with selective antagonists pirenzepine, AF-DX116, methoctramine, and hexahydrosiladifenidol (HHSID) were used to differentiate receptor-binding properties. Receptors could be classified into high-affinity pirenzepine-type receptors, low-affinity pirenzepine-type receptors, and receptors with intermediate affinity for pirenzepine of the type found in exocrine glands (glandular type). Expression of these genes in COS 7 cells demonstrated that pirenzepine displaced [^{3}H]QNB binding with high affinity in cells transfected with M_1, M_3, and M_4, while the human M_2 transfectants had low affinity for pirenzepine consistent with its M_2 classification (116).

2. Specificity of Coupling of a Receptor Subtype to Different Effector Systems

To determine the specificity of coupling of a particular muscarinic receptor subtype to a given effector system, muscarinic receptors were expressed in CHO cells. The ability of the M_2 receptor from pig to mediate inhibition of adenylate cyclase activity and to stimulate phosphoinositide hydrolysis was compared (117). Stimulation of phosphoinositide hydrolysis was significantly less efficient and more dependent on levels of receptors expressed in the transfected cells than the inhibition of adenylate cyclase activity. Both responses were mediated by G-proteins, as evidenced by their inhibition by pertussis toxin. Inactivation of the muscarinic inhibition of adenylate cyclase activity occurred at a 10-fold lower concentration of pertussis toxin than the inactivation of the coupling of muscarinic receptors to PI hydrolysis in these cells. We have recently demonstrated that the IC_{50} for pertussis toxin-catalyzed ADP-ribosylation of α_i was five times greater than that for α_0 (118). One interpretation of these data is that two different G-proteins couple muscarinic receptors to adenylate cyclase and phospholipase C.

Human kidney cells were transfected with each of the four muscarinic receptor subtypes individually and the effects of carbamylcholine on inhibition of adenylate cyclase activity and inositol phosphate production compared (119). It was determined that cells transfected with both Human M_2 and HM3 mediated a carbamylcholine stimulation of inositol phosphate production and an inhibition of forskolin stimulated adenylate cyclase activity with an EC_{50} of 3×10^{-8} M. HM1 and HM4 cells actually stimulated cyclic AMP production in the presence of carbachol while giving a large stimulation of inositol phosphate production. These experiments suggested specificity of coupling of the M_2 and M_3 receptor to inhibition of adenylate cyclase and the M_1 and M_4 receptors to stimulation of phosphilipase C activity. At the fourth international symposium on subtypes of muscarinic receptors the following conventions were adopted in order to correlate pharmacologic subtypes of the muscarinic receptor with the subtypes determined by molecular cloning techniques. By this convention, the M1 or $M_1\alpha$ corresponds to the m_1 receptor cloned from human and rat. M2 or M2α or cardiac form corresponds to the m_2 clone, M_3 or $M_2\beta$ or glandular M_2 corresponds to M_3 cloned from rat or the human M_4, HM_4 (120).

3. Specificity of Coupling of Different G-Proteins to a Given Receptor Subtype

Studies of the specificity of the G-proteins that coupled a given muscarinic receptor subtype to phospholipase C activity suggested that different receptors may be coupled to a similar effector via independent G-proteins (121). Treatment of cells with pertussis toxin resulted in partial inhibition of PI hydrolysis in cells expressing M_1 or M_4 muscarinic acetylcholine receptors, suggesting that both a pertussis-toxin-sensitive G-protein and a pertussis-toxin-insensitive G-protein were involved. In cells expressing M_2 muscarinic receptors, inhibition by pertussis toxin of PI hydrolysis was complete at 10–100 ng/ml. In experiments in which the ability of thrombin, cholecystokinin, and various muscarinic receptor subtypes to stimulate inositol phosphate production were compared, enough muscarinic M_2 receptors were introduced into cells to allow complete saturation of the ability of the cell to respond to carbamylcholine with hydrolysis of phosphatidyl inositol. In these cells the effects of cholecystokinin and carbamylcholine were fully additive. The effects of carbamylcholine and thrombin were not additive, indicating that the carbamylcholine and thrombin coupled to phospholipase C via a common pathway while cholecystokinin activates phosphilipase C via a separate pathway. Thrombin and cholecystokinin curves were likewise fully additive, suggesting that cholecystokinin and thrombin receptors also were coupled to PI hydrolysis via independent pathways or G-proteins. In cells expressing the M_1 receptor, the cholecystokinin response was not additive, with the effects of carbamylcholine indicating that the M_1 receptor and the cholecystokinin receptor are coupled to phospholipase C activity by the same pathway or G-protein. The thrombin response in cells expressing M_1 receptors was likewise not additive with the maximal carbamylcholine dose. These results indicated that M_1 receptors are coupled to PI hydrolysis both by the pathway employed by cholecystokinin and by the pathway employed by thrombin and the M_2 receptor.

IX. CLINICAL IMPLICATIONS OF ALTERATIONS IN MUSCARINIC RECEPTOR G-PROTEIN EFFECTOR COUPLING: FACTORS THAT ALTER AUTONOMIC BALANCE

The balance between sympathetic and parasympathetic responsiveness in the heart plays an important role in establishing the inotropic and chronotropic state of the heart and in the genesis of arrhythmias.

A. Balance Between Stimulation and Inhibition of Adenylate Cyclase Activity

In a recent study Parsons and Stiles (122) suggested that in adipocytes of intact rats perfused for 3 days with adenosine agonists, levels of both adenosine receptors and G_i were decreased whereas beta-adrenergic responsiveness to isoproterenol and levels of cholera toxin substrate appeared to increase. In these cells, stimulation of adenosine receptors resulted in inhibition of adenylate cyclase activity. These data suggested a reciprocal relationship in the regulation of receptors and G-proteins that control levels of adenylate cyclase activity.

Studies by Renaud et al. (123) have demonstrated that growth of cultured embryonic chick heart cells in medium supplemented by serum from which lipoproteins have been removed resulted in elevation of cellular cholesterol and an enhancement of parasympathetic responsiveness in these cells. Total cell cholesterol in cultured embryonic chick atrial cells increased from 23 μg/mg protein in cells grown in control serum to 32 μg/ml protein in cells grown in lipoprotein-depleted serum and was decreased to 20 μg/ml protein in LPDS plus 30 μM mevinolin, an inhibitor of HMG-CoA reductase activity, the enzyme that catalyzes the conversion of HMG-CoA to mevalonic acid (124). Mevinolin is currently being widely used in the treatment of hypercholesterolemia. Growth of chick atrial cells in medium with lipoprotein-depleted serum might constitute a model for a "hypercholesterolemic" state of the cultured myocyte. Studies of cultured chick atrial cells have demonstrated that growth of cells in media containing serum from which lipoproteins have been removed (LPDS) resulted in a 10-fold increase in sensitivity of beating to the muscarinic agonist carbamylcholine, which was reversed by reconstituting the LPDS with the low-density lipoprotein (LDL) fraction of serum during cell growth or by growth with mevinolin. Studies have demonstrated that the enhanced muscarinic cholinergic responsiveness of cells cultured in lipoprotein-depleted serum is associated with an increase in levels of muscarinic receptors and α_o and α_i, the G-proteins that couple the muscarinic receptor to both inhibition of adenylate cyclase activity and to activation of an acetylcholine-sensitive potassium channel (124). It has further been shown that in cells grown in lipoprotein-depleted serum responsiveness to sympathetic stimulation is markedly decreased (125). Thus isoproterenol, which stimulated an increase in contractile state, measured as an increase in amplitude of contraction in control cells, had no significant effect on amplitude of contraction in cells grown in LPDS. This decrease in sympathetic responsiveness was associated with a 50% decrease in the level of beta-adrenergic receptors and a 66% decrease in the level of α_s, the G-protein that couples the beta-adrenergic receptor to stimulation of adenylate cyclase activity. All of these effects of growth of cells in LPDS were reversed by growth with 30 μM mevinolin. Thus, lowering of cellular cholesterol by mevinolin results in enhancement of beta-adrenergic responsiveness and suppression of parasympathetic responsiveness. Regulation of levels of receptors and G-proteins appears to play a critical role in altering autonomic balance under these growth conditions.

B. Role of Changes in Guanine Nucleotide Binding Proteins and Receptors in Congestive Heart Failure and Cardiomyopathy

Cardiomyopathic myocardium has been shown to respond abnormally to neurohumoral stimulation (126). Colucci and Erne (127,128) have shown that the chronotropic response to graded isoproterenol infusion was depressed in patients with congestive heart failure. Studies in patients with idiopathic dilated cardiomyopathic hearts have demonstrated decreased numbers of surface beta-adrenergic receptors and a decreased adenylate cyclase response to isoproterenol and the nonhydrolyzable analogue of GTP, 5 guanylylimidodiphosphate (GppNHp) (129). However, in the same group of patients, the response to forskolin, a direct activator of the catalytic subunit of adenylate cyclase, was preserved, suggesting some postreceptor modification of the adenylate cyclase receptor response. These data are interpreted as suggesting an abnormal response of adenylate cyclase to guanine nucleotide stimulation in the cardiomyopathic human myocardium and further support the hypothesis that this decreased responsiveness may be due to an abnormality in one or more G-proteins. Studies using cholera toxin in genetically cardiomyopathic Syrian hamsters have demonstrated a 50% decrease in G_s activity without a change in immunologically determined G-protein levels (130). In human idiopathic cardiomyopathic cardiac tissue, pertussis toxin labeling has also demonstrated a 36% increase of levels of G_i associated with enhanced inhibition of adenylate cyclase activity by GppNHp (131). These studies suggest that abnormalities in automatic responsiveness in the failing heart are associated with abnormalities in receptor–effector coupling mediated by G-proteins.

C. Effect of Cardiac Denervation on Autonomic Responsiveness of the Heart: A Possible Role in the Autonomic Dysfunction of the Transplanted Heart

Several groups have studied the effects of denervation on the autonomic responsiveness of the heart. Using a model of total surgical cardiac denervation in dogs, Vatner et al. (132) have found that denervation leads to upregulation of beta-adrenergic receptor density and hence isoproterenol-mediated adenylate cyclase activity coincident with downregulation of muscarinic receptor density. Osorio et al. (133) have shown that sympathetic denervation of the heart leads to norepinephrine depletion and the development of adrenergic supersensitivity. Ono (134) has developed a rat model of heterotopic cardiac transplantation in the Lewis rat. Using the established method of Ono, Lurie et al. (135) have demonstrated that in membrane preparations from isographs of rabbit and rat cardiac transplanted myocardium, transplantation is associated with a doubling in beta-adrenergic density and isoproterenol-stimulated adenylate cyclase activity for up to 4 weeks following transplantation.

Following orthotopic human cardiac transplantation, physiological responses to exercise and stress are impaired. Most striking of these is the delay in achieving peak heart rate and the maximum heart rate achieved in response to maximal exercise effort that is seen even years following transplantation (136,137). When one analyzes clinical responses to graded infusions of isoproterenol and exercise response and duration, these abnormalities may appear to be due to lack of sympathetic innervation. Despite this finding in the denervated human transplanted myocardium, beta-adrenergic receptor density and forskolin-stimulated adenylate cyclase response appear to be unchanged from normal human myocardium (138,139). However, the response of adenylate cyclase to GppNHp was depressed in the transplant myocardium. There is no evidence for beta-adrenergic receptor upregulation or supersensitivity in the denervated transplanted human myocardium. These findings suggest that the major abnormality responsible for decreased beta-adrenergic responsiveness may be related to alterations in levels of G-proteins.

Thus, in several model systems in which changes in autonomic balance can be demonstrated changes in levels of receptors and G-proteins may play a role.

Whether these changes involve specific shifts in isoform expression for muscarinic receptors or G-proteins has not been established. Preliminary data on several pathologic states of myocardial function suggest that alterations in the relative levels of G-proteins may play a critical role in both congestive heart failure and in the alterations in autonomic responsiveness associated with denervation and cardiac transplantation.

X. SUMMARY

Muscarinic cholinergic stimulation of the heart has been associated with increasing potassium permeability and the development of a negative chronotropic response. Experiments have demonstrated the role of guanine nucleotide regulatory proteins in coupling muscarinic receptors to potassium channels and to the enhancement of potassium permeability. During embryonic development of the chick heart, the absence of coupling of the muscarinic receptor to a G-protein is associated with decreased ability of muscarinic agonists to mediate a negative chronotropic response and to inhibit adenylate cyclase activity. The development of muscarinic responsiveness in the embryonic chick heart is associated with appearance of increased levels of guanine nucleotide regulatory proteins, suggesting that developmental changes in expression of guanine nucleotide regulatory protein can be related to the appearance of parasympathetic responsiveness in the heart.

The association of the receptor and the guanine nucleotide regulatory protein appears to be critical for the development of the high-affinity state of the muscarinic receptor and coupling the muscarinic receptor to physiologic responses. A ternary complex between muscarinic receptor, G-proteins, and the agonist has been demonstrated. Treatment of cells with pertussis toxin results in uncoupling of the muscarinic receptor from inhibition of adenylate cyclase activity, enhancement of K^+-channel permeability, as well as activation of phosphotidyl inositol hydrolysis and diacylglycerol formation. A pertussis toxin-insensitive G-protein has also been shown to couple muscarinic receptors to phospholipase C activity.

A family of G-proteins has been associated with the coupling of muscarinic receptors to various physiological responses. The specificity of these G-proteins for a given physiological response has not been established. Muscarinic stimulation of K^+ channel activity has been associated with the α_{i-3} isoform of the guanine nucleotide regulatory protein and with the $\beta\gamma$ subunit of the guanine nucleotide regulatory protein. Muscarinic stimulation with inositol phosphate activity is associated with the generation of IP_4 and is coupled to the muscarinic receptor by two separate G-proteins in the chick atrium: one a pertussis toxin substrate and one insensitive to pertussis toxin. During embryonic development of the chick heart, muscarinic stimulation of phospholipase C activity decreases by 50% between days 5 and 15 in ovo. During this time, a pertussis toxin-sensitive muscarinic stimulation of phospholipase C activity appears. Muscarinic stimulation of diacylglycerol formation appears to be associated with both phospholipase C-mediated hydrolysis of phosphatidyl inositol bisphosphate and phospholipase D-mediated hydrolysis of phosphatidyl inositol. Muscarinic stimulation of diacylglycerol formation appears to develop independently of phospholipase C-mediated phosphotidal inositol metabolism in the embryonic chick heart, suggesting that, at least in part, diacylglycerol is produced by a pathway independent from inositol phosphate metabolism.

Following prolonged exposure of embryonic chick heart cells to muscarinic agonist, levels of muscarinic receptors decrease by up to 70%. There is a close correlation between the number of receptors demonstrated on the surface of embryonic chick heart cells and the ability of muscarinic agonist to stimulate a physiological response.

Muscarinic receptors exist in at least five subtypes. These have been demonstrated pharmacologically as well as by molecular biological studies. The M_1, M_3, and M_5 muscarinic receptors appear to be preferentially coupled to phosphatidyl inositol hydrolysis. The M_2 and M_4 receptors appear to be preferentially coupled to inhibition of adenylate cyclase activity. The specific role of guanine nucleotide regulatory proteins in coupling a given muscarinic receptor subtype to a specific physiological response has not been established. However, different G-proteins appear to couple specific muscarinic receptors to a given physiological response.

Alterations in the coupling of muscarinic receptors via G-proteins to a physiological response in the heart have been implicated as a possible mechanism in the abnormalities of autonomic responsiveness seen in both cardiomyopathic hearts and in denervated transplanted hearts in humans. The hypothesis that the relative levels of G-proteins may regulate autonomic balance in the heart and that in pathologic states the relative level of expression of various isoforms of muscarinic receptors and G-proteins may be altered is intriguing.

REFERENCES

1. Levy MN. Sympathetic–parasympathetic interactions in the heart. Circ Res 1971; 29:437–45.
2. Hutter OF. In: Florey F, ed. Nervous inhibition. Ion movements during vagus inhibition of the heart. Elmsford, NY: Pergamon Press, 1961; 114–123.
3. Ten Eick R, Nawrath H, McDonald TF, Trautwein W. On the mechanism of the negative inotropic effect of acetylcholine. Pflugers Arch. 1976; 361:207–13.
4. George WJ, Polson JB, O'Toole AG, Goldberg ND. Elevation of guanosine 3′-5′cyclic phosphate in rat heart after perfusion with acetyl-choline. Proc Natl Acad Sci USA 1970; 66:398–403.
5. Michell RH, Jafferji SS, Jones LM. In: Bazaan H, Brenner R, Giusto H, eds. Advances in experimental medicine and biology. New York: Plenum Press, 1976; 83:447–64.
6. Lindemann JP, Jones LR, Watanabe AM. Effect of muscarinic cholinergic agonist on beta receptor induced increases in membrane protein phosphorylation in intact ventricles. Circ Res 1980; 47:520–32.
7. Carpenter MB, Truzx, RC. In Human neuroanatomy. Baltimore: Williams & Wilkins, 1976.
8. Hirsch EF. The innervation of the vertebrate heart. Springfield, IL: Charles C. Thomas, 1970: 3–24.
9. Loewi O. Uber humorale Uebertragbarkeit der herznervenwirkung. Pflugers Arch Gesamte Physiol 1921; 189:239–42.
10. Feldberg W, Krayer O. Das auftreten eines azetylcholin artigen stoffes in herzvenenblut von warmblutern bei biezung der nervi vagi. Naurnn Scheidebergs Arch Exp Pathol Pharmakol 1933; 172:170–93.
11. Dale HH. The action of certain esters and ethers of choline, and their relation to muscarine. Pharmacol Exp Ther 1914; 6:147–90.
12. Pappano AJ. Onset of chronotropic effects of nicotinic drugs and tyramine on the sinoatrial pacemaker in chick embryo heart; relationship to the development of autonomic neuroeffector transmission. J Pharmacol Exp Ther 1976; 196:676–84.

13. Hutter DF, Trautwein, W. Vagal and sympathetic effects on the pacemaker fibers in the sinus venosus of the heart. J Gen Physiol 1956; 89:715–33.
14. Harris EJ, Hutter OF. The action of acetylcholine on the movement of potassium ions in the sinus venosus of the heart. J Physiol 1956; 133:58–9.
15. Glitsch HG, Pott L. Effects of acetylcholine and parasympathetic nerve stimulation on membrane potential in quiescent guinea pig atria. J Physiol 1978; 279:655–68.
16. Grossman A, Furchgott RF. The effects of various drugs on calcium exchange in the isolated guinea-pig left auricle. J Pharmacol Exp Ther 1964; 145:162–172.
17. Hoditz H, Lullmann H. Der enfluss von actylcholin auf den calcium satz ruhsender und Kontrahierender vonhofnuskulatur in vitro. Experimentia 1964; 20:279–80.
18. Prokopcznk A, Pytkowski B, Lawartowski B. Effect of acetylcholine on calcium efflux from atrial myocardium. Eur J Pharmacol 1961; 70:1–6.
19. Watanabe AM, Besch HR. Jr. Cyclic adenosine monophosphate modulation of slow calcium influx channels in guinea pig hearts. Circ Res 1974; 35:316–24.
20. Tsien RW. Cyclic AMP and contractile activity in the heart. In Greengard P, Robison GA, eds. Advances in cyclic nucleotide research. New York: Academic Press, 1977: 363–420.
21. Jakobs KA. Inhibition of adenylate cyclase by hormones and neurotransmitters. Mol Cel Endocrinol 1979; 16:147–56.
22. Jakobs KA, Aktories K, Schultz G. GTP-dependent inhibition of cardiac adenylate cyclase by muscarinic cholinergic agonists. Naunyn-Schmidebergs Arch Pharmacol 1979; 310:113–19.
23. Abel W. Further observations on the development of the sympathetic nervous system in the chick. J Anat Physiol 1912; 47:35–72.
24. Gardner E, O'Rahilly R. The nerve supply and conducting system of the human heart at the end of the embryonic period proper. J Anat 1976; 121:571–87.
25. Pappano AJ, Loffelholz K. Ontogenesis of adrenergic and cholinergic neuroeffector transmission in chick embryo heart. J Pharmacol Exp Ther 1974; 191:468–78.
26. Galper JB, Klein W, Catterall WA. Muscarinic acetylcholine receptors in developing chick heart. J Biol Chem 1977; 252:8692–9.
27. Coraboeuf E, Le Douarin G, Obrecht-Coutris G. Release of acetylcholine by chick embryo heart before innervation. J Physiol 1970; 206:383–5.
28. Pappano AJ. Ontogenetic development of autonomic neuroeffector transmission and transmitter reactivity in embryonic and fetal hearts. Pharmacol Rev 1977; 29:3–33.
29. Pappano AJ, Skowronek CA. Reactivity of chick embryo hearts to cholinergic agonists during ontogenesis: decline in desensitization at the onset of cholinergic transmission. J Pharmacol Exp Ther 1974; 191:109–18.
30. DuFour JJ, Pasternak JM. Effects chormotropex de l'acetylcholine sur le coeur de l'embryon du poulet. Helv Physiol Pharmacol Acta 1960; 18:563–80.
31. Culver NG, Fishman DA. Pharmacological analysis of sympathetic function in the embryonic chick heart. Am J Physiol 1977; 232:R116–23.
32. Liang BT, Hellmick MR, Neer EJ, Galper JB. Development of muscarinic cholinergic inhibition of adenylate cyclase in embryonic chick heart. J Biol Chem 1986; 261:9011–21.
33. Galper JB, Dziekan LC, O'Hara DS, Smith TW. The biphasic response of muscarinic cholinergic receptors in cultured heart cells to agonists. J Biol Chem 1986; 257:10344–56.
34. Rosenberger LB, Yamamura H, Roeske WR. Cardiac muscarinic cholinergic receptor binding is regulated by Na^+ and guanine nucleotides. J Biol Chem 1980; 255:820–3.
35. Galper JB, Haigh LS, Hart AC, O'Hara DS, Livingston DJ. Muscarinic cholinergic receptors in the embryonic chick heart: interaction of agonist, receptor, and guanine nucleotides studied by an improved assay for direct binding of the muscarinic agonist [^{3}H] cismethyldioxolane. Mol Pharmacol 1987; 32:320–40.

36. Ehlert FJ, Yamamura HI, Triggle D, Roeske WR. The influence of guanyl-5′-yl′imidodiphosphate and sodium chloride on the binding of the muscarinic agonist, [^{3}H] cis-methyldioxolane. Eur J Pharmacol 1980; 61:317–8.
37. Birdsall NJM, Berrie CP, Burgeron ASU, Hulme EC. Modulation of binding properties of muscarinic receptors: evidence for receptor effector coupling. In: Pepeu G, Kuhar MJ, Enna S, eds. Receptors for neurotransmitters and peptide hormones. New York: Raven Press, 1980: 107–16.
38. DeLean A, Stadel JM, Lefkowitz RJ. A ternary complex model explains the agonist-specific binding properties of the adenylate cyclase-coupled β-adrenergic receptor. J Biol Chem 1980; 255:7108–7.
39. Florio VA, Sternweiss PC. Reconstruction of resolved muscarinic cholinergic receptors with purified GTP-binding proteins. J Biol Chem 1985; 260:3477–88.
40. Galper JB, Dziekan LC, Smith TW. The development of physiologic responsiveness to muscarinic agonists in chick embryo heart cell cultures: role of high affinity receptors and sensitivity to guanine nucleotides. J Biol Chem 1984; 259:7382–90.
41. Liang BT, Galper JB. Reconstitution of muscarinic cholinergic inhibition of adenylate cyclase activity in homogenates of embryonic chick hearts by membranes of adult chick hearts. J Biol Chem 1987; 262:2494–2501.
42. Katada T, Ui M. Perfusion of the pancreas isolated from pertussis-sensitized rats: potentiation of insulin secretory responses due to β-adrenergic stimulation. Endocrinology 1977; 101:1247–52.
43. Hazeki O, Ui M. Modification by islet-activating protein of receptor mediated regulation of cyclic AMP accumulation in isolated rat heart cells. J Biol Chem 1981; 256: 28566–72.
44. Lefkowitz R, Stadel J, Caron M. Adenylate cyclase-coupled beta-adrenergic receptors: structure and mechanisms of activation and desensitization. Annu Rev Biochem 1983; 52:159–86.
45. Katada T, Ui M. ADP-ribosylation of the specific membrane protein of C_6 cells by islet-activating protein associated with modification of adenylate cyclase activity. J Biol Chem 1982; 257:7210–6.
46. Katada T, Bokoch GM, Northrup J, Ui M, Gilman AG. The inhibitory guanine nucleotide-binding regulatory component of adenylate cyclase: properties and function of the purified protein. J Biol Chem 1984; 259:3568–77.
47. Katada T, Northrup J, Bokoch GM, Ui M, Gilman AG. The inhibitory guanine nucleotide-binding regulatory component of adenylate cyclase: subunit disassociation and guanine nucleotide-dependent hormonal inhibition. J Biol Chem 1984; 259: 3578–85.
48. Katada T, Bokoch GM, Smigel MD, Ui M, Gilman AG. The inhibitory guanine nucleotide-binding regulatory component of adenylate cyclase: subunit disassociation and the inhibition of adenylate cyclase in S49 lymphoma cyc$^-$ and wild type membranes. J Biol Chem 1984; 259:3586–95.
49. Bokoch GM, Katada T, Northrup JK, Ui M, Gilman AG. Purification and properties of the inhibitory guanine nucleotide-binding regulatory component of adenylate cyclase. J Biol Chem 1984; 259:3560–7.
50. Hildebrandt JD, Codina J, Risenger R, Birnbaumer L. Identification of a gamma subunit associated with the adenylate cyclase regulatory proteins N_s and N_i. J Biol Chem 1984; 259:2039–42.
51. Northrup JK, Smigel MD, Sternweis PC, Gilman AG. The subunits of the stimulatory regulatory component of adenylate cyclase: resolution of the activated 45,000 dalton (α) subunit. J Biol Chem 1976; 258:11369–76.
52. Jones DT, Reed RR. Molecular cloning of five GTP-binding proteins cDNA from rat olfactory neuroepithelium. J Biol Chem 1987; 262:1424–9.

53. Strathmann M, Wilke TM, Simon MI. Diversity of the G-protein family: sequences from five additional α subunits in the mouse. Proc Natl Acad Sci USA, 1989; 86:7407–9.
54. Neer EJ, Clapham DE. Roles of G-protein subunits in transmembrane signaling. Nature 1988; 333:129–34.
55. Kim SY, Ang S-L, Bloch DB, Bloch KD, Ang S-L, Kawahara Y, Tolman C, Lee R, Seidman JG, Neer EJ. Identification of cDNA encoding an additional α subunit of a human GTP-binding protein: expression of three $\alpha 1$ subtypes in human tissue and cell lines. Proc Natl Acad Sci USA 1988; 85:4153–7.
56. Martin JM, Hunter DD, Nathanson NM. Islet activating protein inhibits physiological responsiveness evoked by cardiac muscarinic acetylcholine receptors; role of guanosine triphosphate binding proteins in regulation of potassium permeability. Biochemistry 1985; 24:7521–5.
57. Pfaffinger PJ, Martin JM, Hunter DH, Nathanson NM, Hille B. GTP-binding proteins couple cardiac muscarinic receptors to a K channel. Nature 1985; 317:536–8.
58. Logothetis DE, Kurachi Y, Galper JB, Neer EJ, Clapham DE. The β subunits of GTP-binding proteins activate the muscarinic K^+ channel in heart. Nature 1987; 325:321–6.
59. Logothetis DE, Kim D, Northrup JK, Neer EJ, Clapham DE. Specificity of action of guanine nucleotide-binding regulatory protein subunits on the cardiac muscarinic K^+ channel. Proc Natl Acad Sci USA 1988; 85:5814–18.
60. Kim D, Lewis DL, Graziadei L, Neer EJ, Bar-Sagi D, Clapham DE. G-protein $\beta\alpha$-subunits activate the cardiac muscarinic K^+-channel via phospholipase A_2. Nature 1989; 337:557–60.
61. Kurachi Y, Ito H, Sugimoto T, Shimizu T, Miki I, Ui M. Arachidonic acid metabolites as intracellular modulators of the G-protein-gated cardiac K^+ channel. Nature 1989; 337:555–7.
62. Yatani A, Codina J, Brown AM, Birnbaumer L. Direct Activation of mammalian atrial muscarinic potassium channels by GTP regulatory protein G_k. Science 1987; 235:207–11.
63. Codina J, Olate J, Abramowitz J, Mattera R, Cook RG, Birnbaumer L. α_{i-3} cDNA encodes the γ subunit of G_k, the stimulatory G-proteins of receptor-regulated K^+ channels. J Biol Chem 1988; 263:6746–50.
64. Yatina A, Codina J, Imato U, Reeves JP, Birnbaumer L, Brown AM. Direct regulation of mammalian cardiac channels by a G-protein. Science 1987; 238:1288–92.
65. Yatani A, Codina J, Sekura RD, Birnbaumer L, Brown AM. Reconstitution of somatostatin and muscarinic receptor mediated stimulation of K^+ channels by isolated G_k protein in clonal rat anterior pituitary cell membranes. Mol Endocrinol 1987; 1:283–9.
66. Kirsch GE, Yatani A, Codina J, Birnbaumer L, Brown AM. α-Subunit of G_i activates atrial K^+ channels of chick, rat, and guinea pig. Am J Physiol 1988; 254:H1200–10.
67. Brown AM, Birnbaumer L. Direct G-protein gating of ion channels. Am J Physiol 1988; 254:H401–10.
68. Hokin MR, Hokin LE. Enzyme secretion and incorporation of ^{32}P into phospholipids of pancreas slices. J Biol Chem 1954; 209:549–58.
69. Shears SB. Metabolism of the inositol phosphates produced upon receptor activation. Biochem J 1989; 260:313–29.
70. Berridge MJ. Metabolism of the inositol phosphates produced upon receptor activation. Annu Rev Biochem 1987; 56:159–93.
71. Downes CP, Michell RH. In: Cohen P, MD Houslay, eds. Molecular mechanisms of transmembrane signaling. pp Amsterdam: Elsevier, 1985: 3–56.
72. Irvine RF, Moor RM. Micro-injection of inositol 1,3,4,5-tetrakisphosphate activates sea urchin eggs by a mechanism dependent on external Ca^{2+}. Biochem J 1986; 240:917–20.
73. Morris AP, Gallacher DV, Irvine RF, Petersen OH. Synergism of inositol triphosphate and tetrakisphosphate in activating Ca^+ dependent K^+ channels. Nature 1987; 330:653–65.

74. Parker I, Miledi R. Injecting inositol 1,3,4,5-tetrakisphosphate into *Xenopus* oocytes generates a chloride current dependent upon intracellular calcium. Proc R Soc London [B] 1987; 232:59–70.
75. Vallejo M, Jackson T, Lightman S, Hanley MR. Occurrence and extracellular actions of inositol pentakis- and hexakis-phosphate in mammalian brain. Nature 1987; 330:656–8.
76. Masters SB, Martin NW, Harden TK, Brown JH. Pertussis toxin does not inhibit muscarinic receptor-mediated phosphoinositide hydrolysis or calcium mobilization. Biochem J 1985; 227:993–7.
77. Jones LG, Goldstein D, Brown JH. Guanine nucleotide-dependent inositol trisphosphate for motion in chick heart cells. Circ Res 1988; 62:299–305.
78. Barnett JV, Shamah SM, Griendling KK, Lasseugue B, Galper JB. Muscarinic cholinergic stimulation of inositol phosphate production in cultured embryonic chick atrial cells: evidence for coupling via two independent G-proteins. Biochem. J 1990; 271:443–44.
79. Barnett JV, Shamah SM, Griendling KK, Lasseugue B, Galper JB. The development of muscarinic–cholinergic stimulation of inositol phosphate production in cultured embryonic chick atrial cells: evidence for a switch in G-protein coupling. Biochem. J 1990; 271:437–44.
80. Poggioli J, Sulpice JC, Vassort G. Inositol phosphate production following β-adrenergic, muscarinic or electrical stimulation in isolated rat heart. FEBS Letts 1986; 206:292–8.
81. Schmitz W, Scholz H, Scholz J, Steinfath M, Lohse M, Purunen J, Schwabe U. Pertussis-toxin does not inhibit the α-adrenergic receptor-mediated effect on inositol phosphate products or in the heart. Eur J Pharmacol 1987; 134:377–8.
82. Steinberg SF, Chow YK, Robinson RB, Bilezikian JB. A pertussis toxin substrate regulates $alpha_1$-adrenergic dependent phosphatidyl inositol hydrolysis in cultured rat myocytes. Endocrinology 1987; 120:1889–95.
83. Renaud D, Poggioli J. Pertussis toxin does not inhibit the α_1-adrenoceptor-mediated effect on inositol phosphate production in the heart. FEBS Lett 1987; 217:117–23.
84. Woodcock, EA, Shmank WBL, Smith A, McLeod JK. Stimulation of phosphatidyl inositol metabolism in the isolated perfused rat heart. Circ Res 1987; 61:625–31.
85. Movsesian MA, Thomas AP, Selak M, Williamson JR. Inositol trisphosphate does not release Ca^{++} from permeabilized cardiac myocytes and sarcoplasmic reticulum. FEBS Letts 1985; 185:328–32.
86. Stephan CC, Griendling KK, Galper JB. Muscarinic cholinergic stimulation of diacylglycerol production in cultured chick atrial cells: evidence for a role of phospholipase D and coupling via two G-proteins (submitted).
87. Leatherman GF, Kim D, Smith TW. Effect of phorbol esters on contractile state and calcium flux in cultured chick heart cells. Am J Physiol 1987; 253:H205–9.
88. Galper JB, Smith TW. Agonist and guanine nucleotide modulation of muscarinic cholinergic receptors in cultured heart cells. J Biol Chem 1980; 255:9571–9.
89. Goldstein JL, Anderson RGW, Brown MS. Coated pits, coated vesicles, and receptor-mediated endocytosis. Nature 1979; 279:679–85.
90. Wilson L, Bramburg JR, Mizel SB, Grisham LM, Creswell KM. Interaction of drugs with microtubule proteins. Fed Proc 1974; 33:158–66.
91. Kwatra MM, Hosey MM. Phosphorylation of the cardiac muscarinic receptor in intact chick heart and its regulation by a muscarinic agonist. J Biol Chem 1986; 261:12429–32.
92. Kwatra MM, Leung E, Man AC, McMahon KK, Ptasienski J, Green RD, Hosey MM. Correlation of agonist-induced phosphorylation of chick heart muscarinic receptors with receptor desensitization. J Biol Chem 1987; 262:16314–21.
93. Barlow RB, Berry KJ, Glenton PAM, Nickolaou NM, Soh KS. A comparison of affinity constants for muscarinic-sensitive acetylcholine receptors in guinea pig atrial pacemaker cells at 29° and in ileum at $29^{\circ\circ}$ and 37°C. Br J Pharmacol 1976; 58:613–20.

94. Rattan S, Goyal RK. Evidence of 5-HT participation in vagal inhibitory pathway to opossum LES. Am J Physiol 1978; 234:E273–6.
95. Roszkowski AP. Muscarinic receptor subtypes: an unusual type of sympathetic ganglionic stimulant. J Pharmacol Exp Ther 1961; 132:156–70.
96. Hammer R, Giachetti A. M_1 and M_2 biochemical and functional characterization. Life Sci 1982; 31:2991–8.
97. Birdsall NJ, Burgen ASV, Holme EC, Stockton JM, Zigmond MH. The effect of McN-A343 on muscarinic receptors in the cerebral cortex and heart. Br J Pharmacol 1983; 78:257–9.
98. Goyal RK, Patton S. Neurohumoral, hormonal, and drug receptors from the lower esophageal sphincter. Gastroenterology 1973; 74:593–619.
99. Hammer R, Berrie CP, Birdsall NMJ, Burgen ASV, Hulme EC. Pirenzepine distinguishes between different subclasses of muscarinic receptors. Nature 1980; 283:90–2.
100. Strockbrugger RW, Jaup BH, Dotevall G. The effect of different doses of pirenzepine on gastric secretion stimulated by modified sham feeding in man. Scand J Gastroenterol 1982; 17 (Suppl 72):111–6.
101. Strockbrugger RW, Jaup BP, Abrahmsson H, Dotevall G. Clinical pharmacology of muscarinic antagonists. Trends Pharmacol Sci 1984; 5(Suppl):74–7.
102. Patton WOM, Rang HP. The uptake of atropine and related drugs by intestinal smooth muscle of the guinea-pig in relation to acetylcholine receptors. Proc R Soc London [B] 1965; 163:1–44.
103. Watson M, Yamamura HI, Roeske WR. A unique regulatory profile and regional distribution of [^{3}H]pirenzepine binding in the rat provide evidence for distinct M_1 and M_2 muscarinic receptor subtypes. Life Sci 1983; 32:3001–10.
104. Luthin GR, Wolfe BB. Comparison of [^{3}H]pirenzepine and [^{3}H]-quinuclidinylbenzilate binding to muscarinic cholinergic receptors in rat brain. J Pharmacol Exp Ther 1984; 228:648–55.
105. Luthin GR, Wolfe BB. [^{3}H]pirenzepine and [^{3}H]quinuclidinylbenzilate binding to brain muscarinic cholinergic receptors: differences in measured receptor density not explained by differences in receptor isomerization. J Mol Pharmacol 1984; 26:164–9.
106. Lambrecht G, Linch H, Moser U, Mutschler E, Strecker M, Tacke R, Weiss J. In: Dahlbom R, Nilssan JLG, eds. Proceedings of the VIIIth international symposium on medicinal chemistry. Stockholm: Swedish Pharmaceutical Press, 1985; 2:424–56.
107. Lambrecht G, Moser U, Muschler E, Wess J, Linch H, Strecker M, Tacke R. Hexahydro-sila difenidol: a selective antagonist of ileal muscarinic receptors. Naunyn-Schmidebergs Arch Pharmacol 1984; 325 (suppl):1262.
108. Lambrecht G, Feifel R, Moser U, Waguer-Röder M, Choo LK, Camus J, Tastenoy M, Waelbroeck M, Strohmann C, Tackegh R, Rodrigues de Miranda JF, Christophe J, Mutschler E. Pharmacology of Hexahydro-difenidol, hexahydro-sila-difenidol and related selective muscarinic antagonists. Trends in Pharmacological sciences subtypes of Muscarinic Receptors IV supplement Proceedings of the fourth International Symposium of Muscarinic Receptors 1989, 60–69.
109. Lambrecht G, Mutschler E, Moser U, Riotte R, Wagner M, Wess J, Gmelin G, Tacke R, Zilch H. Heterogeneity in muscarinic recéptors: evidence from pharmacological and physiological studies with selective antagonists in muscarinic cholinergic mechanisms. In: Cohen S, Sokolovsky M, eds. Tel Aviv/London: Freund Publishing House Ltd, 1987.
110. Gil DW, Wolfe BB. Pirenzepine distinguishes between muscarinic receptor-mediated phosphoinositide breakdown and inhibition of adenylate cyclase. J Pharmacol Exp Ther 1985; 232:608–16.
111. Peterson G, Herron G, Yamaki M, Fullerton D, Schimmerlik M. Purification of the muscarinic acetylcholine receptor from porcine atria. Proc Nat Acad Sci USA 1984; 81:4993–8.

112. Peralta EG, Winslow JW, Peterson GL, Smith DH, Ashkenazi A, Ramachandran J, Schimerlik M, Capon DJ. Primary structure and biomechanical properties of an M_2 muscarinic receptor. Science 1987; 236:600–5.
113. Kubo T, Fukada K, Mikami A, Maeda A, Takahashi H, Mishina M, Haga T, Haga K, Ichiyama A, Kangawa K, Kojima M, Matsuo H, Hirose T, Numa S. Cloning, sequencing, and expression of complementary DNA encoding the muscarinic acetylcholine receptor. Nature 1986; 232:411–6.
114. Bonner TI, Buckley NJ, Young AC, Brann MR. Identification of a family of muscarinic acetylcholine receptor genes. Science 1987; 237:527–32.
115. Kubo I, Maeda A, Sugimoto K, Akiba I, Mikami A, Takahashi H, Haga T, Haga K, Ichiyama A, Kangawa K, Matsuo H, Hirose T, Numa S. Primary structure of porcine cardiac muscarinic acetylcholine receptor deduced from the cDNA sequence. FEBS Lett 1986; 209:367–77.
116. Bonner TI, Young AC, Brann MR, Buckley NJ. Cloning and expression of human and rat M_5 muscarinic acetylcholine receptor genes. Neuron 1988; 1:403–10.
117. Ashkenazi A, Winslow JW, Peralta EG, Peterson GL, Schimerlik MI, Capon DJ, Ramachandran J. An M2 muscarinic receptor subtype coupled to both adenylyl cyclase and phosphoinositide turnover. Science 1987; 238:672–5.
118. Liang BT, Galper JB. Differential sensitivity of α_o and α_i ADP-ribosylation by pertussis toxin in the intact cultural embryonic chick myocyte: relationship to the role of G-proteins in the coupling of muscarinic cholinergic receptors to inhibition of adenylate cyclase activity. Biochem Pharmacol 1988; 37:4549–55.
119. Peralta EG, Ashkenzi A, Winslow JW, Ramachandran J, Capon DJ. Differential regulation of PI hydrolysis and adenylatecyclase by muscarinic receptor subtypes. Nature 1988; 334:434–7.
120. Levine RR, Birdsall NJ. Subtypes of muscarinic receptors IV. Trends Pharmacol Sci Suppl 1989; VII.
121. Ashkenazi A, Peralta EG, Winslow JW, Ramachandran J, Capon DJ. Functionally distinct G-proteins selectively couple different receptors to P.I. hydrolysis in the same cell. Cell 1988; 56:487–93.
122. Parson WJ, Stiles GL. Herologous desensitization of the inhibitory A_2 adenosine receptor–adenylate cyclase system in rat adipocytes: regulation of both N_s and N_i. J Biol Chem 1987; 262:841–7.
123. Renaud JF, Scanu AM, Kazazogloa T, Lombart A, Romey G, Lazdunski M. Normal serum and lipoprotein deficient serum give different expressions of excitability, corresponding to different stages of differentiation in chick cardiac cells in culture. Proc Natl Acad Sci USA 1982; 29:7768–72.
124. Haigh LS, Leatherman GF, O'Hara DS, Smith TW, Galper JB. Effects of low density lipoproteins and mevinolin on cholesterol content and muscarinic cholinergic responsiveness in cultured chick atrial cells: regulation of levels of muscarinic receptors and guanine nucleotide regulatory proteins. J Biol Chem 1988; 263:15608–18.
125. Barnett JV, Haigh LS, Marsh JD, Galper JB. Effects of low density lipoproteins and mevinolin on sympathetic responsiveness in cultured chick atrial cells: regulation of β-adrenergic receptors and α_s. J Biol Chem 1989; 264:10779–86.
126. Colucci WS, Denniss RA, Leatherman GF, Quigg RJ, Ludmer PL, Marsh JD, Gauthier DF. Intracoronary infusion of dobutamine to patients with and without severe congestive heart failure. J Clin Invest 1988; 81:1103–10.
127. Colucci WS, Ribiero JP, Rocco MB, Quigg RJ, Creager MA, Marsh JD, Gauthier DF, Hartley LH. Impaired chronotropic response to exercise in patients with congestive heart failure: role of postsynaptic β-adrenergic desensitization. Circulation 1989; 80:314–23.

128. Erne P, Lipkin D, Maseri A. Impaired beta-adrenergic receptors and normal post-receptor responsiveness in congestive heart failure. Am J Cardiol 1988; 61:1132–4.
129. Denniss RA, Marsh JD, Quigg RJ, Gordon JB, Colucci WS. β-adrenergic receptor number and adenylate cyclase function in denervated transplanted and cardiomyopathic human hearts. Circulation 1989; 79:1028–54.
130. Kessler PD, Cates AE, Van Dop C, Feldman AM. Decreased bioactivity of the guanine nucleotide-binding protein that stimulates adenylate cyclase in hearts from cardiomyopathic syrian hamsters. J Clin Invest 1989; 84:244–52.
131. Feldman AM, Cates AE, Veazey WB, Hershberger RE, Bristow MR, Baughman KL, Baumgartner WA, Van Dop C. Increase of the 40,000 mol. wt. pertussis toxin substrate (G-protein) in the failing human heart. J Clin Invest 1988; 82:189–97.
132. Vatner DE, Lavalle M, Amano J, Finizola A, Homcy CJ, Vatner SF. Mechanisms of supersensitivity to sympathomimetic amines in the chronically denervated heart of the conscious dog, Circ Res 1985; 57:55–64.
133. Osorio ML, Stevano JFE, Langer SZ. Heteroptic heart transplanted in the cat. An experimental model for the study of the development of sympathetic denervators and of allograft rejection. Naunyn Schmiedebergs Arch Pharmacol 1974; 283:389–407.
134. Ono K, Lindsey ES. Improved technique of heart transplantation in the rat. J Thorac Cardiovasc Surg 1969; 57:225–9.
135. Luri KG, Bristow MR, Reitz BA. Increased β-adrenergic receptor density in an experimental model of cardiac transplantation. J Thorac Cardiovasc Surg 1983; 86:195–201.
136. Savin WM, Haskell SC, Schroeder JS, Stinson EB. Cardiorespiratory responses of cardiac transplant patients to graded, symptom-limited exercise. Circulation 1980; 62:55–60.
137. Pope SE, Stinson EB, Daughters GT, Schroeder JS, Ingels NB, Alderman EL. Exercise response of the denervated heart in long-term cardiac transplant recipients. Am J Cardiol 1980; 96:213–8.
138. Quigg RJ, Rocco MB, Gauthier DF, Creager MA, Hartley LH, Colucci WS. Mechanisms of the attenuated peak heart rate to exercise after orthotopic cardiac transplantation. J Am Coll Cardiol 1989; 14:338–44.
139. Gilbert EM, Eiswirth CC, Mealey P, Herrick C, Bristow MR. β-Adrenergic supersensitivity of the human heart is presynoptic in origin. Circulation 1989; 79:344–9.

14

Protein Kinase C and Cardiovascular Contractility

ANDRE RUZYCKY

University of Pittsburgh School of Medicine
Pittsburgh, Pennsylvania

I. INTRODUCTION

A parallel consequence of second messenger signaling via the hydrolysis of inositol-containing phospholipids is the concurrent liberation of neutral lipids, most notably diacylglycerol, and fatty acids. These products act as second messengers in their own right and serve to activate an intracellular phospholipid- and Ca^{2+}-dependent protein kinase, termed protein kinase C. Protein kinase C is involved in the phosphorylation of many proteins in the cell and has been implicated as a putative regulator of many diverse cellular functions. With the identification of several activators and substrates of protein kinase C, the role of this enzyme in the regulation of cardiovascular physiology has been the subject of substantial interest in recent years. In this chapter, we will discuss signaling mechanisms involved in the production of second messenger activators of protein kinase C, the current biochemical understanding of this enzyme, describe current observations implicating protein kinase C in the expression of cardiovascular contractile activity, and, in conclusion, discuss potential roles of this signaling pathway in terms of normal and pathologic cardiovascular function. In recent years, the study of apparent protein kinase C-mediated processes has virtually exploded and, as such, for the sake of conciseness, the discussion in this chapter will be limited to the cardiovascular system where possible. For broader based discussions of protein kinase C-mediated events, the reader is referred to several recent reviews (1–3).

II. PRODUCTION OF PROTEIN KINASE C SECOND MESSENGERS

Many neurotransmitters, hormones, growth factors, and some drugs exert their cellular effects through membrane-associated receptors linked to the hydrolysis of inositol-containing phospholipid (Fig. 1). A parallel consequence of the liberation

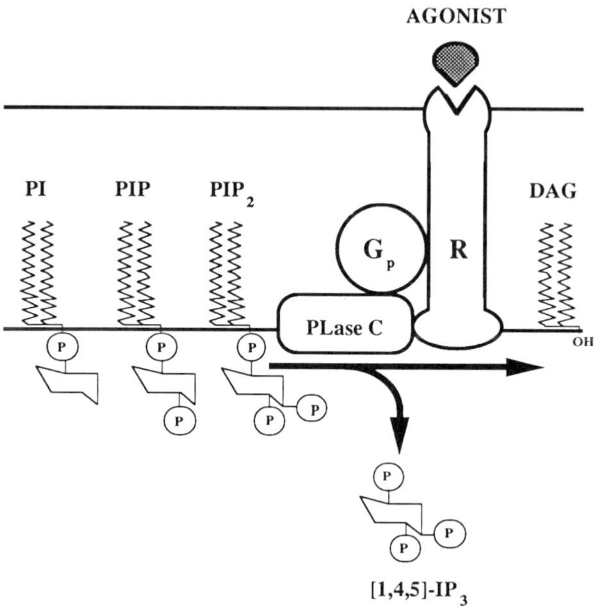

Figure 1 Biochemical pathway of hormone receptor-mediated inositol phospholipid hydrolysis. This transmembrane signaling process involves a hormone receptor (R), a coupling guanine nucleotide-binding protein (Gp), and phospholipase C (PLase C). Biological signal transduction involves receptor-activated stimulation of PLase C resulting in the hydrolysis of phosphatidylinositol bisphosphate (PIP_2) to produce two second messenger molecules: diacylglycerol (DAG) and inositol (1,4,5)-trisphosphate ((1,4,5)IP_3).

of polyphosphoinositides by the action of phospholipase C is the production of neutral lipids, diacylglycerols (DAG). In 1980, Nishizuka and co-workers (4) provided the first evidence that receptor-mediated turnover of phosphoinositides was directly linked to the activation of protein kinase C, suggesting a second messenger role for DAG.

In the resting unstimulated condition, DAG are almost absent from the cellular plasma membrane (5) since this neutral lipid product has a low rate of synthesis under these conditions and can be rapidly metabolized by phosphorylation to phosphatic acid or degraded into component fatty acids by diacylglycerol lipases. DAG formed by the action of phospholipase C are in the 1,2-sn configuration with various fatty acids of differing chain length. DAG species derived from this pathway contain primarily the fatty acid stearic acid in the 1-position and primarily arachidonic acid in the 2-position (6). Other DAG stereoisomers, 2,3-sn species, derived from triacylglycerol by the action of lipoprotein lipase, and the 1,3-sn species, are inactive with respect to protein kinase C (1).

In keeping with the role of a second messenger, the DAG signal must be discretely regulated in terms of synthesis and degradation. DAG are very rapidly and transiently produced (on the order of a few seconds) in many tissues by various stimuli. The metabolic fate of DAG is less well documented, with the relative hydrolysis by either DAG lipase or DAG kinase somewhat variable between tissues and the presence of the original stimulating agonist. DAG kinase enzymes have been found in membrane and cytosolic cellular fractions, with the membrane-bound form exhibiting an apparent selectivity for arachidonoyl-containing DAG species (7). This finding has been proposed as evidence of a selective mechanism for the replenishment of the PIP_2 pool with DAG backbones of acyl specificity. DAG lipase activity has also been found in both membrane and cytosolic cellular fractions. However, the relative contributions and regulation of both metabolic pathways is currently unknown.

Recent reports of temporal and quantitative discrepancies between inositol trisphosphate and DAG liberation have led to speculation regarding other metabolic pathways for DAG production. Kinetic profiles of DAG production have identified early (within 5 sec) and late peaks (5–20 min) of DAG formation, suggesting changes in either substrate pools or pathways of production (8). DAG species have been described to be produced upon receptor activation of other phospholipases such as phospholipase A_2 or D and/or hydrolyzation of other membrane phospholipids such as phosphatidylcholine and phosphatidylethanolamine (9,10). Two such proposed pathways are illustrated in Figure 2. Fatty acid components of these 1,2-sn,DAG species can be oleic, linoleic, palmitoleic, or myristoleic acids (9). Details of the recruitment of these, the classic PIP_2, or other pathways is currently not well understood and may be different between cell types or stimulat-

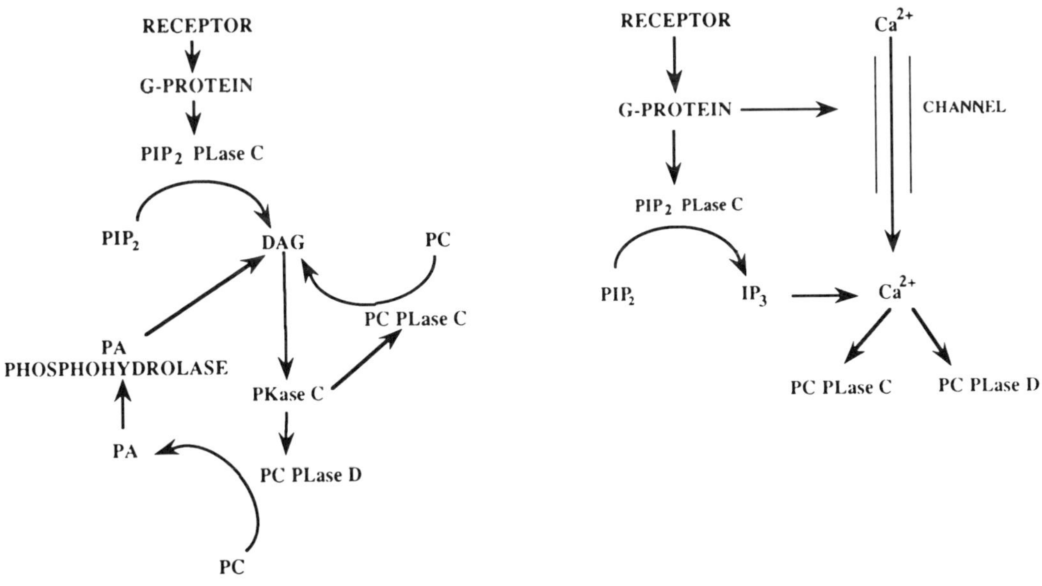

Figure 2 Proposed mechanisms of production of DAG species and the activation of protein kinase C (9). (A) DAG production from the classic PIP_2 pathway activates protein kinase C, which acts on PC phospholipases either directly or indirectly. Sustained production of DAG of varying species could be due to a positive feedback loop through the activation of PC phospholipases, which are most likely differentially regulated by protein kinase C and Ca^{2+}. (B) Sustained DAG production may also occur as a consequence of mobilization of intracellular calcium due to IP_3 production and the opening of membrane calcium channels. Calcium might activate PC phospholipases directly or through a calcium-binding protein or a calcium-dependent protein kinase. The cellular sites of calcium action are currently unknown. (Modified from Ref. 9 with permission.)

ing agents. With the discovery of isozymes of protein kinase C (discussed in the next section) that vary in tissue distribution, substrate specificity, and regulation, different molecular species of DAG may exert differential effects on the various forms of protein kinase C.

III. BIOCHEMISTRY OF THE PHOSPHOLIPID- AND CA^{2+}-DEPENDENT PROTEIN KINASE (PROTEIN KINASE C)

Since the discovery of a phospholipid- and Ca^{2+}-dependent protein kinase activity in 1977 by Nishizuka and co-workers (11), protein kinase C has been the focus of extensive research into the regulation of most stimulus–response coupling pathways in physiology. Today, protein kinase C is recognized as a family of serine/theonine protein kinases found in all mammalian tissues tested (2). Protein kinase C (PKC) is generally recovered from the cellular cytosol as an inactive form. However, upon receptor stimulation PKC is apparently translocated to the cell plasma membrane and the membrane associated form is biochemically active. The enzyme is a single polypeptide with two functional domains: a hydrophobic membrane associated regulatory domain, and a hydrophilic domain containing the catalytic center (1). The regulatory domain contains a secondary structural feature: that of a pseudosubstrate (12). This conserved region of the regulatory domain resembles substrate protein sequences acted upon by PKC and maintain the enzyme in an inactive form in the absence of DAG and cofactor interactions with PKC.

PKC has a biochemical requirement for Ca^{2+} and acidic phospholipids, particularly phosphatidylserine (PS), for activation. The second messenger and PKC agonist, DAG act to increase the affinity for Ca^{2+} by PKC and form a complex of $PS+Ca^{2+}+PKC$ for full stimulation of enzyme activity (13). The mechanism by which DAG and cofactors stimulate PKC activity is still unresolved. It has been suggested that DAG enhances Ca^{2+}-dependent phase separation in PS-rich domains of plasma membranes, allowing association of the PKC protein with PS and DAG (14), while others contend that the delivery and type of PKC substrate are critical in the imparting of PKC cofactor and agonist requirements and extent of activation (15). Furthermore, it appears that PKC may be biochemically but not physiologically dependent on intracelluar Ca^{2+} concentrations, since enzyme activation can occur at measurable yet very low (nanomolar) cytosolic Ca^{2+} levels (16).

With the recent exploitation of molecular biological techniques, investigators have found that PKC is actually a family of isozymes with subtle enzymic characteristics, variable tissue expression and localization, and most likely different functions (2). As shown in Table 1, protein chemistry and molecular cloning techniques have uncovered at least seven isoforms of PKC. Although complementary DNA clones have been found for seven of these isozymes, only four protein isoforms have been purified from mammalian tissue (α, βI, βII, γ) and biochemically characterized (17). The enzymatic properties of the two β species are apparently indistinguishable and result from the alternative splicing of a single RNA transcript. Analyses of the mode and kinetics of activation of the α, β, γ forms found subtle yet discrete differences in enzyme activation by DAG, fatty acids, and metal ions (17). At physiological Ca^{2+} concentrations, the β isoform was found to be the most active of the isozymes when stimulated with DAG. However, both the β and α forms were equally active when stimulated with low concentrations of PIP_2-derived DAG spe-

Table 1 Protein C Isozymes from Mammalian Tissues

	α	βI	βII	γ	δ	ϵ	ζ
Amino acid residues	672	671	673	697	673	737	592
Calculated molecular weight	76,799	76,790	76,933	78,366	77,517	83,474	67,740
Chromosome location (human)	17	16	16	19	?	?	?
Tissue expression	All	Some	Many	Brain, spinal cord	Many	Brain only?	Many
Cell localization	Membrane cytosol	Cytosol granular bodies	Membrane	Golgi body	?	?	?
Activators	PS+DAG+Ca^{2+} AA+Ca^{2+}	PS+DAG+Ca^{2+}	PS+ DAG+Ca^{2+}	PS+DAG+Ca^{2+} AA lipoxyn	PS+DAG +(Ca^{2+})	PS +DAG +(Ca^{2+})	PS +(DAG+Ca^{2+})

AA, arachidonic acid; DAG, diacylglycerol; PS, phosphatidylserine.
Source: Adapted from Ref. 2.

cies, whereas the γ and β forms were equally active when activated with low concentrations of PC-derived (dimyristoylated) DAG species. Although, the PKC-γ was most sensitive to activation by the fatty acid arachidonic acid, its activity decreased with increasing arachidonate concentrations: PKC-β increased and expressed greater activity than PKC-γ at high concentrations of arachidonic acid.

Protein kinase C isozymes have also been found to exhibit tissue-specific expression with distinct cellular localization by cytochemical, Northern blot, and in situ messenger RNA hybridization studies (2,18,19). PKC-γ appears to be only expressed in the brain and spinal cord, while the α form is found in most tissues tested. Most tissues have distinct proportions of multiple isoforms expressed, while in the brain specific isoforms are localized to specific regions; PKC-γ in the hippocampus and amygdaloid complex, PKC-β in the cerebellum (2,18). In addition, PKC α, β, γ isoforms undergo differential developmental expression in the brain (19). Unfortunately, very little is known of the expression and distribution of the δ, ϵ, ζ isozymes.

The expression of one or more PKC isozymes and/or the differential spatial and temporal recruitment of isozymes most likely provide for a very selective and complex level of control of cellular signaling processes. Multiple isozymes may be coupled to specific receptors or class of receptors acting on specific common substrates. They may be activated in sequence to propagate diverse cellular processes or propagate similar processes at different times.

IV. PHARMACOLOGIC MANIPULATION OF PROTEIN KINASE C

The implication of protein kinase C in the regulation of numerous cellular processes has been largely due to the use of specific pharmacologic modulators, both stimulators and inhibitors, to this enzyme. The fortuitous discovery that tumor-promoting phorbol esters mimic the activity of DAG and can directly activate protein kinase C (20,21) was fundamental in leading to the description of apparent protein kinase C-mediated processes. As shown in Figure 3, phorbol esters are structurally similar to DAG. Phorbol esters are potent and full activators of protein kinase C and, like

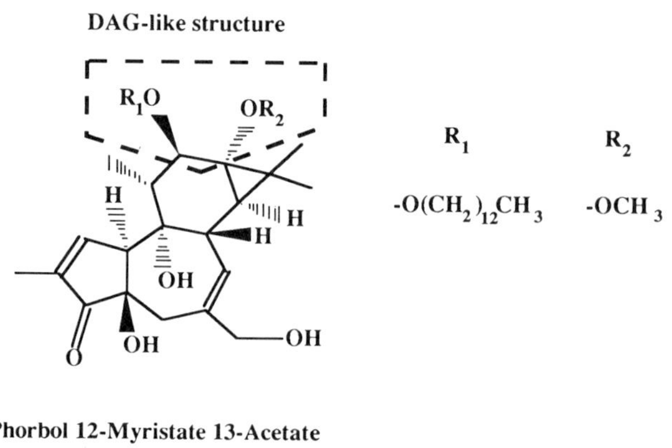

Figure 3 The structure of a tumor-promoting phorbol diester. The hatched box delineates structural homology with diacylglycerols.

DAG, increase the affinity of protein kinase C for calcium under physiological conditions. However, unlike DAG, phorbol esters persistently activate protein kinase C with very little degradation and at higher concentrations may not be solely targeted toward this enzyme. Thus definitive description of phorbol ester-derived protein kinase C-mediated processes has needed to be correlated with the temporal sequence of endogenous events (i.e., production of DAG) during different phases of cellular responses.

Although phorbol esters are now commonly used as protein kinase C-specific activators, the biochemical characterization of phorbol ester specificity for this enzyme and their mechanism of activation are far less well appreciated. Some studies have shown that there are indeed subtle biochemical differences between phorbol esters and DAG in the activation of protein kinase C (22,23). Protein kinase C isozymes may also have differential sensitivities to phorbol ester activation (19,24). When phorbol ester effects were contrasted with cell-permeable synthetic DAG (termed dioleins) and bryostatins, a group of marine toxins that also activate protein kinase C, it was found that all three structurally different activators bound to the same site on protein kinase C (22). However these agents differentially altered apparently protein kinase C-dependent responses with differing selectivities and efficacies (22). Phorbol esters, dioleins, and bryostatins all exhibited similar dose dependencies in enhancing protein kinase C-mediated responses. Bryostatins were found to be full, or partial agonists, and even antagonists to certain responses while dioleins were either partial agonists or inactive compared to the efficacy of phorbol esters in eliciting apparent protein kinase C responses.

Biochemical studies of the effects of DAG and phorbol esters on protein kinase C complexation with membranes and expression of kinase activity have reported that the activation of enzyme kinase activity is a two-step process; an initial reversible and calcium-dependent step with kinase activation by DAG, and a second activated yet irreversible interaction with the cell membrane environment not mediated by DAG (23). Phorbol esters were found to stimulate both the reversible and irreversible membrane interactions, with the latter occurring in the absence of calcium. Studies of the effects of phorbol esters on protein kinase C isozymes have demonstrated that PKC-β downregulates and is degraded more rapidly than PKC-α in response to persistent activation by phorbol esters (19). PKC-ϵ was found to bind phorbol esters with a slightly lower affinity than PKCs α, β, or γ and associate with membrane in a calcium-independent manner (24).

It is becoming increasingly apparent that there exists a sophisticated complexity involving multiple sources of pools of endogenous DAG (and fatty acid), interacting with multiple protein kinase C isoforms, at kinetically distinct time frames during a receptor-mediated response. Thus the past simplistic approach of using phorbol esters as direct selective markers of a protein kinase C involvement is a gross oversimplification and has become insufficient to describe the role of this enzyme in regulating stimulus–response coupling pathways. In addition, the description of other pharmacologic agents such as certain calcium antagonists with indirect stimulatory effects on protein kinase C (25) underscores that the diversity and interaction of protein kinase C isoform-mediated events cannot be resolved by the use of phorbol esters alone.

Protein kinase C activity can also be modulated by specific inhibitors of this enzyme (26–28). As with the use of phorbol esters, these agents have been widely used to apparently identify protein kinase C-mediated cellular processes, even though their mode of inhibitory action or selectivity of action relative to other protein kinase is not well understood. A partial list of such inhibitors is presented in Table 2. The direct protein kinase C inhibitors act directly on the catalytic domain of the enzyme without effect on phorbol ester binding (29). These inhibitors are thought to compete with ATP for a specific site on the catalytic domain (26). The endogenous protein kinase C inhibitor has been sequenced and is thought to interact directly with kinase moiety of the catalytic domain, since it does not interact with substrates or cofactors of protein kinase C (27,30). Other inhibitors of this enzyme, termed indirect inhibitors, act by apparently disrupting hydrophobic interactions between the regulatory domain and phospholipids and calcium cofactors (26,29). Since these type of interactions are relatively common to other protein kinases, the lack of selectivity of these agents for protein kinase C relative to other kinases makes their use difficult and often inconclusive. Furthermore, the effects or selectivity of these inhibitors for the various protein kinase C isoforms are currently unknown. In general, protein kinase C inhibitors have not been used extensively in vivo due to these problems of selectivity. Their relative lack of selectivity predisposes their use due to toxicity resulting from interactions with other cellular processes. For example, tamoxifen

Table 2 Inhibitors of Protein Kinase C

Direct Inhibitors	Isoquinolinesulfonamides
	H-7
	H-9
	Quercetin
	17 kDa protein inhibitor
	Staurosporine
Indirect Inhibitors	Anticalmodulins
	Phenothiazines
	W-7
	Calmidazolium
	Polypeptides
	Cytotoxins
	Polymyxin
	Neurotoxins
	Polyamines
	Spermine
	1,12-Diaminododecane
	Local Anesthetics
	Dibucaine
	Others
	Adriamycin
	Alkylphospholipid
	Calphostin C
	Gangliosides
	Hypericin
	Neomycin
	Sphingosine
	Tamoxifen

Source: Refs. 26–28.

exhibits potent antiestrogenic effects, adriamycin is a toxic antineoplastic agent, and polymyxin is an antibiotic with significant nephrotoxicity.

V. CELLULAR EFFECTS OF PROTEIN KINASE C STIMULATION IN VASCULAR SMOOTH MUSCLE

The description of apparent protein kinase C-mediated cellular processes has arisen largely from the study of the effects of phorbol esters on a particular response cascade. Phorbol esters have been shown to increase or decrease a wide variety of cellular events in as many different tissues. As listed in Table 3, many substrates for protein kinase C phosphorylation have been identified. This discussion, however, will be limited to descriptions of potential protein kinase C involvement in the expression of vascular contractility.

Phorbol esters have been described to have both stimulatory and inhibitory effects on smooth muscle contractility depending on the tissue studied (31). Biochemical studies of protein kinase C-mediated regulation of vascular smooth muscle contractility have generally taken two directions: effects of protein kinase C stimulation on cellular excitation events signaling the muscle to contract (i.e., neurotransmitter release, membrane receptors and transducing proteins, second messenger production pathways, ion channels, intracellular enzymes) and effects on the cellular contractile apparatus allowing the tissue to contract. In vascular smooth muscle, numerous vasoactive hormones, neurotransmitters, and drugs have been described to activate the hydrolysis of inositol-containing phospholipids (32–34) and increase the production of the endogenous protein kinase C activator

Table 3 Partial List of Proposed Substrate Proteins of Protein Kinase C

Receptor proteins:
Epidermal growth factor receptor
β-Adrenoceptor
Nicotinic acetylcholine receptor
Immunoglobulin E receptor
Membrane proteins
Calcium channel
Sodium channel
GTP binding protein
Sodium/potassium ATPase
Calcium-transport ATPase
Contractile proteins
Myosin light chain
Troponin
Caldesmon
Filamin
Enzymes
Glucose phosphorylase kinase
Guanylate cyclase
Myosin light chain kinase
NADPH oxidase

diacylglycerol (8,35). Exogenous stimulation of isolated vascular smooth muscle preparations with synthetic diacylglycerols and phorbol esters leads to a slow developing and sustained contractile response (32,36,37), suggesting that extracellular signals acting through phospholipase C may stimulate vascular contractility via a protein kinase C-dependent pathway.

Since these initial studies, extensive biochemical research has focused on uncovering the mechanism of this regulation. Phorbol esters have been shown to inhibit transmembrane calcium influx through potential-dependent calcium channels (33), modulate neurotransmitter binding of the α1-adrenoceptor (38), increase the activity of the sodium/calcium antiporter (39), and β-adrenoreceptor (38), increase the activity of the sodium/calcium antiporter (39), and β-adrenoreceptor-mediated cAMP production (40). Thus it appears that protein kinase C acts a negative feedback control early after stimulation in the contractile response cascade by modulating the extrusion and limiting influx of a contractile second messenger, calcium, immediately after mobilization and uncoupling receptor signaling via this pathway. Evidence has been obtained that protein kinase C exerts negative feedback control on α1-adrenoreceptors and angiotensin II receptors by uncoupling them from phospholipase C (41,42). Similar feedback control has been proposed for other tissues and cell types (1,3). In other tissue systems, it has been suggested that this receptor uncoupling occurs as a result of phosphorylation of guanine nucleotide-binding proteins (43,44), which functionally link receptors with second messenger-producing enzymes such as phospholipase C or adenylate cyclase. More detailed molecular information of the feedback control or the action of individual protein kinase C isozymes is currently unavailable. However, it appears that this feedback control can be both negative and positive in nature, suggesting different roles for different isozymes found in vascular smooth muscle (45).

One of the most interesting findings with the use of phorbol esters on vascular smooth muscle has been the observation that phorbol esters can stimulate the contractile apparatus of smooth muscle directly and precipitate a contractile response in the absence of receptor stimulation. Phorbol esters have been shown to potently and maximally contract many different blood vessels including the aorta (46,47), coronary (48,49), cerebral (50), carotid (51), and mesenteric arteries (48,52). The magnitude and rate of rise of contractile responses mediated by phorbol esters are enhanced in the presence of increasing intracellular calcium concentrations, suggesting a synergistic interaction with the second messenger calcium on the contractile proteins of smooth muscle (34,53).

The mechanism of phorbol ester or protein kinase C activation in the generation and maintenance of smooth muscle contractile responses is currently not well defined. Furthermore, the role of protein kinase C stimulation in receptor mediated smooth muscle contractility remains the subject of considerable debate. Few studies have directly linked receptor-mediated production of DAG with protein kinase C stimulation leading to contraction. Comparison studies of the temporal patterns of protein phosphorylation induced by receptor agonists and phorbol esters and pharmacologic studies with protein kinase C inhibitors have been used to link these cellular events. Using the protein kinase C inhibitor, H-7, α1-adrenoceptor-mediated responses (phenylephrine stimulation) (53) and prostaglandin receptor-mediated responses (54) have been suggested to elicit vascular smooth muscle contractions via activation of a protein kinase C-dependent pathway.

Comparisons of protein phosphorylation patterns and measurements of intracellular calcium concentrations during receptor and phorbol ester-mediated contractile responses have yielded the most controversial interpretations of the role of protein kinase C in these events (34). These controversies have stemmed largely from discrepancies in the interpretation of biochemical observations during two distinct temporal phases of the vascular smooth muscle contractile response: early force generation and subsequent, late force maintenance. During these phases, receptor and phorbol ester-mediated events have been found to have subtle differences with respect to two major biochemical indices of contractility: intracellular calcium concentrations and myosin light chain phosphorylation. Most contractile agonists increase intracellular calcium concentrations transiently during the early stage of force generation, with levels falling to near resting or resting concentrations during the prolonged period of force maintenance (34,55). Receptor stimulation also results in a similar transient pattern of myosin light chain phosphorylation, with the level of phosphorylation slightly above resting during the temporal phase of contraction maintenance (34,56). In contrast, phorbol ester-mediated vascular smooth muscle contractile responses have been demonstrated to occur in the absence of sustained or transient increases in either intracellular calcium concentration or myosin light chain phosphorylation (47,56).

Initial interpretations of these findings suggested that receptor-mediated vascular smooth muscle contractions are composed of two mechanistically distinct events: force generation and force maintenance. Force generation was suggested to be a transient calcium- and myosin light chain phosphorylation-dependent process involving the formation of cycling actomyosin crossbridges (57). Force maintenance was described as a sustained response characterized by an apparently increased sensitivity of contractile elements to calcium and myosin light chain phosphorylation, leading to the existence of nonphosphorylated force producing crossbridges ("latch bridges") (57). The expression of the force maintenance phase was said to be dependent on the expression of the force generation phase, implying that force maintenance required the initial increase in intracellular calcium and myosin light chain phosphorylation as well. Phorbol ester- or protein kinase C-mediated contractions were thought to activate a mechanism that mimicked a prolonged receptor-mediated force maintenance phase (47,49,51). The relevance of protein kinase C activation in receptor-mediated contractile responses was questioned, however, since phorbol esters were not observed to elicit the force generation phase of a contractile response (e.g., increase in intracellular calcium).

However, recent studies are increasingly arguing that protein kinase C activation may stimulate a novel smooth muscle contractile mechanism in addition to the classic calcium–myosin light chain phosphorylation–actomyosin cross bridge mechanism of force production (34). A "coordinate fibrillar domain model" of smooth muscle contractility has been proposed by Rasmussen and colleagues (34). This model proposes that early increases in intracellular calcium are coincident with the production of DAG from inositol phospholipids and act to enhance protein kinase C activation by DAG. Subsequent kinase activation leads to the phosphorylation of another set of contractile proteins termed actin-binding proteins, which promote force generating and maintaining crossbridges in the presence of low levels of myosin light chain phosphorylation (Fig. 4). This hypothesis is supported by evidence of phorbol ester-mediated phosphorylation of intermedi-

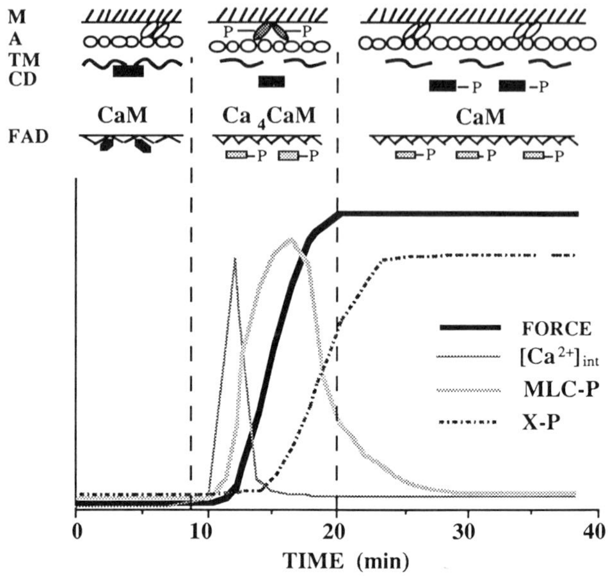

Figure 4 The coordinate fibrillar domain model of smooth muscle contraction involving coordinate processes of the caldesmon–tropomysoin–actin–myosin domain (CD-TM-A-M) and the filamin–actin–desmin domain (FAD). When the smooth muscle is at rest there are few crossbridges between actin and myosin, caldesmon is closely associated with tropomyosin, and filamin is associated with an extended actin–desmin domain and small actin-binding proteins are loosely associated with this domain. Upon smooth muscle cell activation, a rise in intracellular calcium precipitates: (1) an activation of myosin light chain kinase, (2) the calcium-calmodulin dependent dissociation of caldesmon from tropomyosin, and (3) the calcium-dependent solation of the FAD domain. The first two events cooperatively facilitate myosin light-chain phosphorylation. Increasing MLC-P leads to the formation of cycling cross bridges between actin and myosin and tension development. During tension development, the FAD fibrillar domain is reorganized. Concurrently, activation of protein kinase C leads to the phosphorylation of caldesmon, and other actin-binding proteins such as desmin and synemin (X-P). The phosphorylation of myosin light chains is transient and decreases to near resting levels, but tension is maintained due to the stabilization of the FAD domain. Caldesmon phosphorylation permits actin and myosin crossbridge cycling but with a low activity because of low intracellular calcium levels. The low crossbridge cycling rate may be important in the reorganization of the FAD domain. (Adapted from Ref. 34 with permission.)

ate filament actin-binding proteins such as caldesmon (58), desmin, and synemin (59). Temporal profiles of phosphorylation patterns of these proteins in response to receptor- and protein kinase C-stimulation have been compared and found to be similar (59–61). Recent imaging studies of isolated vascular smooth muscle cells employing a fluorescent protein kinase C probe have shown that the translocation of protein kinase C from the cytosol to the cell surface membrane occurs simultaneously with cell shortening (96).

The mechanistic details of protein kinase C-mediated contractility are currently unknown, as are the effects of various protein kinase C isozymes on this response. Functional studies of the effect of phorbol esters on calcium-force relationships have suggested that protein kinase C-activated contractility is calcium independent over a physiological range of intracellular calcium concentrations and is potentiated at higher calcium levels (53). Contractile response studies with sequential receptor agonist and phorbol ester stimulation have found very little additivity of responses, suggesting contractile activation via a common pathway by these different agents (53). Very little is known of the recovery or relaxation mechanisms from protein kinase C-stimulated contractility. Nitrovasodilators and cyclic GMP have been reported to inhibit phorbol ester-mediated contractile responses (46).

In addition to receptor-activated contractility, protein kinase C may also regulate vascular smooth muscle tone at rest or in the presence of mechanical pressures. Phorbol esters have been described to potentiate stretch-induced (myogenic) vascular tone in various blood vessels by apparently increasing the calcium sensitivity of vessel contractile filaments (50,62). In addition, vessel stretching appears to stimulate the hydrolysis of inositol phospholipids by phospholipase C, a source of DAG (63). The protein kinase C inhibitors H-7 and staurosporine have been reported to decrease intrinsic vascular tone in the absence of any stimuli (53,97). Another protein kinase C inhibitor MDL 27,032 has been shown preferentially to dilate large rather than small coronary arteries, suggesting a role for protein kinase C in the expression of myogenic vascular tone (63). These initial findings are especially interesting in that protein kinase C may be implicated in the direct regulation of vascular resistance and, in turn, regional blood flow.

VI. CELLULAR EFFECTS OF PROTEIN KINASE C STIMULATION IN CARDIAC MUSCLE

Even less is known of the effects of protein kinase C stimulation in cardiac muscle than in vascular smooth muscle. Phorbol esters have been generally described to exert negative inotropic and negative chronotropic effects (65–67). However, little else is known of the underlying molecular mechanisms of protein kinase C stimulation in the myocardium or the distribution of protein kinase(s) C within the myocardium. The presence of very strong electromechanical coupling in the heart has made it difficult to identify the relative contributions of electrophysiological and direct contractile effects of protein kinase C stimulation to the end-expression of cardiac function. The assessment of protein kinase C-mediated negative inotropism is further complicated by hypoxia secondary to decreases in coronary blood flow due to vascular smooth muscle effects of this enzyme.

Relatively few studies have described the effects of phorbol esters or DAG on cardiac contractile function or myocardial contractility and fewer still have attempted to investigate the molecular biochemistry of protein kinase C-mediated events in the heart. The negative chronotropic (67,68) and negative inotropic effects of phorbol esters have been described in cultured animal myocardial cells (65,69), isolated animal (67) and human papillary muscles (70), and perfused beating heart preparations (66). In the experimental perfused heart preparation, the negative inotropic effect of phorbol esters has been associated with a increased translocation of protein kinase C from the cytosol to membrane (66), a depression in the rate of force production, and increased resting tension (71). Studies of isolated human trabeculae have reported that phorbol esters concurrently decrease twitch force production, transient peak intracellular calcium concentration elevations, and contractile myofilament sensitivity to intracellular calcium (70).

Recent studies of isolated neonatal and adult cardiomyocytes have described similar results linking the negative inotropic effect of phorbol esters and DAG to diminished mobilization of intracellular calcium from the sarcoplasmic reticulum (spontaneous and stimulated) (68,72) and decreased levels of resting intracellular calcium concentration (72). However, in rat cardiomyocytes, a phorbol ester-mediated decrease in myofilament sensitivity to calcium could not be demonstrated (72). Although it has been known for several years that troponins are substrates for phosphorylation by protein kinase C (73), cardiac troponin T has been reported to be the primary protein kinase C-dependent substrate while β-adrenoreceptor activation stimulates the phosphorylation of troponin I (74,75). Thus, it appears that the functional effects of protein kinase C stimulation of cardiac contractile proteins have yet to be adequately resolved.

Due to the high degree of electromechanical coupling in the heart, phorbol ester effects on membrane ion channels and neurotransmitter receptors can profoundly affect cardiac performance. Phorbol esters have been reported to modulate the function of a number of plasma membrane ion channels, although these effects on the expression of cardiac contractility are currently not well understood. Potential-dependent calcium channels (76,77), sodium channels (78), and muscarinic acetylcholine receptor-activated potassium channels (79) have been shown to be regulated by phorbol esters. In general, electrophysiological analyses of the effects of phorbol esters on channel currents have uncovered different temporal effects on channel function: early and rapid stimulation of ion translocation followed by a later persistent inactivation of current (76–78). The stimulation of calcium channels appears to be mediated by the activation of α_1-adrenoceptors (77). The modulation of muscarinic receptor-stimulated potassium current may also occur at the level of the receptor itself, since ligand binding to membrane muscarinic receptors is increased in the presence of a protein kinase C inhibitor (80).

The modulation of ion channel currents by protein kinase C affects not only cardiac contractility (by altering the level of tissue excitability) but also processes regulating cardiac chronotropy. Thus the differential distribution of protein kinase C isozymes with varying substrates and functions among the different chambers of the heart may play an important role in the control of normal or adaptive cardiac performance. Currently little is known of the organ distribution of protein kinase C isoforms. However, studies of the localization of protein kinase C activity during cardiogenesis described greater and increasing levels of protein kinase C activity in atria than in ventricles during embryonic development (81). This apparent localization of activity may be important in the regulation or development of action potential pathways. Phorbol esters and DAG are known to stimulate norepinephrine release from the sinoatrial node (82) and regulate intercellular communication through gap junctions (83).

Phorbol esters also affect cardiac membrane signaling by the phosphorylation of surface receptors in the heart. The β_2-adrenoceptor (84), α_1-adrenoceptor (41), as well as the cardiac γ-aminobutyric acid A receptor (85) are phosphorylated by phorbol ester-activated protein kinase C. Activation of the α_1-adrenoceptor is followed by protein kinase C-mediated phosphorylation and uncoupling from phospholate C (41,86). The uncoupling of the phosphorylated β_2-adrenoceptor from adenylate cyclase has been suggested to occur at the level of the interaction of the receptor with the transducing guanine nucleotide-binding protein (85). This uncoupling effectively eliminates the sympathetic compensatory reflex to the protein kinase C-mediated negative inotropic effect (87). Thus protein kinase C stimulation in the myocardium can not only have a very important role in the expression of normal cardiac contractility but also affect the capability of the myocardium to adapt and/or recover from pathologic states. Thus the pharmacologic inhibition of protein kinase C may prove to be an attractive therapeutic target in the improvement of inotropic performance in patients with cardiomyopathies and heart failure.

VII. CONCLUSIONS

Since the discovery of protein kinase C in 1977, there is amassing a considerable amount of evidence that it plays a significant role in signal transduction for the activation of numerous cellular processes. Although we are uncovering and beginning to understand more and more protein kinase C-mediated events in the muscle of the cardiovascular system, direct functional understanding of the mechanisms of protein kinase C-mediated regulation of vascular tone, cardiac performance, or the therapeutic manipulation of these processes is still lacking. Some light is being shed on the functional significance of protein kinase C activation in the cardiovascular system by studies of models of disease states and of pathologic conditions.

In animal models of hypertension, increased vascular endogenous protein kinase C activator (DAG) (88) as well as increased vascular reactivity to protein kinase C stimulation with phorbol ester has been reported (52). Recent reports of differential regulation of temporally distinct contractile patterns (tonic vs. phasic) (89,90) by protein kinase C may suggest differential regulation of different vascular beds. The finding that protein kinase C may modulate the expression of inherent vascular tone (62,63) presents the attractive hypothesis that this enzyme pathway may be important in the predisposition of vessels to the development of stenoses or aneurysms. Thus, vascular sensitivity to endogenous vasoactive hormones and neurotransmitters and drugs may also be modulated.

Studies of myocardial injury due to ischemia have described the accumulation of diglycerides during ischemia in cardiac muscle and that these lipids can activate protein kinase C (91). The protein kinase C activated by these lipid species was calcium dependent and apparently different from the isozyme activated by DAG, suggesting that different protein kinase C isoforms may be activated under physiological and pathologic conditions. Myocardial injury resulting from hypoxia or ischemia is thought to involve processes arising from an intracellular overload. This calcium overload has been suggested to be induced by protein kinase C stimulation of sodium entry into the myocardial cell, leading to deranged sodium-calcium exchange (92). In acute myocardial ischemia, protein kinase C-mediated receptor-independent potentiation of adenylate cyclase sensitivity has been also proposed to lead to calcium overload (93).

That protein kinase C may be important in the physiological adaptation processes occurring during the progression of a disease is supported by preliminary studies of idiopathic cardiomyopathies in humans (94). Immunologically detected protein kinase C was found to be expressed in greater quantity in patients with cardiomyopathies than those without the disease. Greater protein kinase C expression was found in patients with hypertrophic than dilated cardiomyopathy. In addition, the amplified expression of protein kinase C was found to be correlated with severity of myocardial hypertrophy. Furthermore, studies in animals have reported increased membrane-associated protein kinase C activity during the progression of the disease (95).

It is now quite evident that protein kinase C is involved in many diverse cellular processes of the heart and blood vessels. However, with diverse complexity of protein kinase C signal transduction with respect to tissue specificity, enzyme isoforms, and cross communication with other signaling pathways the presence of many described protein kinase C-dependent processes remain to be defined in cardiovascular tissue. Most notably, the apparent synergistic interactions of protein kinase C and calcium in metabolic signaling and the expression of contractile function are just beginning to be uncovered. Studies of these processes, the localization and functional characterization of protein kinase C isoforms, along with the definition of the biological importance of DAG and related protein kinase C activators, such as prostaglandins, should provide valuable therapeutic insights into the control of cardiovascular contractility and heart disease.

REFERENCES

1. Nishizuka Y. Studies and perspectives of protein kinase C. Science 1986; 233: 305–12.
2. Nishizuka Y. The molecular heterogeneity of protein kinase C and its implications for cellular regulation. Nature 1988; 334: 661–5.
3. Nishizuka Y. The family of protein kinase C for signal transduction. JAMA 262: 1826–33.
4. Kishimoto A, Takai Y, Mori T, Kikkawa U, Nishizuka Y. Activation of calcium and phospholipid-dependent protein kinase by diacylglycerol. Its possible relation to phosphatidylinositol turnover. J Biol Chem 1980; 255: 2273–6.
5. Hirota K, Hirota T, Aguilera G, Catt KJ. Hormone-induced redistribution of calcium-activated phospholipid-dependent protein kinase in pituitary gonadotrophs. J Biol Chem 1985; 260: 3243–6.
6. Bell RM, Kennady DA, Stanford N, Majerus PW. Diglyceride lipase: a pathway for arachidonate release from human platelets. Proc Natl Acad Sci USA 1979; 76: 3238–41.
7. MacDonald ML, Mack K, Williams BW, King WC, Glomset JA. A membrane-bound diacylglycerol kinase that selectively phosphorylates arachidonoyl-diacylglycerol. Distinction from cytosolic diacylglycerol kinase and comparison with the membrane-bound enzyme from Escherichia coli. J Biol Chem 1988; 263: 1584–92.
8. Griendling KK, Rittenhouse SE, Brock TA, Ekstein LS, Gimbrone MA, Alexander RW. Sustained diacylglycerol formation from inositol phospholipids in angiotensin II-stimulated vascular smooth muscle cells. J Biol Chem 1986; 261: 5901–6.
9. Exton JH. Signalling through phosphatidylcholine breakdown. J Biol Chem 1990; 265: 1–4.
10. Besterman JM, Duronio V, Cuatrecasas P. Rapid formation of diacylglycerol from phosphatidylcholine: a pathway for generation of a second messenger. Proc Natl Acad Sci USA 1986; 83: 6785–9.
11. Takai Y, Kishimoto A, Inoue M, Nishizuka Y. Studies on a cyclic nucleotide-independent protein kinase and its proenzyme in mammalian tissues. I. Purification and characterization of an active enzyme from bovine brain. J Biol Chem 1977; 252: 7603–9.
12. House C, Kemp BE. Protein kinase C contains a psuedosubstrate prototope in its regulatory domain. Science 1987; 238: 1726–8.
13. Kikkawa U, Takai T, Minakuchi R, Inohara S, Nishizuka Y. Calcium-activated, phospholipid-dependent protein kinase from rat brain. Subcellular distribution, purification and properties. J Biol Chem 1982; 257: 13341–8.
14. Ohki K, Yamauchi T, Banno Y, Nozawa Y. A possible role of stimulus-enhanced phosphatidylinositol turnover: calcium-sparing effect of diacylglycerol in inducing

phase separation of phosphatidylcholine/phosphatidylserine mixtures. Biochem Biophys Res Commun 1981; 200: 321–7.
15. Bazzi MD, Nelsestuen GL. Role of substrate imparting calcium and phospholipid requirements to protein kinase C activation. Biochemistry 1987; 26: 1974–82.
16. DiVirgillo F, Lew DP, Pozzan T. Protein kinase C activation of physiologic processes in human neutrophils at vanishingly small cytosolic Ca^{2+} levels. Nature 1984; 310: 691–3.
17. Sekiguchi K, Tsukuda M, Ase K, Kikkawa U, Nishizuka Y. Mode of activation and kinetic properties of three distinct forms of protein kinase C from rat brain. J Biochem 1988; 103: 759–65.
18. Ohno S, Kawasaki H, Imajoh S, Suzuki K, Inagaki M, Yokokura H, Sakoh T, Hidaka H. Tissue-specific expression of three distinct types of rabbit protein kinase C. Nature 1987; 325: 161–6.
19. Huang KP, Huang FL, Nakabayashi H, Yoshida Y. Expression and function of protein kinase C isozymes. Acta Endocrinol (Cophenh) 1989; 121: 307–16.
20. Castagna M, Takai Y, Kaibuchi K, Sano K, Kikkawa U, Nishizuka Y. Direct activation of calcium-activated phospholipid-dependent protein kinase by tumor-promoting phorbol esters. J Biol Chem 1982; 257: 7847–51.
21. Neidel JE, Kuhn LJ, Vandenbark GR. Phorbol diester copurifies with protein kinase C. Proc Natl Acad Sci USA 1983; 80: 36–40.
22. Ramsdell JS, Petit GR, Tashijian AH. Three activators of protein kinase C, bryostatins, dioleins, and phorbol esters, show differing specificities of action on GH_4 pituitary cells. J Biol Chem 1986; 261: 17073–80.
23. Bazzi MD, Nelsestuen GL. Differences in the effects of phorbol esters and diacylglycerols on protein kinase C. Biochemistry 1989; 28: 9317–23.
24. Akita Y, Ohno S, Konmo A, Suzuki K. Expression and properties of two distinct classes of the phorbol ester receptor family, four conventional protein kinase C types, and a novel protein kinase C. J Biol Chem 1990; 265: 354–62.
25. Sutherland C, Walsh MP. Activation of protein kinase C by the blocker dihydropyridine calcium channel blocker, felodipine. Biochem Pharmacol 1989; 38: 1263–70.
26. Hidaka H, Hagiwara M. Pharmacology of the isoquinoline sulfonamide protein kinase C inhibitors. Trends Pharmacol Sci 1987; 8: 162–4.
27. McDonald JR, Groschel-Stewart U, Walsh MP. Properties and distribution of the protein inhibitor (M_r 17000) of protein kinase C. Biochem J 1987; 242: 695–702.
28. Takahashi I, Nakanishi S, Nakano H, Suzuki K, Tamaoki T. Hypericin and pseudohypericin inhibit protein kinase C: possible relation to their antiretroviral activity. Biochem Biophys Res Commun 1989; 165: 1207–12.
29. Nakadate T, Jeng AY, Blumberg PM. Comparison of protein kinase C functional assays to clarify mechanisms of inhibitor action. Biochem Pharmacol 1988; 37: 1541–5.
30. Pearson JD, DeWald DB, Mathews WR, Mozier NM, Zurcher-Neely HA, Heinrikson RL, Morris MA, McCubbin WD, McDonald JR, Fraser ED, Vogel HJ, Kay CM, Walsh MP. Amino acid sequence and characterization of a protein inhibitor of protein kinase C. J Biol Chem 1990; 265: 4583–91.
31. Baraban JM, Gould RJ, Peroutka SJ, Snyder SH. Phorbol ester effects on neurotransmission: Interaction with neurotransmitters and calcium in smooth muscle. Proc Natl Acad Sci USA 1985; 82: 604–7.
32. Legan E, Chernow B, Parillo J, Roth BL. Activation of phosphatidylinositol turnover in rat aorta by α1-adrenergic receptor stimulation. Eur J Pharmacol 1985; 110: 389–90.
33. Galizzi JP, Qar J, Fosset M, VanRenterghem C, Lazdunski M. Regulation of calcium channels in aortic muscle cells by protein kinase C activators (diacylglycerol and phorbol esters) and by peptides (vasopressin and bombesin) that stimulate phosphoinositide breakdown. J Biol Chem 1987; 262: 6947–50.

34. Rasmussen H, Takuwa Y, Park S. Protein kinase C in the regulation of smooth muscle contraction. FASEB J 1987; 1: 177–85.
35. Lee TS, Chao T, Hu KQ, King GL. Endothelin stimulates a sustained 1,2-diacylglycerol increase and protein kinase C activation in bovine aortic smooth muscle cells. Biochem Biophys Res Commun 1989; 162: 381–6.
36. Danthuluri NR, Deth RC. Phorbol ester-induced contraction of arterial smooth muscle and inhibition of α-adrenergic response. Biochem Biophys Res Commun 1984; 125: 1103–9.
37. Forder J, Scriabine A, Rasmussen H. Plasma membrane calcium flux, protein kinase C activation and smooth muscle contraction. J Pharmacol Exp Ther 1985; 235: 267–73.
38. Jagadeesh G, Deth RC. Phorbol ester-induced modulation of agonist binding to Alpha-1 adrenergic receptors in bovine aortic membranes. J Pharmacol Exp Ther 1988; 247: 196–202.
39. Vigne P, Brettmayer JP, Duval D, Frelin C, Lazdunski M. The Na^+/Ca^{2+} antiporter in aortic smooth muscle cells—characterization and demonstration of an activation by phorbol esters. J Biol Chem 1988; 263: 8078–83.
40. Phaneuf S, Berta P, LePeuch C, Haiech J, Cavadore JC. Phorbol ester modulation of cyclic AMP accumulation in a primary culture of rat aortic smooth muscle cells. J Pharmacol Exp Ther 1988; 245: 1042–7.
41. Leeb-Lundberg LMF, Cotecchia S, Lomasney JW, DeBernardis JF, Lefkowitz RJ, Caron MG. Phorbol esters promote alpha 1-adrenergic receptor phosphorylation and receptor uncoupling from inositol phospholipid metabolism. Proc Natl Acad Sci USA 1985; 82: 5651–5.
42. Brock TA, Rittenhouse SE, Powers CW, Ekstein LS, Gimbrone MA, Alexander RW. Phorbol ester and 1-oleoyl-2-acetylglycerol inhibit angiotensin activation of phospholipase C in cultured vascular smooth muscle cells. J Biol Chem 1985; 260: 14158–62.
43. Katada T, Gilman AG, Watanabe Y, Bauer S, Jacobs KH. Protein kinase C phosphorylates the inhibitory guanine-nucleotide-binding regulatory component and apparently suppresses its function in hormonal inhibition of adenylate cyclase. Eur J Biochem 1985; 151: 431–7.
44. Pyne NJ, Murphy GJ, Milligan G, Houslay MD. Treatment of intact hepatocytes with either the phorbol ester TPA or glucagon elicits the phosphorylation and functional inactivation of the inhibitory guanine nucleotide protein Gi. FEBS Lett 1989; 243: 77–82.
45. Kariya K, Kawahara Y, Fukuzaki H, Hagiwara M, Hidaka H, Fukimoto Y, Takai Y. Two types of protein kinase C with different functions in cultured rabbit aortic smooth muscle cells. Biochem Biophys Res Commun 1989; 161: 1020–7.
46. Sybertz EJ, Desiderio DM, Tetzloff G, Chiu PJS. Phorbol dibutyrate contractions in rabbit aorta: calcium dependence to nitrovasodilators and 8-Br-cyclic GMP. J Pharmacol Exp Ther 1986; 239: 78–83.
47. Jiang MJ, Morgan KG. Intracellular calcium levels in phorbol ester-induced contractions of vascular smooth muscle. Am J Physiol 1987; 253: H1365–71.
48. Itoh T, Kanmura Y, Kuriyama H, Sumimoto K. A phorbol ester has dual actions on the mechanical response in the rabbit mesenteric and porcine coronary arteries. J Physiol (Lond) 1986; 375: 515–34.
49. Miller JR, Hawkins DJ, Wells JN. Phorbol diesters alter the contractile responses of porcine coronary artery. J Pharmacol Exp Ther 1986; 239: 38–42.
50. Laher I, Vorkapic P, Dowd AL, Bevan JA. Protein kinase C potentiates stretch-induced cerebral artery tone by increasing intracellular sensitivity to Ca^{2+}. Biochem Biophys Res Commun 1989; 165: 312–8.
51. Chaterjee M, Tejada M. Phorbol ester-induced contraction in chemically skinned smooth muscle. Am J Physiol 1986; 251: C356–61.

52. MacKay MJ, Cheung DW. Increased reactivity in the mesenteric artery of spontaneously hypertensive rats to phorbol esters. Biochem Biophys Res Commun 1989; 145: 1105–11.
53. Ruzycky AL, Morgan KG. Involvement of the protein kinase C system in calcium–force relationships in ferret aorta. Br J Pharmacol 1989; 97: 391–400.
54. Heaslip RJ, Sickels BD. Evidence that prostaglandins can contract the rat aorta via a novel protein kinase C-dependent mechanism. J Pharmacol Exp Ther 1989; 250: 44–51.
55. Morgan JP, Morgan KG. Stimulus-specific patterns of intracellular calcium levels in smooth muscle of the ferret portal vein. J Physiol (Lond) 1984; 351: 155–67.
56. Jiang MJ, Morgan KG. Agonist-specific myosin phosphorylation and intracellular calcium during isometric contractions of arterial smooth muscle. Pflugers Arch 1989; 413: 637–43.
57. Rembold CM, Murphy RA. Myoplasmic calcium, myosin phosphorylation, and the regulation of cross bridge cycling in swine arterial smooth muscle. Circ Res 1986; 58: 803–15.
58. Umekawa H, Hidaka H. Phosphorylation of caldesmon by protein kinase C. Biochem Biophys Res Commun 1985; 132: 56–62.
59. Park S, Rasmussen H. Carbachol-induced protein phosphorylation changes in bovine tracheal smooth muscle. J Biol Chem 1986; 261: 15734–9.
60. Pritchard K, Moody CJ. Caldesmon: a calmodulin-binding actin-regulatory protein. Cell Calcium 1986; 7: 309–28.
61. Tsuda T, Griendling KK, Alexander RW. Angiotensin II and endothelin induce sustained, protein kinase C-mediated protein phosphorylation in cultured vascular smooth muscle cells. Circulation 1989; 80 (Supp 2): II–441.
62. Laher I, Vorkapic P, Dowd AL, Bevan JA. Protein kinase C potentiates stretch-induced cerebral artery tone by increasing intracellular sensitivity to Ca^{2+}. Biochem Biophys Res Commun 1989; 165: 312–8.
63. Kulik TJ, Rothman A, Glennon ET, Underwood RH. Stretching vascular smooth muscle causes inositol phosphates (IP) turnover. Circulation 1989; 80 (Supp 2): II–198.
64. Hsieh CP, Dage RC. Selective dilation of large coronary arteries in the dog by MDL 27,032, a protein kinase C inhibitor. FASEB J 1989; 3: A896.
65. Leatherman GF, Kim D, Smith TW. Effect of phorbol esters on contractile state and calcium influx in cultured chick heart. Am J Physiol 1987; 253: H205–9.
66. Yuan S, Sunahara FA, Sen AK. Tumor-promoting phorbol esters inhibit cardiac functions and induce redistribution of protein kinase C in perfused beating rat heart. Circ Res 1987; 61: 372–8.
67. Teutsch I, Weible A, Siess M. Differential inotropic and chronotropic effects of various protein kinase C activators on isolated guinea pig atria. Eur J Pharmacol 1987; 144: 363–7.
68. Rogers TB, Gaa ST, Massey C, Dosemeci A. Protein kinase C inhibits Ca^{2+} accumulation in cardiac sarcoplasmic reticulum. J Biol Chem 1990; 265: 4302–8.
69. Dosemeci A, Dhallan MRS, Cohen NM, Lederer WJ, Rogers TB. Phorbol ester increases calcium current and stimulates the effects of angiotensin II on cultured neonatal rat heart myocytes. Circ Res 1988; 62: 347–57.
70. Gwathmey JK, Hajjar RJ. Regulation of cardiac function by protein kinase C activation in human myocardium. Circulation 1988 78 (Supp 2): II–266.
71. Watson JE, Karmazyn M. Amiloride attenuates the negative inotropic effect of phorbol 12-myristate 13-acetate: possible role of Na^+/H^+ exchange. Circulation 1989; 80 (Supp 2): II–127.
72. Capograssi M, Kaku T, Filburn CR, Pelto DJ, Hansford RG, Spurgeon HA, Lakatta EG. Phorbol ester and dioctanoylglycerol stimulate membrane association of protein

kinase C and have a negative inotropic effect mediated by changes in cytosolic Ca^{2+} in adult rat cardiac myocytes. Circ Res 1990; 66: 1143–55.
73. Mazzei GJ, Kuo JF. Phosphorylation of skeletal-muscle troponin I and troponin T by phospholipid-sensitive Ca^{2+}-dependent protein kinase and its inhibition by troponin C and tropomyosin. Biochem J 1984; 218: 361–9.
74. Noland TA, Raynor RL, Kuo JF. Identification of sites phosphorylated in bovine cardiac troponin I and troponin T by protein kinase C and comparative substrate activity of synthetic peptides containing the phosphorylation sites. J Biol Chem 1989; 264: 20778–85.
75. Liu JD, Wood JG, Raynor RL, Wang YC, Noland TA, Ansari AA, Kuo JF. Subcellular distribution and immunocytochemical localization of protein kinase C in myocardium, and phosphorylation of troponin in isolated myocytes stimulated by isoproterenol or phorbol ester. Biochem Biophys Res Commun 1989; 162: 1105–10.
76. Lacerda AE, Rampe D, Brown AM. Effects of protein kinase C activators on cardiac Ca^{2+} channels. Nature 1988; 335: 249–51.
77. Iwakura K, Watanabe Y, Hori M, Kusuoka H, Yoshida H. α_1-Adrenergic stimulation attenuates the voltage dependent Ca^{2+} influx through C kinase activation in isolated cardiomyocytes. Circulation 1988; 78 (Suppl 2): II–334.
78. Moorman JR, Kirsch GE, Lacerda AE, Brown AM. Angiotensin II modulates cardiac Na^+ channels in neonatal rat. Circ Res 1989; 65: 1804–9.
79. Brown AM, Yatani A, Codina J, Birnbaumer L. Gating of muscarinic K^+ channels by G proteins. Prog Clin Biol Res 1990; 334: 303–12.
80. Creazzo TL, Wrenn RW. Increased muscarinic receptor binding in heart membranes by an inhibitor of protein kinase C. FEBS Lett 1988; 242: 175–7.
81. Wrenn RW, Barrow MA, Redmond ME. Protein kinase C (calcium/phospholipid-dependent protein kinase) in developing chick heart: selective localization to atrium versus ventricle and changes in activity levels during cardiogenesis. Biochem Biophys Acta 1988; 972: 110–2.
82. Shuntoh H, Tanaka C. Activation of protein kinase C potentiates norepinephrine release from sinus node. Am J Physiol 1986; 251: C833–40.
83. Yada T, Rose B, Loewenstein WR. Diacylglycerol downregulates junctional membrane permeability. TMB-8 blocks this effect. J Membr Biol 1985; 88: 217–32.
84. Sibley DR, Nambi P, Peter JR, Lefkowitz RJ. Phorbol diesters promote beta-adrenergic receptor phosphorylation and adenylate cyclase desensitization in duck erythrocytes. Biochem Biophys Res Commun 1984; 121: 973–9.
85. Browning MD, Bureau M, Dudek EM, Olsen RW. Protein kinase C and cAMP-dependent protein kinase phosphorylate the beta subunit of the purified gamma-aminobutyric acid A receptor. Proc Natl Acad Sci USA 1990; 87: 1315–8.
86. Uglesity A, Sharma VK, Sheu SS. Effects of protein kinase C activation on the inotropic response induced by α-adrenoceptor stimulation in rat myocardium. Biophys J 1987; 51: 264a.
87. Bouvier M, Leeb-Lundberg LM, Benovic JL, Caron MG, Lefkowitz RJ. Regulation of adrenergic receptor function by phosphorylation. II. Effects of agonist occupancy on phosphorylation of alpha 1- and beta 2-adrenergic receptors by protein kinase C and the cyclic AMP-dependent protein kinase. J Biol Chem 1987; 262: 3106–13.
88. Okamura K, Kondo J, Hashimoto H, Ito T. 1,2-Diacylglycerol level in norepinephrine-stimulated aorta of spontaneously hypertensive rats. Circulation 1989 80 (Supp II): II–541.
89. Holzer P, Lippe IT. Protein kinase C may regulate the tonic component of intestinal smooth muscle contraction in response to substance P. Naunyn-Schmeidbergs Arch Pharmacol 1989; 339: 214–20.

90. Sasaguri T, Watson SP. Protein kinase C regulates the tonic but not the phasic component of contraction in the guinea-pig ileum. Br J Pharmacol 1989; 98: 791–8.
91. Ford DA, Gross RW. Activation of myocardial protein kinase C by plasmalogenic diglycerides. Am J Physiol 1990; 258: C30–6.
92. Ikeda U, Arisaka H, Takayasu T, Takeda K, Natsume T, Hosoda S. Protein kinase C activation aggravates hypoxic myocardial injury by stimulating Na^+/H^+ exchange. J Mol Cell Cardiol 1988; 20: 493–500.
93. Strasser RH, Dullaeus RB, Marquetant R. β-Receptor-independent sensitization of adenylyl cyclase by activation of protein kinase C in acute myocardial ischemia. Circulation 1989; 80 (Suppl II): II–442.
94. Adachi K, Sakanashi T, Sako S, Yamamoto K, Mayumi F, Koga Y, Toshima H. Expression of protein kinase C in endomyocardial biopsies in idiopathic cardiomyopathy. Circulation 1989; 80 (Suppl II): II–675.
95. Chambers TC, Elion G. Heart protein kinase C activity during progression of disease in the cardiomyopathic hamster. Biochem Biophys Res Commun 1988; 157: 504–14.
96. Khalil RA, Morgan KG. Imaging of protein kinase C distribution and translocation in living vascular smooth muscle cells. Circ Res 1991; 69: 1626–31.
97. Pawlowski J, Morgan KG. Mechanisms of intrinsic tone in ferret vascular smooth muscle. J Physiol 1992; 448: 121–32.

15

Basic Aspects of Na^+, K^+-ATPase

TAI AKERA

Merck Research Laboratories
Division of Merck & Co., Inc.
West Point, Pennsylvania

YUK-CHOW NG

Pennsylvania State University
Hershey, Pennsylvania

I. STRUCTURES AND FUNCTIONS

Na^+,K^+-ATPase is an enzymatic representation of the sodium pump. The functioning enzyme unit is a dimer consisting of two α-subunits and two β-subunits. The α-subunits have been shown to have at least three isoforms: α-1, α-2, and α-3 (1,2). These isoforms have different sensitivities for inhibition by cardiac glycosides (1,3–6). In addition, differences in activation by Na^+ ions (7,8), or regulation of gene expression responding to thyroid hormone (9,10) changes in intracellular Na^+ or extracellular K^+ concentrations, and during perinatal development (11,12b) have been suggested. The α-subunit is a transmembrane protein. All known functional sites of the enzyme, namely the binding sites for Mg^{2+}, ATP, Na^+, K^+, and also for cardiac glycosides, are associated with α-subunits. The β-subunits also have isoforms: β-1 and β-2 (12a). The β-subunits too are under hormonal regulation (9); however, the functions of the β-subunits are presently unknown.

The α-subunits of Na^+,K^+-ATPase undergo a cycle of conformational transitions, associated with phosphorylation from ATP and subsequent dephosphorylation, as the enzyme hydrolyzes ATP. The conformational transitions are likely to be related to the active transport of Na^+ and K^+ across the cytoplasmic membrane. The reaction cycle of the Na^+,K^+-ATPase as related to the active transport of monovalent cations is depicted schematically in Figure 1. The biological significance of the Na^+,K^+-ATPase is the active transport of monovalent cations (= sodium pump activity), and not the hydrolysis of ATP, even though the name ATPase emphasizes the latter biochemical aspect. In cardiac muscle, the hydrolysis of ATP resulting from Na^+,K^+-ATPase activity is estimated to account for less than 5% of the total ATP utilization under normal conditions (13). The percentage of energy utilization (= ATP hydrolysis) attributable to Na^+,K^+-ATPase activity is greater in neuronal tissues, probably reaching as much as 40% (14). This is because the primary func-

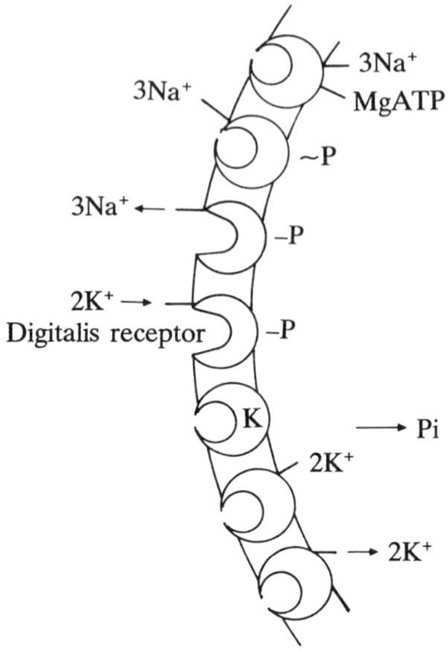

Figure 1 The reaction cycle of Na^+,K^+-ATPase.

tions of neuronal cells (i.e., the conduction of impulses), are associated with transmembrane movements of monovalent cations. In other types of cells in which functions other than transmembrane movements of Na^+ and K^+ are important, the fraction of energy utilization attributable to the sodium pump is smaller. In the cardiac muscle, energy utilization by the sarcoplasmic retaliation calcium pump is calculated to be larger than that for the sodium pump, and the contraction mechanisms uses the largest fraction of energy (13).

The Na^+,K^+-ATPase reaction and sodium pump activity proceed as follow. One unit of enzyme binds 3 molecules of Na^+ and 1 molecule of Mg^{2+}-ATP at the site facing the cytoplasm (Fig. 1). With the transfer of the terminal phosphate of ATP to the enzyme and an associated conformational change, Na^+ ions are transported to the site facing the extracellular space. From these sites, Na^+ ions are released to the extra cellular space, and then 2 K^+ ions combine with the enzyme. With a second conformational change, K^+ ions are transported to the site facing the cytoplasm and released inside the cell. During the transport of K^+, the enzyme takes a form in which K^+ ions are inaccessible from either the extracellular or intracellular medium. This form is called the "occluded" form of the enzyme. Under physiological conditions, the release of K^+ from the enzyme is the rate-limiting step for the reaction cycle.

In Na^+,K^+-ATPase preparations obtained from cell fragments, the sidedness, and the active transport of cations, cannot be observed. The Na^+,K^+-ATPase, however, is apparently undergoing cycles of conformational transitions related to its function. This is apparent from the fact that binding of cardiac glycosides to isolated Na^+,K^+-ATPase observed in vitro is enhanced by Na^+, Mg^{2+}, and ATP, and inhibited by K^+ in the presence of the above ligands. The glycoside-binding site is more easily accessible in the Na^+-induced form than the K^+-induced form of the enzyme (Fig. 1). If K^+ binds to the Na^+-induced form of Na^+,K^+-ATPase before cardiac glycosides, the accessibility of the glycoside binding site becomes less. If K^+ binds to the Na^+-induced form of the sodium pump after glycoside binding, the release of bound glycoside from the enzyme becomes slower. In intact cells, the intracellular Na^+ and extracellular K^+ have these effects.

The stoichiometry of the sodium pump (i.e., 3 Na^+ and 2 K^+ are transported during each functional cycle associated with hydrolysis of one molecule of ATP), would appear flexible (15). In myocardial cells, membrane depolarization is caused by a sudden Na^+ influx. This is followed by Ca^{2+} influx that is essential for maintaining the plateau phase of the action potential. Subsequently, K^+ channels open and K^+ efflux occurs resulting in repolarization of the membrane potential. K^+ efflux increases during phase 3 of the action potential; however, K^+ efflux decreases during the plateau phase of the action potential. Therefore, time-averaged K^+ efflux rate is relatively independent of the frequency of membrane excitations. In contrast, the rate of Na^+ influx is determined by the frequency of membrane depolarizations. As a result, the amount of Na^+ entering the cell during a given period, say 1 min, and hence the amount of Na^+ that has to be pumped out during the same period to maintain overall ionic steady state, is larger when the heart rate is high and is lower when the heart rate is low. Because the amounts of K^+ to be pumped into the cell are relatively independent of the heart rate, the stoichiometry of the Na^+/K^+ exchange must be flexible unless other mechanisms compensate for the flexible Na^+/K^+ ratio.

There are other mechanisms that transport Na^+ and K^+. These are the Na^+/Ca^{2+} exchanger, Na^+/H^+ exchanger, and Na^+,K^+,Cl^- cotransporter. Among these, the first two mechanisms do not appear to play major roles in compensating for the flexible Na^+/K^+ ratio. This is because the amount of Na^+ to be transported to maintain ionic equilibrium (on the order of 4.2 mmoles/kg/min or 50 μmol/kg/beat; 15) would have too large an impact on intracellular Ca^{2+} or H^+ concentrations (= less than 1 μmole/Liter) if equivalent amounts of Ca^{2+} or H^+ are countertransported to compensate for the imbalance between passive Na^+ and K^+ fluxes and the Na^+/K^+ exchange ratio of the sodium pump. The Na^+,K^+,Cl^- cotransporter is the candidate for the mechanism that compensates for the imbalance between the passive Na^+ and K^+ flux ratio and active transport ratio. It is presently unknown whether the imbalance is compensated for by the flexibility of the sodium pump stoichiometry or the activity of the Na^+,K^+,Cl^- cotransporter.

As discussed above, glycoside-binding sites for the sodium pump appear to open and become easily accessible to cardiac glycosides when the enzyme is in the Na^+-induced phosphorylated form. Therefore, glycoside binding to the isolated Na^+,K^+-ATPase is enhanced in the simultaneous presence of Na^+, Mg^{2+}, and ATP (Fig. 1). The simultaneous presence of these ligands, however, is not an absolute requirement. Binding of cardiac glycosides to isolated Na^+,K^+-ATPase is also enhanced in the presence of Mg^{2+} and inorganic phosphate. There are significant differences in the glycoside–enzyme complex formed in the presence of Na^+, Mg^{2+}, and ATP (type I complex) and that formed in the presence of Mg^{2+} and inorganic phosphate (type II complex). The rate of release of bound glycosides from the type I complex is relatively fast and is inhibited by the subsequent addition of K^+. In contrast, the rate of release of glycosides from the type II complex is slow and insensitive to the addition of K^+. Moreover, cardiac glycosides can bind to Na^+,K^+-ATPase in the absence of any ligands or in the presence of Mg^{2+} alone if the concentration of the glycosides is high and the enzyme is incubated with the glycosides for a sufficiently long period of time. Although cardiac glycosides bind to the Na^+,K^+-ATPase under various conditions, the type I complex formed in the presence of Na^+, Mg^{2+}, and ATP appears to represent glycoside binding to the sodium pump in intact cells.

II. FACTORS AND AGENTS THAT MODIFY Na^+,K^+-ATPase ACTIVITY

A. Na^+, K^+, Mg^{2+}, and ATP

When Na^+,K^+-ATPase activity is assayed in vitro using isolated membrane fragments, the rate of ATP hydrolysis is dependent on concentrations of Na^+, K^+, Mg^{2+}, and ATP. In intact cells, the turnover rate of the sodium pump is also affected by these "substrates." The apparent Km value for ATP at the catalytic site, as determined using isolated enzyme preparations, is about 1 μM. The rate of ATP hydrolysis, however, is influenced by the concentration of ATP ranging from 0.1 to 1 mM, which should be saturating at the catalytic site. This is because Na^+,K^+-ATPase has a second binding site for ATP, namely, the regulatory site. Binding of ATP to the regulatory site, which has an apparent Km value in the millimolar range, increases the turnover rate of the Na^+,K^+-ATPase.

Determination of the Km values for Na^+ and K^+ is complicated by the fact that both Na^+ and K^+ have to be present in the assay medium for Na^+,K^+-ATPase activity and that Na^+ and K^+ compete with each other at activating sites for K^+ and Na^+, respectively. In intact cells, intracellular Na^+ and extracellular K^+ activate the sodium pump. Activation by intracellular Na^+ (approximately 10 mM) is antagonized by intracellular K^+ (approximately 150 mM); and activation by extracellular K^+ (approximately 5 mM) is antagonized by extracellular Na^+ (approximately 150 mM). This means that the Na^+ or K^+ activation curve is shifted to the right compared to the position predicted from the theoretical Km values estimated by extrapolating observed values to those in the absence of competing cations. Therefore, sodium pump activity is sensitive to changes in intracellular Na^+ and extracellular K^+ concentrations at levels apparently higher than the reported Km values.

The influence of intracellular Mg^{2+} and ATP on sodium pump activity seems relatively minor in normal cells because concentrations of these ligands are saturating. In tissues exposed to severe ischemia or hypoxemia, however, sodium pump activity may be reduced as the result of low ATP concentrations (16).

B. Specific Inhibitors Acting at the Digitalis Receptor

Before the discovery of Na^+,K^+-ATPase in crab nerve (17), digitalis glycosides had been shown to inhibit the active transport of monovalent cations across the cell membrane. The fact that the cardiac glycoside ouabain inhibits Na^+,K^+-ATPase activity was, therefore, used to show that Na^+,K^+-ATPase represents the sodium pump. Subsequently, Na^+,K^+-ATPase has been shown to be uniquely sensitive to the inhibitory action of pharmacologically active cardiac glycosides. Conversely, Na^+,K^+-ATPase inhibition has been shown to be the only biochemical effect that can be observed with low concentrations of the cardiac glycosides (18). Thus, the digitalis glycosides and related aglycones are specific inhibitors of the Na^+,K^+-ATPase.

The α-subunit of Na^+,K^+-ATPase has binding sites complementary to the steroid nucleus, unsaturated lactone ring, and the first sugar moiety of cardiac glycosides (Fig. 2). The three-point attachment is apparently responsible for high affinity of the enzyme for cardiac glycosides such as digoxin, digitoxin, asnd ouabain. Aglycones lacking the sugar moiety have an affinity about an order of magnitude lower than the corresponding glycoside. Digoxin and digitoxin have three digitoxisoses attached to the lactone–steroid structure. The second and the third sugars do not contribute to stronger binding, indicating that Na^+,K^+-ATPase does not have binding sites complementary to the second and third sugars of the glycosides. Alterations in the lactone ring, such as saturation of the lactone ring (e.g., dihydrodigoxin), or a change in the position of the double bond (e.g., actodigin), markedly reduce the affinity of these compounds.

Structure–activity relationship studies have revealed relatively strict requirements for active cardiac glycosides. These are: 1. an unsaturated lactone ring at C14, 2. a sugar component attached to the C3 position, 3. a steroid nucleus with a *cis* configuration at the C–D junction, and 4. a C14 β-hydroxyl group (Fig. 2). It should be pointed out, however, that several compounds apparently satisfy none of these requirements and yet apparently bind to the glycoside receptor. For example, cassaine is an alkaloid having a relatively flexible structure compared to the rigid structure of pharmacologically active cardiac glycosides. Nevertheless, cassaine is a specific inhibitor of Na^+,K^+-ATPase that binds to the enzyme at the glycoside receptor. Quaternary analogs, cassaine methiodide or ethiodide, do not inhibit

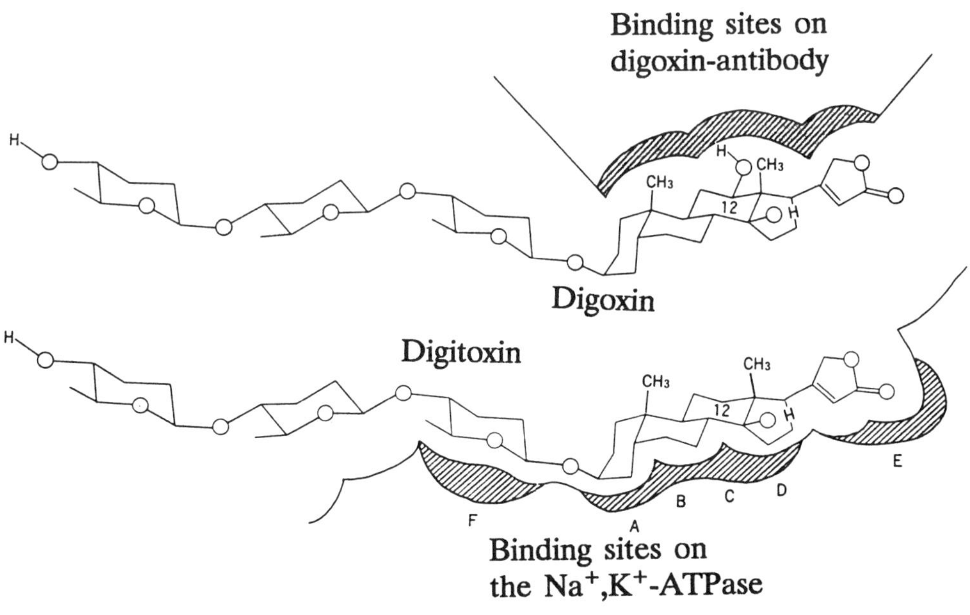

Figure 2 Binding sites on Na^+,K^+-ATPase and digoxin antibodies complementary to digitoxin and digoxin. The digitalis receptor on Na^+,K^+-ATPase does not differentiate between digoxin and digitoxin: the binding site fits the structure common to digoxin and digitoxin. Digoxin-antibodies, however, fail to recognize digitoxin: the binding site on the antibody recognizes the structure on digoxin that is not found on digitoxin.

Na^+,K^+-ATPase (19). Sanguinarine is a quaternary alkaloid shown to inhibit isolated Na^+,K^+-ATPase and produce a positive inotropic effect in isolated heart muscle preparations (20). Its tertiary analog chelidione does not inhibit Na^+,K^+-ATPase. It is presently unknown, however, if sanguinarine binds to the digitalis receptor on Na^+,K^+-ATPase. Benzylaminodihydrodimethoxyimidazoisoquinoline hydrochloride is an example of another flexible compound that inhibits Na^+,K^+-ATPase in low concentrations (21). Again, it is presently unknown if this compound binds at the digitalis receptor.

Corticosteroid hormones have a *trans* configuration at the C–D ring junction. These compounds do not inhibit Na^+,K^+-ATPase. A slight modification, however, enables corticosteroids with a C-D *trans* configuration to inhibit Na^+,K^+-ATPase. Examples of these modifications are prednisolone–bisguanylhydrazone (PBGH), chlormadinone acetate, and megestrol (22). It should be noted that PBGH, for example, loses its activity as a corticosteroid as the result of the modification. It is not well established, however, if all of these compounds inhibit Na^+,K^+-ATPase at the digitalis receptor. The mode of interaction of PBGH with the enzyme is not identical to that of cardiac glycosides. For example, patterns of affinity differences dependent upon the α-isoforms or species from which the enzyme preparations are obtained are remarkably different between PBGH and cardiac glycosides (23,24). The effects of Na^+, K^+, and ATP, however, are similar for glycoside and PBGH binding (23), suggesting that both inhibitors preferentially bind to the site that is more easily accessible in the Na^+-induced phosphorylated form (Fig. 1). The binding sites for digitalis glycosides and PBGH would appear to be closely related.

C. Inhibitors Acting at Other Sites

Several compounds inhibit Na^+,K^+-ATPase, apparently acting at sites other than the digitalis receptor. Among these, sulfhydryl blocking agents inhibit Na^+,K^+-ATPase by acting at the SH group on the cysteine residue near the phosphorylation site. In contrast to Na^+,K^+-ATPase inhibition by the cardiac glycoside, inhibition by sulfhydryl blocking agents is antagonized by the simultaneous presence of Na^+ and ATP in the presence of Mg^{2+} (25,26). The antagonism is partially relieved by K^+. (A recent study by Matsuda and Iwata [27] suggests more complex interactions; however, these investigators examined the effects of Na^+, K^+, or choline added alone in the absence of Mg^{2+} and ATP.) These results indicate that inhibitory site is more easily accessible when the enzyme is in the Ka^+-induced dephosphorylated form. The interaction of sulfhydryl blocking agents with Na^+,K^+-ATPase, however, is not completely understood. For example, both α-1 and α-2 isoforms of Na^+,K^+-ATPase have the cysteine residue near the phosphorylation site. Nevertheless, the α-2 isoform has significantly higher sensitivity to N-ethylmaleimide (NEM) than the α-1 isoform (28; Fig. 3). Moreover, α-1 and α-2 isoforms are equally sensitive to another sulfhydryl blocking agent, p-chloromercuribenzoate. NEM has a higher lipid solubility and hence should have a better access to all sulfhydryl groups. Therefore, inability of NEM to interact with the essential sulfhydryl group on the α-1 isoform of the Na^+,K^+-ATPase is difficult to explain.

Ethacrynic acid inhibits Na^+,K^+-ATPase irreversibly. Inhibition of isolated Na^+,K^+-ATPase by ethacrynic acid, however, is different from that by other sulfhydryl inhibitors because the inhibitory effect of ethacrynic acid is apparently enhanced,

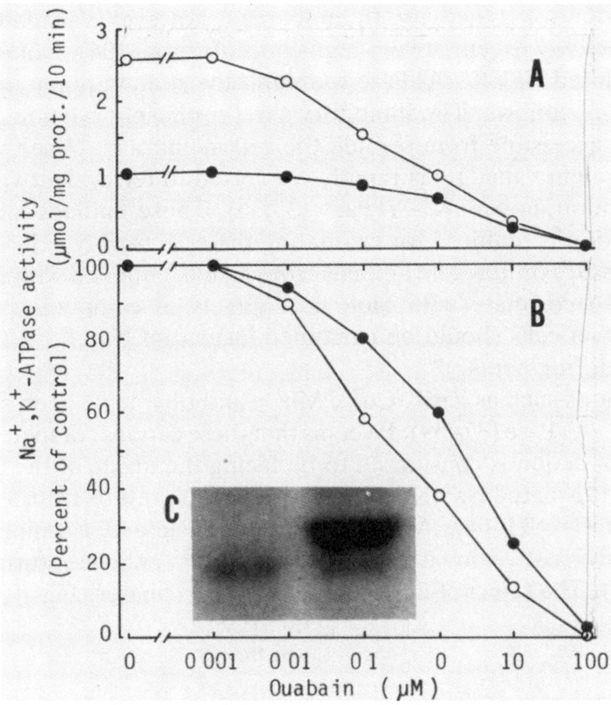

Figure 3 Inhibition of two isoforms of ferret heart Na^+,K^+-ATPase by n-ethylmaleimide (NEM). Partially purified Na^+,K^+-ATPase was pretreated with 1 mM NEM for 15 min (filled circles) and then assayed for enzyme activity. Control preparations were treated in the same manner in the absence of NEM (open circles). *A*. Na^+,K^+-ATPase activity in μmol Pi/mg protein/10 min. *B*. Relative Na^+,K^+-ATPase activity. *C* (*inset*). NEM-pretreated ferret heart Na^+,K^+-ATPase was phosphorylated from [gamma-^{32}P]ATP and separated on sodium dodicyl sulfide (SDS)-polyacrylamide gel. *Right lane*. Control; two isoforms are labeled. *Left lane*. NEM-pretreated preparation; the isoform with higher mobility is not labeled (= inactivated by NEM). (From Ref. 28.)

rather than reduced, by Na^+ and ATP (26). The α-subunit of Na^+,K^+-ATPase has several sulfhydryl groups. It would appear, therefore, necessary to understand which sulfhydryl groups are the target of the sulfhydryl blocking agents, and whether the targets for NEM, p-chloromercuribenzoate, or ethacrynic acid are the same or different.

Vanadate (VO_3^-) has been shown to be a potent inhibitor of isolated Na^+,K^+-ATPase (29). Inhibitory potency (ID_{50} value = approximately 0.6 μM) is not influenced by the source of the enzyme (30), indicating that different isoforms have similar affinity for vanadate. Inhibition is enhanced by Mg^{2+} and K^+, and antagonized by Na^+ and ATP (31–33). These results indicate that vanadate interacts with the dephosphorylated form of Na^+,K^+-ATPase. Vanadate substitutes for inorganic phosphate in supporting ouabain binding to the isolated Na^+,K^+-ATPase observed *in vitro* in the presence of Mg^{2+}. Apparently, vanadate has a very high affinity for the phosphate-binding site on Na^+,K^+-ATPase, and thereby inhibits the turnover of the enzyme that requires formation of the phosphoenzyme and subsequent dephosphorylation for its activity. In intact cells, however, vanadate fails to inhibit sodium pump activity except at very high concentrations (34). Failure of this potent inhibitor of isolated Na^+,K^+-ATPase to inhibit the sodium pump in intact cells has been explained as follows. The inhibitory site (= phosphorylation site on Na^+,K^+-ATPase) is not accessible from outside the cell membrane. When vanadate enters the cell, pentavalent vanadate is rapidly converted to tetravalent vanadyl, which is incapable of inhibiting Na^+,K^+-ATPase (35,36). These findings indicate that cautious extrapolation is required for estimating the effects of Na^+,K^+-ATPase inhibitors on intact tissues or in whole animals from results obtained with isolated enzyme preparations. To correlate with biological effects of compounds, sodium pump inhibition in intact cells should be examined instead of Na^+,K^+-ATPase inhibition with isolated cell fragments.

Divalent cations such as Zn^{2+}, Cu^{2+}, Mn^{2+}, and Pb^{2+} have been shown to inhibit isolated Na^+,K^+-ATPase (37–39). It seems that these cations compete with Mg^{2+}, and hence the site of action is considered to be facing the inside of the cell membrane. Ca^{2+} also inhibits isolated Na^+,K^+-ATPase. Inhibition results from a reduced rate of phosphorylation by ATP (40). When sodium pump activity is estimated in isolated myocyte preparations, removal of extracellular Ca^{2+} enhances turnover of the sodium pump (41). The effect of Ca^{2+} removal has two phases (Fig. 4); a reduction of

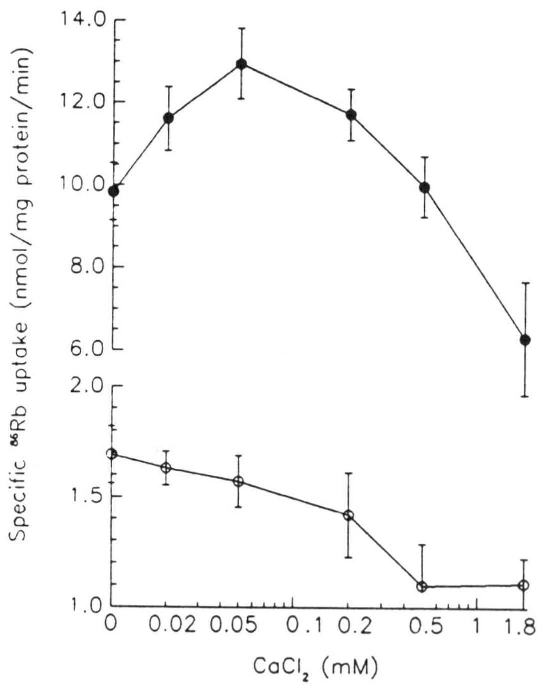

Figure 4 Effects of Ca^{2+} on sodium pump activity. Sodium pump activity was estimated from ouabain-sensitive $^{86}Rb^+$ uptake. Myocytes obtained from guinea pig heart were incubated at 37°C for 10 min with 1 mM ^{86}RbCl in the absence (open circles) or presence (filled circles) of 50 μM monensin. Monensin was used to increase Na^+ influx so that intracellular Na^+ is not the limiting factor for $^{86}Rb^+$ uptake. (From Ref. 42.)

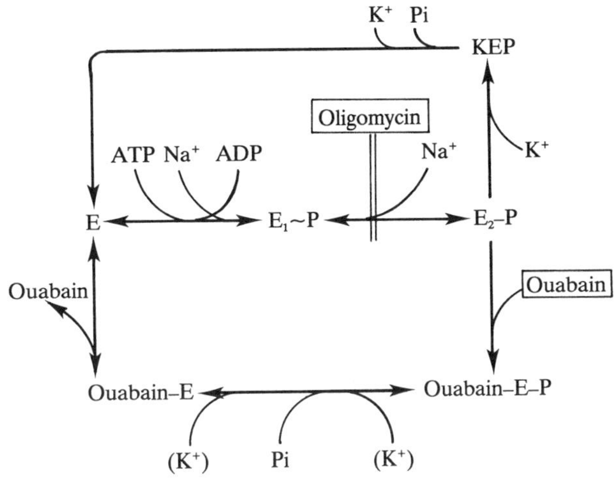

Figure 5 Proposed actions of Na$^+$,K$^+$-ATPase inhibitors, ouabain, oligomycin, and p-chloromercuribenzoate (PCMB). $E_1 \sim P$ and E_2-P represent forms of the phosphylated enzyme that can be dephosphorylated by ADP and K$^+$, respectively.

extracellular Ca^{2+} from 1.8 mM to 0.05 mM causes a significant increase in the ouabain-sensitive $^{86}Rb^+$ uptake and a further decrease causes a slight decrease in sodium pump activity (42). The effect of Ca^{2+} on the sodium pump may depend on the α isoform present in the tissue (43).

Oligomycin has been used to inhibit conversion between two phosphorylated forms of Na$^+$,K$^+$-ATPase: ATP-sensitive form and K$^+$ sensitive form (Fig. 5). It was useful in identifying the two forms of the phosphoenzyme (44). The site of action for oligomycin, however, is unknown. Moreover, the inhibitory effect of this metabolic inhibitor is not selective for Na$^+$,K$^+$-ATPase.

Many compounds have been reported to inhibit isolated Na$^+$,K$^+$-ATPase at relatively high concentrations. Examples of these compounds are diphenylhydantoin, hydroxylamine, chlorpromazine, fusidic acid, dimethylsulfoxide, phlorizin, ethanol, suramine, fatty acids, snake venom cardiotoxin, dichlorodiphenyltrichloroethane, polychlorinated biphenyls, anesthetics, rubratoxin B, quinidine, doxorubicin (Adriamycin), delta-9-tetrahydrocannabinol, and polyamines. Inhibition by these compounds generally requires relatively high concentrations, and their actions at these concentrations are not highly selective for Na$^+$,K$^+$-ATPase.

D. Endogenous Ligands for the Digitalis Receptor

The presence of specific receptors for the plant extract, opiates, lead to the discovery of endogenous ligands for the opioid receptors, enkephalins, and endorphines. The presence of endogenous ligands for the digitalis receptor has likewise been speculated on by many investigators. During the search for endogenous ligands for the digitalis receptor, it was found that lipid peroxidates cause inactivation of Na$^+$,K$^+$-ATPase and inhibit binding of antidigoxin antibodies. Irreversible inactivation of Na$^+$,K$^+$-ATPase or digoxin antibodies, however, does not represent binding of lipid peroxidates to the digitalis receptor. Activity of Na$^+$,K$^+$-ATPase is highly dependent on lipids surrounding the enzyme. Therefore, the direct action of lipid peroxidates on the enzyme protein or perturbation of surrounding lipids by the insertion of peroxidates appears to cause enzyme inhibition unrelated to occupancy of the digitalis receptor. Nevertheless, many papers have been published claiming that lipophilic extracts from plasma, tissues, or urine represent endogenous ligands for the digitalis receptor. Many of these extracts were later found to contain lipid extracts that do not satisfy the criteria for endogenous ligands for the digitalis receptor.

What are the criteria for endogenous ligands for the digitalis receptor? If the endogenous ligands have a mode of interaction similar to digitalis, they should have the following characteristics: 1. inhibition is specific for Na^+,K^+-ATPase, and the endogenous ligand should not inhibit Ca^{2+}-ATPase; 2. binding to the receptor, and ensuing enzyme inhibition, is enhanced by (intracellular) Na^+, Mg^{2+}, and ATP, and antagonized by (extracellular) K^+; 3. The endogenous ligand has a positive inotropic effect at concentrations similar to those required to cause 40–60% inhibition of Na^+,K^+-ATPase obtained from cardiac muscle of the same species; 4. Na^+,K^+-ATPase inhibition and the positive inotropic effect show marked species differences: potent in human or dog heart, intermediate in rabbit or guinea pig heart, and least potent in rat and mouse heart; 5. inhibition is reversible even though the rate of release of potent inhibitors from the digitalis receptor may be very slow. Related to this last point, several investigators have added an additional criterion that the slopes of the concentration–inhibition curves are similar to those observed with digoxin or ouabain. This is because irreversible inhibitors or those that destroy the enzyme have steeper concentration–inhibition curves.

Antibodies for digoxin have been used to detect digitalis-like principles. These antibodies, however, do not recognize digitoxin. The difference between digoxin and digitoxin is that digoxin has a hydroxyl group at the C-12 position (Fig. 2). Digoxin antibodies that do not react with digitoxin apparently recognize the region of digoxin around the C-12 position. This is not the recognition site for Na^+,K^+-ATPase, which does not differentiate between digoxin and digitoxin. Therefore, interaction with digoxin antibodies does not appear to be a valid criterion for endogenous ligands for the digitalis receptor.

There is no a priori reason to believe that endogenous ligands have exactly the same characteristics as the exogenous ligands digitalis glycosides. Nevertheless, the above criterion are related to the fundamental characteristics of Na^+,K^+-ATPase, and are most likely to be applicable to endogenous ligands for the digitalis receptor if the ligands exist. The search for endogenous ligands that satisfy all of the above criteria has been largely in vain; however, several investigators reported recently the presence of endogenous ligands that meet several of the above criteria (45–48).

There may be endogenous regulators of Na^+,K^+-ATPase that affect enzyme activity by mechanisms unrelated to the digitalis receptor. As discussed above, membrane lipids surrounding Na^+,K^+-ATPase influence enzyme and sodium pump activity. Therefore, modification of membrane lipids has been shown to affect Na^+,K^+-ATPase activity. Ca^{2+} ions are another example of physiological substance that may affect sodium pump activity (41–43). More recently, a family of three peptide inhibitors has been purified from procine duodenal extract (49). These peptide inhibitors apparently do not interact with Na^+,K^+-ATPase at the digitalis receptor.

III. MECHANISMS OF DIGITALIS ACTIONS

Even though the digitalis glycosides have been shown to be selective and specific inhibitors of Na^+,K^+-ATPase and the sodium pump (18), the hypothesis that sodium pump inhibition is the cause of the positive inotropic effect of the cardiac glycosides has not been accepted easily. The primary reason for the reluctance of many investigators to accept the above hypothesis is the finding that intracellular Na^+ concentration does not increase, and sometimes even decreases, in isolated heart muscle preparations exposed to positive inotropic concentrations of the glycoside. Apparently the failure to demonstrate the anticipated increase in intracellular Na^+ with the positive inotropic concentration of the cardiac glycoside resulted from technological problems. Estimation of changes in intracellular Na^+ ion activity by biochemical methods is fraught with problems because extracellular space, which accounts for approximately 30% of the tissue volume, has a several-fold higher Na^+ concentration and because more than 60% of the intracellular Na^+ is complexed with macromolecules and does not contribute to Na^+ ion activity. Studies with the Na^+-sensitive microelectrode, however, clearly demonstrated that the development of positive inotropic effect of strophanthidin, and the dissipation of the inotropic effect upon washout of strophanthidin, are associated with an increase, and the return to control levels, of intracellular Na^+ activity (50).

The current hypothesis as to the mechanisms of the positive inotropic effect of digitalis glycosides is as follows. Na^+,K^+-ATPase is the receptor molecule for the positive inotropic effect of digitalis glycosides. The receptor site is on the external surface of the cell membrane. Accessibility of the glycosides to the receptor is increased when the sodium pump transports Na^+ from the cytoplasm to the extracellular space, and the Na^+,K^+-ATPase protein is in the Na^+-induced conformation. When the glycoside binds to this form of the enzyme, the glycoside–enzyme complex may undergo a further conformational change induced by K^+. This conformational change stabilizes the glycoside–enzyme complex, which cannot turn over. Thus, the enzyme ceases to function as the sodium pump until bound glycoside is spontaneously released (Fig. 5).

The rate of spontaneous release of the glycoside from Na^+,K^+-ATPase is determined by temperature and ligand conditions. The absence of Mg^{2+} in a medium with low ionic strength enhances the rate of glycoside release. Under physiological conditions in which ionic strength and Mg^{2+} concentrations are high, the rate of release is determined by the chemical structure of glycosides and the source of the enzyme or, more specifically, the structure of the isoform of the α-subunit. Compounds with high potency have slow rates of release. The Na^+,K^+-ATPase having a α-2 or α-3 subunit has a slow rate of glycoside release and therefore high affinity for the glycosides. The difference in the rate of release of the glycoside from Na^+,K^+-ATPase is related to the rate of washout of the positive inotropic effect observed in isolated heart muscle preparations. (The rate of loss of the positive inotropic effect observed *in vivo* is primarily determined by the rate of metabolism and excretion.)

Inhibition of Na^+,K^+-ATPase, and hence the sodium pump, by cardiac glycosides increases intracellular Na^+ activity from the normal level of approximately 8 mM. The maximal increase in Na^+ observed with nontoxic concentration of the glycosides is about 2 mM. The relationship, however, between intracellular Na^+ concentration and developed tension is steep (Fig. 6). Therefore, a 10–20% increase in intracellular Na^+ may cause more than 100% increase in developed tension.

The preceding increase in intracellular Na^+ concentration during the diastolic phase of the cardiac cycle reduces the rate of Ca^{2+} extrusion by the Na^+/Ca^{2+} exchanger. This exchanger is driven by Na^+ and Ca^{2+} concentration gradients. Because the exchanger countertransports 3 Na^+ and 1 Ca^{2+}, and hence is electrogenic, the rate of cation transport is also affected by the membrane potential. When the membrane is depolarized during membrane excitation, the exchanger mediates Ca^{2+} influx coupled with Na^+ efflux. When the membrane potential is −80–−90 mV, as is the case in the diastolic phase of the cardiac muscle, the exchanger causes Ca^{2+} efflux coupled with Na^+ influx. An elevation of the intracellular Na^+ activity resulting from glycoside-induced sodium pump inhibition reduces the Na^+ concentration gradient and therefore reduces the rate of Ca^{2+} efflux. Intracellular Ca^{2+} ions, which are not extruded by the Na^+/Ca^{2+} exchanger, are taken up into the sarcoplasmic reticulum by the powerful calcium pump. Enhanced Ca^{2+} loading of the sarcoplasmic reticulum increases the amplitude of the Ca^{2+} transients, and thereby enhances the force of contraction.

In addition to the positive inotropic (therapeutic) effect, the digitalis glycosides produce "toxic effects." Clinically important toxic actions of digitalis may be classified into those related to direct action on the heart and those related to neural systems. The direct toxin action of digitalis glycosides on the heart is apparently mediated by sodium pump inhibition. In general, 20–40% inhibition of the sodium pump causes the positive inotropic effect, and that exceeding 60% causes toxicity. The degree of the sodium pump inhibition that triggers toxicity (arrhythmias), however, is affected by many factors (51,52).

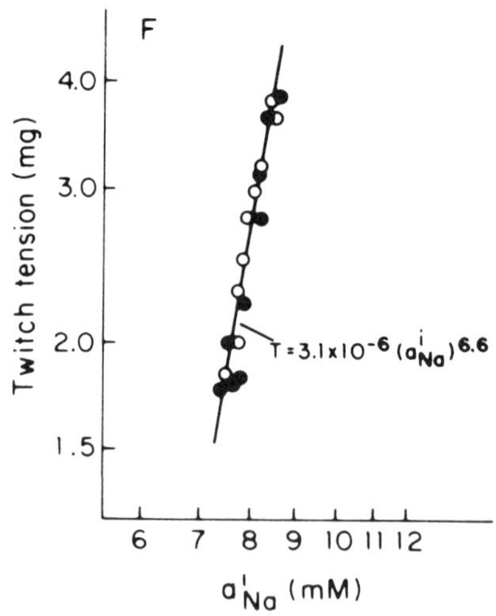

Figure 6 The relationship between intracellular Na^+ activity and developed tension. Strophanthidin, a cardiotonic steroid with rapid onset and offset of action, was used to alter intracellular Na^+ concentration. Canine cardiac Purkinje fibers were exposed to 0.5 μM strophanthidin, and intracellular Na^+ activity, α^{i}_{-Na}, and twitch tension were simultaneously estimated. Filled circles: during the development of the positive inotropic effect. Open circles: during washout (recovery) of the drug effect. (From Ref. 50.)

The relationship between the magnitude of Na^+,K^+-ATPase inhibition and that of the positive inotropic effect may be considered as follows. Under normal conditions, the cardiac sodium pump has a reserve capacity (i.e., the pump is turning over at about 50% of its maximal rate). Intracellular Na^+ concentration is the rate-limiting factor for the sodium pump. Ionic equilibrium of beating cardiac muscle cells can be maintained when the sodium pump extrudes exactly the amount of Na^+ that enters the cell during a cardiac cycle (Fig. 7). In biochemical terms, the concentration of intracellular Na^+ in normal beating heart is significantly lower than that required for full activation of the sodium pump. As the Na^+,K^+-ATPase is inhibited by the cardiac glycoside, the Na^+ activation curve for the enzyme shifts downwards and the rate of Na^+ extrusion decreases (Fig. 7). A 20–40% decrease in sodium pump activity caused by therapeutic concentrations of the cardiac glycoside increases intracellular Na^+ concentration and enhances turnover of the remaining pump units until the overall pump activity of reduced pump units matches the rate of Na^+ influx by turning over at a faster rate. This is caused by a 1–2 mM increase in intracellular Na^+ ion activity. As discussed above, this increase in intracellular Na^+ activity, in turn, increases intracellular Ca^{2+}, and increases Ca^{2+} loading of the sarcoplasmic reticulum.

As the degree of sodium pump inhibition becomes greater, a larger increase in intracellular Na^+ concentration is required to stimulate the sodium pump so that the rate of Na^+ efflux matches the rate of Na^+ influx. Such a large increase in intracellular Na^+, and ensuing increase in Ca^{2+} load the myocytes, causes cellular Ca^{2+} overload

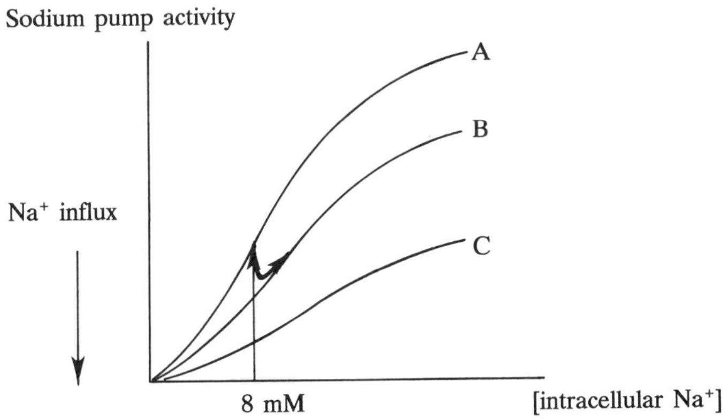

Figure 7 Reserve capacity of the sodium pump and its inhibition by therapeutic and toxic concentrations of the cardiac glycosides. A. Normal condition. At the intracellular Na^+ concentration of approximately 8 mM, the rate of Na^+ efflux by the sodium pump matches the rate of passive Na^+ influx. B. When 20–40% of sodium pump units are inhibited by the therapeutic (positive inotropic) concentration of cardiac glycosides, remaining pump units turn over faster, responding to 1–2 mM increase in intracellular Na^+ concentrations. C. When a toxic concentration of the glycoside inhibits more than 80% of sodium pump units, remaining pump units cannot match the rate of passive Na^+ influx without a large increase in intracellular Na^+, which in turn causes toxic manifestations (arrhythmias) through Na^+/Ca^{2+} exchanger and Ca^{2+} overload. Sodium pump units that can be inhibited without causing excessive increase in intracellular Na^+ concentration may be regarded as "reserve capacity" of the sodium pump.

and toxic manifestations such as increased resting tension, negative inotropic effects, oscillatory after-potentials, and oscillatory after-contractions. This phenomenon may be regarded as follows. When the degree of sodium pump inhibition exceeds the reserve capacity of the sodium pump, cells accumulate Na^+ (and Ca^{2+} though the Na^+/Ca^{2+} exchanger) and lose K^+, resulting in toxic manifestations. From these considerations, it is apparent that the degree of Na^+,K^+-ATPase inhibition afforded by myocytes before the onset of toxicity is determined by the degree of reserve capacity of the sodium pump. Supporting this concept, factors that reduce reserve capacity of the sodium pump (e.g., increases in Na^+ influx rate, decreases in the number of sodium pump units, and decreases in extracellular K^+ concentrations) all reduce the tolerance of the myocardium to the toxic action of digitalis glycosides.

An important point is that the degree of the maximal positive inotropic effect that can be obtained before the onset of toxicity is related to reserve capacity of the sodium pump. As digitalis glycosides inhibit Na^+,K^+-ATPase, developed tension increases resulting from increases in intracellular Na^+ and an ensuing increase in Ca^{2+} loading of the sarcoplasmic reticulum. The degree of the positive inotropic effect increases as the degree of Na^+,K^+-ATPase inhibition increases until reaching the critical point at which the reserve capacity is exhausted. The hypothesis that the maximal positive inotropic effect that can be observed before the onset of toxicity is related to reserve capacity is supported by data obtained in senescent rats (53,54).

It is presently unknown if all toxic manifestations of digitalis glycosides are brought about by Na^+,K^+-ATPase inhibition. In view of the fact that Na^+,K^+-ATPase is the only biochemical effect observed with low concentrations of digitalis glycosides (18), it is not surprising if all actions of digitalis glycosides can be accounted for either by the primary or secondary effect of Na^+,K^+-ATPase inhibition. Whether Na^+,K^+-ATPase inhibition causes dysfunction in a particular group of cells or an organ depends on the affinity of Na^+,K^+-ATPase predominant in the cell, and the reserve capacity of the sodium pump prevailing in those cells at the time they are exposed to the glycoside. If the particular isoform present in a tissue has high affinity for the glycoside, and if the reserve capacity of the sodium pump is small in that tissue, digitalis glycosides may cause toxic manifestations at low concentrations. In the heart, toxic manifestations of the glycosides usually start with Purkinje fibers. For example, concentrations of digitalis glycosides that cause oscillatory after-potentials in isolated dog heart muscle are lowest in Purkinje fibers, intermediate in atrial muscle, and highest in ventricular muscle proper. These results are consistent with the finding that the concentration of Na^+,K^+-ATPase is low in Purkinje fibers (55), and higher in ventricular muscle than in atrial muscle (56).

An additional factor may determine whether digitalis glycosides causes toxic manifestations in a given cell. This is the presence of a system that links an increase in intracellular Na^+ to the dysfunction of cells. A small increase in intracellular Na^+ concentration, or a decrease in intracellular K^+ concentration, *per se* may not cause severe cellular dysfunction. The presence of Na^+/Ca^{2+} exchanger, for example, makes the cell vulnerable to toxic effects of digitalis glycosides because Ca^{2+} overload has markedly greater effect than Na^+ overload for the function of various cells. This may be the reason why pharmacologic and toxic effects of the digitalis glycosides are primarily expressed in the cardiac and neural tissues even though Na^+,K^+-ATPase plays an important function in maintaining intracellular ionic environments in various tissues and organs.

IV. PHYSIOLOGICAL AND PATHOLOGIC CHANGES IN Na^+,K^+-ATPase

A. Changes in α-Isoforms

For a long time, differences in sensitivity of heart muscle to the positive inotropic effects of the cardiac glycosides have been recognized. These differences have been attributed to differences in affinity of Na^+,K^+-ATPase for the cardiac glycosides. The presence of isoforms of the α-subunits of Na^+,K^+-ATPase hving different affinities for the glycosides has subsequently been shown, and it became clear that digitalis sensitivity of the tissue is determined by the particular α-isoform predominant in that tissue. Dog, ferret, and rat heart have at least two α-isoforms. In the dog heart, two isoforms have relatively similar affinities for the cardiac glycosides, whereas affinities of those in the rat heart are different by more than two orders of magnitude. The affinities of two isoforms present in ferret heart differ about 20-fold. In isolated ferret or rat heart muscle preparations, positive inotropic effects of ouabain corresponding to a high- and low-affinity form of the Na^+,K^+-ATPase can be demonstrated (11,57). (Ng and Akera, 1987).

Under physiological and pathologic conditions, the relative abundance of these isoforms may change. In the ferret heart, the α-isoform that has lower affinity for the glycosides is predominant at birth (11). During postnatal development, the relative abundance of the α-1 isoform decreases. The high- and low-affinity forms have about equal abundance in the adult ferret heart. These changes in the relative abundance of high- and low-affinity forms of Na^+,K^+-ATPase are reflected in sensitivity of the heart to the pharmacologic effect of digitalis glycosides. Different isoforms are apparently the products of different genes. The expression of the isoforms may be regulated during development and also by thyroid and glucocorticoid hormones (58). Chronic heart failure and associated hypertrophy have been reported to alter the relative abundance of the α-isoforms of Na^+,K^+-ATPase.

Total amounts of Na^+,K^+-ATPase in a given cell may be regulated by the amount of Na^+ that has to be transported by the sodium pump. It was demonstrated many years ago that the amounts of Na^+,K^+-ATPase in the gill may be up- or down-regulated as fish migrate between fresh and salt water (59). Intracellular Na^+ concentration in cultured cells may be increased by incubating cultured cells in the presence of veratridine, which increases the Na^+ influx, or in a medium containing a low concentration of K^+, which inhibits sodium pump activity. These conditions increase the number of Na^+,K^+-ATPase units (60). Results are controversial as to whether exposure of myocardial cells *in vivo* to inhibiting concentrations of the cardiac glycoside causes an increase in the number of Na^+,K^+-ATPase units. In patients treated with therapeutic doses of digoxin or digitoxin, the degree of sodium pump inhibition and ensuing increase in intracellular Na^+ concentration are probably too subtle to stimulate the synthesis of Na^+,K^+-ATPase.

Quantitative analysis is unavailable as to the relationship between the number or density of the digitalis receptor and the magnitude of response to cardiac glycosides. Signal transduction is the sole function of many receptors. For example, the only known function of β_1-adrenoceptors is to regulate the production of cyclic AMP. For these receptors, an increase in the number of functioning receptor units should increase the size of response observed with a given concentration of the ligand, provided that affinity of the receptor or the efficiency of coupling mechanisms are unchanged. The digitalis receptor is an exception. The primary function of the receptor molecule, Na^+,K^+-ATPase, is the active cation transport. Occupancy of the receptor site by digitalis glycosides inhibits the cation transport but does not generate a specific second messenger. Under these conditions, changes in the number of the sodium pumping units do not necessarily enhance the magnitude of the response observed with a given concentration of digitalis. From the above discussions, the maximal positive inotropic effect of digitalis glycosides that can be observed before the onset of toxic manifestations should be greater if the number of pumping sites is increased resulting in a greater reserve capacity of the sodium pump. Whether this is the case is presently unknown. A decrease in the number of sodium-pumping sites fails to alter digitalis sensitivity of the heart but decreases the maximal positive inotropic effect observed before the onset of toxic manifestations (54).

REFERENCES

1. Shull GE, Greeb J, Lingrel JB. Molecular cloning of three distinct forms of the Na^+,K^+-ATPase α-subunit from rat brain. Biochemistry 1986; 25: 8125–32.
2. Sweadner KJ. Isozymes of the Na^+/K^+-ATPase. Biochim Biophys Acta 1989; 988: 185–220.
3. Shyjan AW, Cena V, Klein DC, Levenson R. Differential expression and enzymatic properties of the Na^+,K^+-ATPase $\alpha 3$ isoenzyme in rat pineal glands. Proc Natl Acad Sci USA 1990; 87: 1178–82.
4. Urayama T, Sweadner KJ. Ouabain sensitivity of the alpha 3 isozyme of rat Na^+,K^+-ATPase. Biochem Biophys Res Commun 1988; 156: 796–800.
5. Hara Y, Nakamoto A, Kojima T, Matsumoto A, Nakao M. Expression of sodium pump activities in BALB/c 3T3 cells transfected with cDNA encoding alpha 3-subunits of rat brain Na^+,K^+-ATPase. FEBS Lett 1988; 238: 27–30.
6. Hara Y, Ohtsubo M, Kojima T, Noguchi S, Nakao M, Kawamura M. Expression of active alpha-3 subunit of rat brain Na^+,K^+-ATPase from the messenger RNA injected into *Xenopus* oocytes. Biochem Biophys Res Commun. 1989; 163: 102–5.
7. Brodsky JL, Guidotti G. Sodium affinity of brain Na^+,K^+-ATPase is dependent on isozyme and environment of the pump. Am J Physiol 1990; 258: C803–11.
8. Lytton J. Insulin affects the sodium affinity of the rat adipocyte (Na^+,K^+)-ATPase. J Biol Chem 1985; 60: 10075–80.
9. Horowitz B, Hensley CB, Quintero M, Azuma KK, Putman D, McDonough AA. Differential regulation of Na^+,K^+-ATPase $\alpha 1$, $\alpha 2$ and β subunit mRNA and protein levels by thyroid hormone. J Biol Chem 1990; 265: 14308–14.
10. Ng YC, Yao AZ, Akera T. Tissue-specific isoform regulation of Na^+,K^+-ATPase by thyroid hormone in ferrets. Am J Physiol 1989; 257: H534–9.
11. Ng YC, Akera T. Relative abundance of two molecular forms of Na^+,K^+-ATPase in the ferret heart: developmental changes and associated alterations of digitalis sensitivity. Mol Pharmacol 1987; 32: 201–5.

12a. Martin-Vasallo P, Dackowski W, Emanuel JR, Levenson R. Identification of a putative isoform of the Na,K-ATPase β subunit. J Biol Chem 1989; 264: 4613–8.

12b. Orlowski J, Lingrel JB. Tissue-specific and developmental regulation of rat Na,K-ATPase catalytic α isoform and β subunit mRNAs. J Biol Chem 1988; **263:** 10436–42.

13. Gibbs CL. Cardiac energetics. In: Langer GA, Brady AJ, eds. The mammalian myocardium. New York: John Wiley and Sons 1974; 105–33.
14. Gubitz RH, Akera T, Brody TM. Control of brain slice respiration by (Na^++K^+)-activated adenosine triphosphatase and the effects of enzyme inhibitors. Biochim Biophys Acta 1977; 459: 263–77.

15. Langer GA. Ionic movements and the control of contraction. In: Langer GA, Brady AJ, eds. The mammalian myocardium. New York: John Wiley and Sons 1974: 193–217.
16. Kim MS, Akera T. O_2 free radicals: cause of ischemia-reperfusion injury to cardiac Na^+,K^+-ATPase. Am J Physiol 1987; 252: H252–7.
17. Skou JC. The influence of some cations on an adenosine triphosphatase from peripheral nerves. Biochim Biophys Acta 1957; 23: 394–401.
18. Lee KS, Klaus W. The subcellular basis for the mechanism of inotropic action of cardiac glycosides. Pharmacol Rev 1971; 23: 193–261.
19. Nix CR, Holland WC, Berry RA. The action of cassaine and two of its alkylated derivatives on atrial contractions. Pharmacol Res Commun 1971; 3: 75–8.
20. Seifen E, Straub KD. Effects of sanguinarine on the isolated mammalian heart. Pharmacologist 1974; 16: 245.
21. Fox AAL, Borchard U, and Greeff K. Digitalisähnliche and antiarrhythmische Wirkung des Isochinolinderivates BIIA. Z Kardiol 1981; 68: 244.
22. Temma K, NG Y-C, Brody TM, Akera T. Effects of progesterone derivatives on sodium pump activity and force of myocardial contraction in isolated guinea pig heart. Res Commun Chem Pathol Pharmacol 1983; 41: 51–63.
23. Yamamoto S, Akera T, Brody TM. Prednisolone-3,20-bisguanylhydrazone: Na^+,K^+-ATPase inhibition and positive inotropic action. Eur J Pharmacol 1978; 49: 121–132.
24. Ng YC, Leung WY, Akera T. Cardiac Na^+,K^+-ATPase isoenzymes: sensitivity to prednisolone bisguanylhydrazone. Eur J Pharmacol 1988; 155: 93–9.
25. Skou JC, Hilberg C. The effect of sulfphydryl-blocking reagents and of urea on the (Na^+,K^+)-activated enzyme system. Biochim Biophys Acta 1965; 110: 359–69.
26. Banerjee SP, Khanna VK, Sen AK. Inhibition of sodium- and potassium-dependent adenosine triphosphatase by ethacrynic acid: ligand-induced modifications. Biochem Pharmacol 1971; 20: 1649–60.
27. Matsuda T, Iwata H. Difference between neuronal and nonneuronal (Na^++K^+)-ATPases in their conformational equilibrium. Arch Biochem Biophys 1988; 263: 323–33.
28. Ng YC, Akera T. Two classes of ouabain binding sites in ferret heart and two forms of Na^+,K^+-ATPase. Am J Physiol 1987; 252: H1016–22.
29. Cantley LC, Josephson L, Warner R, Yanagisawa M, Lechene C, Guidotti G. Vanadate is a potent (Na,K)-ATPase inhibitor found in ATP derived from muscle. J Biol Chem 1977; 252: 7421–3.
30. Borchard U, Fox AAL, Greeff K, Schlieper P. Negative and positive inotropic action of vanadate on atrial and ventricular myocardium. Nature (London) 1979; 279: 339–41.
31. Beauge LA, Glynn IM. Commercial ATP containing traces of vanadate alters response of (Na^++K^+)-ATPase to external potassium. Nature (London) 1978; 272: 551–2.
32. Nechay BR, Saunders JP. Inhibition of Na^+,K^+-ATPase by vanadium pentoxide (V_2O_5). Fed Proc 1978; 37: 240.
33. Quist EE, Hokin LE. The presence of two (Na^+,K^+)-ATPase inhibitors in equine muscle ATP: vanadate and a dithioerythritol-dependent inhibitor. Biochim Biophys Acta 1978; 511: 202–11.
34. Akera T, Takeda K, Yamamoto S, Brody TM. Effects of vanadate on Na,K-ATPase and on the force of contraction in guinea-pig hearts. Life Sci 1979; 25: 1803–12.
35. Cantley LC, Resh MD, Guidotti G. Vanadate inhibits red-cell (Na^++K^+)-ATPase from cytoplasmic side. Nature (London) 1978; 272: 552–4.
36. Myers TD, Boerth RC, Post RL. Effects of vanadate on ouabain binding and inhibition of (Na^+,K^+)-ATPase. Biochim Biophys Acta 1979; 558: 99–107.
37. Donaldson J, St-Pierre T, Minnich J, Barbeau A. Seizures in rats associated with divalent cation inhibition of Na^+,K^+-ATPase. Can J Biochem 1971; 49: 1217–24.
38. Hexum TD. Studies on reaction catalyzed by transport (Na,K)adenosine triphosphatase. I. Effects of divalent meals. Biochem Pharmacol 1974; 23: 3441–7.

39. Siegel GJ, Fogt SM. Inhibition by lead ion of electrophorus electroplax (Na^+,K^+)-adenosine triphosphatase and K^+-p-nitrophenylphosphatase. J Biol Chem 1977; 252: 5201–5.
40. Tobin T, Akera T, Baskin SI, Brody TM. Calcium ion and sodium- and potassium-dependent adenosine triphosphatase: its mechanism of inhibition and identification of the E_1-P intermediate. Mol Pharmacol 1973; 9: 336–49.
41. Stemmer P, Akera T. Sodium pump activity and its inhibition by extracellular calcium in cardiac myocytes of guinea pigs. Biochim Biophys Acta 1988; 940: 188–96.
42. Hagane K, Akera T, Stemmer P. Effects of Ca^{2+} on the sodium pump observed in cardiac myocytes isolated from guinea pigs. Biochim Biophys Acta 1989; 982: 279–87.
43. McGeoch JEM. The α-2 isomer of the sodium pump is inhibited by calcium at physiological levels. Biochem Biophys Res Commun 1990; 173: 99–105.
44. Glynn IM. Transport adenosinetriphosphatase in electric organ. The relation between ion transport and oxidative phosphorylation. J Physiol (London) 1963; 169: 452–65.
45. Cloix JF, Crabos M, Grichois ML, Guicheney P, Meyer P. Klin Wochenschr 1987; 65 (suppl. 8): 146.
46. Goto A, Yamada K, Ishii M, Yoshioka M, Ishiguro T, Eguchi C, Sugimoto T. Purification and characterization of human urine-derived digitalis-like factor. Biochem Biophys Res Commun 1988; 154: 847–53.
47. Hamlyn JM, Harris DW, Clark MA, Rogowski AC, White RJ, Ludens JH. Isolation and characterization of a sodium pump inhibitor from human plasma. Hypertension 1989; 13: 681–9.
48. Hamlyn JM, Harris DW, Ludens JH. Digitalis-like activity in human plasma. Purification, affinity, and mechanism. J Biol Chem 1989; 264: 7395–404.
49. Araki K, Kuroki J, Ito O, Kuwada M, Tachibana S. Novel peptide inhibitor (SPAI) of Na^+,K^+-ATPase from procine intestine. Biochem Biophys Res Commun 1989; 164: 496–502.
50. Im WB, Lee CO. Quantitative relation of twitch and tonic tensions to intracellular Na^+ activity in cardiac Purkinje fibers. Am J Physiol 1984; 247: C478–87.
51. Kennedy RH, Akera T, Brody TM. How increased sodium influx enhances digoxin-induced arrhythmias in guinea-pig atrial muscle. Eur J Pharmacol 1983; 89: 199–209.
52. Kennedy RH, Seifen E, Akera T, Brody TM. Effects of Bay k-8644 on inotropic and arrhythmogenic actions of digoxin. Eur J Pharmacol 1986; 124: 11–20.
53. Katano Y, Akera T, Temma K, Kennedy RH. Enhanced ouabain sensitivity of the heart and myocardial sodium pump in aged rats. Eur J Pharmacol 1984; 105: 95–103.
54. Katano Y, Kennedy RH, Stemmer PM, Temma K, Akera T. Aging and digitalis sensitivity of cardiac muscle in rats. Eur J Pharmacol 1985; 113: 167–78.
55. Rhee HM. Ouabain sensitivity of Rb^+ uptake in canine Purkinje fibre and ventricular muscle. Naunyn-Schmeidebergs Arch Pharmacol 1982; 318: 344–8.
56. Yamamoto S, Akera T, Kim D-H, Brody TM. Tissue concentration of Na^+,K^+-adenosine triphosphatase and the positive inotropic action of ouabain in guinea-pig heart. J Pharmacol Exp Ther 1981; 217: 701–7.
57. Akera T, Ng YC, Hadley R, Katano Y, Brody TM. High affinity and low affinity ouabain binding sites in the rat heart. Eur J Pharmacol 1986; 132: 137–46.
58. Orlowski J, Lingrel JB. Thyroid and glucocorticoid hormone regulate the expression of multiple Na,K-ATPase genes in cultured neonatal rat cardiac myocytes. J Biol Chem 1990; 265: 3462–70.
59. Gallis J-L, Lasserre P, Belloc F. Freshwater adaptation in the euryhaline teleost, Chelon labrosus. I. Effects of adaptation, prolactin, cortisol and actinomycin D on osmotic balance and (Na^+-K^+)ATPase in gill and kidney. Gen Comp Endocrinol 1979; 38: 1–10.
60. Kim D, Marsh JD, Barry WH, Smith TW. Effects of growth in low potassium medium or ouabain on membrane Na,K-ATPase, cation transport and contractility in cultured chick heart cells. Circ Res 1984; 55: 39–48.

16

Endogenous Cardiac Glycoside-Like Factors: Myth or Fact?

JEAN-FRANÇOIS CLOIX

Hôtel Dieu
Paris, France

RALPH A. KELLY

Brigham and Women's Hospital and Harvard Medical School
Boston, Massachusetts

Many mechanisms contribute to the regulation of the contractile state of myocardial tissue, including a number of mechanical and neurohumoral factors discussed in detail elsewhere in this volume. Despite rapid advances in recent years in our understanding of the molecular pharmacology of both endogenous and exogenous inotropic agents, it is possible that other, as yet uncharacterized, mechanisms remain. Indeed, the demonstration that the novel vasoconstrictor peptide of endothelial cell origin, endothelin, is among the most potent inotropic agents ever tested in guinea pig atrial strips (1) and isolated rat ventricular cells is evidence that other hormonal or autocrine regulators of myocardial contractile state may exist.

Of all the positively inotropic pharmaceutical agents yet described that might have an endogenous counterpart, the cardiac glycosides have received by far the greatest scrutiny, and for good reason. The universal presence of a binding site for cardiac glycosides on NaK-ATPase has resulted in much speculation as to whether it also serves as a receptor for an endogenous digitalis-like hormone or autacoid. A number of endogenous compounds that modulate the activity of the sodium pump have been identified, including catecholamines, insulin, thyroxine, mineralocorticoids, and other hormones (2-17, 17a). Most of these compounds affect the sodium pump indirectly by varying the intracellular sodium concentration, the rate-limiting substrate for the pump in vivo, or by increasing the number of pump units in the membrane. Evidence exists, however, that sodium pump activity may be directly affected by several hormones, possibly by altering the affinity of the pump for sodium, although the mechanism by which this occurs is not yet understood. In addition, inorganic ions also may modulate pump function in vivo. For example, vanadate, acting as a pyrophosphate analogue within the cell, can inhibit phosphorylation of several cation-transferring enzymes, including NaK-ATPase (18, 19).

Although all of these compounds may have physiologically important roles in modulating sodium pump activity in vivo, none has been shown to act by binding to the cardiac glycoside-binding site on NaK-ATPase. With the exception of the bufodienolides, cardiac glycoside-like toxins present in certain species of toads, there is as yet no definitive identification of any endogenous factors that bind specifically to the cardiac glycoside-binding site in any animal species (20,21). Despite this, the search for the endogenous digitalis continues with unabated enthusiasm, if recent reports from many laboratories throughout the world serve as an index. This appears to be due largely to two quite different, but equally compelling, arguments that together form the logical foundation for the search for either a hormone or another endogenous agent (autacoid) that is an endogenous ligand for the ouabain-binding site.

I. EVIDENCE FOR THE EXISTENCE OF ENDOGENOUS DIGITALIS-LIKE FACTORS

The first is simply that the binding site has been so highly conserved throughout the phylogeny of eukaryotes as noted above, and also within the ontogeny of individual organisms, from brine shrimp to mammals (22–25). This could, in principle, be due to an absolute requirement for a particular conformation and amino acid sequence within NaK-ATPase that ensures successful ion translocation, having by design nothing to do with binding of any putative extra cytoplasmic ligand but fortuitously divined by certain plants and toads as a means of poisoning animal predators. This formulation, while possible, is not satisfying, for the mere presence of apparent receptors for plant compounds on animal cells does not disqualify the existence of an endogenous ligand and ignores the rationale recently followed in the identification of several classes of hormones and/or hormone receptors based on the example of drug–receptor interactions. The analogy most often cited in the context of the search for the endogenous digitalis has been the discovery of the endogenous opioids (26). Indeed, the recent isolation of nonpeptide opioids in mammalian brain and the characterization of a biosynthetic pathway in mammalian liver analogous to that in the opium poppy has reinforced this comparison, although it is far from proven that these opioids are of endogenous origin (27–29). While the similarities are obvious, they may be more apparent than real, since the mechanism of signal transduction initiated at the cell membrane by the endogenous opioids is typical of most hormones and quite different from that postulated for an endogenous digitalis-like factor, as discussed below.

The second reason for the sustained interest in an endogenous ligand for the ouabain-binding site on NaK-ATPase has centered on speculation about the physiological and pathophysiological effects of such a substance. None of these effects has anything to do, ironically, with the pharmacologic properties responsible for the use of the cardiac glycosides: that is, their positive cardiac inotropic and antiarrhythmic actions. Evidence for the existence of circulating inhibitors of the pump first came from studies suggesting the presence of a natriuretic hormone in the plasma of volume-expanded animals. Since about one-half of renal sodium reabsorption depends on the sodium pumps in the basolateral membrane of renal tubular cells, it would not be surprising if the NaK-ATPase enzyme proved to be a target for a hormonal system that regulates sodium reabsorption (30–35). Evidence supporting this hypothesis has recently been reviewed by deWardener, one of the first investigators to have postulated the existence of a circulating natriuretic hormone 30 years ago (31). Although the discovery of the atrial natriuretic peptides undoubtedly can explain many of the original observations supporting the existence of a natriuretic hormone, these peptides have no direct effect on NaK-ATPase, and their existence does not, a priori, exclude the possibility of a second natriuretic hormone system.

Concurrent with the description of a potential role for endogenous sodium pump inhibitors in the response to extracellular volume expansion, evidence has been presented for the presence of circulating factors that could contribute to the pathogenesis of hypertension. Dahl et al. (36) were the first to suggest the existence of a hormone that might cause vasoconstriction and enhance sodium excretion at the same time. Evidence for the existence of such a vasopressor substance, distinct from known vasopressor hormones, was first supplied by Michelakis and colleagues (37), who demonstrated that small amounts of plasma from hypertensive, uninephrectomized dogs could increase vascular responsiveness to infused norepinephrine or angiotensin II. Subsequently, Haddy and Pamnani (38) published a review in which they suggested that a sodium pump inhibitor might lead to vasoconstriction by inducing depolarization of the vascular cell membrane. Blaustein (39) later codified the hypothesis linking the existence of a possible vasopressor natriuretic hormone to inhibition of the sodium pump in vascular smooth muscle cells. He postulated that NaK-ATPase inhibition in vascular smooth muscle would increase the intracellular sodium concentration and that this might lead to an increase in intracellular calcium by sodium–calcium exchange. Evidence consistent with this hypothesis has come from several sources. Haddy and Pamnani (40) showed that NaK-ATPase activity in vascular smooth muscle is suppressed in rats with volume-expanded forms of hypertension. The ^{22}Na efflux from the leukocytes of patients with essential hypertension was reported to be reduced, and several groups reported a circulating inhibitor of NaK-ATPase in the plasma of patients with essential hypertension (41–43). However, there is disagreement as to whether the sodium–calcium exchange mechanism is physiologically important in vascular smooth muscle of arteriolar resistance vessels (44).

Although a direct effect of sodium pump inhibition on intracellular calcium homeostasis within arteriolar resistance vessels is perhaps the most obvious mechanism of action of an endogenous cardiac glycoside-like hormone, other potential mechanisms have been proposed, and some evidence is presented for each. Perhaps the best characterized is the evidence that indicates that sodium pump inhibitors would potentiate the effect of other vasopressor agents. This would be expected if these inhibitors acted to increase intracellular calcium concentration in vascular smooth muscle. Plasma from patients with essential hypertension and from dogs and rats with experimental hypertension potentiates the constrictor effects of angiotensin II and norepinephrine on isolated rat arterioles (45). Moreover, vascular reactivity to angiotensin II and norepinephrine is enhanced in rats with low-renin, volume-expanded forms of hypertension (46). Ultrafiltrates of plasma from volume-expanded dogs have been reported to potentiate the constrictor responses of isolated arterioles to angiotensin II and norepinephrine (47). Guthrie (48) showed that digoxin, given in therapeutic dosages to normal human subjects, increases vascular responsiveness to exogenously administered angiotensin II and norepinephrine. However, infusions of norepinephrine or ouabain into the brachial artery of hypertensive subjects with or without a low plasma renin level resulted in identical increases in forearm vascular resistance, tending to discount the role of an endogenous inhibitor of NaK-ATPase in the pathogenesis of low renin hypertension (49).

It is also possible that a digitalis-like endogenous sodium pump inhibitor substance acts in the central nervous system to enhance sympathetic nerve activity and thereby indirectly affects peripheral vascular resistance. Infusions of small amounts of ouabain into the cerebral ventricles of rats induce an immediate rise in sympathetic nerve outflow and blood pressure (50). In addition, an extract of human plasma with endogenous digitalis-like activity isolated in our laboratory demonstrated a rise in blood pressure lasting about 1 hr following its injection into the arterioventral third ventricle of anesthetized rats (51,52). The sustained rise in blood pressure and arrhythmogenic effects of a toxic dose of intravenously administered digitalis glycoside can be abolished by selective brainstem lesions (53).

Evidence also exists that the central nervous system either regulates the release, or is the source, of an endogenous NaK-ATPase inhibitor. Disruption of neuronal pathways in the preoptic, hypothalamic, periventricular tissue of an anteroventral third ventricular region (AV3V) of the rat can attenuate or prevent many forms of experimental hypertension, suggesting a role for this anatomical region as a central processing site for sympathetic nervous system control of blood pressure (54,55). AV3V-lesioned rats have higher levels of vascular NaK-ATPase activity after volume expansion than sham-operated rats, consistent with the hypothesis that the levels of circulating pump inhibitor are lower in lesioned animals (56–58). Halperin et al. (59) also described the presence of an endogenous ouabain-like substance in human cerebral spinal fluid (CSF) and demonstrated that acute infusions of saline, but not dextrose, resulted in a rapid rise in CSF levels of this factor (60). The existence of a ouabain-like factor in cerebrospinal fluid was confirmed by Lichstein et al. (61). Recently, Halperin and colleagues have published data further characterizing the ouabain-like activity in CSF as a peptidic, low-molecular-weight compound, although they have not determined its amino acid sequence (62).

In addition to this evidence linking the brain with the origin of an endogenous inhibitor of NaK-ATPase, several groups isolated an inhibitor of active sodium transport from hypothalamic tissue (63–67) or from cultured rat neonatal hypothalamic cells (68). The hypothalamic factor isolated by Haupert et al. (63,64) acts from the cytoplasmic side of the membrane and is a reversible inhibitor of NaK-ATPase. It is not a specific inhibitor of this enzyme, however, and it does not support partial reactions of NaK-ATPase in a manner characteristic of the cardiac glycosides. The active sodium transport inhibitor from cultured rat hypothalamic cells can enhance vascular reactivity to alpha-adrenergic agonists (69).

None of these factors has been shown to be released or to increase in concentration in response to any physiological stimulus. However, Haupert and his colleagues have recently demonstrated that a factor from bovine hypothalamus does inhibit sodium pump-mediated active ^{86}Rb flux in cultured renal endothelial cells, and therefore could potentially have a physiologically relevant action in the kidney (66). The possibility of a biologically important interaction between their hypothalamic factor and atrial natriuretic peptides has been given additional credence due to recent evidence that ANP prevents the release of this factor from rat brain (67,70).

Aside from experimental evidence from animal models, there is evidence in humans that suggests that plasma levels of an inhibitor of NaK-ATPase are increased in primary hypertension. Several studies suggested that plasma levels of an inhibitor of NaK-ATPase are increased in primary hypertension (42,43,71,72). It also was reported that sodium pump-dependent cation flux is abnormal in the erythrocytes and leukocytes of hypertensive patients (73–78). A recent study correlated changes in sodium efflux rates in leukocytes with those from resistance vessels obtained from omental biopsies in humans, suggesting that changes in the electrolyte content of nucleated blood cells reflect similar changes in arteriolar resistance vessels (78).

Another source of speculation about the existence of circulating ouabain-like factors has grown out of the original observations of Welt and co-workers in the 1960s that erythrocytes of some patients with end-stage renal insufficiency demonstrated abnormally high intracellular sodium content and depressed sodium pump activity (reviewed in 79). They also demonstrated that plasma from these uremic patients, but not plasma from equally uremic individuals whose erythrocytes had normal intracellular sodium content, could transfer the defect to normal red cells. Although numerous subsequent reports concerning patients with renal failure or animals with experimental renal insufficiency have confirmed the observation that sodium pump activity is abnormal in some tissues in uremia, it is unclear whether this is due to the multiple metabolic abnormalities characteristic of this syndrome or to the presence in excess of a specific circulating inhibitor of NaK-ATPase (80–85). There are also reports of false-positive results of digoxin radioimmunoassays in the plasma of some patients with chronic renal failure, and a recent finding that plasma levels of endogenous cardiac glycoside-like activity, as defined by digoxin-like immunoreactivity or NaK-ATPase inhibitory activity, are increased in chronic renal failure (83,86–89).

In addition to the finding in patients with chronic renal failure, a number of groups have reported detecting the presence of endogenous substances with immunologic similarities to the cardiac glycosides, particularly to digoxin. Flier et al. (90) were the first to identify an endogenous substance, probably a bufodienolide steroid, in the plasma of toad *Bufo marinus* that cross-reacted with digoxin-specific antibodies and inhibited NaK-ATPase. Gruber and colleagues (91,92) demonstrated the presence of a low-molecular-weight substance in the plasma of volume-expanded dogs that reacted with antidigoxin antibodies and that also appeared to be elevated in the plasma of some subhuman primate species with certain forms of experimental hypertension. Kojima (93,94) reported that rats with deoxycorticosterone acetate–salt hypertension had increased plasma levels of factors with digoxin-like immunoreactivity, and they demonstrated that the infusion of digoxin-specific antibodies into rats with this form of experimental hypertension produced an immediate decline in blood pressure. Nevertheless, despite a number of studies purporting to have documented immunologic cross-reactivity between endogenous NaK-ATPase inhibitors and digitalis glycosides, this issue remains controversial (95–104). Few investigators have used more than one antibody population or rigorously defined the potential artifacts of any given radioimmunoassay technique. Several recent reports reviewed the problems associated with this approach (105–113).

A potential complication of the presence of factors in plasma with digoxin-like immunoreactivity is the problem of properly dosing cardiac glycosides when radioimmunoassay alone is used to quantitate drug levels in some patients. The patient populations at greatest risk appear to be uremic patients, newborn and premature infants, and some pregnant women (114–126). The problem of relying on radioimmunoassay alone for determination of digoxin levels in tissue, plasma, or other biological fluids also has implications for forensic medicine (107,127). Techniques for avoiding this complication and guidelines for determining patients who might have falsely positive plasma levels of digoxin have been discussed at length in the clinical chemistry literature (107).

II. CHARACTERIZATION OF CARDIAC GLYCOSIDE-LIKE FACTORS

With the exception of the bufodienolides as noted above, none of the biologically active endogenous NaK-ATPase inhibitors detected in a wide variety of experimental models and patient samples has been well characterized. Although many potential candidates have been identified, those whose molecular structure has been chemically determined have not been found to be specific, high-affinity ligands for the ouabain-binding site, and any judgment about the numerous remaining potential ouabain-like factors must await their isolation and characterization. To date, two different approaches have been used to provide evidence that endogenous factors exist in vivo that are capable of inhibiting NaK-ATPase directly. Some investigators determined that plasma or urine from hypertensive animals or humans inhibits sodium pump function and cross-reacts with digoxin-specific antibodies to a greater extent than control samples (41,72,90–95, 114–119, 129–134). The identity of these inhibitors remains elusive, however, and plasma levels often do not correlate well with the degree of blood pressure elevation or the extent of disease. A second approach has been to isolate and characterize sodium pump inhibitors from the plasma and tissues of humans and animals (60–62, 64, 65, 135–142). Our laboratory has recently demonstrated that a fraction with endogenous digitalis-like properties derived from a hemofiltrate of plasma can induce a positive inotropic, but negative chronotropic, effect in primary cultures of rat cardiomyocytes, as did ouabain (143). However, the biological relevance of these inhibitors remains to be proved.

Nevertheless, several groups have made considerable progress in isolating and identifying inhibitors of NaK-ATPase from biological sources. English and Cantley (144,145) identified the 68 kDa protein, δ-endotoxin, as a potent inhibitor of NaK-ATPase. These are among the first data suggesting that a protein can directly inhibit NaK-ATPase activity; however, this protein acts from the cytoplasmic side of the cell membrane to inhibit sodium pump activity. Morgan, Mir, and colleagues (68,69) demonstrated that their active sodium transport inhibitor derived from hypothalamus is probably a low-molecular-weight peptide. Haupert and colleagues have continued to characterize the biological effects of their digitalis-like factor derived from bovine hypothalamus (63–67), and Goto et al. have extensively characterized a cardiac glycoside-like factor derived from human plasma and urine (139,140). Rauch and Buckalew have also pursued a digitalis-like compound in rat plasma and tissues (141) and carefully characterized the nature of the interaction between this factor and the NaK-ATPase (142).

The steroid nature of the cardiac glycosides and the bufodienolides has led to a search for endogenous mammalian steroid derivatives that might be relatively specific and for high-affinity inhibitors of NaK-ATPase (146–149). No compounds have yet been identified with the capacity both to bind to the cardiac glycoside-binding site with high affinity and to induce a positive inotropic effect in heart. Nevertheless, recent work on ouabain-like compounds present in amniotic fluid by Graves et al. (114,118) (S.W. Graves, personal communication, 1988) and on similar factors present in human urine by Cloix et al. (137,138) suggests that certain ouabain-like compounds may be structurally similar to steroids.

Finally, Tamura et al. have recently reported that methanol extracts of bovine adrenal, from which virtually all the known inhibitors of NaK-ATPase activity had been rigorously excluded, contains a novel, low-molecular-weight, nonpeptidic compound with sodium pump inhibitor activity (150). Hamlyn et al. (151) have likewise recently reported that following extraction of voluminous amounts of human plasma from normal subjects, they can detect a ouabain-like factor. Both laboratories have demonstrated that, both chemically and in terms of the kinetic interaction between their factors and NaK-ATPase, these ouabain-like substances are remarkably like the digitalis glycosides and may be steroid derivatives. Hamlyn et al. also have preliminary evidence suggesting that their factor is elevated in humans and experimental animals that are volume-overloaded and/or hypertensive, consistent with its possible function as a natriuretic or hypertensinogenic hormone (J.M. Hamlyn, personal communication, 1990).

Several groups have identified a variety of lipid compounds in extracts of tissue or plasma as being cardiac glycoside-like in that they inhibit NaK-ATPase activity, displace [^{3}H]ouabain from its binding site on the enzyme, and even nonspecifically interfere with ligand antibody binding in a digoxin radioimmunoassay. Bidard et al. (152) initially identified free fatty acids as the ouabain-like substances in an extract of the electric organ of the cell. In our laboratory, Kelly et al. isolated and characterized cardiac glycoside-like activity in extracts of plasma from normal humans and determined that most, if not all, of this activity could be attributed to a variety of lysophospholipids and free fatty acids (153,154). Concurrently, Tamura et al. (155) showed that the increase in ouabain-like activity in plasma of hogs acutely volume-expanded with saline could be attributed to oleic and linoleic acids. Recent work from their laboratory also confirmed that this rise in ouabain-like activity in plasma with volume expansion includes a variety of unusual lysophospholipids as well (156). In addition, we recently showed that plasma levels of nonesterified fatty acids increased in Dahl salt-resistant rats in response to dietary salt loading but did not increase in Dahl salt-sensitive rats (157). The increase was predominantly due to a change in plasma levels of arachidonate and arachidonate precursors. Interestingly, Rauch and Buckalew recently demonstrated that lysophosphatidylcholine, given in relatively small amounts intravenously to rats, caused a sustained natriuresis (158). They suggest that this is not due to a nonspecific surfactant effect resulting in inhibition of NaK-ATPase.

The fact that long-chain fatty acids and other amphipathic compounds, such as acylcarnitine and phospholipids, can modulate sodium pump activity has been known for some time (149,160,160a). However, it is very unlikely that these compounds are binding to the ouabain-binding site. The NaK-ATPase, like other membrane-bound cation-transporting enzymes, has an absolute requirement for a specific phospholipid composition of the membrane immediately surrounding the enzyme (161–163). Unsaturated long-chain fatty acids might interact with these membrane lipids, both to influence the affinity of the enzyme for the substrates and to facilitate or restrict the conformational changes the enzyme must undergo during transport of cations from one side of the lipid bilayer to the other. These lipids may influence membrane fluidity as a whole or selectively affect the lipid domain immediately surrounding the enzyme. High concentration of certain phospholipids and fatty acids may also result in loss of enzyme function due to detergent effects. This could explain why low concentrations of phosphatidylserine stimulate NaK-ATPase in phospholipase or detergent-treated membranes, while higher concentrations of the phospholipid inhibit the enzyme (163).

Regardless of the potential of these compounds to induce large changes in NaK-ATPase activity in vitro, little evidence exists that they play an important role in modulating enzyme activity in vivo, except perhaps in certain diseases characterized by abnormalities in lipid metabolism (e.g., hyperlipidemia, chronic renal failure). Several groups, however, recently implicated arachidonic acid metabolites derived from renal tissue and urine as specific high-affinity inhibitors of NaK-ATPase (164–166). Although promising, these results require further confirmation and amplification.

III. NaK-ATPase AS A "RECEPTOR" FOR ENDOGENOUS DIGITALIS-LIKE FACTORS

Despite the diligent efforts of many investigators over the last two decades, and despite the fact that their "receptor" (i.e., NaK-ATPase) has been well characterized, the identity of the endogenous digitalis-like factors remains elusive. It is beyond the scope of this chapter to cite in detail the arguments in support of endogenous cardiac glycoside-like factors or to critique the wide variety of methodologies that have been used to assay for their presence. For this, the reader is referred to several comprehensive reviews of this topic (31,167–176). Recent advances in our knowledge of the molecular biology of the sodium pump have provided a response to a long-standing fundamental objection to the existence of any circulating ouabain-like factor: the potential for nonspecific, toxic effects of such a factor due to the ubiquitous tissue distribution of NaK-ATPase, essential for normal cellular cation homeostasis. The discovery and detailed characterization (177–187) of multiple isoforms of the alpha subunit of the enzyme, first discovered 10 years ago by Sweadner (185) because of differences in their molecular weight and in their sensitivities to the inhibitory effects of ouabain, have lent credence to the possibility of selective enzyme inhibition (187,188). In particular, the recent observation that the sensitivity of renal tubular NaK-ATPase to inhibition by ouabain increases along the nephron, due likely to a gradual shift in the ratio of high-affinity to low-affinity ouabain "receptors," is consistent with the presence of an ouabain-like natriuretic factor acting in the distal nephron to modulate the salt content of the urine (188).

Again, these observations provide only circumstantial evidence for the existence of such a factor. It is entirely possible, perhaps likely, that isoform expression has important cellulra functional correlates that have nothing to do with differential sensitivity to an exogenous toxin: for example, the demonstration that the "alpha+" isoform appears to make up the insulin-responsive subset of NaK-ATPase in rat adipocytes (189). Nevertheless, it raises the possibility of "receptor subtypes" for an ouabain-like factor and an answer to the objection of nonspecific and potentially toxic effects of such a hormone.

IV. IS THE NaK-ATPase "RECEPTOR" PARADIGM APPROPRIATE?

In summary, much of the rationale that underlies the concept of a circulating endogenous ouabain-like factor is based on the fact that its existence would help to explain the persistence of the ouabain-binding site throughout evolution, while providing a convenient and inclusive explanation for a number of physiological and pathophysiological phenomena. Nevertheless, we believe that the proposition that such factors exist rests on unproven assumptions, and that other plausible explanations can be offered for the evolutionary longevity of the cardiac glycoside-binding site, as will be discussed briefly below.

A central assumption in the hypothesis usually advanced is that the NaK-ATPase functions as both a receptor and an effector protein, recognizing and binding an extracellular factor and thereby directly generating an intracellular signal. This signal could be a rise in intracellular sodium or a secondary change in cytosolic calcium activity. Convenient as this explanation may be, there is no hormonal precedent for such a signal transduction mechanism. Hormones, whether autocrine, paracrine, or endocrine, are generally recognized by specific cell-surface or intracellular receptor proteins that subsequently affect the generation of intracellular second messengers and/or the regulation of gene expression (190–193). In each case, modulation of the signal within the cell is possible by a variety of mechanisms, thus allowing for either amplification or feedback inhibition (190). Even the binding of insulin and certain peptide growth factors to their cell-surface receptors, which induces autophosphorylation of the receptor with probable subsequent phosphorylation of other cellular protein, initiates a complex set of intracellular signals that could be modified at any of several points (190–193).

The only examples in eukaryotes of which we are aware in which an extracellular signal induces a conformational change in an integral cell membrane protein, thereby directly affecting transmembrane ion flux, are neurohumoral agents acting at ligand-gated ion channels, such as acetylcholine at nicotinic receptors. In fact, the number of polypeptides, amino acids, amines, and even molecular species such as endothelial-derived relaxing factor (tentatively identified as nitric oxide) involved in polytypic chemical cell-to-cell signaling is quite large and growing rapidly (194,195). Some of these neurohumoral agents act exclusively via distinct cell membrane receptors that subsequently result in modulation of plasmalemmal ion flux, others act only by directly inducing an allosteric modfication in a transmembrane ion channel, while a few, such as gamma aminobutyric acid (GABA), may act by both means, even on the same postsynaptic cell membrane. Such diversity could allow a temporal separation of responses in addition to the specificity of the signal generated by the amplitude and ion selectively of neurotransmitter action, as suggested by Nicoll (195). The search for endogenous ligands for psychotropic drug "receptors" has, indeed, turned up some likely candidates, such as the oligopeptide ligands for the benzodiazepine recognition sites on $GABA_A$ receptors. This has recently been reviewed by Barbaccia et al. (196).

However, in every case, the receptors are located in close apposition at the synaptic junction to the site of neurotransmitter or allosteric neuromodulator release in restricted plasmalemmal domains of specific neurons in specialized areas of the nervous system. Often a high concentration of an appropriate degradative enzyme, such as acetylcholinesterase in the case of nicotinic receptors, is close at hand. Indeed, using the example of acetylcholine acting at nicotonic receptors, the action of cardiac glycosides on NaK-ATPase is more closely analogous to that of alpha-bungarotoxin, a specific high-affinity ligand found in the venom of the snake *Bungarus multicinctus* that interacts noncovalently with the alpha subunit of the nicotinic receptor in skeletal muscle and prevents acetylcholine binding, thereby inhibiting an increase in sodium conductance (197).

If there is an endogenous digitalis that facilitates intracellular communication, by analogy with known neuromodulating agents in neuronal signalling, this native ligand for the cardiac glycoside receptor would likely be produced, released, and inactivated near its target. Since the sodium pump is present in the plasmalemma of every cell in higher eukaryotes, a likely source of such an agent would be adjacent endothelial tissue. While the juxtaposition of vascular and microvascular endothelium would allow local production and vectorial transport of a potent modifier of transmembrane ion flux in target cells, none of the peptides and other vasoactive agents of known endothelial origin has been shown to act directly on plasmalemmal ion transport proteins. Although the recognition of some degree of structural homology between the alpha-scorpion toxins and the novel vasoconstrictor peptide endothelin led to the suggestion, that following its release by endothelial cells, endothelin might act directly on sarcolemmal ion channels, perhaps as an endogenous agonist for the dihydropyridine-sensitive voltage-dependent calcium channel in sarcolemmal membranes, this now appears not to be the case (198,199). More recent evidence indicates that specific, high-affinity receptors for endothelin exist in vascular smooth muscle (200). Also, a newly discovered class of potent cardiotoxic peptides in the venom of the snake *Atractaspis engaddensis* termed sarafotoxins, one of which has almost complete amino acid identity with mammalian endothelin, acts by binding to high-affinity receptors on rat atrial strips and initiating phosphoinositide hydrolysis (201). Endothelin has very recently been shown to be a potent inhibitor of NaK-ATPase on basolateral membranes of rat renal proximal convoluted tubular cells (202). Although a direct allosteric effect of the peptide on sodium pump activity cannot yet be excluded, endothelin's action on the sodium pump in these cells appears to be mediated via a cyclo-oxygenase product (202).

V. NaK-ATPase ISOFORM DIVERSITY: RECEPTOR SUBTYPES?

The concept of a circulating ouabain-like hormone interacting with the NaK-ATPase at its receptor, therefore, seems to run counter to a number of known design criteria for signal transduction at eukaryotic cell membranes. The wide variation in ouabain-binding affinity of the constitutive form of the alpha subunit between some mammalian species also seems inconsistent with a widely shared receptor function for this enzyme among closely related species. Although the existence of multiple isoforms of the NaK-ATPase alpha subunit in mammals, with their differing sensitivities to cardiac glycosides, is consistent with the concept of receptor subtypes with differing affinities for an endogenous ligand, other explanations, none of which are mutually exclusive, are also possible. Changes in the primary structure of the protein at one of the several extracytoplasmic loops that form the ouabain-binding site, or changes in the amino acid sequence elsewhere in the alpha subunit that induce subtle conformational effects, may have evolved to effect changes in protein function unrelated to binding of a cardiac glycoside-like ligand (202a). For example, the "α+" isoform, now referred to as α-2, has been reported to have a $K_{0.5}$ for intracellular sodium of 52 mM, compared to a $K_{0.5}$ for sodium of 17 mM for the a-1 isoform in unstimulated rat adipocytes. In the presence of insulin, the $K_{0.5}$ of the α-2 isoform drops to 33 mM, while that of the α-1 form is unaffected, thus allowing the cells rapidly to increase the velocity of Na^+ and K^+ countertransport (13). The difference in the $K_{0.5}$ values for Na^+ for each isoform was apparent only in intact cells, not in isolated adipocyte membranes, suggesting that the sodium affinity of the α-2 isoform was being modulated by a water- or lipid-soluble effector acting at the cytosolic face of the protein.

Although this is the only report to date of a clear functional difference among the three known isoforms of the alpha subunits, the rapidly accumulating evidence for differential tissue expression of the isoforms during fetal development (203,204) and in response to specific hormonal (11–17) and physiological stimuli (30,205), and their existence as a multigene family, represented in at least three different chromosomes in rat, point to a unique functional role for each isoform (206–212). Recent evidence also points to the existence of isoforms of the β subunit and perhaps a critical role for this small glycoprotein subunit in the regulation of Na pump number in response to rapid changes in intracellular Na^+, among other functions (213,214,218). However, this does not prove that the isoform differ functionally, but only that the mechanisms leading to initiation of transcription and their phenotypic expression differ.

The preceding arguments were not intended to deny the existence of an endogenous ligand for the cardiac glycoside-binding site on NaK-ATPase, but to indicate that such a factor, if it acts as a transcellular signaling mechanism, would be very unusual, perhaps one of the first of a new class of low-molecular-weight, reversible inhibitors that act directly to regulate cell membrane ion-translocating enzyme systems. A spirited search for an endogenous digitalis continues in many laboratories. Recent reports of the isolation and characterization of specific high-affinity, nonpeptidic inhibitors of NaK-ATPase are intriguing and, if confirmed, would begin to dispel many doubts about the existence, if not the biological significance, of such inhibitors. Perhaps there is more than one class of inhibitors, with differential affinity for the several NaK-ATPase isoforms. Complete characterization of any of the numerous candidate compounds described to date has been hampered because of the instability of many of these factors, their apparent heterogeneity of structure, and their lack of specificity (perhaps due to contaminants).

As mentioned above, the possibility that the evolutionary persistence of the cardiac glycoside-binding site is due merely to constraints on the design of an efficient transmembrane ion pump unrelated to any putative endogenous ligand is unsatisfying. But if such a ligand exists, and does not act extracellularly as a hormone or autacoid, what other functions are possible? Advances in the last decade in our understanding of the regulation of intracellular eukaryotic protein trafficking suggests that the answer may lie within the cell. NaK-ATPase, like most integral membrane proteins, after cotranslational insertion of the α and β subunits into the membrane of the rough endoplasmic reticulum: 1. must be targeted through a complex network of intracellular organelles to the correct plasmalemmal domain, and 2. must be monitored for appropriate protein conformation and subunit assembly. In addition, because the ionic milieu of the lumina of these intracellular organelles may favor ATPase activity, the nascent NaK-ATPase units in transit to the plasma membrane, or latent pumps in a subsarcolemmal pool, could have their catalytic function regulated by a digitalis-like ligand before insertion in the cell membrane. Because the lumina of the endoplasmic reticulum, Golgi, and other organelles and vesicles are topologically equivalent to the outside of the cell, all three functions could be subserved by an intraorganellar ligand for the cardiac glycoside-binding site. This "alternative hypothesis" for the evolutionary persistance of the ouabain-binding site on NaK-ATPase has been developed more completely in a recent review (216).

VI. CLINICAL IMPLICATIONS

The clinical implications of the possible existence of endogenous digitalis-like factors depend largely on how the individual interested clinician or scientist interprets the literature. Thorough and well-written reviews of the field have recently appeared, in which the contribution of these agents in the pathophysiology of hypertension (169,171) or chronic renal insufficiency (81) are discussed. For a thoughtful and exhaustive review of the history of the natriuretic hormones and the relationship between atrial natriuretic peptides and digitalis-like factors, the reader is referred to the monograph by deWardener and Clarkson (217). In addition, the implications of the possible existence of two separate natriuretic hormonal systems (as distinct from locally acting natriuretic autacoids in the kidney) are discussed in recent reports by Haupert and colleagues (67,70). Finally, Hamlyn and colleagues have presented evidence recently identifying ouabain itself as an endogenous ligand for the digitalis binding site on NaK-ATPase (218,219). These data are reviewed in a recent editorial (220).

If, however, the reader interprets the evidence supporting the existence of endogenous NaK-ATPase inhibitors or "digitalis-like factors" as being largely indeterminate, as we do, the "clinical implications" narrow only to a discussion of the interpretation of some assay results that might be used to identify the presence or absence of such factors in a clinical population. Perhaps most important, the misinterpretation of results of radioimmunoassays for digoxin due to the presence of apparent digoxin-like immunoreactivity in patients' plasma could lead to inappropriate clinical decisions. Although the exact identity of these interfering substances is as yet unknown, their ability to cross-react in some, but not all, antidigoxin radioimmunoassays may lead to falsely elevated digoxin levels, or the apparent presence of digoxin in plasma when the drug had not been prescribed. Misinterpretation of digoxin radioimmunoassay results has contributed to the erroneous judgment that some patients who had not been prescribed a cardiac glycoside were being poisoned with digoxin (see 106,107). The patient populations most likely to have circulating substances that interfere in a digoxin radioimmunoassay are neonates and fetuses, pregnant women, patients with end-stage renal insufficiency, and, perhaps, acromegalies. Regardless of whether these cross-reacting substances are of interest in the pathophysiology of disease or merely represent known compounds present in unusual concentrations or combinations that result in an artifactually positive analytical signal, the clinician should be aware of the potential for this abnormality in the measurement of cardiac glycoside levels using certain types of analytical techniques.

REFERENCES

1. Ishikawa T, Yanagisawa M, Kimura S, Goto K, and Masaki T. Positive inotropic action of novel vasoconstrictor peptide endothelin on guinea pig atria. Am J Physiol 1988; 255:H970–3.

2. Riozzi A, Heagerty AM, Bing RF, Thurston H, Swales J. Noradrenaline: a circulating inhibitor of sodium transport. Med J 1984; 289:1025–7.
3. Brown MJ, Brown DC, Murphy MB. Hypokalemia from beta-stimulation by circulating epinephrine. N Engl J Med 1983; 309:1414–20.
4. Lytton J, Lin JC, Guidotti G. Identification of two molecular forms of NaK-ATPase in rat adipocytes. J Biol Chem 1985; 260:1177–84.
5. Karin NJ, Cook JS. Regulation of NaK-ATPase by its biosynthesis and turnover. Curr Top Membrane Transport 1983; 1:713–51.
6. Kim D, Smith TW. Effect of thyroid hormone on sodium pump sites, sodium content, and contractile response to cardiac glycosides in cultured chick ventricular cells. J Clin Invest 1984; 74:1481–8.
7. Fagoo M, Braguet P, Robin JP, Esanu A, Godfraind T. Evidence that mammalian ligands show endogenous digitalis-like activities. Biochem Biophys Res Commun 1986; 13:1064–70.
8. Edelman IS, Pressley TA, Hiatt A. Regulation of mammalian Na,K-ATPase. In: Glynn I, Ellory C., eds. The sodium pump. Cambridge: Company of Biologists, 1985: 153–155.
9. Mjuais SK, Chekal MA, Jones WJ, Hayslett JP, Katz A. Modulation of renal sodium-potassium-adenosine triphosphatase by aldosterone: effects of high physiologic levels of enzyme activity in isolated rat and rabbit tubules. J Clin Invest 1985; 76:170–6.
10. Clausen T. Regulation of active Na^+-K^+ transport in skeletal muscle. Physiol. Rev. 1986; 66:542–77.
11. Rosie NK, Standaert ML, Pollet RJ. The mechanism of insulin stimulation of (Na^+,K^+)-ATPase transport activity in muscle. J Biol Chem 1985; 260:6206–12.
12. Schneider-Picard G, Coles JA, Girardier L. Alpha- and beta-adrenergic mediation of changes in metabolism and Na/K exchange in rat brown fat. J Gen Physiol 1985; 86:169–88.
13. Lytton J. Insulin affects the sodium affinity of rat adipocyte (Na^+,K^+)-ATPase. J Biol Chem 1985; 260:10075–80.
14. Johnson JP, Jones D, Wiesmann WP. Hormonal regulation of Na^+K^+-ATPase in cultured epithelial cells. Am J Physiol 1986; 251:C186–90.
15. Barlet-Bas C, Khadouri C, Marsy S, Doucet A. Sodium-independent in vitro induction of Na^+,K^+-ATPase by aldosterone in renal target cells: permissive effect of triiodothyronine. Proc Natl Acad Sci USA 1988; 85:1707–11.
16. Gick GG, Ismail-Beigi F, Edelman IS. Thyroidal regulation of rat renal and hepatic Na,K-ATPase gene expression. J Biol Chem 1988; 263:16610–8.
17. Schmitt CA, McDonough AA. Thyroid hormone regulates alpha and alpha+ isoforms of Na,K-ATPase during development in neonatal rat brain. J Biol Chem 1988; 263:17643–9.
17a. Orlowski J, and Lingrel JB. Thyroid and glucocorticoid hormones regulate the expression of multiple Na,K-ATPase genes in cultured neonatal rat cardiac myocytes. J Biol Chem 1990; 265:3462–70.
18. Norby JG. Ligand interactions with the substrate site of NaK-ATPase: nucleotides, vanadate, and phosphorylation. Curr Top Membrane Transport 1983; 19:281–314.
19. Robinson JD. Effects of cations and modifiers on the hydrolytic steps in the Na,K-ATPase cycle. In: Glynn I, Ellory C, eds. The sodium pump. Cambridge: Company of Biologists, 1985:391–8.
20. Greeff K, ed. Cardiac glycosides: part 1, experimental pharmacology. Berlin/New York: Springer-Verlag, 1981.
21. Shimoni Y, Gotsman M, Deutsch J, Kachalsky S, Lichtstein D. Endogenous ouabain-like compound increases heart muscle contractility. Nature 1984; 307:369–71.
22. Fisher JA, Baxter-Lowe LA, Hokin LE. Regulation of Na,K-ATPase biosynthesis in developing *Artemia saline.* J Biol Chem 1986; 261:515–9.

23. Gonatas JO, Gonatas NK, Stieber A, Fleischer B. Isolation and characterization of an enriched Golgi fraction from neurons of developing rat brains. J Neurochem 1985; 45:497–507.
24. Minuth WW, Gross P, Gilbert P, Kashgarian M. Expression of the alpha-subunit of Na/K-ATPase in renal collecting duct epithelium during development. Kidney Int 1987; 31:1104–12.
25. Sweadner KJ, and Farshi SK. Rat cardiac ventricle has two Na^+,K^++-ATPases with different affinities for ouabain: developmental changes in immunologically different catalytic subunits. Proc Natl Acad Sci USA 1987; 84:8404–7.
26. Gintzler AR, Levy A, Spector S. Antibodies as a means of isolating and characterizing biologically active substances: presence of a non-peptide, morphine-like compound in the central nervous system. Proc Natl Acad Sci USA 1976; 73:2132–6.
27. Kosterlitz HW. Biosynthesis of morphine in the animal kingdom. Nature 1987; 330:606.
28. Weitz CJ, Faull KF, Goldstein A. Synthesis of the skeleton of the morphine molecule by mammalian liver. Nature 1988; 330:674–7.
29. Weitz CJ, Lowney LI, Faull KF, Feistner G, Goldstein A. 6-Acetylmorphine: a natural product present in mammalian brain. Proc Natl Acad Sci USA 1988; 85:5335–8.
30. Katz AI. Renal NaK-ATPase: its role in tubular sodium and potassium transport. Am J Physiol 1982; 242:F207–19.
31. deWardener HE, Clarkson EM. Concept of a natriuretic hormone. Physiol Rev 1985; 65:658–759.
32. Haupert GT Jr. Physiological inhibitors of Na,K-ATPase: Concept and status. In: Skou JC, Norby JG, Maunsbach AB, Esmann M, eds. The Na^+,K^+-pump. Part B: cellular aspects, vol. 2. New York: Alan R. Liss, 1988:297–320.
33. Siegfried BA, Valdes R Jr. Excretion of endogenous digoxin-like immunoreactive factors in human urine is a function of urine flow rate. Clin Chem 1988; 34:960–4.
34. Clerico A. Digoxin-like immunoreactivity, endogenous cardiac glycoside-like factor(s) and natriuretic hormone: more than a hypothesis. J Nucl Med Allied Sci 1987; 31:341–56.
35. Ebara H, Suzuki S, Nagashima K, Kuroume T. Natriuretic activity of digoxin-like immunoreactive substance extracted from cord blood. Life Sci 1988; 42:303–9.
36. Dahl LK, Knudson DKD, Iwai J. Hormonal transmission of hypertension: evidence from parabiosis. Circ Res 1969; 24,25 (suppl I):I-21–33.
37. Michelakis AM, Mizukoshi H, Huang C, Murakami H, Inagami T. Further studies on the existence of a sensitizing factor to pressor agents in hypertension. J Clin Endocrinol Metab 1975; 41:90–6.
38. Haddy FJ, Pamnani MB. The role of humoral agents in volume expanded hypertension. Life Sci 1976; 19:935–48.
39. Blaustein MP. Sodium ions, calcium ions, blood pressure regulation and hypertension: a reassessment and a hypothesis. Am J Physiol 1977; 232:C165–73.
40. Haddy FJ, Pamnani MB. The vascular Na^+,K^+-pump in low renin hypertension. J Cardiovasc Pharmacol 1984; 6:561–74.
41. Hamlyn JM, Ringel R, Schaeffer J, et al. A circulating inhibitor of (Na + K)-ATPase associated with essential hypertension. Nature 1982; 300:650–2.
42. Kelly RA, O'Hara DS, Goldszer RC, Mitch WE, Smith TW. Endogenous digitalis-like inhibitors from human plasma. In: Glynn I, Ellory C, eds. The sodium pump. Cambridge: Company of Biologists, 1985:649–50.
43. Hamlyn JM, Levinson PD, Ringel R, et al. Relationships among endogenous digitalis-like factors in hypertension. Fed Proc 1985; 44:2782–8.
44. Mulvany MJ. Effect of electrolyte transport on the response of arteriolar smooth muscle. J Cardiovasc Pharmacol 1984; 6:582–7.
45. Huang CT, Cardons N, Michelakis AM. Existence of a new vasoactive factor in experimental hypertension. Am J Physiol 1978; 238:E25–31.

46. Marks ES, Bing RF, Thurston H, Russel GI, Swales JD. Responsiveness to pressor agents in experimental renovascular and steroid hypertension: effects of converting enzyme inhibitor and nephrectomy. Hypertension 1982; 4:238–44.
47. Plunkett WC, Hutchins PM, Gruber KA, Buckalew VM Jr. Evidence for a vascular sensitizing factor in plasma of saline-loaded dogs. Hypertension 1982; 4:581–9.
48. Guthrie TP. Effects of digoxin on responsiveness to the pressor actions of angiotensin and norepinephrine. J Clin Endocrinol Metab 1984; 58:76–80.
49. Pedrinelli R, Taddei S, Graziadei L, Salvetti A. Vascular responses to ouabain and norepinephrine in low and normal renin hypertension. Hypertension 1986; 8:786–92.
50. Takahashi H, Iyoda I, Takeda K et al. Centrally induced vasopressin responses to ouabain are augmented in spontaneously hypertensive rats. Clin Exp Hypertension 1984; A6:1499–1515.
51. Devynck MA, Pernollet MG, Cloix JF, de The H, Kamal L, Elghozi JL, Rosenfeld JB, Meyer P. Circulating digitalis-like compounds in essential hypertension. Clin Exp Hypertension 1984; 176:441–53.
52. Elghozi JL, Jacomimile LE, Devynck MA, Cloix JF, Pernollet MG, H. de The, Meyer P. Neurohumoral factor involved in the pathogenesis of hypertension. In: Bailleux RE, Fielding JF, eds. Breakdown in human adaptation to stress. Abbata Martinus Nijkoff Publishers, 1986:1006–12.
53. Somberg JC, Risler T, Smith TW. Neuronal factors in digitalis toxicity: protective effect of C-1 spinal cord transection. Am J Physiol 1978; 235:H531–6.
54. Buggy J, Huot S, Pamnani M, Haddy F. Periventricular forebrain mechanisms for blood pressure regulation. Fed Proc 1984; 43:25–31.
55. Berecek KH, Webb RL, Brody MJ. Evidence for a central role for vasopressin in cardiovascular regulation. Am J Physiol 1983; 244:H852–9.
56. Takahashi H, Matsuzawa M, Okabayashi H, Suga K, Ikegaki I, Yoshimura M, Ijichi H, Okamura H, Murakami S, Ibata Y. Evidence for a digitalis-like substance in the hypothalamopituitary axis in rats: implications in the central cardiovascular regulation associated with an excess intake of sodium. Jpn Circ J 1987; 51:1199–1207.
57. Bealer SL, Hayward JR, Gruber KA et al. Preoptic–hypothalamic periventricular lesions reduce natriuresis to volume expansion. Am J Physiol 1983; 244:R51–7.
58. Songu-Mize E, Bealer SL, Caldwell RW. Effect of AV3V lesions on development of DOCA-salt hypertension and vascular Na^+ pump activity. Hypertension 1982; 4: 575–80.
59. Halperin J, Schaeffer R, Galvey L, Malone S. Ouabain-like activity in human cerebrospinal fluid. Proc Natl Acad Sci USA 1983; 80:6101–4.
60. Halperin JA, Martin Am, Malave S. Increased digitalis-like activity in human cerebrospinal fluid after expansion of the extracellular fluid volume. Life Sci 1985; 37:561–6.
61. Lichtstein D, Minc D, Bourrit KA et al. Evidence for the presence of "ouabain-like" compound in human cerebrospinal fluid. Brain Res 1985; 325:13–9.
62. Halperin JA, Riordan JF, Tosteson DC. Characteristics of an inhibitor of the Na^+/K^+ pump in human cerebrospinal fluid. J Biol Chem 1988; 263:646–51.
63. Haupert GT, Sancho JM. Sodium transport inhibitor from bovine hypothalamus. Proc Natl Acad Sci USA 1979; 76:4658–60.
64. Carilli CT, Berne M, Cantley LC, Haupert GT. Hypothalamic factor inhibits the (Na,K)ATPase from the extracellular surface: mechanism of inhibition. J Biol Chem 1985; 260:1027–31.
65. Haupert GT, Carilli CT, Cantley LC. Hypothalamic sodium transport inhibitor is a high-affinity reversible inhibitor of Na^+-K^+-ATPase. Am J Physiol 1984; 247:F919–24.
66. Cantiello HF, Chen E, Ray S, Haupert GT Jr. Na^+ pump in renal tubular cells is regulated by endogenous Na^+-K^+-ATPase inhibitor from hypothalamus. Am J Physiol 1988; 255:F574–80.

67. Crabos M, Ausiello DA, Haupert GT Jr, Cantiello HF. Atrial natriuretic peptide regulates release of Na^+-K^+-ATPase inhibitor from rat brain. Am J Physiol 1988; 254:F912–7.
68. Morgan K, Lewis MD, Spurlock G et al. Characterization and partial purification of the sodium–potassium ATPase inhibitor released from cultured rat hypothalamic cell. J Biol Chem 1985; 260:13595–600.
69. Mir MA, Chappell SP, Morgan K, Lewis MD, Scanlon MF, Lewis MJ. Hypothalamic sodium transport inhibitor and vascular reactivity. J Hypertension 1986; 4:S233–5.
70. Haupert GT Jr. Endogenous Na,K-ATPase inhibitor(s) and atrial natriuretic peptides: are they interrelated? Prog Biochem Pharmacol 1988; 23:71–6.
71. deMendonca M, Grichois ML, Pernollet MG, Wauquier I, Trouillet-Thorman B, Meyer P, Devynck MA, Garay R. Antihypertensive effect of canrenone in a model where endogenous ouabain-like factors are present. J Cardiovasc Pharmacol 1988; 11:75–83.
72. Devynck MA, Pernollet MG, Rosenfeld JB, Meyer P. Measurement of digitalis-like compound in plasma: application in studies of essential hypertension. Br Med J 1983; 28:631–4.
73. Poston L, Sewell RB, Wilkinson SP et al. Evidence for a circulating sodium transport inhibitor in essential hypertension. Br Med J 1982; 282:847–9.
74. Parker JC, Berkowitz LR. Genetic variants affecting the structure of the human red cell membrane. In: Andreoli TE, Hoffman JF, Fanestil DD, Schultz SG, eds. Physiology of membrane disorders. New York: Plenum Press, 1986:785–814.
75. Ambrosioni E, Costa FV, Montebugnoli L, Targagni F, Magnani B. Increased intra-lymphocytic sodium content in essential hypertension: an index of impaired Na^+ cellular metabolism. Clin Sci 1981; 61:181–6.
76. Walter U, Muller S. Evidence for a Na-K-ATPase inhibitor in erythrocytes of patients with essential hypertension. Eur J Clin Invest 1981; 15:209–14.
77. Oh VMS, Taylor EA. Reversible inhibition of leucocyte sodium pumps by a circulating serum factor in essential hypertension. Br Med J 1986; 292:1551–5.
78. Aalkjaer C, Parvin SD, Bing RF, Heagerty AM, Gell PRF, Swales JD. Cell membrane sodium transport: a correlation between human resistance vessels and leucocytes. Lancet 1986; 1:649–51.
79. Smith EKM, Welt LG. The red blood cells as a model for the study of uremic toxins. Arch Intern Med 1970; 126:827–30.
80. Druml W, Kelly RA, May RC, Mitch WE. Abnormal cation flux in uremia: Mechanisms in adipocytes and skeletal muscle from uremic rats. J Clin Invest 1988; 81: 1197–1203.
81. Kaji D, Kahn T. Na^+-K^+ pumps in chronic renal failure. Am J Physiol 1987; 252:F785–93.
82. Kelly RA, Canessa ML, Steinman TI, Mitch WE. Hemodialysis and red cell cation transport in uremia: role of membrane free fatty acids. Kidney Int 1989; 35:595–603.
83. Kelly RA, O'Hara DS, Canessa ML, Mitch WE, Smith TW. Characterization of digitalis-like factors in human plasma: interactions with NaK-ATPase and crossreactivity with cardiac glycoside-specific antibodies. J Biol Chem 1985; 260:11396–405.
84. Stokes GS, Norris LA, Marwood JF, Monaghan JC, Caterson RJ. An Na^+-K^+-ATPase inhibitor which circulates in renal failure but not in essential hypertension. Prog Biochem Pharmacol 1988; 23:46–54.
85. Boero R, Guarena C, Berto IM, Deabate MC, Rosati C, Quarello F, Piccoli G. Erythrocyte Na,K pump activity and arterial hypertension in uremic dialyzed patients. Kidney Int 1988; 34:691–6.
86. Deray G, Pernollet MG, Devynck MA et al. Plasma digitalis-like activity in essential hypertension or end-stage renal disease. Hypertension 1986; 8:632–8.

87. Lackner TE, Lau BW, Parvin C, Valdes R Jr. Endogenous digoxin-like immunoreactivity in elderly patients with normal serum creatinine concentrations. Clin Pharmacol 1988; 7:449–53.
88. Shimabukuro N, Ebara H, Maruyama K, Tomizawa S, Kuroume T. Demonstration of the presence of digoxin-like immunoreactive substance (DLIS) in the serum and urine in children with nephrotic syndrome. Clin Nephrol 1988; 29:244–7.
89. Skogen WF, Rea MR, Valdes R Jr. Improved interassay correlation of digoxin results in patients with and without renal failure by elimination of digoxin-like immunoreactive factors. Clin Chem 1987; 33:837–9.
90. Flier JS, Maratos-Flier E, Pallotta JA, McIsaac D. Endogenous digitalis-like activity in the plasma of the toad *Bufo marinus*. Nature 1979; 279:341–3.
91. Gruber KA, Whitaker JM, Buckalew VM Jr. Endogenous digitalis-like substance in plasma of volume-expanded dogs. Nature 1980; 287:743–5.
92. Gruber KA, Rudel LL, Bullock BC. Increased circulating levels of an endogenous digoxin-like factor in hypertensive monkeys. Hypertension 1982; 3:348–54.
93. Kojima I, Yoshihara S, Ogata E. Involvement of endogenous digitalis-like substance in genesis of deoxycorticosterone-salt hypertension. Life Sci 1982; 30:1775–81.
94. Kojima I. Circulating digitalis-like substance is increased in DOCA-salt hypertension. Biochem Biophys Res Commun 1984; 122:129–36.
95. Gruber KA, Buckalew VM Jr. Digoxin-like immunoreactivity of a circulating (Na^+-K^+)-ATPase inhibitor. Nature 1983; 305:646.
96. Hamlyn JM, Ringel RR, Hamilton BP, Kowarski AA, Blaustein MP. Digoxin-like immunoreactivity of a circulating (Na^+-K^+)-ATPase inhibitor. Nature 1983; 305:646.
97. Valdes R. Excretion of artifactual endogenous digitalis-like factors. Am J Physiol 1986; 251:H205–9.
98. Yamada K, Goto A, Ishii M, Yoshioka M, Sugimoto T. Dissociation of digoxin-like immunoreactivity and Na^+,K^+-ATPase inhibitory activity in rat plasma. Experientia 1988; 44:992–3.
99. Friedman HS, Heneghan WF, Stern M, Farrer SM, Babb B. Digoxin-like immunoreactivity. Chest 1988; 94:1116–7.
100. Hunt SC, Wu LL, Stults BM, Williams RR. A digoxin-like factor associates with erythrocyte sodium concentration, sodium transport, and ouabain binding. Clin Biochem 1988; 21:183–6.
101. Toseland PA, Oldfield PR, Murphy GM, Lawson AM. Tentative identification of a digoxin-like immunoreactive substance. Ther Drug Monit 1988; 10:168–171.
102. Doris PA. Digoxin-like immunoreactive factor in rat plasma: effect of sodium and calcium intake. Life Sci 1988; 42:783–90.
103. Dasgupta A, Yeo KT, Malik S, Sandu P, Ahmad S, Kenny M. Two novel endogenous digoxin-like immunoreactive substances isolated from human plasma ultrafiltrate. Biochem Biophys Res Commun 1987; 148:623–8.
104. Valdes R, Hagberg JM, Vaughan TE, Lau BW, Seals DR, Ehsani AA. Endogenous digoxin-like immunoreactivity in blood is increased during prolonged strenuous exercise. Life Sci 1988; 42:103–10.
105. Kelly RA. Excretion of artifactual endogenous digitalis-like factors. Am J Physiol 1986; 251:H205–9.
106. Diamandis EP, Papanastasiou-Diamandis A, Soldin SJ. Digoxin immunoreactivity in cord and maternal serum and placental extracts: partial characterization of immunoreactive substances by high-performance liquid chromatography and inhibition of Na^+,K^+-ATPase. Clin Biochem 1985; 18:48–55.
107. Soldin SJ. Digoxin—issues and controversies. Clin Chem 1986; 32:5–12.
108. Stone JA, Soldin SJ. Improved liquid chromatographic/immunoassay of digoxin in serum. Clin Chem 1988; 34:2547–51.

109. Longerich L, Vasdev S, Johnson E, Gault MH. Disposable-column radioimmunoassay for serum digoxin with less interference from metabolites and endogenous digitalis-like factors. Clin Chem 1988; 34:2211–16.
110. Vinge E, Ekman R. Evaluation of crossreactivity of urinary digoxin-like substance in different radioimmunoassay. Ther Drug Monit 1988; 10:316–20.
111. Lau BW, Valdes R Jr. Criteria for identifying endogenous compounds as digoxin-like immunoreactive factors in humans. Clin Chim Acta 1988; 175:67–77.
112. Dasgupta A, Malik S, Ahmad S, Kenny M. Mass spectrometry studies of a novel digoxin-like substance (DLIS-2) isolated from human plasma ultrafiltrate. Biochem Biophys Res Commun 1988; 152:1435–40.
113. Yannakou L, Diamandis EP, Souvatzoglou A. Effect of incubation time and temperature on the interference of digoxin-like immunoreactive substances in digoxin immunoassays. Ther Drug Monit 1987; 9:461–3.
114. Graves SW, Brown B, Valdes R. An endogenous digoxin-like substance in patients with renal impairment. Ann Intern Med 1983; 99:604–8.
115. Kramer HJ, Heppe M, Weiler E, Backer A, Liddiard C, Klingmuller D. Further characterization of the endogenous natriuretic and digoxin-like immunoreacting activities in human urine: effects of changes in sodium intake. Renal Physiol 1985; 8:80–9.
116. Graves SW, Williams GH. An endogenous ouabain-like factor associated with hypertensive pregnant women. J Clin Endocrinol Metab 1984; 59:1070–4.
117. Seccombe DW, Pudek MR, Whitfield MF et al. Perinatal changes in a digoxin-like immunoreactive substance. Pediatr Res 1984; 18:1097–9.
118. Graves SW, Valdes R, Brown BA, Knight AB, Craig HR. Endogenous digoxin-immunoreactive substance in human pregnancies. J Clin Endocrinol Metab 1984; 58:748–51.
119. Vinge E, Helgessen-Rosendal S, Backstrom T. Progesterone, some progesterone derivatives and urinary digoxin-like substances from pregnant women in radioiummuno- and ^{86}Rb uptake assays of digoxin. Pharmacol Toxicol 1988; 63:277–80.
120. Koren G, Farine D, Grundmann H, Heyes J, Soldin S, Taylor J, MacLeod SM. Endogenous digoxin-like substance(s) associated with uneventful and high-risk pregnancies. Dev Pharmacol Ther 1988; 11:82–7.
121. Shrivastav P, Gill DS, D'Souza V, O'Brien PM, Dandona P. Secretion of atrial natriuretic peptide and digoxin-like immunoreactive substance during pregnancy. Clin Chem 1988; 34:977–80.
122. Longerich L, Brent DA, Johnson RL, Vasdev S, Gault MH. Identification of progesterone and cortisol as immunoreactive plasma digitalis-like factors in pregnancy. Res Commun Chem Pathol Pharmacol 1988; 59:383–93.
123. Goodlin RC. Fetal endoxin and pregnancy complication. Am J Obstet Gynecol 1988; 158(Pt.1):529–30.
124. Phelps SJ, Cochran EB, Gonzalez-Ruiz A, Tolley EA, Hammond KD, Sibai BM. The influence of gestational age and preeclampsia on the presence and magnitude of serum endogenous digoxin-like immunoreactive substance(s). Am J Obstet Gynecol 1988; 158:34–9.
125. Weiner CP, Robillard JE. Atrial natriuretic factor, digoxin-like immunoreactive substance, norepinephrine, epinephrine, and plasma renin activity in human fetuses and their alteration by fetal disease. Am J Obstet Gynecol 1988; 159:1353–60.
126. Gonzalez AR, Phelps SJ, Cochran EB, Sibai BM. Digoxin-like immunoreactive substance in pregnancy. Am J Obstet Gynecol 1987; 157:660–4.
127. Seccombe DW, Pudek MR, Humphries KH. Minimizing analytical interferences from digoxin-like immunoreactive substances (DLIS) in cases of digoxin toxicity. J Forensic Sci 1987; 32:650–7.

128. Rafuse PE, Almeida AF, Kwan SF, Smith PA. Effects of mammalian brain extracts and chlormadinone acetate on neuronal Na^+-K^+-ATPase amd electrogenic Na^+,K^+-pump activity in vitro. Brain Res 1985; 344:33–40.
129. Millet JA, Holland SM, Alaghband-Zadeh J, deWardener HE. Na-K-ATPase-inhibiting and glucose-6-phosphate dehydrogenase-stimulating activity of plasma and hypothalamus of the Okamoto spontaneously hypertensive rat. J Endocrinol 1986; 108:69–73.
130. Ebara H, Suzuki S, Nagashima K, et al. Digoxin- and digitoxin-like immunoreactive substances in amniotic fluid, cord blood, and serum of neonates. Pediatr Res 1986; 20:28–31.
131. Lichtstein D, Minc D, Shimoni Y, Deutsch J, Mekler J, Ben-Ishay D. Demonstration of a ouabain-like plasma compound in hypertension prone and hypertensive resistant rats. Hypertension 1985; 7:729–33.
132. Tal DM, Katchalsky S, Lichtstein D, Karlish SJD. Endogenous "ouabain-like" activity in bovine plasma. Biochem Biophys Res Commun 1986; 125:1–8.
133. Masugi F, Ogihara T, Hasegawa T et al. Circulating factor with ouabain-like immunoreactivity in patients with primary aldosteronism. Biochem Biophys Res Commun 1986; 135:41–5.
134. Shimoni Y, Gotsman M, Deutsch J, Kachalsky S, Lichtstein D. Endogenous ouabain-like compound increases heart muscle contractility. Nature 1984; 307:369–71.
135. Whitmer KR, Wallick ET, Epps DE, Lane LK, Collins JH, Schwartz A. Effects of extracts of rat brain on the digitalis receptor. Life Sci 1982; 30:2261–75.
136. Lichtstein D, Samuelov S. Membrane potential changes induced by the ouabain-like compound extracted from mammalian brain. Proc Natl Acad Sci USA 1982; 79:145–6.
137. Crabos M, Wainer IW, Cloix JF. Measurement of endogenous Na^+-K^+-ATPase inhibitors in human plasma and urine using high-performance liquid chromatography. FEBS Lett 1984; 176:223–8.
138. Cloix JF, Crabos M, Wainer IW, Ruegg U, Seiler M, Meyer M. High yield-purification of a urinary Na^+-pump inhibitor. Biochem Biophys Res Commun 1985; 131:1234–40.
139. Goto A, Yamada K, Ishii M, Yoshioka M, Ishiguro T, Eguchi C, Sugimoto T. Purification and characterization of human urine-derived digitalis-like factor. Biochem Biophys Res Commun 1988; 154:847–53.
140. Goto A, Yamada K, Ishii M, Yoshioka M, Ishiguro T, Eguchi C, Sugimoto T. Presence of digitalis-like factor in mammalian plasma. Biochem Biophys Res Commun 1988; 152:322–7.
141. Rauch AL, and Buckalew VM Jr. Tissue distribution of an endogenous ligand to the Na,K-ATPase molecule. Biochem Biophys Res Commun 1988; 152:818–24.
142. Rauch AL, Buckalew VM Jr. Characterization of a competitive and reversible ligand to E_2 conformation of Na,K-ATPase molecule. Biochem Biophys Res Commun 1988; 150:648–54.
143. Grichois ML, Freys M, Milanvoy E, Cloix JF. Eur J Pharmacol (in press).
144. English LJ, Cantley LC. Delta endotoxin is a potent inhibitor of the (Na,K)-ATPase. J Biol Chem 1986; 261:1170–3.
145. English LH, Cantley LC. Delta endotoxin inhibits Rb^+ uptake, lowers cytoplasmic pH and inhibits a K^+-ATPase in *Manduca sexta* CHE cells. J Memb Biol 1985; 85:199–204.
146. Botella J, Paris J, Lahlou B. Steroid regulation of Na^+/K^+-ATPase activity in the rat kidney: effect of a new 19-norprogestagen. J Endocrinol 1986; 110:37–41.
147. Bihler I, LaBella FS, Sawh PC. Chlormadinone acetate, a progesterone derivative that binds to the digitalis receptor and inhibits the sodium pump in the isolated rat diaphragm. Can J Physiol Pharmacol 1985; 63:44–7.
148. Hnatowich M, LaBella F. Endogenous digitalis-like factors: in vitro comparison of biological and immunological activities of peptide and steroid candidates. Eur J Pharmacol 1985; 106:567–75.

149. Vasdev S, Longerich L, Johnson E, Brent D, Gault MH. Dehydroepiandrosterone sulfate as a digitalis-like factor in plasma of healthy human adults. Res Commun Chem Pathol Pharmacol 1985; 49:387–99.
150. Tamura M, Lam TT, Inagami T. Isolation and characterization of a specific endogenous Na^+,K^+-ATPase inhibitor from bovine adrenal. Biochemistry 1988; 29:4244–53.
151. Hamlyn JM, Harris DW, Ludens JH. Digitalis-like activity in human plasma. J Biol Chem 1989; 264:7375–404.
152. Bidard JN, Rossi B, Renaud JF, Lazdunski M. A search for an "ouabain-like" substance from the electric organ of *Electrophorus electricus* which led to arachidonic acid and related fatty acids. Biochim Biophys Acta 1984; 769:245–52.
153. Kelly RA, O'Hara DS, Canessa ML, Mitch WE, Smith TW. Characterization of digitalis-like factors in human plasma: interactions with NaK-ATPase and crossreactivity with cardiac glycoside-specific antibodies. J Biol Chem 1985; 260:11396–405.
154. Kelly RA, O'Hara DS, Mitch WE, Smith TW. Identification of NaK-ATPase inhibitors in human plasma as nonesterified fatty acids and lysophospholipids. J Biol Chem 1986; 261:11704–11.
155. Tamura M, Kawana H, Kinoshita T, Inagami I. Identification of linoleic and oleic acid on endogenous NaK-ATPase inhibitors from acute volume-expanded hog plasma. J Biol Chem 1985; 200:9672–7.
156. Tamura M, Harris TM, Higashimasi K, Sweetman BJ, Blair IA, Inagami T. Lysophosphatidylcholine containing polyunsaturated fatty acids were found as NaK-ATPase inhibitors in acutely volume-expanded hog. Biochemistry 1987; 26:2797–806.
157. Kelly RA, Pfeffer JM, Mitch WE, Smith TW. Plasma nonesterified fatty acids in the Dahl rat: response to salt loading. Hypertension 1987; 10:198–203.
158. Rauch AL, Buckalew VM Jr. Lysophospholipids are natriuretic and diuretic in rats. Am J Physiol 1988; 254:F824–7.
159. Ahmed K, Thomas BS. The effects of long-chain fatty acids on sodium plus potassium ion-stimulated adenosine triphosphatase of rat brain. J Biol Chem 1971; 246:103–9.
160. Pitts BJR, and Okhuysen CH. Effects of palmitoyl carnitine and LPC on cardiac sarcolemmal Na^+-K^+-ATPase. Am J Physiol 1984; 247:H480–6.
160a. Oishi K, Zheng B, Kuo JF. Inhibition of Na,K-ATPase and sodium pump by protein kinase C regulators sphingosine, lysophosphatidylcholine, and oleic acid. J Biol Chem 1990; 265:70–5.
161. Shinitzky M. Membrane fluidity and cellular functions. In: Shinitsky M, ed. Physiology of membrane fluidity, vol. 1. Boca Raton, FL: CRC Press, 1984:1–51.
162. Schmalzing G, Kutschera P. Modulation of ATPase activities of human erythrocyte membranes by free fatty acids or phospholipase A_2. J Membrane Biol 1982; 69:65–76.
163. Roelofsen B. The (non)specificity in the lipid-requirement of calcium- and (sodium plus potassium)-transporting adenosine triphosphatases. Life Sci 1981; 29:2235–47.
164. Schwartzman M, Ferreri NR, Carroll MA, Songu-Mize E, McGiff JC. Renal cytochrome P450-related arachidonate metabolite inhibits (Na+-K+)-ATPase. Nature 1985; 314:620–2.
165. Schueler VJ, Jacobson HR, Siddhanta AW, Pramanik B. Detection of 8,9- and 14,15-epoxyeicosatrienoic acids as endogenous components of rabbit kidney. Kidney Int 1987; 31:269A.
166. Marver D, Schmitz JM. The influence of various lipoxygenase pathway metabolites of arachidonic acid (HPETEs/HETEs) on NaK ATPase activity. Kidney Int 1987; 31:278A.
167. Anner BM. The receptor function of the Na^+,K^+-activated adenosine triphosphatase system. Biochem J 1985; 227:1–11.
168. Buckalew VM, Gruber KA. Natriuretic hormone. In: Epstein M, ed. The kidney in liver disease, 2nd ed. New York: Elsevier Press, 1983:479–99.

169. Graves SW, Williams GH. Endogenous digitalis-like natriuretic factors. Annu Rev Med 1987; 38:433–44.
170. Haber E, Haupert GT. The search for a hypothalamic NaK-ATPase inhibitor. Hypertension 1987; 9:315–24.
171. Haddy FJ. Endogenous digitalis-like factor or factors. N Engl J Med 1987; 316:621–3.
172. Haddy FJ, Pamnani MB, Clough DL. Pathophysiological role of cation transport and natriuretic factors in hypertension. Hypertension 1987; 10:I-101–7.
173. Haupert GT Jr. Physiological inhibitors of Na,K-ATPase: Concept and status. In: Skou JC, Norby JG, Maunsbach AB, Esmann M, eds. The Na^+,K^+-pump, part B: cellular aspects, vol. 2. New York: Alan R. Liss, 1988:297–320.
174. Kim RS, LaBella FS. Endogenous ligands and modulators of the digitalis receptor: some candidates. Pharmacol Ther 1984; 14:391–409.
175. Mir MA. Difficulties in the isolation and identification of endogenous ouabain-like substances. Prog Biochem Pharmacol 1988; 23:1–9.
176. Cloix JF. Endogenous digitalis-like compounds: a tentative update of chemical and biochemical studies. Hypertension 1987; 10:I67–70.
177. Charlemagne D, Mayoux E, Poyard M, Oliviero P, Geering K. Identification of two isoforms of the catalytic subunit of Na,K-ATPase in myocytes from adult rat heart. J Biol Chem 1987; 262:8941–3.
178. Chehab, FF, Kan YW, Law ML, Hartz J, Kao FT, Blostein R. Human placental Na^+,K^+-ATPase alpha subunit: cDNA cloning, tissue expression, DNA polymorphism, and chromosomal localization. Proc Natl Acad Sci USA 1987; 84:7901–5.
179. Felsenfeld DP, Sweadner KJ. Fine specificity mapping and topography of an isozyme-specific epitope of the Na,K-ATPase catalytic subunit. J Biol Chem 1988; 263:10932–42.
180. Herrera VLM, Emanuel JR, Ruiz-Opazo N, Levenson R, Nadal-Ginard B. Three differentially expressed Na,K-ATPase alpha subunit isoforms: structural and functional implications. J Cell Biol 1987; 105:1855–65.
181. Maixent JM, Charlemagne D, de la Chapelle B, Lelievre LG. Two Na,K-ATPase isoenzymes in canine cardiac myocytes. J Biol Chem 1987; 262:6842–8.
182. McDonough AA, Schmitt CA. Isozymes of dog heart Na^+,K^+-ATPase are immunologically similar to isozymes in brain. Am J Physiol 1987; 253:C862–5.
183. Schneider JW, Mercer RW, Gilmore-Hebert M, Utset MF, Lai C, Greene A, Benz EJ Jr. Tissue specificity, localization in brain, and cell-free translation of mRNA encoding the A3 isoform of Na^+,K^+-ATPase. Proc Natl Acad Sci USA 1988; 85:284–8.
184. Shull GE, Green J, Lingrel JB. Molecular cloning of three distinct forms of the Na^+,K^+-ATPase alpha-subunit from rat brain. Biochemistry 1986; 25:8125–32.
185. Sweadner KJ. Two molecular forms of (Na^+-K^+)-stimulated ATPase in brain: separation and difference in affinity for strophanthidin. J Biol Chem 1979; 254:6060–7.
186. Hsu YM, Guidotti G. Rat brain has the alpha-3 form of the (Na^+,K^+)ATPase. Biochemistry 1989; 28:569–73.
187. Maixent JM, and Lelievre LG. Differential inactivation of inotropic and toxic digitalis receptors in ischemic dog heart. J Biol Chem 1987; 262:12458–62.
188. Doucet A, and Barlet C. Evidence for differences in the sensitivity to NaK-ATPase along the nephrons of rabbit kidney. J Biol Chem 1986; 261:993–5.
189. Lytton J. Insulin affects the sodium affinity of rat adipocyte Na^+,K^+-ATPase . J Biol Chem 1985; 260:10075–90.
190. Clark JH, Schrader WT, O'Malley BW. Mechanisms of steroid hormone action; and Roth J, Grunefeld C. Mechanisms of action of peptide hormones and catecholamines. In: Wilson JD, Foster DW, eds. Williams textbook of endocrinology. Philadelphia: W.B. Saunders, 1985:33–122.
191. Kahn CR, and White MF. The insulin receptor and the molecular mechanism of insulin action. J Clin Invest 1988; 82:1151–6.

192. Schlessinger J. Signal transduction by allosteric receptor oligomerization. Trends Biochem Sci 1988; 13:443–7.
193. Yarden Y, and Ullrich A. Growth factor receptor tyrosine kinases. Annu Rev Biochem 1988; 57:443–78.
194. Garthwaite J, Charles SL, Chess-Williams R. Endothelium-derived relaxing factor release on activation of NMDA receptors suggests role as intercellular messenger in the brain. Nature 1988; 336:385–8.
195. Nicoll RA. The coupling of neurotransmitter receptors to ion channels in the brain. Science 1988; 241:545–51.
196. Barbaccia ML, Costa E, Guidotti A. Endogenous ligands for high-affinity recognition sites of psychotropic drugs. Annu Rev Pharmacol Toxicol 1988; 28:451–76.
197. Taylor P. Neuromuscular blocking agents. In: Goodman LS, Gilman AG, Rall TW, Murad F, eds. Goodman and Gilman's the pharmacological basis of therapeutics. New York: MacMillan, 1985:222–35.
198. Gordon J. Put out to contract. Nature 1988; 332:395–6.
199. Yanagisawa M, Kurihara H, Kimura S, Tomobe Y, Kobayashi M, Mitsui Y, Yazaki Y, Goto K, Masaki T. A novel potent vasoconstrictor peptide produced by vascular endothelial cells. Nature 1988; 332:411–15.
200. Hirata Y, Yoshim H, Takata S, Watanabe TX, Kumagai S, Nakajima K, Sakakiboni S. Cellular mechanism of action by a novel vasoconstrictor endothelin in cultured rat vascular smooth muscle cells. Biochem Biophys Res Commun 1988; 155:167–72.
201. Kloog Y, Ambar I, Sokolovsky M, Kochva E, Wollberg Z, Bdolah A. Sarafotoxin, a novel vasoconstrictor peptide: phosphoinositide hydrolysis in rat heart and brain. Science 1988; 242:268–70.
202. Zeidel ML, Kone BC, Brady HR, Gullans SR, and Brenner BM. Endothelin inhibits Na/K-ATPase in kidney collecting duct cells: role of arachidonate derivatives. Kidney Int; 1989 (In Press).
202a. Price EM, Rice DA, and Lingrel JB. Site-directed mutagenesis of a conserved extra-celluar aspartic acid residue affects the ouabain sensitivity of sheep Na,K-ATPase. J Biol Chem 1989; 264:21902–6.
203. Orlowski J, and Lingrel JB. Tissue-specific and developmental regulation of rat Na,K-ATPase catalytic alpha isoform and beta subunit mRNAs. J Biol Chem 1988; 263:10436–42.
204. Orlowski J, and Lingrel JB. Differential expression of the Na,K-ATPase alpha-1 and alpha-2 subunit genes in a murine myogenic cell line. J Biol Chem 1988; 263:17817–21.
205. Herrera VLM, Chobanian AV, and Ruiz-Opazo N. Isoform-specific modulation of Na^+,K^+-ATPase alpha-subunit gene expression in hypertension. Science 1988; 241: 221–3.
206. Herrera VLM, Emanuel JR, Ruiz-Opazo N, Levenson R, Nadal-Ginard B. Three differentially expressed Na,K-ATPase alpha subunit isoforms: Structural and functional implications. J Cell Biol 1987; 105:1855–65.
207. Pressley TA, Ismail-Beigi F. Gick GG, Edelman IS. Increased abundance of Na^+,K^+-ATPase mRNA in response to low external K^+. Am J Physiol 1988; 255:C252–60.
208. Kent RB, Fallows DA, Geissler E, Glaser T, Emanuel JR, Lalley PA, Levenson R, and Housman DE. Genes encoding alpha and beta subunits of Na,K-ATPase are located on three different chromosomes in the mouse. Proc Natl Acad Sci USA 1987; 84:5369–73.
209. Shull MM, and Lingrel JB. Multiple genes encode the human Na^+,K^+-ATPase catalytic subunit (multiple isoforms/genomic library). Proc Natl Acad Sci USA 1987; 84:4039–43.
210. Emanuel JR, Garetz S, Stone L, Levenson R. Differential expression of Na^+,K^+-ATPase alpha- and beta-subunit mRNAs in rat tisuses and cell lines. Proc Natl Acad Sci USA 1987; 84:9030–4.

211. Young RM, and Lingrel JB. Tissue distribution of mRNAs encoding the alpha isoforms and beta subunit of rat Na^+,K^+-ATPase. Biochem Biophys Res Commun 1987; 145:52–8.
212. Urayama O, Shutt H, Sweadner KJ. Identification of three isozyme proteins of the catalytic subunit of the Na,K-ATPase in rat brain. J Biol Chem 1989; 264:8271–80.
213. Taormino JP, Fambrough DM. Pre-translational regulation of the (Na^+ + K^+)-ATPase in response to demand for ion transport in cultured chicken skeletal muscle. J Biol Chem 1990; 265:4116–23.
214. Gloor S, Antonicek H, Sweadner KJ, Pagliusi S, Frank R, Moos M, Schachner M. The adhesion molecule on glia (AMOG) is a homologue of the β subunit of the Na,K-ATPase. J Cell Biol 1990; 110:165–74.
215. Geering K, Theulaz I, Verrey F, Hauptle MT, Rossier BC. A role for the β-subunit in the expression of functional Na^+,K^+-ATPase in Xenopus oocytes. Am J Physiol 1989; 257 (Cell Physiol. 26):C851–58.
216. Kelly RA, and Smith TW. The search for the endogenous digitalis: An alternative hypothesis. Am J Physiol: Cell 1989; C937–50.
217. deWardener HE, and Clarkson EM. Concept of a natriuretic hormone. Physiol Rev 1985; 65:658–759.
218. Hamlyn JM, Blaustein MP, Bova S, DuCharme DW, Harris DW, Mandel F, Mathews WR, Ludens J.H. Identification and characterization of a ouabain-like compound from human plasma. Proc. Natl. Acad. Sci. USA 1991; 88:6259–6263.
219. Gottleib SS, Rogowski AL, Weinberg M, Krichten CM, Hamilton BP, Hamlyn JM. Elevated concentrations of endogenous ouabain in patients with congestive heart failure. Circulation 1992; 86:420–425.
220. Kelly RA and Smith TW. Is ouabain the endogenous digitalis? Circulation 1992; 86:694–697.

17

Inotropic Mechanisms in Heart Muscle: Cardiotonic Steroids—How Do They Work?

W. J. LEDERER, R. W. HADLEY, and M. S. KIRBY

University of Maryland School of Medicine
Baltimore, Maryland

D. A. EISNER

University of Liverpool
Liverpool, England

Heart muscle, like other striated muscle, contracts in response to a calcium signal. Elevated intracellular calcium, $[Ca^{2+}]_i$, is the activator of contraction in heart muscle and it works as a trigger by disinhibiting the troponin/tropomyosin/actin complex. This removal of inhibition allows the myosin heads repetitively to cycle and move the actin filaments with respect to the myosin filament. Thus the neighboring Z-lines of the sarcomeres approach each other and the muscle contracts. The architecture of the myocardium is such that the intraventricular (or intra-atrial) volumes tend to be reduced by this shortening, thereby increasing intraventricular pressure and forcing blood out of the heart. The energy for this work comes from intracellular ATP, which is consumed by the ATPase that is part of the myosin head. In this review, our principal area of interest is the mechanism of action of cardiotonic steroids as inotropic agents. The cardiotonic steroids are a family of drugs widely used in clinical medicine to increase the strength of contraction of the heart, although other important therapeutic uses for these agents exist. While the focus of the presentation is narrow, it will also touch on or allude to diverse areas of cellular physiology and biochemistry including some that cannot be adequately addressed here. In particular, the reader should keep in mind that biochemical features of the intracellular environment (e.g., pH_i, $[Mg^{2+}]_i$, temperature, $[ATP]_i$, [phosphocreatine], inorganic phosphate, etc.) are very important factors in modulating the force of contraction of the heart, as are the diverse other intracellular signalling systems (protein kinase C, protein kinase A, inositol trisphosphate $[IP_3]$, prostaglandins, etc.) and other cellular factors (e.g., sarcoplasmic reticulum Ca-ATPase, mitochondrial state, etc.).

The cardiotonic steroids include a large number of agents identified as chemicals that contain a steroid moiety with a lactone ring and may be linked to sugar(s) (called cardiac glycosides) or not linked to sugars (called cardiac aglycones). They include diverse agents that come from many plants including the common ornamen-

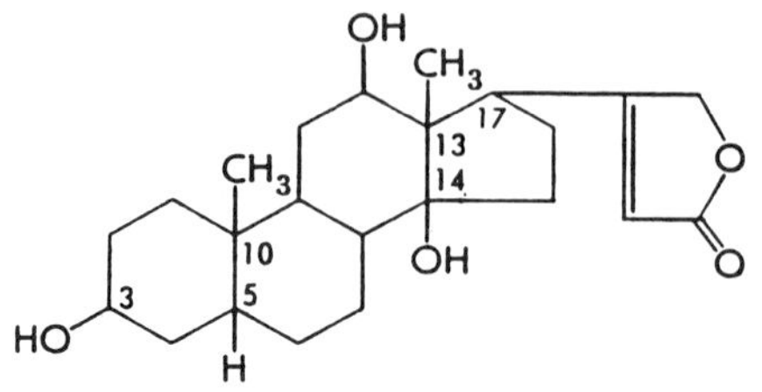

Digoxigenin

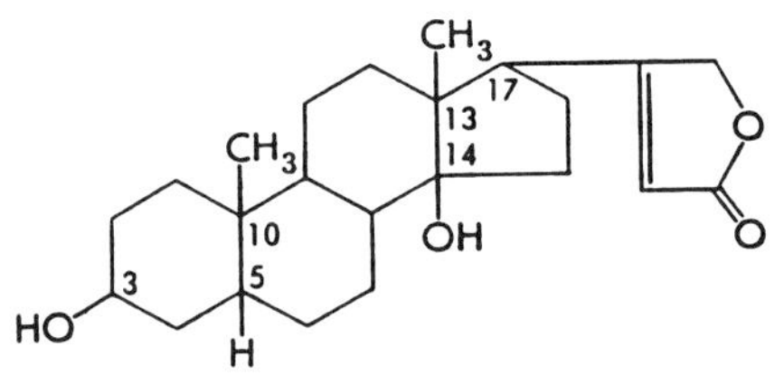

Digitoxigenin

Figure 1 Chemical structures of the aglycones of digoxin and digitoxin, the most frequently prescribed cardiotonic steroids. In both cases the glycoside is the aglycone with three molecules of digitoxose attached at position 3. (Modified from Ref. 91.)

tal foxglove (1) (e.g., *Digitalis pupurea*) and animal sources including certain toads (2). In the clinical arena, the two most widely used forms of this drug are digoxin and digitoxin (see Fig 1). Many other agents are also widely used in research including ouabain and strophanthidin. Recent work has shown that humans themselves synthesize one such agent, ouabain, (3) and that it may be elevated in essential hypertension (4). Many of the studies investigating the mechanism of action of cardiotonic steroids have focused on the ability of these agents to bind to the Na,K-ATPase ("the sodium pump") and inhibit it (5,6). The Na,K-ATPase is found on the plasma membranes of many cells including heart cells, neurons, red blood cells, and virtually every other cell in the body. There are different isoforms of the Na,K-ATPase with varying sensitivity to cardiotonic steroids (7–9). This review will examine the question of how the cardiotonic steroids work to increase the strength of contraction of the heart.

I. BRIEF OVERVIEW

Three simple questions are addressed by this review and one question is addressed that is more complicated. The simple quesions are: 1. Does sodium pump blockade lead to an increase in strength of contraction of the heart? 2. Do cardiotonic steroids produce sodium pump blockade when used at therapeutic levels? 3. Do cardiotonic steroids produce other actions in addition to any sodium pump blockade? The answers to the first two questions are a clear yes. There are few direct data regarding the third question, and those relevant results are either flawed, contradictory or unconfirmed. Consequently, it is still possible that cardiotonic steroids act to increase the strength of contraction of the heart without necessarily involving the sodium pump, but more work needs to be done. The last and most complicated question is: To what extent do other inotropic mechanisms (e.g., those used by catecholamines) and those involving sodium-pump inhibition by cardiotonic steroids interact? Because of the indirect actions of altered calcium metabolism produced by sodium-pump inhibition and because of many common regulatory proteins, there are important interactions.

II. SODIUM PUMP BLOCKADE AND CHANGES IN FORCE

A relationship between force produced by heart muscle and sodium was recognized by Luttgau and Niedergerke 30 years ago (10). However, the first clearly articulated mechanistic discussion dates from the subsequent work by Baker and colleagues (11). Their identification of the Na–Ca exchanger (first shown in heart by Reuter and Seitz [12]) was a key factor in explaining how a change in intracellular sodium could be linked to a change in intracellular calcium, $[Ca^{2+}]_i$, (see also work by Langer [13–15] and below). Following the work by Baker et al. and by Reuter and Seitz, it took about 10 years for a proper investigation of the relationship between intracellular sodium and force in heart muscle to be started because it required measurement of intracellular sodium activity, $[Na^+]_i$, in heart as well as force. The first critical step came from the use of ion-selective microelectrodes in contractile cardiac tissue. Ellis (16) and Deitmer and Ellis (17,18) showed quite clearly that as higher and higher concentrations of cardiotonic steroids were applied, intracellular sodium increased to a greater extent. This work by Ellis and Deitmer represented a real milestone in our ability to investigate how cardiotonic steroids work in heart muscle. Eisner and co-workers showed with the simultaneous measurement of intracellular sodium, contractile force, and electrical activity that a clear relationship between sodium and force was present in the heart (19–24). Furthermore they provided a quantitative description of the relationship that was a power function (23,24). These experiments were carried out using a voltage-clamp method because sodium-pump inhibition by potassium removal or by cardiotonic steroid application produced significant changes in the shape of the action potential and also led to changes in the resting potential of the cardiac preparations. The observed changes in force due to sodium pump inhibition did not require the use of cardiotonic steroids, since other means of Na,K-ATPase inhibition (e.g., reduced extracellular potassium) were equally effective. The important point is that an increase in intracellular sodium was accompanied by an increase in force.

Supporting the overall conclusion that increasing intracellular sodium leads to an increase in contractile force were a number of important experiments by several groups. Sheu and Fozzard showed a clear link between elevated intracellular sodium and calcium (25) (see also below) and that the altered intracellular sodium itself was linked to changes in force. Under voltage-clamp, reducing intracellular sodium led to a clear reduction in force as mentioned above and this was supported by experiments in which intracellular sodium was reduced by treatment with tetrodotoxin (TTX) or with lidocaine (26,27). It did not matter exactly how the reduction or increase of sodium was achieved. Thus Sheu and Lederer (28) showed

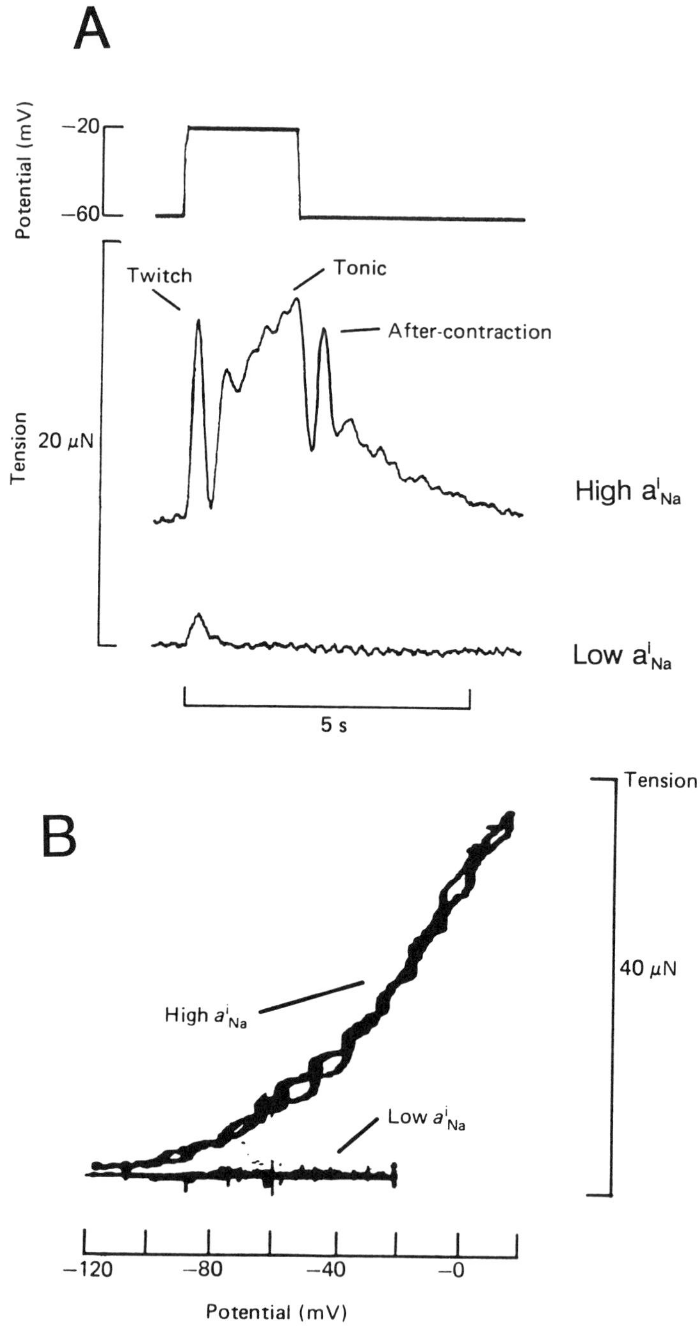

Figure 2 The dependence of tonic force on intracellular sodium in heart. A. A comparison of the effects of high (23.4 mM) and low (9.4 mM) intracellular sodium activity, a^{i}_{Na}, on the development of force in voltage-clamped cardiac Purkinje fibers. B. A comparison of the voltage-dependence of tonic tension at high and low a^{i}_{Na} as in A. (From Ref. 23 with permission.)

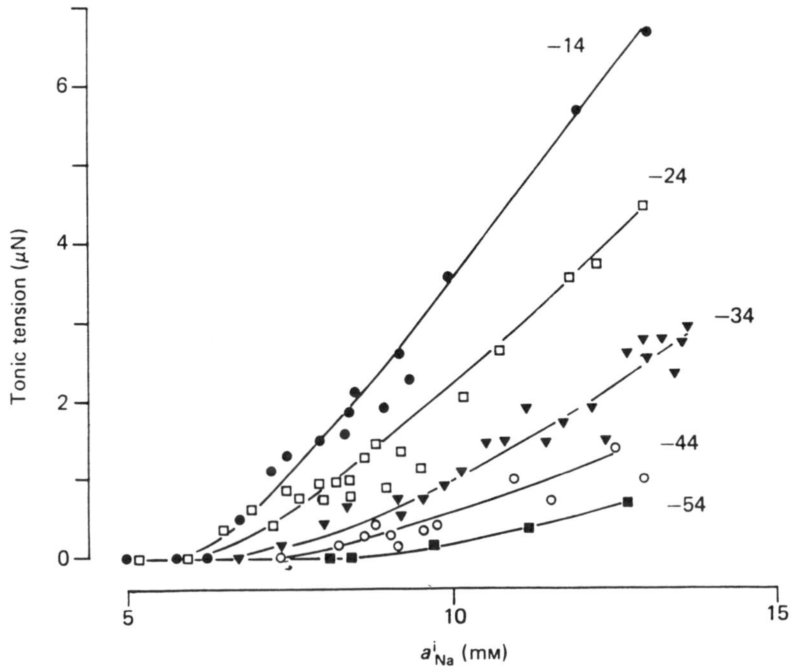

Figure 3 The dependence of tonic force on intracellular sodium in heart. Tonic tension measured in sheep cardiac Purkinje fibers is plotted as a function of a^{i}_{Na} for various membrane potentials. (From Ref. 23 with permission.)

that an increase in intracellular sodium and a concomitant increase in force could also come about simply by increasing the stimulation rate of the cardiac tissue, a finding consistent with Sheu's earlier work. Other papers have confirmed and/or extended these diverse early findings (29–32). The important finding is that a clear (albeit indirect) link exists between resting intracellular sodium in heart muscle and measured contractile force. Both resting force (or cell length) and twitch force (or peak cell shortening) increase as intracellular sodium rises (see Figs. 2 and 3). Three significant factors, however, make direct analysis complicated and should be noted: 1. calcium overload, 2. sodium-force hysteresis, and 3. intracellular acidosis. Although each of these factors complicates the simple monotonic relationship between $[Na^+]_i$ and force, these complexities arise with marked changes in $[Na^+]_i$ and are moderately well understood in terms of altered sarcoplasmic reticulum (SR) function and altered contractile responsiveness of the myofilaments (see below).

Calcium overload is a condition characterized by spontaneous calcium release by the SR (33–37). This condition occurs when the SR is loaded excessively with calcium and is generally seen when intracellular sodium is elevated and intracellular calcium is therefore also elevated. However, other factors can play an important role, such as adrenergic stimulation (38), or altered electrical activity, such as longer than normal action potentials (39,40). Because of the spontaneous calcium release observed during calcium overload, the relationship between intracellular sodium and force is generally altered.

Hysteresis in the relationship between force and $[Na^+]_i$ has been observed when intracellular sodium is rising or falling rapidly. The cause of this hysteresis has not been proven but has been suggested to involve altered intracellular pH or possibly SR function, among other possibilities (41). Thus the rate of change of $[Na^+]_i$ and its history are important factors in evaluating how altered $[Na^+]_i$ may be related to altered force.

Altered intracellular pH may arise for many reasons including altered Na-H exchanger activity (42,43), altered $[Ca^{2+}]_i$ (44), as well as altered metabolism or altered extracellular environment. Changes in intracellular pH produce diverse actions on many systems, including the sodium–calcium exchanger (45,56), but it also can directly alter the sensitivity of the contractile proteins. While the list of factors that can alter the relationship between $[Na^+]_i$ and tension is incomplete, it is important to be aware of such interactions.

The action of $[Na^+]_i$ on force is nevertheless profound and largely mediated by the Na–Ca exchanger because it plays such a dominant role in setting the level of resting $[Ca^{2+}]_i$. Small changes in $[Ca^{2+}]_i$ translate into much larger effects on tension because the SR acts as an amplifier. Thus a slight increase in resting $[Ca^{2+}]_i$ in the cytosol will lead to a significant increase in releasable calcium from the SR. The SR Ca^{2+}-ATPase will continue to pump calcium into the SR and produce an increase in SR Ca-content until the intrinsic efflux of calcium out of the SR (e.g., through Ca^{2+} release channels) equals the influx produced by the Ca^{2+}-ATPase and any other SR Ca-pump.

III. SODIUM–CALCIUM EXCHANGER

The sodium–calcium exchanger plays a critical role in many inotropic mechanisms. Since sarcolemmal processes regulate the steady-state calcium load in the myocyte, their influences on the SR calcium load and on resting $[Ca^{2+}]_i$ are profound. Recent experimental results have provided quantitative evidence showing that the Na–Ca exchanger is the dominant factor in regulating sarcolemmal calcium extrusion (47,48). Being such a central factor in regulating $[Ca^{2+}]_i$, modulation of the Na–Ca exchanger is a means of altering $[Ca^{2+}]_i$, the SR calcium load, and hence inotropy. By reducing the pumping of sodium out of the heart cells, sodium pump inhibition leads to an increase in $[Na^+]_i$. It is this increase of $[Na^+]_i$ that affects the Na–Ca exchanger and hence leads to an increase in $[Ca^{2+}]_i$. This is the hypothesis first articulated by Baker and colleagues and also suggested by Langer (13).

We know a great deal more about the Na–Ca exchanger now than we did in the late 1960s when it was first discovered by Reuter and Seitz (12) and by Baker et al. (11). Its stoichiometry is clearly 3 Na^+ to 1 Ca^{2+} and is consequently electrogenic (49–51), generating inward current under normal conditions. The primary amino acid sequence has been identified (52) as having a number of important physical and chemical properties (53–55) including the transport mechanism, which appears to be consecutive (53,56,57) rather than simultaneous. It is interesting that the Na–Ca exchanger in the retinal rod cells that also serves to extrude intracellular calcium is very different from that in the heart transporting four sodium ions in one direction with the counter-transport of one calcium ion and one potassium ion (58–60). The modulation of the cardiac Na–Ca exchanger by intracellular pH may also be important in our discussion and this feature has been studied. Intracellular acidification inhibits Na–Ca exchange (61). Although the ion-dependence and the voltage-dependence of the Na–Ca exchanger are important for us to understand, the data are incomplete (23,51,62,63). Both features are necessary for us to develop a proper kinetic model of the Na–Ca exchanger. Such a model is needed in order to answer the question of exactly how the Na–Ca exchanger is affected by the elevation of $[Na^+]_i$ produced by Na-pump inhibition. The reversal potential of the Na–Ca exchanger will be altered by changes in $[Na^+]_i$ and this will tend to decrease the extrusion of calcium by the Na–Ca exchanger, if the other kinetic parameters of the Na–Ca exchanger do not change. It is also possible that the Na–Ca exchanger may be affected in other ways by $[Na^+]_i$ or $[Ca^{2+}]_i$ or by extracellular ion activities. Nevertheless, it is clear that the direction of the changes in $[Ca^{2+}]_i$ produced by the increase in $[Na^+]_i$ are those that are expected (25).

Recently a new role was suggested for the Na–Ca exchanger. It was suggested by Leblanc and Hume (64) that the Na–Ca exchanger may also be important in excitation–contraction (EC) coupling even when resting $[Na^+]_i$ is not altered from normal. They provide evidence that depolarization of the cell may produce enough sodium influx through sodium *channels* to activate the Na–Ca exchanger to transport calcium directly into the cell. Quantitative estimates of the amount of sodium and calcium involved and the kinetic, electrical, and anatomical circumstances severely limit how and when such a mechanism can occur and lead to the need for a "fuzzy" space just under the sarcolemmal surface (65–69). *The properties of this "fuzzy" space are equivalent to a 100 Å thick volume under the sarcolemma that has a different diffusion constant for small ions. It must be stressed that such spaces needed to explain the Leblanc and Hume result are not equivalent to those that produce standing ion gradients (over seconds to minutes). The accumulation in this "fuzzy" space is thought to be limited 1–10 msec* (65). Nevertheless, just as the altered behavior of the Na–Ca exchanger leads to an increase in resting $[Ca^{2+}]_i$, when $[Na^+]_i$ increases, its action in EC coupling will almost certainly also be altered when $[Na^+]_i$ is elevated. More work is required to examine how this aspect of Na–Ca exchanger behavior is affected.

It is clear that the Na–Ca exchanger must contribute to a positive inotropic action of any cardiotonic steriod when the Na-pump is inhibited. The question is whether cardiotonic steroids may act to alter some other feature of cell behavior besides the sodium pump (see below). The reasons for raising this doubt is the very small changes in intracellular sodium that are normally produced by sodium pump inhibition. Changes in $[Na^+]_i$ may be around 1 mM (or possibly less) (70) and such small changes are hard to measure reproducibly. In addition, because these changes may take place over minutes to hours, precise measurements become even more difficult. This second factor makes any control experiments equally hard to carry out since the preparations used change over that time-frame due to the experimental procedures. The series of experiments carried out by Eisner et al. (23,24) sought to investigate whether changes in $[Na^+]_i$ could be involved in important inotropic actions even if the changes in $[Na^+]_i$ were very small. The work (see Figs. 2–5) used voltage-clamped cardiac Purkinje fibers and ion-selective microelectrodes to measure intracellular sodium. These investigations showed that there were two important features regulating contractility that must be considered. First, there is a power–function relationship between $[Na^+]_i$ and force. This means that exceedingly small changes in $[Na^+]_i$ were linked to significant changes in force. Second, the manner in which changes in force could be brought about by changes in membrane

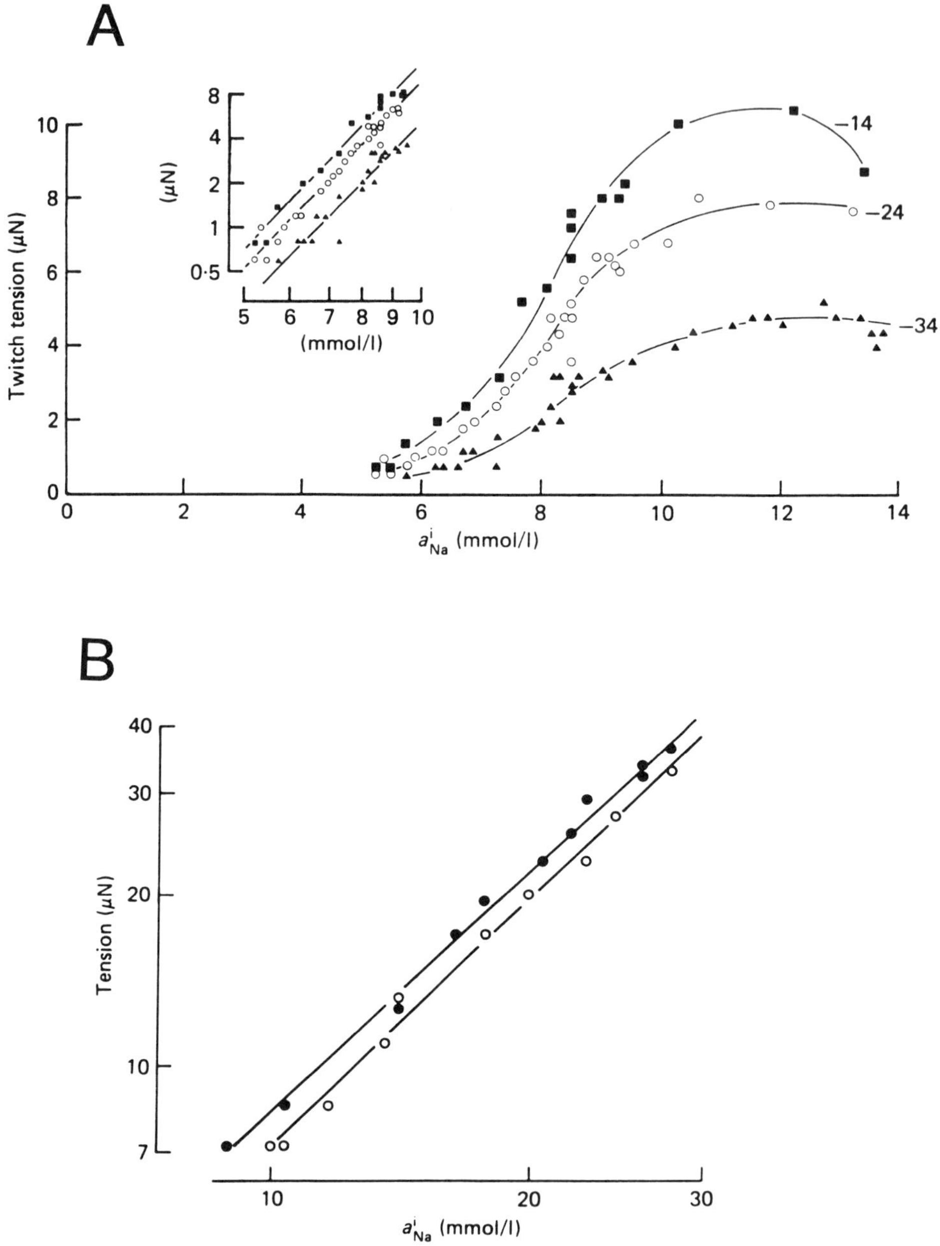

Figure 4 The dependence of twitch force on intracellular sodium in heart. A. Twitch tension is plotted as a function of intracellular sodium activity, a^i_{Na} for three different depolarization potentials. The inset shows the same data (over the range of a^i_{Na} 5–10 mM) plotted on double logarithmic axes. B. A comparison of the elevation of a^i_{Na} on twitch tension when produced by either potassium depletion (open circles) or the application of the cardiotonic steroid strophanthidin (filled circles). (From Ref. 24 with permission.)

potential or by changes in $[Na^+]_i$ suggested that the Na–Ca exchanger was involved. The data suggested that the link between the measured changes in $[Na^+]_i$ and the changes in force arose from changes in $[Ca^{2+}]_i$ attributable to a voltage-dependent Na–Ca exchanger (23).

A number of reports have indicated that the application of very low concentrations of cardiotonic steroids were occasionally linked to a *reduction* of $[Na^+]_i$ (71). However, subsequent studies suggested that when $[Na^+]_i$ was reduced by cardiotonic steroids, so was force (70). Thus the suggestion that another mechanism of cardiotonic steroid inotropy must exist that involves some process other than the sodium pump and the Na–Ca exchanger is not supported. In general, the data in these reports are weak with respect to this point and improved methods and new experiments may be able to address this point better. Some additional reports suggest that cardiotonic steroids can act by means in addition to those that involve the Na-pump and the Na–Ca exchanger. Several reports have suggested that following the application of cardiotonic steroids to cardiac tissue, the calcium current increased (72,73). This increase may be related to the reported increase in I_{Ca} that arises after photorelease of caged calcium (74,75). Although this additional mechanism does not directly depend on either the Na,K-ATPase or on the Na–Ca exchanger, it does secondarily depend on the elevation of $[Ca^{2+}]_i$ that does depend on these two transport systems. This increase may be due to the $[Ca^{2+}]_i$-dependent activation of protein kinase C (PKC), which can phosphorylate diverse proteins and possibly the heteropentameric calcium channel protein. At least one report has suggested that there may be a completely novel mechanism of action of the cardiotonic steroid that involves an intracellular or nuclear binding site (76). Much more data would be needed, however, to support the notion that even a component of the positive inotropic action of cardiotonic steroids arises from intracellular or nuclear binding.

IV. SARCOPLASMIC RETICULUM

Although a direct action of the cardiotonic steroids on the Na,K-ATPase is an undisputed and primary event, the role of all other elements in the story has been challenged over the years. Data presented here and elsewhere provide evidence that the sarcolemmal Na–Ca exchanger is responsible for translating a change in Na-pump activity and hence in $[Na^+]_i$ into a change in $[Ca^{2+}]_i$. Modern techniques to measure $[Ca^{2+}]_i$ using fluorescent indicators and ion-selective microelectrodes have provided a consistent finding: the changes in resting $[Ca^{2+}]_i$ produced by "therapeutic" levels of cardiotonic steroid application are very small. How, then, could a significant change in twitch force still be observed? The simple answer is the "sarcoplasmic reticulum amplifier effect." The SR Ca-ATPase pumps calcium into the intracellular compartment and acts as an amplifier for any change in resting $[Ca^{2+}]_i$. A small change in resting $[Ca^{2+}]_i$ leads to a large change in the amount of calcium stored in the SR. The amplification is a function of the relative high rate of pumping of the cardiac Ca-ATPase and its high affinity for intracellular calcium along with the modest to low leak of the SR calcium release channels. With a very large store of calcium, a large amount of calcium is released when the cardiac myocyte is depolarized and SR calcium release is triggered. It is still not known exactly how calcium is buffered within the cardiac SR, how calsequestrin may be

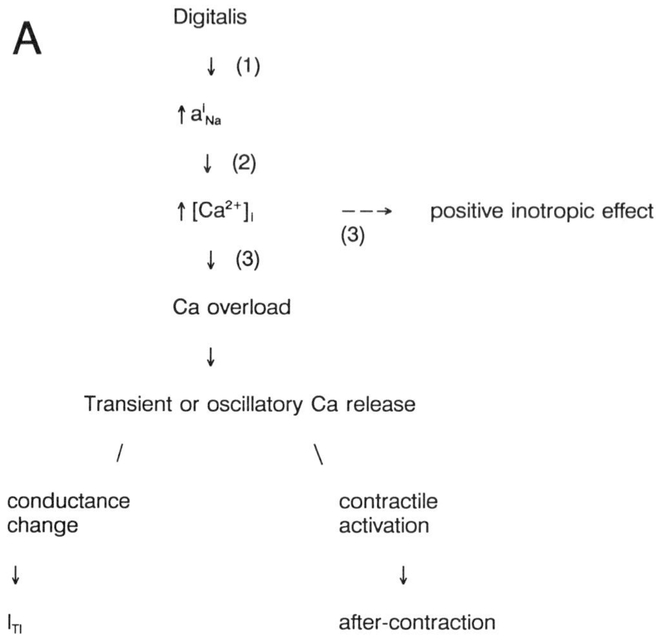

Figure 5 The elevation of a^{i}_{Na} is also associated with a positive inotropic effect and also "calcium overload." The calcium overload gives rise to oscillations of intracellular calcium that are manifest as aftercontractions and arrhythmogenic transient inward currents (I_{TI}). A. Schematic diagram of the process. "Digitalis" is used to mean any cardiotonic steroid. (1) mediated by Na,K ATPase inhibition, (2) mediated by the sarcolemmal Na/Ca exchanger as a^{i}_{Na} increases, (3) mediated by calcium uptake by the sarcoplasmic reticulum as $[Ca^{2+}]_i$ increases. (From Kass Ref. 35.) B. The dependence of twitch tension, tonic tension, the aftercontraction magnitude and I_{TI} magnitude on a^{i}_{Na}. (From Ref. 24 with permission.)

functioning there, how or if intra-SR calcium may itself affect calcium release or exactly how pumping and release functions are spatially distributed in the SR. Nevertheless, these actions are clearly linked to small changes in intracellular sodium brought about by diverse means.

Because of the very high amplification in the system, increases in $[Ca^{2+}]_i$ would be expected to produce a relatively greater increase in the amount of releasable calcium. If, however, the increases in $[Ca^{2+}]_i$ were too high, a condition called "calcium overload" may develop. Although the idea is still somewhat vaguely stated, it means that there is too much calcium in the intracellular compartments for stable handling. Calcium overload is characterized by spontaneous calcium release from the SR. This is associated with a flatenning in the $[Na^+]_i$-tension relationship, as shown in Figure 5, by the development of arrhythmogenic transient inward currents (I_{TI}), the development of membrane electrical "noise" (77), and possibly calcium loading of the mitochondria. The arrhythmogenic transient inward current, I_{TI}, is responsible for activating some triggered extrasystoles and may contribute to both delayed after-depolarizations (also called DADs or transient depolarizations) and early after-depolarizations (also called EADs or transient depolarizations), although other membrane currents are also involved (e.g., I_{Ca}, I_K, and I_{Na}) (33).

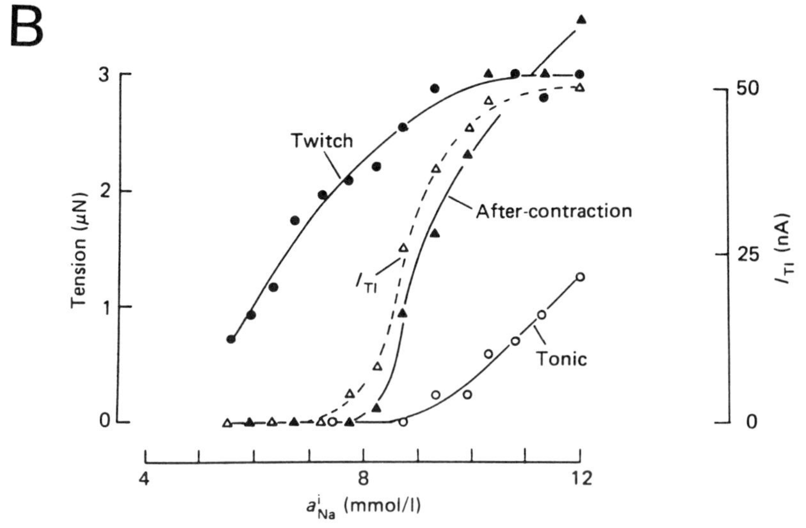

Other inotropic agents that also affect the SR and sarcolemmal currents can affect I_{TI} (e.g., adrenergic agents such as epinephrine). Loss of synchrony of calcium release can affect membrane currents (78) and force (79).

V. SR Ca^{2+}-ATPase, INTRA-SR CALCIUM BUFFERS, AND SR-Ca-RELEASE CHANNEL

The calcium content of the SR depends on the uptake of calcium by the SR (via the SR Ca^{2+}-ATPase), the storage of Ca^{2+} in the SR, and the release mechanisms that control the efflux of Ca^{2+} from the SR. Each of these steps is a potential site of interaction for inotropic agents. There is no evidence to date that cardiotonic steroids have any *direct* action on these processes. The action appears to be mediated indirectly by changes in intracellular calcium. Although we have touched on established features that link Na-pump blockade to altered calcium handling, it should be noted that many other secondary and tertiary factors can also be affected indirectly by Na,K-ATPase inhibition. These other factors may be important in modulating the inotropic action of the cardiotonic steroids and they are only mentioned here because the reader should be aware of the many indirect actions that can arise from Na-pump blockade.

VI. OTHER FACTORS

What "other factors" may mediate or affect contractility following Na-pump inhibition? What do these factors do and how do they get involved? It is the increase in $[Ca^{2+}]_i$ that appears to recruit other signaling mechanisms following Na-pump inhibition. There is Ca^{2+}-activated phosphorylation (e.g., by protein kinase C) as mentioned above (74,75). Such phosphorylation may affect the calcium current, the pumping of calcium by the SR, or the contractile proteins. Ca^{2+}-activated potassium currents have been reported in heart as well as in other tissue (80,81) and may lead to a shorter action potential, just as the recently reported Na-activated potassium currents would (82). Because the Na–Ca exchanger is activated by increasing intracellular calcium and produces more inward current when so activated, its activation will also alter the shape of the cardiac action potential but in the opposite direction to the Ca^{2+}-activated K current. In addition to the possible "upregulation" of the calcium current by protein kinase C phosphorylation, the calcium current has also been shown in many studies (75) to be inactivated by elevated $[Ca^{2+}]_i$. There are diverse short-term and long-term actions of altered $[Ca^{2+}]_i$ and it is not clear now which of these is particularly important regarding inotropic actions of the cardiotonic steroids.

VII. THE CLINICAL DILEMMA: WHICH INOTROPIC AGENT TO USE?

In addition to the cardiotonic steroids, many agents increase the strength of contraction of the heart. For long-term use in patients with heart failure, the preponderance of drugs that have some positive inotropic action are not used because of the diverse side effects. The cardiotonic steroids are also well known because of their toxic side effects, which in the past were reported to affect as many as 25% of hospitalized patients (83). The principal cardiac toxicity is the development of arrhythmias, frequently of ventricular origin. Cellular studies have suggested that the desired increase in intracellular calcium that is part of the positive inotropic effect is also responsible for the development of the arrhythmias. As indicated above, this is characterized by calcium overload, the development of an unstable SR and the spontaneous release of SR calcium. These spontaneous increases in $[Ca^{2+}]_i$ lead to calcium-activated inward current, the appearance of both delayed DADs and early EADs, and even the reduction of contractile force triggered by the cardiac action potential. These arrhythmias are exacerbated by low concentrations of potassium in the blood because of the role of the Na,K-ATPase (36). Indeed lowering extracellular potassium ion concentrations also inhibits the Na-pump and produces effects similar to those produced by cardiotonic steroids. Low magnesium levels also tend to potentiate the toxicity of cardiotonic steroids (35). Because of the linkage between therapeutic action of the cardiotonic steroids and their toxic action and the high prevalence of toxicity, a sustained effort has been made to develop a less toxic and more efficacious inotropic drug. This work has met with mixed success over the years, with a corresponding waxing and waning of support for the use of cardiotonic steroids to treat heart failure. At present, the cardiotonic steroids still appear to be the principal drugs used. It should be noted, however, that the toxic side effects of this family of agents are significant. Recently, the toxicity of digoxin has been effectively treated with digoxin immune Fab fragments (84,85). Of 717 patients treated, 50% responded completely and only 12% showed no response to the antibody therapy. The availability of this effective rapid therapy for digoxin intoxication significantly improves the safety of these agents (86).

Milrinone and amrinone, bipyridine phosphodiesterase inhibitors, have been among the most promising alternative positive inotropic agents to the cardiotonic steroids recently examined (87–89). It is thought that this class of drugs acts by preventing the breakdown of cAMP. The maintained or increased concentrations of these cyclic nucleotides lead to further activation of their respective target kinases, which in turn phosphorylate diverse target proteins. The phosphorylated proteins would be responsible for producing the increased strength of contraction of the heart. It is certainly a challenge to replace a drug that has proven itself for over 200 years. While early results suggested that milrinone produced an excellent positive inotropic effect, these results were not compelling. A recent randomized double-blind study attempted to rectify this matter by studying 230 patients. The patients were in sinus rhythm with heart failure and were treated with milrinone, digoxin, both, or placebo (90). In the population studied, milrinone did produce acceptable increases in strength of contraction of the heart but it offered no advantage over digoxin and was associated with more severe arrhythmias during chronic oral treatment. Milrinone is effective when administered intravenously for acute inotropic support and has recently been approved for this use.

VIII. SUMMARY

The positive inotropic actions of cardiotonic steroid application arise because these agents can inhibit the Na-pump and lead to an increase in $[Na^+]_i$. The increased $[Na^+]_i$ (albeit small) is enough to increase $[Ca^{2+}]_i$ by a small amount as well. The action of the SR to amplify this small signal leads to a large increase in the amount of calcium released by the SR with stimulation. This increased amount of released calcium then activates contraction more and produces a significant increase in the strength of contraction. This positive inotropic effect is effective in treating heart failure but can produce significant toxic side effects.

ACKNOWLEDGMENTS

We would like to thank the American Heart Association and its Maryland affiliate, the National Institutes of Health, the British Heart Foundation, and the Medical Research Council for financial support.

REFERENCES

1. Wray S, Eisner DA, Allen DG. Two hundred years of the foxglove. Med Hist 1985;Suppl. 5:132–50.
2. Shimoni Y, Gotsman M, Deutsch J, Kachalsky S, Lichtstein D. Endogenous ouabain-like compound increases heart muscle contractility. Nature 1984;307:369–80.
3. Hamlyn JM, Blaustein MP, Bova S, DuCharme DW, Harris DW, Mandel F, Mathews WR, Ludens JH. Identification and characterization of a ouabain-like compound from human plasma. Proc Natl Acad Sci USA 1991;88:6259–63.
4. Hamlyn JM, Ringel R, Schaeffer J, Levinson PD, Hamilton BP, Kowarski AA, Blaustein MP. A circulating inhibitor of $(Na^+ + K^+)$ ATPase associated with essential hypertension. Nature 1982;300:650–2.
5. Kaplan JH, DeWeer P. The sodium pump: structure, mechanism, and regulation, New York: The Rockefeller University Press, 1991,
6. Carafoli E, Scarpa A. Transport ATPases 2nd ed. New York: The New York Academy of Sciences, 1982.
7. Berrebi Bertrand I, Maixent JM, Guede FG, Gerbi A, Charlemagne D, Lelievre LG. Two functional Na+/K(+)-ATPase isoforms in the left ventricle of guinea pig heart. Eur J Biochem 1991;196:129–33.
8. Noel F, Wibo M, Godfraind T. Distribution of alpha 1 and alpha 2 (Na+,K+)-ATPase isoforms between the junctional (t-tubular) and non-junctional sarcolemmal domains of rat ventricle. Biochem Pharmacol 1991;41:313–15.

9. Orlowski J, Lingrel JB. Thyroid and glucocorticoid hormones regulate the expression of multiple Na,K-ATPase genes in cultured neonatal rat cardiac myocytes. J Biol Chem 1990;265:3462–70.
10. Luttgau HC, Niedergerke R. The antagonism between Ca and Na ions on the frog's heart. J Physiol 1958;143:486–505.
11. Baker PF, Blaustein MP, Hodgkin AL, Steinhardt RA. The influence of calcium on sodium efflux in squid axons. J Physiol 1969;200:431–58.
12. Reuter H, Seitz N. The dependence of calcium efflux from cardiac muscle on temperature and external ion composition. J Physiol 1968;195:451–70.
13. Langer GA. The role of sodium ion in the regulation of myocardial contractility. J Mol Cell Cardiol 1970;1:203–7.
14. Imanishi S. Calcium-sensitive discharges in canine Purkinje fibers. Jpn J Physiol 1971;21:443–63.
15. Reuter H. Strom-spannungsbeziehungen von Purkinje-fasern bei vershiedenen extracellularen calcium-konzentrationen und unter adrenalineinwirkung. Pflugers Arch 1966;287:357–67.
16. El-Sherif N, Gough WB, Zeiler RH, Mehra R. Triggered ventricular rhythms in 1-day-old myocardial infarction in the dog. Circ Res 1983;52:566–79.
17. Deitmer JW, Ellis D. The intracellular sodium activity of cardiac Purkinje fibres during inhibition and re-activation of the Na-K pump. J Physiol 1978;284:241–59.
18. Deitmer JW, Ellis D. Changes in the intracellular sodium activity of sheep heart Purkinje fibres produced by calcium and other divalent cations. J Physiol 1978;277:437–53.
19. Eisner DA, Lederer WJ, Vaughan-Jones RD. Electrogenic sodium pumping in cardiac muscle: simultaneous measurement of intracellular sodium activity, membrane current and tension. J Physiol 1979;300:42–3.
20. Eisner DA, Lederer WJ. Does sodium pump inhibition produce the positive inotropic effects of strophanthidin in mammalian cardiac muscle. J Physiol 1979;296:75–6.
21. Eisner DA, Lederer WJ. The relationship between sodium pump activity and twitch tension in cardiac Purkinje fibres. J Physiol 1980;303:475–94.
22. Eisner DA, Lederer WJ. Characterization of the electrogenic sodium pump in cardiac Purkinje fibres. J Physiol 1980;303:441–74.
23. Eisner DA, Lederer WJ, Vaughan-Jones RD. The control of tonic tension by membrane potential and intracellular sodium activity in the sheep cardiac Purkinje fibre. J Physiol 1983;335:723–43.
24. Eisner DA, Lederer WJ, Vaughan Jones RD. The quantitative relationship between twitch tension and intracellular sodium activity in sheep cardiac Purkinje fibres. J Physiol (Lond) 1984;355:251–66.
25. Sheu SS, Fozzard HA. Transmembrane Na+ and Ca2+ electrochemical gradients in cardiac muscle and their relationship to force development. J Gen Physiol 1982;80: 325–51.
26. Eisner DA, Lederer WJ, Sheu SS. The role of intracellular sodium activity in the antiarrhythmic action of local anaesthetics in sheep Purkinje fibres. J Physiol (Lond) 1983;340:239–57.
27. Sheu SS, Lederer WJ. Lidocaine's negative inotropic and antiarrhythmic actions. Dependence on shortening of action potential duration and reduction of intracellular sodium activity. Circ Res 1985;57:578–90.
28. Lederer WJ, Sheu S-S. Heart rate-dependent changes in intracellular sodium activity and twitch tension in sheep cardiac Purkinje fibres. J Physiol 1983;345:44.
29. January CT, Fozzard HA. The effects of membrane potential, extracellular potassium, and tetrodotoxin on the intracellular sodium activity of sheep cardiac muscle. Circ Res 1984;54:652–65.
30. Boyett MR, Hart G, Levi AJ. Factors affecting intracellular sodium during repetitive activity in isolated sheep Purkinje fibres. J Physiol 1987;384:405–29.

31. Boyett MR, Hart G, Levi AJ, Roberts A. Effects of repetitive activity on developed force and intracellular sodium in isolated sheep and dog Purkinje fibres. J Physiol 1987;388:295–322.
32. Im W-B, Lee CO. Quantitative relation of twitch and tonic tensions to intracellular NaT+ activity in cardiac Purkinje fibres. Am J Physiol 1984;247:C478–87.
33. Lederer WJ, Tsien RW. Transient inward current underlying arrhythmogenic effects of cardiotonic steroids in Purkinje fibers. J Physiol 1976;263:73–100.
34. Lin CI, Vassalle M. Role of sodium in strophanthidin toxicity of Purkinje fibers. Am J Physiol 1978;234:H477–86.
35. Kass RS, Lederer WJ, Tsien RW, Weingart R. Role of calcium ions in transient inward currents and aftercontractions induced by strophanthidin in cardiac purkinje fibres. J Physiol 1978;281:187–208.
36. Eisner DA, Lederer WJ. Inotropic and arrhythmogenic effects of potassium-depleted solutions on mammalian cardiac muscle. J Physiol 1979;294:255–77.
37. Cannell MB, Vaughan-Jones RD, Lederer WJ. Ryanodine block of calcium oscillations in heart muscle affects the sodium-tension relation. Red Proc 1985;44:2964–2969.
38. Hoffman BF, Rosen MR. Cellular mechanisms for cardiac arrhythmias. Circ Res 1981;49:1–15.
39. Damino BP, Rosen MR. Effects of pacing on triggered activity induced by early afterdepolarizations. Circulation 1984;69:1013–25.
40. Brachmann J, Scherlag BJ, Rosenshtraukh LV, Lazzara R. Bradycardia-dependent triggered activity: relevance to drug-induced multiform ventricular tachycardia. Circulation 1983;68:846–56.
41. Eisner DA, Lederer WJ, Vaughan-Jones RD. The dependence of sodium pumping and tension on intracellular sodium activity in voltage-clamped sheep Purkinje fibres. J Physiol 1981;317:163–87.
42. Vaughan-Jones RD, Eisner DA, Lederer WJ. Effects of changes of intracellular pH on contraction in sheep cardiac Purkinje fibres. J Gen Physiol 1987;89:1015–32.
43. Kaila K, Vaughan Jones RD. Influence of sodium-hydrogen exchange on intracellular pH, sodium and tension in sheep cardiac Purkinje fibres. J Physiol (Lond) 1987;390: 93–118.
44. Vaughan-Jones RD, Lederer WJ, Eisner DA. Ca^{2+} ions can affect intracellular pH in mammalian cardiac muscle. Nature 1983;301:522–4.
45. Philipson KD, Bersohn MM, Nishimoto AY. Effects of pH on Na^{+}-Ca^{2+} exchange in canine cardiac sarcolemmal vesicles. Circ Res 1982;50:287–93.
46. Mullins LJ, Tifferet T, Vassort G, Whittembury J. Effects of internal sodium and hydrogen ions and of external calcium ions and membrane potential on calcium entry in squid axons. J Physiol 1983;338:295–319.
47. Crespo LM, Grantham CJ, Cannell MB. Kinetics, stoichiometry and role of the Na–Ca exchange mechanism in isolated cardiac myocytes. Nature 1990;345:618–21.
48. Bers DM, Bridge JHB. Relaxation of rabbit ventricular muscle by Na–Ca exchange and sarcoplasmic reticulum calcium pump: ryanodine and voltage sensitivity. Circ Res 1989;65:334–42.
49. Reeves JP, Hale CC. The stoichiometry of the cardiac sodium–calcium exchange system. J Biol Chem 1984;259:7733–9.
50. Kimura J, Noma A, Irisawa H. Na–Ca exchange current in mammalian heart cells. Nature 1986;319:596–7.
51. Kimura J, Miyamae S, Noma A. Identification of sodium–calcium exchange current in single ventricular cells of guinea-pig. J Physiol 1987;384:199–222.
52. Nicoll DA, Longoni S, Philipson KD. Molecular cloning and functional expression of the cardiac sarcolemmal Na(+)-Ca2+ exchanger. Science 1990;250:562–5.
53. Niggli E, Lederer WJ. Molecular operations of the sodium–calcium exchanger revealed by conformation currents. Nature 1991;349:621–4.

54. Hilgemann DW. Regulation and deregulation of cardiac Na(+)-Ca2+ exchange in giant excised sarcolemmal membrane patches. Nature 1990;344:242–5.
55. Hilgemann DW. Giant excised cardiac sarcolemmal membrane patches: sodium and sodium–calcium exchange currents. Pflugers Arch 1989;415:247–9.
56. Khananshvili D. Distinction between the two basic mechanisms of cation transport in the cardiac Na–Ca^{2+} exchange system. Biochemistry 1990;29:2437–42.
57. Khananshvili D. Voltage-dependent modulation of ion binding and translocation in the cardiac Na+/Ca2+ exchange system. J Biol Chem 1991;266:13764–9.
58. Yau KW, Nakatani K. Electrogenic Na–Ca exchange in retinal rod outer segment. Nature 1984;311:661–3.
59. Nakatani K, Yau KW. Sodium-dependent calcium extrusion and sensitivity regulation in retinal cones of the salamander. J Physiol (Lond) 1989;409:525–48.
60. Cervetto L, Lagnado L, Perry RJ, Robinson DW, McNaughton PA. Extrusion of calcium from rod outer segments is driven by both sodium and potassium gradients. Nature 1989;337:740–3.
61. Doering AE, Lederer WJ. Cytoplasmic acidity inhibits sodium–calcium exchange in cardiac cells. Biophys J 1991;59.
62. Miura Y, Kimura J. Sodium–calcium exchange current. Dependence on internal Ca and Na and competitive binding of external Na and Ca. J Gen Physiol 1989;93:1129–45.
63. Beuckelmann DJ, Wier WG. Sodium–calcium exchange in guinea-pig cardiac cells: exchange current and changes in intracellular Ca2+. J Physiol (Lond) 1989;414:499–520.
64. Leblanc N, Hume JR. Sodium current-induced release of calcium from cardiac sarcoplasmic reticulum. Science 1990;248:372–6.
65. Lederer WJ, Niggli E, Hadley RW. Sodium–calcium exchange in excitable cells: fuzzy space. Science 1990;248:283.
66. Scheuer T, Auld VJ, Boyd S, Offord J, Dunn R, Catterall WA. Functional properties of rat brain sodium channels expressed in a somatic cell line. Science 1990;247:854–8.
67. Johnson EA, Lemieux RD. Sodium–calcium exchange (technical comment). Science 1991;251:1370–1.
68. Hume JR, Levesque PC, Leblanc N. Sodium–calcium exchange (technical comment). Science 1991;251:1370–1.
69. Lederer WJ, Niggli E, Hadley RW. Sodium–calcium exchange (technical comment). Science 1991;251:1370–1.
70. Sheu S-S, Hamlyn JM, Lederer WJ. Low-dose cardiotonic steroids, intracellular sodium and tension in heart. Circulation 1983;68 (suppl.III):250.
71. Ellis D. The effects of external cations and ouabain on the intracellular sodium activity of sheep heart Purkinje fibres. J Physiol 1977;273:211–40.
72. Lederer WJ, Eisner DA. The effects of sodium pump activity on the slow inward current in sheep cardiac purkinje fibres. Proc R Soc Lond 1982;B 214:249–62.
73. Marban E, Tsien RW. Enhancement of calcium current during digitalis inotropy in mammalian heart: positive feed-back regulation by intracellular calcium? J Physiol 1982;329:589–614.
74. Gurney AM, Charnet P, Pye JM, Nargeot J. Augmentation of cardiac calcium current by flash photolysis of intracellular caged-Ca^{2+} molecules. Nature 1989;341:65–8.
75. Hadley RW, Lederer WJ. Ca^{2+} and voltage inactivate Ca^{2+} channels in guinea-pig ventricular myocytes through independent mechanisms. J Physiol 1991;444:257–68.
76. Isenberg G. Contractility of isolated bovine ventricular myocytes is enhanced by intracellular injection of cardioactive glycosides. Evidence for an intracellular mode of action. In: Erdmann E, ed. Cardiac glycoside receptors and positive inotropy. Darmstadt, 1984:56–71.
77. Kass RS, Tsien RW. Fluctuations in membrane current driven by intracellular calcium in cardiac Purkinje fibers. Biophys J 1982;38:259–69.

78. Berlin JR, Cannell MB, Lederer WJ. Cellular origins of the transient inward current, I_{TI}, in cardiac myocytes: role of fluctuations and waves of elevated intracellular calcium. Circ Res 1989;65:115–26.
79. Cannell MB, Vaughan-Jones RD, Lederer WJ. Ryanodine block of calcium oscillations in heart muscle and the sodium-tension relationship. Fed Proc 1985;44:2964–9.
80. Callewaert G, Vereecke J, Carmeliet E. Existence of a calcium-dependent potassium channel in the membrane of cow cardiac Purkinje cells. Pflugers Arch 1986;406:424–6.
81. Carmeliet E, Biermans G, Callewaert G, Vereecke J. Potassium currents in cardiac cells. Experientia 1987;43:1175–84.
82. Rodrigo GC, Chapman RA. A sodium-activated potassium current in intact ventricular myocytes isolated from the guinea-pig heart. Exp Physiol 1990;75:839–42.
83. Beller GA, Smith TW, Abelmann WH, Haber E, Hood WB Jr. Digitalis intoxication: a prospective clinical study with serum level correlations. N Engl J Med 1971;284(18): 989–98.
84. Hickey AR, Wenger TL, Carpenter VP, Tilson HH, Hlatky MA, Furberg CD, Kirkpatrick CH, Strauss HC, Smith TW. Digoxin Immune Fab therapy in the management of digitalis intoxication: safety and efficacy results of an observational surveillance study. J Am Coll Cardiol 1991;17:590–8.
85. Antman EM, Wenger TL, Butler VP Jr, Haber E, Smith TW. Treatment of 150 cases of life-threatening digitalis intoxication with digoxin-specific Fab antibody fragments. Final report of a multicenter study. Circulation 1990;81:1744–52.
86. Kelly RA. Cardiac glycosides and congestive heart failure. Am J Cardiol 1990;65:10–6E.
87. Wood MA, Hess ML. Long-term oral therapy of congestive heart failure with phosphodiesterase inhibitors. Am J Med Sci 1989;297:105–13.
88. Leier CV. General overview and update of positive inotropic therapy. Am J Med 1986;81:40–5.
89. Packer M. Effect of phosphodiesterase inhibitors on survival of patients with chronic congestive heart failure. Am J Cardiol 1989;63:41–5A.
90. DiBianco R, Shabetai R, Kostuk W, Moran J, Schlant RC, Wright R. A comparison of oral milrinone, digoxin, and their combination in the treatment of patients with chronic heart failure. N Engl J Med 1989;320:677–83.
91. Hoffman BF, Bigger JT Jr. Digitalis and allied cardiac glycosides. In: Gilman AG, Rall TW, Nies AS, Taylor P, eds, The pharmacological basis of therapeutics, 8th ed. New York: Pergamon Press, 1990:814–39.

18

Biochemical and Preclinical Pharmacology of Selective Inhibitors of Cardiovascular Phosphodiesterase Isozymes

PAUL J. SILVER and EDWARD D. PAGANI

Sterling Winthrop Pharmaceuticals Research Division
Rensselaer, New York

I. INTRODUCTION

Cyclic nucleotide phosphodiesterase (PDE) activity was originally described over 20 years ago (1,2). Subsequently, the development of biochemical purification techniques (such as high-resolution diethylaminoethyl (DEAE) and affinity chromatography), immunologic purification techniques (such as use of polyclonal or monoclonal antibodies), and the identification and development of selective pharmacologic inhibitors, has led to the realization that numerous isozymes of PDE exist. These isozymes differ with respect to substrate specificity, tissue/subcellular distribution, and intracellular regulation. For the purpose of this review, emphasis will be focused on cardiac and vascular PDE isozymes, and classified according to primary protein sequence information as recently described (3).

In cardiac muscle, at least four distinct forms of PDE have been identified. These four isozymes vary according to kinetic characteristics, sensitivity to calmodulin, and substrate (cAMP vs. cGMP) specificity (3-6). A calmodulin-sensitive form has a low K_m (0.2–0.5 μM) for cGMP in some species, and V_{max} is stimulated by calmodulin. This isozyme also hydrolyzes cAMP with a slightly lower or equal affinity in most species. A cGMP-stimulated isozyme has a high K_m (10–50 μM) with comparable affinity for cAMP and cGMP, and is insensitive to calmodulin. The V_{max} for this PDE, however, is approximately 10 times greater than the other isozymes. A third PDE isozyme, referred to as cGMP-inhibitable (cGi) or cardiotonic sensitive PDE, is a low K_m form that is specific for cAMP (K_m =0.2–0.3 μM) and insensitive to calmodulin. Cyclic GMP may also be hydrolyzed by this PDE isozyme, but the rate of hydrolysis is extremely low. This PDE is inhibited by cGMP (K_i = 0.2 μM), and by a class of selective PDE isozyme inhibitors that include trequinsin, anagrelide, CI-930, milrinone, imazodan, and numerous other agents. A fourth cAMP-specific PDE (also known as rolipram-sensitive PDE) is a low-K_m cAMP isoform that is not inhibited by cGMP. This isozyme, which often coelutes with cGi PDE, is sensitive to selective inhibition by rolipram.

There are also at least four different PDE isozymes in vascular smooth muscle. A calmodulin-dependent and an independent (zaprinast-sensitive) cGMP PDE have been identified in aortic smooth muscle from human, non-human primate, rodent, and bovine sources (7-9). Zaprinast is a somewhat selective inhibitor of this cGMP PDE, but can also inhibit Ca^{2+}-calmodulin regulated PDE with a relatively higher K_i value. The precise role of these cGMP-PDE isozymes (calmodulin dependent and independent forms) in regulating vascular tone is not yet apparent, and awaits the development of more selective or more potent pharmacologic inhibitors.

Cyclic GMP-inhibitable PDE is the predominant low-K_m cAMP PDE present in aortic vascular smooth muscle (8), although rolipram-sensitive cAMP PDE has been identified in bovine aortic smooth muscle (10).

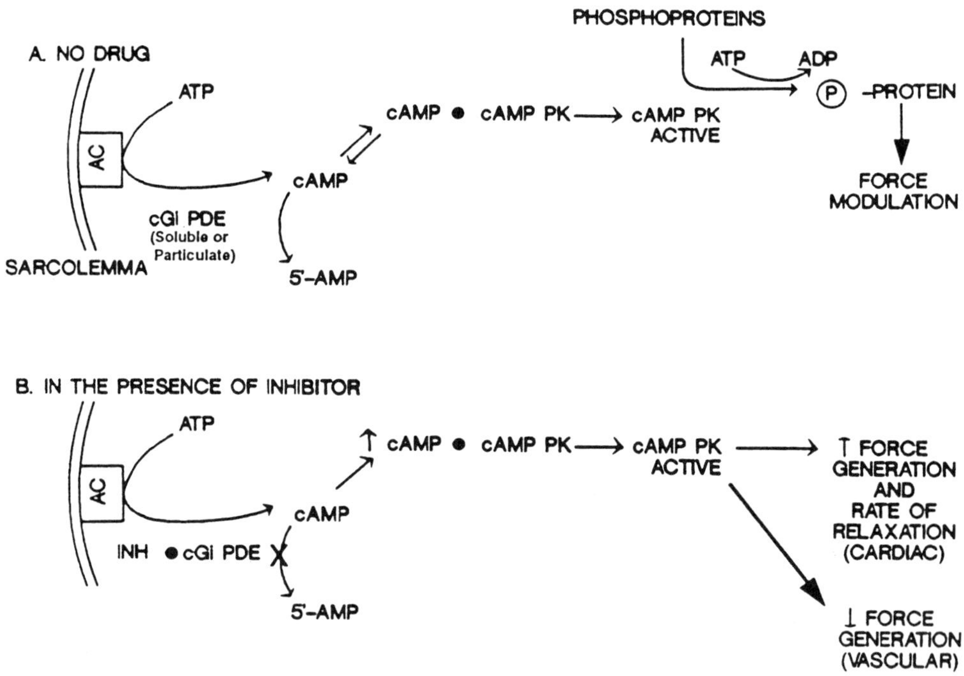

Figure 1 Hypothesis for the cardiovascular mechanism of action of selective cGi PDE inhibitors. A. Events leading to force modulation in cardiac and vascular smooth muscle. In response to stimulation of beta-adrenoceptors in cardiac or smooth muscle, adenylate cyclase (AC) is activated, cAMP is produced, and cAMP-cAMP kinase (cAMP PK) is stimulated. This cascade increases force in cardiac muscle and decreases tone of vascular smooth muscle through the phosphorylation of a number of regulatory proteins. The net concentration of intracellular cAMP formed is determined by the rate of cAMP synthesis by adenylate cyclase and the rate of cAMP hydrolysis to inactive 5'-AMP by cGi PDE in the soluble and/or particulate fractions. B. The same pathways in the presence of a low K_m cAMP cGi PDE inhibitor. Inhibition of cGi PDE will give rise to an accumulation of cAMP, a greater activation of cAMP-cAMP kinase and subsequently to a greater effect on increasing cardiac muscle force and reducing vascular smooth muscle tone.

The majority of this review will focus on the cGi low-K_m cAMP PDE isozyme present in cardiac and vascular smooth muscle, since this is the receptor for the current cardiotonic/vasodilator agents approved for acute intravenous use in the therapy of congestive heart failure (CHF). The consequence of inhibition of this low-K_m cAMP isozyme, in conjunction with constant adenylate cyclase activity, is the accumulation of cAMP within cardiac and vascular smooth muscle cells (Fig. 1). This increase in cAMP subsequently results in an increase in force development and rate of relaxation in cardiac muscle, as well as a reduction in vascular smooth muscle tone.

The low K_m cGMP PDE isozyme is equally interesting as a target for novel CHF therapy. Zaprinast, as well as other selective low-K_m cGMP PDE inhibitors, can potentiate the vasorelaxant and hypotensive actions of guanylate cyclase activators, including endothelial-derived relaxing factor (EDRF), nitrovasodilators, and atrial natriuretic peptide (ANP) (11,12). In addition, zaprinast can lower blood pressure and increase natriuresis following intravenous administration to rats or dogs (13; personal observations). Both activities are consistent with inhibition of the low-K_m cGMP PDE. Given the link between EDRF and ANP-mediated activation of guanylate cyclase and cGMP formation, a selective agent that could prevent the degradation of cGMP offers a new and exciting approach for the discovery of novel agents that may be useful therapy for patients with CHF. Certainly, the aspect of identifying an agent that potentiates the activity of endogenous regulators of vascular tone and sodium balance (such as EDRF and ANP), which ultimately reduces cardiac afterload and produces natriuresis, is of interest. Further development of this hypothesis awaits additional information on the low-K_m cGMP PDE(s) in renal cells, as well as the discovery of nanomolar potent/specific inhibitors of the cGMP PDE isozyme present in vascular smooth muscle.

II. BIOCHEMISTRY OF cGi LOW-K_m cAMP PDE

The cGi low-K_m cAMP, cardiotonic-sensitive PDE has been purified to homogeneity from bovine heart (14). This 120 Kda enzyme is very sensitive to proteolysis and is regulated by both cGMP and cAMP. As previously discussed, this enzyme is inhibited by submicromolar concentrations of cGMP and is stimulated by cAMP protein kinase-mediated phosphorylation. This suggests an interesting synergistic and intracellular feedback mechanism for cyclic nucleotide regulation, with cAMP serving as both the substrate for activation and as the stimulator of activity. Milrinone, enoximone, and amrinone are among the competitive inhibitors of this enzyme. The K_i obtained for milrinone (0.3 μM) with purified bovine ventricular low K_m cAMP PDE (14) is similar to that obtained with DEAE-cellulose isolated canine aortic peak III PDE, or particulate peak III PDE obtained from human cardiac muscle (15). This suggests that DEAE-isolated peak III PDE from some cardiovascular tissues is pharmacologically similar to the enzyme purified to homogeneity.

Low-K_m cAMP cardiotonic-sensitive cGi PDE can be located in either the soluble and/or particulate fractions of cardiac ventricular muscle (15,16). The location and relative amount of this isozyme are species dependent. For example, this PDE is found in the particulate fraction of canine and rat hearts, with only a very small amount of activity present in the rat. Primate hearts (rhesus and cynomolgus monkeys, human) contain cGi PDE activity in both the soluble and particulate fractions, while guinea pig hearts only contain soluble cGi PDE. Further localization studies suggest that the sarcoplasmic reticulum may be the source of the cardiotonic-sensitive form of the cGi PDE in canine hearts (17). It has been hypothesized that the positive inotropic activity of the cardiotonic sensitive PDE inhibitors is dependent upon the presence of cGi PDE in the particulate fraction (16). However, this hypothesis does not account for the well-known positive inotropic activity of cGi PDE inhibitors in isolated guinea pig papillary muscle, which purportedly contains predominantly soluble cGi PDE and no particulate cGi PDE (16). Other factors, including rate of stimulation and external Ca^{2+} concentration, are also prime determinants for efficacy of low-K_m cAMP cGi PDE inhibitors in isolated cardiac muscle (18; personal observations).

Numerous selective cGi PDE inhibitors have been synthesized and tested in recent years. These agents range in potency for inhibition (IC_{50}) from nanomolar (trequinsin, anagrelide), to submicromolar (CI-930, milrinone, medorinone, RGW 2938) and from low (imazodan, pelrinone, enoximone, piroximone, SKF 94120) through middle (amrinone, APP 201-533) micromolar ranges. In general, most of these agents are very selective (at least 30–100X) inhibitors of the cGi PDE relative to other PDE isozymes. However, it has been reported that these compounds are also equally potent inhibitors of the nonproteolyzed cGMP-stimulated (DEAE-peak II) PDE (19). The role that inhibition of this high-K_m, high-V_{max} PDE isozyme plays in mediating the positive inotropic or lusitropic activity of these compounds remains to be identified.

III. ASSESSING INVOLVEMENT OF cGMP-INHIBITABLE cAMP PDE IN POSITIVE INOTROPY OR VASORELAXATION

In general, three types of experiments have been used to link cGi PDE inhibition to positive inotropy or vasorelaxation. These include 1. the demonstration of potentiation of adenylate cyclase stimulators by the cGi PDE isozyme inhibitors, 2. the correlation of potency of cGi PDE inhibition for a series of cGi PDE inhibitors with potency for positive inotropy or vasorelaxation, and 3. the association of activation of the cAMP system (cAMP formation, activation of cAMP protein kinase [cAPK], phosphorylation of relevant substrates) to positive inotropy or vasorelaxation by the cGi PDE inhibitor.

1. There are several examples in the literature in which a number of cGi PDE inhibitors have been shown to potentiate the positive inotropic effects of adenylate cyclase stimulators. These include potentiation of β-adrenergic-mediated force development by milrinone and imazodan in various preclinical models (20,21), as well as potentiation of forskolin by milrinone in preclinical and end-stage failure cardiac muscle preparations (22,23).

2. Positive correlations in potency for positive inotropy or vasorelaxation as a function of cGi PDE inhibition have been reported by many investigators (8,16,24–26). In all cases thus far reported, potency for inhibition of cGi PDE is correlated with positive inotropy in isolated cardiac muscle preparations and in intravenous studies with anesthetized dogs. It is interesting that results obtained in studies with anesthetized dogs indicated that a better correlation exists for inhibition of particulate cGi PDE than for total cGi PDE as the comparator (16). Similar correlations are apparent with vascular (aortic) relaxation as a function of cGi PDE inhibition, although other vascular beds have yet to be carefully examined (25,26).

3. The third way to examine functional translation of cGi PDE inhibition in intact cells or tissues is to correlate activation of the cAMP system with the pharmacologic response mediated by the cGi PDE inhibitor. It is paramount in these studies to make these comparisons on both a concentration–response and temporal basis. It is also important in these studies to include known cAMP-dependent and cAMP-independent reference agents to provide for an accurate comparison of these relationships in each system. Activation of the cAMP system can be assessed in many ways that include measuring the intracellular concentration of cAMP, activation of cAPK by activity–ratio methodology, or by measuring increases in phosphorylation of cellular substrates for cAPK (Fig. 1).

Numerous studies have shown that cGi PDE inhibitors, including milrinone, imazodan, piroximone, and SKF 94120, among others, can increase cAMP content in isolated cardiac muscle (21,24,27–30). In these and other studies, it was clear that increases in cAMP content can be dissociated from increases in force development, especially at low concentrations of these agents or at early time intervals of force development. Moreover, the effect of cAMP-dependent (e.g., forskolin) or cAMP-independent agents (e.g., Bay K 8644) have not been evaluated in the same system. Also not examined was activation of cAPK, which is the next step in the cAMP cascade, which might provide a more sensitive measure of activation of the cAMP system. Therefore studies in our laboratories were initiated with isolated guinea pig papillary muscle and aortic smooth muscle to address these concerns (26,31).

In concentration–response studies, there were correlations in the relationships between increases in isometric force, as a function of either cAMP content or activation of cAPK for the cGi PDE inhibitors medorinone and milrinone, and the β-adrenergic agonist isoproterenol in isolated guinea pig papillary muscles. In isolated guinea pig aortic smooth muscle, similar positive correlations were evident with medorinone, milrinone, papaverine, and forskolin. However, the relationships, as defined by linear regression analysis (i.e., slope), were similar for medorinone, milrinone, and papaverine but different for forskolin. This may be related to "overactivation" of the cAMP system by forskolin, as previously suggested for this agent (32). Non-cAMP-related agents such as ouabain and Bay K-8644 (cardiac muscle) as well as washing out the contractile agonist (aortic smooth muscle) were able effectively to modulate force without changing cAMP or cAMP protein kinase activity.

Studies on the temporal sequences of cAMP formation, activation of cAMP protein kinase, and force modulation further demonstrate the complexities involved in this system. For example, the initial onset of force development and attainment of peak force at 1 min with 100 μM milrinone occurs without significant increases in cAMP content in papillary muscles. However, there is a significant time-dependent increase in the extent of activation of cAPK activity that peaks at 1 min and seems to coincide with changes in isometric force. Similar increases in cAPK activation without cAMP formation are evident with isoproterenol. The same type of response has also been reported with potentiation of forskolin-mediated positive inotropy by milrinone in isolated rabbit papillary muscles (22). It is possible that a very small increase in intracellular cAMP, which is localized to a specific area of the cell and is sufficient to activate cAPK, is too low to be detected using the current radioimmunoassay techniques. In addition, it is also possible that a portion of the cAMP partitions with the regulatory cAMP-binding subunit of cAPK and is thus not detected in the cAMP radioimmunoassay.

In addition to inhibiting cGi PDE isozyme activity, some of the PDE inhibitors have other mechanisms of action. For example, APP 201-533, sulmazole, pimobendan, MCI-154, and other cardiotonics can also directly enhance Ca^{2+} sensitivity of cardiac myofibrils (33). However, assessing the relative contribution of this activity to positive inotropy mediated by these agents has not been easily discernable. Other mechanisms of action of PDE inhibitors involving alteration of ion fluxes have also been proposed. Early studies with milrinone suggested a direct effect on stimulation of Ca^{2+} influx in cardiac muscle (34,35). However, milrinone does not affect Ca^{2+} binding to the voltage-dependent Ca^{2+} channel, nor would this effect be consistent with vasorelaxation. Ca^{2+} entry stimulators, such as Bay K-8644, produce vasoconstriction as well as positive inotropy. Moreover, cAMP-mediated phosphorylation of proteins associated with L-type Ca^{2+} channels can increase the probability of opening of these channels and increase Ca^{2+} influx (36). Thus milrinone may be able to stimulate Ca^{2+} influx in cardiac muscle through voltage-dependent Ca^{2+} channels by cGi PDE inhibition and activation of the cAMP system (37).

It is not possible, at this time, to discern among other cAMP-related mechanisms that may contribute to the efficacy of these agents. It has been suggested (38) that cGi PDE inhibitors, such as sulmazole, may also increase cAMP by inhibiting adenosine binding to A_1 receptors (which inhibits adenylate cyclase), or by directly blocking the G inhibitory protein (G_i) of adenylate cyclase. However, the effects of milrinone on A_1 binding or the G_i-protein occur at concentrations (1–2 mM) beyond the clinical therapeutic micromolar plasma concentration. These effects are probably not relevant to the mechanism of action of milrinone, but may contribute to the efficacy of some of the other less potent cGi PDE inhibitors.

IV. IN VIVO CARDIOVASCULAR EFFECTS OF SELECTIVE cGMP-INHIBITABLE cAMP PDE INHIBITORS

Results from in vitro studies using isolated PDE isozymes and cardiac and smooth muscles have demonstrated that selective inhibition of the low Km cAMP cGi PDE isozyme increases cardiac contractile force and relaxes vascular smooth muscle (Fig. 2), over a similar concentration range, by increasing the concentration of intracellular cAMP. However, the magnitude and the differential effect of selective cGi PDE inhibitors on in vivo cardiac performance and vascular bed resistances are not easily predictable and straightforward. The in vivo pharmacology of cGi PDE inhibitors is dependent upon a number of factors that include 1. both the intracellular and organ distribution of the isozyme, 2. the degree to which cGi PDE is coupled to cellular function, 3. the relative contribution of other PDE isozymes in regulating cardiac performance and vascular relaxation, 4. adenylate cyclase activity (tone) in the respective target tissue and 5. the relative selectivity of the PDE isozyme inhibitor. The concomitant, selective inhibition of cGi PDE in both cardiac and vascular smooth muscle exerts a dual effect on cardiac pump performance. Inhibition of cardiac cGi PDE directly increases maximal contractile force as well as negative and positive dP/dt. Cardiac pump performance is indirectly affected through inhibition of cGi PDE in vascular smooth muscle, which reduces ventricular preload and afterload. Overall, this dual effect of cGi PDE inhibitors enhances cardiac output without significantly increasing cardiac oxygen consumption (39).

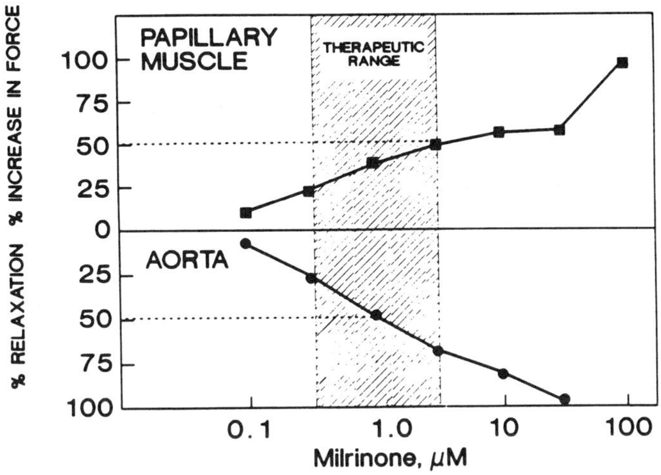

Figure 2 The in vitro concentration–response curve of milrinone for increasing force development by guinea pig papillary muscles and relaxing aortic smooth muscle strips (26,31). The ED_{50} value for papillary muscle force is approximately 3 μM whereas the ED_{50} value for relaxation of phenylephrine-contracted aortic smooth muscle is approximately 1 μM. Both values fall within the clinical therapeutic range (100–500 ng/ml) over which milrinone increases cardiac performance and lowers total peripheral resistance.

In general, the effect of selective cGi PDE inhibitors, like CI 930 (40), piroximone (41), imazodan (42), and milrinone (20,43,44) on in vivo cardiovascular hemodynamics is similar; PDE III inhibitors increase cardiac contractility, lower peripheral resistance, and increase heart rate. However subtle differences can be observed among cGi PDE inhibitors with respect to their maximal and relative effects on heart rate, cardiac output and contractility, total peripheral, pulmonary and renal resistances, and organ perfusion pressures.

To test the effect of selective cGi PDE inhibitors on cardiac performance and systemic, pulmonary, and renal hemodynamics, an anesthetized canine model was developed in which these parameters could be measured simultaneously (44). Intravenous cumulative doses of a selective cGi PDE inhibitor were administered to anesthetized dogs in the presence of the beta-adrenoceptor antagonist nadolol; beta-adrenoceptor blockade was used to eliminate both sympathetic reflex regulation of cardiac contractility and vascular bed resistances that could result from changes in mean arterial blood pressure and vascular bed perfusion pressures. During a 10 min interval following each of four bolus doses of compound or vehicle, maximal changes were recorded for heart rate, positive and negative ventricular dP/dt, cardiac output, left ventricular pressure, total peripheral resistance, mean arterial pressure, renal blood flow and resistance, and pulmonary diastolic and systolic pressures. Milrinone was evaluated in the presence and absence of beta-adrenoceptor blockade; similar results were obtained under both conditions. Compared to vehicle, milrinone induced increases in both positive and negative ventricular dP/dt in a dose-dependent manner (Fig. 3). The effect of milrinone on cardiac positive dP/dt in vivo is similar to that obtained in vitro (Fig. 2) with isolated papillary muscles. As previously described, this effect could result from an elevation in the intracellular concentration of cardiac cell cAMP, activation of cAPK, and phosphorylation of protein components

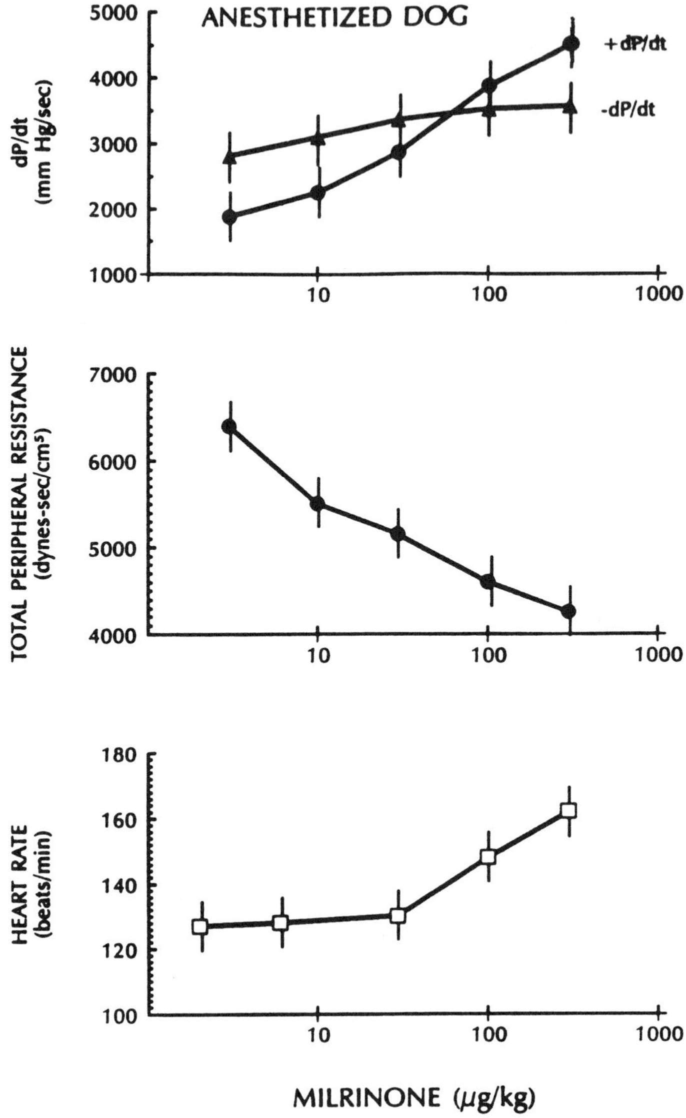

Figure 3 The in vivo cumulative dose–response (3–300 μg/kg) curve of milrinone in a beta-adrenoceptor blocked anesthetized canine model (44). Simultaneous measurements of positive and negative ventricular dP/dt (upper panel), total peripheral resistance (middle panel), and heart rate (lower panel) are shown. The data illustrate the relative potencies of milrinone for having an effect on these cardiovascular parameters.

(e.g., L-type Ca^{2+} channels, sarcoplasmic reticulum phospholamban, myofibrillar troponin-C) that contribute to the regulation of cardiac performance (45). The increase in cardiac negative dP/dt (Fig. 3) that was observed in vivo in response to milrinone may have resulted, in part, from an increase in the rate of calcium uptake by the sarcoplasmic reticulum and from changes in cardiac loading conditions. Relative to other cardiac inotropes, milrinone has been found to enhance cardiac performance without a significant increase in cardiac oxygen consumption (39). One explanation for this observation is that the heart would tend to use less energy if active calcium metabolism by the sarcoplasmic reticulum and sarcolemmal membrane were not stimulated to the same extent relative to other cardiotonic agents or if, at the same time, cardiac afterload was reduced.

Over the same dosage range in which milrinone induced cardiotonic effects in anesthetized dogs, milrinone induced significant reductions in mean renal, systemic, femoral, and pulmonary resistances (Fig. 4). There was also an increase in

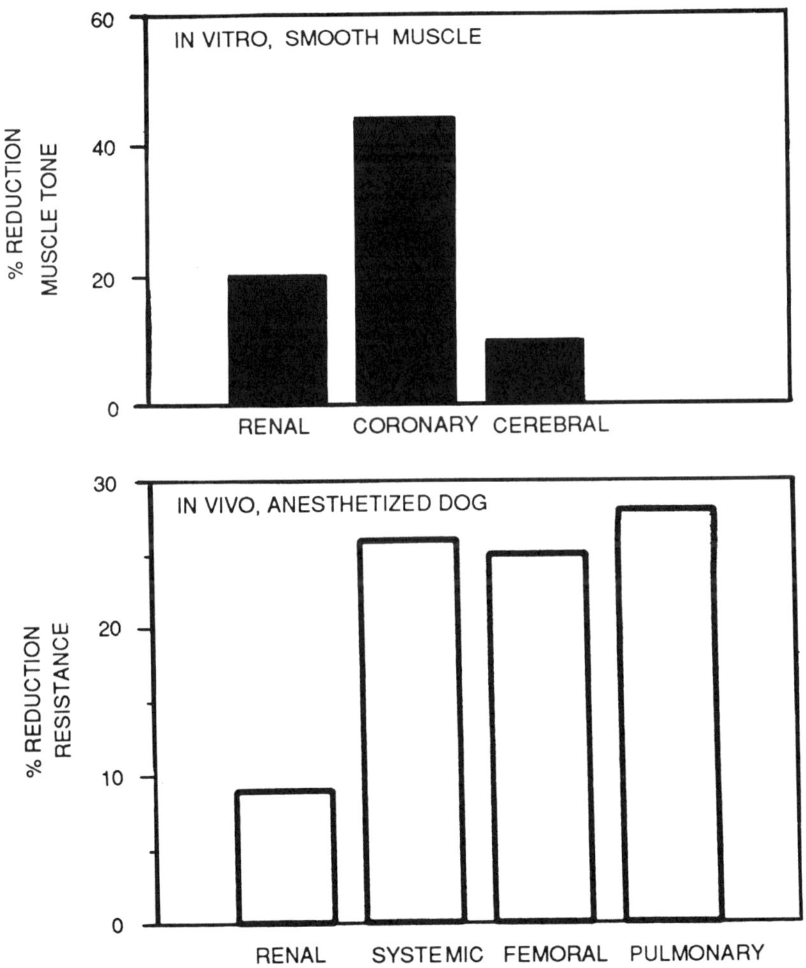

Figure 4 The effect of milrinone on vascular tone in vitro (top panel) and in vivo (bottom panel). In the top panel, canine vascular strips from the indicated vascular beds were contracted with U46619 (a thromboxane A_2 mimetic) and relaxed with milrinone. Data shown were obtained with 3 μM milrinone, a concentration that produced a 50% increase in guinea pig papillary muscle force (Fig. 2). In the bottom panel, reductions in vascular resistance were calculated for the indicated vascular beds at a dosage of milrinone (100 μg/kg) that produced a 50% increase in +dP/dt in anesthetized dogs (Fig. 3). These data demonstrate the differential regional effects of milrinone on vascular tone.

cardiac output that could be attributed to both an increase in cardiac contractility and a reduction in cardiac afterload. Milrinone's concomitant pharmacologic effects on cardiac performance and femoral, systemic, and pulmonary resistances would be expected if inhibition of cGi PDE in canine vascular smooth muscle and cardiac muscle occurred at similar intracellular concentrations of drug. These data are consistent with previous data showing that milrinone is equipotent against cardiac and vascular cGi PDE (26,31).

There was no significant effect of milrinone on renal blood flow in these studies. Similar results were evident in in vitro studies (46), which demonstrated vascular bed specificity (coronary, cerebral, renal) for milrinone (Fig. 4). Reasons for this specificity are not clear but may be related to adenylate cyclase tone or a different role of the low-K_m cAMP PDE in these different vascular beds.

One liability associated with any agent that alters cardiac performance through increasing intracellular concentrations of cAMP in heart cells is the possibility of inducing cardiac arrhythmias. Milrinone (Fig. 3) and other selective cGi PDE inhibitors (47) increase heart rate in a dose-dependent manner. The increase in heart rate most likely due to a direct action of cGi PDE inhibitors on atrial pacemaker cells since the effect occurs in the absence of cardiac sympathetic pathways, although a decrease in parasympathic tone to the heart cannot be ruled out as a possible mechanism. In the case of milrinone, even with the increase in heart rate, arrhythmic events are usually not observed in our preclinical studies. However, we have found that the anesthetized, beta-adrenoceptor blocked canine model is not very sensitive for identifying the proarrhythmogenic potential of cGi PDE inhibitors and other agents. Other parameters, such as atrioventricular (AV) conduction time, effective refractory period, or ventricular fibrillatory threshold, may be more appropriate for assessing proarrhythmic liability of cGi PDE inhibitors.

V. PRECLINICAL PHARMACOLOGY OF cGMP-INHIBITABLE cAMP PDE INHIBITORS IN NORMAL AND MYOPATHIC MODELS

The efficacy of cGi PDE inhibitors in different preclinical models of failure has been well documented, with activity shown in myocardially infarcted rats (48,49), myopathic hamsters (50), rabbits with aortic valve insufficiency (51), and naturally occurring and/or chemically-induced failure in dogs (20,52,53). In general, efficacy of cGi PDE inhibitors is dependent on the species, the amount/subcellular distribution of the cGi PDE isozyme, and adenylate cyclase activity. As previously discussed, the distribution of cGi PDE in cardiac muscle from primates is in both the particulate and soluble fractions, while nonprimates generally have either soluble or particulate cGi PDE. The amount of cGi PDE present in primate myocardium is most similar to what is found in dogs and guinea pigs, although the subcellular distribution is different.

The myocardially infarcted (MI) rat model has proven to be a useful model for the study of a variety of agents for CHF. The model offers the advantage of evaluating effects of these agents on survival, hemodynamics, intact muscle function (cardiac, vascular), and biochemical activity. Moreover, the changes that occur in some hemodynamic variables post-MI resemble some of the clinical manifestations of CHF (49,54,55). Sweet et al. (55) have used this model to evaluate and compare the effects of an ACE inhibitor (enalapril) with a selective low-K_m cAMP PDE inhibitor (milrinone) on long-term survival. Enalapril (mean 50% survival, 233 days), milrinone (297 days), and the combination of both agents (277 days) all increased mean survival relative to no drug intervention (203 days). All treatment groups also reduced cardiac hypertrophy, which is probably reflective of afterload reduction by either enalapril or milrinone. The hemodynamic effects of milrinone in this model have also been studied (48,49). In two separate studies, milrinone produced a reduction in mean arterial blood pressure and in left ventricular end-diastolic filling pressure, and slightly increased left ventricular +dP/dt by 15–18%. The latter study also showed that milrinone increased hepatic and coronary blood flow, while enalapril increased renal blood flow. The separate hemodynamic effects induced by each agent alone were maintained when they were administered together.

Although these studies have demonstrated a moderate effect of milrinone on cardiac +dP/dt, in vivo, a direct effect on cardiac contractility was not proven. Moreover, the purported lack of significant amounts of cardiotonic sensitive cGi PDE in normal rat hearts (16) has led to the conclusion that milrinone may not alter cardiac contractility or inhibit PDE in hearts of rats with myocardial infarction (56). However, no studies have yet been reported that examined the positive inotropic and PDE inhibitory activity of milrinone, or other cGi PDE inhibitors in MI rats. Accordingly, we have carried out these enzymatic and in vitro studies in sham-operated rats and rats 10 weeks after infarction and compared milrinone to other positive inotropes (57). Milrinone alone (0.3–300 nM) did not increase force development or +dF/dt in isolated papillary muscles from either the MI or sham-operated group. The cAMP-related positive inotropes isoproterenol (10 μM) and forskolin (10 μM) both increased force development in papillary muscles from the sham-operated group, while only forskolin was active in the MI group (Fig. 5). These data suggest that cAMP-related agents can function as positive inotropes in this model, but that the beta-adrenergic receptor-linked system is severely attenuated in this model of failure. However, the positive inotropic efficacy of forskolin and Bay K-8644 was also reduced in the MI group. This observation suggests an additional cellular defect in this model of failure, as evidenced by a reduction in pharmacologic activity of these two mechanistically dissimilar positive inotropes.

In patients with end-stage heart failure attributed to idiopathic cardiomyopathy, there is in vitro evidence to suggest that the ventricular beta-adrenoreceptor system is down regulated (58). This defect may involve an increase in the amount of the αG40 subunit of G_i without a decrease in the Gs protein (59), although other sites may also be affected. Although some in vitro studies have suggested that selective inhibitors of cGi PDE are less potent and efficacious in failed human ventricular tissue (23), other studies have demonstrated that the potency and efficacy of contractile force are enhanced in the presence of isoproterenol (60).

Functional cGi PDE isozyme inhibition can also be assessed by demonstrating potentiation of adenylate cyclase activators. Milrinone, at a concentration range (0.3–10 μM) that inhibits cGi PDE activity and was achieved in vivo in the MI rat survival study by Sweet et al. (55), potentiated the forskolin-induced increases in papillary muscle force in both groups and isoproterenol-induced increases in papillary muscle force in the sham-operated group (Fig. 5). These data are similar to those previously published with papillary muscles from hearts of patients with end-stage failure (23) and suggest that the lack of apparent overt activity of cGi PDE inhibitors in in vitro cardiac muscle studies is due to a low turnover of basal

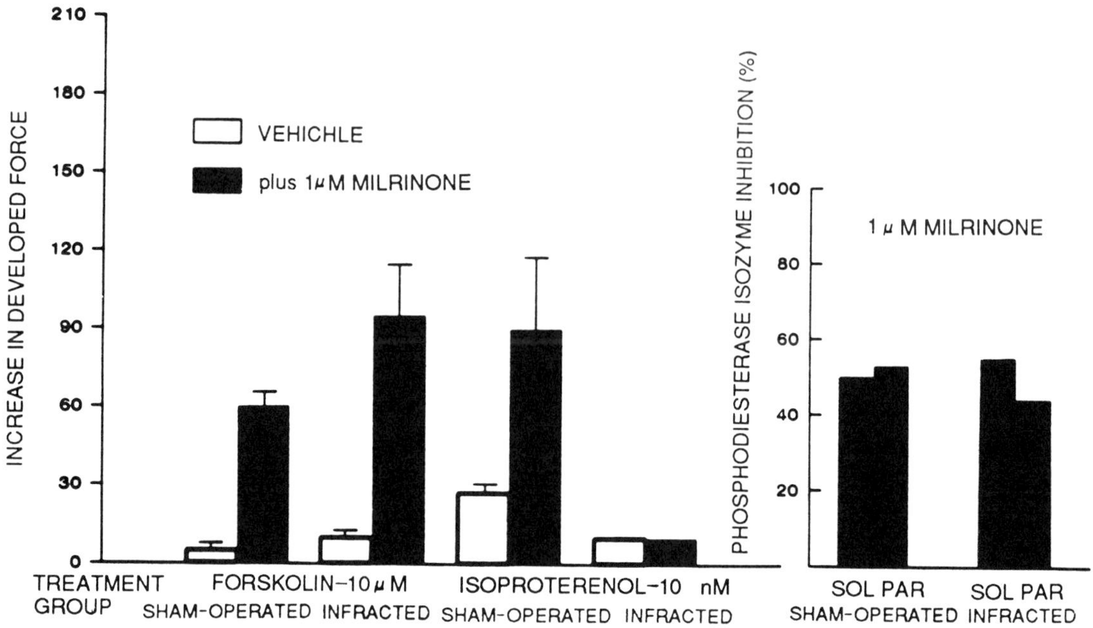

Figure 5 Effects of milrinone on contractile force and PDE isozymes in cardiac muscle from myocardially infarcted and sham-operated control rats. The panel on the left shows the effect of two mechanistically different stimulators of adenylate cyclase (forskolin, 10 μM; isoproterenol, 10 nM) alone or in the presence of 1 μM milrinone (closed bars) or vehicle (open bars) on force development by papillary muscles from rats 10 weeks after myocardial infarction or aged-matched, sham-operated controls (49). In both the sham-operated and infarcted groups, forskolin and isoproterenol alone had little effect on papillary muscle force. However, 1 μM milrinone potentiated the effect of forskolin in both groups and also potentiated isoproterenol in the sham-operated group. Milrinone and isoproterenol together had no effect on papillary muscle force in the infarcted group. The panel on the right shows the the effect of milrinone on inhibiting cAMP (0.2 μM) hydrolysis by the low-K_m cAMP cGi PDE in soluble or particulate ventricular DEAE fractions of sham-operated rats or rats 10 weeks after myocardial infarction. These data indicate that 1 μM milrinone is equally effective (50–55%) in inhibiting the activity of the cGi PDE isozyme from either cardiac fraction in both groups.

adenylate cyclase activity in some species. When the adenylate cyclase system is activated (i.e., with forskolin), efficacy of cGi PDE inhibitors can be demonstrated in vitro. In human heart failure, a loss of beta-adrenoceptor function (probably an increase in G_i) occurs (58,59). Thus, cGi PDE inhibitors have little to no efficacy as positive inotropic agents in end-stage failure because a major system that regulates adenylate cyclase activity (beta-adrenoceptors) is severely downregulated. Although not as extensively studied, preliminary experiments suggest that cGi PDE inhibitors can relax vascular smooth muscle and lower peripheral resistance in the MI rat model. The potency of milrinone as a vasorelaxant against phenylephrine-induced contractions in isolated renal and aortic smooth muscle is similar in MI, control rats, and in other species (A. Harris and P. Silver, personal observations). These observations would be consistent with the concept that cGi PDE inhibitors function as both positive inotropic and vasodilatory agents in the early stages of CHF, but primarily as vasodilatory agents in end-stage CHF. The balance of inotropic to vasodilatory activity will depend in part on the severity of reduction in cardiac beta-adrenoceptor downregulation (i.e., adenylate cyclase tone) and the amount of cardiotonic sensitive cGi PDE in the heart.

The demonstration of functional cGi PDE isozyme inhibition via potentiation of adenylate cyclase stimulators in normal and infarcted myocardium suggests the presence of milrinone-sensitive low-K_m cAMP PDE in this tissue. A previous study (16) concluded that there is no cardiotonic-sensitive low-K_m cAMP PDE in hearts of normal rats. However, a close analysis of the data from that study suggests that normal rat heart most likely contains a mixture of both cGi PDE and rolipram-sensitive PDE isozymes, since flat concentration–response curves for both imazodan (a selective cGi PDE inhibitor) and rolipram were obtained, and the calculated IC_{50} values for these agents as well as cGMP were between the IC_{50} values obtained for either purified PDE isozyme alone. We have obtained similar data when DEAE fractions have contained a mixture of both cGi- and rolipram-sensitive PDEs, as is the case with guinea pig tracheal smooth muscle (61). These results have been further substantiated with the use of rolipram analog and milrinone analog affinity resins that have been used to separate these two isozymes in rat and other cardiac tissues (unpublished observations). We have initiated studies to characterize the low-K_m cAMP PDE isozymes obtained from cardiac muscle from 10 week post-MI and sham-operated rats (Fig. 5). Our data demonstrate the presence of a mixture of both cGi and rolipram-sensitive PDEs in both the particulate and soluble fractions in both groups of animals. The amount of activity is much greater in the soluble fraction, but there is significant activity in the particulate fraction. Moreover, milrinone in the concentration range (0.3–10 μM) used in the previously discussed in vitro and in vivo studies can produce significant inhibition of either PDE fraction. It is of further interest to note that the bipyridines, such as milrinone and amrinone, are not very selective at inhibiting the cGi PDE (IC_{50} for milrinone, 0.5 μM) relative to the rolipram-sensitive PDE (IC_{50}, 8 μM) (62). This is in contrast to other chemical series, such as the pyridazinones (imazodan, CI-930), which are very selective inhibitors of cGi PDE (IC_{50} for CI-930, 0.2 μM vs. IC_{50}, 75 μM for rolipram-sensitive PDE; 62). Thus cGi PDE inhibitors may have different affinities for the rolipram-sensitive PDE. Extrapolation of biochemical data from one inhibitor to in vivo studies with a different inhibitor may lead to erroneous conclusions.

The results of these studies show that milrinone-sensitive cGi PDE is present in the myocardium of normal and MI rats and that functional cGi PDE isozyme inhibition can be demonstrated in intact cardiac muscle via potentiation by milrinone of forskolin-mediated responses. A decreased inotropic response in MI rat myocardium to milrinone is probably related to a decrease in adenylate cyclase activity as well as a reduced efficacy of all positive inotropes, and probably not due to an alteration in the activity or pharmacologic sensitivity of the cGi PDE isozyme.

VI. LOW-K_m cAMP PDE ISOZYMES IN NORMAL AND MYOPATHIC HUMAN MYOCARDIUM

Although numerous studies have been performed with PDE isozymes isolated from nonprimate, nonmyopathic animals, substantially less is known about the cGi PDE isozyme from primates, or in humans with or without cardiac myopathy. Scattered reports with limited sample sizes have appeared in the literature for normal human (one subject) and myopathic (three subjects) cardiac muscle samples (63,64). To our knowledge, there have been no studies reported in which statistically relevant comparisons have been made on the cellular distribution of PDE isozymes with cardiac muscle samples isolated from normal and myopathic subjects. Accordingly, we, in collaboration with Dr. Paul Allen of Brigham and Women's Hospital (Boston, MA), have quantitated and compared the specific activity, apparent K_m for cyclic nucleotide substrate, maximum velocity (V_{max}), and pharmacologic sensitivity ("cardiotonic-sensitive" or "rolipram-sensitive") of PDE isozymes in particulate and soluble fractions prepared from segments of left ventricular muscle obtained from normal subjects as well as from patients with end-stage heart failure due to idiopathic cardiomyopathy or coronary artery disease. Cardiac catheterization data indicated that patients with end-stage heart failure had significant elevations in pulmonary wedge pressure and systemic vascular resistance and a very large reduction (60–70% normal vs. 13% myopathic) in cardiac ejection fraction. Hearts of patients were considered normal in this study based on patient history and physical examination by the attending physician. For all groups, after removal of the heart, the left ventricular wall was dissected free, cut into 3–5 g segments, and frozen within minutes in liquid nitrogen. Samples from the myopathic groups represented noninfarcted ventricular tissue, since there was no visible evidence of gross scarring of the ventricular wall at time of removal. PDE isozymes were isolated from 1–2 g of ventricular muscle via DEAE-Sephacel chromatography or high-performance liquid chromatography (HPLC), as previously described (15,16,62).

Two major findings were noteworthy in this study (Table 1). First, the cardiotonic sensitive/cGMP-inhibitable form of PDE is present in both the particulate and soluble fractions of human myocardium. This is an contrast to the observations that this isozyme is only present in the particulate fraction of canine myocardium or the soluble fraction of guinea pig myocardium (16). Since cGi PDE inhibitors, such as milrinone and CI-930, directly enhance positive inotropy in canine and guinea pig ventricular muscle, it is not possible at this time to discern if clinical cardiotonic efficacy of these agents is related to inhibition of either the soluble cGi PDEs, the particulate cGi PDE isozyme, or both.

Second, this study has shown that there are some significant differences with these low-K_m cAMP PDE isozymes when normal myocardium is compared wtih myocardium from patients with end-stage failure due to idiopathic cardiomyopathy or coronary artery disease. The major difference is a reduction in the specific activity of the particulate cGi PDE in both diseased groups relative to the normal group. This reduction in specific activity of the particulate cGi PDE was observed with no apparent changes in activity of other peak PDEs, suggesting that the reduction in PDE activity was specific for this isozyme. Moreover, this reduced activity as well as a reduced V_{max} of cGi PDE in the idiopathic myopathy group, suggest that degradation of cAMP may be reduced in end-stage heart failure.

Several in vitro studies, including one with segments of heart muscle obtained from the same source as this study, have shown that cGi PDE inhibitors are less potent as positive inotropes in patients with end-stage failure (23). As previously discussed, a reduction in β-adrenoceptor-stimulated adenylate cyclase activity, probably via an increase in G_i, may account for this reduction in potency (23,58–60). While several subcellular sites may contribute to this reduced potency, the

Table 1 Comparison of Low K_m cAMP PDE Isozymes isolated via DEAE-Sepharose Chromatography from Human Cardiac Ventricular Muscle

PDE Isozyme[a]	Specific Activity[b]	K_m[c]	V_{max}[d]	cGMP-Regulated[e]	Pharmacologic Sensitivity[f]	
					Cardiotonic	Rolipram
Soluble peak I						
N	25±7	0.4	0.9	h	−	−
IM	16±2	0.4	0.6	h	−	−
CAD	25±5	0.4	0.9	h	−	−
Soluble peak IIIa						
N	29±5	0.2	2.4	i	+	−
IM	22±5	0.2	1.8*	i	+	−
CAD	24±4	0.2	2.8	i	+	−
Soluble peak IIIb						
N	22±3	0.3	2.0	i	+	+
IM	24±3	0.3	2.8	i	+	+
CAD	27±7	0.4	3.4	i	+	+
Particulate PDE						
N	19±4	0.3	2.3	i	+	−
IM	7±1*	0.3	1.1*	i	+	−
CAD	10±2*	0.3	2.3	i	+	−

[a]The subcellular location of major low K_m cAMP peaks of PDE activity from normal (N), idiopathic myopathy (IM), or coronary artery disease (CAD) cardiac samples is indicated. N=5–6 samples/group.
[b]Specific activity is expressed as pmol cAMP hydrolyzed/mg protein applied to the column/min. The concentration of cAMP was 1 μM; values are the mean ± S.E.M.
[c]Average values (μM) for the apparent K_m for cAMP.
[d]Average values for V_{max} with cAMP as the substrate (pmol hydrolyzed/mg protein/min).
[e]Indicates that the isozyme either hydrolyzed (h) or is inhibited (i) by submicromolar concentrations of cGMP.
[f]Indicates that isozyme is (+) or is not (−) inhibited by submicromolar concentrations of the cardiotonics (milrinone and CI-930) or rolipram.
*Indicates statistical differences ($p<0.05$) when compared with the normal group (Student-Newman-Kuels multiple comparisons test).

reduction in particulate cGi PDE activity in this study is consistent with these previous in vitro findings and suggests that reduced potency of cGi PDE inhibitors in end-stage failure may also be related to decreased amounts of the particulate cGi isozyme. The results from our study suggest that this reduction in in vitro positive inotropic efficacy is probably *not* related to differences in pharmacologic potency of these inhibitors against the isolated isozymes. There were no major differences in potency of either milrinone or CI-930 against particulate cGi or the soluble cGi, thus indicating that these PDE enzymes were cardiotonic-sensitive besides being cGMP-inhibitable. The other soluble peak of activity (IIIb) was also cardiotonic-sensitive and cGMP inhibitable, but also contained a portion of rolipram-sensitive PDE. This activity was not easily separated from cardiotonic sensitive PDE via DEAE-chromatography, but could be resolved pharmacologically with the combined used of selective inhibitors as previously described (61) and by the use of affinity chromatography. This suggests that a rolipram-sensitive PDE isozyme may be present in both myopathic and normal human cardiac muscle samples. These data also suggest that the catalytic site of human cardiac cGi PDE is not substantially altered in hearts of patients with end-stage failure due to cardiomyopathy.

VII. SUMMARY

Within the past decade, numerous selective inhibitors of cGi PDE have been designed and developed as agents useful in acute therapy of congestive heart failure. Efficacy is related to inhibition of cAMP cGi PDE in cardiac and vascular muscle, with subsequent potentiation of adenylate cyclase-mediated cAMP formation, activation of cAMP-dependent protein kinase, and increase in developed force, rate of cardiac ventricular relaxation, and a decrease in peripheral resistance (via vasorelaxation). An additional important concept is the stage of failure during which cAMP PDE inhibitors might be initiated as therapy. Since β-adrenoreceptor/adenylate cyclase activity is decreased in end-stage failure, efficacy of these PDE inhibitors as cardiotonics (but not as vasodilators) is reduced. An additional experimental concept of prevention of downregulation of β-adrenoreceptors with β-adrenoreceptor antagonists in the absence and presence of cAMP PDE inhibitors is interesting as a theoretical approach to maintaining inotropic function at a level distal to the cardiac β-adrenoreceptor. As a concept, this would be an exciting approach to halt the loss of β-adrenoreceptor function that progresses during failure.

Continuing design and development of selective inhibitors of other PDE isozymes, most notably zaprinast-inhibitable cGMP PDE, offer the potential in the future for new therapeutic approaches in heart failure that may lead to ways to potentiate the activity of endogenous modulators of guanylate cyclase activity, such as EDRF and ANP, with simultaneous reduction in peripheral vasoconstriction and enhancement of renal function.

ACKNOWLEDGMENT

The technical assistance of Ms. Peggy Branch in compiling the manuscript is greatly appreciated.

REFERENCES

1. Butcher RW, Sutherland EW. Adenosine 3′, 5′-phosphate in biological materials. J Biol Chem 1962; 237:1244–50.
2. Drummond GI, Perrot-Yee S. Enzymatic hydrolysis of adenosine 3′, 5′-phosphoric acid. J Biol Chem 1961; 236:1126–9.
3. Beavo JA, Reifsnyder DH. Primary sequence of cyclic nucleotide phosphodiesterase isozymes and design of selective inhibitors. Trends Pharmacol Sci 1990; 11:150–5.
4. Appleman MM, Ariano MA, Takemoto DJ, Whitson RH. Cyclic nucleotide phosphodiesterases. Hand Exp Pharmacol 1982; 58:261–300.
5. Weishaar RE, Cain MH, Bristol JA. A new generation of phosphodiesterase inhibitors: Multiple molecular forms of phosphodiesterase and the potential of drug selectivity. J Med Chem 1985; 28:537–45.
6. Beavo JA. Multiple isozymes of cyclic nucleotide phosphodiesterase. Adv Second Messenger Phosphoprotein Res 1988; 22:1–382.

7. Lugnier C, Schoeffter P, LeBec A, Strouthou E, Stoclet JC. Selective inhibition of cyclic nucleotide phosphodiesterases of human, bovine and rat aorta. Biochem Pharmacol 1986; 35:1743–51.
8. Silver PJ, Harris AL. Phosphodiesterase isozyme inhibitors and vascular smooth muscle. In: Halpern W, Brayden J, McLaughlin M, Osol A, Pegram B, Mackey K, eds. Proceedings of the Second International Symposium of Resistance Vessels. Ithaca, NY: Perinatology Press, 1988:284–91.
9. Keravis TM, Wells JN, Hardman JG. Cyclic nucleotide phosphodiesterase activities from pig coronary arteries. Lack of interconvertability of major forms. Biochim Biophys Acta 1980; 613:116–29.
10. Prigent AF, Fougier S, Nemoz G, Anker G, Pacheco H, Lugnier C, LeBec A, Stoclet JC. Comparison of cyclic nucleotide phosphodiesterase isoforms from rat heart and bovine aorta. Separation and inhibition by selective reference phosphodiesterase inhibitors. Biochem Pharmacol 1988; 37:3671–81.
11. Martin W, Furchgott RF, Villian GM, Jothianandan D. Phosphodiesterase inhibitors induce endothelium-dependent relaxation of rat and rabbit aorta by spontaneously released endothelium-derived relaxing factor. J Pharmacol Exp Ther 1986; 237:539–47.
12. Harris AL, Lemp B, Bentley RG, Perrone M, Hamel LT, Silver PJ. Phosphodiesterase isozyme inhibition and the potentiation by zaprinast of endothelium-derived relaxing factor and guanylate cyclase stimulating agents in vascular smooth muscle. J Pharmacol Exp Ther 1989; 249:394–400.
13. Buchholz RA, Dundore RL, Pratt PF, Hallenbeck WD, Wassey ML, Silver PJ. The selective phosphodiesterase I inhibitor zaprinast potentiates the hypotensive effect of nitroprusside in conscious SHR. FASEB J 1989; 3:A1186.
14. Harrison SA, Reifsnyder DH, Gallis B, Cadd GG, Beavo JA. Isolation and characterization of bovine cardiac muscle cGMP-inhibited phosphodiesterase: a receptor for new cardiotonic drugs. Mol Pharmacol 1986; 29:506–14.
15. Silver PJ, Allen P, Hamel LT, Etzler J, Bentley R, Pagani ED. Cellular distribution and pharmacological sensitivity of cyclic nucleotide phosphodiesterase isozymes in cardiac muscle from normal and cardiomyopathic subjects. Second Messengers Phosphoproteins 1990; 13:13–25.
16. Weishaar RE, Kobylarz-Singer DC, Steffen RP, Kaplan HR. Subclasses of cyclic AMP-specific phosphodiesterase in left ventricular muscle and their involvement in regulating myocardial contractility. Circ Res 1987; 61:539–47.
17. Kauffman RF, Crowe VG, Utterback BG, Robertson DW. LY 195115: a potent selective inhibitor of cyclic nucleotide phosphodiesterase located in the sarcoplasmic reticulum. Mol Pharmacol 1987; 30:609–16.
18. Anderson WG. An improved model for assessment of positive inotropic activity *in vitro*. Drug Dev Res 1983; 3:443–51.
19. Price B, Pyne NJ, Houslay MD. Proteolysis of cyclic AMP phosphodiesterase II attenuates its ability to be inhibited by compounds which exert positive inotropic actions in cardiac tissue. Biochem Pharmacol 1987; 36:4047–54.
20. Alousi AA, Canter JM, Montenaro MJ, Fort DJ, Ferrari RA. Cardiotonic activity of milrinone, a new and potent cardiac bipyridine, on normal and failing heart of experimental animals. J Cardiovasc Pharmacol 1983; 5:792–804.
21. Weishaar RE, Quade MM, Schenden JA, Boyd DK, Evans DB. Studies aimed at elucidating the mechanism of action of CI-914, a new cardiotonic agent. Eur J Pharmacol 1985; 119:205–15.
22. Kithas PA, Artman M, Thompson WJ, Strada SJ. Subcellular distribution of high affinity type IV cyclic AMP phosphodiesterase activity in rabbit ventricular myocardium: relations to the effect of cardiotonic drugs. Circ Res 1988; 62:782–9.

23. Feldman MD, Copelas L, Gwathmey JK, Phillips P, Warren SE, Schoen FJ, Grossman W, Morgan JP. Deficient production of cAMP; pharmacologic evidence of an important cause of contractile dysfunction in patients with end-stage heart failure. Circulation 1987; 75:331–9.
24. Ahn HD, Eardley D, Watkins R, Prioli N. Effects of several newer cardiotonic drugs on cardiac cyclic AMP metabolism. Biochem Pharmacol 1986; 35:1113–21.
25. Kauffman RF, Schenck KM, Utterback BG, Crowe VG, Cohen MC. *In vitro* vascular relaxation by new inotropic agents: Relationship to phosphodiesterase inhibition and cyclic nucleotides. J Pharmacol Exp Ther 1987; 242:864–72.
26. Silver PJ, Lepore RE, O'Connor B, Lemp BM, Hamel LT, Bentley RG, Harris AL. Inhibition of the low K_m cAMP phosphodiesterase and activation of the cAMP system in vascular smooth muscle by milrinone. J Pharmacol Exp Ther 1988; 247:34–42.
27. Kariya T, Wille JL, Dage RC. Studies on the mechanism of the cardiotonic activity of MDL 19205: effects on several biochemical systems. J Cardiovasc Pharmacol 1984; 6:50–5.
28. Gristwood RW, English TAH, Wallwork J, Sampford KA, Owens DAA. Analysis of responses to a selective phosphodiesterase III inhibitor, SK & F 94120, on isolated myocardium, including human ventricular myocardium from "end-stage" failure patients. J Cardiovasc Pharmacol 1987; 9:719–27.
29. Endoh M, Yanagisawa T, Taira N, Blinks JR. Effects of new inotropic agents on cyclic nucleotide metabolism and calcium transients in canine ventricular muscle. Circulation 73 1986; (Suppl. III):117–31.
30. Cheng HC, Kariya T, Gleason EM, Dage RC. Studies on the mechanism of the positive inotropic effect of piroximone in cat papillary muscle. J Cardiovasc Pharmacol 1985; 7:747–52.
31. Silver PJ, Harris AL, Canniff PC, Lepore RE, Bentley RG, Hamel LT, Evans DB. Phosphodiesterase isozyme inhibition, activation of the cAMP system and positive inotropy mediated by milrinone in isolated guinea pig cardiac muscle. J Cardiovasc Pharmacol 1989; 13:530–40.
32. Vegesna RVK, Diamond J. Effects of isoproterenol and forskolin on tension, cyclic AMP levels and cyclic AMP-dependent protein kinase activity in bovine coronary artery. Can J Pharmacol Physiol 1985; 62:1116–23.
33. Pagani ED, Silver PJ. Physiological and pharmacological modulation of cardiac contractile proteins. Drug Dev Res 1989; 18:279–293.
34. Farah AE, Canniff PC, Bentley RG, Kaiser LD. Effect of milrinone (Corotrope) on the contractility of isolated dog ventricular muscle. J Cardiovasc Pharmacol 1987; 10:607–15.
35. Gwathmey JK, Morgan JP. The effects of milrinone and piroximone on intracellular calcium handling in working myocardium from the ferret. Br J Pharmacol 1985; 85:97–108.
36. Hess P, Lansman JB, Nilius B, Tsien RW. Calcium channel types in cardiac myocytes: modulation by dihydropyridines and β-adrenergic stimulation. J Cardiovasc Pharmacol 1986; 8 (suppl 9):S11–S21.
37. Olson EM, Kim D, Smith TW, Marsh JD. Mechanism of the positive inotropic effect of milrinone in cultured embryonic chick ventricular cells. J Mol Cell Cardiol 1987; 19:95–104.
38. Parsons WJ, Ramkumar V, Stiles GL. The new cardiotonic agent sulmazole is an A_1 adenosine receptor antagonist and functionally blocks the inhibitory regulator, G_i. Mol Pharmacol 1988; 33:441–8.
39. Kabela E, Barcenas L, Farah A. The effect of milrinone (Win 47203) on coronary blood flow and oxygen consumption of the dog heart-lung preparation. Am Heart J 1986; 111:702–9.

40. Evans DB, Steffan RP, Potoczak RE, Weishaar RE, Kaplan HR. Cardiovascular effects of the novel cardiotonic, CI-930. Pharmacologist 1984; 26:115.
41. Roebel LE, Dage RC, Cheng HC, Woodward JK. *In vitro* and *in vivo* assessment of the cardiovascular effects of the cardiotonic drug MDL 19205. J Cardiovasc Pharmacol 1984; 6:43–9.
42. Steffan RP, Eldon CM, Evans DB. The effect of the cardiotonic imazodan (CI-914) on myocardial and peripheral hemodynamics in the anesthetized dog. J Cardiovasc Pharmacol 1986; 8:520–6.
43. Colucci WS. Observations on the intracoronary administration of milrinone and dobutamine to patients with congestive heart failure. Am J Cardiol 1989; 63:17–22A.
44. Pagani ED, Fort DJ, Ezrin AM, Silver PJ. *In vitro* cardiovascular phosphodiesterase inhibition and *in vivo* cardiovascular activity of milrinone in dogs. FASEB J 1988; 2(4); 406.
45. Silver PJ. Pharmacological modulation of phosphorylation mechanisms in heart and vasculature. Drug Dev Res 1988; 12:93–107.
46. Harris AL, Grant AM, Silver PJ, Evans DB, Alousi AA. Differential vasorelaxant effects of milrinone and amrinone on contractile responses of canine coronary, cerebral and renal arteries. J Cardiovasc Pharmacol 1989; 13:238–44.
47. Naccarelli G, Goldstein RA. Electrophysiology of phosphodiesterase inhibitors. Am J Cardiol 1989; 63:35–40A.
48. Emmert SE, Stabilito II, Sweet CS. Acute and subacute effects of enalaprilat, milrinone and combination therapy in rats with chronic left ventricular dysfunction. Clin Exp Hypertension 1987; A9:297.
49. DeFelice A, Harris AL, Frering R, Horan P. Beneficial hemodynamic effects of milrinone and enalapril in conscious rats with healed myocardial infarction. Eur J Pharmacol 1989; 167:211–20.
50. DesJardins S, Mueller RW. Milrinone treatment of cardiomyopathic hamsters (CHF 147). FASEB J 1988; 2:A366.
51. DeFelice A, Fein S, Daudiss K, Frering R, Horan P. Beneficial hemodynamic effects of milrinone in conscious rabbits with chronic aortic regurgitation. J Cardiovasc Pharmacol 1989; 14:659–65.
52. Kittleson MD, Pipers FS, Knaver KW, Keister DM, Knowlen GG, Miner WS. Efficacy of milrinone in naturally occurring myocardial failure in dogs, In: Braunwald E, Sonnenblick EH, Chakrin LW, Schwarz RP, eds. Milrinone. Investigation of new inotropic therapy for congestive heart failure. New York: Raven Press, 1984; 77–89.
53. Alousi AA, Canter JM, Cicero F, Fort DJ, Helstosky A, Lesher GY, Montenaro MJ, Stankus GP, Stuart JC, Walton LH. Pharmacology of milrinone, In: Braunwald E, Sonnenblick EH, Chakrin LW, Schwarz RP, eds. Milrinone. Investigation of new inotropic therapy for congestive heart failure. New York: Raven Press, 1984; 21–48.
54. Pfeffer J, Pfeffer M, Braunwald E. Influence of chronic captopril therapy on the infarcted left ventricle of the rat. Circ Res 1985; 57:84–95.
55. Sweet CS, Ludden CT, Stabilito II, Emmert SE, Heyse JF. Beneficial effects of milrinone and enalapril on long-term survival of rats with healed myocardial infarction. Eur J Pharmacol 1988; 147:29–37.
56. Packer M. Effect of phosphodiesterase inhibitors on survival of patients with chronic congestive heart failure. Am J Cardiol 1989; 63:41–5A.
57. Harris AL, Van Aller G, DeFelice AF, Horan PJ, Frering R, Pagani ED, Silver PJ. Effect of milrinone on isolated papillary muscles from 10 week post myocardially infarcted and sham-operated rats. FASEB J 1989; 3:A1040.
58. Brodde OE, Zerkowski HR, Doetsch N, Motomura S, Khamssi M, Michel MC. Myocardial beta-adrenoceptor changes in heart failure: concomitant reduction in $beta_1$- and $beta_2$-adrenoceptor function related to the degree of heart failure in patients with mitral valve disease. J Am Coll Cardiol 1989; 14:323–31.

59. Feldman AM, Cates AE, Veazey WB, Hershberger RE, Bristow MR, Baughman L, Baumgartner WA, Dop CV. Increase of the 40,000-mol wt. pertussiss toxin substrate (G protein) in the failing human heart. J Clin Invest 1988; 82:189–97.
60. Böhm M, Diet F, Kemkes B, Erdman E. Enhancement of the effectiveness of milrinone to increase force of contraction by stimulation of cardiac beta-adrenoceptors in the failing human heart. Klin Wochenschr 1988; 66:957–62.
61. Harris AL, Connell MJ, Ferguson EW, Wallace AM, Gordon RJ, Pagani ED, Silver PJ. Role of low K_m cAMP phosphodiesterase inhibition in tracheal relaxation and bronchodilation in the guinea pig. J Pharmacol Exp Ther 1989; 251:199–206.
62. Silver PJ, Hamel LT, Perrone MH, Bentley RG, Bushover CR, Evans DB. Differential pharmacologic sensitivity of cyclic nucleotide phosphodiesterase isozymes isolated from cardiac muscle, arterial and airway smooth muscle. Eur J Pharmacol 1988; 150:85–94.
63. Ito M, Tanaka T, Saitoh M, Masuoka H, Nakano T, Hidaka H. Selective inhibition of cyclic AMP phosphodiesterase from various human tissues by milrinone, a potent cardiac bipyridine. Biochem Pharmacol 1988; 37:2041–4.
64. Reeves ML, Leigh BK, England PJ. The identification of a new cyclic phosphodiesterase activity in human and guinea pig cardiac ventricle. Biochem J 1987; 241:535–41.

19

Clinical Aspects of Phosphodiesterase Inhibitors

RICHARD A. GOLDSTEIN

Cardiac and Vascular Diagnostic Center, Tower Imaging
Los Angeles, California

RICHARD M. FLEMING

University of Texas Medical School
Houston, Texas

The treatment of patients with congestive heart failure has undergone considerable change over the past 20 years. Prior to the 1980s therapy for heart failure primarily consisted of digitalis and diuretics. The recent introduction of angiotensin-converting enzyme (ACE) inhibitors has improved patients' quality of life and long-term survival (1,2). However, digitalis glycosides remain the only inotropic agents approved for oral administration. The search for a new inotropic drug initially included beta-agonists but these drugs were abandoned because of tolerance to their effects and a high death rate, presumably due to aggravation of underlying arrhythmias. In the last 10–15 years, the focus of the effort to develop new inotropic agents has been on phosphodiesterase (PDE) inhibitors.

The first clinical study on the new PDE inhibitors was published in 1978 (3). Since then several agents have been tested with varying results. Amrinone and milrinone are available for use intravenously but none of the PDE inhibitors have been approved by the U.S. Food and Drug Administration (FDA) for oral administration. This chapter will review the results of clinical trials involving these drugs (Table 1).

I. MECHANISM OF ACTION

The contractile state of the heart is regulated in part by the adenyl cyclase (AC)–cyclic adenosine monophosphate system (cAMP). Adenyl cyclase is a membrane-bound protein, which, when stimulated by an appropriate effector (i.e., beta-agonists, prostaglandin E-1, etc.), increases cAMP (4,5). cAMP then phosphorylates an inactive protein kinase to its active form. These activated kinases phosphorylate myocardial slow-calcium channels, which increases the influx of calcium into the cell. This calcium then becomes available for loading of intracellular stores (i.e., predominantly the sarcoplasmic reticulum). Myofilaments are then activated when the cal-

Table 1 PDE Inhibitors (generic names)

Bipyridines	
	Amrinone (WIN 40680)
	Milrinone (WIN 47203)
Imidazolones	
	Enoximone (MDL 17,043)
	Piroximone (MDL 19,205)
Pyridazinones	
	Imazodan (CI-914)
	CI-930

cium stored by the sarcoplasmic reticulum is released and interacts with troponin-C. This causes a conformational change in tropomyosin, resulting in cross-bridging of actin and myosin, which produces myofibril shortening and an increase in force. The release of calcium from troponin-C requires ATP if action–myosin dissociation is to occur.

cAMP is degraded by PDE. Any compound that prevents the degradation of cAMP (e.g., by blocking PDE) will cause an increase in intracellular calcium and, thus, an inotropic effect. The PDE inhibitors exert their positive effects on myocardial contractility via PDE III, which is the form of PDE in the heart (6).

In addition to increasing myocardial contractility, PDE inhibitors also produce arterial vasodilation. The hemodynamic changes occurring in patients include an increase in cardiac output, a decrease in systemic vascular resistance, and a reduction in left and right ventricular filling pressures. Heart rate and blood pressure are usually not affected significantly.

II. THE BIPYRIDINES

A. Amrinone

Amrinone was the first of the new PDE inhibitors to be investigated for the treatment of CHF as a positive inotrope (3,4,7). Amrinone was initially tested as an oral and intravenous drug. The intravenous form of amrinone was approved by the FDA in 1984. However, significant gastrointestinal effects and thrombocytopenia with the oral form of amrinone led to its withdrawal from clinical trials (5). Accordingly, only parenteral amrinone will be reviewed.

1. Pharmacokinetics

Amrinone treatment is initiated by an intravenous loading dosage of 0.75 μg/kg over 2–3 min followed by a maintenance dosage of 5–10 μg/kg/min. A second bolus may be given 30 min after the initial dose if warranted. The daily dosage should not exceed 10 mg/kg/day to avoid thrombocytopenia (8). Amrinone has a half-life of 3.6–5.8 hr. Some recent studies have suggested that the half-life may be as long as 12 hr in patients with congestive heart failure (9,10). Ten to 40% of the drug is excreted unchanged in the urine, while the remainder is conjugated in the liver before urinary excretion (9,10). Accordingly, the effects of the drug should be monitored closely in patients with impaired renal function.

2. Hemodynamic Effects

Like other PDE inhibitors, amrinone is not only a positive inotropic agent but also possesses vasodilatory properties that make it a potent preload and afterload reducer (3,11–17; Table 2). The hemodynamic effects of amrinone in a representative sample of clinical studies are summarized in Table 2. Amrinone has minimal effects on heart rate and mean arterial blood pressure in most patients. However, in patients with left ventricular filling pressures below 10–15 mmHg, reflex tachycardia and hypotension may occur (18). Blood pressure must be closely monitored to adjust the dosage because of amrinone's vasodilatory properties. Although the inotropic effect of the drug would be expected to aggravate pre-existing myocardial ischemia by raising the workload of the heart, myocardial oxygen demand appears to be decreased secondary to a reduction in resting wall tension (14).

3. Electrophysiological Effects

Patients with congestive heart failure have a high incidence of sudden death. The cause of death is usually either pump failure or fatal arrhythmias. Approximately 90% of patients with severe heart failure have frequent multiform ventricular extrasystoles and as many as 70–80% have episodes of ventricular tachycardia (8,16–

Table 2 Hemodynamic Data on Current Phosphodiesterase Inhibiting Drugs: Amrinone and Milrinone

		Mean % Change From Baseline							
Dosage	Pts(n)	CO	PCWP	RA	SVR	PVR	HR	MAP	Ref
Amrinone									
40 μg/kg/min IV	8	+37	−17	−49	−23	–	NS	NS	11
40 μg/kg/min IV	8	+46	−25	−37	−19	–	NS	NS	12
0.75–3.0 mg/kg IV	8	+49	−26	−26	−29	−39	NS	NS	13
0.50–3.5 mg/kg IV	8	+46	−46	−33	−32	−24	NS	NS	3
2.5 mg/kg IV	9	+69	−16	−18	−40	−50	NS	NS	14
1.5–3.5 mg/kg IV	11	+47	−41	–	–	–	NS	NS	15
10–20 mg/kg/min IV	14	+30	−20	−21	−17	−8	NS	NS	16
1.18–1.50 mg/kg IV	6	+13[a]	−17	−18	−18	−5	+8	−2	17
	8	+44	−46	−42	−32	−24	+1	−7	
Milrinone									
125 μg/kg±36 IV	18	+45	−39	−38	−37	–	+8	−13	24
67±13 μg/kg/min IV	10	+50	−29	−38	−34	–	+3	−8	25
50–75 μg/kg LD flu	79	+34	−26	–	−25	–	+7	−6	26
0.5–1.0 μg/kg/min									
12.5 to 75 μg/kg IV	15	+55	−45	−54	−36	–	+11	−15	27
12.5 to 75 μg/kg/min IV	7	+76	–	−53	–	–	+8	−13	28
25 μg/kg LD	11	−49	−40	−42	−33	–	−2	−4	29
7.5 mg po	11	+−	–	–	−34	–	+1	−5	30
25 μg/kg IV	7	+−	−23	–	−29	–	+6	+1	30

HR, heart rate; MAP, mean arterial blood; RA, right artrial pressure; PAP, pulmonary artery pressure; PVR, pulmonary vascular resistance; PCWP, pulmonary capillary wedge pressure; CO/CI, cardiac index; SVR, systemic vascular resistance.

[a]Cardiac output.

19). Since any compound that increases cAMP has the potential to be arrhythmogenic, it is essential to study the electrophysiological properties of these drugs.

Naccarelli and colleagues performed hemodynamic and electrophysiological studies in 15 patients with New York Heart Association (NHYA) class II–IV heart failure before and during infusion with amrinone (16). Vasoactive and anti-arrhythmic drugs were discontinued at least 5 half-lives before the initial baseline study. Amrinone had no significant effect on PR QRS, QTc, AH, or HV intervals. Ventricular effective refractory period and maximal corrected sinus node recovery time also were unaffected. However, there was a statistically significant decrease in atrial effective refractory period, but by only 6%. There was no change in the inducibility of ventricular tachycardia by programmed electrical stimulation.

4. *Side Effects and Drug Interactions*

Intravenous amrinone should not be given in the same tubing as furosemide and must be prepared in solutions not containing dextrose to prevent precipitation. It should be utilized within 24 hr of preparation to optimize effect. Hypotensive episodes have been reported when it is used concomitantly with disopyramide (8). Additional side effects that have been reported include gastrointestinal (GI) intolerance (anorexia, nausea, abdominal pain, and diarrhea), central nervous system manifestations (headache, lightheadedness, and paresthesia), and dose-dependent thrombocytopenia (requiring daily monitoring of platelet counts (5,8).

B. Milrinone

Milrinone is a bipyridine with more than 10 times the potency of amrinone on a per milligram basis (5,20–23). Only the intravenous form of the drug received FDA approval in 1987. However, to date, it has not been made available commercially. Initial results with the oral cogener are still in progress and suggest that the drug is effective and well tolerated.

1. *Pharmacokinetics*

Intravenous milrinone is initiated with a loading bolus of 25–50 μg/kg given over 1 min. The peak effect occurs within 2–5 min. Milrinone has a duration of action that ranges from 30 min to 2 hr and a half-life of approximately 2 hr (5,23). The drug is primarily excreted unchanged in the urine (5).

The oral dosage of milrinone is 7.5–12.5 mg every 4–6 hr to a maximum of 50 mg/day. Onset of action following the oral preparation is between 10 and 30 min. The peak effect of milrinone occurs at 15–20 min and hemodynamic effects persist for approximately 4 hr.

2. *Hemodynamic Effects*

Studies with intravenous milrinone have demonstrated that milrinone, like amrinone, reduces both preload and afterload in addition to increasing contractility (24–30) (Table 2). Heart rate and systemic arterial pressure are not significantly changed. Monrad et al. reported that these hemodynamic effects are not accompanied by an increase in oxygen demand, suggesting that the increased oxygen consumption expected by an increase in contractility is offset by the salutary effect on preload (24). There does not appear to be significant tolerance to the effects of the drug up to at least 48 hr of therapy (26).

3. *Electrophysiological Effects*

Davidenko et al. studied the electrophysiological properties of milrinone in canine cardiac false tendons and found that action potential duration was minimally increased by dosages of 10–20 μg/ml (31). Re-entrant arrhythmias were either blocked or facilitated depending on the initial level of the block. Subsequently, Goldstein et al. studied 10 patients with NYHA class III or IV heart failure who underwent electrophysiological studies before and during infusion of milrinone for 18 hr (32). All cardioactive drugs except diuretics were discontinued at least 5 half-lives before baseline measurements were made. The cardiac rhythm was continuously recorded by Holter monitoring for 48 hr before and during a 48 hr infusion of milrinone. Milrinone enhanced 1:1 maximal atrioventricular conduction but did not significantly affect atrioventricular effective or functional refractory periods. Programmed electrical stimulation induced ventricular tachycardia in 5 of the 10 patients at baseline but none during infusion of milrinone. There was a statistically increased incidence of nonsustained ventricular tachycardia, although no patients were classified as having demonstrated proarrhythmic effects. This study suggests that milrinone could be antiarrhythmic or proarrhythmic depending on the patient.

4. *Studies with Oral Milrinone*

Early studies with oral milrinone have reported improvement in exercise tolerance within a few days to weeks following initiation of the drug (31). However, the results of studies following treatment for several months have been mixed, with some showing a maintained improvement in exercise duration and others no difference from controls (33).

The largest study of oral milrinone included 230 patients with class II or III failure who were randomized to receive milrinone, milrinone and digoxin, digoxin alone, or placebo (33). Diuretics were allowed to supplement therapy in all patients. There was a significant improvement in exercise duration following 3 months with all therapy compared to placebo. However, there was no additive effect of milrinone to digoxin.

A large multicenter trial is currently in progress designed to look specifically at the issue of long-term survival on milrinone as an adjunct to digoxin, diuretics, and captopril in patients with severe failure (34).

5. *Side Effects and Drug Interactions*

Milrinone appears to be well tolerated with few confirmed side effects. The only statistically significant reported side effect appears to be a mild headache in some patients (34). However, because of the vasodilating effects of the drug, hypotension may occur in patients with pulmonary capillary wedge pressures less than 15 mm Hg.

III. THE IMIDALZOLONES

A. Enoximone

Enoximone is an imidazolone being evaluated for intravenous and oral use (35–45). In addition to inhibition of subfraction III PDE, it also appears to activate slow-calcium channels (35).

1. Pharmacokinetics

In most studies, enoximone has been given at a dosage of 0.5–2.0 mg/kg intravenously (IV) at a rate of up to 12.5 mg/min (Table 3). The dosage of oral enoximone is 75–150 mg every 8 hr (37,38). Earlier studies used significantly higher dosages but reported a greater incidence of side effects. The onset of action for the oral dosage is 10 min with a peak effect at 1 hr (44). Enoximone has a half-life of 20 hr and is metabolized to MDL 19,438 with a half-life of 25 hr (44). This metabolite has approximately 20% of the hemodynamic effect of the parent compound in dogs (35).

2. Hemodynamic Effects

Enoximone, like other PDE inhibitors, decreases the left ventricular filling pressure and systemic vascular resistance and increases cardiac output (Table 3). Hemodynamic changes correlate positively with increases in dosage (35,36,39). Heart rate is not significantly changed in most patients except at dosages greater than 1.5 mg/kg (36–40). Arterial systemic pressure is usually unchanged or decreased. Preliminary studies with oral enoximone have reported improvements in exercise capacity and symptoms (37,38). Hemodynamic improvement occurs in approximately 90% of the patients initially. However, only 50% of the patients maintained these effects at 4 weeks and 25% when oral therapy is given for more than 3 months (42). Enoximone also increased plasma renin and decreased plasma norepinephrine levels. Arginine vasopressin was not significantly changed (42).

3. Electrophysiological Effects

Miles et al. studied the electrophysiology of enoximone in a group of patients with heart failure (41). Most patients were receiving therapy with digoxin and antiar-

Table 3 Hemodynamic Data on Current Phosphodiesterase Inhibiting Drugs: Enoximone and Piroximone

		Mean % Change From Baseline							
Dosage	Pts(n)	CO	PCWP	RA	SVR	PVR	HR	MAP	Ref
Enoximone									
3.0 mg/kg IV	44	+55	−29	−30	−33	–	+6	−5	39
10.5 mg/kg IV	44	+68	−42	−46	−44	–	+13	−14	39
150 mg po	12	–	–	–	–	–	−3	+3	37
50–100 mg po	6	+50	−51	–	−42	−68	−5	−4	38
3.7 mg/kg IV	38	+75	−42	−50	−42	−29	+9	−10	40
18.4 mg/kg po	38	+45	−35	−38	−34	−24	+2	−10	40
3–6 mg/kg po	20	+28[a]	−46	−60	−3	–	+9	–	42
1.5 mg/kg IV	16	+76	−48	−50	−52	−29	+10	−19	43
0.5 mg/kg IV q 15–20 4.5 mg kg total	12	+83	−48	−54	−47	−31	+3	−10	44
6 mg/kg po q 6	10	+56	−19	−NS	−35	–	NS	NS	45
IV 0.5 mg/kg q 15–20	13	+76	−27	46	−46	−49	+2	−6	46
po 2 mg/kg	13	+76	−15	−25	−39	−45	+5	−2	46
Piroximone									
1.7 mg/kg po	12	+51	−31	−45	−34	−29	+3	−6	47
1.25 mg/kg IV	8	+74	−36	−67	−43	−33	+4	−8	47

Abbreviations as in Table 2.

rhythmic drugs during the study, making it difficult to interpret the results. They reported a small but statistically significant increase in the sinus cycle length, and a decrease in atrial–His, atrial functional refractory period, atrioventricular (AV) nodal effective and functional refractory period, minimal atrial pacing cycle length maintaining 1:1 AV conduction, ventricular effective and functional refractory period when compared with both amrinone and milrinone.

In a double-blind placebo crossover study with oral enoximone, Choraria et al. evaluated 12 patients with NYHA class II–III heart failure for 6 weeks (37). Holter monitoring 2 weeks into the study revealed an increase in premature ventricular complexes and couplets. No R-on-T phenomenon or sustained runs of ventricular tachycardia longer than 10 beats were noted.

4. *Side Effects and Drug Interactions*

The incidence of adverse effects appears to be dose dependent, increasing considerably when the cumulative dosage exceeds 1.5 mg/kg (35,36,39). Side effects with intravenous enoximone have included hypotension and an increased frequency of new episodes of ventricular tachycardia (39). Up to 7% of the patients had CNS manifestations, 5% had gastrointestinal manifestations, with 4% having other problems. Twenty-eight percent of the patients had > 2 g/dl drop in hemoglobin, which was deemed clinically important (39). Oral enoximone has side effects in as many as 75% of patients although therapy needed to be discontinued in only 7% (44). The major problems affect the gastrointestinal tract and include diarrhea, loose stools, nausea, vomiting, and abdominal cramping (44). Patients may also experience fluid accumulation and thrombocytopenia (5). The absorption of enoximone is reduced in patients taking tetracycline, phenytoin, phenylbutazone, and chlorthiazide (42).

B. Piroximone

Relatively little information is available on this imidazolone compound, which also inhibits PDE III. It has been studied both as an oral preparation and as an intravenous solution. The drug has been given at an intravenous loading dosage of 1.7 mg/kg and then followed by an oral dosage of 0.5 mg/kg (100–400 mg) every 6 hr (48).

Piroximone's hemodynamic effects include an improvement in cardiac output and a reduction in preload and afterload (Table 3). It produces a small but significant decrease in arterial pressure. The drug decreases plasma norepinephrine and raises renin levels. In an initial open-label study, the drug failed to demonstrate any sustained clinical benefits in a group of 11 patients with severe heart failure evaluated over a 2–10 month (mean of 5.6 months) period (48).

The side effects of long-term treatment included diarrhea and worsening of heart failure. Determination of the frequency of this and other side effects will require a greater number of studies in patients.

IV. THE PYRIDAZINONES

A. Imazodan

Few published reports are currently available to determine the usefulness of this drug or its analog CI-930. In vitro it has a potency 10 times that of amrinone (49).

The oral dosage of this medication has ranged from 3 to 30 mg (49,50). Peak plasma levels occur approximately 2 hr after an oral dose is given. There is a

Table 4 Hemodynamic Data on Current Phosphodiesterase Inhibiting Drugs: CI 914 and CI 930

		Mean % Change From Basline							
Dosage	Pts(N)	CO	PCWP	RA	SVR	PVR	HR	MAP	Ref
CI-914									
0.1–30 mg IV	13	+26	−21	−31	−23	−14	+3	+6	49
3.30 mg/kg PO	13	+19	−11	−9	−9	−7	+4	−1	49
CI-930									
0.5–2.1	9	+35	−43	−44	−30	−20	+0	−9	51

Abbreviations as in Table 2.

positive correlation between dosage and maximal blood levels obtained (49). Studies in dogs have demonstrated that imazodan is a coronary vasodilator (50). The drug increases cardiac output and decreases afterload and preload, as do other PDE inhibitors (Table 4).

Oral imazodan appears to be well tolerated with minimal renal, hepatic, or gastrointestinal problems. No significant thrombocytopenia has been noted.

B. CI-930

The initial studies of this drug began in the mid 1980s (50). CI-930 is currently given as an intravenous preparation at a dosage of 0.5–2.1 μg/kg/min. Preliminary data on its hemodynamic effects are shown in Table 4. CI-930 increases plasma atrial natriuretic peptide. There is not sufficient information available to allow us to comment on potential side effects.

V. SUMMARY

The phosphodiesterase inhibitors have inotropic and vasodilator properties. Unlike other drugs that increase contractility, they do not raise myocardial oxygen consumption. However, despite initial optimism about these agents, only intravenous amrinone and milrinone have been approved for use in patients with heart failure to date. The results of trials with oral congeners have not demonstrated clear advantages over other forms of therapy for heart failure. There have also been questions raised about whether these drugs adversely affect patient survival. Trials involving large numbers of patients should provide an answer to this and help to determine whether there is any long-term benefit of therapy with this class of drugs.

REFERENCES

1. Captopril Multicenter Research Group. A placebo-controlled trial of captopril in refractory chronic congestive heart failure. J Am Coll Cardiol 1983;2:755–63.
2. The CONSENSUS Trial Study Group. Effects of enalapril on mortality in severe congestive heart failure: results of the Cooperative North Scandinavian Enalapril Survival Study (CONSENSUS). N Engl J Med 1987;316:1429–35.

3. Benotti J, Grossman W, Braunwald E, Davolos DD, Alousi AA. Hemodynamic assessment of amrinome: A new inotropic agent. N Engl J Med 1978;299 (25):1373–7.
4. Colucci WS, Wright RF, Braunwald E. New positive inotropic agents in the treatment of congestive heart failure: mechanisms of action and recent clinical developments (first of two parts). N Engl J Med 1986;314 (5):290–9.
5. Colucci WS, Wright RF, Braunwald E. New positive inotropic agents in the treatment of congestive heart failure: mechanisms of action and recent clinical developments (second of two parts). Engl J Med 1986;314 (6):349–58.
6. Strada SJ. Cyclic nucleotide phosphodiesterases. Adv Cyclic Nucleotide Protein Phosphoryl Res 1984;16:1–442.
7. Hood W. Controlled and uncontrolled studies of phosphodiesterase III inhibitors in contemporary cardiovascular medicine. Am J Cardiol 1989;63:46–53A.
8. Goldstein R. Clinical effects of intravenous amrinone in patients with congesitve heart failure. Circulation 1986;73 (suppl III):III-191–5.
9. Edelson J, LeJemtel TH, Alousi AA, Biddlecome CE, Maskin CS, Sonnenblick EH. Relationship between amrinone plasma concentration and cardiac index. Clin Pharmacol Ther 1981;29 (6):723–8.
10. Kullberg MP, Freeman GB, Biddlecome C, Alousi AA, Edelson J. Amrinone metabolism. Clin Pharmacol Ther 1981;29(3):394–401.
11. Siskind SJ, Sonnenblick EH, Forman R, Scheuer J, LeJemtel TH. Acute susbstantial benefit of inotropic therapy with amrinone on exercise hemodynamics and metabolism in severe congestive heart failure. Circulation 1981;64:966–73.
12. Klein NA, Siskind SJ, Frishman WH, Sonnenblick EH, LeJemtel TH. Hemodynamic comparison of intravenous amrinone and dobutamine in patients with chronic congestive heart failure. Am J Cardiol 1981;48:170–5.
13. LeJemtel TH, Keung E, Sonnenblick EH, Ribner HS, Matsumoto M, Davis R, Schwartz W, Alousi AA, Davolos D. Amrinone: a new non-glycosidic, non-adrenergic cardiotonic agent effective in the treatment of intractable myocardial failure in man. Circulation 1979;59:1098–104.
14. Benotti J, Grossman W, Braunwald E, Carabello BA. Effects of amrinone on myocardial energy metabolism and hemodynamics in patients with severe congestive heart failure due to coronary artery disease. Circulation 1980;62(1):28–34.
15. Weber, KT, Andrews V, Janicki JS, Wilson JR, Fishman AP. Amrinone and exercise performance in patients with chronic heart failure. Am J Cardiol 1981;48:164–9.
16. Naccarelli GV, Gray EL, Dougherty AH, Hanna JE, Goldstein RA. Amrinone: acute electrophysiologic and hemodynamic effects in patients with congestive heart failure. Am J Cardiol 1984;54:600–4.
17. Benotti J, Lesko LJ, McCue JE. Actue pharmacodynamics and pharmacokinetics of oral amrinone. J Clin Pharmacol 1982;22:425–32.
18. Wilmshurst PT, Thompson DS, Jenkins BS, Coltart DJ, Webb-Peploe MM. Haemodynamic effects of intravenous amrinone in patients with impaired left ventricular function. Br Heart J 1983;49:77–82.
19. Naccarelli GV, Goldstein RA. Electrophysiology of phosphodiesterase inhibitors. Am J Cardiol 1989;63:35–40A.
20. Baim D. Effect of phosphodiesterase inhibition on myocardial oxygen consumption and coronary blood flow. Am J Cardiol 1989;63:23–6A.
21. Alousi AA, Canter JM, Montenaro MJ, Fort DJ, Ferrari RA. Cardiotonic activity of milrinone, a new and potent cardiac bipyridine, on the normal and failing heart of experimental animals. J Cardiovasc Pharmacol 1983;5:792–803.
22. Alousi AA, Stankus GP, Stuart JC, Walton LH. Characterization of the cardiotonic effects of milrinone, a new and potent cardiac bipyridine on isolated tissues from several animal species. J Cardiovasc Pharmacol 1983;5:804–11.

23. Alousi A, Canter JM, Cicero F, Fort DJ, Helstosky A, Lesher GY, Montenaro MJ, Stankus GP, Stuart JC, Walton LH. Pharmacology of milrinone. In: Milrinone: investigation of new inotropic therapy for congestive heart failure. New York: Raven Press, 1984;21–48.
24. Monrad ES, Baim DS, Smith HS, Lanoue A, Braunwald E, Grossman W. Effect of milrinone on coronary hemodynamics and myocardial energetics in patients with congestive heart failure. Circulation 1985;71:972–9.
25. Monrad ES, Baim DS, Smith HS, Lanoue AS. Milrinone, dobutamine, and nitroprusside: comparative effects on hemodynamics and myocardial energetics in patients with severe heart failure. Circulation 1986; 73 (3Pt 2): III 168–74.
26. Biddle TL, Benotti JR, Creager MA, Faxon DP, Firth BG, Fitzpatrick PG, Konstam MA, Krebs C, Walton L, Kershner RP, Jacobsen J, Luczkowec CA, Montenaro MJ, Tandon PK, Fitzpatrick S, Schwarz RP. Comparison of intravenous milrinone and dobutamine for congestive heart failure secondary to either ischemic or dilated cardiomyopathy. Am J Cardiol 1987;59:1345–50.
27. Colucci WS, Wright RF, Jaski BE, Fifer MA, Braunwald E. Milrinone and dobutamine in severe heart failure: differing hemodynamic effects and individual patient responsiveness. Circulation 1986; 73 (3Pt 2): III 175–83.
28. Jaski BE, Fifer MA, Wright RF, Braunwald E, Colucci WS. Positive inotropic and vasodilator actions of milrinone in patients with severe congestive heart failure: Dose-response relationships and comparison to nitroprusside. J Clin Invest 1985; 75(2):643–9.
29. Maskin CS, Sinoway L, Chadwick B, Sonnenblick EH, LeJemtel TH. Sustained hemodynamic and clinical effects of a new cardiotonic agent, WIN 47203, in patients with severe congestive heart failure. Circulation 1983; 67(5):1065–70.
30. LeJemtel, TH, Maskin CS, Mancini D, Sinoway L, Feld H, Chadwick B. Systemic and regional hemodynamic effects of captopril and milrinone administered alone and concomitantly in patients with heart failure. Circulation 1985;72(2):364–9.
31. Davidenko JM, Antzelevitch C. The effects of milrinone on conduction, reflection and automaticity in canine Purkinje fibers. Circulation 1982;65:1026–35.
32. Goldstein R, Geraci SA, Gray EL, Rinkenerger RL, Dougherty AH, Naccarelli GV. Electrophysiologic effects of milrinone in patients with congestive heart failiure. Am J Cardiol 1986;57:524–8.
33. DiBianco R, Shabetai R, Kostuk W, Moran J, Schlant RC, Wright R. Comparison of oral milrinone, digoxin and their combination in the treatment of patients with chronic heart failure. N Engl J Med 1989;320 (11):677–83.
34. Packer M. Effect of phosphodiesterase inhibitors on survival of patients with chronic congestive heart failure. Am J Cardiol 1989;63:41–5A.
35. Dage R, Kariya T, Hsieh CP, Roebel LE, Cheng HC, Schnetler RA, Grisar JM. Pharmacology of enoximone. Am J Cardiol 1987;60:10–4C.
36. Erbel R, Meyer J, Diefenbach C, Delorme G, Bourdarias JP, Vernant P, Lellouche D, Mattioli G, Barbieri A, Installe E, Gonzalez M, Mitrovic V, Nuezner J, Salvade G. A dose–response study of intravenous enoximone in congestive heart failure. Am J Cardiol 1987;59:31–6C.
37. Choraria S, Taylor D, Pilcher J. Double-blind crossover comparison of enoximone and placebo in patients with congestive heart failure. Circulation 1989;76(6):1307–11.
38. Treese N, Erbel R, Pilcher J, Choraria S, Rhein S, Dieterich HA, Meyer J. Long-term treatment with oral enoximone for chronic congestive heart failure: the european experience. Am J Cardiol 1987;60:85–90C.
39. Crawford M. Intravenous use of enoximone. Am J Cardiol 1987;60:42C–5C.
40. Chatterjee K, Kereiakes D, Viquerat C, Podolin R. Potential mechanisms of improved left ventricular function with enoximone in severe congestive heart failure. Am J Cardiol 1987;60:37–41C.

41. Miles WM, Heger JJ, Minardo JD, Prystowsky EN, Zipes DP. Electrophysiologic and hemodynamic effects of intravenous enoximone (abstr.) Circulation 1986;74:Suppl II:II-38.
42. Uretsky B, Generalovich T, Verbalis JG, Valdes AM, Reddy S. MDL 17,043 Therapy in severe congestive heart failure: characterization of the early and late hemodynamic, pharmacokinetic, hormonal and clinical response. J Am Coll Cardiol 1985;5:1414–21.
43. Uretsky BF, Generalovich T, Reddy PS, Spangenberg RB, Follansbee WP. The acute hemodynamic effects of a new agent, MDL 17,043, in the treatment of congestive heart failure. Circulation 1983;67:823–8.
44. Uretsky BF, Valdes AM, Reddy PS. Positive inotropic therapy for short term-support and long-term management of patients with congestive heart failure: hemodynamic effects and clinical efficacy of MDL 17,043. Circulation 1986;73 (Suppl III): III-219–28.
45. Amin DK, Shah PK, Hulse S, Shellock F. Comparative acute hemodynamic effects of intravenous sodium nitroprusside and MDL-17,043, a new inotropic drug with vasodilator effects, in refractory congestive heart failure. Am Heart J 1985;109:1006–12.
46. Rubin SA, Tabak L. MDL 17,043: short-and long-term cardiopulmonary and clinical effects in patients with heart failure. J Am Coll Cardiol 1985;5(6):1422–7.
47. Shah PK, Amin DK, Hulse S, Shellock F, Swan HJC. Inotropic therapy for refractory congestive heart failure with oral fenoximone (MDL-17,043): poor long-term results despite early hemodynamic and clinical improvement. Circulation 1985;7 (2):326–31.
48. Petein M, Levine TB, Cohn JN. Persistent hemodynamic effects without long-term clinical benefits in response to oral piroximone (MDL 19,205) in patients with congestive heart failure. Circulation 1986;73(suppl III):III-230–6.
49. Jafri SM, Burlew BS, Goldberg D, Rogers A, Goldstein S. Hemodynamic effects of a new type III phosphodiesterase inhibitor (CI-914) for congestive heart failure. Am J Cardiol 1986;57:254–9.
50. Steffen RP. The effect of the cardiotonic imazodan (CI-914) on myocardial and peripheral hemodynamics in the anesthetized dog. J Cardiovasc Pharmacol 1986;8(3):520–6.
51. Murali S, Uretsky BF, Valdes AM, Lolesar JA, Reddy S. Acute hemodynamic and hormonal effects of CI-930, a new phosphodiesterase inhibitor, in severe congestive heart failure. Am J Cardiol 1987;59:1356–60.

20

Basic Science Aspects of Angiotensin I Converting Enzyme and Its Inhibitors

RANDAL A. SKIDGEL

University of Illinois College of Medicine at Chicago
Chicago, Illinois

The angiotensin I converting enzyme (ACE; kininase II; EC 3.4.15.1) has been one of the most thoroughly studied peptidases over the last three decades. The synthesis of clinically useful inhibitors of ACE in the late 1970s led to a surge of research on this enzyme that remains unabated today. Although ACE has been studied extensively, many unanswered questions still remain. The most exciting recent findings have come from investigations utilizing the tools of molecular biology to study the structure of ACE. This approach holds the promise of answering many of the unresolved questions about this interesting and important enzyme.

This chapter will focus on the biochemistry, molecular biology, enzymology, and distribution of ACE and how this information relates to the mechanism of action and use of ACE inhibitors in vivo. The development of ACE inhibitors and their use experimentally and clinically have been extensively reviewed elsewhere and will not be considered in detail here.

I. HISTORICAL PERSPECTIVE

A. Discovery of ACE

The study of the renin-angiotensin system and its role in hypertension has a long history. In 1898, Tigerstedt and Bergman discovered a hypertensive factor in saline extracts of rabbit kidney that they called renin (1). Little interest was shown in this discovery until the 1930s, when the pioneering work of Goldblatt and colleagues demonstrated the important role of the kidney in experimental models of hypertension (1). The subsequent search for a hypertensive humoral agent of renal origin led to the 1940 discovery, by two independent groups, that renin is an enzyme that releases a potent vasoconstrictor from a plasma substrate (2,3). Braun-Menendez and his co-workers named the vasoconstrictor hypertensin (2) and Page and Helmer

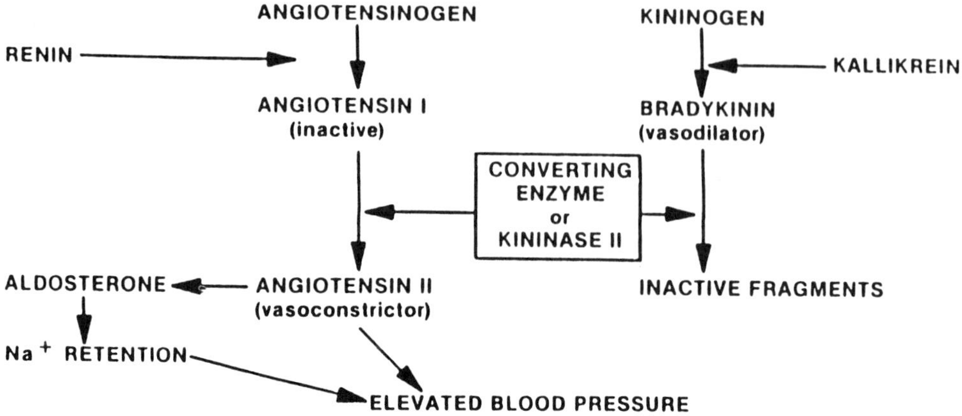

Figure 1 Schematic diagram of the central role ACE plays in the activation of angiotensin II and the inactivation of bradykinin. (From Ref. 153 with permission.)

named it angiotonin (3). It was not until 1958 that they agreed to rename the vasoconstrictor angiotensin (4). Work was begun in the early 1950s by Skeggs and co-workers on the isolation of large quantities of angiotensin in order to characterize it fully. This was accomplished by incubating crude preparations of horse plasma renin substrate (angiotensinogen) with hog kidney renin. The constrictor was purified by countercurrent distribution, resulting in the isolation of a decapeptide, later called angiotensin I (1). The final step in the preparation of both the angiotensinogen and renin involved dialysis against distilled water. For unknown reasons, once the preparations were dialyzed against 0.15 M NaCl. When these were used to prepare angiotensin, a hypertensive agent was isolated that appeared in a different position in the countercurrent apparatus, indicating that angiotensin ocurred in two different forms (1). This somewhat serendipitous finding resulted in the discovery of an enzyme, appropriately named angiotensin-converting enzyme (ACE), which converts angiotensin I to angiotensin II by removal of the C-terminal dipeptide His-Leu (1,5). Experiments on the partially purified enzyme from horse plasma showed that its activity depended on the presence of chloride or other monovalent anions (bromide, fluoride, nitrate) and that it was likely a metalloenzyme, since EDTA or cyanide inhibited it (6,7). It was later shown that the decapeptide angiotensin I has no activity and must be converted to the active octapeptide angiotensin II, emphasizing the critical importance of ACE in the cascade (Fig. 1).

B. Identity of ACE with Kininase II

Independently of these investigations, in the early 1960s Erdös and co-workers began investigating bradykinin metabolism. They initially found a kininase in plasma (carboxypeptidase N; kininase I) that removes the C-terminal arginine residue of bradykinin (8,9). Further studies led to the discovery of another enzyme (named kininase II) in plasma and kidney that inactivates bradykinin by cleaving off the C-terminal Phe^8-Arg^9 dipeptide (8,10,11). In the late 1960s, the studies of Vane and colleagues established that the primary site for conversion of angiotensin I to II was not the plasma, as previously thought, but the pulmonary vascular bed

(12,13). They also found that the pulmonary circulation rapidly inactivates bradykinin and initially speculated that both actions could be due to carboxypeptidase N (13). Later, they and other investigators concluded that bradykinin inactivation and angiotensin conversion were carried out by two different enzymes (14–17). However, a series of papers published by Erdös and co-workers (18–20) clearly established that kininase II is identical with ACE. This was proven by purification of the enzyme and characterization of its substrate specificity and inhibitor profile (18–20). These studies gave rise to the somewhat paradoxical concept that a single enzyme could activate a hypertensive agent (angiotensin) and inactivate a hypotensive agent (bradykinin) and established ACE as an enzyme that could play an important role in the regulation of blood pressure (Fig. 1).

II. DISTRIBUTION OF ACE

Although ACE was initially found in the blood, the discovery that angiotensin I is rapidly converted to angiotensin II in the pulmonary circulation and vascular beds of other organs indicated that it might have a wide distribution. In addition, the initial finding of a high ACE (kininase II) concentration in hog kidney microsomes (10) suggested that ACE is also concentrated in tissues other than the vasculature (Table 1). Indeed, an early survey found ACE activity in crude homogenates of many different tissues (21). Subsequent purification of ACE, first from animal tissues and then from human cadaver tissues (8,22), led to the production of specific antibodies to ACE that were then used to localize it immunohistochemically. The localization of ACE has also been facilitated by the development of sensitive enzyme assays and specific inhibitors which, when labeled, can also be used in histochemical studies.

Table 1 Distribution of ACE

Source of ACE	Form of ACE
Endothelial cells	Membrane-bound
Vasculature of virtually all organs	
Epithelial cells	Membrane-bound
Microvilli; brush border of placenta, kidney proximal tubules, intestine, choroid plexus	
Neuroepithelial cells	Membrane-bound
Subfornical organ, pallidonigral dendrites, median eminence, etc.	
Male genital tract	
testes	Membrane-bound
prostate, epididymides,	Membrane-bound + soluble
seminal plasma	Soluble
Body fluids	Soluble
Blood, urine, lung edema, amniotic fluid, CSF, lymph	

Source: Modified from Erdös EG, Skidgel RA. The unusual substrate specificity and the distribution of human angiotensin I converting enzyme. Hypertension 1986;8:I34–7.

A. Endothelial and Epithelial ACE

ACE is found in all vascular beds, bound to the plasma membranes of endothelial cells (8,23–25) where, as an ectoenzyme, it has access to circulating substrates. This explains the rapid conversion of angiotensin I to II and inactivation of bradykinin in the pulmonary circulation. However, this is not the only physiologically relevant site for ACE action since the enzyme is also highly concentrated on epithelial and neuroepithelial cells (Table 1). In fact, the human kidney contains five to six times more ACE per wet weight than the lung (25,26). In the kidney, most ACE is found in the brush border of the proximal tubules (27,28). Other epithelial brush borders rich in ACE include the small intestine (29), choroid plexus (22,30,31) and placenta (32). ACE is also highly concentrated in tissues of the male reproductive tract including the testes, prostate, and epididymides (21,33–35). Although it was shown that testicles can synthesize a truncated (about 40 kDa lower molecular weight) ACE (36), the size of ACE in prostate and epididymides is similar to that of the lung or kidney enzyme (35,37).

There are many possible functions for ACE outside the vascular endothelium. For example, ACE can release dipeptides for absorption in the intestinal tract (29) or protect the fetus from maternal peptides by inactivating them in the placenta (32). On the renal proximal tubular brush border, ACE may eliminate active peptides that enter the nephron after glomerular filtration (8,27). This can be especially important for kinins, which are thought to be released at the level of the distal tubule where they stimulate prostaglandin synthesis and salt and water excretion. Thus, bloodborne filtered kinins would need to be inactivated before reaching the distal tubule in order for the autoregulatory function of renal kinins to be manifested (8,27). Although these proposed functions of ACE are somewhat speculative, it seems likely that this relatively ubiquitous enzyme has functions other than the conversion of angiotensin I to II or the inactivation of bradykinin. This idea is supported by its presence in discrete areas of the brain and relatively broad substrate specificity (see below).

B. Soluble ACE

Although in tissues ACE is bound tightly to plasma membranes, it also exists in soluble form (Table 1). ACE was first discovered as a bloodborne enzyme and it is also soluble in urine, lung edema fluid, amniotic fluid, seminal plasma, cerebrospinal fluid, and in homogenates of prostate and epididymides (8,26,35,37). Whether soluble ACE has important functions is unclear. In addition, the mechanism of solubilization of ACE from membranes in vivo is still not completely understood. Proteolytic cleavage of the membrane anchor peptide is one possible mechanism of solubilization and, in fact, trypsin solubilization was used to facilitate the first purification of human renal ACE (38). Other possibilities include alternative RNA splicing or posttranslational processing, giving rise to a form of ACE that is directly secreted, or sloughing-off of endothelial ACE into the plasma with its membrane anchor still intact. Recent studies have begun to provide some answers. Utilizing anchor-specific antibody and the techniques of molecular biology, Wei et al (39) showed that the soluble form of ACE is released by proteolytic removal of the C-terminal anchor, although it could not be proven whether this occurs intracellularly immediately after protein synthesis or only after ACE is transported to the plasma membrane.

C. Neuroepithelial ACE

Although there were early reports of ACE activity in homogenates of rat (40) and human (41) brain, these findings were not intensively pursued until other elements of the renin–angiotensin system were detected in the brain and it was hypothesized that the system played a role in some forms of hypertension (42). In the rat brain, high ACE activities were found in the striatum, cerebellum, pituitary gland, subfornical organ, caudate nucleus, nucleus habenularis medialis, area postrema, substantia nigra, and locus ceruleus (31). Possibly the highest concentration of ACE in any tissue was found in the choroid plexus (22,30,31) where it was localized to the ventricular surface of the epithelial cells by immunohistochemistry (43,44). Immunohistochemical studies in rat brain showed no staining of perikaryal cytoplasm but nerve cell bodies and dendrites in cerebral neocortex, hippocampus, hypothalamus, globus pallidus, and substantia nigra were stained superficially, apparently innvervated by nerve terminals containing ACE (44). The only consistently reactive structures in human autopsy brain were the choroid plexus, globus pallidus, and substantia nigra (44).

In addition to the immunohistochemical data, several lines of evidence indicate the probable localization of ACE on nerve terminal membranes. These include findings of high ACE activity in brain synaptosomes and neuroblastoma cell lines (but not glial cell lines), and the reduced ACE activity found in the substantia nigra after kainic acid injection into the ipsilateral striatum (31). The function of ACE in the brain remains unknown, but it may be involved in central blood pressure control and regulation of drinking by converting angiotensin I to II in the central nervous system (42). In brain areas containing ACE but not other components of the renin–angiotensin system, ACE could regulate the activity of other neuropeptides such as substance P, enkephalins, LH-RH, neurotensin, etc. (31; see section on Peptide Substrates of ACE).

III. PROPERTIES OF ACE

ACE has been found in all mammalian species tested. Based on physical properties, enzymatic characteristics, and immunologic cross-reactivity, ACE in different species is quite similar. In fact, when ACE was purified from the electric organ of *Torpedo marmorata* (45), it exhibited all the characteristics of mammalian ACE. It is chloride dependent; inhibited by captopril; cleaves angiotensin I, bradykinin, enkephalins, substance P, and synthetic ACE substrates; has a similar molecular weight; and cross-reacts with antibody to porcine renal ACE (45). Thus, ACE seems to be a well conserved enzyme. The following sections will focus on the properties of the human enzyme whenever possible.

A. Physical Properties

ACE purified from various human tissues is a single-chain polypeptide of M_r 140,000–150,000 as determined by sodium dodecyl sulfate (SDS)-polyacrylamide gel electrophoresis (38,46,47). The enzyme is membrane-bound, with a majority of the protein (including the active site) projecting into the extracellular space. Because it is tightly bound to membranes, it must be solubilized prior to purification, either with detergent (8,10) or by cleaving it from the membrane with trypsin

(38,46). Western blotting of the human enzyme showed that crude, detergent-extracted renal ACE has a slightly higher molecular weight (about 5000 daltons) than purified, trypsin-extracted renal ACE (31,48). This was taken as evidence for the removal of a small hydrophobic anchor peptide from ACE by trypsin. Later studies on porcine renal ACE showed the N-terminal sequences of detergent- and trypsin solubilized ACE to be identical, indicating that the hydrophobic anchor removed by trypsin was at the C-terminus (49). These data are consistent with the deduced amino acid sequence of human ACE (50; see below) and recent studies in which mutant recombinant ACE, truncated at the C-terminus, was not membrane-bound, but was secreted from the transfected cells in a freely soluble form (39).

ACE is heavily glycosylated, with the human renal enzyme containing about 24–28% carbohydrate by weight with a 1.6:3.0:4.5:4.4 ratio of fucose/mannose/N-acetylglucosamine/galactose (46). Based on immunologic studies, the protein portions of ACEs originating from endothelial, epithelial, or neuroepithelial cells are identical (8,25,26,28,38,44,51,52). There are differences, however, in the carbohydrate moieties. For example, human renal ACE has only traces of sialic acid while the human lung enzyme contains an average of 20 sialic acid residues per molecule (46). This is consistent with the hypothesis that the lung is the source of circulating ACE which, with a high sialic acid content, would be protected from uptake by liver lectins. Because of the sialic acid residues, the isoelectric focusing profile of the human lung ACE shows microheterogeneity with pI values ranging from 4.0 to 5.1 whereas human kidney ACE has only one major form at pI=5.2 (38). Another example of carbohydrate heterogeneity is found in pig brain (striatum), which contains two forms of ACE of M_r 180,000 and 170,000 (53). Deglycosylation reduces the size of both brain forms (as well as the M_r 180,000 kidney form) to the same molecular weight of 150,000 (53).

B. General Enzymatic Characteristics

The original studies on ACE by Skeggs and co-workers established its chloride dependence and metalloenzyme nature (6,7). Later studies on the purified enzyme confirmed those results and showed that ACE, like many other peptidases, contains 1 g atom of zinc per mole of enzyme (8). Thus, chelating agents and sulfhydryl compounds inhibit ACE by complexing the active site zinc.

The chloride dependence of ACE is a unique feature that varies with different substrates (8,54). One reason for the slow acceptance of the identity of ACE and kininase II was the fact that angiotensin I conversion is almost absolutely dependent on the presence of chloride ion, while bradykinin hydrolysis still proceeds in the absence of chloride ion at about 30–50% of the maximal rate (8,22,54). Detailed studies on rabbit lung ACE with a series of 26 furylacryloyl-tripeptides showed that anion activation of ACE depends on both the sequence of the substrate and the pH of the medium (55). The substrates tested fell into three classes. Class I substrates are relatively weak binding (K_m=160–4100 μM), show an absolute requirement for chloride, and have activation constants of 75–150 mM chloride ion. Class II substrates are tight binding (K_m=6.5–110 μM), have lower activation constants (2.9–5 mM chloride), and are hydrolyzed by a nonessential activator mechanism. Class III substrates have intermediate binding affinities (K_m=49–520 μM) and activation constants (18–30 mM chloride) and are cleaved by a complex nonessential activator mechanism. The pH dependence (pH 6–9) of the activation constants for chloride varied 60-fold for class I, 3-fold for class II, and 19-fold for class III substrates (55). Angiotensin I could thus be classified as a class I substrate while bradykinin would fit the description of a class II substrate. The mechanism of chloride activation of ACE is unkown but likely involves interaction of the anion with a lysine residue near the active center (54,56,57), which then causes a conformational change that facilitates substrate binding. Spectroscopic techniques have provided evidence of subtle conformational changes upon chloride binding to ACE (51,54). Based on in vitro studies, the in vivo concentration of chloride is sufficiently high to activate ACE fully, although in some tissues chloride ion concentrations may fluctuate enough to regulate ACE activity with some substrates. It is also possible that the membrane-bound enzyme in vivo has a different chloride ion sensitivity from the soublilized, purified enzyme used in the in vitro studies. Indeed, ACE immobilized on Sepharose 4B cleaves angiotensin I at an appreciable rate in the absence of chloride ion (20). Whether the chloride ion requirement is just a biochemical curiosity or has real physiological relevance remains unanswered.

Chemical modification studies have established the importance of at least four functional residues at or near the active site of ACE: tyrosine, arginine, glutamic acid, and lysine (56). Based on the zinc-binding residues determined for other well-studied metallopeptidases and the recently elucidated cDNA sequence of ACE (50), two histidines and a glutamic acid residue coordinate the zinc in ACE (see below). Using carboxypeptidase A as a model, it has been proposed that the active site arginine binds to the C-terminal carboxyl group of substrates, while the amine of the leaving group is protonated by a tyrosine residue (54,58; Fig. 2). Cleavage of the scissile amide bond is thought to involve the electrophilic effect of Zn^{++} and nucleophilic attack by the gamma-carboxylate group of the active site glutamic acid (54,58; Fig. 2).

As is expected for a plasma membrane-bound ectopeptidase, ACE has a pH optimum in the neutral range (pH 7–8). The activity falls off rapidly at acid pH due, in large part, to dissociation of Zn^{++} from the active center (59), likely caused by protonation of the Zn^{++} binding histidine residues. In the presence of added Zn^{++}, near maximal activity can be maintained down to about pH 5.5 (59). Replacement of the active site Zn^{++} with Co^{++} results in modest stimulation (20–60%) with some substrates, although it is inhibitory with others (54).

IV. PEPTIDE SUBSTRATES OF ACE

The hydrolysis of physiologically active peptides by ACE will be considered in this section. Much of the data come from in vitro studies with purified ACE. It must be remembered, however, that ACE functions in vivo mostly as a membrane-bound enzyme (with the exception of some biological fluids such as, blood, seminal plasma, and cerebrospinal fluid [CSF]) and the enzymatic properties demonstrated with purified enzyme in vitro may not all be operative under physiological conditions. For example, it has been observed that ACE bound to a solid support is less chloride dependent than the soluble enzyme (20,60,61). Nevertheless, a growing body of evidence indicates that ACE may be involved in the hydrolysis of a variety of peptides in vivo (see section on ACE Inhibitors).

Studies over the years have indicated that ACE is not specific for angiotensin I or bradykinin: it releases C-terminal dipeptides from a variety of synthetic and naturally occurring peptide substrates, providing they do not have a penultimate proline

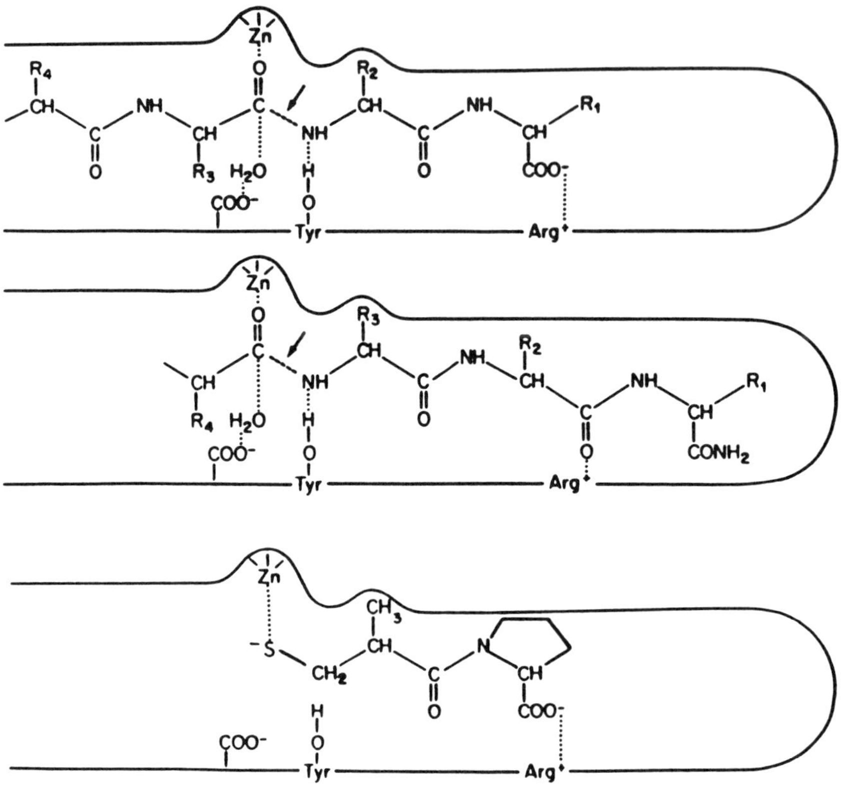

Figure 2 Model of the binding of substrates and inhibitors to the active site of ACE. Top. Binding of a substrate with a free C-terminal carboxyl group. Middle. Binding of a substrate with a blocked (amidated) C-terminal amino acid. Bottom. Binding of the inhibitor captopril. Arrow denotes the peptide bond cleaved. (Modified from Ref. 64; active site model based on data from Ref. 58.)

residue (8,18–20; Table 2). Until the early 1980s, it was thought that ACE only cleaved substrates containing a free carboxyl group on the C-terminal amino acid. Evidence that this is not the case was obtained by Hersh et al. (62), who reported that ACE could cleave peptides in which the last amino acid is replaced with nitrobenzylamine. Subsequent studies showed that ACE can cleave a C-terminal tripeptide from peptides with blocked C-terminal amino acids and even an N-terminal tripeptide (63). Thus, the substrate specificity of ACE is rather broad and raises the possibility that this ubiquitous enzyme regulates the activity of a variety of peptide hormones in vivo.

A. Angiotensin I and Bradykinin

Because they were the first active peptide substrates described, the hydrolysis of bradykinin and angiotensin I by homogeneous human and animal ACE has been studied extensively (8,20,22,38,54,63). It is well known that ACE converts the inactive angiotensin I to the active angiotensin II by removing the C-terminal dipeptide, His^9-Leu^{10} and that it inactivates bradykinin by cleaving off the C-terminal Phe^8-Arg^9 (Table 2). With purified human renal ACE, the turnover number of bradykinin and

Table 2 Peptide Substrates of ACE

Peptide	Amino Acid Sequence
Angiotensin I	Asp-Arg-Val-Tyr-Ile-His-Pro-Phe-His-Leu
Bradykinin	Arg-Pro-Pro-Gly-Phe-Ser-Pro-Phe-Arg
des-Arg^9-bradykinin	Arg-Pro-Pro-Gly-Phe-Ser-Pro-Phe
Opioid peptides	
Enkephalin	Tyr-Gly-Gly-Phe-Met/Leu
Heptapeptide	Tyr-Gly-Gly-Phe-Met-Arg-Phe
Octapeptide	Tyr-Gly-Gly-Phe-Met-Arg-Gly-Leu
β-Neo-endorphin	Tyr-Gly-Gly-Phe-Leu-Arg-Lys-Tyr-Pro
Dynorphin$_{1-8}$	Tyr-Gly-Gly-Phe-Leu-Arg-Arg-Ile
Dynorphin$_{1-6}$	Tyr-Gly-Gly-Phe-Leu-Arg
Neurotensin	<Glu-Leu-Tyr-Glu-Asn-Lys-Pro-Arg-Arg-Pro-Tyr-Ile-Leu
Chemotactic peptide	fMet-Leu-Phe
Substance P	Arg-Pro-Lys-Pro-Gln-Gln-Phe-Phe-Gly-Leu-Met-NH_2
LHRH	<Glu-His-Trp-Ser-Tyr-Gly-Leu-Arg-Pro-Gly-NH_2
CCK-8	Asp-Tyr(SO_3H)-Met-Gly-Trp-Met-Asp-Phe-NH_2
[Leu^{15}]Gastrin$_{11-17}$	Ala-Tyr-Gly-Trp-Leu-Asp-Phe-NH_2

Arrows denote primary (↑) and secondary (↑) sites of cleavage by ACE.

angiotensin I is the same ($k_{cat}=500\ min^{-1}$), but bradykinin has a higher affinity for ACE (8,22); thus, the specificity constant (k_{cat}/K_m) of bradykinin is higher than that of angiotensin I (38,64).

Because angiotensin II contains a penultimate proline (Pro^7-Phe^8), it is not cleaved further by ACE. Des-Arg^9-bradykinin, the product of bradykinin hydrolysis by carboxypeptidase N or kininase I (8,9), has the same C-terminal sequence, Pro^7-Phe^8, but, in contrast, ACE cleaves it. However, instead of removing the C-terminal dipeptide, it acts as a peptidyl tripeptidase to release the C-terminal Ser^6-Pro^7-Phe^8 (Table 2; 65).

B. Enkephalins and Related Opioid Peptides

The potential involvement of ACE in the metabolism of neuropeptides was suggested by the finding that ACE cleaves enkephalins (66). ACE purified from hog kidney or in intact human endothelial cells cleaves both Leu- and Met-enkephalin to release the C-terminal dipeptide (Table 2; 66). ACE purified from human lung or kidney gave similar results when enkephalins were used as substrates (38,67). The action of purified ACE on enkephalin was not due to a contaminant enzyme, since antibodies to ACE and the specific inhibitor enalaprilat both inhibited the reaction.

Kinetic studies with human ACE showed that Met-enkephalin has the highest turnover number (3500 min^{-1}) of any substrate tested (38). The K_m (1 mM) is also high; thus, the specificity constant (k_{cat}/K_m) would seem to be unfavorable for in vivo metabolism. However, the effect of membrane binding on the kinetics must be considered. Benuck and Marks (61) reported that with purified rat brain ACE bound to an immunoaffinity support, the K_m for Met-enkephalin was 100 μM, 10-fold lower than that with the solubilized, purified human ACE.

Enkephalin peptides extended at the C-terminus possess opioid activity and are also substrates for ACE. For example, ACE from bovine striatum (68) and rabbit brain or kidney (69) rapidly converts Met-enkephalin-Arg^6-Phe^7 to Met-enkephalin by cleaving the C-terminal Arg^6-Phe^7 (Table 2). Because Met-enkephalin-Arg^6-Phe^7 is a better substrate for ACE than Met-enkephalin (68,70), this metabolic route could be a way of generating Met-enkephalin. As an alternative, the conversion could be viewed as an inactivation step because the heptapeptide is more potent than Met-enkephalin in some tests.

Other opioid peptides can also be substrates for ACE (Table 2). Ulrich and Hersh (71) reported that β-neo-endorphin (Leu-enkephalin-Arg^6-Lys^7-Tyr^8-Pro^9) is cleaved by partially purified rat brain ACE or homogeneous human kidney ACE. High-performance liquid chromatographic (HPLC) analysis showed that ACE sequentially removes the dipeptides Tyr-Pro, Arg-Lys and Phe-Leu (Table 2). When one compares the relative affinities of these substrates for human ACE, β-neo-endorphin and Leu-enkephalin-Arg^6-Lys^7 have much higher affinities than Leu-enkephalin (71). α-Neo-endorphin (Leu-enkephalin-Arg^6-Lys^7-Tyr^8-Pro^9-Lys^{10}) is totally resistant to hydrolysis by ACE (71), because of the penultimate proline residue (18,19). Rat brain ACE cleaves $dynorphin_{1\text{-}8}$ (Leu-enkephalin-Arg^6-Arg^7-Ile^8), $dynorphin_{1\text{-}6}$, and Met-enkephalin-Arg^6-Gly^7-Leu^8 (Table 2) but not $dynorphin_{1\text{-}13}$ and $dynorphin_{1\text{-}17}$ (72), probably due to the large size of the peptides, as discussed below.

C. Neurotensin

It was shown many years ago that one of the factors that determines the rate of hydrolysis of peptide substrates by ACE is the length of the peptide chain (8). For example, Met^1-Lys^2-bradykinin, an undecapeptide, is hydrolyzed more slowly than kallidin (Lys^1-bradykinin) or bradykinin (8). Although ACE can cleave a dipeptide from the C-terminal end of the B chain of insulin, the reaction is very slow and the B chain is more of an inhibitor than a substrate of ACE (20). Human ACE cleaves neurotensin, a tridecapeptide, at Tyr^{11}-Ile^{12} (Table 2), releasing the C-terminal Ile^{12}-Leu^{13} (64). The remaining $neurotensin_{1\text{-}11}$ is not hydrolyzed because ACE does not hydrolyze the imide bond of proline (18,19). The rate of hydrolysis of neurotensin by human ACE is relatively slow (0.2 μmol/min/mg at a substrate concentration of 0.1 mM). This is likely due to the size of the substrate, since the C-terminal hexapeptide ($neurotensin_{8\text{-}13}$) was hydrolyzed 6.5 times faster than the tridecapeptide (64). Because of the slow rate of hydrolysis, it is questionable whether ACE metabolizes neurotensin in vivo. However, ACE activity could be important after neurotensin is initially cleaved by another enzyme(s). For instance, in studies of the degradation of neurotensin by rat brain synaptic membranes, conversion of neurotensin$_{1\text{-}13}$ to neurotensin$_{1\text{-}10}$ was followed by rapid conversion of neurotensin$_{1\text{-}10}$ to neurotensin$_{1\text{-}8}$ (73). The latter step was inhibited by a low concentration of captopril, indicating that it was due to the action of ACE.

D. Chemotactic Peptide fMet-Leu-Phe

The chemotactic peptide, fMet-Leu-Phe, is another active peptide substrate cleaved by ACE. This short protected tripeptide was cleaved by human ACE with a K_m of 82 μM and a turnover number (k_{cat}) of 270 min^{-1} (63). Because monocytes contain ACE, it may play a role in these cells of metabolizing chemotactic peptides. In addition, endothelial ACE might inactivate chemotactic peptides at sites of inflammation.

E. Substance P and Tachykinins

Reports that ACE inhibitors prevented the inactivation of substance P and that substance P inhibited the hydrolysis of other substrates by ACE were difficult to reconcile with the dogma that ACE only cleaves peptides with free carboxyl termini (31,63). It was thus concluded that these effects were not due to hydrolysis of substance P by ACE because this peptide has a blocked C-terminal amino acid (Met^{11}-NH_2) that should render it resistant to hydrolysis. In this light, the colocalization of ACE and substance P in the substantia nigra and globus pallidus was also puzzling (44,67). This mystery was solved when three different groups independently reported the hydrolysis of substance P by rat brain (74), rabbit lung (75), or human kidney (64) ACE.

Homogeneous human ACE cleaves substance P at Phe^8-Gly^9 and at Gly^9-Leu^{10}, to release either the C-terminal tri- or dipeptide (Table 2; 64). The release of the tripeptide is clearly favored by a ratio of 4:1. This unusual reaction was proven to be due to ACE and not to a trace contaminant in the preparation because chloride ion stimulated the hydrolysis and captopril inhibited it (64). After initial removal of the C-terminal di-or tripeptide, ACE sequentially cleaves dipeptides from the remaining N-terminal fragment. When, instead of the amidated peptide, substance P methyl ester (Met^{11}-OCH_3) was used as substrate, the major product of the initial cleavage was again the C-terminal tripeptide. While ACE can hydrolyze C-terminal amidated peptides, the form with a free C-terminus is still preferred. Thus, the free acid of substance P is hydrolyzed about seven times faster (at 0.1 mM concentration) than substance P and only the C-terminal dipeptide is released (64). Shorter C-terminal fragments of substance P (i.e., substance $P_{4\text{-}11}$, substance $P_{5\text{-}11}$, substance $P_{6\text{-}11}$) are also hydrolyzed by human ACE but the tetrapeptide, substance $P_{8\text{-}11}$, is not cleaved (64). When substance P and the free acid derivative were used as competitive inhibitors of furylacryloyl-Phe-Gly-Gly hydrolysis by human ACE, the K_i was 25 μM for substance P and 2 μM for the free acid. Thus, substance P free acid interacts more favorably with the active site than native amidated substance P. As discussed above, chemical modification studies indicated that the active site of ACE contains a positively charged arginine that is presumed to interact with the negatively charged carboxyl group of most substrates (Fig. 2; 56,58). To determine whether the hydrolysis of substance P (which lacks a free carboxyl group) requires a functional active site arginine, the arginine residues of ACE were blocked with cyclohexanedione or butanedione. After this chemical modification, the hydrolysis of bradykinin, benzoyl-Gly-Phe-Arg, or substance P was inhibited by 80–93% (64). This indicates that the active site arginine is required for hydrolysis of substrates with both free and blocked C-terminal amino acids. A hypothetical scheme has been proposed to explain these data (Fig. 2). In this model, the active site arginine interacts with the carbonyl oxygen of Leu^{10}, which, according to the proposed model of the active site (58), may allow the active site zinc to complex the carbonyl oxygen of Phe^{8}. This would result in the hydrolysis of the Phe^{8}-Gly^{9} bond and release of the C-terminal tripeptide (Fig. 2; 64). The small amount of dipeptide released may come from a similar interaction of the active site arginine with the carbonyl oxygen of Met^{11}-NH_2.

Independent studies using purified rat brain (74) or lung (76) ACE, or rabbit lung ACE (75) also demonstrated that the hydrolysis of substance P is due primarily to release of the C-terminal tripeptide. However, more recently, Strittmatter et al. (77) reported the isolation of a presumably unique ACE isozyme from rat striatum that differs in its specificity from rat lung ACE. They found that rat striatal ACE hydrolyzed substance P by preferential release of the C-terminal dipeptide over the tripeptide (ratio of 1.4:1), while the rat lung ACE gave results similar to those found by us and others. In contrast, Yokosawa et al. (74,76) found no difference between rat lung and rat brain ACE in the hydrolysis of substance P. Hooper and Turner (53) likewise reported identical patterns of substance P hydrolysis by purified pig striatal or kidney ACE. In the studies of the latter two groups (53,74,76), ACE from all sources released predominantly the C-terminal tripeptide from substance P, as found with the human enzyme (64).

Because substance P is a member of the tachykinin peptide family, which all have a common C-terminal sequence (-Phe-Xxx-Gly-Leu-Met-NH_2), it was logical to assume that ACE could cleave other tachykinins. However, the interaction of ACE with these substrates turned out to be more complex. Porcine renal or striatal ACE does not cleave neurokinin A (substance K; His-Lys-Thr-Asp-Ser-Phe-Val-Gly-Leu-Met-NH_2) or neurokinin B (neuromedin K; Asp-Met-His-Asp-Phe-Phe-Val-Gly-Leu-Met-NH_2), even with prolonged incubation (53). In contrast, Strittmatter et al. (77), reported that rat striatal ACE cleaves neurokinin A while rat lung ACE does not. The reason for this discrepancy is not apparent, but species differences may play a role. Preliminary evidence indicates that rat lung or striatal ACE can cleave physalaemin (76,77) but not eledoisin or kassinin (77).

The ability of ACE to cleave some tachykinins, but not others, is somewhat unexpected and may relate to the unusual binding of amidated peptides which allows the release of the C-terminal tripeptide (Fig. 2). In this case, the P_1 residue (the fourth amino acid from the C-terminus) may play a critical role in binding of the peptide to the active site of ACE. In this regard, it is of interest that tachykinins susceptible to ACE (substance P, physalaemin) have aromatic residues (Phe or Tyr, respectively) in the P_1 position while those resistant to ACE (neurokinin A, neurokinin B, eledoisin, kassinin) have an aliphatic hydrophobic amino acid (Val or Ile). Whether this explains the difference in susceptibility of tachykinins to ACE will require further experimentation.

F. Luteinizing Hormone-Releasing Hormone

The decapeptide luteinizing hormone-releasing hormone (LHRH) is another hormone with a blocked C-terminal amino acid (and a blocked NH_2-terminus as well) present in tissues containing ACE. It was thus tested as a substrate for human ACE. ACE quite unexpectedly cleaved LHRH in vitro by attack at both the N- and C-terminal ends to release several peptides (78). A major product was the N-terminal tripeptide, <Glu^1-His^2-Trp^3; another was $LHRH_{4\text{-}10}$ heptapeptide, suggesting that the Trp^3-Ser^4 bond is cleaved to release the NH_2-terminal tripeptide (Table 2). ACE also released the C-terminal tripeptide, Arg^8-Pro^9-Gly^{10}-NH_2, and then sequentially the dipeptides Gly^6-Leu^7 and Ser^4-Tyr^5, leaving <Glu^1-His^2-Trp^3 intact (Table 2). Thus, <Glu^1-His^2-Trp^3 is a product of both N- and C-terminal hydrolysis. The cleavage of LHRH was prevented by specific ACE inhibitors and by antibody to ACE but not by inhibitors of other enzymes, proving that the hydrolysis was not due to a contaminant (78). In the absence of chloride, the rate of hydrolysis was only 16% of the maximal rate (established in 500 mM NaCl), but it increased to 64% at a relatively low (10 mM) NaCl concentration (78). In 500 mM NaCl, 86% of the hydrolysis was due to the release of the N-terminal tripeptide, whereas in 10 mM NaCl, cleavage at the C- and N-terminus occurred about equally. In 500 mM NaCl, the K_m was 167 μM and the k_{cat} was 210 min^{-1} (78).

This very atypical pattern of hydrolysis of LHRH by ACE was later confirmed in studies using purified pig kidney or striatal ACE (53) or purified rat brain or mouse neuroblastoma cell ACE (79).

A location for enzymes that may inactivate LHRH is the median eminence (31). The major products of LHRH degradation in extracts of the rat median eminence are $LHRH_{1\text{-}5}$, $LHRH_{6\text{-}10}$, and <Glu^1-His^2-Trp^3 (80). The first two products result from cleavage of the bond between Tyr^5 and Gly^6 by the "LHRH endopeptidase," but the enzyme that releases <Glu-His-Trp was not identified. Since ACE was found in the median eminence (44), it might be responsible for the production of <Glu-His-Trp in this tissue.

G. Other Amidated Peptides

The ability of ACE to cleave amidated peptide substrates seems to be a general property of the enzyme, rather than just an exception, since it has recently been shown to cleave several other amidated peptides. This may indicate an important role for ACE: about half of all biologically active peptides contain a C-terminal amide (81).

Bunnett et al. (82) obtained evidence that ACE in membranes of the pig gastric corpus could cleave a gastrin-releasing peptide fragment, GRP10 (Gly-Asp-His-Trp-Ala-Val-Gly-His-Leu-Met-NH_2), representing the C-terminal sequence of GRP27, although they did not identify the peptide bonds cleaved.

Purified rabbit lung ACE was also reported to cleave other amidated gastric peptides: cholecystokinin-8 (CCK-8) and several gastrin analogs (Table 2; 83). However, the major initial cleavage product was the C-terminal dipeptide instead of the C-terminal tripeptide found with other amidated peptides (Table 2). The reason for this difference is not readily apparent although the penultimate aspartic acid residue in the gastric peptides may influence binding of the peptide to the active center. The K_m values for CCK-8 and [Leu[15]]gastrin-(11-17)-peptide were 115 and 420 μM and the k_{cat} values were 33 and 115 min^{-1} (83).

V. MOLECULAR CLONING AND SEQUENCING OF ACE

Very exciting new developments in studies on ACE came from investigations employing the tools of molecular biology to determine the sequence of the enzyme. This was a somewhat difficult task, given the relatively large size of the protein, but the unexpected and intriguing findings have proven the effort to be worthwhile.

A. Endothelial ACE

The first full-length cDNA sequence for ACE was determined by Soubrier et al., who cloned it from a human endothelial cell cDNA library (50). The nucleotide sequence of human ACE, obtained by sequencing three overlapping clones, comprises 4024 nucleotides with an open reading frame encoding 1306 amino acids (50). Based on the N-terminal protein sequence of the purified enzyme, the first 29 amino acids represent the signal peptide, yielding a calculated molecular weight for the mature enzyme of 146,600 daltons (50). As expected for the heavily glycosylated ACE, the enzyme contains 17 potential Asn-linked glycosylation sites (Fig. 3). In order to determine which region serves as the transmembrane anchor, hydropathic analysis of the deduced protein sequence was carried out and revealed two significantly hydrophobic regions: one at the N-terminus and one near the C-terminus (Fig. 3; 50). Because the N-terminal hydrophobic sequence represents the

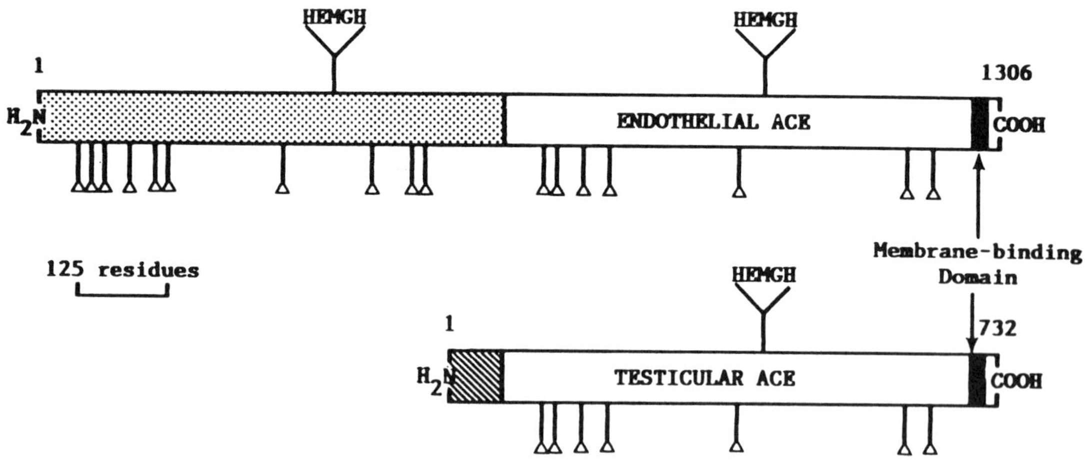

Figure 3 Schematic diagram of the primary structure of human endothelial and testicular ACE. The locations of the putative active sites are indicated by HEMGH, representing the amino acids His-Glu-Met-Gly-His. Potential sites for attachment of Asn-linked carbohydrate are marked with open triangles. Hydrophobic membrane spanning region is represented by the shaded box near the C-terminus. Sequences identical in the two forms of ACE are shown by the open rectangles whereas the domain unique to each form is indicated by either the stippled (endothelial ACE) or hatched (testicular ACE) region. (Based on data from Refs. 50 and 86.)

signal peptide, the C-terminal hydrophobic region is responsible for anchoring ACE to the plasma membrane, as proven in biochemical studies (49) and in recent experiments using recombinant DNA technology (39; see above).

The most striking feature of the sequence is the presence of two putative active centers located within two highly homologous domains (Fig. 3; 50). The sequence identity between positions 198-554 (nucleotides 700-1770) and 796-1152 (nucleotides 2495-3565) is 67.7% at the amino acid level and 70.1% at the nucleotide level (50). The maximal identity was found in the central portion of each domain surrounding the putative active site residues. Here, the identity at the amino acid level is 89% for amino acids 361-404 and 959-1002. Although the overall sequence is not similar to that of any known protein, there are short regions of sequence similarity to the zinc binding/active site domains of other metalloenzymes (Table 3). The sequence His-Glu-Met-Gly-His appears twice in human ACE (residues 361-365 and 959-963) and suggests the presence of two putative active centers in the enzyme (Table 3, Fig. 3). The full-length cDNA for mouse kidney ACE also contains two homologous domains and exhibits significant sequence identity (83% at both the DNA and amino acid level) with human endothelial ACE (84). The identity between mouse and human ACE is highest in the two homologous domains and lowest in the region joining the two domains. The mouse ACE sequence contains 15 potential Asn-linked glycosylation sites compared with the 17 found in the human enzyme (50,84).

The presence of two homologous domains making up the majority of the ACE molecule implies that the enzyme arose via gene duplication (50,85). The finding that testicular ACE contains only one of these domains and may represent the

Table 3 Comparison of the Sequence of Putative Active Site Residues in ACE with Those of Other Metalloenzymes.

Enzyme	Source	Sequence		
ACE	Human, mouse, rabbit	His Glu	Met Gly	His
Neutral endopeptidase 24.11	Human, rat, rabbit	His Glu	Ile Thr	His
Fibroblast collagenase	Human	His Glu	Leu Gly	His
Stromelysin	Human	His Glu	Ile Gly	His
Gelatinase	Human	His Glu	Phe Gly	His
Stromelysin, transin 1 and 2	Rat	His Glu	Leu Gly	His
Aminopeptidase N	Human	His Glu	Leu Ala	His
Digestive protease	Crayfish	His Glu	Leu Met	His
Thermolysin	*B. stearothermophilus*	His Glu	Leu Thr	His
Surface protease	*Leishmania* sp.	His Glu	Met Ala	His
Neutral protease	*B. subtilis*	His Glu	Met Thr	His
Neutral protease	*Serratia* sp.	His Glu	Ile Gly	His
Peptidase N	*E. coli*	His Glu	Tyr Phe	His

Identical amino acid residues are boxed. The sequence shown for ACE is identical in the two putative active site domains. Based on the x-ray crystal structure of thermolysin, the boxed Glu residue acts as a general base in catalysis and the two conserved His residues bind the zinc. The third zinc binding residue is a more distant glutamic acid C-terminal to the sequence shown above. It is located 20 amino acids away from the second His residue in thermolysin and 24 amino acids away in ACE (50).

Source: Data from Jongeneel CV, Bouvier J, Bairoch A. A unique signature identifies a family of zinc-dependent metallopeptidases. FEBS Lett 1989;242:211–4 and Refs. 50, 84–87.

ancestral form of the enzyme (see below) lends further support to this conclusion. Southern blot analysis of human genomic DNA (cleaved with Hind III) probed with a 300 base pair restriction fragment of the human ACE cDNA detected a single 9.5 kilobase band, consistent with the presence of a single gene for human ACE (50).

B. Testicular ACE

Earlier studies (36,54) that had demonstrated the presence of a unique form of ACE (at both the protein and mRNA level) in testicles were proven correct when testicular ACE was cloned and sequenced from human (86,87) or rabbit (88) testicular cDNA libraries. The open reading frame of the human testicular cDNA encodes a protein of 732 amino acids with a calculated molecular weight of 83 kDa, which is in good agreement with biochemical studies (86,87). The first 67 amino acids (containing a 31 residue signal peptide) are unique to the human testicular ACE but the last 665 amino acids (and the DNA sequence encoding this region) are identical with the C-terminal (or 3′) region of endothelial ACE (Fig. 3; 86,87). This region includes the second putative active center in endothelial ACE. Testicular ACE contains seven potential Asn-linked glycosylation sites (Fig. 3) and the N-terminal-specific sequence contains a high concentration of serine and threonine residues, which are possible sites for O-linked glycosylation (86).

C. Genomic Structure

Analysis of the genomic structure of human ACE revealed a single gene which spans 21 kilobases, made up of 26 exons ranging in size from 88 to 481 base pairs (88a). The larger (4.3 kb) endothelial type ACE mRNA [the exclusive type in all tissues (except testes) where ACE is synthesized] is transcribed from exon 1 to exon 26 except for exon 13 which is treated as an intron and spliced out (88a). The shorter, testicular ACE mRNA (3 kb) is transcribed from exon 13 (which codes for the unique 67 N-terminal amino acids of the testicular enzyme) through exon 26 (88a). In addition to these differences, the promoters and polyadenylation signals are unique for the endothelial and testicular forms of ACE. Whereas the promoter for the endothelial form is in the 5′ flanking region of exon 1, the testicular promoter is in intron 12 (88a) and the polyadenylation site for endothelial ACE is 628 bp downstream from that of the testicular form (88b).

D. Functional Significance of Two Active Sites in ACE

Whether both of the putative active sites are catalytically active cannot be determined from the sequence alone. Previous findings of one zinc atom per molecule of ACE (8,54) and binding studies with radiolabeled inhibitors (89,90) indicated that only one active site is functional. However, recent investigations reevaluating these properties have revealed the presence of two zinc and inhibitor binding sites per molecule, indicating there are two functional active sites (90a,90b). The most convincing data was obtained by Wei et al. (90c) who transfected mutant ACE cDNAs (either lacking one of the two domains, or containing point mutations of active site residues in one domain) into CHO cells, and found that both domains were independently active. The two domains have similar K_m values with substrates but the turnover number (k_{cat}) with the C-terminal domain is about 3–10 fold higher than with the N-terminal domain, depending on the substrate (90c). The N-terminal domain is less dependent on the presence of chloride, because maximal activity was obtained at 3 to 80-fold lower chloride concentration than the C-terminal domain (90c). These data are consistent with earlier work by Iwata, et al., (91) who isolated an M_r = 82,000 N-terminal fragment of rabbit ACE that had only 23% of the activity of the native enzyme and was much less dependent on chloride. Although the hydrolysis of many substrates (e.g., angiotensin I, bradykinin) by ACE is due predominantly to the C-terminal domain, the unusual release of the N-terminal tripeptide from LH-RH by ACE (78) depends almost exclusively on the presence of the N-terminal domain (90a). Differences between the two domains in inhibitor binding (90a, 90b), chloride sensitivity (90c) and substrate hydrolysis (90a,90c) indicate that each domain has unique structural characteristics that could play a role in determining their functions in vivo.

VI. ACE INHIBITORS

The development, design, and effects of ACE inhibitors have been the subject of numerous review articles (see, for example, 92–97) and the clinical use of ACE inhibitors is reviewed elsewhere in this volume. This section summarizes the putative effects of ACE inhibitors that are not necessarily due to inhibition of the peripheral renin–angiotensin system and points out aspects of inhibitor therapy that relate to some basic properties of ACE already discussed.

A. Background

Because ACE plays a central role in the activation of the vasoconstrictor angiotensin II and inactivation of the vasodilator bradykinin (Fig. 1), it seemed reasonable to assume that inhibitors of the enzyme would be effective antihypertensive agents. In early experiments, before the identity of ACE and kininase II was known, Erdös and Wohler (98) administered several compounds to guinea pigs with the idea of lowering blood pressure by inhibiting the degradation of bradykinin. Blood pressure reductions of 10–42% were achieved with a number of compounds, most containing a free sulfhydryl group, such as dimercaptopropanol (BAL), disulfiram (Antabuse), and penicillamine (98). Although the target of the inhibitors was not identified, based on current knowledge, and on the fact that guinea pigs have a very high concentration of plasma ACE (22), it was very likely this enzyme.

Many peptides and proteins were subsequently found to inhibit ACE, most notably peptides derived from snake venom containing C-terminal proline residues (92,93,99). However, these peptides had to be administered intravenously and they had very short half-lives. Thus, the search was begun for more stable enzyme inhibitors. Development of the first potent, orally active ACE inhibitor utilized the concept that carboxypeptidase A (whose structure was known) and ACE (whose structure was unknown) have similar active sites based on some similarities in enzymatic characteristics. The carboxypeptidase A inhibitor D-2-benzylsuccinic acid served as a model for the first synthetic inhibitor of ACE, succinyl-L-proline (92,93,95,96). Although we now know that carboxypeptidase A has no sequence similarity to ACE (50,85), the concept was useful because it led to the eventual development of the potent specific inhibitor captopril (92–94). The important features of captopril that allow it to bind with high affinity to ACE are 1. a C-terminal proline residue (based on the venom peptides), 2. a free C-terminal carboxyl group to interact with the active site arginine, 3. a zinc-binding sulfhydryl group, and 4. a side chain methyl group next to proline (Fig. 2; 92–94). More recently developed inhibitors (95,96) have either a zinc-binding carboxylic acid (e.g., enalaprilat) or a phosphinic acid group (e.g., fosinopril) in place of the sulfhydryl group.

B. Effects of ACE Inhibitors on Angiotensin II Formation

ACE inhibitors turned out to be very effective antihypertensive agents, not only in high-renin forms of hypertension, as would be expected, but in many other forms as well, especially in combination with diuretics (97). ACE inhibitors are also valuable in the treatment of congestive heart failure (100,101). Many of the beneficial effects of ACE inhibitors can be attributed to inhibition of the conversion of angiotensin I to angiotensin II, at least theoretically. However, in some cases it has been difficult to correlate long-term changes in blood pressure with persistent decreases in levels of circulating angiotensin II (102–104). This may be due to several factors, including the antibody employed in radioimmunoassays, which may cross-react with angiotensin I or angiotensin fragments (105), or the presence of another enzyme(s) that could convert angiotensin I to II (e.g., by carboxypeptidase action; 106–110) but is not inhibited by ACE inhibitors. In addition, circulating levels of angiotensin II may not reflect the activity of local renin–angiotensin systems, which may be more important.

Although measurement of plasma or serum ACE activity has been used as a convenient method for assessing the effectiveness of ACE inhibitors, this can result in misleading conclusions (111). ACE inhibitors are competitive and reversible, so when plasma or serum samples are diluted in the enzyme assay the inhibitor will also be diluted and be less effective. This could lead to the erroneous conclusion that ACE was not inhibited in vivo when it actually was. In addition, the original studies of Vane and co-workers (12,13) showed that plasma ACE is much less important in the conversion of angiotensin I to II than that taking place in the vascular beds of the lung and other tissues. "Tissue ACE" has recently been emphasized as the target of ACE inhibitors (112–114). Based on what we know about the major sites of ACE action (i.e., the endothelium of vessels in various tissues), ACE inhibitors must inhibit "tissue ACE" to be effective. Whether subendothelial (i.e., epithelial or neuroepithelial) ACE in various tissues is also an important component of "local" renin–angiotensin systems (and therefore an important target for ACE inhibitors) is less clear (112–114).

C. ACE Inhibitors and Kinins

Some of the antihypertensive effects of ACE inhibitors could be due to elevating the levels of vasodilator kinins. Both positive and negative results have been obtained when trying to correlate plasma kinin levels with decreases in blood pressure caused by ACE inhibitors (92–94,115,116). However, many confounding factors can make it difficult to determine precisely the contributions of kinins. These include difficulties in assaying plasma kinin levels, the stimulation of second messenger systems by kinins (e.g., prostaglandins, phospholipase C, endothelial-derived relaxing factor/nitric oxide), and the fact that kinins are synthesized and function mainly as local paracrine hormones and not as circulating hormones (117). In addition, many different enzymes can degrade kinins (8). Nevertheless, high-titer antibodies against kinins were able to block partially the antihypertensive effect of captopril in spontaneously hypertensive and two-kidney, one-clip renovascular hypertensive rats (118). The recently developed kinin receptor antagonists (119) have allowed more definitive determinations of the role of kinins in various physiological responses to ACE inhibitors. A few studies have shown that at least some of the antihypertensive effects of ACE inhibitors can be blocked by kinin receptor antagonists (117,120).

Much stronger evidence has been obtained for the involvement of kinins in the cardioprotective effects of ACE inhibitors in the ischemic myocardium (121–127). Whereas bradykinin has beneficial effects on myocardial flow and metablolism and decreases the incidence and duration of postischemic reperfusion arrhythmias, angiotensin I and II have the opposite effects (124,127). ACE inhibitors have the same actions as bradykinin (121–127) and bradykinin receptor antagonists block these effects (126,127). These data suggest that the cardioprotective effects of ACE inhibitors are due to enhancement of endogenous kinin levels. This may be relevant clinically as recent large-scale trials in patients with asymptomatic left ventricular dysfunction after myocardial infarction demonstrated that long term (up to 4 years) administration of ACE inhibitors is associated with a reduction in morbidity and mortality due to major cardiovascular events (127a,127b).

A rare but potentially serious side effect of ACE inhibitors is angio-edema, which may be associated with the protection of endogenous kinins in certain individuals (97,128).

D. ACE Inhibitors and Neuropeptides

The role of the brain renin–angiotensin system in various forms of hypertension has been the subject of many studies (42). Angiotensin II injected intracerebroventricularly (i.c.v.) is a potent dipsogen and it also triggers a pressor response (42). Angiotensin I injected i.c.v. mimics the effects of angiotensin II due to its conversion by ACE and the effects can be blocked by i.c.v. injections of ACE inhibitors (31,42). However, whether any of the effects of ACE inhibitors are due to inhibition of the central renin–angiotensin system is still controversial. There have been conflicting reports about the ability of ACE inhibitors to penetrate the central nervous system. Recent studies indicate that certain ACE inhibitors can cross the blood–brain barrier, but the most widely used drugs, captopril and enalapril, generally do not (114,129).

Because ACE is localized in the brain, it is tempting to speculate that it may be involved in the metabolism of neuropeptides such as the opioid enkephalins (31,66). Inhibition and kinetic studies suggest that in the CNS, aminopeptidases and endopeptidase 24.11 are more important in enkephalin metabolism than ACE (31). Nevertheless, ACE could be the in vivo inactivator of enkephalins in some locations. For example, in cerebrospinal fluid, ACE is the major enzyme hydrolyzing enkephalyl peptides (130). In another study, i.c.v. administration of captopril inhibited the metabolism and potentiated the analgesic action of Met-enkephalin (131).

In addition, i.c.v. injected captopril itself induced a rapid-onset, short-lasting analgesia that was blocked by prior administration of the opioid antagonist naltrexone (131). Another opioid peptide, Met-enkephalin-Arg^6-Phe^7, was eight times more potent than Met-enkephalin in producing analgesia in the mouse tail-flick test (132). ACE inhibitors potentiated the analgesic response to Met-enkephalin-Arg^6-Phe^7 (133) and blocked the conversion of the heptapeptide to Met-enkephalin in rat brain synaptosomes (134) and in rabbit plasma (135).

ACE may also be involved in the degradation of enkephalins peripherally. ACE inhibitors reduce enkephalin degradation in mouse vas deferens (136), guinea pig ileum (137), isolated perfused rat lungs (138), and they potentiate the vasodepressor action of Met-enkephalin in anesthetized rats (139).

Some interesting human studies have suggested that ACE inhibitors may have central actions involving opioid peptides (140). A double-blind clinical trial involving 626 men taking various antihypertensive medications showed a significant enhancement in the quality of life (a general feeling of well-being and an increase in life satisfaction index) in patients taking captopril (141). Although some have attributed this to relief from side effects of previously used antihypertensive drugs (97), other reports suggest that ACE inhibitors can have central effects. For example, captopril administration was associated with substantial mood elevation in depressed patients (142,143) and, in one patient, induced acute psychosis that was reversed by the opioid antagonist naloxone (144). ACE inhibitor therapy also brought about pronounced mental deterioration in a patient with Huntington's disease (145), a disorder in which the ACE concentration in certain brain regions is abnormally low (31). In other studies, a reduction in voluntary alcohol consumption in rats treated with ACE inhibitors points to the potential use of these drugs in the treatment of alcoholism (146,147). Whether these central effects of ACE inhibitors result from blocking the metabolism of opioid or other peptides in unknown. The relative lack of obvious central side effects in most patients might be due to the relative inaccessibility of the CNS to captopril or enalapril (114,129). The few individuals who do exhibit side effects involving the CNS might have a compromised blood–brain barrier. It will be interesting to see if these central effects become more prominent with the use of lipophilic ACE inhibitors that can more easily distribute into the brain.

Although ACE is localized in brain areas containing high concentrations of substance P, there is so far no evidence for the involvement of CNS ACE in the metabolism of substance P *in vivo*. However, ACE can participate in the metabolism of substance P peripherally. In the rat, ACE inhibitors potentiated the sialogogue action of intravenous (i.v.) substance P (75), increased the renal clearance of endogenous substance P fourfold (120), and partially blocked the metabolism of both neurotensin and substance P in the stomach wall in vivo (148). In the guinea pig, captopril considerably enhanced the recovery of injected substance P and potentiated the bronchoconstrictor effects of substance P in lung (149). This last study is interesting since one of the class-specific side effects of ACE inhibitors is a persistent dry cough (97,150), especially in patients who exhibit bronchial hyperreactivity (151,152). Because substance P and bradykinin are both stimulators of the cough response, the protection of one or both of these peptides by ACE inhibition may be responsible for this side effect.

VII. CONCLUSION

It should be clear from this review that ACE has a much wider distribution and a broader substrate specificity than originally thought. Although great strides have been made in understanding the structure and functions of this important enzyme, many questions still remain (153). We are only beginning to explore the possible functions of the enzyme beyond the conversion of angiotensin I to II or bradykinin inactivation. Even its physiological role in the metabolism of these well-studied peptides is not completely understood, especially outside of the vasculature. In addition, the functions of ACE in the central nervous system and male genital tract remain to be explored. Many interesting questions are raised by the presence of two active sites in ACE and by the testicular ACE isozyme, which represents a nonduplicated, ancestral form of the enzyme. Future studies utilizing ACE inhibitors and specific peptide antagonists, as well as investigations employing the tools of molecular biology, hold the promise of answering many of these provocative questions.

REFERENCES

1. Skeggs LT, Dorer FE, Kahn JR, Lentz KE, Levine M. Experimental renal hypertension: the discovery of the renin–angiotensin system. In: Soffer RL, ed. Biochemical regulation of blood pressure. New York: John Wiley & Sons, 1981: 3–38.
2. Braun-Menendez E, Fasciolo JC, Leloir LF, Munoz JM. The substance causing renal hypertension. J Physiol (London) 1940;98:283–98.
3. Page IH, Helmer OM. Angiotonin-activator, renin- and angiotonin-inhibitor and the mechanism of angiotonin tachyphylaxis in normal, hypertensive and nephrectomized animals. J Exp Med 1940;71:485–519.
4. Braun-Menendez E, Page IH. Suggested revision of nomenclature–angiotensin. Science 1958;127:242.
5. Lentz KE, Skeggs LT, Woods KR, Kahn JR, Shumway NP. Amino acid composition of hypertensin II and its biochemical relationship to hypertensin I. J Exp Med 1956;104:183–91.
6. Skeggs LT, Marsh WH, Kahn JR, Shumway NP. Existence of two forms of hypertensin. J Exp Med 1954;99:275–82.
7. Skeggs LT, Kahn JR, Shumway NP. Preparation and function of the hypertensin-converting enzyme. J Exp Med 1956;103:295–99.
8. Erdös EG: Kininases. In: Erdös EG, ed. Bradykinin, kallidin and kallikrein; Handbook of experimental pharmacology. Heidelberg: Springer-Verlag, 1979: 427–87.
9. Erdös EG, Sloane EM. An enzyme in human blood plasma that inactivates bradykinin and kallidins. Biochem Pharmacol 1962;11:39–43.
10. Erdös EG, Yang HYT. An enzyme in microsomal fraction of kidney that inactivates bradykinin. Life Sci 1967;6:569–74.
11. Yang HYT, Erdös EG. Second kininase in human blood plasma. Nature 1967;215: 1402–3.
12. Ng KKF, Vane JR. Conversion of angiotensin I to angiotensin II. Nature 1967;216:762–6.
13. Ng KKF, Vane JR. Fate of angiotensin I in the circulation. Nature 1968;218:144–50.
14. Vane JR. The release and fate of vaso-active hormones in the circulation. Br J Pharmacol 1969;35:209–42.
15. Bakhle YS. Conversion of angiotensin I to angiotensin II by cell-free extracts of dog lung. Nature 1968;220:919–20.

16. Freer RJ, Stewart JM. In vivo pulmonary metabolism of bradykinin, angiotensin I and 5-hydroxytryptamine in the rat. Arch Int Pharmacodyn 1975;217:97–109.
17. Scholz HW, Biron P. Non-identity between pulmonary bradykininase and converting-enzyme activity. Rev Can Biol 1969;28:197–200.
18. Yang HYT, Erdös EG, Levin Y. A dipeptidyl carboxypeptidase that converts angiotensin I and inactivates bradykinin. Biochim Biophys Acta 1970;214:374–76.
19. Yang HYT, Erdös EG, Levin Y. Characterization of a dipeptide hydrolase (kininase II; angiotensin I converting enzyme). J Pharmacol Exp Ther 1971;117:291–300.
20. Igic R, Erdös EG, Yeh HSJ, Sorrells K, Nakajima T. Angiotensin I converting enzyme of the lung. Circ Res 1972;31(suppl II):II-51–61.
21. Cushman DW, Cheung HS. Concentrations of angiotensin-converting enzyme in tissues of the rat. Biochim Biophys Acta 1971;250:261–5.
22. Erdös EG. Angiotensin I converting enzyme. Circ Res 1975;36:247–55.
23. Ryan US, Ryan JW, Whitaker C, Chiu A: Localization of angiotensin converting enzyme (kininase II). II. Immunocytochemistry and immunofluorescence. Tissue Cell 1976;8:125–45.
24. Johnson AR, Erdös EG. Metabolism of vasoactive peptides by human endothelial cells in culture: angiotensin I converting enzyme (kininase II) and angiotensinase. J Clin Invest 1977;59:684–95.
25. Erdös EG, Skidgel RA. Structure and functions of human angiotensin I converting enzyme (kininase II). Biochem Soc Trans 1985;13:42–4.
26. Erdös EG, Skidgel RA. Editorial: the angiotensin I converting enzyme. Lab Invest 1987;56:345–8.
27. Ward PE, Schulz W, Reynolds RC, Erdös EG. Metabolism of kinins and angiotensins in the isolated glomerulus and brush border of rat kidney. Lab Invest 1977; 36:599–606.
28. Skidgel RA, Schulz WW, Tam L-T, Erdös EG. Human renal angiotensin I converting enzyme and neutral endopeptidase. Kidney Int 1987;31(suppl. 20):S45–8.
29. Ward PE, Sheridan MA, Hammon KJ, Erdös EG. Angiotensin I converting enzyme (kininase II) of the brush border of human and swine intestine. Biochem Pharmacol 1980;29:1525–9.
30. Igic R, Robinson CJG, Erdös EG. Angiotensin I converting enzyme activity in the choroid plexus and in the retina. In: Buckley JP, Ferrario CM, eds. Central actions of angiotensin and related hormones. New York: Pergamon Press, 1977, 23–7.
31. Skidgel RA, Defendini R, Erdös EG. Angiotensin I converting enzyme and its role in neuropeptide metabolism. In: Turner AJ, ed. Neuropeptides and their peptidases. Chichester: Ellis-Horwood, 1987: 165–82.
32. Johnson AR, Skidgel RA, Gafford JT, Erdös EG. Enzymes in placental microvilli: angiotensin I converting enzyme, angiotensinase A, carboxypeptidase, and neutral endopeptidase ("enkephalinase"). Peptides 1984;5:789–96.
33. Yokohama M, Hiwada K, Kokubu T, Takada M, Takeuchi M. Angiotensin-converting enzyme in human prostate. Clin Chim Acta 1980;100:253–8.
34. Hohlbrugger GH, Schweisfurth H, Dahlheim H. Angiotensin I converting enzyme in rat testis, epididymis and vas deferens under different conditions. J Reprod Fertil 1982;65:97–103.
35. Erdös EG, Schulz WW, Gafford JT, Defendini R. Neutral metalloendopeptidase in human male genital tract. Comparison to angiotensin I-converting enzyme. Lab Invest 1985;52:437–47.
36. El-Dorry HA, Pickett CB, MacGregor JS, Soffer RL. Tissue-specific expression of mRNAs for dipeptidyl carboxypeptidase isoenzymes. Proc Natl Acad Sci USA 1982;79: 4295–7.
37. El-Dorry HA, MacGregor JS, Soffer RL. Dipeptidyl carboxypeptidase from seminal

fluid resembles the pulmonary rather than the testicular isoenzyme. Biochem Biophys Res Commun 1983;115:1096–100.
38. Stewart TA, Weare JA, Erdös EG. Purification and characterization of human converting enzyme (kininase II). Peptides 1981;2:145–52.
39. Wei L, Alhenc-Gelas F, Soubrier F, Michaud A, Corvol P, Clauser E. Expression and characterization of recombinant human angiotensin I-converting enzyme. J Biol Chem 1991;266:5540–6.
40. Yang HYT, Neff NH. Distribution and properties of angiotensin converting enzyme of rat brain. J Neurochem 1972;19:2443–50.
41. Poth MM, Heath RG, Ward M. Angiotensin-converting enzyme in human brain. J Neurochem 1975;25:83–5.
42. Ganten D, Printz MP, Phillips MI, Schölkens BA (eds). The renin angiotensin system in the brain. Heidelberg: Springer-Verlag, 1982.
43. Rix E, Ganten D, Schüll B, Unger T, Taugner R. Converting-enzyme in the choroid plexus, brain, and kidney: Immunocytochemical and biochemical studies in rats. Neurosci Lett 1981;22:125–30.
44. Defendini R, Zimmerman EA, Weare JA, Alhenc-Gelas F, Erdös EG. Angiotensin-converting enzyme in epithelial and neuroepithelial cells. Neuroendocrinology 1983; 37:32–40.
45. Turner AJ, Hryszko J, Hooper NM, Dowdall MJ. Purification and characterization of a peptidyl dipeptidase resembling angiotensin converting enzyme from the electric organ of Torpedo marmorata. J Neurochem 1987;48:910–6.
46. Weare JA, Gafford JT, Lu HS, Erdös EG. Purification of human kidney angiotensin I converting enzyme using reverse immunoadsorption chromatography. Anal Biochem 1982;123:310–9.
47. Lanzillo JJ, Stevens J, Dasarathy Y, Yotsumoto H, Fanburg B. Angiotensin-converting enzyme from human tissues. Physicochemical, catalytic and immunological properties. J Biol Chem 1985;260:14938–44.
48. Erdös EG, Gafford JT. Human converting enzyme. Clin Exp Hypertension 1983; A5:1251–62.
49. Hooper NM, Keen J, Pappin JC, Turner AJ. Pig kidney angiotensin converting enzyme. Purification and characterization of amphipathic and hydrophilic forms of the enzyme establishes C-terminal anchorage to the plasma membrane. Biochem J 1987; 247:85–93.
50. Soubrier F, Alhenc-Gelas F, Hubert C, Allegrini J, John M, Tregear G, Corvol P. Two putative active centers in human angiotensin I-converting enzyme revealed by molecular cloning. Proc Natl Acad Sci USA 1988;85:9386–90.
51. Oshima G, Gecse A, Erdös EG. Angiotensin I converting enzyme of the kidney cortex. Biochem Biophys Acta 1974;350:26–37.
52. Alhenc-Gelas F, Weare J, Johnson RL Jr, Erdös EG. Measurement of human converting enzyme level by direct radioimmunoassay. J Lab Clin Med 1983;101:83–96.
53. Hooper NM, Turner AJ. Isolation of two differentially glycosylated forms of peptidyl-dipeptidase A (angiotensin converting enzyme) from pig brain: a re-evaluation of their role in neuropeptide metabolism. Biochem J 1987;241:625–33.
54. Ehlers MRW, Riordan JF. Angiotensin-converting enzyme. Biochemistry and molecular biology. In: Laragh JH, Brenner BM, eds. Hypertension: pathophysiology, diagnosis and management. New York: Raven Press, 1990: 1217–31.
55. Shapiro R, Holmquist B, Riordan JF. Anion activation of angiotensin converting enzyme: dependence on nature of substrate. Biochemistry 1983;22:3850–7.
56. Bünning P, Holmquist B, Riordan JF. Functional residues at the active site of angiotensin converting enzyme. Biochem Biophys Res Commun 1978;83:1442–9.
57. Weare JA. Activation/inactivation of human angiotensin I converting enzyme following

chemical modifications of amino groups near the active site. Biochem Biophys Res Commun 1982;104:1319–26.
58. Bünning P, Holmquist B, Riordan JF. Characterization of the active site of angiotensin converting enzyme. In: Holzer H, Tschesche H, eds. Biological functions of proteinases. Heidelberg: Springer-Verlag, 1979: 269–75.
59. Bünning P, Holmquist B, Riordan JF. Substrate specificity and kinetic characteristics of angiotensin converting enzyme. Biochemistry 1983;22:103–10.
60. Igic R, Nakajima T, Yeh HSJ, Sorrells K, Erdös EG. Kininases. In: Acheson G, ed. Pharmacology and the future of man, vol 5. Proceedings of the 5th International Congress of Pharmacology. Basel: Karger, 1972: 307–19.
61. Benuck M, Marks N. Co-identity of brain angiotensin converting enzyme with a membrane bound dipeptidyl carboxypeptidase inactivating Met-enkephalin. Biochem Biophys Res Commun 1979;88:215–21.
62. Hersh LB, Gafford JT, Powers JC, Tanaka T, Erdös EG. Novel substrates for angiotensin I converting enzyme. Biochem Biophys Res Commun 1983;110:654–9.
63. Skidgel RA, Erdös EG. The broad substrate specificity of human angiotensin I converting enzyme. Clin Exp Hypertension 1987;A9:243–59.
64. Skidgel RA, Engelbrecht S, Johnson AR, Erdös EG. Hydrolysis of substance P and neurotensin by converting enzyme and neutral endopeptidase. Peptides 1984;5:769–76.
65. Inokuchi J-I, Nagamatsu A. Tripeptidyl carboxypeptidase activity of kininase II (Angiotensin-converting enzyme). Biochim Biophys Acta 1981;662:300–7.
66. Erdös EG, Johnson AR, Boyden NT. Hydrolysis of enkephalin by cultured human endothelial cells and by purified peptidyl dipeptidase. Biochem Pharmacol 1978;27:843–8.
67. Defendini R, Zimmerman EA, Weare JA, Alhenc-Gelas F, Erdös EG. Hydrolysis of enkephalins by human converting enzyme and localization of the enzyme in neuronal components of the brain. In: Costa E, Trabucchi M, eds. Regulatory peptides: from molecular biology to function. New York: Raven Press, 1982:271–80.
68. Yang HYT, Majane E, Costa E. Conversion of [Met^5]-enkephalin-Arg^6-Phe^7 to [Met^5]-enkephalin by dipeptidyl carboxypeptidase. Neuropharmacology 1981;20:891–4.
69. Benuck M, Berg MJ, Marks N. Met-enkephalin-Arg^6-Phe^7 metabolism: conversion to Met-enkephalin by brain and kidney dipeptidyl carboxypeptidases. Biochem Biophys Res Commun 1981;99:630–6.
70. Benuck M, Berg MJ, Marks N. Separate metabolic pathways for Leu-enkephalin and Met-enkephalin-Arg^6-Phe^7 degradation by rat striatal synaptosomal membranes. Neurochem Int 1982;4:389–96.
71. Ulrich C, Hersh LB. Degradation of α and β neo-endorphin by rat brain membrane peptidases. Peptides 1985;6:475–82.
72. Benuck M, Berg MJ, Marks N. Membrane-bound enzymes and their role in processing of the dynorphins and of the proenkephalin octapeptide Met-enkephalin-Arg-Gly-Leu. Neurochem Res 1984;9:733–49.
73. Checler F, Vincent J-P, Kitabgi P. Degradation of neurotensin by rat brain synaptic membranes: involvement of a thermolysin-like metalloendopeptidase (enkephalinase), angiotensin-converting enzyme, and other unidentified peptidases. J Neurochem 1983; 41:375–84.
74. Yokosawa H, Endo S, Ogura Y, Ishii S. A new feature of angiotensin-converting enzyme in the brain: hydrolysis of substance P. Biochem Biophys Res Commun 1983;116:735–42.
75. Cascieri MA, Bull HG, Mumford RA, Patchett AA, Thornberry NA, Liang T. Tripeptidyl carboxyl-terminal hydrolysis of substance P by purified rabbit lung angiotensin-converting enzyme and the potentiation of substance P activity *in vivo* by captopril and MK-422. Mol Pharmacol 1984;25:287–93.

76. Yokosawa H, Endo S, Ohgaki Y, Maeyama J, Ishii S. Hydrolysis of substance P and its analogs by angiotensin-converting enzyme from rat lung. Characterization of endopeptidase activity of the enzyme. J Biochem 1985;98:1293–9.
77. Strittmatter SM, Thiele EA, Kapiloff MS, Snyder SH. A rat brain isozyme of angiotensin-converting enzyme. Unique specificity for amidated peptide substrates. J Biol Chem 1985;260:9825–32.
78. Skidgel RA, Erdös EG. Novel activity of human angiotensin I converting enzyme: release of the N- and C-terminal tripeptides from the luteinizing hormone-releasing hormone. Proc Natl Acad Sci USA 1985;82:1025–9.
79. Yokosawa H, Fujii Y, Ishii S. Degradation of luteinizing hormone-releasing hormone by neuroblastoma cells and their membrane: evidence for the involvement of a thiol protease and angiotensin-converting enzyme. J Neurochem 1987;48:293–8.
80. Advis JP, Krause JE, McKelvy JF. Luteinizing hormone-releasing hormone peptidase activities in the female rat: characterization by an assay based on high-performance liquid chromatography. Anal Biochem 1982;125:41–9.
81. Fisher JM, Scheller RH. Prohormone processing and the secretory pathway. J Biol Chem 1988;263:16515–8.
82. Bunnett NW, Kobayashi R, Orloff MS, Reeve JR, Turner AJ, Walsh JH. Catabolism of gastrin releasing peptide and substance P by gastric membrane-bound peptidases. Peptides 1985;6:277–83.
83. Dubreuil P, Fulcrand P, Rodriguez M, Fulcrand H, Laur J, Martinez J. Novel activity of angiotensin-converting enzyme. Hydrolysis of cholecystokinin and gastrin analogues with release of the amidated C-terminal dipeptide. Biochem J 1989;262:125–30.
84. Bernstein KE, Martin BM, Edwards AS, Bernstein EA. Mouse angiotensin-converting enzyme is a protein composed of two homologous domains. J Biol Chem 1989;264: 11945–51.
85. Alhenc-Gelas F, Soubrier F, Hubert C, Allegrini J, Lattion AL, Corvol P. The angiotensin I-converting enzyme (kininase II): Progress in molecular and genetic structure. J Cardiovasc Pharmacol 1990;15(suppl. 6):S25–9.
86. Lattion A-L, Soubrier F, Allegrini J, Hubert C, Corvol P, Alhenc-Gelas F. The testicular transcript of the angiotensin I-converting enzyme encodes for the ancestral, non-duplicated form of the enzyme. FEBS Lett 1989;252:99–104.
87. Ehlers MRW, Fox EA, Strydom DJ, Riordan JF. Molecular cloning of human testicular angiotensin-converting enzyme: the testis isozyme is identical to the C-terminal half of endothelial angiotensin-converting enzyme. Proc Natl Acad Sci USA 1989;86:7741–5.
88. Kuman RS, Kusari J, Roy SN, Soffer RL, Sen GC. Structure of testicular angiotensin-converting enzyme. A segmental mosaic enzyme. J Biol Chem 1989;264:16754–8.
88a. Hubert C, Houot A-M, Corvol P, Soubrier F. Structure of the angiotensin I-converting enzyme gene. Two alternate promoters correspond to evolutionary steps of a duplicated gene. J Biol Chem 1991;266:15377–83.
88b. Thekkumkara TJ, Livingston W, Kumar RS, Sen GC. Use of alternative polyadenylation sites for tissue-specific transcription of two angiotensin-converting enzyme mRNAs. Nucl Acids Res 1992;20:683–7.
89. Cumin F, Vellaud V, Corvol P, Alhenc-Gelas F. Evidence for a single active site in the human angiotensin I-converting enzyme from inhibitor binding studies with [^{3}H]RU 44 403: Role of chloride. Biochem Biophys Res Commun 1989;163:718–25.
90. Strittmatter SM, Snyder SH. Characterization of angiotensin converting enzyme by [^{3}H]captopril binding. Mol Pharmacol 1986;29:142–8.
90a. Ehlers MRW, Riordan JF. Angiotensin-converting enzyme: zinc- and inhibitor-binding stoichiometries of the somatic and testis isozymes. Biochemistry 1991;30: 7118–26.

90b. Wei L, Clauser E, Alhenc-Gelas F, Corvol P. The two homologous domains of human angiotensin I-converting enzyme interact differently with competitive inhibitors. J Biol Chem 1992;267:13398–405.
90c. Wei L, Alhenc-Gelas F, Corvol P, Clauser E. The two homologous domains of human angiotensin I-converting enzyme are both catalytically active. J Biol Chem 1991;266:9002-8.
91. Iwata K, Blacher R, Soffer RL, Lai C-Y. Rabbit pulmonary angiotensin-converting enzyme: the NH_2-terminal fragment with enzymatic activity and its formation from the native enzyme by NH_4OH treatment. Arch Biochem Biophys 1983;227:188–201.
92. Cushman DW, Ondetti MA. Inhibitors of angiotensin converting enzyme. Prog Med Chem 1980;17:42–104.
93. Ondetti MA, Cushman DW. Angiotensin-converting enzyme inhibitors: biochemical properties and biological actions. Crit Rev Biochem 1984;16:381–411.
94. Antonaccio MJ. Angiotensin converting enzyme (ACE) inhibitors. Annu Rev Pharmacol Toxicol 1982;22:57–87.
95. Wyvratt MJ, Patchett AA. Recent developments in the design of angiotensin-converting enzyme inhibitors. Med Res Rev 1985;5:483–531.
96. Thorsett ED, Wyvratt MJ. Inhibition of zinc peptidases that hydrolyse neuropeptides. In Turner AJ, ed. Neuropeptides and their peptidases. Chichester: Ellis-Horwood, 1987: 229–95.
97. Gavras I, Gavras H. The use of ACE inhibitors in hypertension. In: Kostis JB, DeFelice EA, eds. Angiotensin converting enzyme inhibitors. New York: Alan R. Liss, 1987: 93–122.
98. Erdös EG, Wohler JR. Inhibition *in vivo* of the enzymatic inactivation of bradykinin and kallidin. Biochem Pharmacol 1963;12:1193–9.
99. Ferreira SH. A bradykinin-potentiating factor (BPF) present in the venom of *Bothrops jararaca*. Br J Pharmacol 1965;24:163–9.
100. Davis R, Ribner HS, Keung E, Sonnenblick EH, LeJemtel T. Treatment of chronic congestive heart failure with captopril, an oral inhibitor of angiotensin-converting enzyme. N Engl J Med 1979; 301:117–21.
101. Cody RJ, Covit AB, Schaer GL, Laragh JH. Evaluation of a long-acting enzyme inhibitor (enalapril) for the treatment of chronic congestive heart failure. J Am Coll Cardiol 1983;1:1154–9.
102. Boillaz J, Brunner H, Gavras I, Waeber B, Gavras H. Antihypertensive therapy with MK421: angiotensin II-renin relationships to evaluate efficacy of converting enzyme blockade. J Cardiovasc Pharmacol 1982;4:966–72.
103. Wilkes BM. Evidence for a vasodepressor effect of the angiotensin-converting enzyme inhibitor, MK421 (enalapril), independent of blockade of angiotensin II formation. J Cardiovasc Pharmacol 1984;6:1036–42.
104. Mento PF, Wilkes BM. Plasma angiotensins and blood pressure during converting enzyme inhibition. Hypertension 1987;9(suppl. III):III-42–8.
105. Brunner HR, Nussberger J, Waeber B. Effects of angiotensin converting enzyme inhibition: a clinical point of view. J Cardiovasc Pharmacol 1985; 7(Suppl. 4):S73–81.
106. Snyder RA, Watt KWK, Wintroub BU. A human platelet angiotensin I-processing system: identification of components and inhibition of angiotensin-converting enzyme by product. J Biol Chem 1985;260:7857–60.
107. Miller JJ, Changaris DG, Levy RS. Conversion of angiotensin I to angiotensin II by cathepsin A isoenzymes of porcine kidney. Biochem Biophys Res Commun 1988;154: 1122–9.
108. Drummer OH, Kourtis S, Johnson H. Formation of angiotensin II and other angiotensin peptides from des-Leu 10-angiotensin I in rat lung and kidney. Biochem Pharmacol 1988;37:4327–33.

109. Okunishi H, Miyazaki M, Noboru T. Evidence for a putatively new angiotensin II-generating enzyme in the vascular wall. J Hypertension 1984;2:277–84.
110. Jackman HL, Tan F, Tamei H, Beurling-Harbury C, Li X-Y, Skidgel RA, Erdös EG. A peptidase in human platelets that deamidates tachykinins: Probable identity with the lysosomal "protective protein." J Biol Chem 1990;265:11265–72.
111. Erdös EG. Evolution of concepts and use of converting enzyme inhibitors. In: Mechanisms of action of antihypertensive drugs. Rahway: Merck, Sharp and Dohme, 1983: 121–9.
112. Unger T, Ganten D, Lang RE, Schölkens BA. Is tissue converting enzyme inhibition a determinant of the antihypertensive efficacy of converting enzyme inhibitors? Studies with the two different compounds Hoe498 and MK421, in spontaneously hypertensive rats. J Cardiovasc Pharmacol 1984;6:872–80.
113. Unger T, Ganten D, Lang RE. Effect of converting enzyme inhibitors on tissue converting enzyme and angiotensin II: therapeutic implications. Am J Cardiol 1987;59:18–22D.
114. Cushman DW, Wang FL, Fung WC, Harvey CM, DeForrest JM. Differentiation of angiotensin-converting enzyme (ACE) inhibitors by their selective inhibition of ACE in physiologically important target organs. Am J Hypertension 1989;2:294–306.
115. Odya CE, Wilgis FP, Walker JF, Oparil S. Immunoreactive bradykinin and [des-Arg^9]-bradykinin in low-renin essential hypertension—before and after treatment with enalapril (MK421). J Lab Clin Med 1983;102:714–21.
116. Iimura O, Shimamoto K. Role of kallikrein–kinin system in the hypotensive mechanisms of converting enzyme inhibitors in essential hypertension. J Cardiovasc Pharmacol 1989;13(Suppl.3):S63–6.
117. Carretero OA, Scicli AG: Kinins paracrine hormone. In: Fritz H, Schmidt I, Dietze G, eds. The Kallikrein–kinin system in health and disease. Munich: Limbach, Druch-and Verlagshaus Braunschweig, 1989: 63–78.
118. Carretero OA, Miyazaki S, Scicli AG. Role of kinins in the acute antihypertensive effect of the converting enzyme inhibitor, captopril. Hypertension 1981;3:18–22.
119. Stewart JM, Vavrek RJ. Kinin antagonists: design and activities. J Cardiovasc Pharmacol 1990;15(suppl. 6):S69–74.
120. Kramer HJ, Glänzer K, Meyer-Lehnert H, Mohaupt M, Predel HG. Kinin- and non-kinin-mediated interactions of converting enzyme inhibitors with vasoactive hormones. J Cardiovasc Pharmacol 1990;15(suppl. 6):S91–8.
121. Ertl G, Kloner RA, Alexander RW, Braunwald E. Limitation of experimental infarct size by an angiotensin-converting enzyme inhibitor. Circulation 1982; 65:40–8.
122. Hock CE, Ribeiro LGT, Lefer AM. Preservation of ischemic myocardium by a new converting enzyme inhibitor, enalaprilic acid, in acute myocardial infarction. Am Heart J 1985;109:222–8.
123. Ertl G. Coronary vasoconstriction in experimental myocardial ischemia. J Cardiovasc Pharmacol 1987; 9(Suppl.2):S9–17.
124. Schölkens BA, Linz W, Lindpaintner K, Ganten D. Angiotensin deteriorates but bradykinin improves cardiac function following ischaemia in isolated rat hearts. J Hypertension 1987; 5(Suppl.5):S7–9.
125. Tio RA, van Gilst WH, Rett K, Wolters K, Dietze GJ, Wesseling H. The effects of bradykinin and the ischemic isolated rat heart. In Pfeiffer EF, Reaven GM, eds. Effects of antihypertensive treatment on glucose metabolism. New York: Thieme Medical Publishers, 1990: 85–8.
126. Linz W, Martorana PA, Grötsch H, Qi B-Y, Schölkens BA. Antagonizing bradykinin (BK) obliterates the cardioprotective effects of bradykinin and angiotensin-converting enzyme (ACE) inhibitors in ischemic hearts. Drug Dev Res 1990;19:393–408.

127. Linz W, Martorana PA, Schölkens BA. Local inhibition of bradykinin degradation in ischemic hearts. J Cardiovasc Pharmacol 1990;15(suppl. 6):S99–109.
127a. Pfeffer MA, Braunwald E, Moye LA, Basta L, Brown EJ Jr, Cuddy TE, Davis BR, Geltman EM, Goldman S, Flaker GC, Klein M, Lamas GA, Packer M, Rouleau J, Rouleau JL, Rutherford J, Wertheimer JH, Hawkins CM, on behalf of the SAVE investigators. Effect of captopril on mortality and morbidity in patients with left ventricular dysfunction after myocardial infarction. N Engl J Med 1992;327:669–77.
127b. The SOLVD Investigators. Effect of enalapril on mortality and the development of heart failure in asymptomatic patients with reduced left ventricular ejection fractions. N Engl J Med 1992;327:685–91.
128. Slater EE, Merrill DD, Guess HA, Roylance PJ, Cooper WD, Inman WHW, Ewan PW. Clinical profile of angioedema associated with angiotensin converting-enzyme inhibition. JAMA 1988;260:967–70.
129. Gohlke P, Urbach H, Schölkens B, Unger T. Inhibition of converting enzyme in the cerebrospinal fluid of rats after oral treatment with converting enzyme inhibitors. J Pharmacol Exp Ther 1989;249:609–16.
130. Lantz I, Terenius L. High enkephalyl peptide degradation, due to angiotensin-converting enzyme-like activity in human CSF. FEBS Lett 1985;193:31–4.
131. Stine SM, Yang HYT, Costa E. Inhibition of in situ metabolism of [^{3}H] (Met^5)-enkephalin and potentiation of (Met^5)-enkephalin analgesia by captopril. Brain Res 1980;188:295–9.
132. Inturrisi CE, Umans JG, Wolff D, Stern AS, Lewis RV, Stein S, Udenfriend S. Analgesic activity of the naturally occurring heptapeptide [Met]-enkephalin-Arg^6-Phe^7. Proc Natl Acad Sci USA 1980;77:5512–4.
133. Norman JA, Autry WL, Barbaz BS. Angiotensin-converting enzyme inhibitors potentiate the analgesic activity of [Met]-enkephalin-Arg^6-Phe^7 by inhibiting its degradation in mouse brain. Mol Pharmacol 1985;28:521–6.
134. Demmer W, Brand K. Processing and degradation of Met-enkephalin by peptidases associated with rat brain cortical synaptosomes. Arch Biochem Biophys 1983;227: 310–20.
135. Chou J, Tang J, Costa E. Met^5-enkephalin-Arg^6-Phe^7 content of human and rabbit plasma. Life Sci 1983;32:2589–95.
136. Aoki K, Kajiwara M, Oka T. The inactivation of [Met^5]-enkephalin by bestatin-sensitive aminopeptidase, captopril-sensitive peptidyl dipeptidase A and thiorphan-sensitive endopeptidase-24.11 in mouse vas deferens. Jpn J Pharmacol 1986;40: 297–302.
137. Aoki K, Kajiwara M, Oka T. The role of bestatin-sensitive aminopeptidase, angiotensin converting enzyme and thiorphan-sensitive "enkephalinase" in the potency of enkephalins the guinea-pig ileum. Jpn J Pharmacol 1984;36:59–65.
138. Manwaring D, Mullane K. Disappearance of enkephalins in the isolated perfused rat lung. Life Sci 1984;35:1787–94.
139. DiNicolantonio R, Hutchinson JS, Takata Y, Veroni M. Captopril potentiates the vasodepressor action of Met-enkephalin in the anaesthetized rat. Br J Pharmacol 1983;80:405–8.
140. Etienne PE, Zubensko GS: Does captopril elevate mood? TIPS 1987;8:329–30.
141. Croog SH, Levine S, Testa MA, Brown B, Bulpitt CJ, Jenkins CD, Klerman GL, Williams GH. The effects of antihypertensive therapy on the quality of life. N Engl J Med 1986;314:1657–64.
142. Zubenko GS, Nixon RA. Mood-elevating effect of captoril in depressed patients. Am J Psychiatry 1984;141:110–1.
143. Deicken RF: Captopril treatment of depression. Biol Psychiatr 1986;21:1425–8.

144. Gillman MA, Sandyk R. Reversal of captopril-induced psychosis with naloxone. Am J Psychiatry 1985;142:270.
145. Goldblatt J, Bryer A: Huntington's disease: deterioration in clinical state during treatment with angiotensin converting enzyme inhibitor. Br Med J 1987; 294:1659–60.
146. Spinosa G, Perlanski E, Leenen FHH, Stewart RB, Grupp LA. Angiotensin converting enzyme inhibitors: Animal experiments suggest a new pharmacological treatment for alcohol abuse in humans. Alcohol Clin Exp Res 1988; 12:65–70.
147. Lingham T, Perlanski E, Grupp LA. Angiotensin converting enzyme inhibitors reduce alcohol consumption: some possible mechanisms and important conditions for its therapeutic use. Alcohol Clin Exp Res 1990;14:92–9.
148. Orloff MS, Turner AJ, Bunnett NW. Catabolism of substance P and neurotensin in the rat stomach wall is susceptible to inhibitors of angiotensin converting enzyme. Regul Peptides 1986;14:21–31.
149. Shore SA, Stimler-Gerard NP, Coats SR, Drazen JM. Substance P-induced bronchoconstriction in the guinea pig. Enhancement by inhibitors of neutral metalloendopeptidase and angiotensin-converting enzyme. Am Rev Respir Dis 1988;137:331–6.
150. Morice AH, Lowry R, Brown MJ, Higenbottam T. Angiotensin-converting enzyme and the cough reflex. Lancet 1987;2:1116–8.
151. Bucknall CE, Neilly JB, Carter R, Stevenson RD, Semple PF. Bronchial hyperreactivity in patients who cough after receiving angiotensin converting enzyme inhibitors. Br Med J 1988;296:86–8.
152. Kaufman J, Casanova JE, Riendl P, Schlueter DP. Bronchial hyperreactivity and cough due to angiotensin-converting enzyme inhibitors. Chest 1989; 95:544–8.
153. Erdös EG. Angiotensin I converting enzyme and the changes in our concepts through the years. Hypertension 1990;16:363–70.

21

Clinical Aspects of the Renin–Angiotensin System and Its Inhibitors in Cardiovascular Disease

HERIBERT SCHUNKERT

Regensburg University
Regensburg, Germany

The recognition of the renin–angiotensin system and its functional significance in the regulation of blood pressure, as well as fluid and sodium homeostasis, originates in the discoveries of Tigerstedt and Bergmann in 1898 (1). Since then, the enzymatic cascade leading to the activation of angiotensin II, the effector peptide of the renin–angiotensin system, has been elucidated, and the components of the system have been characterized utilizing biochemical as well as molecular biological methodologies (2, 3). Furthermore, a broad scale of angiotensin II effects, such as vasoconstriction, fluid and sodium retention, stimulation of aldosterone release, and growth induction of cardiac and vascular smooth muscle cells, has been studied extensively (2, 4, 5). The potential importance of the renin–angiotensin system in pathologic conditions was emphasized by early clinical studies demonstrating that angiotensin converting enzyme (ACE) inhibitors produced significant hemodynamic improvement in patients with hypertension and heart failure (6–8). Furthermore, a number of controlled and uncontrolled trials identified major therapeutic benefits of ACE inhibition in patients with high, normal, or low plasma renin levels (9–15), suggesting that the participation of the renin–angiotensin system is more complex than previously expected (16). In turn, results from clinical investigations have stimulated further basic research to characterize the various actions and interactions of the renin–angiotensin system in cardiovascular disease.

This chapter summarizes the results from clinical trials employing ACE inhibitors in patients with cardiovascular diseases and discusses the role of the renin–angiotensin system in the cardiovascular abnormalities of these patients. Furthermore, the potential pharmacodynamic mechanisms of ACE inhibitors will be discussed.

I. RENIN–ANGIOTENSIN SYSTEM

Epithelioid cells of afferent renal arterioles are the predominant site of renin synthesis (17). Within these specialized cells preprorenin, the translational product of the renin gene, is enzymatically processed to prorenin or renin, both of which reach the circulation via regulated and/or constitutive intracellular pathways of secretion (18). The physiological role of circulating *prorenin* remains controversial. *Renin* cleaves angiotensin I from its high-molecular-weight precursor angiotensinogen, which is synthesized in the liver, as well as many other tissues (19). Angiotensin converting enzyme, predominantly located in pulmonary and systemic blood vessels (20, 21), splits two amino acids from angiotensin I to yield angiotensin II, which binds to membrane-bound receptors to elicit its various effects. This enzymatic cascade can be interrupted pharmacologically by blockade of the catalytic sites of renin and converting enzyme, as well as by blockade of angiotensin II receptor-binding sites.

A. Circulating Renin–Angiotensin System

According to the concept of an endocrine system, plasma angiotensin II is presumably produced via the angiotensinogen–renin–angiotensin-converting enzyme biochemical cascade in the systemic and pulmonary circulation. The short-lived peptide angiotensin II (118) is then delivered to target tissues to elicit its various effects. Renin is thought to be the rate-limiting component of the circulating renin–angiotensin system (119). Synthesis and release of this enzyme are regulated in a complex fashion (120, 121).

1. Regulation of Plasma Renin in Heart Failure

Several factors that can increase plasma renin activity are typically altered in decompensated or severe heart failure. Enhanced sympathetic nervous system activity, decreased renal perfusion pressure, and impaired sodium delivery to the macula densa may all stimulate plasma renin levels (119). However, other factors that are activated in heart failure, such as angiotensin II (121, 123) and atrial natriuretic peptide (ANP) (122), downregulate plasma renin activity. Therapeutic interventions in patients with heart failure further complicate the regulation of renin. Diuretic treatment or sodium restriction cause a marked increase of plasma renin activity (12). Digitalis, on the other hand, suppresses plasma renin and aldosterone (124). The net effect of the various regulatory mechanisms is a wide scatter of plasma renin levels in patients with chronic heart failure, especially those with mild or moderate disease (12, 10). However, in patients with acute or decompensated heart failure plasma renin activity is often increased (10). The extent of sodium retention correlates with plasma renin activity in these patients (210). Pharmacologic blockade of the renin–angiotensin system by ACE inhibitors elicits hemodynamic effects in patients with low, normal, or high-renin heart failure (10–15, 85). However, the first dose effect is much more pronounced when the circulating renin–angiotensin system is activated (e.g., plasma renin activity is high) (211). Whether patients with heart failure who have high plasma renin levels benefit more from chronic ACE inhibition than those with normal plasma levels remains to be elucidated.

2. Regulation of Plasma Renin in Hypertension

The impact of the circulating renin–angiotensin system on blood pressure regulation is well documented for patients with renin-producing tumors as well as in those with renovascular or Goldblatt hypertension (125, 46). ACE inhibitors can cause a dramatic fall in arterial blood pressure in such patients. However, not all patients with renal artery stenosis present with an increased plasma renin activity (84), raising the question of how hypertension is maintained in these patients. Pharmacologic interruption of the presumed negative feedback by angiotensin II increases plasma renin levels in all patients with renovascular hypertension, suggesting that intrarenal renin levels and inducibility of renin release are increased in these patients (84). The role of the circulating renin–angiotensin system in essential hypertension is more difficult to define, since most patients present with normal plasma renin activity. Nevertheless, ACE inhibition can normalize blood pressure in this group as well (11). Even more surprising is that ACE inhibitors cause a significant fall of blood pressure in patients with low renin hypertension, which occurs after bilateral nephrectomy (14, 15). Finally, Bravo et al. demonstrated that long-term efficacy of ACE inhibitors in the treatment of hypertensive patients is not a function of pretreatment plasma renin levels (85).

B. Tissue Renin–Angiotensin Systems

It is well established that in patients with acute myocardial infarction (95) or acute cardiac decompensation (10) plasma levels of renin are increased. However, in the chronic phase of congestive heart failure plasma levels are often normal (10, 126) and cannot account for the various hemodynamic and renal effects of ACE inhibitors (9). Increasing evidence suggests the existence of several renin–angiotensin systems in target tissues of angiotensin II. Biochemical and molecular biological studies have demonstrated local renin, angiotensinogen, and angiotensin-converting enzyme synthesis in vasculature, heart, and kidney, as well as in many other tissues (3). Furthermore, angiotensin II has been found to be generated in cultured endothelial and mesangial cells in the absence of plasma, suggesting that the full enzymatic cascade can take place within a single cell (127, 128).

1. Cardiac Renin–Angiotensin System

Renin, angiotensinogen, and angiotensin-converting enzyme mRNAs are all found in the heart (21, 129–131). Renin enzymatic activity has been demonstrated in isolated cardiac myocytes (129). ACE activity is located throughout the myocardium, with highest concentrations found in the atria, vasculature, and cardiac valves (130). The conversion of angiotensin I to angiotensin II has been demonstrated in isolated rat hearts and has been blocked by ACE inhibitors (131). Other non-angiotensin-converting enzyme peptidases found in normal and failing human hearts may contribute to local angiotensin II synthesis as well (132).

a. Regulation of the Cardiac Renin–Angiotensin System in Heart Failure The activity of the cardiac renin–angiotensin system can be modulated by various physiological perturbations. For example, the expression of renin and angiotensinogen genes is stimulated in hearts of sodium-depleted or corticosteroid-treated animals (134, 135). Cardiac angiotensin-converting enzyme is elevated in chronic, compensated experimental heart failure in the rat (136). Angiotensin-converting enzyme mRNA level and enzymatic activity are increased in the right ventricle and interventricular septum of rats with left ventricular myocardial infarction, and correlate with the extent of cardiac dilatation (136). High concentrations of angiotensin-converting enzyme are found in the infarcted myocardium, as well (137). In the same animal model Drexler et al. have demonstrated an induction of angiotensinogen mRNA levels (138). At present, no data are available concerning renin gene expression in failing hearts. However, the increase of cardiac angiotensinogen and ACE mRNA levels suggests that local angiotensin II synthesis might be induced under these conditions. Local inhibition of cardiac ACE by intracoronary infusion of an ACE inhibitor has been studied in patients with idiopathic dilated cardiomyopathy (108). Enalaprilat caused a significant reduction of coronary resistance as well as a decline of ejection fraction (108). Furthermore, local ACE inhibition decreased end-systolic stress/end-systolic volume ratio in these patients (108). End diastolic pressure decreased as well without change in end-diastolic volume (108). Another study, carried out in patients with ischemic heart disease, confirmed the slight negative inotropic effects of ACE inhibition. Furthermore, diastolic distensibility slightly improved in patients treated with ACE inhibitors (97).

b. Regulation of the Cardiac Renin–Angiotensin System in Hypertension The status of the cardiac renin–angiotensin system has been studied in left ventricles of rats exposed to chronic pressure overload. Hearts of spontaneously hypertensive rats (SHR) develop severe hypertrophy, which can be prevented by ACE inhibition (113). Plasma renin and plasma angiotensin II levels are normal in the SHR; however angiotensinogen mRNA and angiotensin II tissue levels in the hearts of spontaneously hypertensive rats are significantly increased (139, 140). Another animal model of hypertensive heart disease is induced by chronic banding of the ascending or abdominal aorta of Wistar rats. Severe left ventricular hypertrophy (LVH) develops over a period of 2–8 weeks after aortic banding (105). ACE inhibition has been shown to prevent pressure overload LVH in the aortic banded rats (112). It is interesting that cardiac hypertrophy can be prevented, even when ACE inhibitors are given at a dosage not affecting blood pressure (141). The plasma renin activity is only transiently increased in this model of hypertensive heart disease, thus the circulating renin–angiotensin system cannot account for the beneficial effects of ACE inhibitors (115). However, both angiotensinogen and ACE mRNAs are induced in rat hearts with left ventricular hypertrophy (LVH) exposed to aortic banding (115, 105). Cardiac ACE activity increased in several regions of the pressure-overloaded left ventricle, whereas ACE activity in the normal right ventricle was unchanged (105). Isolated buffer-perfused rat hearts with LVH generated more angiotensin II than control hearts when exposed to angiotensin I (105). Furthermore, hypertrophied hearts displayed a marked deterioration of diastolic function when perfused with angiotensin I, suggesting that intracardiac conversion can affect cardiac function (105). In another study, hypertrophied rat hearts were perfused in an isolated organ chamber with washed red cells but no exogenous angiotensins. When exposed to low-flow ischemia, LVH hearts displayed a marked improvement of diastolic dysfunction when cardiac ACE was blocked with enalaprilat (142). This result is even more remarkable, since no exogenous substrate is given (e.g., the cardiac renin–angiotensin system has to account for these effects) (142).

2. *Renal Renin–Angiotensin System*

All components of the renin–angiotensin system are found intrarenally (17). This local or paracrine renin–angiotensin system might be regulated independently from the circulating system (143–145) and might be activated even when plasma levels of renin and angiotensin II are normal (145). The demonstration of intrarenal synthesis of renin, angiotensinogen, and converting enzyme messenger RNAs by Northern blotting (146, 147) and the localization of the production sites by in situ hybridization (148, 149) provided strong evidence for a tissue renin–angiotensin system within the kidney. In fact, angiotensin II levels in crude homogenates of the kidney or in proximal tubule fluid by far exceeded plasma concentrations (150, 151).

a. Regulation of the Renal Renin–Angiotensin System in Heart Failure It has been shown that renal and circulatory renin–angiotensin systems can be regulated differently after various experimental pertubations such as sodium depletion or genetic hypertension (19, 145, 146, 149, 152, 157). Increasing evidence suggests that in experimental models of heart failure the intrarenal renin–angiotensin system is activated earlier than the circulating system (153). For example, rats with mild to moderate chronic heart failure lose the capability to respond to volume load by adequate increase of urinary flow (154). This maladaptation, can be corrected by intrarenal administration of ACE inhibitors (155), despite the fact that the circulating levels of renin and angiotensin II are normal in these animals (156). Kastner et al. have demonstrated that during reduction of renal perfusion pressure, locally formed angiotensin II modifies glomerular filtration rate and filtration fraction. Furthermore, studies concerning angiotensinogen messenger RNA levels in animals with heart failure with myocardial infarctions demonstrated a tissue-selective increase of angiotensinogen mRNA in the kidneys (157), indicating an activation of the intrarenal renin–angiotensin system. Chronic treatment of the heart failure rats with ACE inhibitors attenuated the activation of angiotensinogen mRNA, suggesting that angiotensin II might stimulate the system by a positive feedback mechanism (157, 158).

Although tools to study the renal renin–angiotensin systems in human subjects with heart failure are limited, there is indirect evidence that the intrarenal system might be activated in patients with heart failure (13). Patients with heart failure are characterized by increased renal vascular resistance, which can be markedly reduced by ACE inhibition. In parallel, urinary sodium excretion can be substantially increased by blockade of the system, even when plasma renin activity is normal (13). Furthermore, there are striking similarities between the symptoms in chronic congestive heart failure and nonmodulating salt-sensitive hypertension (76).

b. Regulation of the Renal Renin–Angiotensin System in Hypertension Patients with “nonmodulating” hypertension display impaired sodium excretion and positive fluid balance after salt administration (76). The renal maladaptation can be corrected by administration of a low dosage of an ACE inhibitor into the renal artery, suggesting that the primary cause for hypertension in nonmodulators is a selective defect of the tissue renin–angiotensin system in the kidney. Spontaneously hypertensive rats, which are a genetic model of hypertension, in which blood pressure can be normalized by ACE inhibition, are characterized by an alteration of intrarenal angiotensinogen mRNA synthesis (152). Renovascular hypertension is a classic example of the importance of the circulating renin–angiotensin system. However, the intrarenal renin–angiotensin system might be activated as well, since kidneys of patients with renal artery stenosis release more angiotensin into the circulation than kidneys with normal blood supply (159). Experimental studies in rats or dogs with renovascular hypertension have shown a biphasic stimulation of the renin–

angiotensin system. Initially after banding of the renal artery, renal renin synthesis and release are increased. In the chronic phase of the disease, when plasma renin is normal, hypertension may be maintained by an induction of local vascular or renal ACE activity (160, 161).

II. ANGIOTENSIN II EFFECTS IN CARDIOVASCULAR DISEASE

Regardless of whether the main source of angiotensin II synthesis is the circulating or the various tissue renin–angiotensin systems, angiotensin II has a wide variety of direct and indirect physiological effects (Table 2). Angiotensin II receptors are widely distributed throughout the vascular tree. Furthermore, angiotensin II receptors are found in virtually all organs involved in cardiovascular regulation such as the heart, kidney, adrenal, and brain (162–165). In patients with heart failure or hypertension, the net result of an activated renin–angiotensin system is detrimental. The higher angiotensin II levels in patients with heart failure before onset of treatment, the better the improvement in prognosis when they are treated with ACE inhibitors (166).

A. Direct vs. Indirect Angiotensin II Effects

1. Direct Cardiac Angiotensin II Effects

Angiotensin II causes a marked vasconstriction of the coronary arteries as well as many other vascular beds (167–169). Thereby, angiotensin II decreases cardiac oxygen supply and increases cardiac afterload and workload. Angiotensin II also displays a positive inotropic effect, which might increase the mismatch between oxygen supply and demand of the heart (170–173). Both vasoconstriction and positive inotropic effect are partially mediated by activation of protein kinase C (174). Other important cardiac effects of angiotensin II include activation of voltage-sensitive slow Ca^{2+} channels and G-protein-coupled second messengers such as inositol phosphates and cAMP (173, 175). There is emerging evidence that angiotensin II impairs diastolic function of the heart as well. Hypertrophied rat hearts displayed a marked increase in left ventricular end-diastolic pressure when exposed to angiotensin II (105). ACE inhibition, on the other hand, may improve diastolic function (142, 97). Angiotensin II receptors are found in high density along the conduction system of the heart, and it was hypothesized that angiotensin II might have arrhythmogenic effects as well (176). In fact, when isolated rat hearts are exposed to ischemia, ACE inhibitors can prevent reperfusion arrhythmia (177, 191). Whether this applies to humans remains to be elucidated. Finally, angiotensin II might be a potent growth stimulus for cardiac and vascular smooth muscle cells. Protooncogenes, such as *c-fos* and *c-jun,* can be activated by angiotensin II and might be involved in this process (178, 179).

2. Direct Renal Angiotensin II Effects

Angiotensin II effects on renal hemodynamics and function serve two principal goals: regulation of blood pressure and preservation of fluid and salt homeostasis (2, 180). As in other vascular beds, angiotensin II causes a strong vasoconstriction in the kidney and increases renal vascular resistance (181). By acting mainly on the efferent arteriole of the glomerulus, the peptide increases intraglomerular hydrostatic pressure and filtration fraction (39). This mode of action allows maintenance of a stable filtration rate even when renal blood flow is decreased. However, angiotensin II is also capable of changing glomerular capillary surface area by contracting glomerular mesangial cells and thereby influencing the ultrafiltration coefficient, K_f (40).

Within the proximal tubules, angiotensin II stimulates sodium reabsorption by activating the Na^+/H^+ antiporter (182, 183). In addition, Liu et al. have shown that angiotensin II may enhance proximal tubule bicarbonate reabsorption (184).

3. *Indirect Angiotensin II Effects*

The direct cardiac and renal effects of angiotensin II are modified by close interaction between the renin–angiotensin system as well as other endocrine and paracrine hormonal systems and sympathetic nerve activity. Furthermore, angiotensin II controls its own production by negative feedback regulation of renal renin and pulmonic angiotensin-converting enzyme mRNA synthesis (185, 186). Angiotensinogen mRNA synthesis, on the other hand, is upregulated by angiotensin II (123). Angiotensin II has been shown to stimulate catecholamine release from noradrenergic nerve endings, further increasing vascular tone (187, 188). β_2-Adrenoreceptor activation, on the other hand, can increase angiotensin II release and potentiate its effects (189). The interaction of the two neuroendocrine systems might play a role in vascular and cardiac remodeling by activation of protooncogenes such as *c-myc* (190). The dysrhythmic effects of angiotensin II might be caused by coactivation of β_2-adrenoreceptor and angiotensin II receptors as well (192). Angiotensin II also stimulates endothelin mRNA synthesis, further augmenting vasoconstriction (193). These multiple effects favoring vasoconstriction may be blunted to some extent by parallel activation of vasodilating systems. For example, angiotensin II can increase prostacyclin synthesis and the release of endothelium-derived relaxing factor (194–196).

The direct renal effects of angiotensin II may be potentiated by interaction with other endocrine systems as well. Antidiuretic hormone (ADH) (197) and aldosterone secretion (198) are stimulated by angiotensin II, thereby amplifying fluid and salt retention. Renal prostaglandins are also increased after administration of angiotensin II (199) and might contribute to the maintenance of glomerular filtration rate by lowering afferent vascular resistance (200). The kinin system is related to the renin–angiotensin system by common use of the angiotensin converting enzyme (see chapter on basic aspects of ACE). Finally, angiotensin II has been shown to be important for full functional effects of alpha-adrenergic nerve stimulation on vascular resistance and antinatriuresis (201, 202).

III. CLINICAL PHARMACOLOGY OF ACE INHIBITORS

All currently available ACE inhibitors are characterized by competitive inhibition of the catalytic site of angiotensin-converting enzyme, also called kininase II. Consequently, both angiotensin I conversion and bradykinin degradation are slowed by these agents. Several pharmacologic differences among ACE inhibitors merit consideration. Some drugs (e.g., captopril, zofenopril, and alacepril) contain a sulfhydryl group that might function as a scavenger of O_2-derived free radicals (22). Such effects may be particularly important during reperfusion after myocardial ischemia (23).

Adverse reactions, such as dry cough and rash, have been attributed to the sulfhydryl group (24), although ACE inhibitors without the sulfhydryl group provoke these symptoms as well (25). The affinity of ACE inhibitors to the catalytic site of the angiotensin-converting enzyme varies, which requires different dosing to allow for completel inhibition of serum ACE. Perhaps more importantly, tissue ACE may be differentially inhibited by the various drugs. The other major differences among ACE inhibitors are due to the distinct pharmacokinetic properties of these compounds (Table 1).

A. Pharmacokinetics

Commonly used ACE inhibitors are efficiently absorbed from the gastrointestinal tract, with 60–75% of an oral dose being absorbed (26, 27). Oral bioavailability of lisinopril and fosinopril is somewhat lower and averages about 30% (28, 29). Several orally active ACE inhibitors such as enalapril, ramipril, pentopril, quinapril, perindopril, and alacepril are so called "prodrugs" (25, 27). After enteric absorption, these compounds are de-esterified in the liver to form the active metabolite. Thereby, the onset of action of such drugs might be delayed. For example, peak plasma levels of captopril are measured 45–60 min after ingestion; in contrast, plasma levels of active metabolites (enalaprilat, ramiprilat, etc.) of the respective prodrugs (i.e., enalapril, ramipril, etc.) peak 2–6 hr after oral intake (25). Some ACE inhibitors in both immediate acting and prodrug groups (e.g., captopril, ramipril, etc.) undergo further metabolism forming multiple, mostly inactive, metabolites (30, 31).

With the exception of fosinopril, which is also excreted by the liver, the kidney is the major route of eliminatation for all ACE inhibitors. Whether ACE inhibitors are excreted by glomerular filtration or whether tubular transport mechanisms account for the renal excretion remains unclear, with the exception of captopril, which is excreted by tubular secretion (32). The elimination plasma half-lives of

Table 1 Pharmacokinetic Characteristics of Several ACE Inhibitors

Drug	Active Form	Dosage[a] (mg)	Onset of Action (min)	Duration of Action (hr)
Captopril	Captopril	6.25–150	15	6–10
Enalpril	Enalprilat	2.5–40	60	18–48
Lisinopril	Lisinopril	2.5–40	60	18–48
Alacepril	Captopril	6.25–150	30	6–12
Benazapril	Benazaprilat	2.5–40	30	12–24
Cilazapril	Cilazaprilat	0.5–20	60	24–72
Fosinopril	SQ 27,519	2.5–40	n.a.	>24
Pentopril	Pentoprilat	50–750	30	10–24
Perindopril	Perindoprilat	1–16	n.a.	24–72
Quinapril	Quinaprilat	2–40	30	18–48
Ramipril	Ramiprilat	2.5–40	30	24–96
Zofenopril	Zofenoprilat	7.5	n.a.	n.a.

[a]Represents dosages most commonly used in clinical trials
n.a., Not available.

ACE inhibitors range between 1.7 hr (captopril) (27) in patients with normal renal functions and 15.5 hr (ramiprilat) (31) in patients with low creatinine clearance. Accordingly, the dosage of most ACE inhibitors has to be adapted to renal function to avoid overtreatment (31). Age and heart failure increase the plasma half-life of several ACE inhibitors as well. Thus, the dosage should be reduced in elderly patients with chronic heart failure (33). Hepatic dysfunction might alter the pharmacokinetics of some ACE inhibitors as well, but changes are small and not considered to be clinically significant.

Plasma levels of ACE inhibitors display a multiphasic concentration–time curve. First, there is a rapid initial decline from high concentrations, followed by a slow terminal elimination rate of up to 3–4 weeks (ramiprilat) after the last dose (31). This latter phase of the multiphasic concentration–time curve might be determined by a slow release of the agent from ACE binding (34). The affinity of various ACE inhibitors for the catalytic site of the converting enzyme varies markedly, affecting the duration of action (e.g., 6–12 hr after 6.25–75 mg captopril and 12–60 hr after 2–10 mg ramipril). The binding affinity of the drug for the ACE enzyme may also determine the dosage required to achieve maximal effects.

ACE inhibitors can be differentiated by high and low lipophilicity. Like captopril and enalapril, most ACE inhibitors have poor lipophilicity and may not penetrate the blood–brain barrier, although this finding has not been confirmed by all investigators (35). Ramipril and SA 466, on the other hand, have high lipophilicity and inhibit central nervous system ACE activity (36). This might affect the local renin–angiotensin system in the brain, which is involved in regulation of sympathetic nervous activity and thirst (37). However, at the present time, no clinically significant effects have been be attributed to differences in lipid solubility of ACE inhibitors.

B. Adverse Effects/Side Effects

In general, ACE inhibitors are well tolerated drugs and adverse reactions are rare (25, 33) (see warning in full prescription information provided for each compound). Most side effects are functional and relate to inhibition of renin–angiotensin system activity or bradykinin degradation (25). These adverse reactions are limited by the duration of ACE inhibition. Therefore, it has been suggested that the longer the action of ACE inhibitors, the more frequent and more severe their side effects (25, 38). Specific problems that may occur in patients treated with ACE inhibitors include those detailed below.

1. Renal Hemodynamics

In patients with heart failure or those with renal artery stenosis, glomerular filtration rate is partially maintained by the renin–angiotensin system. Angiotensin II mediates constriction of the efferent arteriole causing an increase in filtration fraction (39, 40). ACE inhibition reverses this effect. Consequently, ACE inhibition increases renal plasma flow, which reflects a decline of renal vascular resistance. While filtration fraction decreases in this situation, the response of glomerular filtration rate can vary (9, 43). Some investigators have observed *acute* improvement of renal function (9) but others have noted no change (42) or decrease of glomerular filtration rate (43, 44). Increase of serum creatinine levels or acute renal failure have been reported in some patients with chronic heart or renal failure after treatment with ACE inhibitors was initiated (45). Especially in patients with bilateral renal artery stenosis these drugs should be avoided (46–48). Effects of *chronic* treatment with captopril or enalapril in patients with chronic heart failure or chronic renal failure may result in progressive improvement of both glomerular filtration rate and renal plasma flow (49, 50), but deterioration of renal function has been noted in other investigations (38).

2. Proteinuria

The effects of ACE inhibitors on proteinuria vary widely. In patients treated with high dosages of captopril, new onset of proteinuria, or, in rare cases, nephrotic syndrome has been observed (51). Since lower dosages are now recommended, these events occur less frequently. In patients with diabetic nephropathy, proteinuria can be reduced by long-term treatment with ACE inhibitors (52, 53).

3. Hyperkalemia

Another functional side effect of ACE inhibitors is hyperkalemia. By lowering aldosterone secretion or blocking renal angiotensin II effects, serum potassium levels increase slightly in most patients (54). However, serious hyperkalemia can occur during ACE inhibition in patients with chronic renal failure, especially when treated concurrently with potassium-sparing diuretics or potassium supplementation (55).

4. Hypotension

Excessive hypotension after initiation of treatment with an ACE inhibitor is rarely seen in hypertensive patients, but can be a serious complication in sodium- or volume-depleted patients. In these patients maintenance of blood pressure is more dependent on the renin–angiotensin system. About 50% of patients with heart failure treated with an ACE inhibitor experience a decrease in blood pressure (56). This side effect can be minimized by slow induction of treatment or use of low dosages of short-acting ACE inhibitors (57).

5. Angioedema

Angioedema occurs in approximately 1: 1000 patients (58). Fatal cases have been reported (58). Usually this side effect occurs shortly after induction of treatment and may require subcutaneous injection of epinephrine and hospitalization.

6. Neutropenia/Agranulocytosis

Neutropenia occurs in about 1: 10,000 patients (58). However, in patients with impaired renal function, and especially those with lupus erythematosus or scleroderma, this adverse reaction was observed in up to 4 % of cases.

7. Rash/Dry Cough/Dizziness/Headache/Fatigue/Diarrhea

These symptoms are the most frequent side effects. They are usually mild and disappear after dosage reduction or discontinuation of treatment in most patients (25).

8. Drug Interactions

Patients treated with drugs that stimulate the renin–angiotensin system, such as diuretics, are more likely to develop hypotension or renal failure after induction of ACE inhibition. Therefore, diuretics should be reduced before ACE inhibition is initiated or small dosages of short-acting ACE inhibitors should be used at the start of therapy. As mentioned above, the combination of potassium-sparing diuretics, potassium supplementation, and ACE inhibitors can cause severe hyperkalemia (55), and should be avoided especially in patients with renal failure.

9. *Lipid Profile*

Patients with hypertension or heart failure often present with coronary or peripheral atherosclerosis. Since metabolic side effects of pharmacotherapy might affect plasma lipids in these patients, Pollare et al. compared the effects of hydrochlorothiazide with chronic ACE inhibition (captopril) on glucose and lipid metabolism (59). In their study, captopril improved insulin-mediated disposal of glucose. The ACE inhibitor had no effect on serum lipids, whereas hydrochlorothiazide treatment worsened both glucose and lipid metabolism (59). In fact, it has been shown that ACE inhibitors (captopril) can effectively decrease atherosclerosis in hyperlipidemic normotensive rabbits or monkeys (60, 61).

10. *Quality of Life*

Subjective well-being has rarely improved and often has deteriorated in patients treated for hypertension with conventional therapy. Thus, subjective quality of life is another criterion for comparison of various antihypertensive agents. Patients treated with ACE inhibitors have presented better scores for work performance and visual motor functioning as well as better measures of life satisfaction, compared with those treated with methyldopa or propranolol (62). A possible mechanism for this unexpected finding is the interaction of ACE inhibitors with central nervous enkephalin metabolism (63).

IV. ROLE OF ACE INHIBITORS IN CARDIOVASCULAR DISEASE

A. Treatment of Hypertension

1. *Essential Hypertension*

ACE inhibitors are an effective treatment modality at all stages of essential hypertension. Recently, the Joint National Committee of Detection, Evaluation and Treatment of High Blood Pressure considered ACE inhibitors to be equal to beta-blockers and diuretics as first-step treatment in mild to moderate hypertension (64).

Monotherapy with ACE inhibitors has been shown to normalize systolic and diastolic blood pressure in 35–70% of hypertensive patients (25). These results are equally good, or better, than those with any other antihypertensive agent used as monotherapy (65). When ACE inhibitors have been used as monoagents, systolic blood pressure decreased by 15–25% on average, with a slightly larger drop in diastolic pressure. ACE inhibition in patients with essential hypertension has been even more successful when dietary sodium intake was concomitantly reduced (66). Numerous controlled as well as uncontrolled studies have been designed to compare antihypertensive and adverse effects of various ACE inhibitors. Many comparisons between short- and long-acting ACE inhibitors have been attempted (38). In available studies, differences in pharmacokinetics and definition of equally effective (equipotent) dosages have hampered these comparisons. However, long-acting ACE inhibitors have tended to have more profound and persistent effects on lowering blood pressure and improving symptoms in heart failure. These beneficial effects may be offset by a slightly higher incidence of hypotension and potassium retention in patients with CHF or renal failure (38, 68–71).

Combination therapy with diuretics or calcium channel blockers appears to enhance the blood-pressure-lowering effect of ACE inhibitors markedly (72, 73). On such a regimen, normotension has been achieved in more than 90% of patients with mild to moderate hypertension (25, 72, 73). The high effectiveness of combination therapy can, in part, be explained by the synergistic effects of these agents. Combination of ACE inhibitors and beta-blockers appears to be less effective. However, when blood pressure control has been poor under a combination of diuretics and beta blockers, addition of captopril normalized blood pressure is 85% of the patients (74, 75). In fact, several studies have shown that triple therapy that includes ACE inhibitors is more effective than other triple-therapy regimens.

2. *Nonmodulators*

ACE inhibitors decrease blood pressure and increase renal plasma flow in virtually all hypertensive patients on a low-sodium diet. Hollenberg et al. have identified a subgroup of patients with essential hypertension who are more sensitive to ACE inhibition, even when salt intake is high. These patients, so-called nonmodulators, show a blunted natriuresis in response to sodium loading, which can be corrected by ACE inhibition. Furthermore, when nonmodulators are treated with ACE inhibitors, renal blood flow in these individuals shows a disproportionate increase. The primary defect in these patients is thought to be located in the kidney, since local infusion of ACE inhibitors into the renal artery has normalized natriuresis. Plasma levels of renin and angiotensin II, on the other hand, are normal in nonmodulators (76).

3. *Renal Parenchymal Hypertension*

ACE inhibitors are very effective in lowering blood pressure in hypertensive patients with various forms of renal disease (77, 78). However, a second therapeutic effect of ACE inhibitors may be even more important in patients with chronic renal parenchymal disease and hypertension. In chronic renal disease, those nephrons that remain normal have an increased "workload," characterized by glomerular hypertension. Angiotensin II-mediated constriction of the efferent arteriole may partially cause this intrarenal hypertension as well as hyperfiltration of the remaining glomeruli, which is thought to lead ultimately to progressive deterioration of renal function (79). Therefore, local and systemic ACE inhibition may have additional effects on preserving glomerular filtration rate in these patients. However, ACE inhibition carries more risks in patients with renal disease as well (80). Since ACE inhibitors and their active or inactive metabolites are mainly excreted by the kidney, plasma concentrations may accumulate and exceed therapeutic levels (31). Drug side effects such as neutropenia, agranulocytosis, proteinuria, and hyperkalemia are observed more often in patients with impaired renal function (80). Therefore, frequent evaluations of electrolytes, creatinine, and white blood cell counts are required in patients with renal insufficiency treated with ACE inhibitors.

4. *Diabetic Nephropathy*

Deterioration of renal function in diabetic subjects, especially those with hypertension, may be partially mediated by the renin–angiotensin system. Glomerular hyperfiltration might play a crucial role in this process (81). Some experimental studies in animals have shown that ACE inhibitors are superior to other antihypertensive agents in preserving renal function, even when similar blood pressure control is achieved (82). Furthermore, ACE inhibitors may slow down the onset of proteinuria, which often complicates diabetic nephropathy (52, 53).

5. Renovascular Hypertension

The renin–angiotensin system is intimately involved in the pathophysiology of renovascular hypertension (83). Low perfusion pressure distal to a renal artery stenosis stimulates renin synthesis and secretion (83). Plasma renin levels often are high but can be normal in about 50% of patients with renal artery stenosis (84). Acute ACE inhibition, or blockade of the negative angiotensin II feedback on renin synthesis, is followed by a large increase in plasma renin levels in virtually all patients with hemodynamic renal artery stenosis (84). Since elevated blood pressure is highly dependent on angiotensin II in patients with renovascular hypertension, blood pressure can be normalized by angiotensin II receptor blockade or ACE inhibition. However, in patients with renovascular hypertension, glomerular filtration is critically dependent on angiotensin II-mediated efferent arteriole vasoconstriction. Therefore, ACE inhibition can be complicated by acute renal failure or anuria (48), especially in patients with bilateral renal artery stenosis, renal artery stenosis of a single kidney, or of a transplanted kidney (46). Since surgical repair or angioplasty allows anatomical correction of the lesion, drugs are not the prefered treatment modality in patients with renovascular hypertension. However, ACE inhibitors or other oral antihypertensive agents might be warrented (46, 77) if there are contraindications to interventional therapy, or persistent severe hypertension.

B. Treatment of Heart Failure

1. Severe Heart Failure

The renin–angiotensin system is important in the maintenance of elevated systemic vascular resistance in patients with chronic heart failure (CHF). Blockade of angiotensin II production by ACE inhibitors reverses this effect (Table 2). The beneficial results of ACE inhibition are best documented in patients with severe CHF. These benefits were evident even though many patients in the clinical trials were receiving concomitant therapy with digitalis and diuretics (9, 38, 69, 90).

a. Acute Hemodynamic Effects. Acute administration of ACE inhibitors in patients with CHF decreased systemic vascular resistance by 20–45% on average (8, 56, 86), as well as mean arterial blood pressure (10–20 mmHg; 8, 56, 86). Average heart rate remained stable or slightly decreased after acute administration of ACE inhibitors (8, 56, 86). Concomitant with the decrease in afterload, an increase of ejection fraction and cardiac output was observed (15–25%; 8, 13). Pulmonary wedge pressure fell sharply in most patients with severe CHF (5–10 mmHg; 8). Pulmonary arterial pressure and right atrial pressure decreased as well (87). The onset of action ranged between 30 and 60 min (depending on the route of administration and the kinetics of the ACE inhibitors) and lasted for 8 hr on average (56).

b. Acute Renal Effects. The resistance vessels of the kidney are most sensitive to angiotensin II. Consequently, acute ACE inhibitors in patients with severe heart failure decreased renal perfusion pressure and glomerular filtration fraction (13).

Table 2 Potential Effects of Angiotensin II or ACE Inhibition in Patients with Cardiovascular Disorders

Target Organ	Angiotensin II	ACE Inhibition
Heart		
Myocardium	Positive inotropy:	Negative inotropy:
	Oxygen demand ↑	Oxygen demand ↓
	? Diastolic dysfunction	? Positive lusitropy
	Proto-oncogene induction	?
	Growth induction	Regression of hypertrophy
		Prevention of remodeling
Conduction system	? Dysrhythmia induction	?
Neuroendocrine systems	? Sympathetic activation:	?
	Positive inotropy	
	Dysrhythmia induction	?
Vasculature	Coronary vasoconstriction:	Coronary vasodilatation:
	Oxygen supply ↓	Oxygen supply ↑
Systemic Circulation	Systemic vasoconstriction:	Systemic vasodilatation:
	Afterload ↑	Afterload ↓
	Cardiac output ↓	Cardiac output ↑
Kidney	Sodium reabsorption ↑:	Sodium reabsorption ↓:
	Plasma volume ↑	Plasma volume ↓
	Preload ↑	Preload ↓
	Efferent arterial vasoconstriction:	Efferent arterial vasodilatation:
	Renal blood flow ↓	Renal blood flow ↓
	Glomerular filtration rate ↓ ↑	Glomerular filtration rate ↓ ↑

Creatinine clearance is usually preserved in these patients. Some patients show a moderate improvement of renal function after ACE inhibition (9). However, profound decrease of blood pressure must be avoided in order to prevent prerenal azotemia (38). Sodium excretion increases after initiation of ACE inhibition, causing a further decrease in cardiac workload (13). Furthermore, ACE inhibitors appear to reverse dilutional hyponatremia in heart failure patients with extensive fluid retention (67).

c. *Chronic Effects.* The acute changes seen after ACE inhibition are sustained during chronic treatment in most patients with severe CHF (87, 88). About 80 % of patients with severe heart failure improved their New York Heart Association (NYHA) functional class value when studied after 6–12 month of treatment (9,88,89). Ejection fraction, cardiac output, cardiac index, or exercise performance continue to improve during the first months of ACE inhibition in most patients treated chronically (8, 88). Furthermore, systemic vascular resistance and pulmonary wedge pressure remain improved during continuous blockade of the renin–angiotensin system. Most important is that the mortality of patients with severe CHF was reduced significantly by chronic treatment with ACE inhibitors (90). The CONSENSUS I study demonstrated a 40% reduction of overall mortality after 6 months and 31% reduction after 12 months of treatment in patients with severe heart failure (NYHA IV). This clear benefit was accompanied by a reduction in heart size and reduced requirement for other medication for heart failure in the enalapril treated patients.

2. *Mild to Moderate Heart Failure*

Although patients with severe heart failure may benefit the most from ACE inhibition, hemodynamic improvement is documented in patients with mild to moderate heart failure as well. Left ventricular ejection fraction and cardiac output increase and systemic vascular resistance usually decreases in these patients. Acute hemodynamic improvements are maintained during long-term treatment with ACE inhibitors in patients with mild to moderate heart failure as well. Improved exercise tolerance, a very sensitive marker for effectiveness of treatment, was noted after about 1 week of ACE inhibition and was still evident after 1 year of follow-up (69, 91, 92). The beneficial effects on hemodynamics are reflected by a decrease in NYHA functional class value in about 85% of patients with mild CHF treated with ACE inhibitors, whereas deterioration was noted only in 1.5% (93). Similar to the effects in severe heart failure, ACE inhibition can improve survival in patients with mild to moderate heart failure (213,214). In patients with an ejection fraction of less than 30% (mostly NYHA II and III), enalapril reduced the mortality after 4 years of follow up by 16% and number of hospitalizations for worsening heart failure by 26% (213). Interestingly, the benefit of ACE inhibition is also evident when compared with other vasodilating agents. The V-HeFT I and II trials demonstrated two year mortality rates in patients with congestive heart failure of 34% when treated with conventional therapy, 28% when treated with hydralazine and isosorbide dinitrate, but 18% when treated with enalapril, demonstrating a clear benefit of long term ACE inhibition in patients with mild to moderate heart failure.

C. Treatment of Myocardial Disease

1. *Ischemic Heart Disease*

Neuroendocrine systems as well as the renin angiotensin system are often activated acutely after myocardial infarction, causing increased circulating levels of renin and angiotensin II (95). Since angiotensin II affects cardiac performance as well as systemic and cardiac circulation, direct and indirect cardiac effects of ACE inhibitors might be of great clinical importance. However, the therapeutic efficacy of ACE inhibition after acute myocardial infarction is not, as yet, proven.

Unless myocardial infarction is complicated by acute, decompensated heart failure, plasma levels of renin and angiotensin II return to normal within weeks (95). However, patients with stable coronary artery disease might still benefit from ACE inhibition by improvement of systemic and pulmonary hemodynamics. As shown by Chatterlee et al., the decrease of cardiac workload by captopril can reduce myocardial oxygen consumption significantly in these patients (96). Direct myocardial effects of ACE inhibition in patients with coronary artery disease include a slight negative inotropic effect, which is not considered to be clinically significant since afterload decreases as well, leading to an overall increase in cardiac output (97). ACE inhibition may alter diastolic function as well, causing improved diastolic distensibility of the left ventricle and accelerated ventricular filling in patients with ischemic heart disease (97, 98).

Whether ACE inhibitors, administered immediately after onset of coronary occlusion, can decrease infarct size remains an open question. Data from experimental studies are inconsistent (99, 100) and clinical data are not available so far. ACE inhibitors may diminish arterial reocclusion after endothelial injury in an experimental model (101). However, unfortunately, the drug had no effect on restenosis after percutaneous transluminal coronary angioplasty in human subjects (212). More favorable data are available with regard to cardiac dilatation that occurs after myocardial infarction (209). Pfeffer et al. studied the effects of captopril in patients with a recent myocardial infarction but with no evidence of heart failure in a placebo-controlled study. Left ventricular filling pressures and end-diastolic volumes increased less in treated patients than in the placebo group, suggesting that ACE inhibition might prevent or delay cardiac remodeling or overt heart failure in patients with myocardial infarction (102). These data were recently confirmed by a large multicenter study (SAVE). In addition, the SAVE trial clearly indicates that long term ACE inhibition can significantly reduce overall mortality as well as cardiovascular mortality in patients following myocardial infarction.

2. *Cardiac Hypertrophy*

In patients with systemic hypertension, the presence of left ventricular hypertrophy contributes to morbidity from symptoms of pulmonary congestion as well as excess mortality (103, 104). Angiotensin II may contribute to this process in a complex fashion, since acute administration of angiotensin II has been shown to worsen diastolic function acutely in experimental cardiac hypertrophy in the rat heart (105). Angiotensin II administered may contribute chronically to excessive myocyte growth by its growth-promoting properties (106, 107). Both of these angiotensin II effects might be relevant for the efficacy of ACE inhibitors in hypertensive cardiomyopathy. Indeed, local inhibition of cardiac ACE can improve diastolic filling in patients with dilated cardiomyopathy (108). Furthermore, pharmacologic reduction of left ventricular hypertrophy can contribute to improvement of diastolic function (109, 103). Numerous clinical and laboratory investigations have shown that cardiac mass can be decreased by ACE inhibition (111–115). Furthermore, patients with arterial hypertension demonstrate significant improvement of left ventricular hypertrophy when treated with ACE inhibitors (116). Effects of ACE inhibition on regression of hypertrophy were particularly more prominent than those of antihypertensive agents that stimulate the renin–angiotensin system (e.g., diuretics; 117). These data suggest that ACE inhibitors might affect cardiac hypertrophy by a second mechanism in addition to afterload reduction.

V. SUMMARY

A large number of trials has accumulated over the last 10 years consistently documenting the efficacy of ACE inhibitors in the therapy of hypertension. Furthermore, in connection with the evolving clinical experience from the use of other afterload-reducing agents (204, 205), the concept of pharmacologic heart failure treatment has been revised since ACE inhibitors first became available (206). In parallel, laboratory investigations have expanded our understanding of the renin–angiotensin system and its role in the pathophysiology of hypertension and congestive heart failure. However, neither the full spectrum of angiotensin II effects nor the precise pharmacodynamic actions of ACE inhibitors in the setting of hypertension or heart failure are fully understood. New physiological concepts, such as the potential role of tissue renin–angiotensin systems in hypertension and heart failure as well as the pharmacologic implications (207, 208) of these systems need to be tested.

REFERENCES

1. Tigerstedt R, Bergmann PG. Niere und Kreislauf. Scand Arch Physiol 1898;8:223–71.
2. Oparil S, Haber E. The renin angiotensin system. N Engl J Med 1974;291:389–401.
3. Dzau VJ, Burt DW, Pratt RE. Molecular biology of the renin angiotensin system. Am J Physiol 1988;255:F563–73.
4. Campbell-Boswell M, Robertson AL. Effects of angiotensin II and vasopressin on human smooth muscle cells in vitro. Exp Mol Pathol 1981;35:265–76.
5. Geisterfer AAT, Peach M, Owens GK. Hypertrophic response of cultured vascular smooth muscle cells to angiotensin II. Circ Res 1988;62:749–56.
6. Gavras H, Brunner HR, Laragh JH, Sealey JE, Gavras I, Vukovich RA. An angiotensin converting enzyme inhibitor to identify and treat vasoconstriction in hypertensive patients. N Engl J Med 1974;291:817–21.
7. Ferguson RK, Turini GA, Brunner HR, Gavras H, McKinstry DN. A specific orally active inhibitor of angiotensin-converting enzyme in man. Lancet 1977;1:775–8.
8. Curtiss C, Cohn JN, Vrobel T, Francioza JA. The role of the renin–angiotensin system in the systemic vasoconstriction of chronic congestive heart failure. Circulation 1978; 58:763–70.
9. Dzau VJ, Colucci WS, Williams GH, Curfman G, Meggs L, Hollenberg NK. Sustained effectiveness of angiotensin-converting enzyme inhibition in patients with severe congestive heart failure. N Engl J Med 1980;302:1373–9.
10. Dzau VJ, Colucci WS, Hollenberg NK, Williams GH. Relation of the renin-angiotensin-aldosterone system to clinical state in congestive heart failure. Circulation 1981; 63:645–51.
11. Brunner HR, Gavras H, Waeber B, Kershaw GR, Turini GA, Vukovich RA, McKinstry VN. Oral angiotensin-converting enzyme inhibitor in long-term treatment of hypertensive patients. Ann Intern Med 1979;90:19.
12. Kubo SH, Clark M, Laragh JH, Borer JS, Cody RJ. Identification of normal neurohormonal activity in mild congestive heart failure and stimulating effect of upright posture and diuretics. Am J Cardiol 1987;60:1322–8.
13. Creager MA, Faxon DP, Halperin SL, et al. Determinants of clinical response and survival in patients with congestive heart failure treated with captopril. Am Heart J 1982;104:1147–53.
14. Wenting GJ, Blankestijn PJ, Poldermans D, van Geelen J, Derkx FHM, Man in't Veld M, Schalekamp MADH. Blood pressure response of nephrectomized subjects and patients with essential hypertension to ramipril: indirect evidence that inhibition of tissue angiotensin converting enzyme is important. Am J Cardiol 1987;59:92–7D.
15. Man In T' Veld AJ, Schicht I, Derkx FHM. Effects of angiotensin-converting enzyme inhibitor (captopril) on blood pressure in anephric subjects. Br Med J 1980:288–90.
16. Hirsch AT, Pinto Y, Schunkert H, Dzau VJ. Potential role of the tissue renin angiotensin system in the pathophysiology of congestive heart failure. Am J Cardiol 1990;66 (Suppl): 22–32D.
17. Taugner R, Hackenthal E, Helmchen U, Ganten D, Kugler P, Marin-Grez M, Nobiling R, Unger T, Lockwald I, Keilbach R. The intrarenal renin–angiotensin system. An immunocytochemical study on the localization of renin, angiotensinogen, converting enzyme, and the angiotensins in the kidney of mouse and rat. Klin Wochenschr 1982;60:1218–22.
18. Pratt RE, Carleton JE, Richie JP, Heusser C, Dzau VJ. Human renin biosynthesis and secretion in normal and ischemic kidneys. Proc Natl Acad Sci USA 1987;84:7837–40.
19. Campbell DJ, Habener JF: Angiotensinogen gene is expressed and differentially regulated in multiple tissues of the rat. J Clin Invest 1986;78:31–9.
20. Ng KKF, Vane JR. Fate of angiotensin I in the circulation. Nature 1968;218:144–150.

21. Paul M, Schunkert H, Allen PD, Dzau VJ. Evidence for widespread expression of angiotensin converting enzyme mRNA in human tissues. J Hypertens 1990;8 (Suppl 3):S36 (abstr.).
22. van Gielst W, Scholtens E, deGraeff PA, deLangen CDJ, Wesseling H. Differential influences of angiotensin converting enzyme inhibitors on the coronary circulation. Circulation 1988;77:I-24–9.
23. Westlin W, Mullane K. Does captopril attenuate reperfusion induced myocardial dysfunction by scavenging free radicals. Circulation 1988;77:I-30–9.
24. Jaffe IA. Adverse effect profile of sulfhydryl compounds in man. Am J Med 80:471–6.
25. Williams GH. Converting enzyme inhibitors in the treatment of hypertension. N Engl J Med 1988;319:1517–25.
26. Duchin KL, McKinstry DN, Cohen AI, Migdalof BH. Pharmacokinetics of captopril in healthy subjects and in patients with cardiovascular diseases. Clin Pharmacokinet 1988;14:241–59.
27. Kubo SH, Cody RJ. Clinical pharmacokinetics of angiotensin converting enzyme inhibitors. A review. Clin Pharmacokinet 1985;10:377–91.
28. Dickstein K. Hemodynamic, hormonal and pharmacokinetic aspects of treatment with lisinopril in congestive heart failure. J Cardiovasc Pharmacol 1987 (Suppl 3):S73–81.
29. van Schaik BA, Geykes GG, van der Wouw PA, Rooij HH, Porsius AJ. Pharmacokinetics of lisinopril in hypertensive patients with normal and impaired renal function. Eur J Clin Pharmacol 1988;34:61–5.
30. Duchin KL, Singhvi SM, Willard DA, Migdalof BH, McKinstry DN. Captopril kinetics. Clin Pharmacol Ther 1982;31:452–8.
31. Schunkert H, Kindler J, Gassmann M, Lahn W, Irmisch R, Ritz E, Debusmann ER, Ocón-Pujadas J, Koch KM, Sieberth HG. Pharmacokinetics of ramipril in hypertensive patients with renal insufficiency. Eur J Clin Pharmacol 1989;37:249–56.
32. Singhvi SM, Duchin KL, Willard DA, McKinstry DN, Migdalof BH. Renal handling of captopril; Effect of probenecid. Clin Pharmacol Ther 1982;32:182–9.
33. Cody RJ. Pharmacology of angiotensin converting enzyme inhibitors as a guide to their use in congestive heart failure. Am J Cardiol 1990;66 (Suppl):7–13D.
34. Belz GG, Kirch W, Kleinbloesem CH. Angiotensin converting enzyme inhibitors. Relationship between pharmacodynamics and pharmacokinetics. Clin Pharmacokinet 1988; 15:295–318.
35. Geppetti P, Spillantini MG, Frilli S, Pietrini U, Fanciullacci M, Sicuteri F. Acute oral captopril inhibits angiotensin converting enzyme activity in human cerebrospinal fluid. J Hypertension 1987;5:151.
36. Unger T, Moursi M, Ganten D, Hermann K, Lang E. Antihypertensive action of the converting enzyme inhibitor perindopril in spontaneously hypertensive rats: comparison with enalapril and ramipril. J Cardiovasc Pharmacol 1986;8:276.
37. Unger T, Bodoer E, Ganten D, Lang E, Rettig R. Brain angiotensin: pathways and pharmacology. Circulation 1988;77 (suppl I):I40–54.
38. Packer M, Lee WH, Yushak M, Medina N. Comparison between captopril and enalapril in patients with severe chronic heart failure. N Engl J Med 1986;315:847–53.
39. Myers BD, Deen WM, Brenner BM. Effects of norepinephrine and angiotensin II on the determinants of glomerular ultrafiltration and proximal tubule fluid reabsorption in the rat. Circ Res 1975;37:101–10.
40. Blantz RC, Konnen KS, Tucker BJ. Angiotensin II effects upon the glomerular microcirculation and ultrafiltration coefficient of the rat. J Clin Invest 1976;57: 419–34.
41. Click RL, Joyner WL, Gilmore JP. Reactivity of glomerular afferent and effeerent arterioles in renal hypertension. Kidney Int 1979;15:109–15.
42. Creager MA, Halperin JL, Bernard DB, Faxon DP, Melidossian CD, Gavras H, Ryan

TJ. Acute regional circulatory and renal hemodynamic effects of converting enzyme inhibition in patients with severe congestive heart failure. Circulation 1981;64:483–9.
43. Pierpont G, Francis GS, Cohn JN: Effect of captopril on renal function in patients with congestive heart failure. Br Heart J 1981;46:522–7.
44. Cleland JGF, Dargie HJ, Ball SG. Effects of enalapril in heart failure: a double blind study of effects on exercise performance, renal function, hormones and metabolic state. Br. Heart J 1985;54:305–12.
45. Mujais SK, Fouad FM, Textor SC, Tarazi RC, Bravo EL, Hart N, Gifford RW. Transient renal dysfunction during initial inhibition of converting enzyme in congestive heart failure. Br Heart J 1984;52:63–71.
46. Jackson B, McGrath BP, Matthews PG, Wong C, Johnston CI. Differential renal function during angiotensin converting enzyme inhibition in renovascular hypertension. Hypertension 1986;8:650–4.
47. Hricik DE, Browning PJ, Kopelman R, Goorne WE, Madias NE, Dzau VJ. Captopril induced functional renal insufficiency in patients with bilateral renal artery stenoses or renal artery stenosis in a solitary kidney. N Engl J Med 1983;308:373–6.
48. Anderson WP, Woods RL: Intrarenal effects of angiotensin II in renal artery stenosis. Kidney Int 1987;31 (Suppl 30):S157–67.
49. Anderson S, Rennke HG, Garcia DL, Brenner BM. Therapeutic advantage of converting enzyme inhibitors in arresting progressive renal disease associated with systemic hypertension. J Clin Invest 1986;77:1993–2000.
50. Reisch C, Mann J, Ritz. Konversionsenzymhemmer in der antihypertensiven Behandlung niereninsuffizienter Patienten. Dtsch Med Wochenschr 1987;112:1249–52.
51. Prins EJ, Hoorntje SJ, Weening JJ, Donker AJ. Nephrotic syndrome in patient on captopril. Lancet 1979;2:306–7.
52. Heeg JE, deJong PE, van der Hem GK, deZeeuw D. Reduction of proteinuria by angiotensin converting enzyme inhibition. Kidney Int 1987;32:78–83.
53. Taguma Y, Kitamoto Y, Futaki G. Effect of captopril on heavy proteinuria in azotemic diabetics. N Engl J Med 1985;313:1617–20.
54. Nicholls MG, Espiner EA, Ikram H. Angiotensin II is more potent than potassium in regulating aldosterone in cardiac failure: evidence during captopril therapy. J Endocrinol Metab 1981;52:1253–6.
55. Hess B, Keusch G, Neftel K, Margelist F, Bansky G. Severe electrolyte disorders during the therapy of heart failure with the ACE inhibitor enalapril. Schweiz Med Wochenschr 1986;116:1331–6.
56. Ader R, Chatterjee K, Ports T, Brundage B, Hiramatsu B, Parmley W. Immediate and sustained hemodynamic and clinical improvement in chronic heart failure by an oral angiotensin converting enzyme inhibitor. Circulation 1980;61:931–7.
57. Sharpe DN, Coxon RJ, Douglas JE. Low-dose captopril in chronic heart failure: acute hemodynamic effects andlong term treatment. Lancet 1980;2:1154–7.
58. Suarez M, Ho PW, Johnson ES, Perez G. Angioneurotic edema, agranulocytosis, and fatal septicemia following captopril therapy. Am J Med 1986;81:336–8.
59. Pollare T, Lithell H, Berne C. A comparism of the effects of hydrochlorothiazide and captopril on glucose and lipid metabolism in patients with hypertension. N Engl J Med 1989;321:868–73.
60. Chobanian AV: The effects of ACE inhibitors and other antihypertensive drugs on cardiovascular risk factors and atherogenesis. Clin Cardiol 1990;13 (6 Suppl 7):VII43–8.
61. Aberg G, Ferrer P: Effects of captopril on atherosclerosis in cynomolus monkeys. J Cardiovasc Pharmacol 1990;15 (Suppl 5):S65–72.
62. Croog SH, Levine S, Testa MA, Brown B, Bulpitt CJ, Jeenkins CD, Klerman GL, Williams GH. The effects of antihypertensive therapy on quality of life. N Engl J Med 1986;314:1657–64.

63. Zubenko GS, Nixon RA. Mood elevating effect of captopril in depressed patients. Am J Psychiatry 1984;141:110–11.
64. The 1988 report of the Joint National Committee on Detection, Evaluation and Treatment of High Blood Pressure. Arch Intern Med 1988;148:1023–38.
65. Herrick AL, Waller PC, Berkin KE, Pringle SD, Callender JS, Robertson MP, Findlay JG, Murray GD, Reid JT, Lorimer AR, et al. Comparison of enalapril and atenolol in mild to moderate hypertension. Am J Med 1989;86:421–6.
66. Shoback DM, Williams GH, Swartz SL, Davies RO, Hollenberg NK. Time course and effect of sodium intake on vascular and hormonal responses to enalapril (MK 421) in normal subjects. J Cardiovasc Pharmacol 1983;5:1010–8.
67. Packer M, Medina N, Yusak M. Correction of dilutional hyponatremia in severe congestive heart failure by converting enzyme inhibition. Ann Intern Med 1984;199:782–9.
68. Schnaper HW: Comparisn of the efficacy and safety of quinapril vs. captopril in treatment of moderate to severe hypertension. Angiology 1989;40:389–95.
69. Giles TG, Katz R, Sullivan JM, Wolfson P, Haugland M, Kirlin P, Powers E, Rich S, et al. Short- and long-acting angiotensin converting enzyme inhibitors: a randomized trial of lisinopril versus captopril in the treatment of congestive heart failure. J Am Coll Cardiol 1989;13:1240–7.
70. Drexler H, Banhardt U, Meinertz T, Wollschlager H, Lehmann M, Just H. Contrasting peripheral short-term and long-term effects on converting enzyme inhibition in patients with congestive heart failure. Circulation 1989;79:491–502.
71. Taylor SH. A comparison of the efficacy and safety of quinapril with that of enalapril in treatment of mild to moderate essential hypertension. Angiology 1989;40:382–8.
72. Morlin C, Baglivo H, Boeijinga JK. A comparative trial of lisinopril and nifedipine in mild to severe essential hypertension. J Cardiovasc Pharmacol 1987;9 (Suppl 3):S49–52.
73. Pool JL, Gennari J, Goldstein R, Kochar MS, Lewin AJ, Maxwell MH, McChesney JA, Metha J, Nash DT, Nelson EB, et al. Controlled multicenter study of the antihypertensive effects of lisinopril, hydrochlorothiazide, and lisinopril plus hydrochlorothiazide in the treatment of 394 patients with mild to moderate hypertension. J Cardiovasc Pharmacol 1987;9 (Suppl 3):S36–42.
74. Muiesan G, Alicandri C, Agabiti-Rosei E, et al. A multicenter trial of low dose captopril administered twice daily in patients with essential hypertension unresponsive to beta blocker-diuretic treatment. J Clin Hypertens 1987;3:144–52.
75. Drayer JI, Weber MA, Lipson JL, Megaffin BB. Differential effects of diuresis and beta-adrenoreceptor blockade during ACE inhibition in patients with severe hypertension. J Clin Pharmacol 1982;22:179–86.
76. Hollenberg NK, Williams GH. Angiotensin and the renal circulation in hypertension. Circulation 1988;77 (Suppl I):I-59–63.
77. Björck S, Herlitz H, Nyberg G, Granerus G, Aurell M. Effect of captopril on renal hemodynamics in the treatment of resistant renal hypertension. Hypertension 1983;5 (Suppl III):III 152–3.
78. Vetter W, Wehling M, Foerster EC, Kuhlmann U, Boerlin HJ, Greminger P, Vetter H. Long term effect of captopril on kidney function in various forms of hypertension. Klin Wochenschr 1984;62:731–7.
79. Hostetter TH, Olson JL, Rennke HG, Venkatachalan MA, Brenner BM. Hyperfiltration of remnant nephrons: a potentially adverse response to renal ablation. Am J Physiol 1981;241:F85–93.
80. Izzo JL, Larrabee PS, Scandling JD. Hyperkalemia with enalapril in advanced renal failure. JAMA 1986;215:2605–6.
81. Hostetter TH, Rennke HG, Brenner BM. The case for intrarenal hypertension in the initiation and progression of diabetic and other glomerulopathies. Am J Med 1982; 72:375–80.

82. Anderson S, Rennke HG, Garcia DL, Brenner BM. Short term and long term effects of antihypertensive therapy in the diabetic rat. Kidney Int 1989;36:526–36.
83. Laragh JH: The pathophysiology and diagnosis of renovascular hypertension. In: Glorioso N, Laragh JH, Rapelli A, eds. Renovascular hypertension, pathophysiology, diagnosis, and treatment. New York: Raven Press, 1987:237–57.
84. Muller, FB, Sealey JE, Case DB, Atlas SA, Pickering TG, Pecker MS, Preibisz JJ, Laragh JH. The captopril test for identifying renovascular disease in hypertensive patients. Am J Med 1986;80:633–44.
85. Bravo EL, Tarazi RC. Converting enzyme inhibition with an orally active compound in hypertensive man. Hypertension 1979;1:39–46.
86. Uretsky BF, Shaver JA, Liang CS, Amin DK, Shah PK, Levine TB, Walinsky P, LeJemtel T, Linnemeier TJ. Lisinopril for congestive heart failure. Am J Cardiol 1989;63:8–11D.
87. Stone CK, Uretsky BF, Linnemeier TJ, Shah PK, Amin DK, Snapinn SM, Rush JE, Langendorfer A, Liang CS. Hemodynamic effects of lisinopril after long term administration in congestive heart failure. Am J Cardiol 1989;63:567–70.
88. Captopril Multicenter Research Group. A placebo controlled trial of captopril in refractory chronic congestive heart failure. J Am Coll Cardiol 1983;2:755–63.
89. Levine TB, Franciosa JA, Cohn JN. Acute and long term responseto an oral of converting enzyme inhibitor, captopril, in congestive heart failure. Circulation 1980;62:35–41.
90. The CONSENSUS Trial Study Group: Effects of enalapril on mortality in severe heart failure. N Engl J Med 1987;316:1429–31.
91. Magnani B, Magelli C. Captopril in mild heart failure: preliminary observations of a long term, double blind, placebo controlled multicenter trial. Postgrad Med J 1986;62 (Suppl 1):153–9.
92. Borgi C, Magelli C, Costa FV, Magnani B, Ambrosioni E. Captopril improves hemodynamic response to static exercise in patients with congestive heart failure. Clin Cardiol 1990;13:329–34.
93. Romankiewicz JA, Brogden RN, Heel RC: Captopril: an update review of its pharmacological properties and therapeutic efficacy in congestive heart failure. Drugs 1983; 25:6–40.
94. Studies of left ventricular dysfunction (SOLVD)—rationale, design and methods: two trial that evaluate the effect of enalapril in patients with reduced ejection fraction. Am J Cardiol 66:315–22.
95. Dargie HJ, McAlpine HM, Morton JJ. Neuroendocrine activation in acute myocardial infarction. J Cardiovasc Pharmacol 1987;9 (Suppl 2):S21–4.
96. Chatterlee K, Rouleau JL, Parmley WW. Hemodynamic and myocardial metabolic effects of captopril in chronic heart failure. Br Heart J 1982;47:233–8.
97. Rousseau MF, Gurne O van Eyll C, Benedict CR, Pouleur H. Effects of benazeprilat on left ventricular systolic and diastolic function and neurohumoral status in patients with ischemic heart disease. Circulation 1990;81 (Suppl II):III123–9.
98. Marmor A, Green T, Krakuer J, Szucs T, Schneeweis A. A single dose of cilazapril improves diastolic function in hypertensive patients. Am J Med 1989;87:61–3S.
99. Ertl G, Kloner RA, Alexander RA, Braunwald E. Limitation of experimental infarct size by an angiotensin converting enzyme inhibitor. Circulation 1982;65:40–48.
100. Liang CS, Gavras H, Black J, Sherman LG, Hood WB. Renin angiotensin system inhibition in acute myocardial infarction in dogs. Effects on systemic hemodynamics, myocardial blood flow, segmental myocardial infarction and infarct size. Circulation 1982;66:1249–55.
101. Powell JS, Clozel JP, Muller RK, Kuhn H, Hefti F, Hosang M, Baumgartner HR. Inhibitors of angiotensin converting enzyme prevent myointimal proliferation after vascular injury. Science 1989;245:186–8.

102. Pfeffer MA, Lamas GA, Vaughn DE, Parisi AF, Braunwald E. Effect of captopril on progressive ventricular dilatation after anterior myocardial infarction. N Engl J Med 1988;319:80–6.
103. Lorell BH, Grossman. Cardiac hypertrophy: consequences for diastole. J Am Coll Cardiol 1987:1189–93.
104. Levy D, Garrison RJ, Savage DD, Kannel WB, Castelli WP. Prognostic implications of echocardiographically determined left ventricular mass in the Framingham Heart Study. N Engl J Med 1990;322:1561–6.
105. Schunkert H, Dzau VJ, Tang SS, Hirsch AT, Apstein C, Lorell B. Increased rat cardiac angiotensin converting enzyme activity and mRNA levels in pressure overload left ventricular hypertrophy: effects on coronary resistance, contractility and relaxation. J Clin Invest 1990;86:1913–20.
106. Khairallah PA, Kanabus. Angiotensin and myocardial protein synthesis. Perspect Cardiovasc Res 1983;8:337–47.
107. Komuro I, Katoh Y, Shibasaki Y, Yamaguchi H, Yazaki Y. Angiotensin II induces hypertrophy and oncogene expression in cultured rat heart myocytes (abstr) Circulation 1989;80 (Suppl II):II–450.
108. Foult JM, Tavolaro O, Antony I, Nitenberg A. Direct myocardial and coronary effects of enalaprilat in patients with dilated cardiomyopathy: assessment by a bilateral intracoronary infusion technique. Circulation 1988;77:337–44.
109. Schulman SP, Weiss JL, Becker LC, Gottlieb SO, Woodruff KM, Wiesfeldt ML, Gerstenblith G. The effects of antihypertensive therapy on left ventricular mass in elderly patients. N Engl J Med 1990;322:1350–6.
110. Tarazi RC, Fouad FM. Reversal of cardiac hypertrophy in humans. Hypertension 1984;6 (Suppl III):III 140–5.
111. Wakashima Y, Fouad FM, Tarazi RC: Regression of left ventricular hypertrophy from systemic hypertension by enalapril. Am J Cardiol 1984;53:1044–9.
112. Kromer EP, Riegger GA. Effects of long-term angiotensin converting enzyme inhibition on myocardial hypertrophy in experimental aortic stenosis in the rat. Am J Cardiol 1988;62:161–3.
113. Pfeffer JM, Pfeffer MA, Mirsky I, Braunwald E. Regression of left ventricular hypertrophy and prevention of left ventricular dysfunction by captopril in the spontaneously hypertensive rat. Proc Natl Acad Sci USA 1982;79:3310.
114. Gay RG. Captopril reduces left ventricular enlargement induced by chronic volume overload. Am J Physiol 1990;259:H796–803.
115. Baker KM, Cherin MI, Wixson SK, Aceto JF: Renin angiotensin system involvement in pressure overload hypertrophy in rats. Am J Physiol 1990;259:H324–32.
116. Garavaglia GE, Messerli FH, Nunez BD, Schmieder RE, Frohlich ED. Immediate and short term cardiovascular effects of a new angiotensin converting enzyme inhibitor (lisinopril) in essential hypertension. Am J Cardiol 1988;62:912–6.
117. Drayer JIM, Gardin JM, Weber MA, Arronow WS. Changes in ventricular septal thickness during diuretic therapy. Clin Pharmacol Ther 1982;32:283.
118. Al-Merani SA, Brooks DP, Chapman BJ, Munday KA. The half-lives of angiotensin II, angiotensin II-amide, angiotensin III, Sar1-Ala8-angiotensin II and renin in the circulatory system of the rat. J Physiol (Lond) 1978;278:471–90.
119. Cody RJ, Laragh JH: The renin angiotensin aldosterone system in chronic heart failure: pathophysiology and implications for treatment. In: Cohn JN, ed. Heart failure, 2nd edition. Secaucus: Advanced Therapeutical Communications International, 1988:79–104.
120. Davis JO, Freeman RH. Mechanisms regulating renin release. Physiol Rev 1976; 56(1):1–56.
121. Gibbons GH, Dzau VJ, Farhi ER, Barger AC. Interaction of signals influencing renin release. Annu Rev Physiol 1984;46:291–308.

122. Cody RJ, Atlas SA, Laragh JH, Kubo SH, Covit AB, Ryman KS, Shaknovich A, Pondolfino K, Clark M, et al. Atrial natriuretic factor in normal subjects and heart failure patients: plasma levels and renal, hormonal, and hemodynamic responses to peptide infusion. J Clin Invest 1986;78:1362–74.
123. Schunkert H, Ingelfinger JR, Jacob H, Bouyounes B, Jackson B, Dzau VJ. Angiotensin II causes reciprocal regulation of intrarenal renin and angiotensinogen gene expression. Clin Res 1990;38:443A (abstr).
124. Covit AB, Schaer GL, Sealey JE, Laragh JH, Cody RJ. Suppression of the renin angiotensin system by intravenous digoxin in chronic congestive heart failure. Am J Med 1983;75:445–7.
125. Galen FX, Devaux C, Houot AM, Menard J, Corvol P, Corvol MT, Gubler MC, Mounier F, Camilleri JP. Renin biosynthesis by a tumoral juxtaglomerular cells. Evidences for a renin precursor. J Clin Invest 1984;73:1144–55.
126. Watkins IJ, Burton JA, Haber E, Cant JR, Smith FM, Barger AC. The renin-aldosterone system in congestive heart failure in conscious dogs. J Clin Invest 1976; 57:1606–17.
127. Tang SS, Stevenson L, Dzau. Endothelial renin angiotensin pathway. Adrenergic regulation of angiotensin secretion. Circ Res 1990;66:103–8.
128. Inagami T, Kawamura M, Naruse K, Okamura T. Localisation of components of the renin angiotensin system within the kidney. Fed Proc 1986;45:1414–9.
129. Dzau VJ, Re RN. Evidence for the existence of renin in the heart. Circulation 1987;73(Suppl I):I-134–6.
130. Yamada H, Fabris B, Allen AM, Jackson B, Johnston C, Mendelsohn FAO. Localization of angiotensin converting enzyme in the rat heart. Circ Res 1991;68:141–9.
131. Lindpaintner K, Jin M, Wilhelm MJ, Susuki F, Linz W, Schoelkens BA, Ganten D. Intracardiac generation of angiotensin and its physiologic role. Circulation 1988 (Suppl I); I18–24.
132. Urata H, Healy B, Stewart RW, Bumpus FM, Husain A. Angiotensin II-forming pathways in normal and failing human hearts. Circ Res 1990;66:883–90.
133. Urata H, Kinoshita A, Misono KS, Bumpus FM, Husain A. Identification of a highly specific chymase as a major angiotensin II-forming enzyme in the human heart. J Biol Chem 1990;265:22348–57.
134. Dzau VJ, Ellison KE, Ouellette AJ. Expression and regulation of renin in the mouse heart. Clin Res 1985;33:181A (abstr).
135. Lindpaintner K, Jin M, Niedermaier N, Wilhelm MJ, Ganten D. Cardiac angiotensinogen and its local activation in the isolated perfused beating heart. Circ Res 1990;67:564–573.
136. Hirsch AT, Talsness CE, Schunkert H, Paul M, Dzau VJ: Tissue-specific activation of cardiac angiotensin converting enzyme in experimental heart failure. Circ Res 1991: 69:475–82.
137. Jackson B, Fabris B, Kohzuki M, Mendelsohn FAO, Johnston C. Angiotensin converting enzyme in the myocardium of rats with heart failure following myocardial infarct. J Hypertension 1990;8 (Suppl 3):S40.
138. Drexler H, Lindpainter K, Lu W, Schieffer B, Ganten D. Transient increase in the expression of cardiac angiotensinogen in rat model of myocardial infarction and failure. Circulation 1989;80 (Suppl II):II459.
139. Nagano M, Nakamura M, Tabuchi Y, Raguki H, Higashimori K, Katahira K, Tsunetoshi T, Otsuka A, Higaki J, Mikami H, Ogihara T. Role of cardiac Angiotensin II in left ventricular hypertrophy of spontaneously hypertensive rats. Circulation 1990;82 (Suppl III):III-616.
140. Li C, Prakash O, Re RN. Altered regulation of angiotensin gene expression in the left ventricles of the hypertensive rats. Circulation 1989;80 (Suppl II):II-616.

141. Ganten D, Todt M, Niedermeyer N, Linz W, Lindpaintner K, Schölkens B. The cardiac renin angiotensin system and its possible role in cardiac hypertrophy. J Mol Cell Cardiol 1989;21 (Suppl III):S9.
142. Eberli FR, Apstein CS, Ngoy S, Lorell BH. Enalaprilat decreases ischemic diastolic dysfunction in pressure overload hypertrophy. Circulation 1990;82 (Suppl III):III 161.
143. Levens NR, Peach MJ, Carey RM. Role of intrarenal renin angiotensin system in the control of renal function. Circ Res 1981;48:157–67.
144. Kastner PR, Hall JE, Guyton AC. Control of glomerular filtration rate: role of intrarenally formed angiotensin II. Am J Physiol 1984;246:F897–907.
145. Schunkert H, Ingelfinger JR, Dzau VJ. Molecular biology of the intrarenal renin angiotensin system. Renal Physiol Biochem 1991;14:146–54.
146. Ingelfinger JR, Pratt RE, Ellison K, Dzau VJ. Sodium regulation of angiotensinogen mRNA expression in rat kidney cortex and medulla. J Clin Invest 1986;78:1311–5.
147. Soubrier F, Alhenc-Gelas F, Hubert C, Allegrini J, John M, Tregear G, Corvol P. Two putative active centers in human angiotensin I converting enzyme revealed by molecular cloning. Proc Natl Acad Sci USA 1988;85:9386–90.
148. Ingelfinger JR, Fon EA, Ellison KE, Dzau VJ. Localization of the intrarenal renin angiotensin system (RAS) by in situ hybridization of renin and angiotensinogen (Ang-n) mRNAs. Kidney Int 1988;33:269 (abst).
149. Ingelfinger JR, Zuo WM, Fon EA, Ellison KE, Dzau VJ. In situ hybridization evidence for angiotensinogen messenger RNA in the rat proximal tubule. J Clin Invest 1990;85:417–23.
150. Mendelsohn FAO: Evidence for the local occurrence of angiotensin II in rat kidney and its modulation by dietary sodium intake and converting enzyme blockade. Clin Sci 1979;57:173–9.
151. Seikaly MG, Arant BS Jr, Seney FD Jr: Endogenous angiotensin concentrations in specific intrarenal fluid compartments in the rat. J Clin Invest 1990;86:1352–7.
152. Pratt RE, Zuo WM, Naftilan A, Ingelfinger JR, Dzau VJ. Altered sodium regulation of renal angiotensinogen in the spontaneously hypertensive rat. Am J Physiol 1989; 256:S 469–74.
153. Stanton RC, Brenner B. Role of kidney in congestive heart failure. Acta Med Scand 1986;707 (Suppl):21–5.
154. Hostetter TH, Pfeffer JM, Pfeffer MA, Dworkin LD, Braunwald E, Brenner BM. Cardiorenal hemodynamics and sodium excretion in rats with myocardial infarction. Am J Physiol 1983;245:H98–103.
155. Ichikawa I, Pfeffer JM, Pfeffer MA, Hostetter TH, Brenner BM. Role of angiotensin II in the altered renal function of congestive heart failure. Circ Res 1984;55:669–75.
156. Hodsman GP, Kohzuki M, Howes LG, Sumithran E, Tsunoda K, Johnston CI. Neurohormonal responses to chronic myocardial infarction in rats. Circulation 1988; 78:376–81.
157. Schunkert H, Hirsch AT, Mankadi S, Talsness C, Dzau VJ. Renal angiotensinogen gene expression in experimental heart failure: effect of angiotensin converting-enzyme inhibition. Clin Res 1989;37:584A.
158. Iwao H, Fukui K, Kim S, Nakayama K, Ohkubo H, Nakanishi S, Abe Y. Sodium balance effects on renin angiotensinogen and atrial natriuretic polypeptide mRNA levels. Am J Physiol 1988;255:E129–36.
159. Admiraal PJJ, Derkx FHM, Jan Danser AH, Pieterman H, Schalenkamp MADH. Metabolism and production of angiotensin I in different vascular beds in subjects with hypertension. Hypertension 1990;15:44–55.
160. Miyasaki M, Okunishi H, Okamura T, Toda N. Elevated vascular angiotensin converting enzyme in chronic two kidney, one clip hypertension in the dog. J Hypertens 1987;5:155–60.

161. Okamura T, Miyasaki M, Inagemi T, Toda N. Vascular renin angiotensin system in two-kidney, one clip hypertensive rates. Hypertension 1986;8:560–5.
162. Urata H, Healy B, Stewart RW, Bumpus FM, Husain A. Angiotensin II receptors in normal and failing human hearts. J Clin Endocrinol Metab 1989;69:54–66.
163. Douglas JG: Angiotensin receptor subtypes of the kidney cortex. Am J Physiol 1987;253:F2–7.
164. Belluci A, Wilkes BM. Mechanism of sodium modulation of glomerular angiotensin receptors in the rat. J Clin Invest 1984;74:1593–1600.
165. McQueen J, Semple PF. Cation dependent and cation independent stages in the regulation of the vascular angiotensin receptor after alteration of sodium balance in the rat. Endocrinology 1987;121:1256–64.
166. Swedberg K, Eneroth P, Kjekshus J, Wilhelmsen L. Hormones regulating cardiovascular function in patients with severe congestive heart failure and their relation to mortality. CONSENSUS Trial Study Group. Circulation 1990;82:1730–6.
167. Longnecker DI, Durcus MI, Donovan KR, Miller ED, Peach MJ. Saralasin dilates arterioles in SHR but not WKY rats. Hypertension 1984;1 (Suppl 1):106–10.
168. Simon ACH, Levenson JA, Bouther JI, Safar ME. Comparison of oral MK 421 and propranolol in mild to moderate hypertension and their effects on arterial and venous vessels of the forearm. Am J Cardiol 1984;53:781–3.
169. Dzau VJ, Safar MI. Large conduit arteries in hypertension; role of the vascular renin angiotensin system. Circulation 1988;77:947–54.
170. Koch-Weser J. Nature of the inotropic action of angiotensin on ventricular myocardium. Circ Res 1965;16:230–7.
171. Koch-Weser J. Myocardial actions of angiotensin II. Circ Res 1964;14:337–44.
172. Dempsey PJ, McCallum ZT, Kent, KM, Cooper T. Direct myocardial effects of angiotensin II. Am J Physiol 1971;220:477–81.
173. Freer R, Pappano A, Peach M, Bing K, McLean M, Vogel S, Sperelakis N. Mechanism for the positive inotropic effect of angiotensin II on isolated cardiac muscle. Circ Res 1976;39:178–83.
174. Urabe Y, Kent RL, Mann DL. The positive inotropic effect of angiotensin II is modulated by protein kinase C. Circulation 1990;82 (Suppl III):III 216.
175. Baker KM, Singer. Identification and characterization of guinea pig angiotensin II ventricular and atrial receptors: coupling to inositol phosphate production. Circ Res 1988;62:896–904. ;176. Saito K, Gutkind JS, Saavedra JM. Angiotensin II binding sites in the conduction system of rat hearts. Am J Physiol 1987;253:H1618-22.
177. van Gilst WH, deGraeff PA, Wessling H, deLangen CDJ. Reduction of reperfusion arrhythmias in the ischemic isolated rat heart by angiotensin converting enzyme inhibitors: a comparison of captopril, enalapril and HOE 498. J Cardiovasc Pharmacol 1987;9:254–5.
178. Naftilan AJ, Pratt RJ, Eldridge CS, Lin HL, Dzau VJ. Angiotensin II induces c-fos expression in smooth muscle via transcriptional control. Hypertension 1989;13:706–11.
179. Katoh Y, Komuro I, Shibasaki Y, Yamaguchi H, Yazaki Y. Angiotensin II induces hypertrophy and oncogene expression in cultured rat heart myocytes (abstr) Circulation 1989;80 (Suppl II):II–450.
180. Hall JE, Guyton AC, Smith MJ Jr, Coleman TG. Blood pressure and renal function during chronic changes in sodium intake; role of angiotensin. Am J Physiol 1980;239: F271–80.
181. Steele TH, Gottstein JH, Challoner-Hue L, Underwood JL. Actions of angiotensin II on the isolated spontaneously hypertensive rat kidney. Kidney Int 1982;21:466–70.
182. Schuster VL, Kokko JP, Jacobsen HR. Angiotensin II directly stimulates sodium transport in rabbit proximal convoluted tubules. J Clin Invest 1984;73:507–15.
183. Harris PJ, Navar LG. Tubular transport responses to angiotensin. Am J Physiol 1985;248:F621–30.

184. Liu FY, Cogan MG: Angiotensin II: a potent regulator of acidification in the rat early proximal convoluted tubule. J Clin Invest 1987;80:273–5.
185. Fyhrquist F, Forslund T, Tikkanen I, Gronhagen-Riska C. Induction of angiotensin I converting enzyme in rat lung with captopril (SQ 14225). Eur J Pharmacol 1980;67: 124–8.
186. Schunkert H, Hirsch AT, Pinto Y, Pelletier P, Jacob H, Remme WJ, Ingelfinger JR, Dzau VJ. Feedback regulation of angiotensin converting enzyme mRNA and activity by angiotensin II. Circulation 1990;82 (Suppl III):III–230.
187. Ziogas J, Story DF, Rand MJ. Effects of locally generated AII on noradrenergic transmission in guinea pig isolated atria. Eur J Pharmacol 1985;106:11–18.
188. Malik KU, Masjletti A. Facilitation of adrenergic transmission by locally generated angiotensin II in rat mesenteric arteries. Circ Res 1976;40(3):422–8.
189. Nakamura M, Jackson EK, Inagami T. Beta adrenoreceptor mediated release of angiotensin II from mesenteric arteries. Am J Physiol 1986;250:H144–8.
190. Starksen NF, Simpson PC, Bishopric N, Coughlin SR, Lee WMF, Escobedo JA, Williams LT. Cardiac myocyte hypertrophy is associated with c-myc protooncogene expression. Proc Natl Acad Sci USA 1986;83:8348–50.
191. Linz W, Scholkens BA, Han YF. Beneficial effects of the converting enzyme inhibitor, ramipril, in ischemic rat hearts. J Cardiovasc Pharm 1986;8 (Suppl 10):S91–9.
192. Ziang J, Linz W, Becker H, Ganten D, Lang RE, Schoelkens B, Unger T. Effects of converting enzyme inhibitors: ramipril and enalapril on peptide action and sympathetic neurotransmission in the isolated rat heart. Eur J Pharmacol 1984;113:215–23.
193. Dohi Y, Lüscher T. Angiotensin II causes endothelium dependent potentiation of contractions to norephinephrine in hypertensive rats: role of endothelin. Circulation 1990;82 (Suppl III):III 261.
194. Gimbrone RM, Alexander RW. Angiotensin II stimulation of prostaglandin production in cultured human vascular endothelium. Science 1975;189:219–20.
195. Toda N: Endothelium-dependent relaxation induced by angiotensin II and histamine in isolated arteries of dog. Br J Pharmacol 1984;81:301–7.
196. Yamaguchi K, Nishimura H. Angiotensin II-induced relaxation of fowl aorta. Am J Physiol 1988;255:R591–9.
197. Brooks VL, Keil LC, Reid IA. Role of the renin–angiotensin system in the control of vasopressin secretion in conscious dogs. Circ Res 1986;58:829–38.
198. Muller J, Lund EG, Hofstetter L, Brunner DB, Haldy P. Stimulation of aldostrone biosynthesis by sodium sequestration: role of angiotensin II. Am J Physiol 1982;243: E450–7.
199. Diz DI, Baer PG, Nasjletti A. Angiotensin II-induced hypertension in the rat. Effects on the plasma concentration, renal excretion, and tissue release of prostaglandins. J Clin Invest 1983;72:466–77.
200. Packer M. Interaction of prostaglandins and angiotensin II in the modulation of renal function in congestive heart failure. Circulation 1988;77 (Suppl):I64–73.
201. Pelayo JC, Ziegler MG, Blantz RC. Angiotensin II in adrenergic-induced alterations in glomerular hemodynamics. Am J Physiol 1984;247:F799–807.
202. Persson PB, Ehnke H, Kogler U, Kinchheim H. Modulation of natriuresis by sympathetic nerves and angiotensin II in conscious dogs. Am J Physiol 1989;256:F485–9.
203. Tucker BJ, Mundy CA, Maciejewski AR, Printz MP, Ziegler MG, Palayo JC, Blantz RC: Changes in glomerular hemodynamic response to angiotensin II after subacute renal denervation in rats. J Clin Invest 1986;78:680–8.
204. Cohn JN, Archibald DG, Ziesche S, Franciosa JA, Harston WE, Tristani FE, Dunkman WB, Jacobs W, Francis GS, Flohr KH, Goldman S, et al. Effect on vasodilator therapy on mortality in chronic congestive heart failure. Results of a Veterans Administration Cooperative Study (V-HeFT). N Engl J Med 1986;314:1547–52.

205. Svedberg K, Hjalmarson A, Waagstein F, Wallentin I. Prolongation of survival in congestive cardiomyopathy by beta receptor blockade. Lancet 1979,2:1374–6.
206. Packer M: Therapeutic options in the management of chronic heart failure. Is there a drug of first choice? Circulation 1989;79:198–204.
207. Hirsch AT, Talsness CE, Smith AD, Schunkert H, Ingelfinger JR. Captopril vs. enalapril: differential effects on tissue converting enzyme in experimental heart failure. Circulation 1990;82 (Suppl III):III-274.
208. Johnston CI, Fabris B, Yamada H, Mendelsohn FAO, Cubela R, Sivell D, Jackson B. Comparative studies of tissue inhibition by angiotensin converting enzyme inhibitors. J Hypertension 1989;7 (Suppl 5):S11–6.
209. Pfeffer MA, Pfeffer JM, Steinberg C, Finn P. Survival after an experimental myocardial infarction: beneficial effects of long-term therapy with captopril. Circulation 1985;72:406–12.
210. Cody RJ, Covit AB, Schaer GL, Laragh JH. Sodium and water balance in chronic congestive heart failure. J Clin Invest 1986;77:1441–52.
211. Cody RJ, Laragh JH. Use of captopril to estimate renin angiotensin aldosterone activity in pathophysiology of chronic heart failure. Am Heart J 1982;104:1184–8.
212. The MERCATOR Study Group. Does the new angiotensin converting enzyme inhibitor cilazapril prevent restenosis after percutaneous transluminal coronary angioplasty? Circulation 1992;86:100–110.
213. The SOLVD Investigators. Effect of enalapril in patients with reduced left ventricular ejection fractions and congestive heart failure. N Engl J Med 1991;325:293–032.
214. Cohn JN, Johnson G, Ziesche S, Cobb F et al. A comparison of enalapril with hydralazine-isosorbit dinitrate in the treatment of congestive heart failure. N Engl J Med 1991;325:303–310.

22

Calcium-Sensitizing Positive Inotropic Drugs

JOHANN CASPAR RÜEGG

University of Heidelberg
Heidelberg, Germany

R. JOHN SOLARO

University of Illinois College of Medicine at Chicago
Chicago, Illinois

I. INTRODUCTION

Rational approaches to the design of inotropic agents in one way or another involve myocardial Ca^{2+} metabolism. Normal changes in ventricular pressure and ejection during systole depend on an intracellular release of Ca^{2+} ions and a binding of Ca^{2+} to the myofilaments that promotes the reaction of myosin cross-bridges with the thin filaments (1,2). Diastolic events are, in turn, related complexly to removal of Ca^{2+} from the myofilaments and diminished cross-bridge activity. It is apparent that when hearts fail, mechanisms regulating intracellular Ca^{2+} are altered and there are associated defects in the processes by which the myofilaments are activated and relaxed. It is reasonable, therefore, that thinking about how one might pharmacologically restore cardiac function to levels compatible with alleviation of the symptoms of heart failure has focused on manipulation of Ca^{2+} delivery to the myofilaments. In fact, digitalis and related drugs, the most widely used agents for the treatment of heart failure, appear to work by increasing Ca^{2+} delivery to the myofilaments by an indirect action on intracellular Na^{+} levels. However, digitalis compounds are toxic and have a relatively narrow range of therapeutic concentrations. Thus there has been a search for a "digitalis substitute," and one avenue of approach has been the investigation of compounds that increase delivery of Ca^{2+} to the myofilaments, but that have a more satisfactory pharmacologic profile than digitalis (3–5). An example of new inotropic agents that apparently fit into this category are the phosphodiesterase inhibitors (6,7), which appear to work by elevating intracellular cAMP, thus mimicking the increases in Ca^{2+} flow to the myofilaments associated with adrenergic stimulation of the heart.

Although approaches involving an increase in Ca^{2+} flows to the myofilaments are important and proven, recent thinking (5,8) about the design of cardiotonic agents includes what might be considered a novel approach: mechanisms involving an altered response of the myofilaments to Ca^{2+}. The term *altered response* is used generically here to mean a change in level of free Ca^{2+} associated with 50% activation of myofilament activity (ATPase or tension) normalized to the maximum at saturating levels of free Ca^{2+}, a change in the shape of the pCa-normalized myofilament activity relation, a change in maximal activity, or a combination of these alterations. Here we will be mainly concerned with decreases in half-maximally activating free Ca^{2+}, which we refer to as Ca^{2+}-sensitization. Some agents with cardiotonic activity appear to have a Ca^{2+}-sensitizing effect as part of their mechanism of action (9,10), and there is convincing evidence that physiological alterations in inotropic state of the myocardium are associated with alterations in the response of myofilaments to Ca^{2+} (1,2).

Is it reasonable to target cardiac myofilaments for the action of inotropic agents? This is an important issue in the search for a digitalis substitute, and we consider this question here from the perspective of current knowledge of structure–function relations in the regulation of cardiac myofilament activity by Ca^{2+}. It is important to realize that drugs affecting the myofilament response to Ca^{2+} may act at the Ca^{2+}-receptor, troponin C (TNC), itself, or may affect downstream mechanisms of the Ca^{2+} signaling cascade. Many drugs having Ca^{2+}-sensitizing action have also been found to have other effects such as a calmodulin-antagonistic or phosphodiesterase (PDE)-inhibiting activity. We will also consider the advantage and importance of the Ca^{2+}-sensitizing principle compared with the more classic positive inotropic mechanisms.

II. CARDIAC MYOFILAMENT STRUCTURE/FUNCTION RELATIONS AND THE PRINCIPLE OF CALCIUM SENSITIZER ACTION

Figure 1 depicts a current concept of the basic functional unit of the cardiac myofilaments. In general, thick and thin filaments are similar among various stri-

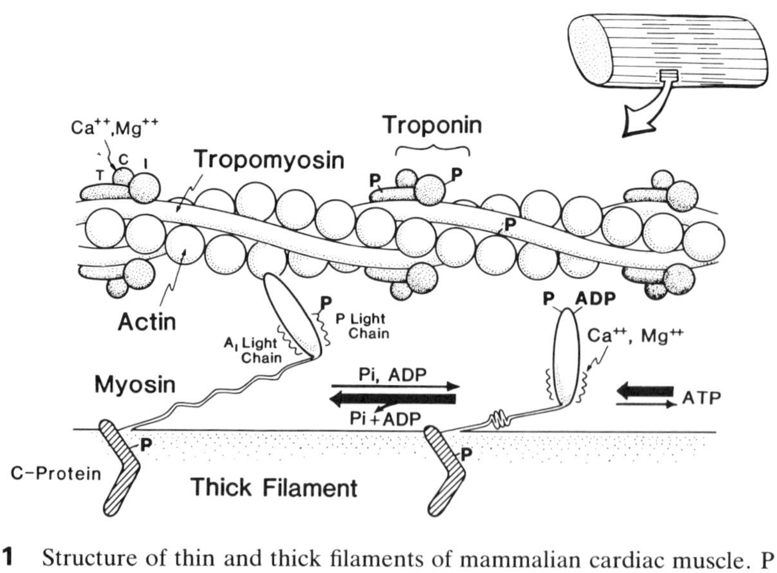

Figure 1 Structure of thin and thick filaments of mammalian cardiac muscle. P indicates sites of covalent phosphorylation.

ated muscles, and it is likely that the contractile process involves a similar, fundamental energy transduction process in which ATP hydrolysis is coupled to an actin–myosin reaction that impels the thin filaments toward the center of the sarcomere. Physiological regulation of the actin–myosin reaction in striated muscle depends on the presence of a set of thin-filament-associated proteins that contain troponin C (TNC), the receptor for Ca^{2+}; TnI, an inhibitory protein; and TnT-Tropomyosin, a set of proteins that together with TnI and TNC serve to transduce the intracellular Ca^{2+} signal into an increase in actin cofactor activity as an activator of myosin ATPase activity and cross-bridge cycling (1,2). In cellular Ca^{2+} concentrations associated with mechanical relaxation, it is believed that the TnI–TNC interaction is weak, and that the inhibitory action of TnI dominates the regulatory complex. When intracellular Ca^{2+} rises, Ca^{2+} binding to TNC promotes a relatively strong interaction between TNC and TnI, which overcomes the inhibitory activity of TnI. Exactly how activation of cross-bridge cycling occurs is the subject of controversy. There is evidence that the activation may involve steric factors associated with tropomyosin movement on the thin filament. However, there is also evidence that tropomyosin does not compete directly with cross-bridge attachment, but acts through an effect on one of the elementary kinetic steps in the hydrolysis of ATP. Activation may also depend on the light-chain components of myosin. It may well be that all three elements are important in the physiological regulation of contraction, and that various experimental approaches reveal different aspects of the process. In any case, it is apparent that when the inhibitory effect of troponin-I on tropomyosin–actin is abolished, the rate constant of cross-bridge attachment to actin (f) is enhanced whereas the apparent rate constant of cross-bridge detachment (g) is not affected (11).* In this way, force development and ATP splitting by actomyosin are stimulated by Ca^{2+} since they are proportional to the expression f/f+g and fg/f+g, respectively. The rate of force development (contractility or dP/dt) is likewise also increased since dP/dt depends on (f+g).

An important aspect of regulation of cardiac function is that force can be graded by increasing the myoplasmic free Ca^{2+} ion concentration, a maximum being reached at about 10^{-5}M. During basal activity, myoplasmic free Ca^{2+} apparently does not reach values above 10^{-6}M during systole (12). As a result Ca^{2+} bound to myofilament TNC is sufficient to induce less than half-maximal activation (13). Thus the heart has a large contractile reserve that might be exploited by applying drugs, such as dobutamine, digitalis, and PDE inhibitors, that increase the amount of Ca^{2+} released into the myoplasm. In principle, however, it should also be possible to develop agents that increase force by enhancing the sensitivity of the contractile proteins to Ca^{2+} ions rather than by increasing the Ca^{2+} ion concentration per se. Such agents have been called Ca^{2+} sensitizers (8).

A. Sulmazole: Prototype of Calcium Sensitizer Drugs

In investigating the mechanism of action of sulmazole (AR-L 115BS), Herzig and colleagues (3) were the first to identify explicitly a Ca^{2+} sensitizer action in a

*In a multistate cross-bridge model (strictly speaking), f is an apparent rate constant at which cross-bridges enter the strongly bound state, while g is the rate constant describing the transition from the strongly bound to the weakly bound cross-bridge state. Thus, f and g stand for the apparent rate constants f app. and g app. in the denotation of Brenner (11).

clinically utilized cardiotonic drug. To demonstrate the sensitizer effect, they used cardiac muscle fibers in which the cell membrane was removed by a "skinning" procedure. In this way conditions surrounding the myofilaments could be controlled. If the Ca^{2+} ion concentration in the bathing medium was raised to new steady-state levels in a cumulative manner, steady-state force increased in steps reaching a maximum at about 10^{-5}M. This procedure was repeated in the presence of AR-L 115BS and, at submaximally activating concentrations of Ca^{2+}, force was increased. Thus, the resulting Ca^{2+}–force relationship was shifted to the left of the control curve and half-maximal activity was achieved at a lower free Ca^{2+} ion concentration. Solaro and Rüegg (4) showed also that the relationship between myofibrillar Mg-dependent ATPase activity and free Ca^{2+} ion concentration is also shifted to the left by AR-L 115BS. Using the aequorin technique to measure Ca^{2+}-transients in intact muscle preparations, Blinks and Endoh (14) showed a similar effect of AR-L 115BS on myofilament Ca^{2+}-sensitivity. The relation between peak light (maximum Ca^{2+} in the twitch) and peak force (generated by varying the extracellular Ca^{2+} concentration) was shifted to the left by relatively low concentrations of AR-L 115BS.

B. Sensitizers May Alter Calcium Occupancy of TNC

The simplest hypothesis to account for the effects of AR-L 115BS on myofilament Ca^{2+}-sensitivity is that exposure to this drug increases the affinity of TNC for Ca^{2+}. Indeed, Solaro and Rüegg (4) were able to show that in the range of Ca^{2+} ion concentrations in which AR-L increased force there was also an increase in the amounts of Ca^{2+} bound to myofilament TNC. According to their concept, an increase in myofibrillar activity could be achieved simply by increasing the Ca^{2+} occupancy of TNC no matter whether this occurs with an increase in free Ca^{2+} ion concentration or with an increase in the affinity of TNC for Ca^{2+}.

Since the discovery of sulmazole as a Ca^{2+} sensitizer, many other drugs (discussed below) have been found to exert a Ca^{2+}-sensitizer action on myofibrils. One of these drugs, perhexiline, has also been shown to have a pronounced Ca^{2+}-sensitizer action on skinned fibers from skeletal muscle (15). As shown in Figure 2, this drug increases the force of skinned fibers simply by increasing the Ca^{2+} affinity of TNC; the unique relationship between Ca^{2+} occupancy of TNC and force production is not altered by the drug. In these experiments, Ca^{2+} occupancy of TNC was measured in skeletal muscle fibers (rabbit psoas rather than in the heart) by incorporating DANZ-labeled TNC into skinned fibers and measuring the Ca^{2+}-dependent fluorescence of the label as well as force under various experimental conditions, as described by Zot et al. (16). Troponin-C of cardiac muscle unlike fast skeletal muscle troponin-C has only one Ca^{2+} specific binding site, which is in equilibrium with free Ca^{2+}:

$$\begin{aligned} &Ca^{2+} + TNC \rightleftarrows Ca\text{-}TNC \\ &CaTNC = 1/K\,[Ca^{2+}]\,[TNC] \end{aligned} \qquad (1)$$

where K is the dissociation constant of the TNC–Ca^{2+} complex, that is, the ratio of the off-rate k_{-1}/on-rate k_{+1}. Although the dissociation constant of the Ca^{2+}-TNC complex is decreased by Ca^{2+}-sensitizer drugs, it is increased by cAMP-dependent

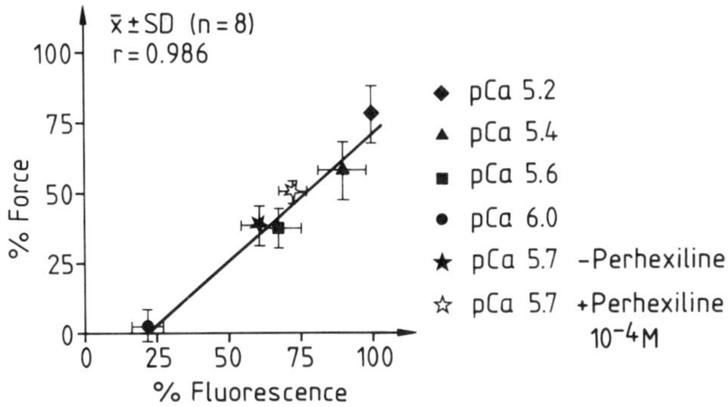

Figure 2 Relationship between apparent calcium occupancy of troponin-C (measured as DANZ-TNC fluorescence on the abscissa) and relative force of skinned psoas fibers in ATP salt solution. The calcium occupancy and force were increased by enhancing the free calcium ion concentration in the medium or by addition of perhexiline (10^{-4}M) at a given calcium ion concentration. The fluorescence of DANZ-labeled troponin-C incorporated into skinned psoas fibers was determined according to the method of Zot et al. (16). Note the correlation (r=0.98) of calcium-dependent force and DANZ fluorescence (at 460 nm) in skinned rabbit psoas fibers at various Ca^{2+} concentrations.

phosphorylation of troponin-I (17). These effects on the Ca^{2+} sensitivity are brought about by altering the Ca^{2+} off-rate constant (k_{-1}) rather than the on-rate, which is very high and diffusion limited. Consequently, phosphorylation of TNC by cAMP-dependent protein kinase would be expected to accelerate the process of Ca^{2+}-TNC dissociation and thus relaxation, whereas a Ca^{2+} sensitizer increasing Ca^{2+} affinity would retard these processes, thus prolonging the active state. As will be shown below, there is experimental evidence to support this idea (cf. also Fig. 3).

C. Calcium Sensitizers May Alter the Duration of Active State

We have assumed above that force development would depend on the Ca^{2+} occupancy of TNC at any one moment. Thus, force would be high as long as TNC is occupied by Ca^{2+}. Under these conditions, the thin filaments are "turned on" and reactive with myosin cross-bridges: muscle is in the "active state." It is important to realize, however, that, ultimately, force production depends not only on the degree of Ca^{2+} occupancy of TNC at any one moment but also on the duration of Ca^{2+} occupancy or the active state. This statement holds for skeletal muscle as well as cardiac muscle. In skeletal muscle, for example, Ca^{2+} occupancy reaches a maximum 20 msec after the onset of tetanic stimulation (18), while force continues to rise over a period of 50–100 msec. The reason for this discrepancy is that considerable time is required for cross-bridge attachment. It is clear, therefore, that in a twitch in which the Ca^{2+} transient and the time of Ca^{2+} occupancy is short, the force-generating process is interrupted long before it reaches a maximum. Twitch tension, therefore, is much smaller than tetanic twitch tension. It can be increased, however, when the active state is prolonged (e.g., after an intervention with twitch potentiators). One such twitch potentiator is sulmazole (19) which, as a Ca^{2+} sensitizer, slows down off rate for Ca^{2+} exchange with TNC, thereby prolonging the life time of the Ca^{2+}-TNC complex even though the Ca^{2+} transient is short. In this way, twitch force of skeletal muscle is increased by sulmazole whereas the tetanic tension is only slightly affected (19).

In cardiac muscle, there is also evidence that force depends on the duration of active state. Yue et al. (20) have shown that tetanic force is larger than twitch force although the steady Ca^{2+} concentration in the myoplasm, as determined by aequorin, may be similar to the peak of the Ca^{2+} transient. In other words, the apparent Ca^{2+} responsiveness is increased in tetanus, as compared with the twitch. A Ca^{2+} sensitizer such as sulmazole, which inhibits the Ca^{2+} off-rate for TNC and, therefore, prolongs the active state, would be expected to increase force. Yet it is important to realize that a Ca^{2+} sensitizer may have such a force-enhancing effect via prolonging the active state even if the Ca^{2+} occupancy of TNC were not increased. This is probably the case in the intact myocardiac cell where, unlike in skinned fibers, the amount of Ca^{2+} bound to TNC is limited by the amount of Ca^{2+} supplied by the sarcoplasmic reticulum to the contractile machinery. Thus, a Ca^{2+}-sensitizing twitch potentiator would increase the twitch force. However, since the Ca^{2+} occupancy of TNC may stay constant, the rate of force development would then not necessarily be increased, for reasons discussed below. This is why in the intact heart a "pure" Ca^{2+} sensitizer may not necessarily increase contractility, as determined by dP/dt. As discussed below, it may, therefore, be an advantage to combine the Ca^{2+} sensitizer action with other positive inotropic mechanisms, such as inhibition of PDE, which increases the Ca^{2+} delivery to the myofilaments.

D. Many Calcium Sensitizers Also Inhibit Phosphodiesterase

Many of the Ca^{2+} sensitizers such as pimobendan and sulmazole have, in addition to a Ca^{2+}-sensitizing action, an inhibitory effect on phosphodiesterase (PDE). The question, therefore, arises as to how much of the inotropic effect is due to PDE inhibition and how much to Ca^{2+}-sensitization. Associated with inhibition of PDE is an increase of intracellular cAMP, activation of cAMP-dependent protein kinase, and phosphorylation of substrates. Among these substrates for cAMP-dependent protein kinase are Ca^{2+}-channels of the sarcolemma, phospholamban in the sarcoplasmic reticulum (SR), and TNI and C-protein of the myofilaments. An important result of the phosphorylation is the increase in open probability of Ca^{2+}-channels, enhanced transsarcolemmal Ca^{2+}-movements, enhanced loading and release of Ca^{2+} from the SR, and thus increased release of Ca^{2+} to myofilament TNC.

An agent acting solely as a PDE-inhibitor could be expected to increase not only Ca^{2+}–TNC interaction but also the peak of the Ca^{2+}-transient. Figure 3 shows results comparing the effects of pimobendan, an inotropic agent with activity as a PDE-inhibitor and Ca^{2+}-sensitizer, with isoproterenol. Brenner (11) showed that a rise in Ca^{2+} occupancy of TNC enhances the probability of cross-bridge attachment in a force-generating state, that is, the rate constant f in the terminology of A.F. Huxley (21). However, the normalized rate of force production or cross-bridge attachment (dP/dt/P) will also be enhanced. This means that contractility is increased for the same reason that the rate constant of force development is probably related to the sum of apparent cross-bridge attachment and detachment rate constant (f+g), whereas steady-state force is proportional to f/f+g, according to Brenner's analysis (11).

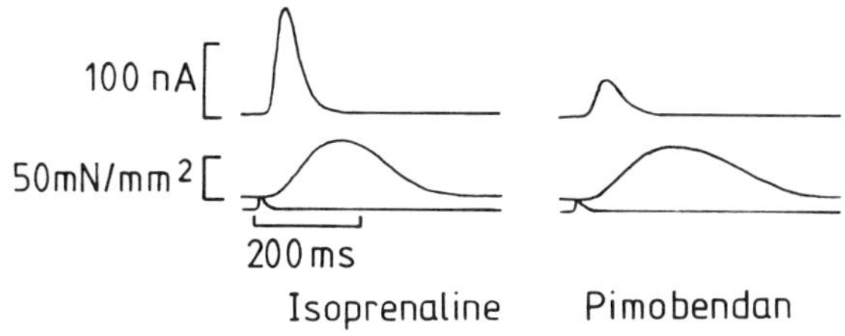

Figure 3 Twitch force and calcium transients determined by aequorin luminescence in ferret papillary muscle in the presence of isoprenaline (10^{-7}M) or pimobendan (20 μM). (Adapted from Ref. 48.)

As pointed out above, the Ca^{2+} occupancy of TNC is largely determined by the amount of Ca^{2+} released from the SR, since most of it appears to be bound to TNC. A drug with a "pure" Ca^{2+}-sensitizing action would, therefore, not be expected to increase Ca^{2+} occupancy of TNC and dP/dt in vivo, unless it had the additional effect of enhancing the rate constant f directly or causing the release of more Ca^{2+} from the SR. Although a "pure" Ca^{2+}-sensitizer may not increase contractility as determined by dP/dt, it would nevertheless increase force in heart muscle by prolonging the active state, as discussed above. In the intact heart, this effect would presumably increase the ejection fraction even without alteration in dP/dt. If, however, a Ca^{2+}-sensitizing drug also had PDE-inhibiting activity, Ca^{2+} release from the SR and thus Ca^{2+} binding to TNC would be increased. Thus, contractility "dP/dt" would be enhanced essentially via a cAMP-dependent mechanism. What then would, under these circumstances, be the competitive advantage of such a drug?

Consider that the Ca^{2+}–TNC complex is in equilibrium with TNC and Ca^{2+} (Eq. 1). The free Ca^{2+} ion concentration is, therefore, proportional to the Ca^{2+} occupancy and the dissociation constant. Any increase in the occupancy of TNC by Ca^{2+} supplied by the SR would, therefore, necessarily cause a dramatic increase in the free Ca^{2+} ion concentration, unless the dissociation constant were, at the same time, decreased. By raising the affinity of TNC for Ca^{2+}, the disadvantages of high intracellular free Ca^{2+} ion levels causing Ca^{2+} overload could be avoided. This goal may be achieved by a drug, which, on the one hand, promotes an increased Ca^{2+} release of Ca^{2+} from the SR, thereby increasing the Ca^{2+} occupancy of TNC, but which, on the other hand, also reduces the dissociation constant of the Ca^{2+}–TNC complex. For this reason positive inotropic drugs that combine a PDE-inhibitory action with a Ca^{2+}-sensitizing action may be more useful and safer than drugs that are solely PDE inhibitory. Such drugs, unlike "pure Ca^{2+} sensitizers," would increase contractility, but, in contrast to a pure PDE-inhibitor or β-agonist, this increase in contractility would not be offset by a greatly increased free Ca^{2+} ion concentration. On the contrary, as shown in Figure 3, a given force would be achieved at a lower level of free Ca^{2+} than in the presence of a drug that acts solely by raising the cyclic AMP level. In the experiment shown in Figure 3, the Ca^{2+} transients of ferret papillary muscle were determined by aequorin luminescence after increasing contractility with either isoproterenol, which acts solely by raising the cAMP level, or by pimobendan, which is a phosphodiesterase inhibitor as well as a Ca^{2+}-sensitizer.

E. Contractile and Regulatory Proteins as Targets of Drug Action

The site(s) of action of Ca^{2+}-sensitizer drugs is (are) far from being clear, and may involve multiple, diverse domains on the thin and thick filaments. In principle, all of the subunits of troponin as well as actin and myosin may be target sites. Specific interactions among all these proteins have been shown to be involved in Ca^{2+} activation of the contractile machinery. Thus, Ca^{2+}-binding to TNC strengthens the interaction between TNC and TNI whereas the TNI–actin interaction is weakened. However, the reverse is also true. If TNI interacts with TNC, the Ca^{2+} affinity of the latter increases, but it is reduced again if actin is permitted to interact with TNI. It is possible that drugs binding to sites remote from TNC itself may affect protein interactions and thus would also modulate Ca^{2+} sensitivity. Some compounds with Ca^{2+}-sensitizing action, such as trifluoperazine, seem to bind to TNC directly. The binding domain is the stretch of the peptide chain lying between the upper helical domain containing the low-affinity binding sites and the domain containing the high-affinity Ca^{2+}–Mg^{2+} sites. Binding is assumed to change the conformation of TNC, thereby altering the Ca^{2+} affinity of the EF-hand structure involved in Ca^{2+} binding. Since many of the Ca^{2+}-sensitizer drugs have a PDE-III inhibitory action, or a calmodulin antagonistic effect in addition to binding to TNC, the question arises as to whether all these proteins contain a common structural domain recognized by the drug.

The interaction between TNI and TNC seems to be particularly important for Ca^{2+} sensitivity. El-Saleh and Solaro (22) have shown, for example, that the effect of acidic pH to inhibit Ca^{2+}-activated ATPase activity of myofibrils is related to an inhibition of the TNI–TNC interaction as well as to a direct effect of protons on TNC Ca^{2+}-binding. The interaction between TNI and TNC involves the amino acid residues 89–100 of TNC and 104–115 of TNI. Synthetic peptides, which contain the corresponding sequence of TnI, therefore, compete with this protein for the complementary recognition site on TNC, thereby inhibiting TnI–TNC interaction and Ca^{2+} activation. This inhibition has been demonstrated directly in circular dichroism studies investigating the effect of a synthetic peptide of TNC-TnI interaction in vitro (23). The peptides have also been found to inhibit the Ca^{2+}-induced force production of skinned cardiac and skeletal muscle fibers in a Ca^{2+}-dependent manner. Thus the Ca^{2+}–force relationship is shifted towards higher Ca^{2+} concentration (to the right). On the other hand, peptides containing the sequence 1–40 of actin, which is thought to interact with TNI, apparently inhibit TNI–actin interaction. In any case, these peptides increase Ca^{2+} sensitivity of skinned fibers. Peptides affecting actin–myosin interaction might also influence Ca^{2+} responsiveness, since the attachment of cross-bridges to actin has been found to increase the Ca^{2+}-activated force and Ca^{2+}-binding to TNC (13). The interaction of actin and myosin depends on the rate constants f (attachment rate constant) and g (detachment rate constant), inasmuch as the extent of interaction (the number of cross-bridges attached at any one time) is proportional to $f/f+g$. As a consequence, an increase in actin–myosin interaction associated with a concomitant increase in force could be due either to an increase in the rate constant f or to a decrease in the rate constant g. Since peptides having the amino acid sequence 700–740 of myosin (23) have been found to affect Ca^{2+} responsiveness of skinned fibers, it would seem that this domain of myosin is very important in determining the apparent Ca^{2+} sensitivity. This stretch of the peptide chain may be implicated in the regulation of Ca^{2+} sensitivity when cycling cross-bridges interact with actin or when regulatory myosin light chains become phosphorylated (23).

Indeed, the phosphorylation of the regulatory light chain increases the rate constant of cross-bridge attachment (f) at a given Ca^{2+} ion concentration and, therefore, Ca^{2+} sensitivity (24; private communication). Since the contractility parameter dP/dt depends on the sum of the rate constants f and g, it is clear that phosphorylation of light chains could also be an important principle of increasing contractility. Drugs that increase phosphorylation by inhibiting phosphatase or by activating myosin light chain kinase would be expected to have a cardiotonic effect.

After having discussed some general principles of the possible effects and modes of action of drugs acting on myofilament, we now compare the basic pharmacologic properties of some Ca^{2+}-sensitizing drugs that are currently being developed.

III. BASIC PHARMACOLOGY OF CALCIUM-SENSITIZING DRUGS

Several compounds structurally related to sulmazole were synthesized and had a positive inotropic action that combined Ca^{2+} sensitizer effects with the capacity to increase the availability of Ca^{2+} in the myocardium (5). These compounds will be discussed here in relation to sulmazole.

A. Sulmazole

As already described, sulmazole (AR-L 115 BS, Thomae, Biberach/Riss, Germany) is the first compound suggested to act directly on the contractile proteins by increasing the Ca^{2+} sensitivity (3,4). However, other mechanisms have also been discussed. Thus, sulmazole is said to enhance the open probability of Ca^{2+} release channels in the sarcoplasmic reticulum (25), and it may increase cyclic AMP levels. The latter effect may be mediated via an increase in adenylate cyclase activity due to an antagonism with adenosine receptors and/or the inhibitory G-protein (26) or by inhibiting phosphodiesterase, type 3. The concentrations required to inhibit the latter enzyme, however, are much larger than those required for the positive inotropic effect (27). Furthermore, although while (+) and (−) isomers of sulmazole are equipotent in their phosphodiesterase inhibitory effect, only the (+) enantiomere has significant Ca^{2+} sensitizer action on the contractile proteins in vitro and a positive inotropic effect (28). On the other hand, the vasodilator effect showed no stereoselectivity. A Ca^{2+}-sensitizing effect has also been demonstrated in intact cardiac muscle by experiments in which sulmazole produced a leftward shift in the relationship between force and myoplasmic free Ca^{2+} (29). In closed-chest dogs, this drug given at a dosage of 1 mg/kg body weight increased the dP/dt_{max} without increasing the heart rate and myocardial oxygen consumption, while reducing the peripheral resistance (30,31). However, the further development of this promising drug had to be discontinued when it was found to have toxic effects. A related compound is pimobendan (UDCG 115 BS), which, in the liver, is rapidly metabolized into UDCG 212 (see below).

B. Adibendan

Adibendan (Boehringer Mannheim, Germany) has a strong positive inotropic effect in anesthetized rats and cats as well as in conscious dogs. It increases the cardiac output and stroke volume, and lowers peripheral resistance. Left ventricular dP/dt is also increased as well as the force of isolated papillary muscle (32). These effects are at least partly mediated by an increase in cellular cyclic AMP levels, thereby causing an increase in the slow inward current (33). The increase in cyclic AMP levels is due to an inhibition of phosphodiesterase, the half maximal effect being about 1 μm (34). In skinned cardiac muscle fibers, the Ca^{2+}-activated force was also increased by 100 μm adibendan (35). Adibendan is a positive inotropic and vasorelaxing agent, which effects are associated with an increase in cyclic AMP rather than with a Ca^{2+}-sensitizing effect on the myofibril. Because of this agent's toxic effects, clinical tests (36) had to be discontinued.

C. EMD 53998

EMD 53998 (Merck, Darmstadt, Germany) is a thiadiazinone derivative with pronounced positive inotropic action. In micromolar and submicromolar concentrations, it increases the force of skinned cardiac muscle fibers and lowers the EC_{50} for Ca^{2+} by as much as 1.5–1 pCa units (observations by Merck). In isolated myocytes, it stimulates shortening without increasing the Ca^{2+} transient and it shifts the relationship between twitch shortening and free Ca^{2+} level to the left, that is, towards a lower Ca^{2+} ion concentration (37). In ferret papillary muscle, twitch force is likewise approximately doubled by 10 μM EMD, while the aequorin Ca^{2+} transients remain unaffected or are only slightly decreased (38). Thus, the increase in twitch force may be ascribed to the increase in Ca^{2+} sensitivity of the myofilaments rather than to an inhibition of phosphodiesterase-3, which has also been observed (Merck Pharmaceuticals). The kinetics of the Ca^{2+} transients and of the twitch contraction are not affected (Fig. 4). The latter effect suggests that the compound does not act by lowering the Ca^{2+} off-rate from TNC or the apparent detachment rate constant g of cross-bridges.

D. MCI 154

MCI (Mitsubishi Kasai, Japan) is one of the most potent new cardiotonic agents with a pronounced Ca^{2+} sensitizing action on the myofibrils in vitro. It is a pyridazonone derivative, which has a nonsympathomimetic and nonglycosidic action, and increases dP/dt_{max} in anesthetized open-chest dogs, while reducing atrial

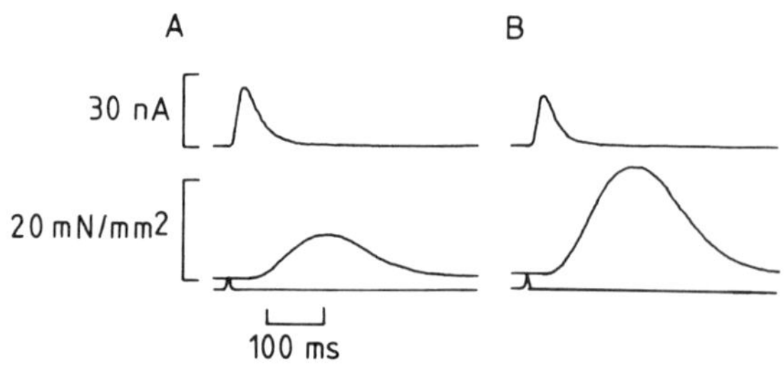

Figure 4 Twitch force and calcium transients determined with aequorin luminescence in ferret papillary muscle in the absence (A) and presence (B) of EMD 53998 (10 μM). (Adapted from Ref. 38.)

pressure and total peripheral resistance. Furthermore, it improves cardiac function in dogs with experimental heart failure induced by either verapamil and/or propanolol (39), after pentobarbital-induced heart failure (40), or during reperfusion injury (41). Kitada et al. (42) demonstrated a very pronounced sensitizing action of Ca^{2+} on skinned cardiac muscle fibers with 1–10 μM MCI 154, the shift of the Ca^{2+} force relationship being approximately 0.2 pCa units. At a given submaximal Ca^{2+} ion concentration, force was increased by up to 300% with 100 μmol MCI (42). These pronounced effects of MCI on Ca^{2+} sensitivity could, however, not be confirmed by Sellin et al. (43), who also reported an inhibitory effect of MCI on phosphodiesterase type 3, thus postulating the action via cyclic AMP.

E. Pimobendan

This drug is a congener of AR-L 115BS and is a benzimidazole–pyridazinone derivative with potent cardiotonic and vasodilatory activity (44). A major metabolite of the agent is UD-CG 212, which also has these activities (45). The mechanism of action of the parent compound and the metabolite appear to be different, however. Both are PDE inhibitors and thus elevate cAMP concentrations, yet pimobendan has activity as a Ca^{2+} sensitizer (46,10) and UD-CG 212 apparently does not. ATP hydrolysis and force of skinned fiber preparations at submaximally activating concentrations of Ca^{2+} were both stimulated by pimobendan in a dose-dependent manner (10). Fujino et al. (47) showed that this effect of pimobendan on myofilament Ca^{2+} sensitivity is related to a stereo-specific effect on Ca^{2+} binding to myofilament TNC. The Ca^{2+}-sensitizing action could also be demonstrated in the intact muscle. Honerjager et al. (7) and Fujino et al. (10) showed that treatment of partially depolarized muscle preparations with pimobendan caused an increase in force, with little or no effect on the "slow" action potentials that reflect activity of the Ca^{2+} channels. Moreover, it was shown that pimobendan caused a further elevation of force with no effect on contours of the action potential when added to these preparations maximally stimulated with isoproterenol. Studies on papillary muscle preparations microinjected with aequorin for determination of intracellular Ca^{2+} transients have revealed some interesting aspects of the effects of pimobendan in situ. Lee et al. (48) reported that although pimobendan increased force of skinned fibers, addition of this agent to intact preparations resulted in an increase in force accompanied by an increase in the Ca^{2+} transient. Relations between the peak of the light transient and the force transient generated by varying the extracellular Ca^{2+} were unaffected by pimobendan. Studies comparing the effect of pimobendan with isoproterenol indicated that the sensitizing effect was masked by the desensitization that occurs with an increase in cAMP concentration due to PDE inhibition. Convincing evidence that the effect of pimobendan on contractility involved Ca^{2+} sensitization came from comparison of the effects of pimobendan and isoproterenol on twitch dynamics and the Ca^{2+} transient. In the case of isoproterenol the increase in cAMP is associated with an abbreviation and increase in peak of the both force and the Ca^{2+} transient. In the case of the positive inotropic effect of pimobendan, there was an increase in peak and abbreviation of the Ca^{2+} transient, but the twitch was prolonged, as expected from an agent that would enhance Ca^{2+} binding to TNC by depressing the off rate for Ca^{2+} exchange, as predicted by the work of Fujino et al. (10).

F. Isomazole

Isomazole is another compound structurally related to sulmazole that increases cardiac contractility and decreases peripheral resistance (49). This effect seems to be mediated at least in part through a cyclic cAMP-dependent mechanism, since this compound inhibits phosphodiesterase type III (7). In addition, however, isomazole causes a further increase in contractility in concentrations higher than those required for completely inhibiting phosphodiesterase. Thus, isomazole seems to have additional mechanisms that are not mediated via cyclic AMP. Indeed, experiments with skinned cardiac muscle fibers have demonstrated an increase in Ca^{2+} responsiveness of these preparations (50). These latter studies also demonstrated interesting species differences. Thus, the Ca^{2+}–force relationships were different in skinned fibers from rat, guinea pig, and human heart, and the effects of the drugs were largest on skinned fibers from guinea pig papillary muscles. In these preparations, the dose–response relationship were similar to those in the living papillary muscle (50).

G. APP 201-533

APP 201-533 (3-amino-6-methyl-5-phenyl-2(1H)-pyridinone; Sandoz AG, Basel, Switzerland) was also one of the earlier compounds to demonstrate pharmacologic actions as a positive inotropic agent with direct effects on Ca^{2+} sensitivity of cardiac myofilaments. APP 201-533 increased dp/dt in several species with an associated mild increase in heart rate (51). These effects were dose-dependent and unchanged when measured in the presence of alpha, beta, or histamine receptor blockers. In guinea pig ventricular muscle, APP 201-533 had no effect on parameters of the normal action potential. Moreover APP 201-533 had no effect on myocardial Na/K ATPase activity (52). Although its action as an inhibitor of cAMP phosphodiesterase had a relatively high IC_{50}, this activity may be related to the inotropic effect. Yet APP 201-533 was shown to be equipotent to amrinone, a more potent PDE inhibitor, in its inotropic effect. This suggests a mechanism different from pure PDE inhibition. In studies with isolated myofibrils and skinned fibers from heart muscle, APP 201-533 increased submaximal Ca^{2+}-dependent force and ATPase activity and increased Ca^{2+}-binding to myofibrillar TNC (52,53). It is interesting that the effect of APP 201-533 on force did not occur in parallel with an increase of ATP hydrolysis and it is apparent that APP 201-533 may increase the efficiency of chemomechanical transduction process by an as yet unexplained mechanism (51).

H. DPI 201-106

DPI (Sandoz AG, Switzerland) is a piperazinyl-indole and a novel cardioactive agent that combines a cAMP-independent positive inotropic effect with negative chronotropy and vasodilatory properties. DPI does not change the cAMP levels in the heart, nor does it inhibit phosphodiesterase activity. It does, however, increase the duration of the action potential in papillary muscle and the Ca^{2+} sensitivity of skinned cardiac fibers (54). As with APP-201-533 (9), the myofibrillar ATPase was little affected by the compound. Most interesting was that in skinned fibers of ventricles from cardiomyopathic patients, Ca^{2+} sensitivity is also increased by 1 μmol DPI whereas this compound had little effect on the Ca^{2+} responsiveness of skinned fibers from control human hearts (55). These authors also found an increase in Ca^{2+} responsiveness in intact human papillary muscle following treatment with DPI. The increase in Ca^{2+} sensitivity may contribute to a positive inotropic action of this compound. However, an increase in the availability of intracellular free Ca^{2+} may also be of importance. Thus, the positive inotropic effect of DPI may also be induced via an increase in intracellular sodium concentration (56), caused by a prolongation of the open time of sodium channels (57) and prolongation of the action potential (54).

In summary, then, all the compounds described so far are not pure Ca^{2+} sensitizers acting only by an increase in the sensitivity of the contractile proteins to Ca^{2+}, but they also have other effects that increase the availability of Ca^{2+}. These include effects on intracellular free sodium and the inhibition of phosphodiesterase III.

IV. CONCLUSIONS

Cardiac contractile force may be elevated by increasing the amount of Ca^{2+} released by the SR and delivered to the myofilaments, for instance, by PDE inhibitors. Some PDE inhibitors also have a Ca^{2+}-sensitizing action, that is, they lower the dissociation constant of the Ca^{2+}–TNC complex. Because of this effect, the advantage of increased Ca^{2+} occupancy and force production is not offset by the disadvantage of increasing the free Ca^{2+} ion concentration, since the latter is related not only to the Ca^{2+} occupancy of TNC but also to the dissociation constant of the Ca^{2+}–TNC complex. The decrease of the dissociation constant of the Ca^{2+}–TNC complex is most likely related to a decrease in the "off-rate constant" for Ca^{2+} exchange. This means that in a twitch contraction, Ca^{2+} occupancy of TNC would be prolonged, an effect that might itself increase force production. In addition to these effects mediated by manipulating the Ca^{2+} occupancy of TNC, Ca^{2+} responsiveness might also be influenced by drugs that affect the other subunits of troponin or the contractile system. Such drugs might enhance contractile responses either by increasing the cross-bridge rate constant f or by decreasing the rate constant g. We propose that drugs that, in addition to inhibiting PDE, also have a Ca^{2+}-sensitizer action, are better suited for the treatment of cardiac failure than pure PDE inhibitors, since they would avoid a Ca^{2+} overload of the heart.

ACKNOWLEDGMENTS

Work described here was supported in part by the Deutsche Forschungsgemeinschaft, the Fonde fúr Chemie, and by National Institutes of Health Grants R01 HL 22231 and P01 HL 22619 (III B).

REFERENCES

1. Rüegg JC. In: Calcium in muscle contraction, 2nd ed. Berlin/Heidelberg: Springer-Verlag, 1992: 165–199; 268–285.
2. Solaro RJ, Pan B-S. Control and modulation of contractile activity of cardiac myofilaments. In: Sperelakis N, ed. Physiology and pathophysiology of the heart, 2nd ed. Kluwer Academic Publishers, 1988: 291–303.
3. Herzig JW, Feile K, Rüegg JC. Activating effects of AR-L 115 BS on the Ca^{2+} sensitive

force, stiffness and unloaded shortening velocity (V_{max}) in isolated contractile structures from mammalian heart muscle. Arzneim Forsch/Drug Res 1981; 31:188–91.
4. Solaro RJ, Rüegg JC. Stimulation of Ca^{2+} binding and ATPase activity of dog cardiac myofibrils by AR-L 115 BS, a novel cardiotonic agent. Circ Res 1982; 51:290–4.
5. Wetzel B, Hauel N. New cardiotonic agents—promising approach for treatment of heart failure. TIPS 1988; 9:166–70.
6. Alousi AA, Canter JM, Montenaro MJ, Fort DJ, Ferrari RA. Cardiotonic activity of milrinone, an new and potent cardiac bipyridine on the normal and failing heart of experimental animals. J Cardiovasc Pharmacol 1983; 5:792–803.
7. Honerjäger P, Heiss A, Schäfer-Korting M, Schönsteiner G, Reiter M. UD-CG 115—a cardiotonic pyridazinone which elevates cyclic AMP and prolongs the action potential in guinea-pig papillary muscle. Naunyn Schmiedebergs Arch Pharmacol 1984; 325:259–69.
8. Colucci WS, Wright RF, Braunwald E. New positive inotropic agents in the treatment of congestive heart failure. Mechanisms of action and recent clinical developments. N Engl J Med 1986; 314:290–358.
9. Herzig JW, Bormann G, Botelho L, Erdmann E, Salzmann R, Solaro RJ. App 201-533, a novel cardiotonic agent: increase in Ca^{++} sensitivity and economization of the myocardial contractile process. J Mol Cell Cardiol 1983; 15 (Suppl 1):244.
10. Fujino K, Sperelakis N, Solaro RJ. Sensitization of dog and guinea pig cardiac myofilaments to Ca^{2+}-activation and the inotropic effect of pimobendan: Comparison with milrinone. Circ Res 1988; 63:911–22.
11. Brenner B. Effect of Ca^{2+} on cross-bridge turnover kinetics in skinned single rabbit psoas fibers. Proc Natl Acad Sci 1988; 85:3265–9.
12. Fabiato A. Myoplasmic free calcium concentration reached during the twitch of an intact isolated cardiac cell and during calcium-induced release of calcium from the sarcoplasmic reticulum of a skinned cardiac cell from the adult rat or rabbit ventricle. J Gen Physiol 1981; 78:457–97.
13. Pan B-S, Solaro RJ. Calcium binding properties of troponin C in detergent skinned heart muscle fibers. J Biol Chem 1987; 262:7339–49.
14. Blinks JR, Endoh M. Sulmazole (AR-L 115 BS) alters the relation between Ca^{2+} and tension in living canine ventricular muscle. J Physiol 1984; 353:63.
15. Silver PJ, Dachiw J, Ambrose JM, Pinto PB. Effects of calcium antagonists perhexiline and cinnarizine on vascular and cardiac contractile protein function. J Pharmacol Exp Ther 1985; 234:629–33.
16. Zot HG, Güth K, Potter JD. Fast skeletal muscle skinned fibers and myofibrils reconstituted with N-terminal fluorescent analogues of troponin C. J Biol Chem 1986; 261: 15883–90.
17. Solaro RJ, Robertson SP, Johnson JD, Holroyde MJ, Potter JD. Troponin-I phosphorylation: a unique regulator of the amounts of calcium required to activate cardiac myofibrils. Cold Spring Harb Conf Cell Prolif 1981; 8:901–11.
18. Kress M, Huxley HE, Faruqi AR, Hendrix J. Structural changes during activation of frog muscle studied by time-resolved X-ray diffraction. J Mol Biol 1986; 188:325–42.
19. Cecchi G, Lombardi V, Menchetti G. Development of force–velocity relation and rise of isometric tetanic tension measure the time course of different processes. Pflügers Arch 1984; 401:396–401.
20. Yue PT, Marban E, Weir WG. Relationship between force and intracellular $[Ca^{2+}]$ in tetanized mammalian heart muscle. J Gen Physiol 1986; 87:223–42.
21. Huxley AF. Muscle structure and theories of contraction. Prog Biophys Chem 1957; 7:255–318.
22. El-Saleh S, Solaro RJ. Troponin I enhances acidic pH induced depression of Ca-binding to the regulatory sites in skeletal troponin C J Biol Chem 1988; 263:3274–8.
23. Rüegg JC, Zeugner C, Van Eyk JE, Hodges RS, Trayer IP. Myosin and troponin

peptides affect calcium sensitivity of skinned muscle fibres. In: Rüegg JC, ed. Peptides as probes in muscle research, Springer, Berlin Heidelberg, New York, 1991; pp 95–110.
24. Morano I, Hofmann F, Zimmer F, Rüegg JC. The influence of P-light chain phosphorylation by myosin light chain kinase on the calcium sensitivity of chemically skinned heart fibres. FEBS Lett 1985; 189:221–4.
25. Ashley RH, and Williams AJ. Activation of the sheep cardiac muscle sarcoplasmic reticulum membrane Ca^{2+} channel by AR-L 115 (sulmazole). J Physiol (Lond) 1988; 406:213.
26. Parsons WJ, Ramkumar V, Stiles GL. The new cardiotonic agent sulmazole is an A_1 adenosine receptor antagonist and functionally blocks the inhibitory regulator, G_1. Mol Pharmacol 1988; 33:441–8.
27. Bristol JA, Sircar J, Moos WH, Evans DB, Weishaar RE. Cardiotonic agents. 1. 4,5-dihydro-6-(4-(1H-imidazol-1-yl)phenyl)-3(2H)-pydridazinones: novel positive inotropic agents for the treatment of congestive heart failure. J Med Chem 1984; 27:1099–01.
28. von Meel JCA, Zimmermann R, Diederen W, Erdmann E, Mrwa U. Increase in calcium sensitivity of cardiac myofibrils contributes to the cardiotonic action of sulmazole. Biochem Pharmacol 1988; 37:213–20.
29. Endoh M, Yanagisawa T, Taira N, Blinks JR. Effects of new inotropic agents on cyclic nucleotide metabolism and calcium transients in canine ventricular muscle. Circulation 1986; 73(Suppl III):117–33.
30. Dämmgen J, Kadatz R, Diederen W. Action of AR-L 115 BS on myocardial oxygen consumption, cardiac performance and vascular resistance capacitance. Arzneim-Forsch/Drug Res 1981; 31:151–4.
31. Hellige G, Baller D, Ensink FBM, Zipfel J, Wolpers HG, Bretschneider HJ. Effects of AR-L 115 BS on hemodynamics, myocardial oxygen consumption and cardiac pumping efficiency. Arzneim-Forsch/Drug Res 1981; 31:155–6.
32. Müller-Beckmann B, Freund P, Honerjäger P, Kling L, Rüegg JC. In vitro investigations on a new positive inotropic vasodilating agent (BM 14.478) that increases myocardial cyclic AMP content and myofibrillar calcium sensitivity. J Cardiovasc Pharmacol 1988; 11:8–16.
33. Müller-Beckmann B, Sponer G, Strein K, Bartsch W. Hemodynamic profile of BM 14.478: a new positive inotropic and vasodilating agent. J Cardiovasc Pharmacol 1988; 11:1–7.
34. Bethke T, Brunkhorst D, V der Leyen H, Meyer W, Nigbur R, Scholz H. Mechanism of action and cardiotonic activity of a new phosphodiesterase inhibitor, the benzimidazole derivative adibendan (BM 14.478), in guinea-pig hearts. Naunyn-Schmiedebergs Arch Pharmacol 1988; 337:576–82.
35. Rüegg JC, Morano I. Calcium-sensitivity modulation of cardiac myofibrillar proteins. J Cardiovasc Pharmacol 1989; 14 (Suppl 3):S20–3.
36. Neugebauer G, Akpan W, Hagena C, v Möllendorf E, Schröter E. Hemodynamic effects of the new positive inotrope adbendan after oral administration in healthy subjects. Br J Clin Pharmacol 1988; 25:655.
37. Ferroni C, Spurgeon HA, Klockow M, Lakatta EG, Capogrossi MC. Contractile potentiation without increasing cytosolic calcium in single rat ventricular myocytes. 1989; FASEB, in press.
38. Allen DG, Lee JA. EMD 53998 increases tension with little effect on the ampitude of calcium transients in isolated ferret ventricular muscle. J Physiol 1989; 416: 43P.
39. Narimatsu A, Kitada Y, Satoh N, Suzuki R, Okushima H. Cardiovascular pharmacology of 6-(4-(4′-pyridyl)aminophenyl)-4,5-ihydro-3(2H)-pyridazinone hydrochloride, a novel and potent cardiotonic agent with vasodilator properties. Arzneim-Forsch/Drug Res 1987; 37:398–9.
40. Satoh K, Nunoki K, Goto T, Hosono M, Hashimoto H, Sato Y, Taira N. Improvement

of pentobarbital-induced heart failure by MCI-154, a novel and potent cardiotonic agent, in the dog heart-lung preparation. Jpn J Pharmacol 1988; 47:189–95.
41. Wynsen JC, Shimshak TM, Preuss KC, Gross GJ, Brooks HL, Warltier DC. Stimulation of myocardium during reperfusion injury by a new inotrope-vasodilator agent, MCI-154. Fundam Clin Pharmacol 1987; 1:335–45.
42. Kitada Y, Narimatsu A, Matsumura N, Endo M. Increase in Ca^{++} sensitivity of the contractile system by MCI-154, a novel cardiotonic agent, in chemically skinned fibers from the guinea pig papillary muscles. Eur J Pharmacol 1987; 134:229–31.
43. Sellin LC, Alajoutsijärvi A, Törnquist K, Fraser M, Pippuri A, Ojala I. Inhibition of cardiac phosphodiesterase III by the novel cardiotonic agent 6-(4-(4′-pyridyl)aminophenyl)-4,5-dihydro-3(2H)-pyridazinone hydrochloride. Arzneim-Forsch/Drug Res 1988; 38:1787.
44. von Meel JCA. Cardiovascular effects of the positive inotropic agents pimobendan and sulmazole in vivo. Arzneim-Forsch/Drug Res 1984; 35:284–8.
45. Kitzen JM, Winbury MM. Pimobendan Cardiovasc Drug Rev 1989; 6:265–91.
46. Rüegg JC, Pfitzer G, Eubler D, Zeugner C. Effect on contractility of skinned fibers from mammalian heart and smooth muscle by a new benzimidazole derivative, 4,5-dihdro-6-[2-(4-methoxyphenyl)-1H-benzimidazol-5-yl]-5-methyl-3 (2H)=pyridazinone. Arzneim-Forsch/Drug Res 1984; 34:1736–8.
47. Fujino K, Sperelakis N, Solaro RJ. Differential effects of stereoisomers of pimobendane on myofibrillar Ca-sensitization and cardiac inotropic effects. J Pharmacol Exp Ther 1988; 247:519–23.
48. Lee JA, Rüegg JC, Allen DG. The effects of pimobendan, a novel inotropic agent, on intracellular calcium and tension in isolated ferret ventricular muscle. J Clin Invest 1989; in press.
49. Hayes JS, Pollock GD, Wilson H, Bowling N, Robertson DW. Pharmacology of LY 175326: a potent cardiotonic with vasodilator activities. J Pharmacol Exp Ther 1985; 233:318–26.
50. Lues I, Siegel R, Harting J. Effect of isomazole on the responsiveness to calcium of the contractile elements in skinned cardiac muscle fibers of various species. Eur J Pharmacol 1988; 146:145–53.
51. Salzmann R, Bormann G, Herzig JW, Markstein R, Scholtysik G. Pharmacological actions of APP 201-533, a novel cardiotonic agent. J Cardiovasc Pharmacol 1985; 7:588–96.
52. Herzig JW, Bormann G, Botelho L, Erdmann E, Salzmann R, Solaro RJ. Intracellular acitons of APP 201-533, a novel cardiotonic agent: increase in Ca^{++} sensitivity and economization of the myocardial contractile process. J Mol Cell Cardiol 1983; 15 (Suppl 1):244.
53. Herzig JW, Botelho LH, Solaro RJ. Myofibrillar Ca^{++} activation and heart failure—Ca^{++} sensitization of the cardiotonic agent APP 201-533. In: Just HJ, Holubarsch C, Scholz H, eds. Inotropic stimulation and myocardial energetics. Basic Res Cardiol 1989; 84 (Suppl 1):117–24.
54. Scholtysik G, Salzmann R, Berthold R, Herzig JW, Quast U, Markstein R. DPI 201-106, a novel cardioactive agent. Combination of cAMP-independent positive inotropic, negative chronotropic, action potential prolonging and coronary dilatory properties. Naunyn-Schmiedeberg's Arch Pharmacol 1985; 329:316–25.
55. Hajjar RJ, Gwathmey JK, Briggs GM, Morgan JP. Differential effect of DPI 201-106 on the sensitivity of the myofilaments to Ca^{2+} in intact and skinned trabeculae from control and myopathic human hearts. J Clin Invest 1988; 82:1578–84.
56. Gwathmey JK, Slawsky M, Briggs GM, Morgan JP. Role of intracellular sodium in the regulation of intracellular calcium and contractility. Effects of DPI 201-106 on

excitation-contraction coupling in human ventricular myocardium. J Clin Invest 1988; 82:1592–1605.
57. Romey G, Quast U, Pauron D, Frelin C, Renaud JF, Lazdunski M. Na^+ channels as sites of action of the cardioactive agent DPI 201-106 with agonist and antagonist enantiomers. Proc Natl Acad Sci USA 1987; 84:896–900.

23

Clinical Aspects of Drugs Affecting Contractile Proteins and Myosin Ca^{2+} Sensitivity—of the β-Stimulator Denopamine (TA-064), and of the Recent Phosphodiesterase Inhibitor Drugs Amrinone, Enoximone, and Piroximone

JOCHEN THORMANN

Kerckhoff-Klinik der Max-Planck-Gesellschaft, Bad Nauheim, Germany

HANS ARMIN DIETERICH

Marion Merrell Dow Research, Rüsselsheim, Germany

I. INTRODUCTION

Heart failure in dilated cardiomyopathy results from depression of myocardial contractility and is usually inadequately controlled by standard therapy consisting of digitalis, diuretics, and afterload-reducing substances. In this situation, drugs found capable of combining nonglycosidic-based inotropic effects, and having the advantages of dobutamine-like action, as well as being effective both intravenously and orally, would be most welcome to the clinician. In view of the rather limited clinical success with the existing inotropic agents (1,2), there is a demand for new compounds to treat cardiac failure more adequately.

It was over two centuries after digitalis was introduced that other drugs with inotropic properties, the β-adrenergic agonists, dopamine and dobutamine, became available, as well as the phophodiesterase inhibitor amrinone in 1978. The clinician is confronted with the glycosides' limited inotropic potential and their unfavorable therapeutic/toxic ratio. This and the renewed scrutiny into the pharmacologic management of heart failure have accelerated the search for new inotropic drugs within the last decade, while our comprehension of the mechanism of cardiac pump function has improved considerably. The interaction of the myofilaments during the contraction process is dependent on the presence of energy in the form of ATP and the binding of calcium to troponin. Both the concentration of intracellular calcium and the affinity of troponin for calcium regulate the development of force by the myocyte (3). The action of the new inotropic agents propagates the above mechanism.

This chapter reviews the clinical aspects of a group of new inotropes that exert their inotropic effects at least in part via increasing the activating potency of calcium ions at the myofibrils. These are DPI 201-106 (4,5), AR-L 115 BS (sulmazole) (6), UD-CG 115 BS (pimobendan) (7,8), and MCI-154 (9). This chapter also discusses the beta-1-stimulator TA-064 (denopamine) (10,11). And finally, we deal with the effects of the most recent phosphodiesterase inhibitor drugs, amrinone, enoximone, and piroximone. Their influence on clinical hemodynamics and (end-systolic) pressure–volume relationship is presented.

II. DPI 201-106

The cardiotonic agent DPI 201-106's mechanism of action is not related to cAMP, beta-adrenergic or histaminic receptor stimulation, liberation of catecholamines, glycoside-like action (12,13), or phosphodiesterase inhibitory activity (14). DPI 201-106 increases cardiac performance by enhancing sodium influx into the myocardial cell by inhibiting inactivation of the sodium channel (15). The drug may also increase the sensitivity of the contractile proteins to calcium (16).

The impression has been that DPI 201-106 produces marked increases in cardiac output with minimal decreases in right and left ventricular filling pressures, accompanied by a notable prolongation of the QT_c interval (via prolonged activation of the sodium channel). This proarrhythmic potential has raised concerns that DPI 201-106 may predispose to serious ventricular arrhythmias in patients with heart failure.

A. General Hemodynamics

The results of the eight relevant clinical studies (4,5,17–22) (Table 1) involving patients with comparable ages and dosages of DPI 201-106 (administered both intravenously and orally) can be summarized as follows. Drug-induced increases of cardiac index ranged from 17 to 25%, ejection fraction from 27 to 42%, stroke work index from 21 to 24%, while heart rate, arterial pressure, myocardial oxygen consumption, and coronary sinus flow did not change significantly. A reduction in preload was suggested by a considerable fall in left ventricular filling pressure, as expressed by a reduction in left ventricular end-diastolic pressure of 41–50% and of pulmonary capillary wedge pressure by 45%. In addition, a moderate decline in peripheral vascular resistance, ranging from 14 to 17%, was registered.

These results could account for a DPI 201-106-induced improvement of left ventricular performance, as summarized in Table 1. However, a direct inotropic effect is suggested by a drug-induced rise in dP/dt_{max}, ranging from 16 to 45% and a decline in systolic time intervals (PEP by 26% and PEP/LVET by 30%). This is supported also by the drug-induced motions of the pressure/volume loops leftward and downward (Fig. 1) in patients with congestive heart failure (5).

B. Hemodynamics After Oral Administration

Oral administration of the drug about matched hemodynamic changes achieved by the intravenous route. Oral DPI 201-106 in single dosages (80 and 100 mg) administered to 15 patients with severe congestive heart failure (and still symptomatic when receiving conventional treatment), significantly increased cardiac index by an average of 18 and 25% (21). A dose-dependent increase in left ventricular stroke work (by 24%), left ventricular stroke volume (by 32%), and QT_c (by 7%) was also observed. There were no effects on heart rate and left ventricular pressure. Maximum changes occurred in about 4 hr after the administration of DPI 201-106 and lasted 8 hr. The DPI 201-106 plasma level, as well as the parameters of stroke work and ventricular ectopic activity, did not correlate significantly with the QT_c interval.

Table 1 Hemodynamic Alterations (% change) Induced by DPI 201-106

Reference	Patients (n)	NYHA Class	Dosage (mg) Intravenous	Dosage (mg) Oral	LV Filling pressure	dP/dt_{max}	SVR	CI	SVI	EF
17	16	1/2	20	—	—	—	—	—	—	—
18	10	2/3	20	—	−40	—	—	17	44	42
19	6	2/3	25–40	—	−50	45	−14	22	25	—
5	15	2/3	25	—	41	32	−17	18	12	27
20	9	3/4	25	—	−18	16	—	22	—	—
21	15	3	—	80–100	—	—	−14	25	25	—
22	18	2/3	—	30	—	—	—	—	—	21
4	10	1/2	—	30–60	−40	—	—	—	—	42

LV, left ventricular; SVR, systemic vascular resistance; CI, cardiac index; SVI, stroke volume; EF, ejection fraction.

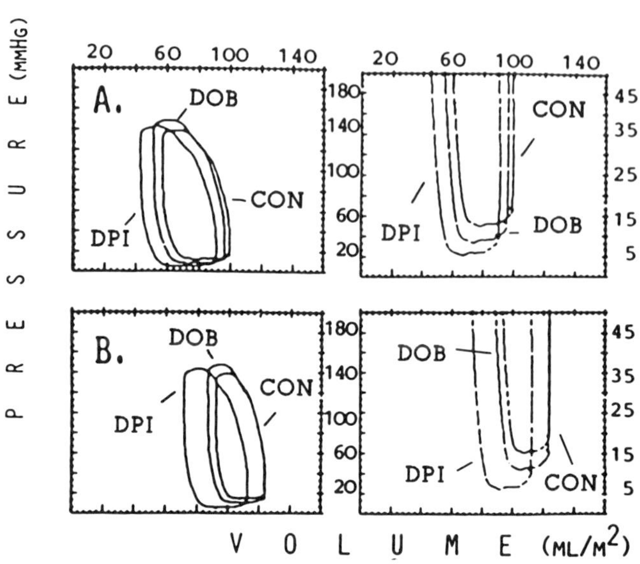

Figure 1 Summarized computer printout shows pressure–volume (PV) relationships of the maximal average drug effects vs. controls (CON) for group A (**top**) and group B (**bottom**); the expanded diastolic portions of the PV- loops appear on the **right.** The drug-induced rise in contractility is expressed by a leftward motion of the PV loops, which appears more pronounced with DPI 201-106 (**DPI**) than with dobutamine (**DOP**) and maximal for group B (47% vs. 32%). Increases in stroke index (group B: 29% vs. 18%) are due to a decrease in end-diastolic volume (group B:−22% vs.−6%), and end-diastolic pressure declines simultaneously, more so than during DOB therapy. (Modified from Ref. 5.)

C. Hemodynamics After Intravenous Administration

In seven patients with cardiomyopathy with normal (group A) and eight patients with abnormal (group B) left ventricular function, serial analysis of pressure–volume effects was performed comparing acute hemodynamic alterations of DPI 201-106 (30 μg/kg/min × 10 min) with dobutamine (10 μg/kg/min × 10 min) (5). A microtip catheter was used for left ventricular catheterization and pressure assessments and $[^{99m}]T_c$ scintigraphy for continuous volume analysis. Comparative hemodynamic alterations are listed in Table 2.

Contractility (dP/dt_{max}) improvement was greater ($p < 0.05$) with DPI 201-106 (group A by an average of 23%, $p<0.05$; group B by 47%, $p<0.05$) than with dobutamine (group A by 21%,$p<0.05$; group B by 32%, $p<0.05$), as was the simultaneous left ventricular end-diastolic pressure (i.e., preload) decrease, for DPI 201-106 (group A by −39%, $p<0.5$; group B by −42%, $p<0.05$). The average decrease in afterload (expressed as peripheral vascular resistance) was more marked ($p>0.05$) with DPI 201-106 (by −17%, $p>0.05$) than with dobutamine (by −7%, $p>0.05$). Left ventricular efficiency increased with DPI 201-106 (group A by 22%, $p<0.05$; group B by 55%, $p>0.05$), but myocardial oxygen consumption (indirectly assessed) did not change significantly. Five of the 15 patients showed an increase in dP/dt_{max} with DPI 201-106 only; with this drug there were fewer nonresponders than with dobutamine.

Table 2 Clinical Characteristics and Hemodynamic Alterations with Dobutamine (DOB) and DPI 201-106 (DPI)

	Group A (n = 7)			Group B (n = 8)		
Parameters (mean ± SD)	Control	DOB	DPI	Control	DOB	DPI
HR (liters/min)	88 ± 17	96 ± 31	92 ± 15	74 ± 14	77 ± 21	69 ± 14
LVSP (mmHg)	139 ± 16	149 ± 21	142 ± 19	139 ± 17	148 ± 28	143 ± 23
LVEDP (mmHg)	17.3 ± 6.4	13.7 ± 6.8*	10.6 ± 4.6*	20.0 ± 7	16.3 ± 9.4*	11.5 ± 4.9*
dP/dt_{max} (mmHg/sec)	2,096 ± 575	2,535 ± 965*	2,579 ± 946*	1,096 ± 322	1,450 ± 809*	1,606 ± 571*
dP/dt_{min} (mmHg/sec)	1,497 ± 401	1,542 ± 392	1,500 ± 343	1,149 ± 317	1,263 ± 403	1,188 ± 371
MVO_2 (ml/min/100 g)	8.3 ± 1.3	9.6 ± 3.8	8.7 ± 1.7	7.4 ± 0.9	7.5 ± 1.7	6.9 ± 1.3
EDVI (ml/m^2)	100 ± 38	97 ± 43	91 ± 39	124 ± 50	125 ± 59	113 ± 49
ESVI (ml/m^2)	57 ± 30	52 ± 32	43 ± 21	92 ± 49	87 ± 56	72 ± 46
SVI (ml/m^2)	43 ± 12	45 ± 16	48 ± 15	32 ± 15	38 ± 17*	42 ± 14*
EF (%)	45 ± 10	49 ± 15	57 ± 18*	29 ± 16	35 ± 19*	42 ± 21*
CI (L/min/m^2)	3.8 ± 1.6	4.4 ± 2.4	4.5 ± 1.8*	2.3 ± .97	2.8 ± 1.1*	2.8 ± .94*
LVSWI (g/m/m^2)	477 ± 112	555 ± 161	575 ± 180*	344 ± 180	475 ± 295*	517 ± 214*
LV_{eff} (%)	46 ± 13	52 ± 19	56 ± 17*	29 ± 14	40 ± 21*	45 ± 20*
SCI (ml/m^2)	0.87 ± 0.42	0.72 ± 0.41*	0.58 ± .034*	1.2 ± 0.67	1.07 ± 0.86	0.7 ± 0.38*
SVR (dyne/sec/cm^3)	1,263 ± 473	1,313 ± 719	1,090 ± 436	2,178 ± 988	1,895 ± 738	1,787 ± 681

HR, heart rate; LVSP, left ventricular systolic pressure; LVEDP, left ventricular end-diastolic pressure; MVO_2, myocardial oxygen consumption; EDVI, end-diastolic volume index; ESVI, end-systolic volume index; SVI, stroke volume index; EF, ejection fraction; CI, cardiac index; LVSWI, left ventricular stroke work index; LV_{eff}, cardiac efficiency; SCI, compliance index; SVR, systemic vascular resistance.

* = Significant vs. control, $p<0.05$ at least

Source: Modified from Ref. 5.

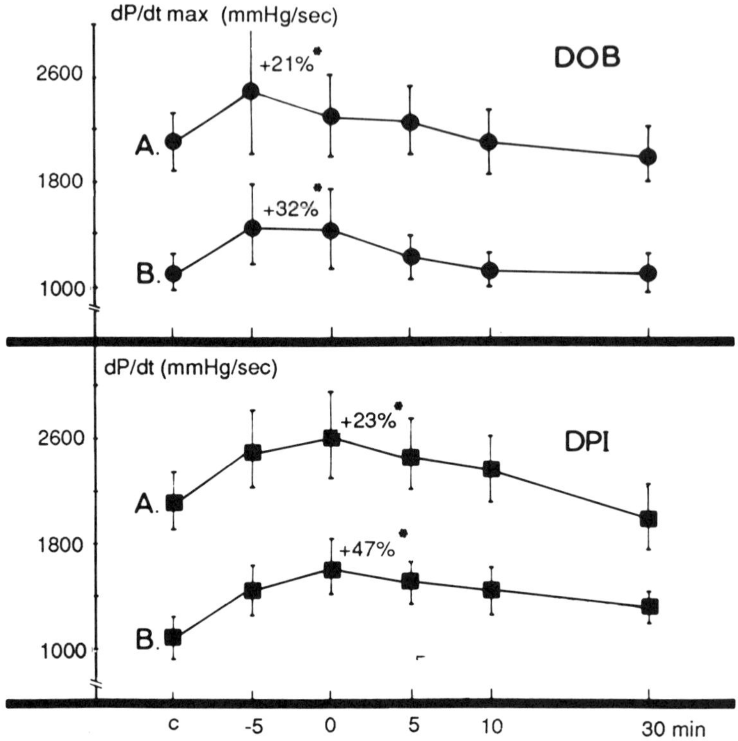

Figure 2 Drug-induced changes of contractility parameters (mean ± SEM) for the following phases in group A and B: control (C); 5th (−5), 10th (0), and 30th (+30) min after the end of infusion. For further details see text. DOB, dobutamine; DPI, DPI 201-106. *Significant vs. control. (Modified from Ref. 5.)

D. Improved Left Ventricular Contractility vs. Function

DPI 201-106 induced higher dP/dt_{max} values than dobutamine, especially in group B (with a primarily more reduced left ventricular pump function) (Fig. 2); this condition also applied to all other relevant parameter changes (Table 2). The more pronounced increase of left ventricular pump function during DPI 201-106 treatment compared with dobutamine treatment was further indicated by average increases of the cardiac index and the ejection fraction, and was also apparent in the shift leftward and up in the Frank-Starling type correlogram (Fig. 3). In contradistinction to dobutamine, inotropic improvement due to DPI 201-106 did not result in a significant rise in myocardial oxygen consumption ($p>0.05$). Increases in left ventricular pump function were accompanied (more pronounced with DPI 201-106 than with dobutamine) by a decrease in preload (left ventricular end-diastolic pressure) and afterload (systemic vascular resistance), while left ventricular pump efficiency rose, again more markedly with DPI 201-106 than with dobutamine.

The effects generated by DPI 201-106 generally induced pressure–volume loops to shift slightly to the left, and downward in the diastolic portion (Fig. 1), which primarily points to an improvement in left ventricular pump function. This DPI

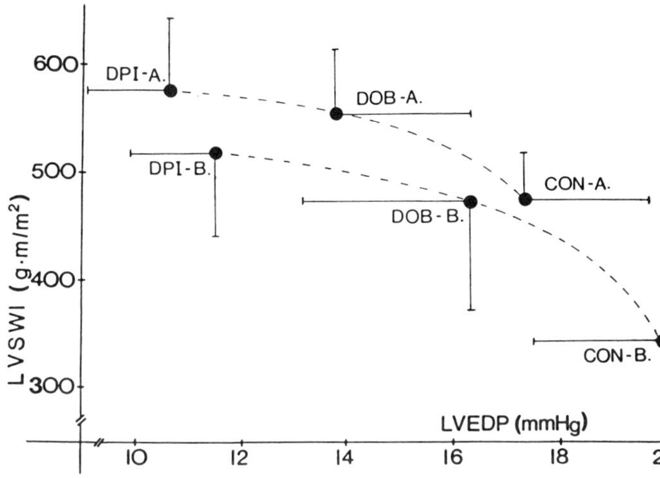

Figure 3 For two groups of patients with dilated cardiomyopathy (NYHA II/III), the drug-induced changes in left ventricular pump function are defined by the relationship of filling pressure (LVEDP) to stroke work (LVSWI). After the administration of dobutamine (DOB) or DPI 201-106 (DPI), more stroke work is achieved at lower preload levels. The drug-induced characteristic motion of the mean values away from the control position leftward and up also signifies increases in contractility that appear to be more pronounced for DPI than DOB. (Modified from Thormann Ref. 5.)

201-106-induced improved contractility is influenced, at least in part, by preload changes.

Thus, DPI 201-106 increases contractility in patients with dilated cardiomyopathy while reducing preload and afterload rather than causing higher metabolic costs. Such beneficial hemodynamic effects appear to be stronger in the more impaired myocardium (group B patients) and quantitatively superior to those induced by dobutamine.

E. Side Effects

DPI 201-106-induced hemodynamic effects were accompanied by significant prolongations of the QT_c-interval. Boutrous et al. (17) reported a QT_c prolongation of 20%, after the loading dose DPI 201-106 (1.8 mg/kg × 10 min, intravenously), as well as during atrial pacing at 600 msec, and of 12% with ventricular pacing at 600 msec. Kostis et al. (21) found that DPI 201-106, after a single oral dose (80 and 100 mg), increased the QT_c interval by 7% and observed a correlation between QT_c interval and DPI 201-106 plasma level. Scholtysik et al. (4,23) also reported a dose-dependent prolongation of the QT_c-interval (Fig. 4), In addition, the electrocardiograms (ECGs) showed dose-related alterations in the morphology of the repolarization, with reduction in amplitude of the T wave.

The mechanism responsible for these side effects is thought to stem from drug-induced increased vagal tone as well as the finding that DPI 201-106 has a calcium channel antagonistic effect (15,24). The fact that there was a slight but significant

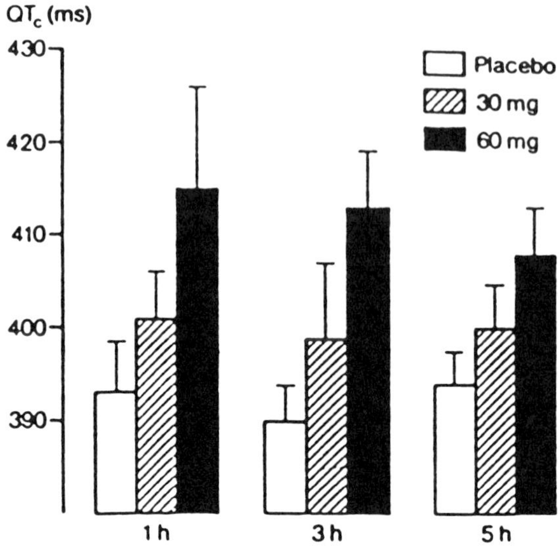

Figure 4 Average QT$_c$ intervals after single oral dosages of 30 and 60 mg DPI 201-106 and placebo in 10 healthy volunteers. The results indicate a drug-induced QT$_c$-prolongation in dosage-related fashion ($p<0.05$). (Modified from Ref. 4.)

prolongation of the atrioventricular nodal conduction during fixed-rate atrial pacing (17) supports the hypothesis of a DPI 201-106-induced increased vagal activity.

These finding imply that close monitoring of the QT interval may be advised in clinical follow-up and dosage adjustment with DPI 201-106 treatment. Although in none of the clinical studies have proarrhythmic effects been observed, one has to keep in mind that QT$_c$ prolongation has been associated with ventricular arrythmias and sudden death (25,26). On the other hand, the potential proarrhythmic effect of inotropic agents used in patients with severe congestive heart failure is difficult to determine because of the high density of ventricular ectopic activity in these patients and the great spontaneous variability of arrhythmias (27).

Despite the beneficial hemodynamic effects demonstrated with DPI 201-106, the associated prolongation of the QT-interval (i.e., its proarrhythmic potential) finally set the limit for the clinical usefulness of this agent. The concentration-related increase in ventricular ectopic beats, as observed in a clinical study (21), prompted the withdrawal of DPI 201-106 from clinical investigation.

III. AR-L 115 BS (SULMAZOLE, VARDAX)

Recent experimental and clinical data (28–34) have revealed the action of AR-L 115 BS (sulmazole) to be similar to that of amrinone (35–37) although there is no structural relation. In general, the drug exhibits positive inotropic effects and cause reduction of preload and afterload, thus meeting the requirement for the treatment of congestive heart failure. With respect to its positive inotropic action, the drug may be compared with catecholamines (38). Catecholamines augment left ventricular function and concomitantly lower anginal threshold by increasing myocardial oxygen consumption. However, the newly developed drug sulmazole increases left ventricular pump function without inducing angina in patients with documented coronary artery disease, even though myocardial oxygen consumption was found to be increased (34). Elevated left ventricular end-diastolic pressure is a distinct feature of the vicious cycle in hemodynamic alterations that result in the clinical state of angina.

A. General Hemodynamics

The hemodynamic alterations after use of application of sulmazole in 14 relevant clinical studies (Table 3) (6,33,39–49) involving patients with comparable ages and dosages of sulmazole (administered both intravenously and orally) can be summarized as follows. Drug-induced increases in cardiac index showed a mean of 27% (range, 5–65%), ejection fraction 23% (range, 14–35%), stroke work index of 23% (range, 9–75%), myocardial oxygen consumption 25% (range, 14–41%), coronary sinus flow 39%, while heart rate and left ventricular pressure did not change significantly.

A reduction in preload was suggested by a fall in left ventricular filling pressure as expressed by a reduction in left ventricular end-diastolic pressure (Table 3) by an average of 33% (range, 19–57%) and pulmonary capillary wedge pressure by 29% (range, 10–64%). In addition, a moderate decline in peripheral vascular resistance by an average of 22% (10–64%) was registered. These results could account for a sulmazole-induced improvement of left ventricular performance as summarized in Table 3. However, a direct inotropic effect also is suggested by a drug-induced rise in DP/DT max of 22% (range, 19–30%) and a decline in systolic time intervals (PEP, 15%).

B. Hemodynamics After Oral Administration

Eighteen patients with dilated cardiomyopathy (New York Heart Association [NYHA] class III/IV) were investigated (6,46). They had a mean serum digoxin level of 1.4 μg/ml and exhibited reduced ventricular function as demonstrated by the following averaged hemodynamic values: cardiac index, 2.03 liters/min; pulmonary artery mean pressure, 31 mmHg; ejection fraction, 33%; and mean circumferential fiber shortening rate, 0.67 circ/sec. Sulmazole, 200 mg, was given orally every 8 hr. According to the results of a pilot study, measurable effects of the drug set in between 40 and 60 min and were maximal between 60 and 120 min after oral intake (serum levels >500 μg/ml). Thus measurements in all 18 patients (over 4 continuous days) were carried out prior to and 120 and 300 min after oral administration of sulmazole.

All but two patients responded with improvement in hemodynamics after sulmazole was given orally (Fig. 5). At 120 min, the time at which the maximal effect was to be expected, the following hemodynamic values were measured. Heart rate and arterial pressure did not change significantly. However, cardiac output increased significantly by an average of 31%, from 4.2 to 5.5 liters/min, while mean pulmonary artery pressure decreased by 29% from 31 to 22 mmHg. Ejection fraction increased by 35%, from 33.1 to 45.2%. Circumferential fiber shortening rate increased by an average of 25%, from 0.67 to 0.84 circ/sec. Fractional posterior wall thickening increased by 32%, from 33 to 44%. At 300 min after

Table 3 Hemodynamic Alterations (% change) Induced by Sulmazole

Reference	Patients (n)	NYHA Class	Dosage: Intravenous (mg/kg)	Dosage: Oral (mg)	LV Filling pressure	dP/dt_{max}	SVR	CI	SVI	EF	VCF
39	19	2/3	0.45	—	−42	25	—	24	—	14	65
40	10	2/3	0.70	—	−10	—	−19	25	—	—	—
41	10	4	0.15	—	−64	—	−40	63	25	—	—
42	7	2	0.70	—	−18	19	−31	34	18	—	—
43	8	2/3	0.75	—	−30	—	—	21	19	—	—
44	13	3/4	0.75	—	−31	—	−16	5	—	—	—
45	18	2/3	0.75	—	−43	—	—	21	8	—	—
46	11	3/4	3.00	—	−28	—	−18	27	—	—	—
6	30	2	2.00	—	−50	26	−16	24	—	25	36
47	14	2	0.75	—	−29	19	−17	12	—	—	—
48	10	3/4	—	100	−38	—	—	33	—	—	—
49	6	2/3	—	150	−19	—	—	—	—	16	26
33	18	3/4	—	200	−29	—	—	31	39	35	25

LV, left ventricular; SVR, systemic vascular resistance; CI, cardiac index; SVI, stroke volume index; EF, ejection fraction; VCF, velocity of circumferential fiber shortening.

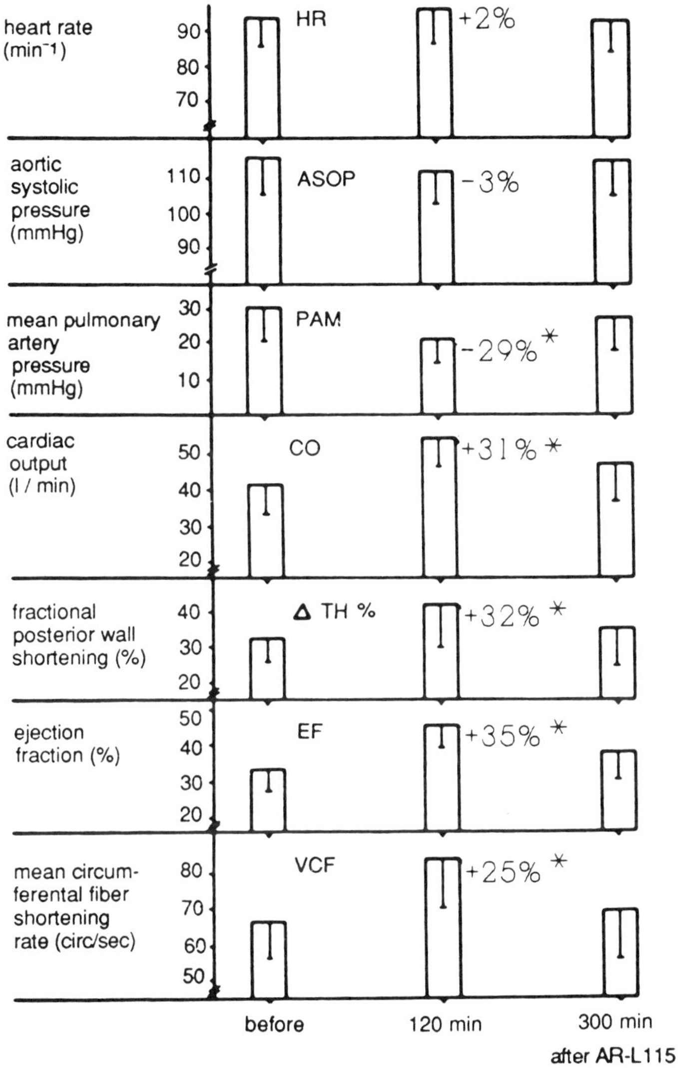

Figure 5 All but 2 of 18 patients (dilated cardiomyopathy, NYHA class III/IV) responded with maximal hemodynamic alterations at 120 min after receiving 200 mg oral sulmazole. Percent changes are given. At 300 min after sulmazole, all parameters had reached the control level, so that at this time a drug effect could no longer be ascertained. *Significantly different, $p < 0.05$, at least. (Modified from Ref. 6.)

sulmazole was administered orally, all parameters had reached the control levels, so that at this time a drug effect could no longer be ascertained.

Improved cardiac performance is also represented by correlating accumulated results (18 patients) of stroke index with ventricular filling pressure (Fig. 6). At 120 min after oral administration of sulmazole, 200 mg, a considerably (by 38%) increased stroke volume was transported at a reduced (by 29%) filling pressure.

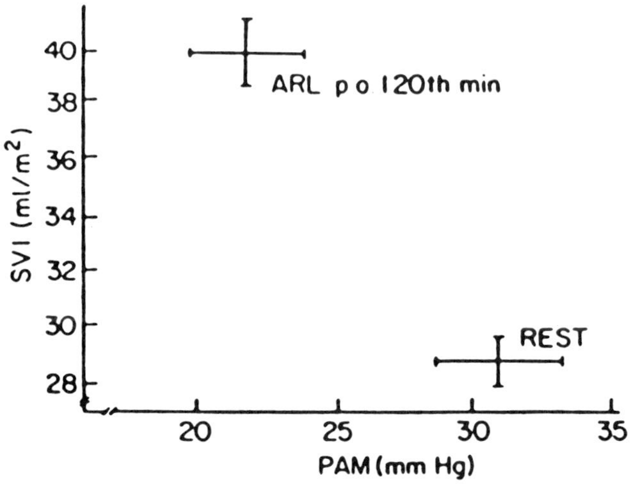

Figure 6 For 18 patients with dilated cardiomyopathy (NYHA III/IV), the drug-induced changes of left ventricular pump function are defined by the relation of stroke index (SVI) to ventricular filling pressure (PAM). After 200 mg oral sulmazole, greater stroke volume (+38%) was achieved at considerably decreased (−29%) preload levels. (Modified from Ref. 6.)

Two (NYHA class IV) of 18 patients did not exhibit any improvement in ventricular function after the administration of sulamzole; their results are included in the mean values given. The percentile improvement of left ventricular performance after sulmazole in patients with relatively little myocardial impairment was less than the improvement exhibited by patients who had a higher degree of left ventricular functional impairment.

From these results it was concluded that residual contractile reserves can be mobilized by sulmazole in the digitalized heart of patients with dilated cardiomyopathy.

C. Hemodynamics After Intravenous Administration

The clinical use of sulmazole could be limited by inducing myocardial ischemia on account of its experimentally proven positive inotropic properties. Therefore, drug-induced hemodynamics and myocardial oxygen consumption were investigated in 30 patients with coronary ischemic disease (6). In these patients pacing-induced myocardial ischemia was signified by angina, typical ST-T changes, a rise in left ventricular filling pressure, and lactate production. The total patient population presented was organized into two groups that did not differ in their characteristic clinical parameters: age, cardiac functional parameters, NYHA class, reproducibly effort-induced myocardial ischemia, scars of myocardial infarction, absence of aneurysm and mitral insufficiency, and distribution of one to three-vessel disease. The objective of the study was to assess sulmazole's hemodynamic efficacy and the associated metabolic expenditure as well as its influence on regional wall motion.

1. Group 1

Pacing-induced ischemia was confirmed in 13 patients in group 1 (6). Heart rate, arterial pressures, ejection period and systolic period, dP/dt_{max}, thermodilution coronary sinus flow (50), myocardial oxygen consumption calculated directly and indirectly (51,52), as well as thermodilution cardiac output were assessed at rest, at the 50th second of paced ventricular tachycardia, in the immediate postpacing period, and at the 9th, 14th, and 19th min after the administration of sulmazole, 2 mg/kg intravenously (i.v.).

The drug's peak effect was established for the 14th min after injection, without inducing ischemia. Sulmazole-induced changes in left ventricular pump function were defined by the relationship of the average cardiac index to left ventricular filling pressure. During pacing-induced ischemia, pump function declined, but during the drug's peak action an average increase in cardiac index of 25% was achieved, while filling pressure fell by an average of 44% without angina being induced.

The evidence for improved left ventricular pump function during sulmazole's peak action (Fig. 7) was as follows. Cardiac index rose by 25%, cardiac work by 17%, dP/dt_{max} by 30%, coronary sinus flow by 39% and heart rate by 18%. Simultaneously, preload declined (i.e., left ventricular filling pressure by 44%), as did afterload (i.e., arterial pressure by 13%). These sulmazole-induced beneficial hemodynamic changes required an average rise of myocardial oxygen consumption by 41%, and no myocardial ischemia could be ascertained.

2. Group 2

Figure 8 demonstrates schematically the investigational procedures carried out in the 17 group 2 patients with coronary artery disease (53). Here, in addition to all parameters derived from arterial pressure curves, angiographic parameters were assessed (i.e., stroke volume, ejection fraction, mean circumferential fiber shortening rate, and regional wall motion), so that comparisons of the hemodynamic situations could be carried out as listed at the bottom of the scheme. In this case the postpacing period without medication compared with the postpacing period with sulmazole peak influence was of primary importance, indicated here as "3" for the pressure-derived parameters and as "5" for the angiographic parameters. Regional wall motion was determined from biplane ventriculograms, calculated as fractional reductions of eight-wall segments (as shown in Fig. 9) using a computer-assisted procedure based on a radial model.

a. Regional Wall Motion The computer printouts of patient 17 are shown in a semischematic fashion in Figure 9. The conditions are resting conditions at the top, nonmedicated postpacing phase in the middle, and the postpacing phase under sulmazole's peak influence at the bottom. A marked decrease in left ventricular pump function accompanies reduced regional wall motion during the postpacing phase while the obvious improvement in regional wall motion in the sulmazole-medicated postpacing phase is accompanied by a rise in cardiac index up to and somewhat above resting levels, and left ventricular filling pressure is similar to the resting condition.

Comparison of the medicated postpacing phase (i.e., drug-abolished ischemia) with the postpacing phase without medication (i.e., pacing-induced ischemia) indi-

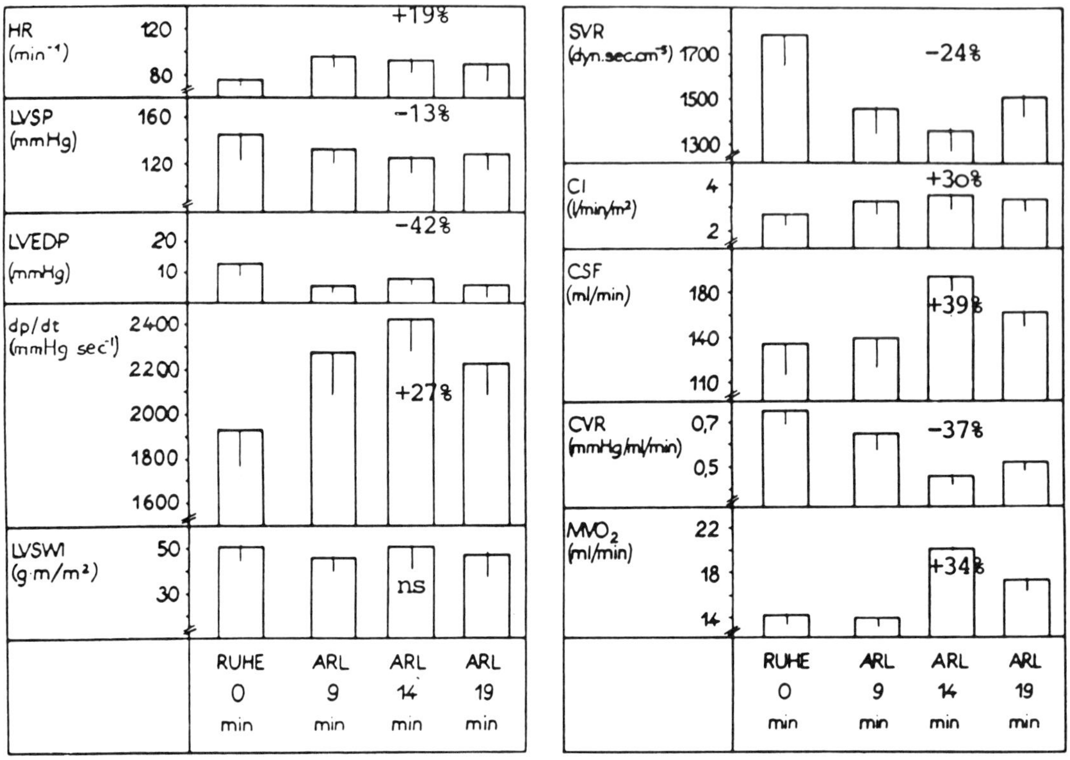

Figure 7 Peak parameter changes were registered 14 min after the administration of sulmazole, 2 mg/kg i.v. in group 1 patients with proven ischemic coronary artery disease. Drug-induced percentage parameter changes are given for heart rate (HR), left ventricular pressure (LVSP), filling pressure (LVEDP), contractility (dP/dt_{max}), stroke work (LVSWI), systemic vascular resistance (SVR), cardiac index (CI), coronary sinus flow (CSF), coronary vascular resistance (CVR), and directly estimated (Fick) myocardial oxygen consumption (MVO_2). The hemodynamic improvements registered with sulmazole were achieved with moderate increases in MVO_2 and without myocardial ischemia being induced. (Modified from Ref. 34.)

cated that regional wall motion generally improved with sulmazole (by an average of 26%). However, the resulting changes in regional wall motion presented in this manner neglect the rather differing degree of coronary obstructive disease in individual cases and the modifications of individual contractile patterns.

Only from the analysis of all areas does it become apparent that 86 of 136 areas (63%) showed a reduction in fractional shortening during the postpacing phase without medication, while 18 of these segments showed a smaller decrease or even improvement after sulmazole; these may have been potentially ischemic segments. Further analysis revealed that 50 of 136 (37%) showed an increase in regional wall motion after pacing without the drug. Of these areas, which may well have been normal, 33 showed a further small increase after medication, presumably because of the inotropic effect of sulmazole, or did not increase regional wall motion as

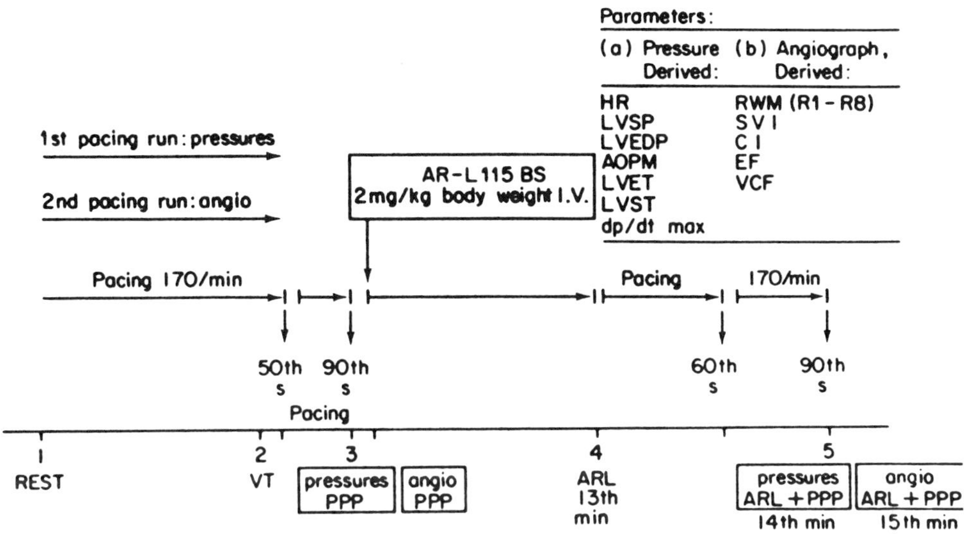

Figure 8 Schematic outline of the investigational procedures carried out in 17 patients with ischemic coronary artery disease (group II). Here, in addition to all parameters derived from arterial pressure curves, angiographic parameters were assessed, including regional wall motion (RWM), so that comparisons for the hemodynamic situations could be achieved as listed at the bottom of the scheme. In this investigation the postpacing period (PP) without and the PPP with sulmazole (AR-L 115 BS) are of primary importance, indicated in the scheme as "3" for the pressure-derived parameters and as "5" for the angiographic parameters. (For further abbreviations, see legend to Fig. 7).

much as without the drug, possibly because abnormal wall motion elsewhere in the ventricle was less marked after administration of sulmazole.

b. Hemodynamics As regards the other variables (comparing the postpacing phase with and without medication), significant mean alterations were as follows: heart rate +19%, aortic mean pressure 6%, cardiac index +24%, stroke index by 17%, and ejection fraction by 25%.

It was concluded from the results of these 2 studies (involving 30 patients with ischemic coronary artery disease) that sulmazole improves left ventricular pump function and regional wall motion in patients with coronary artery disease without inducing ischemia, probably by means of a drug-induced reduction in preload and extravascular resistance.

3. Healthy Volunteers

In a study group of 10 volunteers (54,55) the following changes were achieved with sulmazole (infusion of 1.4–4.2 mg/min over 45 min). Arterial pressure and heart rate remained unchanged ($p>0.05$), ejection fraction rose by an average of 26%, fiber shortening rate by 40%, and the rate-corrected electromechanical systole (QS_2) index was reduced by 7%. Thus, sulmazole exhibited beneficial hemodynamic effects, combining positive inotropy and vasodilation (cardiac unloading: reduction of preload and afterload) in healthy hearts.

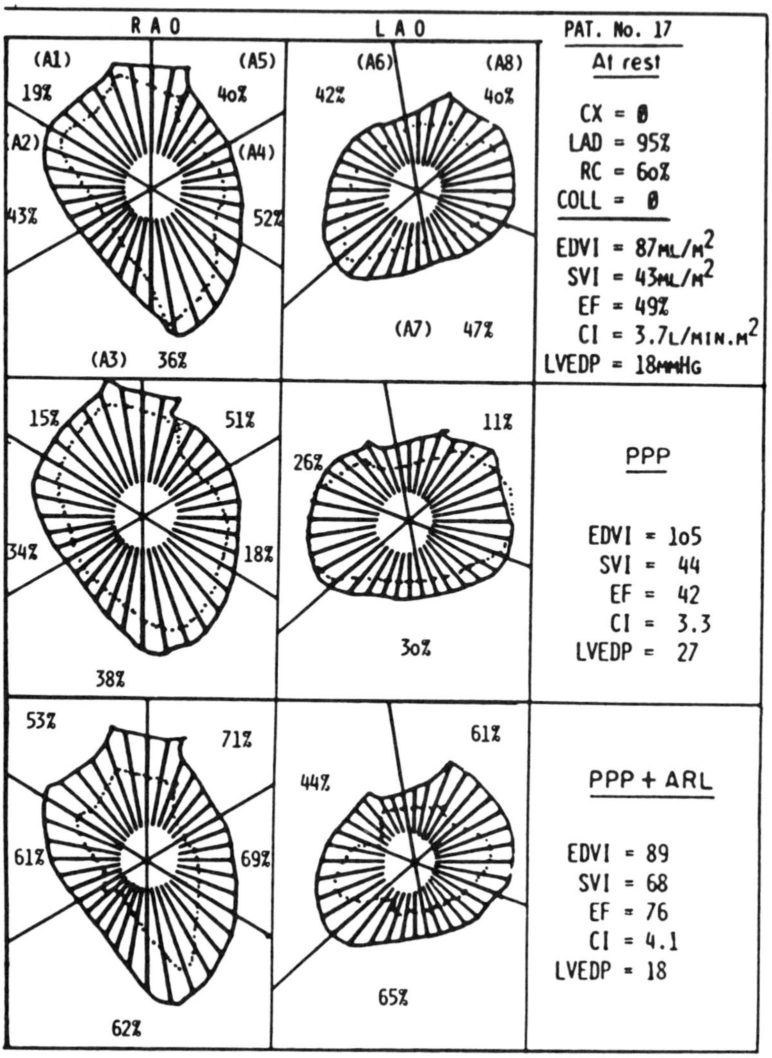

Figure 9 Computer printout displays individual alterations in left ventricular regional wall motion (RWM) (patient 17 with ischemic coronary artery disease). Eight percentile fractional surface reductions are indicated for each of the three investigational phases. The conditions are, from top to bottom: REST, PPP, the immediate postpacing phase without medication; PPP+ARL, the postpacing phase under sulmazole's (= AR-L 115 BS) peak influence. A marked decrease in left ventricular pump function accompanies the reduced RWM and myocardial ischemia during the PPP, while the obvious improvement of RWM in the sulmazole-medicated PPP is accompanied by a rise in cardiac index (CI) up to and somewhat above resting levels. The left ventricular filling pressure (LVEDP) reveals a level as if at rest, and ischemia was no longer present (for further abbreviations see legend to Fig. 7). (Modified from Ref. 53.)

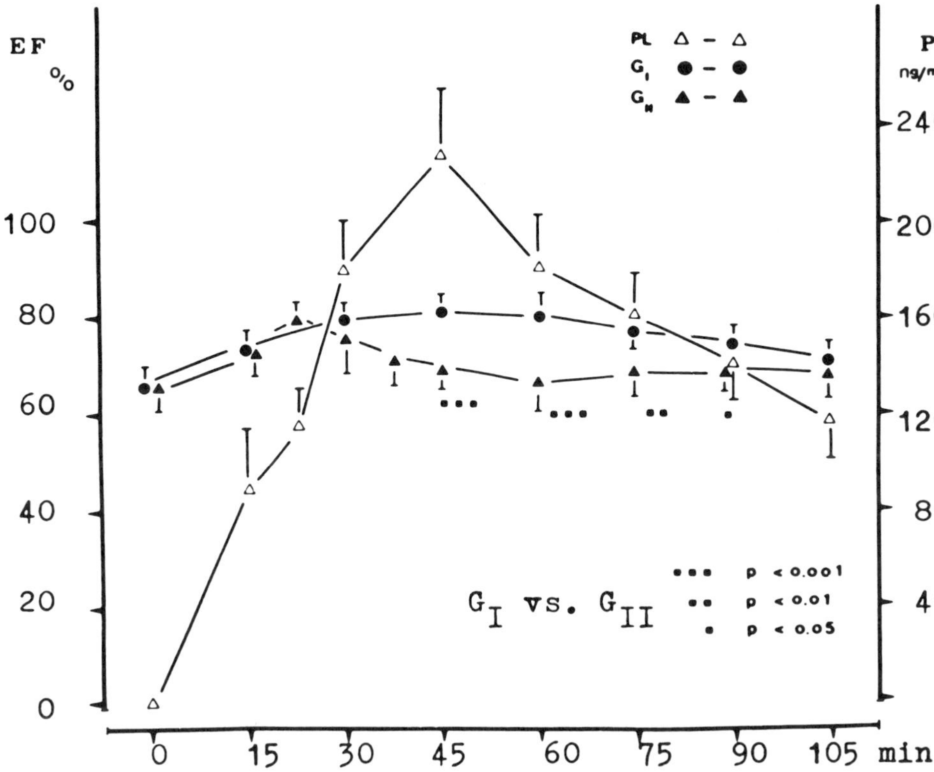

Figure 10 Sulmazole-induced alterations of ejection fraction (EF) in healthy volunteers and average plasma levels (PL) following the infusion of sulmazole without verapamil (group I, G_I and with the additional application of verapamil (group II, G_{II}). Conclusions: alterations of left ventricular performance in group I correspond to the increase of plasma levels up to 1800 ng/ml; further elevations do not result in an additional increase in efficiency: beyond a certain plasma level of sulmazole, a dosage/efficiency relationship no longer exists. The sulmazole-induced increases in ejection fraction in group II are abolished with the influence of verapamil setting in: sulmazole effects are blocked with verapamil. (Modified from Ref. 55.)

a. Effects vs. Serum Levels With increasing dosages (Fig. 10) (infusion of 1.4–2.8 mg/min over 45 min) at 1.5 hr an increase in contractility still was present (improved fractional shortening: +34%, sulmazole serum level: 1097 ng/ml) (55). Up to a dosage of 2.8 mg/min (serum level, 1800 ng/ml) hemodynamic effects correlated well (r=0.91), but no further rise in left ventricular performance could be ascertained with dosages increasing up to 4.2 mg/min. On a speculative basis, this could indicate a full saturation of drug-specific "receptors" for sulmazole at a serum level of 1800 ng/ml.

The conclusion is that alterations in left ventricular performance correspond with the increase of serum levels up to 1800 ng/ml; further elevations do not result in an additional increase in ejection fraction (i.e., beyond a certain serum level of sulmazole, a dosage/efficacy relationship no longer exists).

b. Effects Blocked by a Ca^{2+} Antagonist Healthy volunteers (54,55) received verapamil, 0.15 mg/kg i.v., 30 min after the start of the sulmazole infusion (Fig. 10). Comparison at 1 hr revealed a fractional shortening of 41 ± 6% vs. 33 ± 3%; verapamil inhibited the sulmazole-induced augmentation of ejection fraction, fractional shortening, and a reduction of the total electromechanic systolic (QS_2) index.

The conclusion is that sulmazole-induced increases in left ventricular pump function are abolished as soon as the influence of verapamil commences. Verapamil and sulmazole effects somehow interfere at the cellular level. The observed antagonistic effect is supported by experimental results demonstrating that sulmazole enhances intracellular Ca^{2+} availability by means of Ca^{2+} release from and inhibition of its uptake by the sarcoplasmic reticulum (56,57).

D. Side Effects

Occasional nausea, headaches, and temporary dizziness were encountered with administration of sulmazole (54,55); this, however, occurred at a time when higher serum levels did not induce further changes in hemodynamic parameters. As reported in other studies (34,40,54,55), the only clinical manifestation encountered was transient visual disturbances involving light-dark vision. During the intravenous injection of sulmazole, in dosages of 3 mg/kg (33) and 2 mg/kg (34), patients experienced visual "dimming effects" over a period of a few seconds.

Specific ophthalmologic studies of this phenomenon (54,55,58) revealed that the drug caused an increase in amplitude of the visual-evoked cortical potential in response to contrast stimulation, which correlated with an increase in visual acuity. Higher dosages of sulmazole were found to have a specific effect on the visual system, causing reversible color vision deficiencies, which strongly correlated with the drug's serum level. In contrast to studies on patients, who are usually still receiving digitalis medication when studied, the above-mentioned ophthalmologic investigations were carried out in volunteers without the potential interaction of any other drug.

It should be remembered that disturbances in color vision have also been reported in patients with therapeutic serum levels of digoxin and derivatives of the methylxanthines (59). Again all side effects encountered appeared minor when weighed against this agent's therapeutic effects. However, sulmazole has recently been reported to produce severe gastrointestinal side effects in many patients. It was withdrawn from further clinical investigation because of the development of hepatic neoplasms in long-term toxicologic studies (48).

IV. PIMOBENDAN

Pimobendan is a phosphodiesterase inhibitor with Ca^{2+}-sensitizing properties. Pimobendan increases (as does sulmazole) calcium sensitivity in isolated tissues derived from normal and failing hearts (60,61). However, inotropic action of these agents is achieved by their ability to increase cAMP via inhibition of type III phophodiesterase (60), and also by interfering with the inhibitory regulator of adenyl cyclase. As a consequence, only about 50% of pimobendan's (or sulmazole's) effect on cAMP accumulation can be attributed to phosphodiesterase inhibition; the remaining production of cAMP involves stimulation of adenylate cyclase activity (61).

A. General Hemodynamics

The following hemodynamic alterations were obtained in several patient groups after pimobendan was given, both intravenously and orally. Drug-induced increases of cardiac index ranged from 25 to 90% (mean, 43%), and of stroke index 44%, while heart rate, left ventricular pressure, and therefore myocardial oxygen consumption did not change significantly.

A pimobendan-induced reduction in preload was suggested by a fall in left ventricular filling pressure as expressed by a reduction in left ventricular end-diastolic pressure of an average of 47% (range, 26–65%). In addition, a decline in peripheral vascular resistance of 30% was registered, ranging from 22 to 37%.

These results could account for a pimobendan-induced improvement of left ventricular performance. However, a direct inotropic effect is also suggested by an average drug-induced rise in dP/dt_{max} of 17%, without an inappropriate rise in metabolic expenditure (myocardial oxygen consumption) being ascertained.

B. Hemodynamics After Oral Administration

In 10 patients with congestive heart failure (NYHA class 2/3) pimobendan, 2.5–10 mg, induced the following average percentile alterations in hemodynamic parameters (28): an increase in cardiac index of 43% and in heart rate of 9%, while arterial pressure fell by 12% and left ventricular filling pressure by 52%. These hemodynamic benefits lasted up to 12 hr. After chronic therapy over 4 weeks, functional capacity had improved in all patients.

These results correspond well with those obtained in five other patient groups (7,62–65) treated with pimobendan, 10 mg orally. They all exhibited reduced left ventricular pump function, representing NYHA class 3/4 in the control state. The respective average hemodynamic alterations after pimobendan were as follows: left ventricular filling pressure decreased by 42%, systemic vascular resistance by 30%, while cardiac index increased by 48%. Again, these reactions are indicative of drug-induced improved left ventricular function clearly mediated by vasodilative action.

C. Hemodynamics After Intravenous Administration

Six patients with heart failure (NYHA 2/4) were investigated before 1–2 hr after administration of intravenous pimobendan (2.5 and 5 mg) (66). There was a reduction in left ventricular filling pressure by an average of 65%, and in end-diastolic volume by 24%. Left ventricular end-systolic volume decreased by 20% while the mean velocity of shortening rose by 30%. The isovolumic index of inotropic state (dP/dt)dP40 increased by 21% and the rate of isovolumic left ventricular relaxation was reduced by 31%, indicating improvement. The diastolic pressure/volume relation was shifted downward and to the left. The results also indicated that the inotropic responses were not caused by reflex activation of the sympathetic nervous system alone.

The authors concluded from the above results that pimobendan was a positive inotropic and vasodilator agent that induces beneficial hemodynamic changes in patients with moderate to severe heart failure, refractory to conventional treatment, at least in short-term therapy.

D. Side Effects

Serious side effects with pimobendan have not been encountered so far (7,63,64). Walter et al. (65) observed a transient decrease of thrombocytes in four patients, which was severe in one patient. However, since these patients also were treated with heparin (which in itself can be the cause of blood platelet reduction) the validity of this finding has to be questioned.

For the chronic oral administration of pimobendan (i.e., after 4 weeks of 5 mg twice daily [b.i.d.] and 10 mg b.i.d.) a partial tolerance seemed to be evident, since significant hemodynamic drug effects originally obtained could not be ascertained after 1 month (67). This is in contrast to findings by others (63). Indeed, larger-scale evidence is needed in this regard.

V. MCI-154

The cardiotonic agent MCI-154 is thought to exert its positive inotropic effect by increasing myofibrillar Ca^{2+} sensitivity, as has been demonstrated with sulmazole. While the hemodynamic profile of MCI-154 has been studied extensively, there are no results of clinical evaluations available. In anesthetized open-chest dogs, dose-dependent increases in dP/dt_{max} and cardiac output have been achieved, as well as decreases in arterial pressure and total peripheral resistance, with only moderate increases in heart rate. The cardiovascular profile of MCI-154 was similar to that of amrinone and milrinone, and its positive inotropic effect was found to be more potent than the two other drugs. In anesthetized intact-chest dogs, infusion of MCI-154, 0.3–3 μg/kg/min i.v., also exerted a positive inotropic effect. Oral administration of MCI-154 (10–300 μg/kg) increased dP/dt_{max} in conscious beagle dogs. Furthermore, the cardiotonic effect of MCI-154 was not attenuated by blockade of autonomic receptors, catecholamine depletion, and prostaglandin synthesis inhibition. In hindlimbs, 0.3–30 μg intra-arterially (i.a.) produced direct vasodilatation (68).

The potent cardiotonic and vasodilator activities of MCI-154 revealed by the above (68) and other studies (99) in dog models suggest that the drug would be effective in the treatment of heart failure. Clinical trials of the drug are pending.

VI. DENOPAMINE (TA-064)

TA-064 has the advantage over dobutamine of being effective when administered both intravenously and orally. Its effects have been proven both experimentally (69–71) and clinically (10,11,72–74). TA-064 is capable of influencing adrenal metabolism directly, and its inotropic effect is not mediated by the release of intrinsic catecholamines. Although the exact mechanism remains to be determined, TA-064 is thought to act on the beta-adrenergic receptors; in fact, it is thought to be relatively selective for β_1-receptors, and its action is inhibited by β-blocking agents (69–71). Its oral effectiveness and lack of significant toxicity (11,72,73) have made TA-064 potentially important for clinical use as a cardiotonic agent.

A. General Hemodynamics

Table 4 provides a synopsis of the results in several clinical studies, involving patients with comparative ages and dosages of TA-064 (administered both, intrave-

Table 4 Hemodynamic Alterations (% change) Induced by TA-064

Reference	Patients (n)	NYHA Class	Dosage (mg) Intravenous	Dosage (mg) Oral	LV Filling pressure	dP/dt_{max}	SVR	CI	SVI	EF
75	23	2/3	1	—	—	—	−14	15	9	—
10	6	2	30	—	−65	56	−33	8	−13	—
76	7	3	35	—	−25	—	−28	41	32	—
11	7	2/3	60	—	−39	34	−34	82	40	48
11	9	3/4	60	—	−35	34	−23	28	23	38
72	8	1/2	—	10	—	—	−9	19	9	6
10	9	2/3	—	10	—	—	−14	10	21	21
77	11	3/4	—	20	−16	—	—	50	—	—
77	11	3/4	—	40	−20	—	—	41	—	—
73	9	2/3	—	20	−18	—	−18	22	12	—
78	15	3	—	10	−51	15	−23	—	—	—
76	6	3	—	20–30	−18	—	−29	—	46	—
76A	8	3/4	—	20	−35	—	−30	56	48	—

Abbreviations as in Table 1.

nously and orally) (10,11,72,73,75–78). The following results were obtained. Drug-induced mean values for increases in cardiac index were 27% (range, 8–28%), ejection fraction 30% (range, 10–48%), and stroke work index 26% (range, 12–40%), while heart rate, left ventricular pressure, and myocardial oxygen consumption did not change significantly.

A reduction in preload was suggested by a fall in left ventricular filling pressure as expressed by a reduction in left ventricular end-diastolic pressure by an average of −39%, ranging from 18 to 64%. In addition, a moderate decline in peripheral vascular resistance by an average of −21% (range, 9–34%) was registered. These results could account for a TA-064-induced improvement of left ventricular performance, as summarized in Table 4. However, a direct inotropic effect is also suggested by a drug-induced rise in dP/dt_{max}, mean value 31%, ranging from 16 to 56%.

B. Hemodynamics After Oral Administration

After a single oral dose of TA-064, 10 mg, the plasma level reached its peak at 90 min (16±9 ng/ml) in 17 patients investigated echocardiographically (10). A positive inotropic effect was confirmed in both healthy volunteers (n = 8) and patients with congestive heart failure (n = 9) who were maximally treated with conventional medications. Maximal percentile TA-064-induced changes in patients with heart failure compared with healthy volunteers were as follows: 9% vs. 21% for stroke index, 19% vs. 18% for cardiac index, 21% vs. 14% for fractional shortening. This improved ventricular function was accompanied by a reduction in afterload, as expressed by systemic vascular resistance (by −14% vs. −9%) and preload, as expressed by a reduction in end-systolic volume (by −13% vs. −23%).

In a different study (11), 16 patients with more or less reduced ejection fraction (group A:41 ± 16%; group B:20 ± 10%) were investigated. After the administration of TA-064, 20 mg orally, maximum serum levels were obtained at the first hour for group A patients (23.8 ± 12 ng/ml) and at the second hour for group B patients (26.4 ± 20 ng/ml). These levels corresponded with those of the 1–2 μg/kg/min phase of TA-064 infusion and again with those measured towards 10 min after infusion (Fig. 11), under which application none of these parameter changes had attained significant alterations ($p>0.05$). Mean parameter changes at the peak serum level after TA-064, 20 mg orally, were as follows for group A vs. B, respectively: an increase in heart rate by an average of 10% and 6%, a rise in stroke index by 10% and 12%, an increase in cardiac index by 17% for both groups, and a rise in ejection fraction by an average of 9% and 14%; none of these hemodynamic alterations attained significance ($p>0.05$). Thus, the reactive parameter changes are comparable to those relating to similar TA-064 serum levels of the intravenous study on the first day.

Whereas Kino et al. (10) found changes in ejection phase parameters that were small but still significant, the above study (11) produced similar changes that were even smaller and not significant. Such discrepancies may be explained by methodologic variances in both studies. What may be stated with reasonable assurance, however, after comparing, in the study of Thormann et al. (11), serum levels and parameter changes subsequent to intravenous and oral application in one identical patient collective, is that massively higher oral dosages are required if beneficial

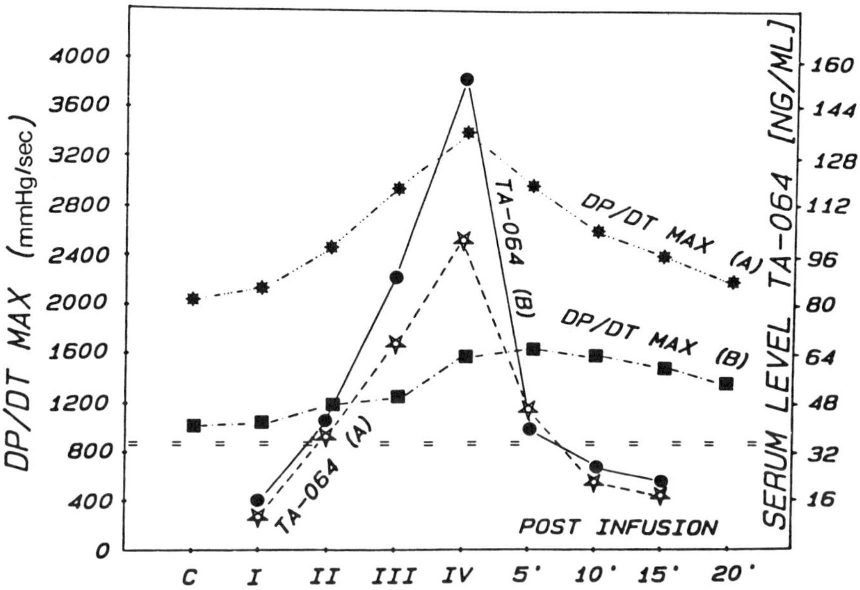

Figure 11 Dosage responses of mean contractility changes during administration of TA-064, 1,2,4, and 8 μg/kg/min (5 min periods), and up to 20 min after the infusion in 16 patients with dilated cardiomyopathy (group A moderately and group B with more drastically impaired ventricular function). With higher serum levels for group B, there was less increase in dP/dt_{max} compared to group A. The interrupted (horizontal) line indicates maximal serum levels achieved with TA-064, 20 mg orally, which stayed below those that had caused alterations of hemodynamic parameters. C, control; I, TA-064, 1 μg/kg/min i.v. over 5 min; II, TA-064, 2 μg/kg/min i.v. over 5 min; III, TA-064, 4 μg/kg/min over 5 min; IV, TA-064, 8 μg/kg/min over 5 min; 5′,10′,15′,20′, 5–20 minutes after the end of infusion. (Modified from Ref. 11.)

hemodynamic changes of the same order as those following intravenous administration are to be achieved. The dose–response rate of TA-064 being established, further discussion of this may be foregone. On the other hand, with different parameters contractility increases were identified at dosage levels that produced no relevant increases in either heart rate or arterial pressures. From the results obtained one can conclude that TA-064, if administered orally but in adequate dosages three to four times daily, can be expected to induce beneficial hemodynamic effects comparable to those resulting from intravenous application; experimental proof for this is available (70,71).

C. Hemodynamics After Intravenous Administration

In 16 patients with dilated cardiomyopathy with moderately decreased ejection fraction (41 ± 16%) in group A, and drastically decreased ejection fraction (20 ± 10%) in group B, serial analysis of left ventricular function and of pressure–volume effects was carried out to assess acute hemodynamic alterations of TA-064 given intravenously, starting with a dosage of 1 μg/kg/min over a 5-minute infusion period. The dosage was doubled in four steps up to 8 μg/kg/min at the end of each steady-state period of 3 min duration (11). Left ventricular catheterization used microtip catheter for pressure assessments and $^{99m}T_c$ scintigraphy for continuous volume analysis.

TA-064-induced improvement of left ventricular function in percentile average was greater in group A compared to group B; parameters increased as follows: cardiac index by 82% vs. 28%, respectively; stroke work by 65% vs. 47%; ejection fraction by 48% vs. 38%; and stroke volume by 40% vs. 23%. Left ventricular end-diastolic pressure (the preload) decreased simultaneously by −39% vs. 35%. The average decrease in afterload (expressed as peripheral vascular resistance) was −34% vs. −23%. Left ventricular efficiency increased with TA-064 by 62% vs. 53%, but myocardial oxygen consumption (indirectly assessed) increased significantly by 31% in group A but not in group B (11%; $p>0.05$).

D. Improved Left Ventricular Function vs. Contractility

The TA-064-induced increase of dP/dt_{max} (by 60%) was equal for both groups. However, the more pronounced increase of left ventricular pump function during drug treatment in group A than in group B was represented by average increases of the cardiac index and the ejection fraction. This was also apparent from the TA-064-induced leftward shift in the Frank-Starling-type correlogram (Fig. 12): with the medication considerably more stroke work was produced at a lower filling pressure.

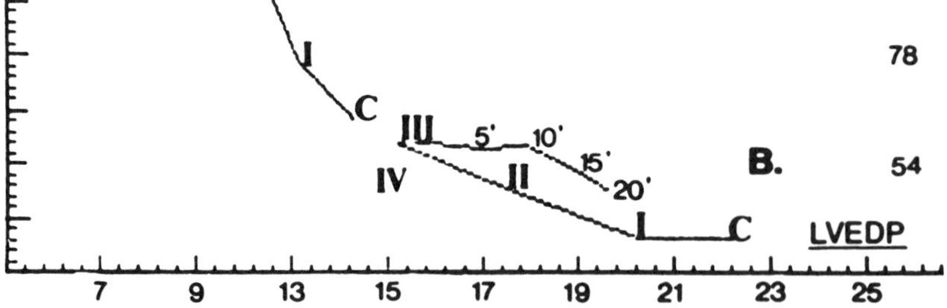

Figure 12 Computer printout relates left ventricular filling pressure with left ventricular work during the nine phases of intravenous TA-064 intervention in group A and B patients. The drug-induced characteristic motion of the average left ventricular work values, away from the control position C, leftward and up toward the maximum infusion step IV, also signifies an increase in contractility. This motion is retrograde, starting at 5 min after infusion, without reaching the control position C. This indicates continued TA-064 effects after the end of infusion. Abbreviations as in legend for Figure 11. (Modified from Ref.11.)

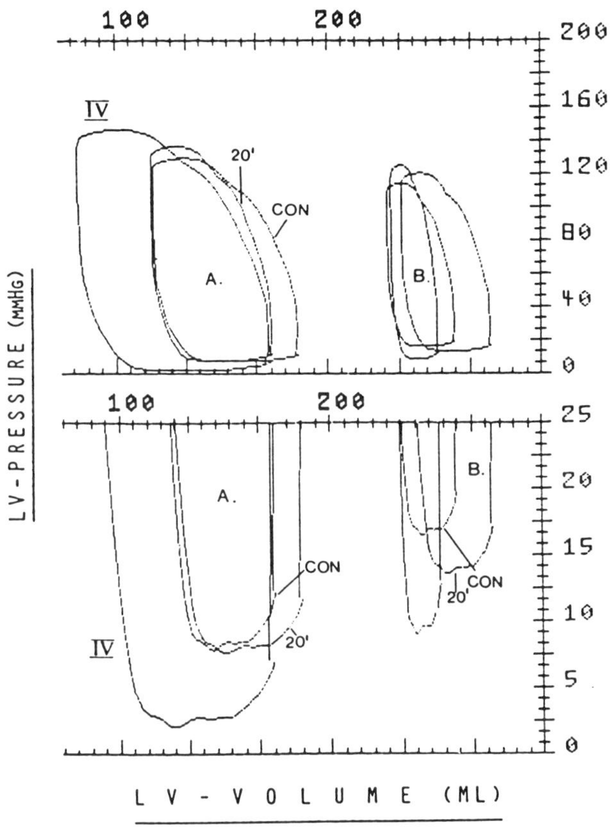

Figure 13 Computer printout displays a summation of pressure–volume relationships of the following phases: control (CON), phase IV of TA-064 infusion (IV), and 20 min after the end of infusion (20′). With maximal drug effects (IV) pressure–volume loops for groups A and B show a motion upward and to the left (i.e., contractility increase top) with a downward motion of the left ventricular end-diastolic portion of the loop (i.e., decline of filling pressure). Bottom, Blown-up portion of the loops shown above. (Modified from Ref. 11.)

Inotropic improvement due to TA-064 did not lead to a significant rise in either heart rate (26% vs. 9%; $p>0.05$) or arterial pressure (13% vs. 15%; $p>0.05$). Increases in myocardial oxygen consumption (31% vs. 11%) were significant for group A only. Increases in left ventricular pump function were accompanied by a decrease in preload (left ventricular end-diastolic pressure) and of afterload (systemic vascular resistance) while left ventricular pump efficiency rose.

The effects generated by TA-064 generally induced pressure–volume loops to shift slightly to the left, and downward in the diastolic portion (Fig. 13), which primarily points to an improvement in left ventricular pump function. The TA-064-induced increase in contractility is influenced, at least in part, by preload changes.

Thus, according to the results of this study, TA-064 increases contractility in patients with dilated cardiomyopathy while reducing preload and afterload without causing higher metabolic costs. Such beneficial hemodynamic effects appear to be stronger in the more impaired myocardium (group B patients).

E. Comparable Studies

With certain restrictions, comparisons are possible between the results provided by a patient group with congestive heart failure, as reported by Kino et al. (10), and group B of the above study (11). With a dosage of 4 μg/kg/min, comparable serum levels of TA-064 were measured (Kino et al.:82 ng/ml; group B:90 ng/ml). In Kino's study, however, increases in heart rate and dP/dt_{max} and decline in left ventricular end-diastolic pressure were certainly more marked, whereas ejection phase parameters did not change significantly. No conclusions can be drawn here as to the existence of basic differences in the drug's effect on the two collectives; other factors seem to be more determinant. Kino's group was smaller in number, clinically not homogeneous, and had better initial left ventricular functions. Also the method of parameter assessment differed: while the TA-064 dosage was the same up to the 4 μg/kg/min level, parameters in Kino's study were assessed at 10 min rather than 5 min intervals.

F. Metabolic Expenditure

Although the exact mechanism is unclear, there are indications that TA-064 does directly influence adrenal metabolism and that its inotropic effect is not mediated by the release of intrinsic catecholamines. Its β_1-adrenergic action was blocked by practolol in animal experiments (69,70), and digitalis in connection with TA-064 produced synergistic but no additional arrhythmogenic effects (71). It is to be expected that with TA-064-induced positive inotropy, myocardial ischemia will be induced through a rise in myocardial oxygen consumption. On the other hand, in the failing heart with a dilated left ventricular cavity, the inotropy-induced increase in myocardial oxygen consumption may be offset by a reduction in left ventricular chamber size (i.e., systolic wall tension). In the above investigations, TA-064 was found to induce a reduction in left ventricular volumes and systolic time interval (both being determinants of myocardial oxygen consumption), accompanied by a decrease in left ventricular filling pressures. Thus it may be thought that it was by this mechanism that metabolic expenses were kept in proportion, which is in keeping with similar assumptions relating to the effects of amrinone and vardax (AR-L 115 BS) under comparable circumstances (11,37).

G. Side Effects

In all studies quoted, TA-064 was well tolerated and was without noteworthy adverse effects. Indeed, no subject with coronary artery disease had chest pain, palpitations, or ECG changes. No dysrhythmia was recorded under the influence of TA-064. Thus, it may be stated that the drug can be safely administered in patients with coronary artery disease and that beneficial effects can be expected in patients with congestive heart failure. Documentation of a lack of chronic toxicity in human subjects will be necessary before the drug can be considered for long-term administration.

H. Clinical and Therapeutic Implications

We conclude from the results of the two major clinical investigations with TA-064 (10,11) that the drug improves left ventricular function and contractility in patients with dilated cardiomyopathy while reducing pre- and afterload (filling pressures and total vascular resistance, respectively). Also, an additional positive inotropic component can be more safely assumed, since it has been proven not just by increases in dP/dt_{max} but more appropriately by using the analysis of continuous systolic pressure volume relations (11). Neither arrhythmias nor other untoward or toxic effects could be observed. Beneficial hemodynamic effects were achieved without any disproportional increase in myocardial oxygen consumption. TA-064-induced metabolic costs were probably partially offset by a decrease in left ventricular wall tension. Since, subject to its use in adequate dosages, the drug is effective orally as well, this cardiotonic agent seems to offer promising potential in the therapy of dilated cardiomyopathy.

VII. GENERAL IMPLICATIONS

Beneficial hemodynamic effects surely can be attested to for all cardiotonic agents reviewed in this chapter. This is true especially for the dramatic short-term hemodynamic benefits. The enthusiasm about such new agents must be restrained, however, until their true potentials have been evaluated in long-term controlled trials. Up to 1988 the majority of the controlled trials completed (of the 80 novel vasodilators and inotropic drugs) have been unable to demonstrate that these therapeutic interventions have advanced the treatment of chronic cardiac failure. On the other hand, with respect to the agents discussed in this chapter, DPI 201-106 had to be withdrawn from clinical investigation since a concentration-related increase in ventricular ectopic beats was observed as a proarrhythmic potential. Sulmazole was also withdrawn from further clinical studies because of the development of hepatic neoplasms in long-term toxicologic studies. The two other cardiotonic agents pimobendan and MCI-154 are still in the race, while the promising hemodynamic profile of MCI-154 is as yet known only experimentally.

Recent research has focused on the pathophysiological abnormalities of heart failure: positive inotropic drugs for depressed contractility and vasodilator action for the excessively constricted systemic vessels in heart failure fail consistently to make patients feel better or prolong life. However, this must remain the ultimate goal. Nevertheless, the research along these lines (involving some 80 novel cardiotonic drugs) has not been futile. It rather teaches us to understand why certain drugs fail and others succeed, and most certainly helps to amplify our understanding of heart failure and makes us consider the altered hemodynamic state as a factor rather than the most important pathophysiological abnormality. Eminent investigators have rightly stated that research has been promising when it tried to modify physiological derangements in heart failure rather than merely correct the hemodynamic abnormalities that can easily be measured. This is an approach that we can also subscribe to.

VIII. THE RECENT PHOPHODIESTERASE III-INHIBITOR DRUGS (AMRINONE, ENOXIMONE, PIROXIMONE): DO THEY GENERATE INOTROPIC EFFECTS? ANALYSIS OF END-SYSTOLIC PRESSURE-VOLUME RELATIONS (CONDUCTANCE TECHNIQUE)

A. Introduction

We analyzed the end-systolic pressure–volume relations (ESPVR), using the conductance technique, to study the potential inotropic effects of phosphodiesterase–inhibitor drugs.

The question of contractility involvement is of clinical importance, since with the inotropy-induced rise of myocardial oxygen consumption there is a risk of myocardial ischemia, should anyone of the cardiotonic drugs (amrinone, enoximone, piroximone) be used in patients with coronary artery disease. Accordingly, we analyzed their hemodynamic effects and identified improved contractility as one factor of these drugs' mode of action and we proved their inability to induce myocardial ischemia.

An important prerequisite of clinical pharmacotherapy is to achieve as close as possible an insight into a drug's mechanism of action, its hemodynamic effects. This notion is going to be exemplarily corroborated by the methodologically problematic analysis of the complex mechanism of action of the PDE drugs, which were developed with high hopes of potentially aiding the (insufficient) present therapeutic concept of chronic heart failure.

1. Inodilator Drugs (PDE-Inhibitors)

Do the new noncatechole, nonglycosidic, cardiotonic agents (such as the PDE-inhibitor drug enoximone) improve left ventricular function by mere changes in load? Is contractility involved? These have been controversial questions ever since the advent of one of the first of this type of cardiotonic drug having been developed: amrinone. For, with the inotropy-induced rise of myocardial oxygen consumption there is a risk of ischemia, should anyone of these new "positive inotropic" drugs be used in patients with cardiac failure due to CAD.

Aside from the hemodynamics, accurate assessments of contractility alterations are needed in any of the given examples. In addition to conventional hemodynamic parameter changes, we, therefore, analyzed end-systolic pressure–volume relationships (using the conductance technique) during the above clinical interventions in order to appropriately define their potential influence on ventricular contractility.

B. Methods

1. The Conductance (Volume) Catheter System

We used the analysis of the end-systolic pressure–volume relationship (ESPVR), since presently it is considered the most sensitive index of LV contractility (79), on account of its near load insensitivity.

For all ventriculodynamic investigations the conductance technique was applied which has been dealt with elsewhere (80,81,82,90,100,101). The special catheter supplies the continuous sectorial volume signals, which are then assembled by computer assistance to form the total volume signal and, in addition, supplies the ventricular pressure. The synchronization of both parameters then provides the pressure–volume diagrams, the beat-to-beat loops of the end-systolic pressure–volume relationship (ESPVR).

2. Caval Balloon Occlusion for Rapid Load Changes

The construction of the line of the isometric maxima was achieved by using temporary balloon occlusion in the vena cava inferior (81,83,84,85), since multiple loops under different loading conditions are required (79). The ESPVR–loop motion of the initial cycles, as induced by the sudden and temporary preload changes via balloon occlusion in the vena cava inferior, determines the course of the isometric maxima line (the ESPVR) for a given interventional condition. Acutely induced changes in the slope k (mmHg/ml) of this line of ESPVR, then indicate an altered contractile state.

3. *Course of the Investigations*

The analysis of the hemodynamic effects consisted of the computer-assisted assessment of serial phasic pressure–volume diagrams prior and after the acute intervention in each patient. Following routine diagnostic cardiac catheterization an 8F conductance catheter was percutaneously advanced, until its tip reached the left ventricular apex (via an 8F introducer with sideport). From the antecubital vein, a pacer electrode was placed into the right atrium for maintaining constantly paced heart rates and also periods of tachycardia.

4. *Investigational Protocols*

Aside from conventional hemodynamic parameters, for the analysis of the ESPVR during the above interventions the following representative measuring phases were registered and fed into the computer: (1) values at rest, the control; (2) during constant atrial pacing (CAP 90 bpm), the control; (3) temporary balloon occlusion of the v.cava inf. (BOVCI) during CAP, the control; (4) phase of paced atrial tachycardia (PAT 160 bpm), the control; (5) temporary BOVCI during PAT, the control; (6) return to control during CAP; (7) measurements during CAP and during maximal influence of an intervention (INT), i.e. drugs: 3 PDE-inhibitors; (8) temporary BOVCI during INT and CAP; (9) PAT during INT; (10) temporary BOVCI during PAT.

C. Results

1. *Inotropic Effects of the Inodilators*

The new positive inotropic agents, like the phosphodiesterase (PDE)-inhibitors acutely improve hemodynamics in congestive heart failure (86). Whether or not the improved LV function might be induced by mere changes in load or also (at least in part) by contractility, has been controversial ever since the advent of amrinone in 1979 (87). This is of clinical importance since, with the inotropy-induced rise of MVO2, there is a risk of ischemia, when one of these new cardiotonics should be used in patients with cardiac failure due to CAD. On the other hand, a PDE-inhibitor drug-induced positive inotropic action altogether has seriously been questioned (88,89). Therefore, the following clinical investigations were designed to identify some of the PDE-inhibitor drugs' true inotropy with appropriate methodology, versus the drugs' vasodilator actions.

2. *Amrinone*

We analyzed end-systolic pressure–volume relations (ESPVR) in 19 patients with still normal LV function (study I) (81). Amrinone 1.5 mg/kg i.v. failed to induce alterations in ESPVR but rather caused load changes, resembling those seen with nitroprusside. During constant atrial pacing (90/min) brief infusion phases with nitroprusside and phenylephrine provided the required load changes of this study.

The analysis of ESPVR and LVF in 11 patients (study II) (81) with impaired LV function revealed the following changes (Fig. 14): Amrinone 2.5 mg/kg i.v induced increased contractility, which was even further improved after the additional appli-

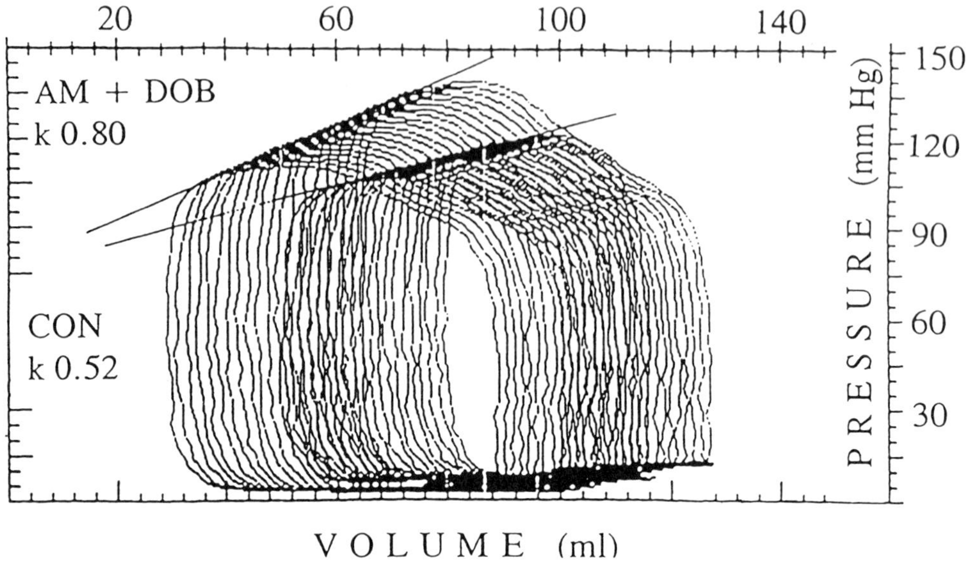

Figure 14 Demonstrated is the summed series of diagrams from 11 patients: before (CON) and after the application of amrinone plus dobutamine (AM+DOB). The loop of the ESPVR is shifted to the left by the drug effect, while slope k increases from 0.52 to 0.8 mmHg/ml, both indicating inotropic effects. Thus, amrinone's positive inotropic effects in these groups II patients (impaired LV function) are shown to be further augmented by added dobutamine.

cation of dobutamine, 10 ug/kg/min: slope k increased from 0.52 to 0.8 mmHg/ml and the loop of the ESPVR moved leftward, both indicating an increase in inotropic effects. dP/dt_{max} rose by 39% after amrinone and by 57% with both, amrinone and added dobutamine. Transient vena cava inferior balloon occlusion provided the required rapid load changes for this study.

Thus, amrinone's contractility-increasing effects were demonstrated in a dose-related fashion; they are generated probably (at least in part) via an increase in heart rate; inotropic effects further increased when dobutamine was added.

3. *Enoximone*

We analyzed ESPVR and LV function in 12 of 18 CAD patients after enoximone, 0.75 mg/kg i.v. (90). The slope k increased (7 patients; Table 5) and loops of the ESPVR (12 patients;) moved leftward with enoximone by an average of 32% and downward 19%, in the diastolic portion (Fig. 15). The delta percent changes in enoximone versus control (18 patients; Table 6) indicated an improved LVF via load changes: LV-filling pressure fell by 50% and end-systolic volume by 28%, while dP/dt_{max} rose by 25%, LV work by 10% and ejection fraction by 11%. Lastly, in precatheterization studies, the pacing-induced anginal threshold increased from an average of 58±18 sec to 89± 12 sec after enoximone, while ischemic postpacing LV-filling pressure and ST-segment changes normalized under the drug's influence.

Table 5 ESPVR Before and After Enoximone

Pat. no.	LVEDP mmHg	dP/dt mmHg/s	Slope of the ESPVR k mmHg/ml	V_0	r	EF (%)	EDV (ml)
ESPVR before enoximone							
1	12	1800	1.32	−66.00	0.92	71	145
2	9	1700	1.64	−37.00	0.91	56	147
4	16	2000	1.20	−80.00	0.88	62	133
5	18	1800	1.02	−12.10	0.90	55	137
6	18	1600	1.87	−16.20	0.91	69	77
8	10	1500	1.08	−55.00	0.87	51	148
11	18	1300	2.61	−9.60	0.98	61	110
Mean	14.40	1672	1.53			60.7	128
± SD	3.90	229	0.57			7.4	26
ESPVR after enoximone							
1	6	2100	2.31	−33.00	0.98	76	124
2	4	2300	2.92	−23.00	0.98	68	127
4	8	2700	1.41	−86.00	0.91	71	120
5	6	2400	1.35	−8.40	0.90	60	134
6	2	2800	2.68	−9.90	0.86	86	74
8	6	1850	1.51	−31.00	0.93	76	98
11	6	1500	3.08	−7.70	0.97	66	83
Mean	5.40*	2236*	2.18*			71.9*	109*
±SD	1.90	461	0.75			8.4	24

*Significant vs. control, $p < 0.05$ at least.

Thus, enoximone improved left ventricular function, both by unloading and by true positive inotropy. Lack of enoximone-induced angina and an increased anginal theshold indicate that the drug can be used safely in CAD patients as well.

4. *Piroximone*

Piroximone is one of the new PDE-III inhibitor drugs, which is known to display beneficial hemodynamic effects in severe congestive heart failure (91), probably via direct inotropic and vasodilator actions. We analyzed LV function and ESPVR after piroximone (0.75 μg/kg i.v.) in 16 patients with CAD and still normal ejection fraction (100). Slope E_{max} increased by 39% (Table 7; Fig. 16) and the loops of the ESPVR moved leftward, indicating improved contractility. The delta% changes piroximone vs. control showed an improved LV function via load changes (Table 8): LV volumes decreased (end-systolic volume by 37%, end-diastolic volume by 19%), LV-filling pressure by 35% and systemic vascular resistance by 19%, dP/dt_{max} increased by 28%, ejection fraction by 13%, while MVO_2 remained unchanged.

In their precatheterization evaluation of the 16 patients, pacing-induced anginal threshold had increased after piroximone, and during the analysis of the ESPVR no angina had developed in any of the patients investigated. Thus, summing up all results of this study, piroximone improved LV function both, by unloading and by an increase in contractility without inducing myocardial ischemia. The results indi-

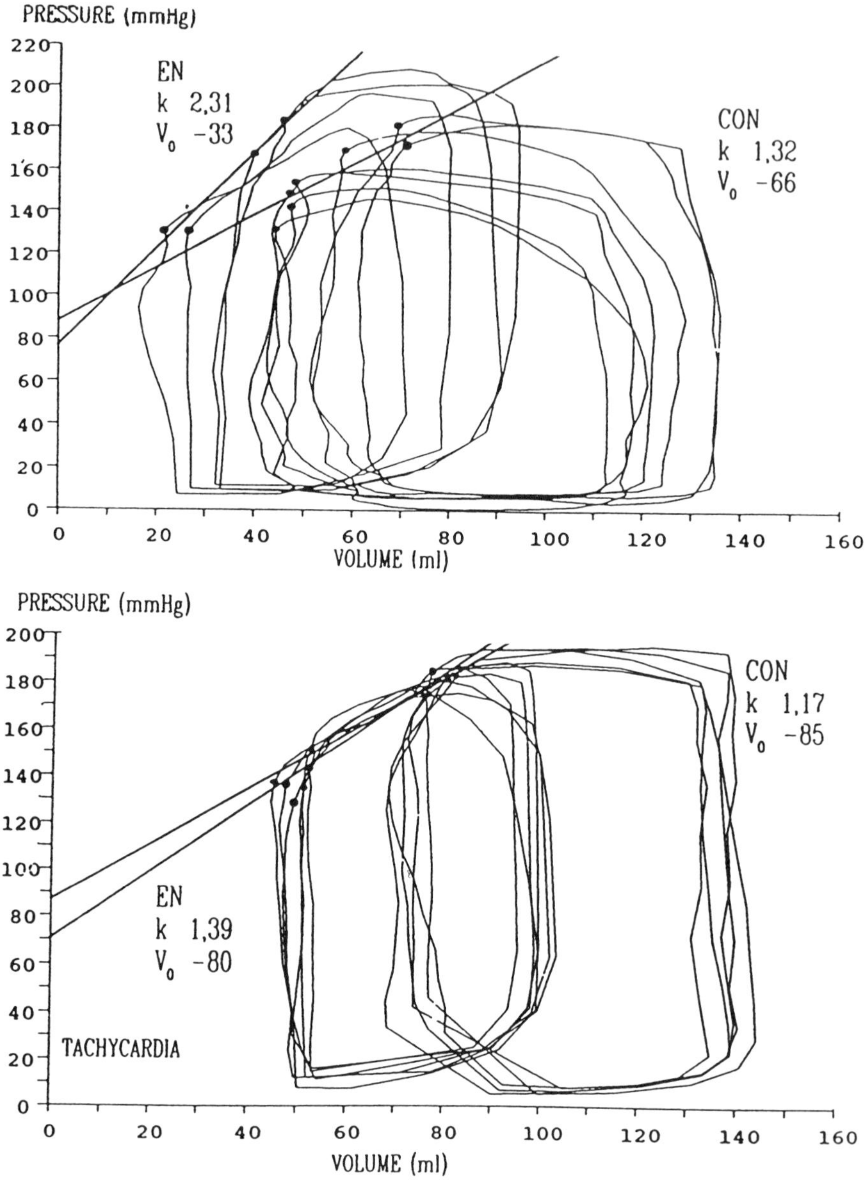

Figure 15 In the example of patient no. 2 the enoximone-induced increase in contractility is demonstrated both at resting conditions (above) and during tachycardia (below). This is indicated by the leftward shift of the loop of the ESPVR and by an increase in slope k (E_{max}) at rest and is less marked during tachycardia with a rate of 160 bpm.

Table 6 Hemodynamic Alterations

	Without enoximone	With enoximone
LV end-diastolic pressure (mmHg)	14.8 ± 5.3	7.4 ± 3.5*
LV systolic pressure (mmHg)	140 ± 27	140 ± 31
dP/dt_{max} (mmHg/s)	1719 ± 311	2147 ± 562*
End-diastolic volume index (ml/m²)	76.5 ± 15	63.9 ± 17*
End-systolic volume index (ml/m²)	30.8 ± 9	22.1 ± 10*
Stroke index (ml/m²)	45.7 ± 11	41.9 ± 11
Ejection fraction (%)	59.9 ± 8	66.6 ± 11*
LV work (kg · m)	80.5 ± 28	87.9 ± 28*
Systemic vascular resistance (dyne·s·cm⁻⁵)	1477 ± 540	1469 ± 532
Myocardial oxygen consumption (ml/min/100 g)	7.8 ± 1.5	8.1 ± 1.9
LV efficiency (%)	2.1 ± 0.6	2.2 ± 0.6

Values: mean ± standard deviation.
LV = left ventricular.
*$p < 0.05$, at least, without versus with enoximone.

Table 7 Piroximone-Induced Alterations in Hemodynamics and the ESPVR

Patient No.	LVEDP (mmHg)	dP/dt_{max} (mmHg/s)	EDV (ml)	EF (%)	E_{max} (ml/mmHg)	V_0	r
Control							
2	17	2100	250	52	0.55	−248.4	0.92
4	14	1800	178	65	1.81	−9.8	0.99
6	9	1900	170	70	0.68	−39.8	0.89
7	10	1600	184	61	1.71	−10.6	0.96
8	22	2200	199	66	0.89	−74.4	0.99
11	8	2400	234	63	0.81	−46.5	0.94
12	12	2400	239	69	2.48	2.2	0.91
13	12	2400	143	62	2.03	−7.9	0.93
14	17	1300	116	49	0.73	−52.4	0.91
mean	13.4	2011	190.3	61.9	1.31		
± SD	4.5	392	45.1	7.2	0.72		
Piroximone							
2	4	2400	197	51	0.88	−97.7	0.93
4	8	2400	127	80	3.52	−4.0	0.94
6	8	2300	166	80	1.27	−4.3	0.92
7	7	2000	133	46	2.27	−5.3	0.91
8	12	2800	174	72	1.05	−66.9	0.87
11	11	2800	220	75	1.21	−3.49	0.84
12	8	3400	192	78	2.92	6.01	0.88
13	9	3000	123	61	2.06	10.2	0.97
14	11	1650	102	60	1.22	−7.5	0.89
mean	8.7•	2528•	159.3•	67•	1.82		
± SD	2.5	532	40	12.9	0.93		

• = significant vs. control, $p<0.05$ at least. (See Table 2 for abbreviations.)

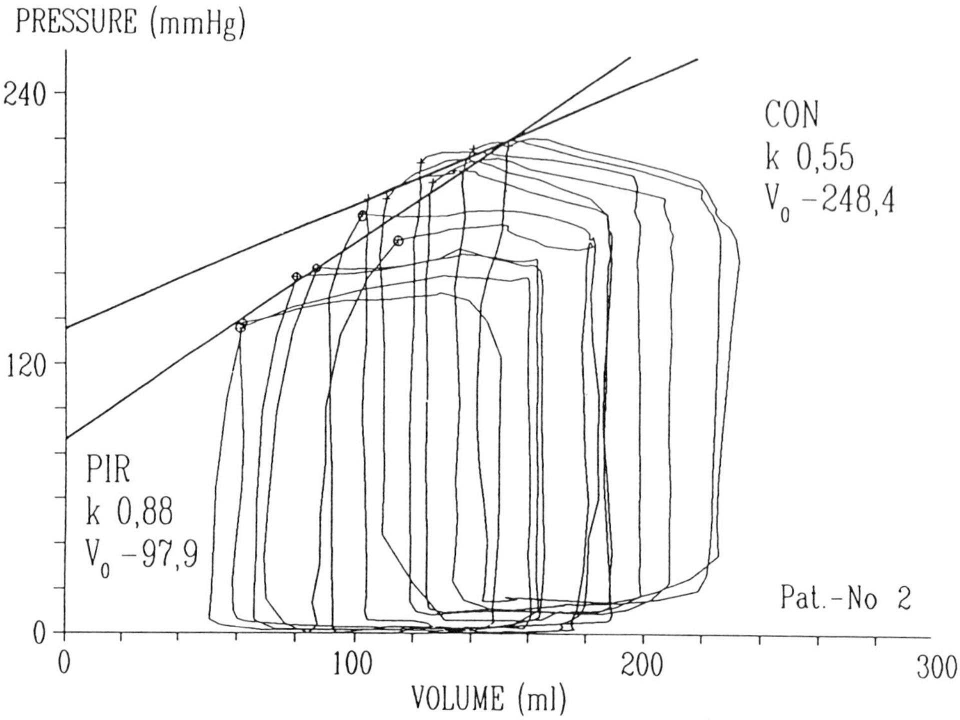

Figure 16 In this example piroximone, the new PDE-III inhibitor drug improves LV function by unloading and by positive inotropic effects as indicated by leftward motion of the loop and increase in slope k (E_{max}) of the ESPVR from 0.55 to 0.88 mmHg/ml.

Table 8 Hemodynamic Parameter Changes with and Without the Influence of Piroximone at Rest and During Tachycardia

		Rest		Tachycardia	
		Without PIR	With PIR	Without PIR	With PIR
LVEDP	(mmHg)	14.1 ± 4.3	9.3 ± 3.5•	10 ± 4.8	5.8 ± 3.0•
LVSP	(mmHg)	155 ± 29	147 ± 21	147 ± 22	144 ± 19
dP/dt_{max}	(mmHg/s)	1938 ± 398	2409 ± 559•	2100 ± 390	2500 ± 534•
dP/dt_{min}	(mmHg/s)	1803 ± 349	1803 ± 32	1922 ± 458	2000 ± 430
ESV	(ml)	69.8 ± 35	44.2 ± 24	61.7 ± 37	53.1 ± 43
EDV	(ml)	176.3 ± 43	143.5 ± 38•	131.4 ± 58	130.8 ± 58
LV eff	(%)	2.16 ± 0.71	2.67 ± 0.91•	2.5 ± 1.1	2.7 ± 1.1
EF	(%)	61.6 ± 10.1	69.6 ± 13.1•	53.4 ± 14.8	60.8 ± 18
CI	(L/min/m2)	4.02 ± 1.3	4.89 ± 1.7•	5.3 ± 2.4	5.9 ± 2.5
LVW	(kg·m)	109.1 ± 48.4	124.7 ± 47.6•	151 ± 76.9	160.1 ± 72
SVR	(dyne·s·cm^{-5})	1297 ± 425	1050 ± 384•	1233 ± 879	1081 ± 812

• = Significant, $p<0.05$ at least. (See table 2 for abbreviations.)

cate that the drugs' combined beneficial hemodynamic effects can be used safely also in CAD.

5. Synopsis: Hemodynamic Effects of PDE-Inhibitors

a. Contractility Improving Components PDE-inhibitors' positive effects on contracility in the human heart have largely been assumed on account of methodological insufficient proof, and the results are equivocal. There is considerable data that the agents, such as the 3 PDE-inhibitors we have analyzed, increase cardiac index and reduce filling pressures in patients with heart failure (86), but it has been demonstrated that similar effects can be produced by pure vasodilators as well (92).

Increase in dP/dt_{max} achieved with these agents, averaging 15-42% (93,94), could also have been induced by increases in heart rate or changes in preload and afterload (95). In a study of 14 patients with heart failure due to cardiomyopathy, dP/dt_{max} failed to be changed by the administration of amrinone, and the otherwise drug-induced beneficial hemodynamic effects were attributed to vasodilator effects exclusively (88). In patients with heart failure, an increase in dP/dt_{max} and stroke volume index was achieved at intracoronary applied dosages of milrinone that had few systemic effects (96). This strongly suggested a positive inotropic action of the drug, but also that increased contractility alone does not confer any hemodynamic benefit.

The production of evidence of PDE-inhibitors' positive inotropic effect is further hampered by other issues: Since these agents have the potential to increase catecholamine levels (97), an augmentation of the heart rate and contractility might also have been induced indirectly by an altered sympathetic tone. In our 3 studies, presented here, however, inotropy and LV-pump function improved, while heart rate was kept constant (a methodologic requirement for correct analysis of the ESPVR).

In addition, there is proof that myocardium from patients with severe heart failure has little or no inotropic responsiveness to PDE-inhibitors and β-adrenergic agonists (98). In studies 2 and 3 presented here this argument for nonresponders is invalid, since in the precatheterization study anginal threshold was raised by enoximone in all patients having taken part in the analysis of the ESPVR. The enoximone and piroximone study groups each consisted of patients with ischemic CAD, but symptomatic cardiac failure was not present in any of them.

b. Effects on Inotropy and LV-Pump Function Although many studies have shown improved hemodynamics after the acute administration of PDE-inibitor drugs in congestive heart failure (86,94) it has been difficult to demonstrate a positive inotropic effect of the drug in vivo because of their concomitant vasodilator properties. Using only the conventional left ventricular output parameters as employed in the investigations of others, the influences of preload (ventricular filling), afterload (ventricular wall stress and arterial pressure), and heart rate can hardly be evaluated separately. Output indices, such as ejection fraction and cardiac index are unfit for proving inotropic drug action, since they are significantly influenced by changes in afterload.

There is only one study (99) that succeeded in assessing enoximone's significant positive inotropy by analyzing its effects on the ESPVR. In other studies, the assessment of LV-contractile function has been based merely on measurements of the peak positive left ventricular dP/dt, which amounted to an average of 30% after the intravenous administration of enoximone in patients with heart failure (94,99). Although an increase in dP/dt_{max} suggests improved contractility, this may also be the result of increases in heart rate and changes in LV-preload and/or afterload (95).

c. PDE-Inhibitor Effects on Myocardial Ischemia In a recent study 2 out of 9 patients with CAD developed angina after enoximone with an estimated rise in myocardial oxygen consumption of greater than 30% (99). The ischemia in these patients could have occurred because of an increase in myocardial consumption resulting from the increases in heart rate and arterial pressure, along with improved contractility in these cases (the counterbalance provided by a fall in wall tension due to a decrease in ventricular chamber size was probably missing). However, in the present study, the administration of enoximone increased the pacing-induced anginal threshold, while LV function improved. The mechanism responsible for these results has to be multifold. It seems to consist of a decrease in preload (end-diastolic pressure fell by 50%, end-systolic volume by 28%) and inotropic activity (increases in dP/dt_{max} and slope k of the ESPVR and leftward motion of the loops) without a significant rise in MVO_2, while the metabolic balance was probably provided by reduced wall stress, which was not measured in our study. Thus, in this study enoximone improved LV function, both by unloading and by true positive inotropy. The lack of PDE-inhibitor drugs'-induced angina and an increased anginal threshold indicate that they can be used beneficially and safely in patients with CAD as well.

D. Discussion

1. Methodological Aspects

The aim of this study was to identify potential inotropic effects inherent in the mechanism of action of PDE-inhibitor drug intervention. Appropriately, analysis of the end-systolic pressure–volume relations (ESPVR) was chosen, relying on previous experiences with the conductance catheter technique (81,82,90,100,101,102, 113). The ESPVR at present is considered to be the most sensitive index of LV contractility since it is virtually load independent (79,103,104).

Volume assessment using the conductance system represents a definite improvement in the methodology of analyzing ESPVR. It offers the possibility of producing any number of the beat-to-beat pressure–volume diagrams over a wide range of load changes; all this is achieved in connection with the technique of rapid load changes with temporary balloon occlusion in the v.cava inf. Investigations using this combined technique are experimentally sound, have been brought to maturity (84,105,106,107), and have proven their reliability and practicability in our catheterization laboratory for the past 7 years (81,82,90,100,101,102,113).

2. Limitations and Critique

a. Volume measurements Volume assessments of the conductance technique correlate sufficiently with stroke volume (thermodilution, angiography) of the human (80) and the isolated heart (106). The claim for absolute volume measurements meets its major obstacle in form of the *parallel conductance volume* (107), i.e., the volume of structures outside the blood filled LV cavum, and cannot be accurately determined. It is automatically included into the conductance volume measuring process and renders the actual measurement incorrect as an absolute volume. Special methods of correction which had been developed previously (80) were recently classified as being too variable in relation to the actual volume dimension (107), i.e., increasingly unreliable, the larger the ventricular size. The usefulness of the method to measure relative volume changes, however, has not been questioned (107). In previous investigations (82,101,102) as well as in the ones presented here (81,90,100) we did not use the above correction method for parallel conductance volume, but accepted, like other investigators (84) that the conductance technique reliably assesses relative but not absolute volumes based on the angiographic volume of the control phase. These individual angiograms served as a volume reference for all further volume measurements using the conductance technique in each particular case of our studies.

b. End-Systolic Pressure–Volume Relationship (ESPVR) We did not succeed in assessing drug-induced changes of slope k (E_{max}) of the ESPVR in all patients of each study group. In the majority drug effects caused the ESPVR loops to move rightward and up (antiarrhythmic agents) and leftward down (PDE-inhibitor drugs), respectively. This, like in other studies (104,108), has been accepted to primarily indicate negative inotropic or positive inotropic effects of the drug. The ajmaline-induced changes of slope k of the ESPVR (101), for instance, could be achieved in 6/12 patients only (due to the self-imposed time limitations for the conduct of the study). The preload-dependent parameter dP/dt_{max} was not available for adequate comparison of contractility effects. On the other hand, enoximone (90), for instance, did induce an increase of slope k of the ESPVR in 7 patients (Table 1), and piroximone (100) in 9 patients (Table 7), indicating drug-induced positive inotropy. However, statistically relevant comparative or quantifying statements cannot be made from the accumulated results.

The slope k of the ESPVR showed a weak correlation only with parameters of LV systolic function (for instance, r=0.67 for LVP/ESV). It should be considered, however, that inotropic interventions are known to induce variable effects on the slope k and intercept V_0 of the ESPVR (109). These discrepancies might be due to the fact that theoretical (110) and experimental arguments (104,111) have given rise to doubt the linearity of the ESPVR. The exact ESPVR analysis depends on the reliability of data collected during programmed load changes, which are required for the construction of the line of the isometric maxima, and on the quality of their linear correlation. But even in case all requirements are fulfilled (as in the present studies), the statistical reliability of the values for slope k and V_0 (the intercept) of the ESPVR is regarded as not ufficient under all circumstances by some investigators (110,112). Therefore, it presently has become customary for clinical studies to rather rely primarily on form and motion of the loops of the ESPVR and regard changes of the slope k as an adjunct parameter (104,108) if at all aviable.

E. Conclusions

Being well aware of the above methodological limitations, the presented studies then aimed for the assessment of changes in myocardial contractility and not of its absolute state. PDE-inhibitor drugs' positive inotropic components were defined. However, their effects did not induce angina in CAD patients, which is of importance for the clinical use of these drugs. The conductance technique proved to be useful, sensitive, and safe in the assessment of inotropic effects by analyzing the ESPVR within the routine of the cardiac catheterization procedure.

REFERENCES

1. Johnston GD. Alternatives to the digitalis glycosides for heart failure. Br Med J 1985; 290:803–4.
2. Packer M, Medina N, Yusahk M. Hemodynamic and clinical limitations of longterm inotropic therapy with amrinone in patients with severe chronic heart failure. Circulation 1984; 70:1038–47.
3. Feldman AM. A biochemical base for the use of inotropic drugs. Heart Failure 1988; 3/6:223–9.
4. Scholtysik G, Rüegg P. DPI 201-106. In: Scriabine A, ed. New cardiovascular drugs. New York: Raven Press, 1987; 5:173–88.
5. Thormann J, Kramer W, Kindler M, Kremer FP, Schlepper M. Comparative efficacy of the new cardiotonic agent DPI 201-106 versus dobutamine in dilated cardiomyopathy: analysis by serial pressure/volume relations and "on-line" MVO_2 assessment. J Cardiovasc Pharmacol 1986; 8:749–57.
6. Thormann J, Kramer W, Schlepper M, Gottwick M. ARL-115 BS in the treatment of heart failure. Eur Heart J 1982; 3(suppl D):87–95.
7. Brand HJ, Hagemeijer F. Hemodynamic effects of pimobendan given orally to patients with severe heart failure. Eur Heart J 1987; 8:(suppl 2):73/276.
8. Katz SD, Forman R, Giustino SR, Sonneblick EH, LeJemtel TH. Double-blind randomized evaluation of pimobendan, a new inotrope and vasodilator agent for refractory heart failure. Circulation 1987; 76(suppl IV):IV-178–707.
9. Shibata S, Satake N, Hester RK, Kurahashi K, Ito M. The mode of vasoinhibitory action of a pyridazione derivative (MCI-154), a new cardiotonic agent, on contractile responses induced by alpha- adrenoceptor agonists and ^{45}Ca influx in isolated vascular smooth muscles. Eur J Pharmacol 1988; 145:113–21.
10. Kino M, Hirota Y, Yamamoto S Sawada K, Moriguchi M, Kotaka M, Kubo C, Kawamura K. Cardiovascular effects of a newly synthesized cardiotonic agent (TA-064) on normal and diseased hearts. Am J Cardiol 1983; 51:802–10.
11. Thormann J, Kramer W, Kindler M, Neuss H, Bahawar H, Schlepper M. Analysis of the efficacy of the new cardiotonic agent TA-064. Am Heart J 1985; 110:426–38.
12. Petein M, From AHL, Frances GS, Pierpoint GL. DPI 201-106: a new non-adrenergic inotropic agent with possible beta adrenergic blocking activity. Circulation 1985; 72:(suppl III) III-304.
13. Scholtysik G, Salzmann R, Berthold R, Herzig JW, Quast U, Markstein R. DPI 201-106, a novel cardioactive agent. Combination of cAMP-independent positive inotropic, negative chronotropic, action potential prolonging and coronary dilatory properties. Naunyn Schmiedebergs Arch Pharmacol 1985; 329:316–25.
14. Takahashi K, Endoh M, Taira N. Inotropic versus chronotropic, dromotropic, and coronary vasodilator actions of DPI 201-106, a novel positive inotropic agent, in the dog heart. J Cardiovasc Pharmacol 1987; 9:451–60.
15. Siegl PK, Garcia ML, Kling VF, Scott AL, Morgan G, Kaczorowski GJ. Interactions of DPI 201-106, a novel cardiotonic agent, with cardiac calcium channels. Naunyn Schmiedeberg's Arch Pharmacol 1988; 338:684–91.
16. Buggish D, Isenberg G, Ravens U, Scholtysik G. The role of sodium channels in the effects of the cardiotonic compound DPI 201-106 on contractility and membrane potentials in isolated mammalian heart preparations. Eur J Pharmacol 1985; 118:303–11.

17. Butrous CS, Debbas NMG, Erwin J, Davies DW, Keller HP, Lunnon MW, Nathan AW, Camm AJ. Clinical cardiac electrophysiologic evaluation of the positive inotropic agent, DPI 201-106. Eur Heart J 1988; 9:489–97.
18. Hogan JC, Greenbaum RA, Lunnon MW, Hilson AJW, Evans TR. Hemodynamic effects of DPI 201-106, following single intravenous dose administration to patients with moderate cardiac failure. Eur Heart J 1988; 9:498–501.
19. Linderer T, Heineking M, Schroeder R. The effects of DPI 201-106, a cardiotonic agent with negative chronotropic activity, on hemodynamics and myocardial metabolism. Z Kardiol 1987; 76: suppl 1–79.
20. Uretsky BF, Murali S, Reddy PS, Valdes AM, Kolesar JA. Hemodynamic and electrocardiographic effects of the fast channel activator, DPI 201-106. J Am Coll Cardiol 1987; 9/2:161A.
21. Kostis JB, Lacy CR, Raia JJ, Dworkin JH, Warner RG, Casazza LA. DPI 201-106 for severe congestive heart failure. Am J Cardiol 1987; 60:1334–9.
22. Morganroth J, Horowitz LN, Mulhern C. The effects of Sandoz DPI 201-106, a new inotropic and antiarrhythmic agent, on ventricular function and arrhythmias. Clin Res 1986; 34/2:328A.
23. Rüegg JC, Nüesch E. The effect of a new inotropic agent, DPI 201-106, on systolic time intervals and the electrocardiogram in healthy subjects. Br J Clin Pharmacol 1987; 24:453–8.
24. Hof RP, Hof A. Mechanism of the vasodilator effects of the cardiotonic agent DPI 201-106. J Cardiovasc Pharmacol 1985; 7:188–92.
25. Haynes RE, Hallstrom AP, Cobb LA. Repolarization abnormalities in survivors of out-of-hospital ventricular fibrillation. Circulation 1978; 57:654.
26. Schwartz PJ, Wolf S. QT interval prolongation as predictor of sudden death in patients with myocardial infarction. Circulation 1978; 57:1074–7.
27. Pratt CM, Slyman DJ, Wierman AM, Young JB, Francis MJ, Seals AA, Quinones MA, Roberts R. Analysis of the spontaneous variability of ventricular arrhythmias: consecutive ambulatory electrocardiographic recordings of ventricular tachycardia. Am J Cardiol 1985; 56:67–72.
28. Dämmgen J, Kadatz R, Diederen W. Action of AR-L 115BS on myocardial oxygen consumption, cardiac performance and vascular resistance and capacitance. Arzneim Forsch (Drug Res) 1981; 31:151–4.
29. Diederen W, Kadatz R. Effects of AR-L 115, a new cardiotonic compound, on cardiac contractility, heart rate and blood pressure in anaesthetized and conscious animals. Arzneim Forsch (Drug Res) 1981; 31:146–50.
30. Hellige G, Baller D, Ensink FBM, Zipfel J, Wolpers HG, Bretschneider HJ. Effects of AR-L 115 on hemodynamics, myocardial oxygen consumption in cardiac pumping efficiency. Arzneim Forsch (Drug Res) 1981; 31:155–6.
31. Herzog H, Grube E, Sarrasch V, Simon H, Schaede A. Linksventrikuläre Funktionsparameter unter ARL-115 bei Myokardinsuffizienz im Akutversuch. Z Kardiol 1981; 70:271/60.
32. Klein G, Sauer E, Bauer R, Wirtzfeld A, Sebening H, Schmidt G. Vergleich von AR-L115 mit Dobutamin bei schwerer Herzinsuffizienz. Z Kardiol 1980; 69/10:706–72.
33. Thormann J, Kramer W, Schlepper M. AR-L 115:a new nonglycosidic, non-adrenergic cardiotonic agent; hemodynamic proof fot its effectiveness, both intravenously and by oral application, Circulation 1980; 61(suppl III):III-233.
34. Thormann J, Kramer W, Schlepper M. Changes of hemodynamics, coronary flow and myocardial energy metabolism in patients with coronary artery disease after the application of the new cardiotonic agent AR-L 115. Am Heart J 1982; 104:1294–302.
35. Benotti JR, Grossman W, Braunwald E, Davolis DD, Alousi AA. Hemodynamic assessment of amrinone, a new inotropic agent. N Engl J Med 1978; 299:1373–7.

36. LeJemtal TH, Keung E, Sonnenblick E. Amrinone:a new glycosidic, non-adrenergic, cardiotonic agent effective in the treatment of intractable myocardial failure in man. Circulation 1979; 59:1038–41.
37. Thormann J, Kramer W, Kindler M, Kremer P, Schlepper M. Assessment of the effective components of amrinone by continuous analysis of the pressure–volume relationship; use of the conductance (volume) catheter technique and of the transient vena cava inferior ballon occlusion for rapid load changes. Z Kardiol 1987; 76:530–40.
38. Tuttle RR, Mill J. Development of a new catecholamine to selectively increase cardiac contractility. Circ Res 1975; 36:185–96.
39. Colle JP, Ohayon J, Ledain L, Besse P. Effects hemodynamique d'un nouvel agent inotrope positif (AR-L 115BS) dans les myocardopathies ischémiques et non ischémiques. Arch Mal Coeur 1984; 77/13:1532–9.
40. Drexler H. Wollschläger H, Löllgen H, Just H. Study of the acute effect of AR-115 BS, a new positive inotropic agent in patients with exercise-induced heart failure. Arzneim Forsch (Drug Res) 1981; 31(I),1a:259–62.
41. Hagemeijer F, Segers A, Schelling A. Cardiovascular effects of sulmazol administered intravenously to patients with severe heart failure. Eur Heart J 1984; 5/2:158–67.
42. Pozenel H. Ergometric and hemodynamic studies on a new cardiotonic agent AR-L115 BS. Arzneim Forsch (Drug Res) 1981; 31 (I), 1a:263–6.
43. Nebel W, Sabin G, Szurawitzki G. Influence on hemodynamic parameters after parenteral administration of AR-L 115 BS in patients with acute myocardial infarction. Arzneim Forsch (Drug Res) 1981; 31(I)/1A:251.
44. Simoons ML, Muskens G, Hugenholtz PG. Hemodynamic effects of sulmazol (ARL-115BS), a new vasodilator and positive inotropic agent, in patients with cardiogenic shock. Herz 1983; 8/1:34–40.
45. Stauch M, Nechwatal W. Effects of AR-L115 BS on hemodynamics and contractility of the heart in cardiac patients. Arzneim Forsch (Drug Res) 1981; 31(I),1a:267–71.
46. Thormann J, Kramer W, Schlepper M. A new non-glycoside, non-adrenergic cardiotonic agent AR-L 115 BS. Hemodynamic proof of its efficacy after both i.v. and oral administration. Arzneim Forsch (Drug Res) 1981; 31(I),1a:273–8.
47. Weikl A, Kohlschütter S, Durst OE, Lang E. Hemodynamic effects of single-dose administration of AR-L115 BS in patients with coronary artery disease. Arzneim Forsch (Drug Res) 1981; 31(I),1a:244–7.
48. Berkenboom GM, Sobolski JC, Depelchin PE, Contu E, Dieudonne PM, Degre SG. Clinical and hemodynamic observations on orally administered sulmazol (AR-L 115 BS) Cardiology 1984; 71/6:323–30.
49. Ruffmann KD, Mehmel HC, Kübler W. A new orally active positive inotropic substance: AR-L 115 BS. Arzneim Forsch (Drug Res) 1981; 31(I),1a:271–3.
50. Ganz W, Tamura K, Marcus HS, Donosi R, Yoshida S, Swan HJC. Measurements of coronary sinus blood flow by continuous thermodilution in man. Circulation 1971; 44:181–7.
51. Baller D, Bretschneider HJ, Hellige G. A critical look at currently used indirect indices of myocardial oxygen consumption. Basic Res Cardiol 1981; 76:163–81.
52. Schaper W. Determinants of myocardial oxygen consumption and coronary blood flow. In: Schaper W, ed. The pathophysiology of myocardial perfusion. Amsterdam: Elsevier/North-Holland Biomedical Press, 1979: 173–6.
53. Thormann J, Schlepper M, Kramer W, Gottwik M, Kindler M. Effects of AR-L 115 BS (Sulmazol), a new cardiotonic agent, in coronary artery disease: improved ventricular wall motion, increased pump function and abolition of pacing-induced ischemia. J Am Coll Cardiol 1983; 2:332–7.
54. Kramer W, Thormann J, Schlepper M, Zrenner E. Aktivitätsprofil von AR-L 115 BS bei therapierefraktärer kongestiver Kardiomyopatzhie und Herzgesunden: Wirkungsverlust durch Ca^{2+}-Antagonisten. Verh Dtsch Ges Inn Med 1982; 87:446–50.

55. Kramer W, Thormann J, Schlepper M. Effects of the new cardiotonic agent AR-L115 in normal hearts and loss of its effectivity by the Ca^{++}antagonist verapamil. Eur Heart J 1981; 2 (suppl A):56–103.
56. Diederen W, Weisenberger M. Studies on the mechanism of the positive-inotropic action of AR-L115BS, a new cardiotonic drug. Arzneim Forsch/Drug Res 1981; 31(I),1a:177–82.
57. Hasselbach W. Calcium transport of the sarcoplasmic reticulum in the presence of AR-L 115 BS. Arzneim Forsch (Drug Res) 1981; 31(I),1a:191–3.
58. Zrenner E, Kramer W, Bopp M, Schlepper M. Rapid effects on colour vision, following intravenous injection of a new, non-glycoside positive inotropic substance (AR-L115BS). Docum Ophthalmol 1982; 33:493–507.
59. Towbin EJ, Pickens WS, Doherty JE. The effects of digoxin upon colour vision and the electroretinogram. Clin Res 1967; 60:583–90.
60. Endoh M, Yanagisawa T, Taira N, Blinks JR. Effects of new inotropic agents on cyclic nucleotide metabolism and calcium transients in canine ventricular muscle. Circulation 1986; 73(suppl III):III- 117–31.
61. Ruegg JC. Effects of new inotropic agents on Ca^{2+} sensitivity of contractile proteins. Circulation 1986; 73(suppl III): III- 82–7.
62. Baumann G, Ningel K, Permanetter B, Busch U, Wirtzfeld A. Effects of UDCG-115 BS (pimobendan) on hemodynamics in patients with advanced congestive cardiomyopathy. Z Kardiol 1985; 74 (suppl 3):85/308.
63. Renard M, Walter M, Liebens I, Dresse A, Bernhard R. Pimobendane (UD-CG 115 BS) in chronic congestive heart failure. Short-term and one-month effects of a new inotropic vasodilating agent. Chest 1988; 93:1159–64.
64. Spitzer W. Hemodynamic effects of UCDG-115, a new not glycosidic, not adrenergic but positively inotropic compound. Z Kardiol 1985; 74 (suppl 5):31–82.
65. Walter M, Liebens I, Goethals H, Renard M, Dresse A, Bernard R. Pimobendane (UDCG-115 BS) in the treatment of severe congestive heart failure. An acute hemodynamic cross-over and double-blind study with two different doses. Br J Clin Pharmacol 1988; 25:323–9.
66. Rousseau MF, Hanet C, Etienne J, Leonard J, Mengeot P, Pouleur H. Effects of UDCG-115 on inotropic state and left ventricular diastolic function in patients with heart failure. Acta Pharmacol Toxicol 1986; 59 (suppl 5/2): 182–1173.
67. Permanetter B, Sebening H, Busch U, Lutilsky L, Klein G, Baumann G. Improvement of left ventricular function by UDCG 115 BS in idiopathic dilative cardiomyopathy. Eur Heart J 1987; 8 (suppl 2):37–127.
68. Narimatsu A, Kitada Y, Satoh N, Suzuki R, Okushima H. Cardiovascular pharmacology of 6-[4-(4-Pyridyl)aminophenyl]-4,5-dihydro-3(2H)-pyridazinone hydrochloride, a novel and potent cardiotonic agent with vasodilator properties. Arzneim Forsch (Drug Res) 1987; 37(I)/4:398.
69. Ikeo T, Nagao T, Suzuki T, Yabana H, Nkajima H. Effects of TA-064, a new positive inotropic agent, on left ventricular function in conscious instrumented dogs (abstr). Tokyo, Proceedings, 55th General Meeting, Japanese Pharmacological Society, p. 20.
70. Nagao T, Ikeo T, Sato M, Nakajima H, Kiyomoto A. Positive inotropic effect of (-)alpha-(3,4-dimethoxyphenetyl amino- methyl)-4- hydroxybenzyl (TA-064) in the dog (abstr). Tokyo, 1981, Proceedings of the 8th International Congress on Pharmacology p 921.
71. New Product Information TA-064. Osaka, Japan, Tanabe Seiyaku, 1982.
72. Kino M, Hirota Y, Saitoh T, Nakayama A, Hara M, Sawada K. Yamamoto S, Suwa M, Kubo S, Kawamura K. Cardiovascular effects of a new inotropic agent, denopamine (TA-064); with reference to its effects on cardiac hemodynamics and metabolism. Jpn Circ J 1986; 50/7:644–51.
73. Nakajima H, Yoshiki Y, Chuichi K. Hemodynamic effects of a new oral inotropic

agent, TA-064, on patients with congestive heart failure (abstr). J Am Coll Cardiol 1983; 2:676.
74. Takarada A, Yokota Y, Fukuzaki H. Effects of a new cardiotonic agent, TA-064, in patients with dilated cardiomyopathy-relationship between cardiac effect of TA-064 and severity of myocardial lesion. Jpn Circ J 1987; 51/3:251–8.
75. Bito K, Kinoshita M, Mashiro I, Ozaki N, Sakoda S, Tsutamoto T, Motomura M, Mitsunami K, Fukuhara T, Kawakita S. Clinico-pharmacological studies of a newly synthesized cardiotonic agent (TA-064) in patients with congestive heart failure. Clin Cardiol 1988; 11/5:334–9.
76. Kusama Y, Munakata K, Tanaka K, Katch T, Takano T, Hayakawa H. Hemodynamic and clinical effects of denopamine, a new cardiotonic agent, in patients with congestive heart failure. Acta Pharmacol Toxicol 1986; 59(suppl 5):Pt2, 184.
76A. Takatsu Y, Yui Y, Hattori R, Sagaguchi K, Susawa T, Yui N, Kawai C. Hemodynamic effects of oral TA-064 after dobutamine in congestive heart failure. Jpn Circ J 1987; 51/6:611–6.
77. Matsumoto N, Matsumura K, Takahashi S, Kimata S, Hirosawa K. Hemodynamic and clinical effects of a new inotropic agent TA-064 in patients with refractory heart failure due to cardiomyopathy with special reference to dose–response effects. Heart Vessels 1985; 1: suppl 1:187–94.
78. Kobayashi Y, Nakamura M, Yazawa T, Baba T, Mukai H, Twasaki S, Takeyama Y, Niitani H. Effect of TA-064 on bradyarrhythmias. Kokyo To Junkan 1986; 34/8:857–82.
79. Suga H, Sagawa K. Instantaneous pressure volume relationships and their ratio in the excised, supported canine left ventricle. Circ Res 1974; 35:117–123.
80. Baan J, Van de Velde ET, DeBruin HG, Smeenk GJ, Koops J, VanDuk AD, Temmerman D, Senden J, Buis B. Continuous measurement of left ventricular volume in animals and humans by conductance catheter. Circulation 1984; 70:812–823.
81. Thormann J, Kramer W, Kindler M, Kremer P, Schlepper M. Bestimmung der Wirkkomponenten von Amrinon durch kontinuierliche Analyse der Druck-Volumenbeziehung; Anwendung der Conductance- (Volumen-) Kathetertechnik und der schnellen Laständerung durch Ballonokklusion der Vena cava inferior. Z Kardiol 1987; 76:530–540.
82. Thormann J, Kramer W, Kremer P, Schlepper M. Influence of the new class I antiarrhythmic agent diprafenone on the end-systolic pressure–volume relationship (conductance technique). Cardiovasc Drugs and Therapy 1989; 3:145–154.
83. Bashore TM, Walker S, Fossen DV, Fontana ME, Magorien RD. Use of inferior vena caval occlusion to acutely alter preload in man. Circulation 1985; 72(suppl III):III–43.
84. McKay RG, Miller MJ, Ferguson JJ, Momomura SL, Shahagian B, Grossman W, Pasternak RC. Assesment of left ventricular end-systolic pressure–volume relations with an impedance catheter and transient inferior vena cava occlusion: Use of this system in the evaluation of the cardiotonic effects of dobutamine, milrinone. AM J Coll Cardiol 1986; 8:1152–1160.
85. Van Fossen D, Fontana ME, Unverferth DV, Walker S, Kolibash AJ, Bashore TM. Safety and efficacy of inferior vena caval occlusion to rapidly alter ventricular loading conditions in idiopathic dilated cardiomyopathy. Am J Cardiol 1987; 59:937–942.
86. Kereiakes D, Chatterjee K, Parmley WW, et al. Intravenous and oral MDL 17043 (a new inotropic–vasodilatoragent) in congestive heart failure: Hemodynamic and clinical evaluation in 38 patients. Am J Coll Cardiol 1984; 4:884–889.
87. Alousia AA, Farah AE, Lesher CY, Opalka CJ. Cardiotonic activity of amrinone WIN 40680, 5-amino-3,4'bipyridine-6(1H)-one. Circulation Res 1979; 45:666–677.
88. Wilmshurst PT, Thompson DS, Suhl SM et al. Comparison of the effects of amrinone and sodium nitroprusside on hemodynamics, contractility, and myocardial metabolism in patients with cardiac failure due to coronary artery disease and dilated cardiomyopathy. Br Heart J 1984; 52:38–48.

89. Hermiller JB, Leithe ME, Magorien RD et al. Amrinone insevere congestive heart failure: Another look at an intriguing new cardioactive drug. J Pharmac Exp Ther 1984; 228:319–326.
90. Thormann J, Hüting J, Kremer P, Wissemann J, Mitrovic V, Dietrich HA, Schlepper M. Enoximone: True inotropic effects? Do they cause ischemia? Analysis of end-systolic pressure–volume relations using the conductance (volume) catheter technique. Cardiovasc Drugs Ther 1990; 4:1403–1416.
91. Axelrod RJ, DeMarco T, Dae M, Botvinick EH, Chatterjee K. Hemodynamic and clinical evaluation of piroximone, a new inotrope–vasodilator agent, in severe congestive heart failure.J Am Coll Cardiol 1987; 9:1124–1130.
92. Thompson DS, Juul SM, Wilmshurst P. Effects of sodium nitroprusside upon cardiac work, efficiency and substrate extraction in severe left ventricular failure. Br Heart J 1981; 46:394–400.
93. Jaski BE, Fifer MA, Wright RF et al. Positive inotropicand vasodilator actions of milrinone in patients with sereve congestive heart failure. J Clin Invest 1985; 75:643–649.
94. Strain J, Grose R, Maskin CS, LeJemtel TH. Effects of anew cardiotonic agent,, MDL 17043 on myocardial contractility and left ventricular performance in congestive heart failure. Am Heart J 1985; 110:91–96.
95. Quinones MA, Gaasch WH, Alexander JK. Influence of acute changes in preload, afterload, contractile state and heart rate on ejection and isovolumetric indices of myocardial contractility in man. Circulation 1976; 53:293–302.
96. Ludmer PL, Wright RF, Arnold MO et al. Separation of the direct myocardial and vasodilator actions and milrinone administered by an intracoronary infusion technique. Circulation 1986; 73:130–137.
97. Cody RJ, Kubo SH, Covit AB. Regional blood flow and neurohumoral response to chronic milrinone in CHF. Circulation 1984; 70: II 192.
98. Bristow MR, Ginsberg R, Minobe W. Decreased catecholamine sensitivity and beta–adrenergic receptor density in failing human hearts. N Engl J Med 1982; 397:205–211.
99. Herrmann HC, Ruddy TD, Dec W et al. Inotropic effect of enoximone in patients with severe heart failure: Demonstration by left ventricular end-systolic pressure–volume analysis. J Am Coll Cardiol 1987; 9:1117–1123.
100. Thormann J, Wissemann J, Liebrich A, Mitrovic' V, Dieterich HA, Schlepper M: Proof for piroximone's inotropic influence; can it be safely used in coronary artery disease? Analysis of end-systolic pressure–volume relations (conductance technique). J Cardiovasc Pharm 1992; 20/1:50–62.
101. Thormann J, Hüting J, Kremer P, Wissemann J, Bahawar H, Schlepper M. Do class 1 antiarrhythmic drugs impair myocardial contractility? The class 1A example of ajmaline. J Cardiovasc Pharm 1990; 16:182–190.
102. Thormann J, Kramer W, Kindler M, Neuss H, Schlepper M. Linksventrikuläre Funktionsdiagnostik mit Analyse serieller Druck-Volumenbeziehungen: Erster Einsatz der Conductance (Volumen-) Kathetertechnik. Z Kardiol 1985; 74 (suppl 5) 5:124.
103. Sagawa K. The ventricular pressure–volume diagram revisited. Circ Res 1978; 43:677–6874.
104. Kass DA, Maughan WL. From "Emax" to pressure–volume relations: a broader view. Circulation 1988; 77:1203–1212.
105. Kass Da, Midei M, Brinker J, Maughan WL. Influence of coronary occlusion during PTCA on end-systolic and end-diastolic pressure–volume relations in humans. Circulation 1990; 81:447–460.
106. Burkhoff D, Van der Velde E, Kass D, Baan J, Maughan WL, Sagawa K Accuracy of volume measurement by conductance catheter in isolated, ejecting canine hearts. Circulation 1985; 72:440–447.
107. Boltwood CM, Appleyard RF, Glantz SA. Left ventricular volume measurement by

conductance catheter in intact dogs. Parallel conductance volume depends on left ventricular size. Circulation 1989; 80:1360–1377.

108. Hermann HC, Ruddy TD, Dec W, Strauss HW, Boucher CA. Inotropic effect of enoximone in patients with severe heart failure: Demonstration by left ventricular end-systolic pressure–volume analysis. J Am Coll Cardiol 1987; 9:1117–1123.
109. Crottogini AJ, Willshaw P, Barra JG, Armientano R, Fischer EIC, Pichel RH. Inconsistency of the slope and the volume intercept of the end-systolic pressure–volume relationships as indl indexes of inotropic state in conscious dogs: presentation of an index combining both variables. Circulation 1987; 76:1115–1126.
110. Mirsky I, Tajimi T, Peterson KL. The development of the entire end-systolic pressure–volume and ejection fraction–afterload relation: a new concept of systolic myocardial stiffness. Circulation 1987; 76:343–356.
111. Burkhoff D, Sugiura S, Yue DT, Sagawa K. Contractility dependent curvilinearity of end-systolic pressure–volume relations. Am J Physiol 1987; 252H:1218–1227.
112. Spratt JA, Tyson GS, Glower DD, David JW, Muhlbaier LH, Olsen CO, Rankin JS. The end-systolic pressure–volume relationship in conscious dogs. Circulation 1987; 75:1295–1302.
113. Thormann J. The influence of clinical intervention on pressure-volume relationships—the conductance (volume) technique. Europ J Cardiol 1992;13(suppl E):69–79.

24

Endothelial Cell-Derived Vasoactive and Inotropic Paracrine Factors

THOMAS MICHEL, BERNHARD K. KRÄMER, and RALPH A. KELLY

Brigham and Women's Hospital and Harvard Medical School
Boston, Massachusetts

The vascular endothelium forms the lining of the circulatory system in all vertebrates, forming a dynamic interface between the surrounding vascular cells and the soluble and cellular components of the blood. In response to a number of hormonal, metabolic, and mechanical stimuli, the vascular endothelium has been shown to synthesize and secrete compounds of disparate biological activity, including cytokines, mitogens, pro- and antithrombogens, as well as vasoactive agents that control vascular tone (1–4). Recent experiments have identified vasoactive agents such as endothelin (5) and nitric oxide (˙N=O) (6–8) as important endothelial products regulating vascular tone. Nevertheless, relatively little is known about the regulation of endothelin release, or about the structure and regulation of the enzyme system that synthesizes ˙N=O.

In addition to the vascular endothelium within the large epicardial and penetrating coronary arteries, with its documented ability to control the release of vasodilator and vasoconstrictor agents, the cardiac microvascular and endocardial endothelium may also control the contractile state of cardiac myocytes. It has long been assumed that the primary influences regulating cardiac contractility are the extent of mechanical loading of muscle fibers and the activity of the automatic nervous system. However, there is growing evidence that locally elaborated paracrine factors, perhaps derived from the microvascular endothelium or the endocardium, also are important in modifying cardiac function. In larger blood vessels, endothelial cells have been identified as the source of a number of biologically active factors that act in a paracrine fashion to influence the behavior of both bloodborne elements and subjacent vascular tissue. Within the heart, the role of the endocardium in normal cardiac physiology has been noted in recent reports documenting that this endothelium regulates the inotropic response of subjacent cardiac myofibrils to changes in extracellular Ca^{2+}, as reviewed by Brutsaert (9).

In this chapter, we examine the vasodilating action of nitric oxide and its synthesis, describe the vasoconstrictor and inotropic action of endothelin, and consider evidence that the cardiac microvascular endothelium and/or endocardial endothelium regulates cardiac muscle function. Finally, the role of G proteins in initiating transduction of the endothelin signal at the sarcolemma, as well as those of many other neurohumoral and paracrine agents, will be briefly reviewed.

I. ENDOTHELIAL CELL CONTROL OF VASCULAR SMOOTH MUSCLE TONE

Organic nitrates, including the clinically important compounds sodium nitroprusside and trinitroglycerin, have long been known to induce vasodilatation (7,8,10). These nitrovasodilator compounds undergo nonenzymatic transformations to produce nitric oxide in vivo, and numerous studies have documented that nitric oxide formation is an important component of their pharmacologic response (10,11). Nitric oxide induces vasorelaxation primarily via its activation of soluble guanylate cyclase (7,8), leading to increased cyclic GMP levels in vascular smooth muscle cells (10). Soluble guanylate cyclase is a heme-containing protein, and the catalytic activity of the enzyme is markedly increased by the formation of a $^{\bullet}N{=}O$ heme adduct (8,12). Increased cyclic GMP levels in vascular smooth muscle cells are correlated with decreased developed tension and may inhibit smooth muscle mitogenesis in vitro (8,13). Other tissues and cells also are influenced by administration of organic nitrates; for example, platelet function is attenuated by $^{\bullet}N{=}O$-induced increases in cyclic GMP (7,14–16).

The observations of Furchgott (6,13) were the first to document the critical role of the endothelium in the control of vascular smooth muscle tone. Furchgott and colleagues demonstrated that arterial preparations denuded of endothelium would contract in response to acetylcholine, whereas a vasodilatory response was observed when the vascular endothelial layer was left intact. He proposed the existence of an "endothelium-derived relaxing factor" (EDRF) that was responsible for this intercellular signal. Several laboratories have subsequently identified EDRF as nitric oxide (17; summarized in 3,8,13), and the identification of other endothelium-derived vasoactive substances has been an active area of investigation. It is clear that $^{\bullet}N{=}O$ (or $^{\bullet}N{=}O$-derived adducts) form quantitatively the most important endothelium-derived vasorelaxant substance (13), and that this molecule thus represents the "endogenous nitrovasodilator" (8,10). Other vasoactive substances secreted by endothelial cells include the peptide endothelin, which is a potent smooth muscle vasoconstrictor and, as noted below, a potent cardiac inotropic agent as well, and prostacyclin, another potent vasodilating agent (3,18). Thus, the balance between vascular constriction and relaxation can be modulated by products of the vascular endothelium.

The role of endothelium-dependent vascular relaxation in pathyphysiological states has been explored in a variety of experimental systems and clinical contexts. In all mammalian systems studied to date, the characteristic response to an arterial infusion of acetylcholine is vasodilatation; this response is dependent on the presence of an intact endothelial layer (13,19). Abnormalities in endothelium-dependent vascular relaxation have been documented in experimental models of atherosclerosis (20,21), hypertension (22), and diabetes (23–25). In hypercholesterolemic animals, acetylcholine-induced endothelium-dependent vasorelaxation is markedly impaired, but the vasorelaxation induced by nitroglycerin remains intact (21,26). This suggests that the locus for impaired vasorelaxation in hypercholesterolemic animals is at the level of the endothelial cell. This endothelial dysfunction may reflect impaired signal transduction from endothelial cell-surface receptors to stimulation of EDRF synthesis. As an alternative, the catalytic properties of the enzyme system responsible for EDRF synthesis and release may be altered, substrate or cofactor availability might be impaired, or there may be perturbations in the subsequent biotransformations or intercellular transport of EDRF. The clinical relevance of this endothelial cell dysfunction has been established by the observation that the usual dilatation of human coronary arteries to acetylcholine is markedly impaired in the presence of coronary atherosclerosis (27), and indeed may reflect an early state in the development of an atherosclerotic lesion. Recently, Lefer et al. reported that the peptide signaling factor/cytokine, tumor growth factor beta (TGFβ), can protect either buffer-perfused or blood-perfused hearts from injury due to ischemia and subsequent reperfusion (28). They noted that TGFβ maintained the vasodilatory response to acetylcholine in coronary arteries and reduced infarct size, possibly by suppressing the production of superoxide anions and by inhibiting the production and activity of the cytokine tumor necrosis factor alpha (TNFα) (28). This evidence suggests that the dynamic regulation of this pathway may be altered in pathophysiological states.

II. VASODILATION: REGULATION OF NITRIC OXIDE SYNTHESIS IN ENDOTHELIAL CELLS

Nitric oxide is rapidly produced and/or released from endothelial cells in response to the activation of a large variety of cell surface receptors, including ADP, thrombin, adenosine, ATP, bradykinin, acetylcholine, epinephrine, histamine, and vasopressin (reviewed in reference 13). Interactions among these multiple receptor pathways, either to potentiate or desensitize $^{\bullet}N{=}O$ synthetase activity, may be the most important mechanisms regulating the generation of $^{\bullet}N{=}O$ by multiple ligands. Autoinduction of $^{\bullet}N{=}O$ synthesis, possibly mediated by endothelial cell guanylate cyclase, might represent another control mechanism. The roles of these regulatory pathways remain incompletely understood, but almost certainly will be relevant to our understanding of the mechanisms of endothelial dysfunction in several disease states.

The diversity of receptors which, in response to ligand activation, lead to the generation of $^{\bullet}N{=}O$ in endothelial cells, indicates that $^{\bullet}N{=}O$ release provides a common pathway for the generation of intercellular intravascular signals. It is less clear how these receptors are coupled to the activation of $^{\bullet}N{=}O$ release. Coupling of endothelial cell plasma membrane receptor occupancy to activation of the $^{\bullet}N{=}O$ synthetase appears to be mediated by an increase in intracellular Ca^{2+}, possibly involving the G protein-dependent activation of phospholipase C (reviewed in reference 7). The calcium ionophore A23187 also stimulates $^{\bullet}N{=}O$ production in the presence of extracellular Ca^{2+} (7,28). Purified preparations of the cerebellar and endothelial $^{\bullet}N{=}O$ synthetases are activated in vitro by Ca^{2+}-calmodulin (29), but other pathways may exist that regulate enzyme activity in situ.

The existence of other intracellular pathways for the activation of $^{\bullet}N{=}O$ release is suggested by experiments with the wasp venom, mellitin (30). Mellitin is a potent activator of endothelial cell $^{\bullet}N{=}0$ synthesis, an effect probably unrelated to its well-characterized activation of phospholipase A_2. However, the effects of mellitin, like those of other insect venoms, are pleiotropic, and include the activation of phospholipase C. Another effect of mellitin seen at similar venom concentrations is an inhibition of Ca^{2+}-calmodulin (31). The fact that a calmodulin inhibitor (albeit one with pleiotropic effects) can nevertheless stimulate ˙N=O release that other pathways exist for the activation of ˙N=O synthetase in the cell, aside from its activation by Ca^{2+}-calmodulin. Whether ˙N=O synthetase is regulated, directly or indirectly, by reversible phosphorylation by second messenger-dependent protein kinases, a common mechanism for regulating the production and/or release of other endothelial and nonendothelial cell paracrine regulatory factors, is an open question.

III. BIOSYNTHESIS OF NITRIC OXIDE

The biochemical pathway for the synthesis of nitric oxide was first demonstrated in macrophages, and subsequently in endothelial cells. The amino acid L-arginine is required for synthetic activity, resulting in the production of ˙N=O and L-citrulline, and this pathway is common to both cell types. However, the tissue-specific regulatory and enzymologic features of ˙N=O synthesis activities reflect heterogeneity in biochemical pathways leading to ˙N=O synthesis among different cell types. For example, in macrophages ˙N=O synthesis in response to a stimulus takes place over several hours and requires new protein synthesis (32). By contrast, the ˙N=O synthetase in endothelial cells is activated within seconds by the stimulation of cell surface receptors (13). In both cell types, ˙N=O synthetase appears to be predominantly a cytosolic enzyme, but cofactor requirements differ markedly between macrophages and endothelial cells. Cell-free synthesis of ˙N=O by macrophage extracts is dependent upon NADPH and tetrahydrobiopterin (33), and the endothelial ˙N=O synthetase is dependent on NADPH (34). Calcium ionophores such as A23187 are potent activators of endothelial cell ˙N=O synthesis but have little effect on the macrophage enzyme. These regulatory differences are likely to reflect the vastly different physiological roles for ˙N=O in the two cell types: in the macrophage, high local concentrations of secreted ˙N=O probably play a role in that cell's cytotoxic activity, whereas the primary role of endothelial ˙N=O appears to be the regulation of vascular smooth muscle tone.

Over the past year, arginine-dependent ˙N=O synthesis has been documented in a wide variety of tissues, including the central nervous system (29,35,36) and adrenal gland, as well as in various cultured cell lines derived from kidney and neuroblastoma cells. The functional consequences of the synthesis of ˙N=O in these diverse tissues are unknown, but have attracted much interest (35). The first purification to homogeneity of an ˙N=O synthetase, from rat cerebellum, was recently reported (29). The rat cerebellar enzyme requires NADPH and Ca^{2+}-calmodulin for production of L-citrulline plus ˙N=O from L-arginine. This enzyme shares many features with the ˙N=O synthetase present in the bovine cerebellum and in bovine aortic endothelial cells.

IV. VASOCONSTRICTION: RELEASE OF ENDOTHELIN BY VASCULAR ENDOTHELIUM

In addition to the vasodilatory actions of EDRF, and of eicosanoids such as prostacyclin that had been recognized to exist by the mid-1980s, a vasoconstrictor activity had also been noted in the supernatant of cultured endothelial cells (37–40). In 1988, Yanagisawa et al. (41) isolated a vasoconstrictor peptide containing 21 amino acids from the supernatant of cultured porcine endothelial cells, determined the amino acid sequence, and called it "endothelin." These isoforms of endothelin have since been identified, each with four cysteine residues forming two disulfide bonds with a molecular weight of 2492 (42). Endothelin caused vasoconstriction of porcine coronary arteries with an EC_{50} of 400 pM and a maximum tension comparable to potassium chloride (KCl)-induced contraction (41). Sarafatoxins within the venom of the burrowing asp *Atractaspis engaddensis* were contemporaneously identified and noted to have remarkable homology to endothelin (43).

Endothelin has since been shown to be a ubiquitous autacoid: it is released from both endothelial and numerous nonendothelial tissue sources. These include aortic (41,44–47), bovine pulmonary (48), bovine carotid (49,50), bovine adrenal cortical capillary (51), and human umbilical vein (49,52) endothelial cells, and also from several cell lines (canine MDCK, $LLCPK_1$, rabbit RK-13, rat NRK-52E, hamster BHK-21, monkey COS-7) (53,54), canine airway epithelial cells (55), and rabbit endometrial cells in primary culture (56). Using immunohistochemical techniques, it has also been found in relatively high levels in the central and peripheral nervous system, where its role has yet to be determined (57–59). Unlike $^{\bullet}N{=}O$, which has yet to be found in the microvascular circulation of any organ, endothelin production has been documented in low-resistance vessels and capillaries in some tissues. Endothelin gene transcription can be modulated in endothelial cells at the mRNA level by a diverse number of neurohumoral, paracrine, and mechanical stimuli, including thrombin, epinephrine, angiotensin II, arginine vasopressin, TGFβ, interleukin-1, the calcium ionophores A23187 and ionomycin, phorbol esters and shear stress, and its release can be inhibited by nitric oxide (41,44,46–49,51,52).

A propeptide mRNA encodes the 203 amino acid endothelin precursor preproendothelin, indicating that endothelin is produced by de novo synthesis in a manner similar to that of various peptide hormones and neuropeptides (41). "Big endothelin," a 39 amino acid residue intermediate, is cleaved from preproendothelin by dibasic-pair-specific endopeptidase(s) and endothelin is subsequently generated through an unusual, previously unknown, proteolytic process by a putative "endothelin-converting enzyme" (45,48,50,51,60). Recently, endothelin-converting enzyme has been purified and characterized, and shown to be a cathepsin D-like aspartic protease. Concomitant release of "big endothelin," endothelin, and a C-terminal fragment (amino acid 22-39) from endothelial cells has been demonstrated (45,50). The endothelin-1 gene (encoding the 212 amino acid precursor preproendothelin) gene was localized to human chromosome 6 and has been shown to contain 5 exons, with nucleotide sequences encoding the mature 21-amino acid endothelin-1 contained within the second exon (61). Subsequently, three distinct human endothelin-related genes (ET-1, ET-2, ET-3) have been cloned by screening a human genomic DNA library (42).

In rats and dogs, endothelin administered intravenously has a characteristic bimodal effect on blood pressure. Typically, there is a transient, dose-dependent decrease in mean arterial pressure and increase in heart rate, detectable within 5–10 sec and maximal at 1–2 min, followed by a prolonged increase in blood pressure and decrease in heart rate due to an initial decrease and subsequent increase in total peripheral resistance. Cardiac output decreases or remains unchanged in comparison to baseline following a transient increase, while maximum upstroke velocity (max dP/dt) may increase for 5–10 min and then decreases to baseline (41,62–82).

No transient initial depressor response was demonstrated in guinea pigs, and a sustained decrease in blood pressure, total peripheral resistance, and increase in cardiac output has been demonstrated in cats (83,84), pointing to species differences in the effects of endothelin on systemic circulation following intravenous administration. The precursor protein, "big endothelin," has been reported to have a less marked pressor effect (69) than endothelin-1, but did not demonstrate the transient, initial depressor effect in the anesthetized rat (77). Calcium antagonists (e.g., verapamil, diltiazem, nicardipine) have been shown to attenuate the sustained pressor, but not the initial depressor actions of endothelin (71,72,75,84).

The effects of endothelin in the systemic circulation are reflected in the pharmacodynamics of the peptide's action in the coronary arteries. A decrease in coronary perfusion pressure and ischemia following intracoronary administration of endothelin has been demonstrated in the Langendorff-perfused rat and rabbit heart (85,86), and in the anesthetized dog (87–90) at concentrations below 1 nM. Calcium channel blockers again reversed partially endothelin's effects on coronary blood flow in the above studies, shifting the dose–response curve to the right. Watanabe et al. (91) reported that infarct size could be reduced by administration of an antiendothelin antibody in an ischemic rat heart model, although this preliminary report has yet to be confirmed.

V. CORONARY FLOW, ENDOTHELIAL CELLS, AND MYOCARDIAL FUNCTION

Shortly after endothelin was identified as an endothelium-derived vasoconstrictor factor (EDCF), Masaka and colleagues noted that endothelin also had a potent inotropic activity in guinea pig atrial strips (92). Subsequently, high-affinity receptors were identified in mammalian atria and ventricles (93–95), and endothelin was also found to be a potent secretogogue for atrial natriuretic peptide (ANP) (96–102). A number of laboratories have now confirmed these original reports, documenting endothelin to be one of the most potent inotropic agents yet described in mammalian myocardium.

The origin of the endothelin responsible for mediating the peptide's action on myocardium (as opposed to vascular smooth muscle) is unknown. However, the work of Brutsaert and colleagues on the role of the endocardial endothelium as a source of positively inotropic paracrine factors that influence the subjacent myocardium suggests that release of endothelin by the endocardial and microvascular endothelium is one possibility (9,103,104).

The cardiac microvasculature may contribute importantly to the regulation of cardiac function. For example, the importance of coronary flow rates per se as a determinant of cardiac contractile state, and distinct from low-flow rates that could result in relative tissue ischemia, was originally identified by the cardiac physiologist, Gregg, in 1958, and has since been the source of much controversy, as was reviewed by Feigl (105) and recently re-examined by Kitakaze and Marban (106). The latter authors also showed that increasing coronary flow rate per se modifies cardiac contractile state by documenting that a significant change in end-diastolic length with increased flow did *not* occur and could not be a cause of Gregg's phenomenon. Because the effect can easily be demonstrated in denervated, buffer-perfused hearts, and neither autonomic, metabolic, nor mechanical influences could be implicated, the release of local paracrine factors by vascular tissue, either the large epicardial arteries or the microvasculature, or both, is a reasonable explanation. A second line of evidence supporting a role for local, paracrine influences on blood flow, and secondarily on myocyte function, has been the well-documented temporal and spatial heterogeneity of flow over small regions of ventricular muscle, (reviewed recently in references 107 and 108). The heterogeneity in microvessel flow and in the anatomical networking of capillaries becomes greater as one looks at smaller and smaller sections of any portion of the ventricular wall, a relationship best described by fractal equations (107,108). Bassingthwaite and colleagues (108) speculated that although the "natural expectation is that metabolism drives flow," the fractal character of flow patterns that change over time could "influence the local capacity for metabolism within working ventricular muscle."

Further evidence for control of myocardial function by endothelium has come from pharmacologic studies of peptides and other autacoids of presumed endothelial origin. Perhaps the best studies are angiotensin II and endothelin itself (see below). The role of angiotensin II in modifying cardiac function is being reexamined with the recent detection, by biochemical, immunologic, and in situ molecular biology techniques, of components of the renin–angiotensin system within the heart (i.e., renin, angiotensinogen, and angiotensin-converting enzyme [ACE]), as reviewed by Lindpainter et al. (109). Despite the clear documentation of both positive inotropic and other unique effects of angiotensin II on isolated mammalian heart muscle or ventricular myocytes, the role of the renin–angiotensin system in normal and abnormal cardiac physiology remains unclear.

VI. MECHANISM OF POSITIVE INOTROPIC EFFECT OF ENDOTHELIN

The positive inotropic effect of endothelin has been documented in isolated hearts (85), in isolated cardiac muscle preparations (64,80,92,110–116), and isolated adult rat (117) and rabbit (118) ventricular cells. As with the vasoconstrictor effects of the peptide, calcium channel blockers shift the dose–response curve to the right, and adrenergic, serotonergic, and histaminergic antagonists have no effect (92,117). In similar fashion, the pharmacokinetics of endothelin's action in heart resembles that of vascular smooth muscle, with a delayed onset of action and a maximal effect at 5–8 min in isolated cell preparations that is quite prolonged, lasting 5–15 min after washout of the peptide. Kelly et al. reported that in isolated adult rat ventricular myocytes paced at 1.5 Hz, endothelin, at concentrations below 1 nM that nevertheless yielded a maximal inotropic response of about 100% above baseline, did not increase cytosolic calcium, thus appearing to sensitize the myofilaments to calcium (117). Lauer et al. did find an increase in calcium transients and transmembrane calcium current in isolated rabbit cells at 20 nM endothelin (118), although contractility was not measured. Kelly et al. did find a variable increase in cytosolic calcium in isolated rat cardiocytes at concentrations of endothelin in the 10–100 nM range, well above the dose eliciting a maximal inotropic effect of the peptide (i.e., 0.5–1.0 nM). As shown in Figure 1, when the calcium activity of the buffer superfusing isolated single fura-2-loaded myocytes paced at 1.5 Hz was varied from

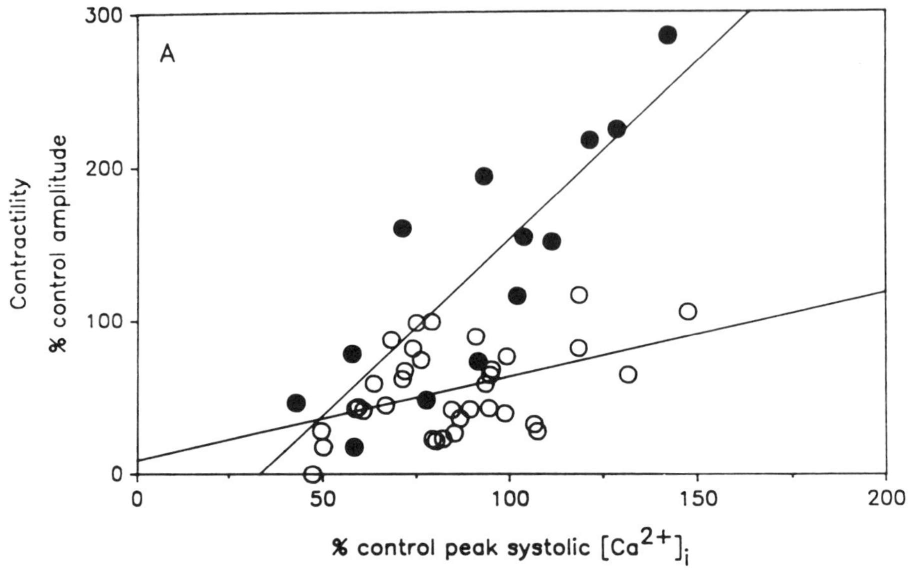

Figure 1 Endothelin enhances the contractile response to intracellular calcium ($[Ca^{2+}]_i$). The values are given for contractile amplitude and peak systolic $[Ca^{2+}]_i$ in 6 cells loaded with the Ca^{2+}-selective fluorescent probe fura-2, initially exposed to 0.9 mM external Ca^{2+} in physiological buffer and then stepped down to 0.1 mM Ca^{2+} with sufficient time at each step to allow contractile amplitude and $[Ca^{2+}]_i$ to stabilize, in the absence (open circles) or presence (closed circles) of 100 pM endothelin. Note that for any given level of systolic $[Ca^{2+}]_i$, expressed as a percentage of initial control values for $[Ca^{2+}]_i$, contractile amplitude was always higher in endothelin-treated cells. (From Ref. 117, with permission.)

0.1 to 0.9 mM Ca^{2+} outside, 100 pM endothelin increased contractile amplitude with little or no change in either the systolic value of the Ca^{2+} transient (117). Prior exposure to pertussis toxin completely abolished the positive inotropic effect of the peptide (Fig. 2), implicating the involvement of a pertussis toxin-sensitive G protein in the initial signal transduction steps following endothelin binding to its sarcolemmal receptor (117).

Having demonstrated that endothelin's inotropic effect was due, in part, to an apparent sensitization of the myofilaments to intracellular calcium (117), we determined whether this could be due to a rise in intracellular pH (pH_i), since a rise in pH_i has been well documented to increase contractile amplitude with little or no change in $[Ca^{2+}]_i$ (119–121). As shown in Figure 3, 100 pM endothelin increased pH_i by 0.07 $\pm$ 0.02 ($n = 8$) and contractile amplitude to 190 $\pm$ 26% of baseline, while 1 nM endothelin increased pH_i by 0.13 $\pm$ 0.03 with little further increase in contractility (122). The Na^+/H^+ exchange blocker amiloride completely prevented the intracellular alkalinization response to endothelin at doses (10^{-4} M) that had no baseline effect on isolated adult rat myocyte contraction paced at 1.5 Hz. Nonspecific inhibitors of protein kinase C (H-7 and sphingosine) also diminished or abolished the rise in pH_i with endothelin (Fig. 4) (122). However, neither amiloride nor inhibitors of protein kinase C could completely suppress the positive inotropic response, which

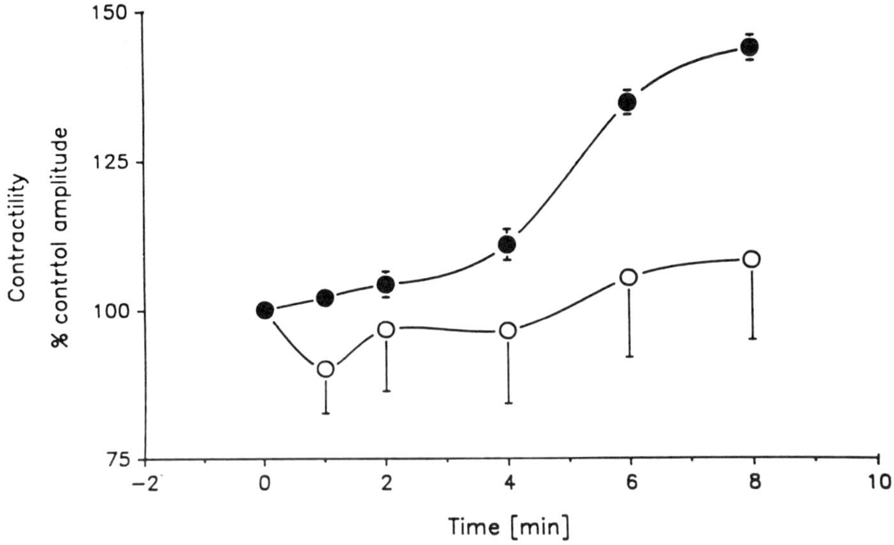

Figure 2 Pertussis toxin abolishes the contractile reponse to endothelin. Isolated rat ventricular myocytes were exposed to 100 pM endothelin either after a 3 hr preincubation in 100 ng/ml pertussis toxin (open circles; n = 9) or after preincubation at 37°C in control media (solid circles; n = 5), and the change in contractile amplitude was recorded. (From Ref. 117, with permission.)

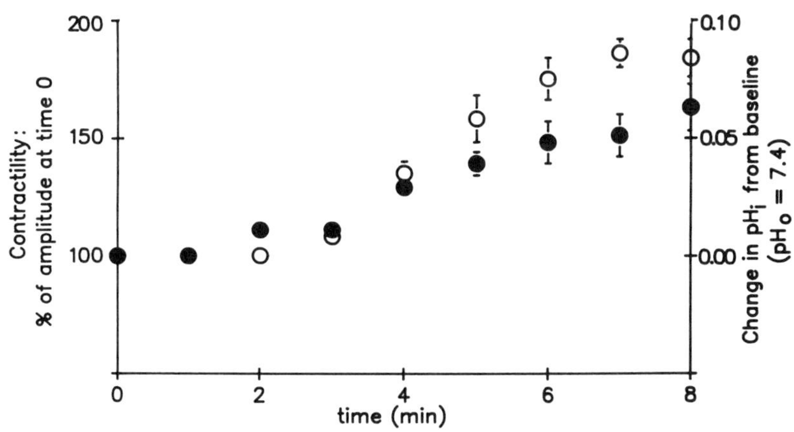

Figure 3 Time course of changes in pH_i and contractile amplitude with endothelin. Freshly isolated ventricular myocytes superfused with physiological buffer at pH_o 7.4, loaded with the pH-sensitive dye BCECF, and stimulated at 1.5 Hz, were exposed to 100 pM endothelin at time 0. A change in contractile amplitude (open symbols) or pH_i (closed symbols) was not apparent for about 4 min ($p < 0.05$ at 4 min; n = 6). (From Ref. 122, with permission.)

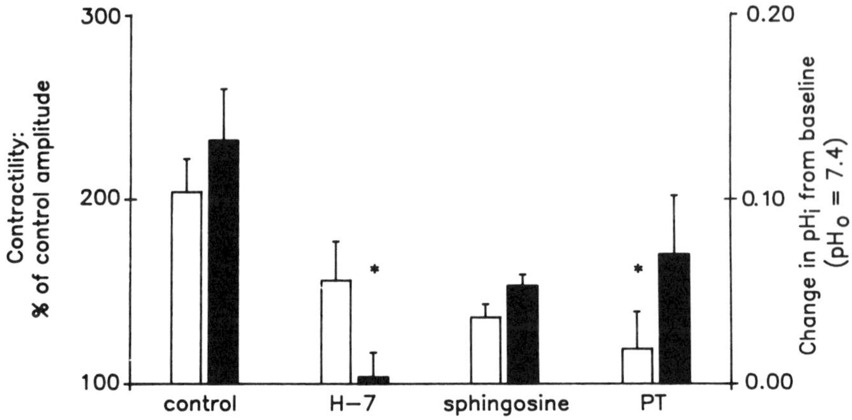

Figure 4 Role of protein kinase C and resistance to pertussis toxin in the pH_i response to endothelin. Freshly isolated rat ventricular myocytes were exposed to 1 nM endothelin, and contractility (open bars) and pH_i (filled bars) were recorded at 8 min in BCECF-loaded cells. Eight cells were preincubated with either 50 μM H-7 or 200 μM sphingosine. H-7 completely blocked the rise in pH_i with 1 mM endothelin, but there was no significant fall in contractility. In contrast, as shown in Figure 2, pertussis toxin (PT) effectively blocked the inotropic effect of the peptide ($p < 0.01$), but did not significantly affect the change in pH_i with 1 nM endothelin. (From Ref. 122, with permission.)

was reduced by about 50% by each drug. In contrast, pretreatment with pertussis toxin, which had been documented to abolish the inotropic response to endothelin (117), only partially reduced the intracellular alkalinization (Figs. 2, 4).

Endothelin has had inconsistent effects on heart rate and cardiac output when injected into intact animals. Most reports document a transient increase followed by a sustained decrease in heart rate, accompanied by an early increase, followed by a sustained decrease in cardiac output. These changes can be explained, in part, by a slowly developing systemic (and coronary) vasoconstriction due to the unusual pharmacokinetics and pharmacodynamics of endothelin's action. As noted above, endothelin has been documented to stimulate release of ANP (96–102), and this may be responsible for the initial transient hypotension associated with the systemic endothelin infusions (102). Endothelin also inhibits renin release (123–125) and stimulates aldosterone secretion (126,127). Endothelin also acts in an autocrine fashion to induce the release of eicosanoids from endothelial cells, including thromboxane A_2 and prostacyclin (64,86,128–133), as well as $^{\cdot}N{=}O$ (63,134), which may also be responsible for the transient hypotensive effects of endothelin. Other modulating and countervailing actions to systemic endothelin include the release of catecholamines from adrenal chromaffin cells (112,135) and a change in the responsiveness of the postsynaptic α-adrenergic receptor (136–140). Finally, the effects of endothelin on blood pressure will also be mediated by the well-known renal effects of the peptide, including dose-dependent changes in glomerular filtration rate, decreases in renal plasma flow, and increases in filtration fraction at the glomerulus. The fractional excretion of sodium is usually unaffected or only slightly increased depending on the dose of endothelin and the animal model employed (67,76,141–147).

VII. ENDOTHELIN'S ROLE IN CARDIAC MYOCYTE CELL BIOLOGY AND FUNCTION

Intracellular alkalinization could have other roles in normal myocyte physiology aside from the effects on contractility described above. A rise in pH_i is clearly associated with a mitogenic response in many cells and with hypertrophy in vascular smooth muscle (148–150). In addition, endothelin has been shown to have mitogenic effects in vascular smooth muscle cells (151), as well as other cell types (152–155). The mitogenic effects of endothelin and, where they have been measured, the effects of endothelin on pH and on the expression of certain protooncogenes, such as c-*fos* and c-*jun* associated with some forms of hypertrophic growth in cardiac myocytes (156), occur at relatively low concentrations (i.e., <1 nM), comparable to the concentrations used by Kelly et al. (117) and Kramer et al. (122) that induced maximal increases in contractile amplitude and pH_i. Activation of phospholipase C by endothelin has been well documented in both established cell lines and primary cultures of vascular smooth muscle cells (157), endothelial cells (154), and glial cells (158), although only at higher concentrations, typically with an EC_{50} of 10 nM or higher.

The response of a variety of cell lines and primary cultures pretreated with pertussis toxin and then exposed to endothelin also implicates a complex and perhaps tissue-specific signal transduction mechanism for this peptide, comprising several independently-regulated pathways. In freshly isolated rat ventricular cells, as described above, pertussis toxin completely inhibited the inotropic effect following endothelin, while variably reducing the concomitant intracellular alkalinization by no more than 50%. In contrast, pertussis toxin had no effect on the endothelin-induced rise in IP_3 (EC_{50}, 10 nM) in freshly dissociated rat atrial cells (159). A dissociation between phospholipase C and significant phospholipase A_2 activation in vascular smooth muscle cells has been noted based on their response to pertussis toxin (105), and a similar large increase in phospholipase A_2 activation with endothelin was seen in mesangial cells, but only at concentrations near 0.1 μM (155). This is well above the dose range necessary for IP_3 generation (1–10 nM), or for the induction of mitogenesis, intracellular alkalinization, and the stimulation of c-*fos* (<1 nM) (160).

Thus, it is possible that other actions of endothelin on ventricular myocytes might be demonstrable at concentrations greater than 1 nM. It is unknown what local tissue concentrations of endothelin are relevant. Although the reported K_d for receptor binding of endothelin-1 to cardiac tissue is in the subnanomolar range (93–95), much higher concentrations could occur under pathologic conditions. Nevertheless, the data reported by Krämer et al. (122) indicate that endothelin, in amounts well below 1 nM, will result in increased contractile function and an intracellular alkalinization that could facilitate the development of myocyte hypertrophy.

VIII. GTP-BINDING PROTEINS AND SIGNAL TRANSDUCTION AT THE SARCOLEMMAL MEMBRANE

The evidence that pertussis toxin blocks the increase in contractile amplitude with endothelin, but only diminishes the concomitant intracellular alkalinization, at least in isolated rat cardiocytes, points to a complex signal transduction mechanism that may employ more than one GTP binding or G protein.

The G proteins are a ubiquitous and versatile family of proteins that play a central role in transducing hormonal and sensory signals across eukaryotic plasma membranes, and have been the subject of several recent reviews (161–163). G proteins are heterotrimers consisting of α, β, and γ subunits. Over the past several years, work from a number of laboratories has revealed an unexpected structural diversity in the G protein α, β, and γ subunits. At present, more than 15 α subunits have been identified by cDNA cloning. Their structures are extremely similar, ranging from approximately 50% amino acid identity among the most distant to 95% amino acid identity among the most closely related members of the subunit groups.

The G protein α subunits bind GTP, and can be grouped into four families according to their structure and sensitivity to bacterial toxins (161,164). One group, composed of G_s (of which there are several isoforms due to alternative splicing [165]) and G_{olf}, is covalently modified by cholera toxin, which ADP-ribosylates an arginine residue. This group of G proteins stimulates adenylyl cyclase and regulates ion channels. The second group, which includes G_i (isoforms 1–3) and G_o (for "other"), is covalently modified by pertussis toxin, which ADP-ribosylates a cysteine near the carboxyl terminus (166). The functions of this group of proteins include inhibition of adenylyl cyclase, activation of phospholipase A_2, activation of phospholipase C, and regulation of ion channels. The three $G_i\alpha$ subtypes differ by 15% or less, while $G_o\alpha$ differs from the $G_i\alpha$ by 30%. The α_o subunit also exists in two forms due to alternative splicing (167,168). A third group includes the two retinal G proteins, transducin 1 and transducin 2 (95% identical), which can be modified by both cholera toxin and pertussis toxin. Transducin couples photoactivated rhodopsin to a cGMP phosphodiesterase. These proteins are more similar structurally to the G_i/G_o group than to the G_s group. There is a fourth group of G proteins, which, according to their structure, are predicted not to be substrates either for cholera or for pertussis toxin (169–174). One member of this group, G_z, has been purified. It is found predominantly in the brain, but it is a minor fraction of the brain G protein α subunits and its function is not known (171). The structural diversity of the α subunits thus reflects both the presence of multiple distinct genes and the differential processing of mRNA transcribed from these genes, although the functional properties of the various differentially spliced mRNA products are very similar.

Like the α subunits, the $\beta\gamma$ subunits are also heterogenous, with three very closely related forms of β having been identified and several forms of γ, at least one of which appears to be specific for the retina (172–179). Since $\beta\gamma$ does not dissociate under native conditions, different combinations of β and γ will form stable dimers.

Signal transduction by cell surface receptors coupled to G proteins appears to involve the receptor-promoted binding of GTP to the $\alpha\beta\gamma$ heterotrimer (reviewed in 161–163). The binding of GTP promotes the dissociation of a heterotrimer into two components. The GTP-liganded α subunit appears to interact directly with several effectors within the plasma membrane, with a specificity dictated primarily, but not exclusively, by the individual α subtype involved. For example, the α_s subunit activates adenylate cyclase directly, but the three α_i isoforms have yet to be clearly differentiated by distinct functional phenotypes in regulating effector systems in the membrane. The $\beta\gamma$ subunits liberated from the heterotrimer as a consequence of GTP binding to the α subunit exert both direct and indirect effects on cellular signaling systems. The generation of "free" $\beta\gamma$ subunits may serve to attenuate the pharmacologic response to activation of a cell surface receptor as a consequence of the "free" α subunits by promoting the formation of the $\alpha\beta\gamma$ heterotrimer. The α, β, and γ subunits each show considerable structural heterogeneity within their class, and yet further functional heterogeneity might be generated by the vast number of possible combinations of individual subunits in the G protein heterotrimer.

The role of the G proteins in the function of endothelial vasomediators is a subject of active investigation. The majority of the cell surface receptors linked to the activation of endothelial $^{\bullet}N{=}O$ release are coupled to G proteins. Endothelin's effects are, at least in part, dependent on a pertussis toxin-sensitive pathway, implicating a role for G proteins. The alteration of G protein function in different pathophysiological states might profoundly influence the role of endothelial vasomediators in the control of vascular tone and inotropic state.

IX. FUTURE DIRECTIONS

The vascular endothelium serves as both a source of vasoactive paracrine mediators, and as a transducer of intravascular signals derived from chemical and mechanical factors. The roles of the endothelium reflect a complex interplay of its vasorelaxant and vasoconstrictor products. Some of the same autacoids that promote endothelin release (via G-protein coupled receptors) also promote nitric oxide release in vitro. How these counterregulatory mechanisms operate in vivo to achieve hemodynamic and inotropic homeostasis remains an area of active investigation. It seems likely that future work will result in the isolation of yet other vasoactive endothelial products, and that novel short-term and longer-term regulatory mechanisms will be identified. An integrated model of endothelial function will derive from a more thorough understanding of these regulatory mechanisms, and of the differential importance of the diverse endothelial vasomediator substances.

ACKNOWLEDGMENTS

RAK is supported by grants HL-19259 and HL-36141 from the National Institutes of Health and by a Faculty Development Award from the Pharmaceutical Manufacturers Association. TMM is the recipient of a Clinician–Scientist Award from the American Heart Association. BKK was supported by a grant from the Paul-Martini-Stiftung, Bonn, Germany. The authors thank Dr. Eva J. Neer for invaluable advice in writing the sections on G proteins.

REFERENCES

1. Osborn L. Leukocyte adhesion to endothelium in inflammation. Cell 1990; 62:3–6.
2. Murphy-Ullrich JE, Höök M. Thrombospondin modulates focal adhesions in endothelial cells. J Cell Biol 1989; 109:1309–19.

3. Vane JR, Anggard EE, Botting RM. Regulatory functions of the vascular endothelium. N Engl J Med 1990; 323:27–36.
4. Pober JS, Cotran RS. Cytokines and endothelial cell biology. Physiol Rev 1990; 70: 427–51.
5. Simonson MS, Dunn MJ. Cellular signaling by peptides of the endothelin gene family. FASEB J 1990; 4:2989–3000.
6. Furchgott RF: The role of endothelium in the response of vascular smooth muscle to drugs. Annu Rev Pharmacol Toxicol 1984; 24:175–97.
7. Ignarro LJ. Biological actions and properties of endothelium-derived nitric oxide formed and released from artery and vein. Circ Res 1989; 65:1–21.
8. Ignarro LJ. Biosynthesis and metabolism of endothelium-derived nitric oxide. Annu Rev Pharmacol Toxicol 1990; 30:535–60.
9. Brutsaert DL. The endocardium. Annu Rev Physiol 1989; 51:263–73.
10. Murad F. Cyclic guanosine monophosphate as a mediator of vasodilation. J Clin Invest 1986; 78:1–5.
11. Ignarro LJ. Endothelium-derived nitric oxide: actions and properties. FASEB J 1989; 3:31–6.
12. Marletta MA. Nitric oxide: biosynthesis and biological significance. TIBS 1989; 14: 488–92.
13. Furchgott RF, Vanhoutte PM. Endothelium-derived relaxing and contracting factors. FASEB J 1989; 3:2007–18.
14. Radomski MW, Palmer RMJ, Moncada S. Comparative pharmacology of endothelium-derived relaxing factor, nitric oxide and prostacyclin in platelets. Br J Pharmacol 1987; 92:181–7.
15. Azuma H, Ishikawa M, Sekizaki S. Endothelium-dependent inhibition of platelet aggregation. Br J Pharmacol 1986; 88:411–5.
16. Mellion BT, Ignarro LJ, Meyers CB, Ohlstein EH, Ballot BA, Hyman AL, Kadowitz PJ. Inhibition of human platelet aggregation by S-nitrosothiols. Heme-dependent activation of soluble guanylate cyclase and stimulation of cyclic GMP accumulation. Mol Pharmacol 1983; 23:653–64.
17. Palmer RMJ, Ferrige AG, Moncada S. Nitric oxide release accounts for the biological activity of endothelium-derived relaxing factor. Nature 1987; 327:524–6.
18. Moncada S, Gryglewski R, Bunting S, Vane JR. An enzyme isolated from arteries transforms prostaglandin endoperoxides to an unstable substance that inhibits platelet aggregation. Nature 1976; 263:663–5.
19. Furchgott RF, Zawadzki JV. The obligatory rule of endothelial cells in the relaxation of arterial smooth muscle by acetylcholine. Nature 1980; 288:373–6.
20. Forstermann U, Mugge A, Alheid U, Haverich U, Frolich JC. Selective attenuation of endothelium-mediated vasodilation in atherosclerotic human coronary arteries. Circ Res 1988; 62:185–90.
21. Freiman PC, Mitchell GG, Heistad DD, Armstrong ML, Harrison DG. Atherosclerosis impairs endothelium-dependent vascular relaxation to acetylcholine and thrombin in primates. Circ Res 1986; 58:783–9.
22. Gryglewski RJ, Botting RM, Vane JR. Mediators produced by the endothelial cell. Hypertension 1988; 12:530–48.
23. Kamata K, Miyata N, Kasuya Y. Impairment of endothelium-dependent relaxation and changes in levels of cyclic GMP in aorta from streptozotocin-induced diabetic rats. Br J Pharmacol 1989; 97:614–8.
24. Harris KH, MacLeod KM. Influence of the endothelium on contractile responses of arteries from diabetic rats. Eur J Pharmacol 1988; 153:55–64.
25. Saenz de Tejada I, Goldstein I, Azadzoi K, Krane RJ, Cohen RA. Impaired neurogenic

and endothelium-mediated relaxation of penile smooth muscle from diabetic men with impotence. N Engl J Med 1989; 320:1025–30.
26. Harrison DG, Freiman PC, Armstrong ML, Marcus ML, Heistad DD. Alterations of vascular reactivity in atherosclerosis. Circ Res 1987; 61 (Suppl II):II-74–80.
27. Ludmer PL, Selwyn AP, Shook TL, Wagner RW, Mudge GH, Alexander RW, Ganz P. Paradoxical vasoconstriction induced by acetylcholine in atherosclerotic coronary arteries. N Engl J Med 1986; 315:1046.
28. Lefer AM, Tsao P, Aoki N, Palladino MA Jr. Mediation of cardioprotection by transforming growth factor-β. Science 1990; 249:61–4.
29. Bredt DS, Snyder SH. Isolation of nitric oxide synthetase, a calmodulin-requiring enzyme. Proc Natl Acad Sci USA 1990; 87:682–5.
30. Forstermann U, Neufang B. Endothelium-dependent vasodilation by melittin: are lipoxygenase products involved? Am J Physiol 1985; 249:H14–9.
31. Milner PG, Izzo NJ, Saye J, Lock AL, Johns RA, Peak MJ. J Clin Invest 1988; 81:1795.
32. Stuehr DJ, Marletta MA. Mammalian nitrate biosynthesis: mouse macrophages produce nitrite and nitrate in response to *Escherichia coli* lipopolysaccharide. Proc Natl Acad Sci USA 1985; 82:7738–42.
33. Tayeh MA, Marletta MA. Macrophage oxidation of L-arginine to nitric oxide, nitrite, and nitrate. J Biol Chem 1989; 264:19654–8.
35. Gally JA, Montague PR, Reeke GN Jr, Edelman GM: The NO hypothesis: possible effects of a short-lived, rapidly diffusible signal in the development and function of the nervous system. Proc Natl Acad Sci USA 1990; 87:3547–51.
36. Knowles RG, Palacios M, Palmer RMJ, Moncada S. Formation of nitric oxide from L-arginine in the central nervous system: a transduction mechanism for stimulation of the soluble guanylate cyclase. Proc Natl Acad Sci USA 1989; 86:5159–62.
37. Gillespie MN, Owasoyo JO, McMurtry IF, O'Brien RF. Sustained coronary vasoconstriction provoked by a peptidergic substance released from endothelial cells in culture. J Pharmacol Exp Ther 1986; 236:339–43.
38. Hickey KA, Rubanyi G, Paul RJ, Highsmith RF. Characterization of a coronary vasoconstrictor produced by cultured endothelial cells. Am J Physiol 1985; 248:C550–6.
39. O'Brien FJ, Robbins FJ, McMurtry IF. Endothelial cells in culture produce a vasoconstrictor substance. J Cell Physiol 1987; 132:263–70.
40. Rubany GM, Vanhoutte PM. Hypoxia releases a vasoconstrictor substance from the canine vascular endothelium. J Physiol 1985; 364:45–56.
41. Yanagisawa M, Kurihara H, Kimura S, Tomobe Y, Kobayashi M, Mitsui Y, Yazaki Y, Goto K, Masaki T. A novel potent vasoconstrictor peptide produced by vascular endothelial cells. Nature 1988; 332:411–5.
42. Inoue A, Yanagisawa M, Kimura S, Kasuya A, Miyauchi T, Goto K, Masaki T. The human endothelin family: three structurally and pharmacologically distinct isopeptides predicted by three separate genes. Proc Natl Acad Sci USA 1989; 86:2834–67.
43. Kloog Y, Ambar I, Sokolovsky M, Kochva E, Wollberg Z, Bdolah A. Sarafotoxin, a novel vasoconstrictor peptide: phosphoinositide hydrolysis in rat heart and brain. Science 1988; 242:268–70.
44. Boulanger C, Luscher TF. Release of endothelin from the porcine aorta. Inhibition by endothelium-derived nitric oxide. J Clin Invest 1990; 85:587–90.
45. Matsumura Y, Ikegawa R, Takaoka M, Morimoto S. Conversion of porcine big endothelin to endothelin by an extract from the porcine aortic endothelial cells. Biochem Biophys Res Commun 1990; 167:203–10.
46. Yoshizumi M, Kurihara H, Sugiyama T, Takaku F, Yanagisawa M, Masaki T, Yazaki Y. Hemodynamic shear stress stimulates endothelin production by culture endothelial cells. Biochem Biophys Res Commun 1989; 161:859–64.

47. Yoshizumi M, Kurihara H, Morita T, Yamashita T, Oh-hashi Y, Sugiyama T, Takaku F, Yanagisawa M, Masaki T, Yazaki Y. Interleukin 1 increases the production of endothelin-1 by cultured endothelial cells. Biochem Biophys Res Commun 1990; 166:324–9.
48. Ohlstein EH, Arleth A, Ezekiel M, Horohonich S, Ator MA, Caltabiano MM, Sung C-P. Biosynthesis and modulation of endothelin from bovine pulmonary arterial endothelial cells. Life Sci 1990; 46:181–8.
49. Emori T, Hirata Y, Ohta K, Shichiri M, Marumo F. Secretory mechanisms of immunoreactive endothelin in cultured bovine endothelial cells. Biochem Biophys Res Commun 1989; 160:93–100.
50. Emori T, Hirata Y, Ohta K, Shichiri M, Shimokado K, Marumo F. Concomitant secretion of big endothelin and its C-terminal fragment from human and bovine endothelial cells. Biochem Biophys Res Commun 1989; 162:217–23.
51. Hexum TD, Hoeger C, Rivier JE, Baird A, Brown MR. Characterization of endothelin secretion by vascular endothelial cells. Biochem Biophys Res Comm 1990; 167:294–300.
52. Yanagisawa M, Inoue A, Takuwa Y, Mitsui Y, Kobayashi M, Masaki T. The human preproendothelin-1 gene: Possible regulation by endothelial phosphoinositide turnover signaling. J Cardiovasc Pharmacol 1989; 13:S13–7.
53. Kosaka T, Suzuki N, Matsumoto H, Itoh Y, Yasuhara T, Onda H, Fujino M. Synthesis of the vasoconstrictor peptide endothelin in kidney cells. FEBS Lett 1989; 249:42–6.
54. Shichiri M, Hirata Y, Emori T, Ohta K, Nakajima T, Sato K, Sato A, Marumo F. Secretion of endothelin and related peptides from renal epithelial cell lines. FEBS Lett 1989; 253:203–6.
55. Black PN, Ghatei MA, Takahashi K, Bretherton-Watt D, Krausz T, Dollery CT, Bloom SR. Formation of endothelin by cultured airway epithelial cell. FEBS Lett 1989; 255:129–32.
56. Orlando C, Brandi ML, Peri A, Giannini S, Fantoni G, Calabresi E, Serio M, Maggi M. Neurohypophyseal hormone regulation of endothelin secretion from rabbit endometrial cells in primary culture. Endocrinology 1990; 126:1780–2.
57. Yoshizawa T, Shinmi O, Giaid A, Yanagisawa M, Gibson SJ, Kimura S, Uchiyama Y, Polak JM, Masaki T, Kanazawa I. Endothelin: a novel peptide in the posterior pituitary system. Science 1990; 247:462–4.
58. Shinmi O, Kimura S, Yoshizawa T, Sawamura T, Uchiyama Y, Sugita Y, Kanazawa I, Yanagisawa M, Goto K, Masaki T. Presence of endothelin-1 in porcine spinal cord: Isolation and sequence determination. Biochem Biophys Res Commun 1989; 162: 340–6.
59. Hirata Y, Matsunaga T, Ando K, Furukawa T, Tsukagoshi H, Marumo F. Presence of endothelin-1-like immunoreactivity in human cerebrospinal fluid. Biochem Biophys Res Commun 1990; 166:1274–8.
60. Takaoka M, Takenobu Y, Miyata Y, Ikegawa R, Matsumura Y, Morimoto S. Pepsin, an aspartic protease, converts porcine big endothelin to 21-residue endothelin. Biochem Biophys Res Commun 1990; 166:436–2.
61. Bloch KD, Friedrich SP, Lee M-E, Eddy RL, Shows TB, Quertermous T. Structural organization and chromosomal assignment of the gene encoding endothelin. J Biol Chem 1989; 264:10851–7.
62. Inoue A, Yanagisawa M, Kimura S, Kasuya Y, Miyauchi T, Goto K, Masaki T. The human endothelin family: three structurally and pharmacologically distinct isopeptides predicted by three separate genes. Proc Natl Acad Sci USA 1989; 86:2863–7.
63. De Nucci G, Thomas R, D'Orleans-Juste P, Antunes E, Walder C, Warner TF, Vane JR. Pressor effects of circulating endothelin are limited by its removal of the pulmonary circulation and by the release of prostacyclin and endothelium-derived relaxing factor. Proc Natl Acad Sci USA 1988; 85:9797–800.

64. Eglen RM, Michel AD, Sharif NA, Swank SR, Whiting RL. The pharmacological properties of the peptide endothelin. Br J Pharmacol 1989; 97:1297–307.
65. Hinojosa-Laborde C, Osborn JW, Cowley AW. Hemodynamic effects of endothelin in conscious rats. Am J Physiol 1989; 256:H1742–6.
66. Hoffman A, Grossman E, Ohman KP, Marks E, Keiser HR. Endothelin induces an initial increase in cardiac output associated with selective vasodilation in rats. Life Sci 1989; 45:249–55.
67. King AJ, Brenner BM, Anderson S. Endothelin: a potent renal and systemic vasoconstrictor peptide. Am J Physiol 1989; 256:F1051–8.
68. Kohno M, Murakawa K, Yasunari K, Yokokawa K, Horio T, Kurihara N, Takeda T. Prolonged blood pressure elevation after endothelin administration in bilaterally nephrectomized rats. Metabolism 1989; 38:712–3.
69. McMahon EG, Fok KF, Moore WM, Smith CE, Siegel NR, Trapani AJ. In vitro and in vivo activity of chymotrypsin-activated big endothelin (porcine 1-40). Biochem Biophys Res Commun 1989; 161:406–13.
70. Gardiner SM, Compton AM, Bennett T. Regional haemodynamic effects of endothelin-1 and endothelin-3 in conscious Long Evans and Brattleboro rats. Br J Pharmacol 1990; 99:107–12.
71. Le Monnier de Gouville AC, Mondot S, Lippton H, Cavero I. Hemodynamic and pharmacological evaluation of the vasodilator and vasoconstrictor effects of endothelin-1 in rats. J Pharmacol Exp Ther 1990; 252:300–11.
72. Miyauchi T, Ishikawa T, Tomobe Y, Yanagisawa M, Kimura S, Sugishita Y, Ito I, Goto K, Masaki T. Characteristics of pressor response to endothelin in spontaneously hypertensive and Wistar-Kyoto rats. Hypertension 1989; 14:427–34.
73. Mortensen LH, Fink GD. Hemodynamic effect of human and rat endothelin administration into conscious rats. Am J Physiol 1990; 258:H362–8.
74. Rohmeiss P, Photiadis J, Rohmeiss S, Unger T. Hemodynamic actions of intravenous endothelin in rats: comparison with sodium nitroprusside and methxamine. Am J Physiol 1990; 258:H337–46.
75. Cao L, Banks RO. Cardiovascular and renal actions of endothelin: effects of calcium-channel blockers. Am J Physiol 1990; 258:F254–8.
76. Lopez-Farre A, Montanes I, Milles I, Lopez-Novoa JM. Effect of endothelin on renal function in rats. Eur J Pharmacol 1989; 163:187–9.
77. Kashiwabara T, Inagaki Y, Ohta H, Iwamatsu A, Nomizu M, Morita A, Nishikori K. Putative precursors of endothelin have less vasoconstrictor activity in vitro but a potent pressor effect in vivo. FEBS Lett 1989; 247:73–6.
78. Goetz KL, Wang BC, Madwed JB, Zhu JL, Leadley RJ Jr. Cardiovascular, renal, and endocrine responses to intravenous endothelin in conscious dogs. Am J Physiol 1988; 255:R1064–8.
79. Herman F, Magyar K, Chabrier P-E, Braquet P, Filep J. Prostacyclin mediates anti-aggregatory and hypotensive actions of endothelin in anesthetized beagle dogs. Br J Pharmacol 1989; 98:38–40.
80. Watanabe T, Kusumoto K, Kitayoshi T, Shimamoto N. Positive inotropic and vasoconstrictive effects of endothelin-1 in in vivo and in vitro experiments: Characteristics and the role of L-type calcium channels. J Cardiovasc Pharmacol 1989; 13 (Suppl 5):S108–11.
81. Tsuchiya K, Naruse M, Sanaka T, Naruse K, Kato Y, Zeng ZP, Nitta K, Shizume K, Demura H, Sugino N. Effects of endothelin on renal hemodynamics and excretory function in anesthetized dogs. Life Sci 1990; 46:59–65.
82. Kitayoshi T, Watanabe T, Shimamoto N. Cardiovascular effects of endothelin in dogs: positive inotropic action in vivo. Eur J Pharmacol 1989; 166:519–22.
83. Lippton HL, Hauth TA, Summer WR, Hyman AL. Endothelin produces pulmonary vasoconstriction and systemic vasodilation. J Appl Physiol 1989; 66:1008–12.

84. Li L, Ishikawa T, Miyauchi T, Yanagisawa M, Kimura S, Goto K, Masaki T. Pressor response to endothelin in guinea pigs. Jpn J Pharmacol 1989; 49:549–52.
85. Baydoun AR, Peers SH, Cirino G, Woodward B. Effects of endothelin-1 on the rat isolated heart. J Cardiovasc Pharmacol 1989; 13:S193–6.
86. Reynolds EE, Mok LLS. Role of thromboxane A_2/prostaglandin H_2 receptor in the vasoconstrictor response of rat aorta to endothelin. J Pharmacol Exp Ther 1990; 252:915–21.
87. Igarashi Y, Aizawa Y, Tamura M, Ebe K, Yamaguchi T, Shibata A. Vasoconstrictor effect of endothelin on the canine coronary artery: is a novel endogenous peptide involved in regulating myocardial blood flow and coronary spasm? Am Heart J 1989; 118:674–8.
88. Kurihara H, Yamaoki K, Nagai R, Yoshizumi M, Takaku F, Satoh H, Inui J, Yazaki Y. Endothelin: a potent vasoconstrictor associated with coronary vasospasm. Life Sci 1989; 44:1937–43.
89. Larkin SW, Clarke JG, Keogh BE, Araujo L, Rhodes C, Davies GJ, Taylor KM, Maseri A. Intracoronary endothelin induces myocardial ischemia by small vessel constriction in the dog. Am J Cardiol 1989; 64:956–8.
90. Nichols AJ, Koster PF, Ohlstein EH. The effect of diltiazem on the coronary haemodynamic and cardiac functional effects produced by intracoronary administration of endothelin-1 in the anesthetized dog. Br J Pharmacol 1990; 99:597–601.
91. Watanabe T, Suzuki N, Shimamoto N, Fujino M, Imada A. Endothelin in myocardial infarction. Nature 1990; 344:114.
92. Ishikawa T, Yanagisawa M, Kimura S, Goto K, Masaki T. Positive inotropic action of a novel vasoconstrictor peptide endothelin in guinea pig atria. Am J Physiol 1988; 255:H970–3.
93. Gu X-H, Casley D, Nayler W. Specific high-affinity binding sites for ^{125}I-labelled porcine endothelin in rat cardiac membranes. Eur J Pharmacol 1989; 167:281–90.
94. Galron R, Kloog Y, Bdolah A, Sokolovsky M. Functional endothelin/sarafotoxin receptors in rat heart myocytes: structure–activity relationships and receptor subtypes. Biochem Biophys Res Commun 1989; 163:936–43.
95. Hirata Y. Endothelin-1 receptors in cultured vascular smooth muscle cells and cardiocytes of rats. J Cardiovasc Pharmacol 1989; 13:S157–8.
96. Stasch J-P, Hirth-Dietrich C, Kazda S, Neuser D. Endothelin stimulates release of atrial natriuretic peptides in vitro and in vivo. Life Sci 1989; 45:869–75.
97. Fukuda Y, Hirata Y, Yoshimi H, Kojima T, Kobayahi Y, Yanagisawa M, Masaki T. Endothelin is a potent secretagogue for atrial natriuretic peptide in cultured rat atrial myocytes. Biochem Biophys Res Commun 1988; 155:167–72.
98. Fukuda Y, Hirata Y, Takentani S, Kojima T, Oikawa S, Nakazato H, Kobayashi Y. Endothelin stimulates accumulations of cellular atrial natriuretic peptide and its messenger RNA in rat cardiocytes. Biochem Biophys Res Commun 1989; 164:1431–6.
99. Ru Hu J, Berninger UG, Lang RE. Endothelin stimulates atrial natriuretic peptide (ANP) release from rat atria. Eur J Pharmacol 1988; 158:177–8.
100. Lew RA, Baertschi AJ. Endothelial cells stimulate ANF secretion from atrial myocytes in co-culture. Biochem Biophys Res Commun 1989; 163:701–9.
101. Mantymaa P, Leppaluoto J, Ruskoaho H. Endothelin stimulates basal and stretch-induced atrial natriuretic peptide secretion from the perfused rat heart. Endocrinology 1990; 126:587–95.
102. Winquist RJ, Scott AL, Vlasuk GP. Enhanced release of atrial natriuretic factor by endothelin in atria from hypertensive rats. Hypertension 1989; 14:111–4.
103. Brutsaert DL, Meulemans AL, Sipido KR, Sys SU. Effects of damaging the endocardial surface on the mechanical performance of isolated cardiac muscle. Circ Res 1988; 62:358–66.

104. Shah AM, Meulemans AL, Brutsaert DL. Myocardial inotropic responses to aggregating platelets and modulation by the endocardium. Circulation 1989; 79:1315–23.
105. Feigl EO. Coronary physiology. Physiol Rev 1983; 63:1.
106. Kitakaze M, Marban E. Cellular mechanism of the modulation of contractile function by coronary perfusion pressure in ferret hearts. J Physiol 1989; 414:455–72.
107. Hoffman JIE, Spaan JAE. Pressure–flow relations in coronary circulation. Physiol Rev 1990; 70:331–90.
108. Bassingthwaighte JB, King RB, Roger SA. Fractal nature of regional myocardial blood flow heterogeneity. Circ Res 1989; 65:578–90.
109. Lindpainter K, Jin M, Wilhelm MJ, Suzuki F, Linz W, Schoelkens BA, Ganten D. Intracardiac generation of angiotensin and its physiologic role. Circulation 1988; 77 (Suppl I):I-18.
110. Vigne P, Lazdunski M, Frelin C. The inotropic effect of endothelin-1 on rat atria involves hydrolysis of phosphatidylinositol. FEBS Lett 1989; 249:143–6.
111. Ru Hu J, Von Harsdorf R, Lang RE. Endothelin has potent inotropic effects in rat atria. Eur J Pharmacol 1988; 158:275–8.
112. Borges R, Von Grafenstein H, Knight DE. Tissue selectivity of endothelin. Eur J Pharmacol 1989; 165:223–30.
113. Volkmann R, Bokvist K, Wennmalm A. Endothelin has no positive inotropic effect in guinea-pig atria or papillary muscle. Acta Physiol Scand 1990; 138:345–8.
114. Tohse N, Hattori Y, Nakaya H, Endou M, Kanno M. Inability of endothelin to increase Ca^{2+} current in guinea-pig heart cells. Br J Pharmacol 1990; 99:437–8.
115. Shah AM, Lewis MJ, Henderson AH. Inotropic effects of endothelin in ferret ventricular myocardium. Eur J Pharmacol 1989; 163:365–7.
116. Schomisch Moravec C, Reynolds EE, Stewart RW, Bond M. Endothelin is a positive inotropic agent in human and rat heart in vitro. Biochem Biophys Res Commun 1989; 159:14–8.
117. Kelly RA, Eid H, Kramer BK, O'Neill M, Liang BT, Reers M, Smith TW. Endothelin enhances the contractile responsiveness of adult rat ventricular myocytes to calcium by a pertussis toxin-sensitive pathway. J Clin Invest 1990 (in press).
118. Lauer MR, Gunn MD, Clusin W. Effect of endothelin on cytosolic calcium and membrane current in single ventricular myocytes. Circulation 1989; 80:II-194.
119. Fabiato A, Fabiato F. Effects of pH on the myofilaments and the sarcoplasmic reticulum of skinned cells from cardiac and skeletal muscles. J Physiol 1978; 276:233–55.
120. Allen DG, Orchard CH. The effects of changes of pH on intracellular calcium transients in mammalian cardiac muscle. J Physiol 1983; 335:555–67.
121. Ruegg JC. Calcium in muscle activation. A comparative approach. New York: Springer-Verlag, 1988.
122. Kramer BK, Smith TW, Kelly RA. Endothelin and increased contractility in adult rat ventricular myocytes: role of intracellular alkalosis induced by activation of the protein kinase C-dependent Na^+-H^+ exchanger. Circ Res 1991 (in press).
123. Matsumura Y, Nakase K, Ikegawa R, Hayashi K, Ohyama T, Morimoto S. The endothelium-derived vasoconstrictor peptide endothelin inhibits renin release in vitro. Life Sci 1989; 44:149–57.
124. Takagi M, Matsuoka H, Atarashi K, Yagi S. Endothelin: a new inhibitor of renin release. Biochem Biophys Res Commun 1988; 157:1164–8.
125. Takagi M, Tsukuda H, Matsuoka H, Yagi S. Inhibitory effect of endothelin on renin release in vitro. Am J Physiol 1989; 257:E833–8.
126. Cozza EN, Gomez-Sanchez CE, Foecking MF, Chiou S. Endothelin binding to cultured calf adrenal zone glomerulosa cells and stimulation of aldosterone secretion. J Clin Invest 1989; 84:1032–5.
127. Morishita R, Higaki J, Ogihara T. Endothelin stimulates aldosterone biosynthesis by

dispersed rabbit adreno-capsular cells. Biochem Biophys Res Commun 1989; 160: 628–32.

128. Karwatowska-Prokopczuk E, Wennmalm A. Effects of endothelin on coronary flow, mechanical performance, oxygen uptake, and formation of purines and on outflow of prostacyclin in the isolated rabbit heart. Circ Res 1990; 66:46–54.
129. Reynolds EE, Mok LLS, Kurokawa S. Phorbol ester dissociates endothelin-stimulated phosphoinositide hydrolysis and arachidonic acid release in vascular smooth muscle cells. Biochem Biophys Res Commun 1989; 160:868–73.
130. Resink TJ, Scott-Burden T, Buhler FR. Activation of phospholipase A_2 by endothelin in cultured vascular smooth muscle cells. Biochem Biophys Res Commun 1989; 158:279–86.
131. Takayasu M, Kondo K, Terao S. Endothelin-induced mobilization of Ca^{2+} and the possible involvement of platelet activating factor and thromboxane A_2. Biochem Biophys Res Commun 1989; 160:751–7.
132. Rakugi H, Nakamura M, Tabuchi Y, Nagano M, Mikami H, Ogihara T. Endothelin stimulates the release of prostacyclin from rat mesenteric arteries. Biochem Biophys Res Commun 1989; 160:924–8.
133. Zoja C, Benigni A, Renzi D, Piccinelli A, Perico N, Remuzzi G. Endothelin and eicosanoid synthesis in cultured mesangial cells. Kidney Int 1990; 37:927–33.
134. Luscher TF, Yang Z, Tschudi M, Von Segesser L, Stulz P, Boulanger C, Siebermann R, Turina M, Buhler FR. Interaction between endothelin-1 and endothelium-derived relaxing factor in human arteries and veins. Circ Res 1990; 66:1088–94.
135. Boarder MR, Marriott DB. Characterization of endothelin-1 stimulation of catecholamine release from adrenal chromaffin cells. J Cardiovasc Pharmacol 1989; 13:S223–4.
136. Han S-P, Knuepfer MM, Trapani AJ, Fok KF, Westfall TC. Endothelin and sarafotoxin S6b have similar vasoconstrictor effects and post-synaptically mediated mechanisms. Eur J Pharmacol 1990; 177:29–34.
137. Reid JJ, Wong-Dusting HK, Rand MJ. The effect of endothelin on noradrenergic transmission in rat and guinea-pig atria. Eur J Pharmacol 1989; 168:93–6.
138. Tabuchi Y, Nakamaru M, Rakugi H, Nagano M, Ogihara T. Endothelin enhances adrenergic vasoconstriction in perfused rat mesenteric arteries. Biochem Biophys Res Commun 1989; 159:1304–8.
139. Tabuchi Y, Nakamaru M, Rakugi H, Nagano M, Mikami H, Ogihara T. Endothelin inhibits presynaptic adrenergic neurotransmission in rat mesenteric artery. Biochem Biophys Res Commun 1989; 161:803–8.
140. Wong-Dusting HK, Reid JJ, Rand MJ. Paradoxical effects of endothelin on cardiovascular noradrenergic neurotransmission. Clin Exp Pharmacol Physiol 1989; 16:229–33.
141. Badr KF, Murray JJ, Breyer MD, Takahashi K, Inagami T, Harris RC. Mesangial cell, glomerular and renal vascular responses to endothelin in the rat kidney. J Clin Invest 1989; 83:336–42.
142. Ferrario RG, Foulkes R, Salvati P, Patrono C. Hemodynamic and tubular effects of endothelin and thromboxane in the isolated perfused rat kidney. Eur J Pharmacol 1989; 171:127–34.
143. Loutzenhiser R, Epstein M, Hayashi K, Horton C. Direct visualization of effects of endothelin on the renal microvasculature. Am J Physiol 1990; 258:F61–8.
144. Nitta K, Naruse M, Sanaka T, Tsuchiya K, Naruse K, Zeng Z-P, Demura H, Sugino N. Natriueretic and diuretic effects of endothelin in isolated perfused rat kidney. Endocrinol Jpn 1989; 36:887–90.
145. Perico N, Dadan J, Gabanelli M, Remuzzi G. Cyclooxygenase products and atrial natriuretic peptide modulate renal response to endothelin. J Pharmacol Exp Ther 1990; 252:1213–20.

146. Stacy DL, Scott JW, Granger JP. Control of renal function during intrarenal infusion of endothelin. Am J Physiol 1990; 258:F1232–6.
147. Kon V, Yoshioka t, Fogo A, Ichikawa I. Glomerular actions of endothelin in vivo. J Clin Invest 1989; 83:1762–7.
148. Griendling KK, Tsuda T, Alexander RW. Endothelin stimulates diacylglycerol accumulation and activates protein kinase C in cultured vascular smooth muscle cells. J Biol Chem 1989; 264:8237–0.
149. Grinstein S, Rotin D, Mason MJ. Na^+-H^+ exchange and growth factor-induced cytosolic pH changes. Role in cellular proliferation. Biochem Biophys Acta 1989; 988:73–97.
150. Soltoff SP, Cantley LC. Mitogens and ion fluxes. Ann Rev Physiol 1988; 50:207–23.
151. Bobik A, Grooms A, Millar JA, Mitchell A, Grinpukel S. Growth factor activity of endothelin on vascular smooth muscle. Am J Physiol 1990; 258:C408–15.
152. Brown KD, Littlewood CJ. Endothelin stimulates DNA synthesis in Swiss 3T3 cells. Synergy with polypeptide growth factors. Biochem J 1989; 263:977–80.
153. Takuwa N, Takuwa Y, Yanagisawa M, Yamashita K, Masaki T. A novel vasoactive peptide endothelin stimulates mitogenesis through inositol lipid turnover in Swiss 3T3 fibroblasts. J Biol Chem 1989; 264:7856–61.
154. Vigne P, Marsault R, Breittmayer JP, Frelin C. Endothelin stimulates phosphatidylinositol hydrolysis and DNA synthesis in brain capillary endothelial cells. Biochem J 1990; 266:415–20.
155. Simonson MS, Dunn MJ. Endothelin-1 stimulates contraction of rat glomerular mesangial cells and potentiates β-adrenergic-mediated cyclic adenosine monophosphate accumulation. J Clin Invest 1990; 85:790–7.
156. Simpson PC. Proto-oncogenes and cardiac hypertrophy. Annu Rev Physiol 1988; 51:189–202.
157. Takauwa Y, Kasuya Y, Takuwa N, Kudo M, Yanagisawa M, Goto K, Masaki T, Yamashita K. Endothelin receptor is coupled to phospholipase C via a pertussis toxin-insensitive guanine nucleotide-binding regulatory protein in vascular smooth muscle cells. J Clin Invest 1990; 85:653–8.
158. MacCumber MW, Ross CA, Snyder SH. Endothelin in brain: receptors, mitogenesis and biosynthesis in glial cells. Proc Natl Acad Sci USA 1990; 87:2359–63.
159. Vigne P, Breittmayer J-P, Marsault R, Frelin C. Endothelin mobilizes Ca^{2+} from a caffeine- and ryanodine-insensitive intracellular pool in rat atrial cells. J Biol Chem 1990; 265:6782–7.
160. Simonson MS, Wann S, Mene P, Dubyak GR, Kester M, Nakazato Y, Sedor JR, Dunn MJ. Endothelin stimulates phospholipase C, Na^+/H^+ exchange, c-fos expression, and mitogenesis in rat mesangial cells. J Clin Invest 1989; 83:708–12.
161. Neer EJ, Clapham DE. Roles of G protein subunits in transmembrane signalling. Nature 1988; 333:129–34.
162. Lochrie MA, Simon MI. G protein multiplicity in eukaryotic signal transduction systems. Biochemistry 1988; 27:4957–65.
163. Freissmuth M, Casey PJ, Gilman AG. G proteins control diverse pathways of transmembrane signaling. FASEB J 1989; 3:2125–31.
164. Kaziro Y, Itoh H, Kozasa T, Toyama R, Tsukamoto T, Matsuoka M, Nakafuku M, Obara T, Takagi T, Hernandez R. Structures of the genes coding for G-protein α subunits from mammalian and yeast cells. Cold Spring Harbor Symp Quant Biol 1988; 103:209–20.
165. Bray P, Carter A, Simons C, Guo V, Puckett C, Kamholtz J, Spiegel A, Nirenberg M. Human cDNA clones for four species of G-alpha$_s$ signal transduction protein. Proc Natl Acad Sci USA 1986; 83:8893–7.

166. West RE Jr, Moss J, Vaughan M, Liu T, Liu T-Y. Pertussis toxin-catalyzed ADP-ribosylation of transducin. J Biol Chem 1985; 260:14428–30.
167. Hsu WH, Rudolph U, Sanford J, Bertrand P, Olate J, Nelson C, Moss LG, Boyd AE, Codina J, Birnbaumer L. Molecular cloning of a novel splice variant of the α subunit of the mammalian G_o protein. J Biol Chem 1990; 265:11220–6.
168. Strathmann M, Wilkie TM, Simon MI. Alternative splicing produces transcripts encoding two forms of the α subunit of GTP-binding protein G_o. Proc Natl Acad Sci USA 1990; 87:6477–81.
169. Matsuoka M, Itoh H, Kozasa T, Kaziro Y. Sequence analysis of cDNA and genomic DNA for a putative pertussis toxin-insensitive guanine nucleotide-binding regulatory protein α subunit. Proc Natl Acad Sci USA 1988; 85:5384–8.
170. Fong HKW, Yoshimoto KK, Eversole-Cire P, Simon MI. Identification of a GTP-binding protein α subunit that lacks an apparent ADP-ribosylation site for pertussis toxin. Proc Natl Acad Sci USA 1988; 85:3066–70.
171. Casey PJ, Fong HK, Simon MI, Gilman AG. G_z, a guanine nucleotide-binding protein with unique biochemical properties. J Biol Chem 1990; 265:2383–90.
172. Fong HKW, Amatruda TT, Birren BW, Simon MI. Distinct forms of the β subunit of GTP-binding regulatory proteins identified by molecular cloning. Proc Natl Acad Sci USA 1987; 84:3792–6.
173. Gao B, Gilman AG, Robishaw JD. A second form of the β subunit of signal-transducing G proteins. Proc Natl Acad Sci USA 1987; 84:6122–5.
174. Levine MA, Feldman AM, Robishaw JD, Ladenson PW, Ahn TG, Moroney JF, Smallwood PM. Influence of thyroid hormone status on expression of genes encoding G protein subunits in the rat heart. J Biol Chem 1990; 265:3553–60.
175. Amatruda TT III, Fong HKW, Birren BW, Simon MI. Molecular cloning of a distinct form of the β subunit of GTP-binding regulatory proteins. In: Signal transduction in cytoplasmic organization and cell motility. New York: Alan R. Liss, 1988; 339–51.
176. Gautam N, Baetscher M, Aebersold R, Simon MI. A G protein gamma subunit shares homology with ras proteins. Science 1989; 244:971–4.
177. Robishaw JD, Kalman VK, Moomaw CR, Slaughter CA. Existence of two γ subunits of the G proteins in brain. J Biol Chem 1989; 264:15758–61.
178. Lerea CL, Somers DE, Hurley JB, Klock IB, Bunt-Milam AH. Identification of specific transducin α subunits in retinal rod and cone photoreceptors. Science 1986; 234:77–80.
179. Grunwald GB, Giershik P, Nirenberg M, Spiegel A. Detection of alpha-transducin in retinal rods but not cones. Science 1986; 231:856–9.

25

Calcium Channels in the Heart: Biophysics, Physiology, and Clinical Significance

C. WILLIAM BALKE

University of Maryland at Baltimore
Baltimore, Maryland

I. INTRODUCTION

Calcium channels are composed of several closely associated proteins and are found in the surface membranes of virtually all excitable cells (1–5). These sarcolemmal proteins form a functional unit or pore that is both highly permeable to and highly selective for calcium ions (Ca^{2+}). By regulating the transmembrane flux of Ca^{2+}, calcium channels play a crucial role in coupling the electrical events of the cell surface membrane to a wide variety of cellular functions, such as excitability, contraction, secretion, and gene expression. The transduction of electrical signals to cellular function is initiated by the opening of voltage-gated calcium channels in response to depolarization of the surface membrane. Calcium ions flow into the cell down a steep electrochemical gradient from an extracellular calcium concentration in the millimolar (10^{-3} M) range to an intracellular free calcium concentration ($[Ca^{2+}]_i$) in the nanomolar range (10^{-9} M) range (for reviews, see Refs. 6 and 7). The subsequent rise in $[Ca^{2+}]_i$ as a result of sarcoplasmic reticulum release is transient (micromolar range) and is terminated not only by closure of the sarcolemmal calcium channels but also by the sequestration of Ca^{2+} by the sarcoplasmic reticulum and extrusion of Ca^{2+} from the cytoplasm by multiple cellular processes that maintain Ca^{2+} homeostasis.

In cardiac cells, the inward calcium current (influx of positive charge) influences the duration of the action potential and the refractory period (8–10). Calcium current underlies the upstroke of the action potential of the sinus and atrioventricular nodes (11,12) and contributes to the pacemaker potential of sinoatrial cells (13,14). Calcium current has also been implicated in the generation of arrhythmias under certain pathologic conditions (15,16). In addition to the influx of positive charge, calcium ions function as "second messengers" that regulate a variety of cellular functions. Several intracellular enzyme systems are sensitive to changes in the concentration of $[Ca^{2+}]_i$, including the Ca^{2+} binding proteins calmodulin and troponin (17,18) and the Ca^{2+}-ATPase of the sarcoplasmic reticulum Ca^{2+} pump (19). Furthermore, the transient influx of Ca^{2+} through the sarcolemmal calcium channels both initiates and grades the contractile response of heart cells via control of the release of Ca^{2+} from the sarcoplasmic reticulum (see Chap. 2) (20–25).

The importance of Ca^{2+} for the electrical and contractile properties of the heart has been recognized for many years (26), and voltage-clamp studies on multicellular preparations provided the initial insights into the biophysical characteristics of calcium channels. However, numerous technical limitations associated with these methods hampered the quantitative characterization of calcium channel properties (27). For example, the variety of calcium channels was not anticipated, the complexities of calcium channel kinetics were not appreciated, and calcium channel permeability and selectivity were poorly understood. In the early 1980s, the development of several new techniques sustained continued advancements in the understanding of the properties of calcium channels. The availability of single myocytes obtained from the enzymatic digestion of hearts from a variety of species overcame the difficulties of voltage clamping large multicellular preparations (28,29). The introduction of the patch-clamp technique (30) allowed manipulation of the intracellular solution and provided the means for recording currents from both the whole cell and from single calcium channels (for historical review, see Ref. 5). The synthesis of radioactive probes with a high affinity for calcium channels has led to the elucidation of the biochemical structure of the protein subunits of the calcium channel (see Ref. 31 and, for review, Ref. 28). Recent advances in molecular biology have led to the cloning of the α_1 subunit of the L-type calcium channel of skeletal muscle (32,33) and the sequencing of the cardiac L-type calcium channel (34). The development of Ca^{2+}-selective fluorescent probes has led to a more refined understanding of the cellular processes that regulate intracellular Ca^{2+} homeostasis, including calcium channels (7,35).

The objective of this review is to summarize the salient features of the biophysical and pharmacologic properties of the two types of calcium channels found in the surface membranes of heart cells. An understanding of the properties of cardiac T- and L-type calcium channels is essential for clarifying their different physiologic roles. In addition, this foundation provides the rationale for anticipating the possible involvement of L-type calcium channels in the mechanisms of altered contractility associated with several pathologic conditions, such as ischemia, hypertrophy, and failure. As such, this chapter is not intended to be an encyclopedic review (14,27) of the topic of calcium channels in heart. It focuses on investigations in which the experimental conditions mimic as closely as possible the conditions encountered in both physiologic and pathophysiologic situations (e.g., identity and concentration of divalent charge carrier). Original data are presented when appropriate.

II. TYPES OF CALCIUM CHANNELS

With the demonstration of two types of calcium channels in starfish eggs, Hagiwara and coworkers (36) were the first to challenge the traditional notion that calcium channels belonged to a single homogeneous class of membrane channels. Tsien and coworkers (37) identified three types of calcium channels in dorsal root ganglion cells, including the L-type calcium channel (large conductance and long-lasting current), the T-type calcium channel (tiny conductance and transient duration relative to L-type calcium channels), and the intermediate N-type calcium channel. It is now well established that at least two types of calcium channels coexist in heart cells from a variety of species (for reviews, see Refs. 4, 14, 38, and 39). The predominant type of calcium channel found in most cardiac cells is the L-type calcium channel (40). L-type calcium channels are now known to be the channels that have been classically recognized in heart muscle as the mediators of the "slow inward calcium current" (I_{si}). The T-type calcium channel has been identified in many types of cardiac cells, but the N-type calcium channel has been found only in neurons. In addition, there is evidence for the existence of different subtypes of channels within the family of L-type calcium channels (6). For example, L-type calcium channels from smooth muscle and cardiac muscle have markedly different sensitivities to calcium channel antagonists. Although both cardiac T- and L-type calcium channels are highly permeable to and selective for Ca^{2+}, they can be separated by their different kinetics and voltage dependence, single-channel properties, ion selectivity, and pharmacology (4,38).

A. Differences in Kinetics and Voltage Dependence

At the whole-cell level, T- and L-type calcium currents can be distinguished on the basis of the large difference in their ranges of steady-state inactivation (4,41). Since L-type calcium channels are fully reprimed (i.e., inactivation is removed and the channels are available to open) at a holding potential of −50 mV and T-type calcium channels are fully reprimed at holding potentials of −80 or −90 mV, currents elicited from a holding potential of −90 mV contain both components. However, currents elicited from a holding potential of −50 mV contain only the component from L-type calcium channels. Figure 1 illustrates the separation of T- and L-type calcium currents in a guinea pig ventricular cell with physiologic concentrations of external Ca^{2+} (2 mM). In Figure 1A and B the voltage protocol and superimposed currents from holding potentials of −90 and −50 mV are shown. As shown in Figure 1A, a 200 ms depolarization of 0 mV from holding potentials of −90 and −50 mV elicits an inward current with a peak amplitude of 567 pA. In this case, a depolarization to 0 mV does not recruit any additional current from a more negative holding potential of −90 mV compared with a holding potential of −50 mV. Because the currents elicited by depolarization to 0 mV from both holding potentials are superimposable, they must represent current exclusively through L-type calcium channels. As shown in Figure 1B, a 200 ms depolarization to −40 mV elicits an inward current of 142 pA from a holding potential of −90 mV but no inward current from a holding potential of −50 mV. Since this additional rapidly inactivating inward current is elicited only by depolarization from a holding potential of −90 mV, it must represent current exclusively through T-type calcium channels. Since currents elicited by depolarizations from −90 mV contain both T- and L-type components and currents elicited from a holding potential of −50 mV have only the L-type component, the calculated difference between the currents obtained at each holding potential represents the T-type component of the calcium current at that test potential. Figure 1C shows pooled data from 12 cells illustrating the current-voltage relations for combined T- and L-type calcium currents elicited from a holding potential of −90 mV, L-type calcium current from a holding poten-

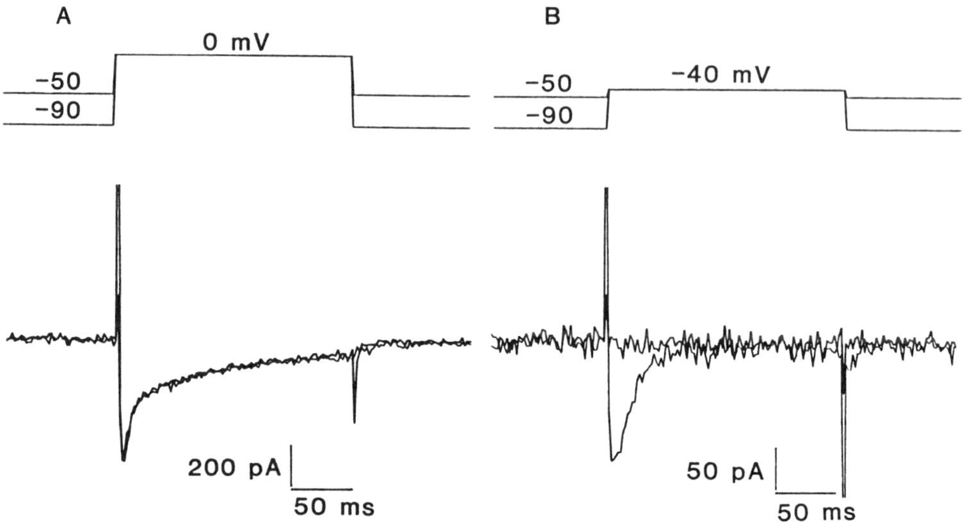

Figure 1 Two components of calcium current in a guinea pig ventricular cell with 2 mM Ca^{2+} as the charge carrier. Sodium current was blocked by equimolar replacement of Na^+ with Tetraethylammonium chloride (TEA) (140 mM) in the presence of 30 μM tetrodotoxin (TTX); potassium currents were blocked by 10 mM CsCl in both the external and pipette solutions. Currents were elicited by steps to (A) 0 and (B) −40 mV from holding potentials of −90 and −50 mV. The peak current-voltage relation (C) was obtained from currents elicited from holding potentials of −90 mV (filled circles), at which both T- and L-type calcium channels are available to open with depolarization and −50 mV (open circles), in which only L-type calcium channels are fully available to open. The T-type current-voltage relation (triangles) was calculated as the difference between currents elicited from a holding potential of −90 mV and currents elicited from a holding potential of −50 mV. (Modified from Balke et al., Ref. 41.)

tial of −50 mV, and T-type current (difference current). Consistent with the current records in Figure 1A and B, L-type calcium currents were maximal during depolarizing pulses to 10 mV (peak current density = 4.7 ± 0.3 nA nF^{-1}), and T-type calcium currents were maximal during depolarizing pulses between −30 and −40 mV (peak current density of 0.62 ± 0.21 nA nF^{-1}). At test potentials positive to 0 mV, the current-voltage relations from each holding potential are superimposable and the component of T-type current becomes immeasurably small (41).

It is clear that the accurate separation of the T- and L-type components of calcium current depends upon the appropriate choice of holding potential. If a holding potential is used when L-type calcium channels are not fully reprimed (e.g., −40 mV), the calculated T-type calcium current component can be greatly overestimated by inclusion of some L-type calcium current. Since the density of L-type calcium current in guinea pig ventricular cells (42) is on average fivefold greater than that of T-type calcium current (41), the inclusion of even a small fraction of L-type current can dramatically alter the calculated T-type current, especially at positive test potentials. Unrecognized overlap with L-type calcium channels may explain why previous work has reported sizable T-type calcium currents at test potentials positive to 0 mV (38,43,44). This may also explain why some workers have shown that β-adrenergic agents (43) and dihydropyridines (44) affect whole-

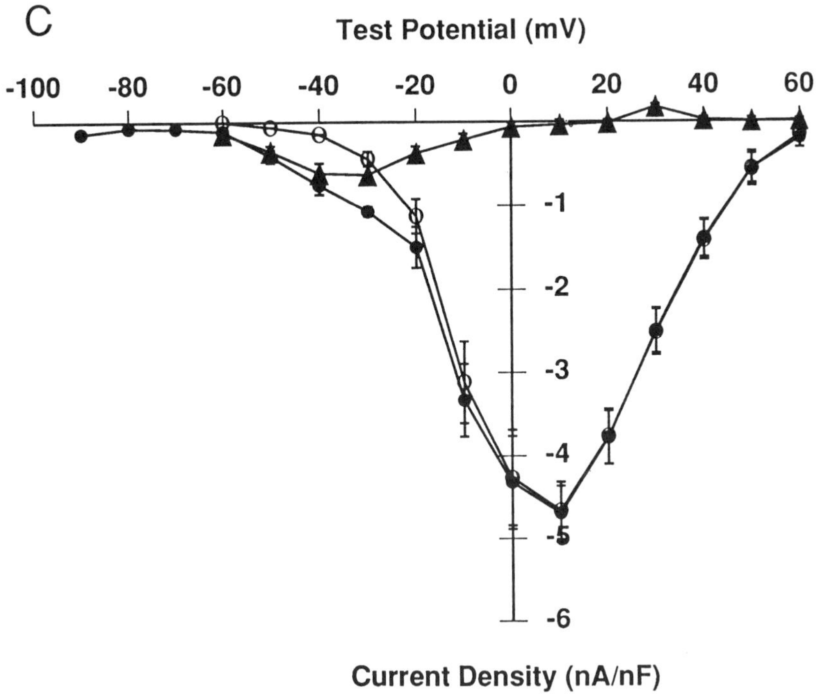

Figure 1 Continued

cell T-type calcium current despite the absence of any clear effects of either agent at the single-channel level (40,45).

The results in Figure 1 imply that test pulses to −40 mV elicit only T-type calcium current but test pulses to 10 mV elicit exclusively L-type calcium current. This distinction can be exploited to determine the voltage dependence of steady-state inactivation of each component. Figure 2 shows the steady-state inactivation curves derived from currents elicited at test potentials of −40 and 10 mV from more negative conditioning potentials. The inactivation ranges of T- and L-type calcium current are very clearly separated. L-type currents first measurably inactivate at −45 mV and reach 50% inactivation only at −25 mV; in contrast, T-type calcium currents begin to inactivate at −75 mV and are 50% available at −61 mV (41,46).

The kinetic differences between T- and L-type calcium channels are accentuated by the substitution of Ba^{2+} for Ca^{2+} as the divalent charge carrier (4). The inactivation of L-type calcium current involves at least two mechanisms, including a fast Ca^{2+}-dependent component and a slower voltage-dependent component (47–49). Since Ba^{2+} does not substitute well for Ca^{2+} in supporting calcium-dependent inactivation, L-type calcium current inactivates much more slowly in the presence of Ba^{2+}. In contrast, the kinetics of T-type calcium current are unaffected by the substitution of Ba^{2+} for Ca^{2+} as the charge carrier (4). Therefore, the mechanism of T-type calcium channel inactivation does not appear to involve a Ca^{2+}-dependent process. Even under physiologic conditions (2 mM external Ca^{2+}), striking differences are evident in the activation and decay of whole-cell T- and L-type calcium currents, as shown in Fig. 1A and B. At test potentials that elicit the largest T-type

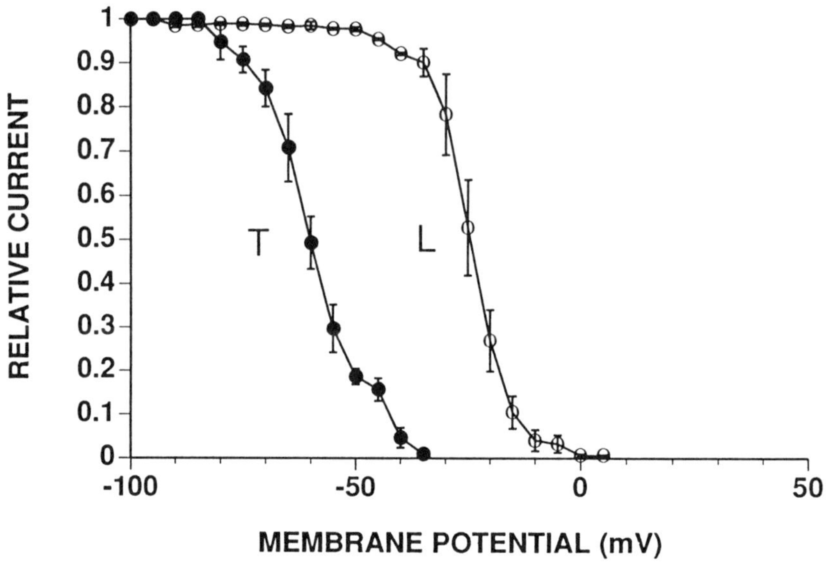

Figure 2 Steady-state inactivation curves for T- and L-type calcium current. Experimental conditions were identical to those described in Fig. 1. T-type calcium currents (filled circles) were elicited by a test potential of −40 mV as a function of holding potential. L-type calcium currents (open circles) were elicited by a test potential of 10 mV as a function of holding potential. Steady-state inactivation curves were generated from normalized peak current amplitudes as a function of holding potential. The inactivation curves were not characterized by a Boltzmann distribution function because of the upturn of current at positive holding potentials (not shown). $N = 12$. (Modified from Balke et al., Ref. 41.)

calcium current (−40 and −30 mV), the current peaks within 10 ms and then decays completely within 50–100 ms (Fig. 1B) (41). This time course is consistent with previous recordings of T-type calcium current under different ionic conditions (50,51). With progressive depolarization, the current turns on more rapidly and the duration of the entire current transient shortens even more dramatically (41,50–52). In contrast, the decay of L-type calcium current is slower than that of the T-type component. As shown in Figure 1A, peak L-type calcium current is elicited at a test potential of 10 mV, slowly decays over the 200 ms duration of the depolarization, and is not complete at the time of repolarization. This incomplete inactivation or "current pedestal" distinguishes this current from the T type (Fig. 1B), which inactivates completely over this time scale.

B. Differences in Single-Channel Properties

At the single-channel level, T- and L-type calcium channels can be distinguished by differences in the way that they respond to voltage ("gating") and in how they pass ions ("permeation"). These differences are exaggerated with the use of surrogate divalent charge carriers, such as Ba^{2+} (4,38,40,52). When 110 mM Ba^{2+} replaces Ca^{2+} as the charge carrier, the decay of L-type calcium currents becomes much slower but the decay of T-type calcium currents remains rapid and is complete within 100 ms. Under these conditions, L-type calcium channels reopen many times, leading to a pedestal of maintained inward current lasting the duration of a 200 ms depolarization. Since T-type calcium channel gating is not influenced by replacing Ba^{2+} for Ca^{2+}, the decay of current is not sensitive to the identity of the divalent charge carrier. In the presence of high external Ba^{2+} concentrations (110 mM), T-type calcium channels have a relatively small single-channel conductance of 6–8 pS (37,40,50) compared with a single-channel conductance of L-type calcium channels of 15–25 pS (40,43,53).

Despite superficial similarities, the two channel types can be distinguished even when Ca^{2+} is the charge carrier. Figure 3 shows single-channel recordings from a guinea pig ventricular cell in the cell-attached configuration (30) obtained with high concentrations of Ca^{2+} (70 mM) as the charge carrier. Figure 3A shows the voltage protocol, selected single sweeps, and the ensemble average current from 101 con-

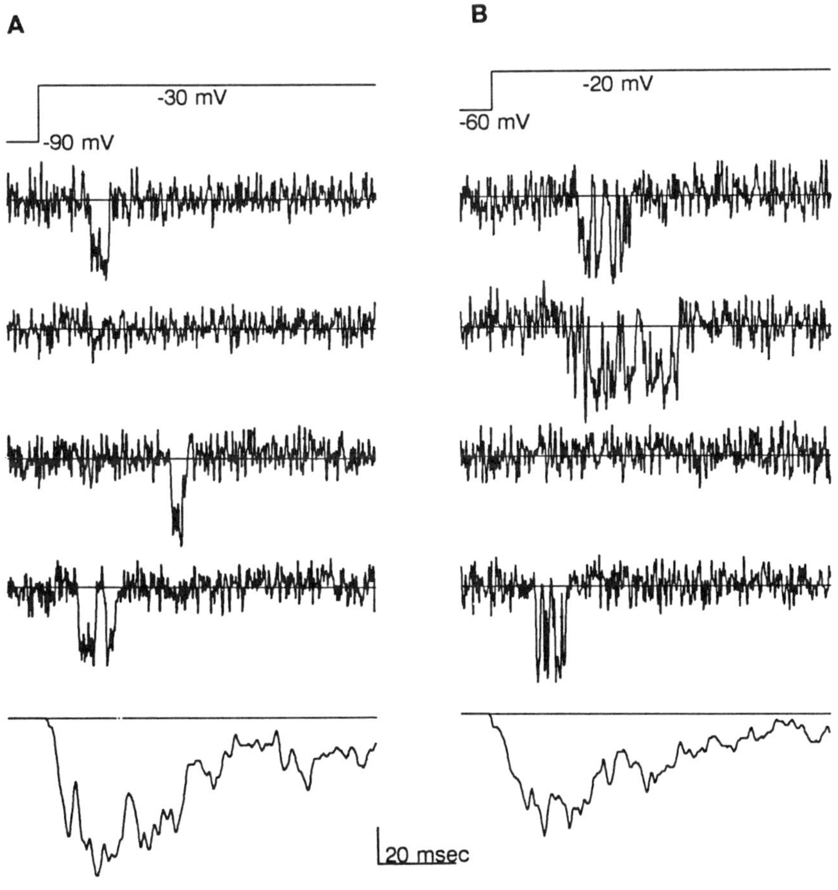

Figure 3 Representative single-channel records and ensemble average currents from a T- and L-type calcium channel in 120 mM KCl with 70 mM Ca^{2+} as the charge carrier. Vertical scale bar indicates 0.2 pA for single-channel currents and 0.01 pA for ensemble average currents. (A) T-type calcium channel: holding potential = −90 mV; test potential = −30 mV; ensemble average from 101 consecutive depolarizations. (B) L-type calcium channel: holding potential = −60 mV; test potential = −20 mV; ensemble average from 257 consecutive depolarizations. (From Balke et al., Ref. 54.)

secutive sweeps of a channel whose activity was evoked by a depolarization to −30 mV from a holding potential of −90 mV. This channel opened during approximately 50% of the sweeps (e.g., Fig. 3A, sweeps 1, 3, and 4) at this test potential. As predicted from the steady-state inactivation relation for T-type calcium channels (Fig. 2), T-type channels are inactivated at holding potentials positive to −60 mV. Indeed, this channel opened during only 6% of the sweeps at a holding potential of −50 mV (not shown). This channel therefore displays the activity characteristic of a T-type calcium channel. A subtly different pattern of activity is evident in the channel in Figure 3B. Compared with the T-type channel activity shown in Figure 3A, this channel retains robust activity at a holding potential of −60 mV (e.g., Fig. 3B, sweeps 1, 2, and 4), tends to have longer bursts of activity (e.g., Fig. 3B, sweeps 1 and 2), has a greater amplitude of opening, and increased its activity in the presence of a L-type calcium channel agonist (Bay K8644; not shown). These features allow assignment of this channel to the L-type family with confidence (42,54).

Because of technical considerations, the biophysical characterization of T- and L-type calcium channels has generally relied on the use of relatively high concentrations of divalent charge carriers, such as Ca^{2+} or Ba^{2+}. Therefore, these approaches provide little information about the function of T- and L-type calcium channels when physiologic concentrations of Ca^{2+} support the flux through the channels. Such information is particularly important for understanding the unitary mechanisms underlying the decay of current (i.e., macroscopic inactivation), especially considering that the decay of L-type calcium current is strongly influenced by both the identity and the concentration of the permeant ion (47,49,55). Recent studies have attempted to characterize and contrast the properties of physiologic ion flux through T- and L-type calcium channels by correlating whole-cell and single-channel currents recorded under comparable conditions (2–10 mM external Ca^{2+}). (41,42). With respect to T-type channels, unitary currents obtained with 10 mM Ca^{2+} in the pipette in the cell-attached configuration (30) exhibited a single-channel conductance of 4–5 pS. The ensemble average currents through a single channel of this conductance accurately reproduced the time course of whole-cell T-type calcium current recorded with the same voltage protocol under identical ionic conditions. The agreement between whole-cell and unitary ensemble average currents is consistent with the traditional notion that all T-type channels are alike and independent (56).

The absence of whole-cell T-type calcium currents at test potentials positive to 0 mV was attributed to changes in channel gating rather than to peculiar permeation properties, for several reasons. First, outward currents through T-type channels were never recorded during test potentials positive to 0 mV. Second, a clearly positive reversal potential was predicted by extrapolation from the current-voltage relation generated from single-channel currents over a limited range of depolarizations from −40 to −10 mV (41). Third, convolution analysis revealed that the decay of T-type calcium current was shaped predominantly by transitions among open and closed states, rather than by single openings of variable duration. Specifically, the waveform of T-type calcium current was profoundly influenced by the latencies to first opening and reopening, and the open times were sufficiently brief that they did not contribute significantly to the shape of the current decay (41). These results are entirely consistent with studies of T-type channels using high concentrations of divalent charge carriers (50,51). Investigations using both physiologic and elevated concentrations of divalent charge carriers support the view that microscopic activation is the principal voltage-dependent process and microscopic inactivation is voltage dependent only to the extent that it is determined by differences in the probabilities that individual channels will reach the open state at any given test potential (41). These observations are in obvious disagreement with traditional gating schemes, which suggest that current decay is a function of the time that channels remain open before entering an absorbing inactivated state (56). However, they support the idea that T-type channels shuttle back and forth between open and closed states before finally entering an absorbing inactivated state (42,57,58). Therefore, the decay of T-type calcium currents during maintained depolarizations (macroscopic inactivation) largely reflects rate-limiting microscopic activation events. Consistent with studies using high divalent ion concentrations (50,51), these results support the notion that T-type channel gating is primarily voltage dependent and is not significantly influenced by the identity or concentration of the permeant ion (4).

Even at 2–10 mM Ca^{2+} concentrations, the pattern of activity of L-type calcium channels is distinctly different from that of T-type channels (42). Unlike T-type channel activity, the L-type channel opens infrequently throughout the depolarization pulse and each channel opens several times during a single depolarization. Unitary recordings in 10 mM Ca^{2+} revealed a single-channel conductance of 6.9 pS (42,59,60). The single-channel ensemble average currents accurately reproduced the features of whole-cell L-type Ca^{2+} current, including the rapid rise to peak current, the initial rapid decay, and the pedestal of maintained current. As with T-type channels, convolution analysis revealed that the decay of the macroscopic and ensemble average current did not reflect the duration of opening of single channels since the mean open time is much shorter than the decay of the current waveform. The peak inward current was shaped largely by first openings, but the rapid component of the current decay was due to a combination of decreased first latency density and to a decay of the conditional open probability. The pedestal of maintained inward current characteristic of both the macroscopic and ensemble average L-type current was due to reopenings of the channel during a single depolarization. This type of behavior cannot be accounted for by simple Markov models, which describe current decay (inactivation) as a consequence of the successive entry of channels in a long-lived inactivated state (61). As an alternative, Marban and coworkers (42) tested the hypothesis that the pedestal of maintained current arises from the existence of multiple distinct gating patterns, as has been proposed by Plummer and Hess (62) with regard to N-type channel gating in neurons. Sweeps with single-channel activity were sorted among two kinetically distinct patterns of gating. The "active-early" pattern of gating described sweeps with an early opening (within the first 15–30 ms of the depolarization pulse), and the "active-late" pattern of gating described sweeps with a late opening (after 30 ms of the depolarization pulse). These patterns of activity were not randomly distributed and tended to cluster over time. The active-early pattern accounted for the initial transient current, and the active-late pattern described the pedestal of maintained inward current. The active-late pattern of gating could be predicted by a Markov model that lacked an inactivated state. Apart from its intrinsic interest, the information on single-channel gating has important implications for the physiologic relevance of both T- and L-type calcium channels, as discussed subsequently.

C. Differences in Permeation and Ion Selectivity

In contrast to the T-type calcium channel, the properties of permeation and selectivity of the L-type calcium channel have been studied extensively. The goal of this section is to present the prevailing model of L-type calcium channel permeation and to use this model to formulate hypotheses regarding the functional structure of cardiac T-type calcium channels. As such, a detailed discussion of the experimental basis for L-type calcium channel permeation is not included in this review (3,14,63). Experimental results that emphasize some of the important similarities and differences in permeability and selectivity between T- and L-type calcium channels are described.

L-type calcium channels are far more important than being merely biophysical curiosities, and their physiologic relevance derives from the functional consequences conveyed by their biochemical structure. L-type calcium channels have two seemingly incompatible properties: (1) they are highly selective for Ca^{2+} over other divalent and monovalent cations commonly present in physiologic external solutions, and (2) they allow passage of ions at a rate that is meaningful physiologically, that is, millions per second. The selective permeability of the L-type calcium channel is inconsistent with simple models that describe the pore structure as a molecular sieve for Ca^{2+}. However, this selectivity can be accounted for by a model originally proposed by Hess and Tsien (63,64) in which Ca^{2+} passes through the pore of the channel by interacting with multiple binding sites. The selectivity of the channel is determined by the high affinity of Ca^{2+} to the binding sites within the channel pore, and rapid permeation of Ca^{2+} depends on double occupancy of the intrapore binding sites and electrostatic ion-ion repulsion (42,53).

Although support for this model has largely come from experiments using high concentrations of divalent charge carriers, recent work with physiologic concentrations of Ca^{2+} (2–10 mM) is also consistent with features of this model. A unitary conductance of 6.9 pS was calculated from single-channel currents obtained from guinea pig ventricular cells bathed in 10 mM Ca^{2+} (42). Remarkably, this is only slightly smaller than the single-channel conductance of 9 pS obtained in 110 mM Ca^{2+} (59,62). Although the 6.9 pS conductance is similar to estimates of unitary current under similar conditions obtained by others (59,60), it is disproportionately high compared to predictions from single-site saturation estimates (65) or from nonstationary fluctuation analysis (63). This again suggests that Ca^{2+} permeation involves multiion occupancy of the L-type calcium channel pore (53).

Although detailed information about the selectivity and permeability of T-type calcium channels is not yet available, some structural characteristics of T-type calcium channels can be inferred from a comparison of the permeation properties of both channels. In single guinea pig ventricular cells, a unitary conductance of 4.7 pS at 10 mM calcium (41) is surprisingly high compared with the conductance of 6.8 pS obtained with 110 mM Ca^{2+} as the charge carrier (50). The finding of relatively high unitary conductance with low permeant ion concentrations suggests that T-type calcium channels, like L-type channels, may involve multiion occupancy of the channel pore (41,53). The possibility that T-type channels are multiion pores is also suggested by the observation that, like L-type channels, T-type calcium channels support the flux of monovalent cations (e.g., Na^{+}) in the absence of divalents. (66,67).

Despite these similarities, T- and L-type calcium channels may not have identical transmembrane pore structures, as evidenced by striking differences in their selectivity for divalent charge carriers and in their sensitivity to block by inorganic cations (13,37,38,40). For example, L-type calcium channels are highly permeable to Ba^{2+} as the charge carrier. Both whole-cell (38) and unitary Ba^{2+} currents (40) carried through L-type channels are much larger than currents carried by equimolar concentrations of Ca^{2+}. On the other hand, T-type calcium channels are equally permeable to Ba^{2+} and Ca^{2+}. Consequently, whole-cell and single-channel currents carried through these channels are relatively insensitive to the identity of the charge carrier.

Both T- and L-type calcium channels have different sensitivities to block by such inorganic ions as nickel (Ni^{2+}) and cadmium (Cd^{2+}). Figure 4 shows the effects of

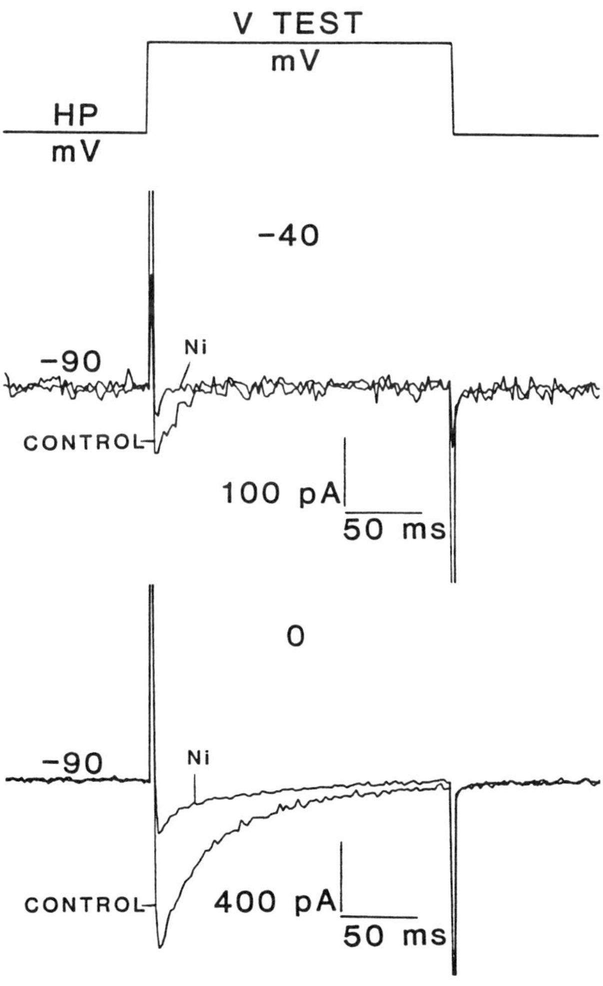

Figure 4 Nonselective inhibition of T- and L-type calcium current by Ni^{2+}. Exposure to 200 μM Ni^{2+} reduces T-type calcium current (upper record) to 30% of control, and L-type calcium current (lower record) was reduced to 40% of control. Experimental conditions and voltage protocol were identical to those described in Figure 1. (From Balke et al., Ref. 54.)

Ni^{2+} (200 μM) on whole-cell T- and L-type calcium currents that were separated on the basis of differences in the voltage dependence of steady-state inactivation as described earlier (Fig. 2). The voltage protocol, superimposed T-type currents before and after exposure to Ni^{2+}, and superimposed L-type currents before and after exposure to Ni^{2+} are shown in Figure 4. Although nonselective, Ni^{2+} is slightly more effective in blocking peak T-type current than peak L-type current (13,54). Figure 5 shows the effect of Cd^{2+} (50 μm) on whole-cell T- and L-type calcium currents. In contrast to Ni^{2+}, Cd^{2+} blocks L-type current more effectively (approximately 20% of control) than T-type calcium current (nearly 60% of control) (40,43,54). Although the differences in selectivity predict some differences in the

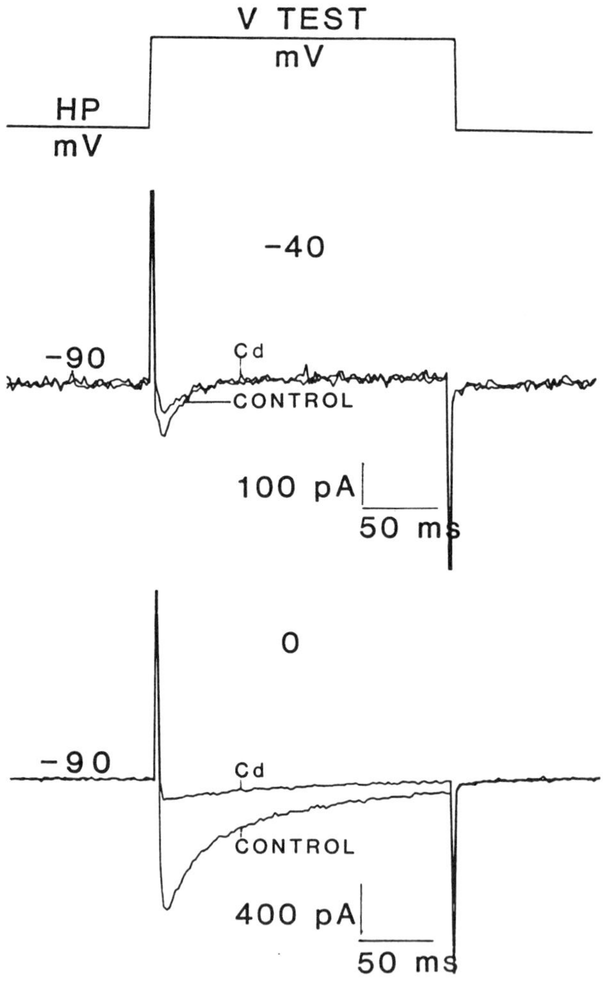

Figure 5 Nonselective effects of Cd^{2+} on T- and L-type calcium channels. After exposure to 50 μM Cd^{2+}, T-type calcium current (upper record) was reduced to 60% of control and L-type calcium currents (lower record) were reduced to 20% of control. Experimental conditions and voltage protocol were identical to those described in Figure 1. (Balke et al., Ref. 54.)

permeation pathway, T- and L-type calcium channels probably share some common structural features since both types are highly permeable for Ca^{2+} and since most of the inorganic ions are not entirely specific for either channel type (13).

D. Differences in Pharmacology

In addition to differences in kinetics, single-channel properties, and ion selectivity, T- and L-type calcium channels can also be distinguished by differences in their respective sensitivity to a variety of pharmacologic compounds. Since a detailed discussion of the pharmacology of L-type calcium channels is contained in the chapter on calcium channel antagonists, only the pharmacologic properties pertinent to the distinction of T- and L-type calcium channels are briefly reviewed here.

Cardiac L-type calcium channels are exquisitely sensitive to the 1,4-dihydropyridine (DHP) class of calcium channel activators and blockers. The high-affinity binding of the tritiated DHP calcium antagonist, [^{3}H]nitrendipine, to channel receptors was prerequisite for the isolation and partial purification of the α_1 subunit of the skeletal muscle L-type calcium channel(31). This work has enabled the L-type calcium channel of skeletal muscle to be cloned (32) and expressed (68) and has led to the sequencing of the cardiac L-type calcium channel (34). In contrast to L-type channels, cardiac T-type calcium channels are relatively insensitive to the DHP class of calcium channel antagonists [whole-cell currents (41) and single-channel currents (40,45)]. Figure 6 shows the effects of nitrendipine (10 μM) on whole-cell T- and L-type calcium currents from a guinea pig ventricular cell. In Figure 6A, peak T-type calcium current elicited by a 200 ms depolarization to −40 mV from a holding potential of −90 mV (upper current trace) was not altered by nitrendipine. In contrast, peak L-type calcium current elicited by a depolarization to 0 mV from a negative holding potential of −90 mV (middle trace) was substantially reduced. Consistent with the voltage dependence of DHP binding to calcium channels (4), peak L-type calcium current elicited by a depolarization to 0 mV from a more positive holding potential of −50 mV (bottom trace) was almost completely blocked. Figure 6B shows the full current-voltage relation during control and after exposure to nitrendipine from holding potentials of −90 mV (both T- and L-type components of calcium current) and −50 mV (L-type component of calcium current). Only currents elicited at test potentials positive to −30 mV (L-type calcium currents) are sensitive to the blocking effects of nitrendipinc. As noted in Section II.A, inaccurate separation of T- and L-type components of calcium current may explain why some workers have reported T-type channel sensitivity to dihydropyridines (44).

L-type calcium channels are also sensitive to a variety of DHP calcium channel agonists. Bay K8644 enhances L-type calcium current by markedly increasing the single-channel open times (63,69). In contrast, T-type calcium channels are unaffected by DHP calcium channel agonists. This property can be exploited to separate both types of channels under experimental conditions (Ca^{2+} as the charge carrier) in which they can display remarkably similar behaviors (e.g., Fig. 1).

β-Adrenergic stimulation with such compounds as isoproterenol has been shown to enhance cardiac calcium current via a cytoplasmic pathway involving cAMP-mediated increases in calcium channel phosphorylation (28,70,71) and, more recently, via a direct membrane-delimited G protein pathway (72,73). Only L-type

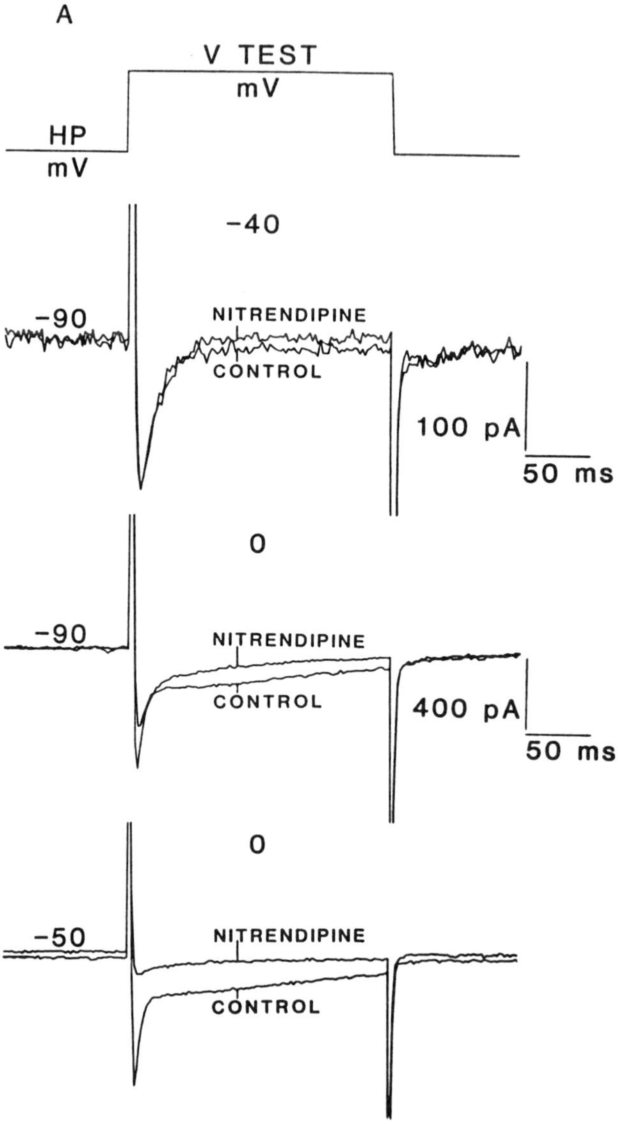

Figure 6 Effect of nitrendipine (3 μM) on T- and L-type calcium current. Experimental conditions were identical to those described in Fig. 1, except for the absence of 30 μM TTX. (A) Voltage protocol and currents elicited from a holding potential of −90 mV by a 200 ms test depolarization to −40 mV (upper record, T-type calcium current) and to 0 mV (middle record, L-type calcium current). L-type calcium currents elicited by a test depolarization to 0 mV from a more positive holding potential of −50 mV (lower record) show the voltage dependence of DHP block of L-type calcium channels. (B) Peak current-voltage relations for currents elicited from each holding potential before (squares, −90; plus signs, −50 mV) and after (diamonds, −90; triangles, −50 mV) the addition of 3 μM nitrendipine. (From Balke et al., Ref. 41.)

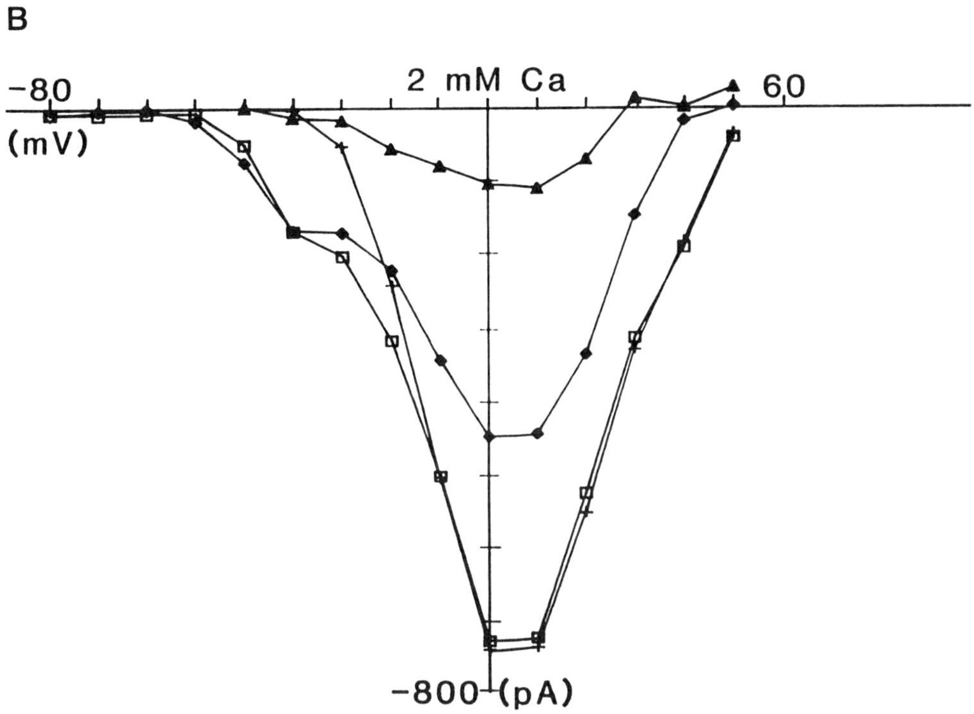

Figure 6 Continued

calcium current appears to be enhanced by isoproterenol (38,40,70,73). The effects of isoproterenol on whole-cell T- and L-type calcium currents in a guinea pig ventricular myocyte are shown in Figure 7. T- and L-type calcium currents were separated by differences in their respective voltage dependence of inactivation, as described earlier (Fig. 1). Peak L-type calcium current elicited by a depolarization to 0 mV (bottom current record) from a holding potential of −50 mV was increased over twofold, but peak T-type calcium current elicited by a depolarization to −50 mV from a holding potential of −90 mV was unaffected.

III. STRUCTURAL CHARACTERIZATION OF THE L-TYPE CALCIUM CHANNEL

Recent developments in the fields of biochemistry and molecular biology have led to significant advances in the understanding of the molecular mechanisms involved in the physiologic function of ion channels. L-type calcium channels are exquisitely sensitive to the dihydropyridine class of calcium channel antagonists, such as nitrendipine. Because these agents bind to channel proteins with high selectivity and affinity, radiolabeled derivatives of dihydropyridine calcium channel antagonists (e.g., [^{3}H]nitrendipine) have been used as molecular probes for the identification and isolation of the L-type calcium channel. Since the density of dihydropyridine receptors in the T tubule membranes of skeletal muscle is several orders of magnitude greater than in cardiac membranes, experimental work initially

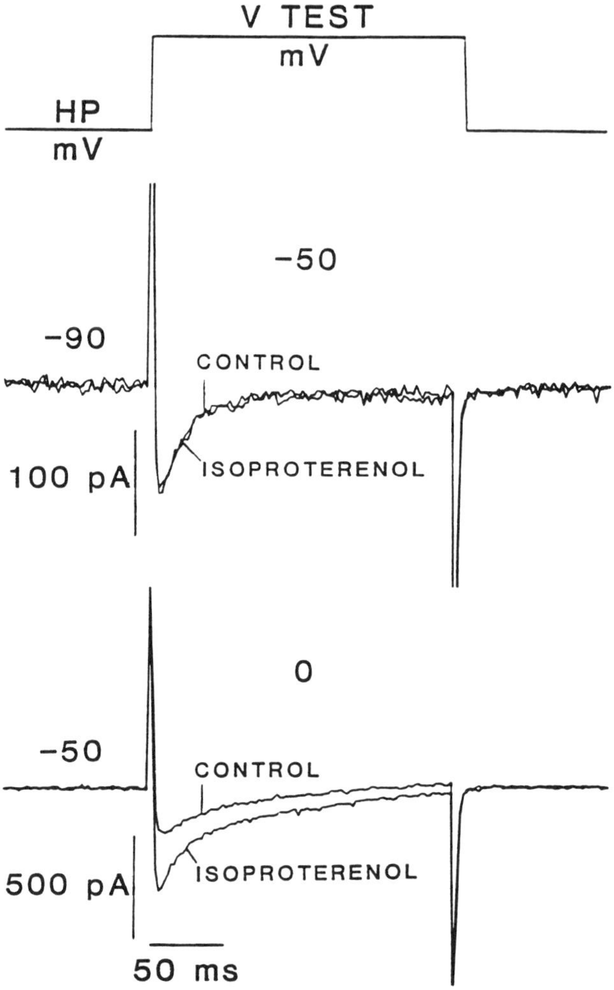

Figure 7 Selective enhancement of L-type calcium current by the β-adrenergic agonist, isoproterenol. Experimental conditions are identical to those described in Figure 1. Peak T-type calcium currents (upper record) and L-type calcium currents (lower record) before and after the addition of 1 μM isoproterenol. Peak T-type current was unaffected, but peak L-type calcium current increased over twofold. (From Balke et al., Ref. 54.)

focused on the structural characterization of the L-type calcium channel purified from skeletal muscle. As described by Catterall and coworkers (31,74), the skeletal muscle L-type calcium channel is a complex composed of five polypeptide subunits (α_1, α_2, β, γ, and δ, Fig. 8). The α_1 subunit appears to be responsible for the principal functional characteristics of the L-type calcium channel. That is, the α_1 subunit is characterized by extensive hydrophobic domains expected of a channel protein that spans the sarcolemmal membrane (31); it contains the receptor sites for calcium channel antagonists (75,76); it is phosphorylated by cAMP-dependent protein kinase (31,77); it supports dihydropyridine-sensitive and voltage-dependent calcium current in a cell line transformed with complementary

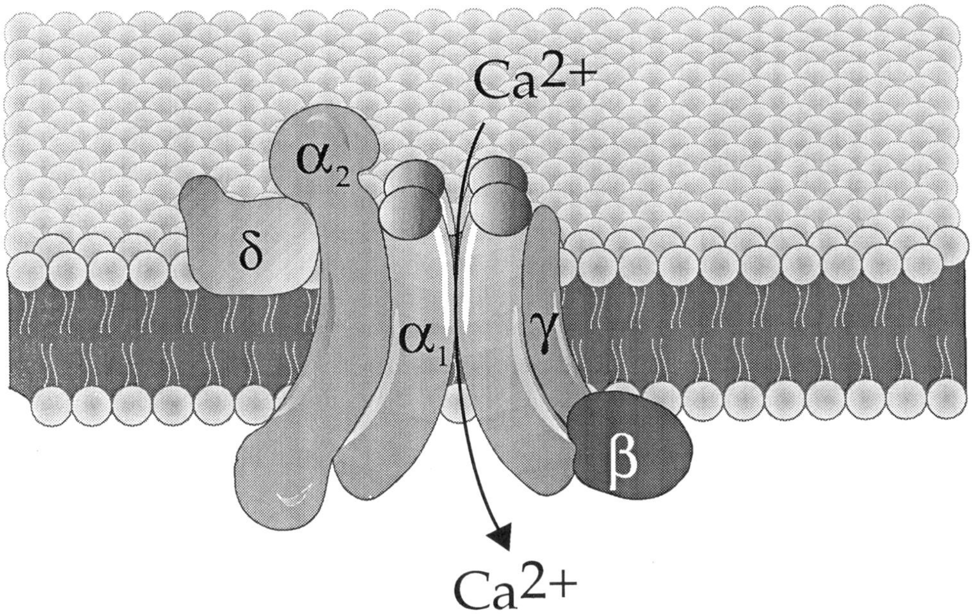

Figure 8 The putative structure of a skeletal muscle L-type calcium channel. The ion pore appears to be formed by the four transmembrane domains of the α_1 subunit. This is the principal component of the L-type calcium channel and conveys the main characteristics of the channel, such as voltage dependence and dihydropyridine binding. Several other discrete proteins (α_2, β, γ, and δ) are associated with the pore protein and may modulate channel activity (see text for discussion).

DNA of the α_1 subunit (68); and it functions as a voltage-dependent calcium channel when reconstituted in lipid bilayers (78). Although the additional subunits are not essential for ion channel function, the α_2, β, γ, and δ components may modulate the activity of the α_1 subunit (34).

Similar to the α subunit of the sodium channel (79,80), the primary structure of the α_1 subunit of the skeletal muscle calcium channel appears to be composed of four homologous domains, each of which is composed of six α-helical structures (32). The six α-helical segments of each domain are linked by a pattern of hydrophobic and hydrophilic residues, which is consistent with a membrane-spanning orientation (79,80). A putative transmembrane structure for the α_1 subunit of the skeletal muscle calcium channel has been proposed in which the four domains of the α_1 subunit fold around a central region, which may function as the channel pore (Fig. 8) (32,79).

Recently, Numa and colleagues (34) described the primary structure of the α_1 subunit of the L-type calcium channel in rabbit cardiac muscle. Although slightly larger than its skeletal muscle counterpart, the cardiac α_1 subunit also contains four homologous domains, each of which is composed of five hydrophobic and one hydrophilic segment. The overall amino acid homology between the cardiac and the skeletal muscle dihydropyridine receptor was 66%. The regions corresponding to the four domains were highly conserved, but the cytoplasmic spanning regions were less well conserved. Based on these structural similarities, Numa and coworkers proposed that the cardiac dihydropyridine receptor has a transmembrane topology similar to that of the skeletal muscle dihydropyridine receptor and to sodium channels (34). In addition, *Xenopus* oocytes injected with messenger RNA derived from the cloned cDNA of the cardiac dihydropyridine receptor showed a sustained inward current in the presence of Ba^{2+} (40 mM) characteristic of a dihydropyridine-sensitive calcium channel (34). This inward current had many of the features typical of barium current through L-type calcium channels. The current-voltage relation of the barium current resembled that of a cardiac L-type calcium channel in the presence of barium. The inward barium current was completely suppressed by Cd^{2+} (0.2 mM) and by nifedipine in a concentration-dependent manner. The dihydropyridine agonist Bay K8644 increased the peak inward barium current severalfold.

Tanabe and coworkers recently injected an expression plasmid (pCARD1) carrying the rabbit cardiac receptor cDNA into the nuclei of myotubes from mice with muscular dysgenesis (81). Normally, dysgenic myotubes do not show excitation-contraction coupling or L-type calcium current (82). Dysgenic myotubes that were injected with pCARD1 displayed both spontaneous and electrically evoked contractions. These myotubes also expressed an inward current similar to the L-type calcium channel of cardiac muscle. Like the cardiac L-type calcium current, the inward current in injected myotubes was voltage dependent, was rapidly activating and slowly inactivating, increased with Ba^{2+} as the charge carrier, was dihydropyridine sensitive, and was blocked by Cd^{2+}. Also like cardiac muscle, contraction in pCARD1-injected myotubes was dependent on external Ca^{2+} and blocked by Cd^{2+}. In addition, excitation-contraction coupling in pCARD1-injected myotubes appeared to depend on calcium entry from the expressed L-type calcium channels to trigger the release of calcium from the sarcoplasmic reticulum (81).

IV. PHYSIOLOGICAL ROLE OF T- AND L-TYPE CALCIUM CHANNELS

While two types of calcium channels have been clearly identified in many heart cells, the L-type channel is the principal calcium channel found in cardiac cells from most species. Because of its specific biophysical and pharmacologic properties, the L-type calcium channel determines the electrophysiological characteristics of all cardiac cells and of the specialized pacemaking and conduction tissues in particular. Because of its inactivation kinetics, the L-type calcium channel provides the inward current that contributes to the plateau of the action potential in all cardiac cells (9,10,60). In pacemaker cells from the sinoatrial (SA) (83) and atrio-ventricular (AV) (84) nodes, L-type calcium channels alone determine the upstroke of the action potential (85). The threshold for activation of the L-type calcium channel is in the same voltage range as the slow inward current of SA and AV node cells. These pacemaker cells are exquisitely sensitive to the dihydropyridine calcium channel antagonists that preferentially block L-type calcium channels. In addition, L-type calcium channels are important for both normal and abnormal cardiac automaticity. They are responsible for the normal phase 4 diastolic depolarization characteristic of these pacemaker cells. They may contribute to the automaticity observed in partially depolarized cells of the atrium, ventricle, and Purkinje fibers, which normally do not show automatic behavior (86,87). This may contribute to the development of certain clinically observed arrhythmias, such as those that arise from abnormalities of impulse formation and triggered activity (15,16).

In cardiac muscle, L-type calcium channels play a crucial role in coupling membrane excitability to subsequent contractions. It is well established that the principal mechanism of excitation-contraction coupling in cardiac muscle involves Ca^{2+}-induced Ca^{2+}-release (for review, see Ref. 88). The influx of Ca^{2+} through L-type channels both triggers (20–22) and grades the release of Ca^{2+} from the sarcoplasmic reticulum (SR), although the precise mechanism by which L-type calcium current grades SR release is unknown (20–22,24,25). The transient rise in $[Ca^{2+}]_i$ from the combined influx of Ca^{2+} via L-type calcium channels and SR Ca^{2+} release activates the myofilaments and initiates contraction. The importance of L-type calcium channels as the source of the "Ca^{2+} trigger" is supported by several lines of experimental evidence, including (1) a similar voltage dependence for L-type calcium current, contraction, and $[Ca^{2+}]_i$ (23,89,90); (2) the observation of contractions and $[Ca^{2+}]_i$ elicited by calcium tail currents (23,89); (3) the independence of contraction and $[Ca^{2+}]_i$ from charge movement through the L-type channel (91); (4) the initiation of contraction and $[Ca^{2+}]_i$ with rapid increases in intracellular calcium by photolysis of "caged" calcium (24); (5) the ubiquitous presence of L-type calcium channels in virtually all cardiac cells (4); and (6) the larger ratio of functional L-type calcium channels to DHP binding sites in cardiac muscle compared with skeletal muscle (42,92). In addition to supplying the Ca^{2+} trigger for the release of Ca^{2+} from the sarcoplasmic reticulum, L-type calcium channels support excitation-contraction coupling in several other important ways. By contributing to $[Ca^{2+}]_i$, influx of Ca^{2+} via L-type calcium channels is an important source of Ca^{2+} for the replenishment of the sarcoplasmic reticulum by the Ca^{2+}-ATPase pump. Under certain conditions, Ca^{2+} influx through L-type calcium channels is sufficient to directly activate the myofilaments. For example, contractions can be sustained in frog ventricular cells by Ca^{2+} entry through L-type calcium channels in the presence of ryanodine, which effectively abolishes sarcoplasmic reticulum function (93).

The physiologic role of T-type calcium channels is less well understood. Unlike L-type calcium channels, T-type channels are not universally distributed throughout the heart. They are found only in specific cell types from certain species (94). The density of T-type calcium channels relative to the density of L-type calcium channels also varies between species. For example, T-type calcium currents are not found in rabbit or bovine atrial cells or bovine, canine, or bullfrog ventricular cells (4). Therefore, it appears that T-type calcium channels do not have a large role in the generation of the action potential or in excitation-contraction coupling in normal myocardial cells (see Ref. 43). T-type calcium channels may be important in cells that normally display automaticity, such as the pacemaking cells of the sinoatrial node or the specialized conduction fibers of the Purkinje system. T-type calcium channels have a relatively negative range of activation and may therefore be inactivated at normal resting membrane potentials. They may be activated by small depolarizations in well-depolarized cells and by recovery from a hyperpolarization that follows a depolarization (85). In many cells in which both types of calcium channels can be separated [guinea pig ventricular cells (40,41,43) frog atrial cells (95), canine atrial cells (38), and rabbit sinoatrial cells (13)], peak T-type calcium current is typically only a small fraction of the peak L-type calcium current (41,42). The amount of T-type current relative to L-type current is greater in cell types that have specialized pacemaker functions. In rabbit sinoatrial cells and canine Purkinje cells, peak T current can be of similar magnitude as peak L-type current (13,44,46).

V. CLINICAL SIGNIFICANCE OF CARDIAC CALCIUM CHANNELS

Experimental work has focused almost exclusively on L-type Ca^{2+} channels. It is clear that knowledge of their biophysical and physiologic properties is essential for understanding their role in cardiovascular disease and for planning rational therapeutic strategies. As Ca^{2+} channel antagonists have been instrumental in separating the two types of cardiac Ca^{2+} channels and clarifying their respective physiologic functions, these compounds have also played a key role in identifying the involvement of Ca^{2+} channels in the pathogenesis of a variety of cardiovascular disorders. Therefore, much of the subsequent discussion will rely heavily on experimental and clinical experience with specific Ca^{2+} channel antagonists.

The clinical success of Ca^{2+} channel antagonists in the treatment of a variety of cardiovascular disorders depends on the interaction of a number of factors. As noted earlier, T- and L-type channels have different sensitivities to several Ca^{2+} channel blockers. In addition, different subtypes of L-type channels have markedly different sensitivities to particular Ca^{2+} channel blockers. For example, verapamil preferentially affects the myocardium compared with vascular smooth muscle and is clinically useful as an antiarrhythmic agent. The dihydropyridines, on the other hand, act primarily on vascular smooth muscle and have relatively little direct effect on the myocardium. The enhanced sensitivity of L-type channels in vascular smooth muscle to dihydropyridine calcium channel antagonists explains in part why the dihydropyridines cause potent peripheral and coronary vasodilation in the absence of significant effects on impulse conduction or myocardial contractility. The clinical response to dihydropyridine calcium channel antagonists can also involve a reflex stimulation of the sympathetic nervous system, which can predominate over their direct effects on the L-type channel. For this reason, the dihydropyridines have no important antiarrhythmic action since the direct inhibition of the sinus node is outweighed by the chronotropic response mediated by reflex stimulation of the sympathetic system triggered by vasodilation (96). These observations may help to reconcile the compelling evidence for the role of intracellular Ca^{2+} in the pathogenesis of arrhythmias with the somewhat restricted clinical success with calcium channel antagonists.

A. Role of Ca^{2+} Channels in Ischemic Heart Disease

Acute myocardial ischemia is associated with a loss in myocardial viability. The degree of myocardial injury depends on the duration of ischemia (e.g., "stunned myocardium"). Reperfusion following short periods ($\leq$15 minutes) is associated with recovery of myocardial function; reperfusion following prolonged periods of ischemia ($>$40 minutes) is associated with irreversible injury and myocardial dysfunction (97–99). Although the precise cellular mechanisms involved in ischemic injury are unclear, several lines of evidence suggest that disruptions of $[Ca^{2+}]_i$ homeostasis are important in both reversible and irreversible myocardial cell injury (for review, see Ref. 100). In particular, clinical and experimental studies have shown an association between elevations in $[Ca^{2+}]_i$ (calcium overload) and irreversible ischemic injury (101–104), as well as reversible ischemic injury (105–107). Reperfusion with low concentrations of extracellular Ca^{2+} improves recovery of "stunned myocardium." These studies support the hypothesis that Ca^{2+} overload may be the common cellular abnormality through which numerous factors contribute to myocardial dysfunction in ischemia.

Increased Ca^{2+} influx through L-type Ca^{2+} channels is a potential mechanism for causing Ca^{2+} overload. In several in vivo models of irreversible injury, pretreatment with Ca^{2+} channel antagonists has been shown to attentuate ischemia-induced injury (108–110). However, studies in isolated myocardial cells have failed to show that block of L-type Ca^{2+} channels prevents Ca^{2+} accumulation (111). It therefore seems likely that the protective effects of Ca^{2+} channel antagonists observed in models *in vivo* are not due to an inhibition of L-type Ca^{2+} channels but rather to their effects on afterload reduction and myocardial contractility. In irreversible ischemic injury, it is more likely that the massive amounts of Ca^{2+} overload are associated with enhanced Na^{+}/Ca^{2+} exchange and/or sarcolemmal membrane defects (100). In contrast, in models of reversible injury, pretreatment with Ca^{2+} channel antagonists preserves myocardial function after reperfusion in the absence of hemodynamic effects (112,113). This suggests the possibility that L-type Ca^{2+} channels may contribute to the elevations of $[Ca^{2+}]_i$ that are seen early in ischemia (105–107). These studies also suggest that the time course of $[Ca^{2+}]_i$ elevations seen in early ischemia precedes the massive Ca^{2+} overload associated with irreversible injury. Taken together, the observations of the protective effect of Ca^{2+} channel antagonists and the early time course of $[Ca^{2+}]_i$ elevations support the central role of disruptions in $[Ca^{2+}]_i$ regulation in the mediation of ischemic injury. Although the cellular mechanisms that underlie the transition from reversible to irreversible injury are unknown, these two observations permit the formulation of a hypothesis for a mechanism of progressive cellular injury in which the L-type Ca^{2+} channel may have a prominent role (100). The onset of ischemia stimulates numerous biochemical responses, including a fall in intracellular pH, depletion of energy substrates, such as high-energy phosphates, accumulation of metabolites, and activation of lipases. These biochemical derangements could affect intracellular pathways involved in maintaining the stability of the sarcolemma, as well as in regulating membrane constituent proteins, such as L-type Ca^{2+} channels (114). Increased Ca^{2+} flux across the L-type channel could elevate $[Ca^{2+}]_i$ and activate Ca^{2+}-dependent proteases and phospholipases. With increasing durations of ischemia, the Ca^{2+}-dependent degradative processes coupled with multiple other mechanisms could alter the Ca^{2+} permeability of the sarcoplasmic reticulum as well as the sarcolemma. Therefore, the massive increases in $[Ca^{2+}]_i$ that accompany irreversible ischemia may come from both SR calcium release and calcium entry from the extracellular space.

Flux of Ca^{2+} through L-type channels may also contribute to the rise in $[Ca^{2+}]_i$ following a period of ischemia (115). Several investigators have suggested that free radicals (116,117) from a variety of sources (for review, see Ref. 100) may rapidly increase membrane permeability, possibly via peroxidation of membrane lipids (118). In addition to their direct effects on the lipid bilayer, lipid peroxides may indirectly contribute to Ca^{2+} overload by affecting membrane-delimited enzyme systems, such as adenylate cyclase, which regulates L-type Ca^{2+} channels.

B. Role of Ca^{2+} Channels in Heart Failure

Although the cellular mechanisms of heart failure are unknown, several lines of experimental and clinical investigation support the hypothesis that the contractile dysfunction of the failing heart is due to abnormalities in the regulation of $[Ca^{2+}]_i$ (for reviews, see Refs. 119–121). As discussed earlier, $[Ca^{2+}]_i$ homeostasis in normal heart cells depends upon the complex interactions of many intracellular processes. Abnormalities in many or all of these constitutive processes can be expected to contribute to the disruption of $[Ca^{2+}]_i$ regulation. Since Ca^{2+} influx from inward calcium current affects $[Ca^{2+}]_i$, alterations in the function of L-type Ca^{2+} channels may partially explain the contractile abnormalities observed in some types of heart failure.

Gwathmey and coworkers (122,124) were the first to demonstrate abnormalities in $[Ca^{2+}]_i$ homeostasis in ventricular cells from patients with congestive heart failure. They studied action potential characteristics and $[Ca^{2+}]_i$ in isometrically contracting papillary muscle preparations injected with the calcium indicator aequorin. Compared with controls from normal hearts, the resting $[Ca^{2+}]_i$ was elevated. In addition, the decay of the $[Ca^{2+}]_i$ was markedly prolonged and biphasic compared with the monophasic decline of the $[Ca^{2+}]_i$ of normal cardiac cells. They also showed that the duration of the action potential was prolonged. From these results, they ascribed the defects in calcium homeostasis to the combination of an impaired reuptake of Ca^{2+} by the SR and an altered trigger signal for SR calcium release (e.g., influx of Ca^{2+} from L-type calcium channels). The possibility that the abnormalities of $[Ca^{2+}]_i$ observed in myopathic cells is a consequence, in part, of alterations in the L-type calcium channels is also supported by experiments in certain animal models of failure. Although the relationship between the number of functional L-type calcium channels and DHP binding sites is uncertain, there is evidence for alterations in the density of DHP receptors in the cardiomyopathic hamster (125) and in the rat with heart failure (126). However, recent studies on DHP binding in normal and myopathic human myocardium suggest that the number of L-type calcium channels is unchanged (127).

Beuckelmann et al. (128,129) studied L-type calcium currents and $[Ca^{2+}]_i$ in single ventricular cells isolated from hearts obtained from patients with end-stage heart failure undergoing transplantation and from organ donors without heart disease. Action potentials and calcium currents were recorded by the whole-cell variation of the patch-clamp technique (30). Calcium transients were obtained by internal perfusion of the cell with the fluorescent calcium indicator fura-2. In cells from both normal and myopathic hearts, the amplitude and voltage dependence of the L-type calcium current and the $[Ca^{2+}]_i$ was bell shaped and peaked at test potentials of 10 mV. Calcium tail currents could also trigger SR calcium release. Consistent with the multicellular studies of human papillary muscle (122–124), isolated myopathic cells had a markedly prolonged action potential, a higher resting $[Ca^{2+}]_i$, and a markedly slowed (although not biphasic) declining phase of the $[Ca^{2+}]_i$. However, the peak $[Ca^{2+}]_i$ in single myopathic cells was significantly smaller than the peak $[Ca^{2+}]_i$ recorded in normal cells. Beuckelmann and coworkers (129) proposed two possible mechanisms to explain the reduction in the peak $[Ca^{2+}]_i$. An impaired reuptake of Ca^{2+} by the SR could deplete the amount of Ca^{2+} available for release, resulting in a smaller peak $[Ca^{2+}]_i$. Alternatively, the transduction of a normal trigger signal (e.g., normal L-type calcium current) to the SR calcium release channel could be "partially uncoupled." Although some of the disparities between the results obtained in multicellular preparations (121,124) and single cells (128, 129) may be partially explained by differences in the preparations and techniques, both studies together provide compelling evidence that cellular mechanism(s) for the contractile abnormalities seen clinically involve profound abnormalities in the regulation of $[Ca^{2+}]_i$. However, calcium current does not appear to play a dominant role in the abnormalities of $[Ca^{2+}]_i$ (128).

ACKNOWLEDGMENTS

I thank E. Marban, W. J. Lederer, and S. S. Gottlieb for their helpful reviews of the manuscript. This work was supported in part by National Institutes of Health Grant 1-K11-HL02466-01 and by a Grant-in-Aid from the American Heart Association, Maryland Affiliate.

REFERENCES

1. Hagiwara S. *Membrane potential-dependent ion channels in cell membrane.* New York: Raven Press, 1983; 5–47.
2. Reuter H. Calcium channel modulation of neutrotransmitters, enzymes and drugs. *Nature* 1983; 301:569–74.
3. Tsien RW, Hess P, McCleskey EW, Rosenberg RL. Calcium channels: mechanisms of selectivity, permeation, and block. *Annu Rev Biophys Biophys Chem* 1987; 16:265–90.
4. Bean B. Classes of calcium channels in vertebrate cells. *Annu Rev Physiol* 1989; 51:367–84.
5. Hille B. *Ionic channels of excitable membranes,* 2nd ed. Sunderland, MA: Sinauer, 1992; 83–114.
6. Partridge LD. The physiology of calcium channels: an overview. In: Hurwitz L, Partridge LD, Leach JK, eds. *Calcium channels: their properties, functions, regulation, and clinical significance.* Boston: CRC Press, 1991; 63–7.
7. Wier WG. $[Ca^{2+}]_i$ transients during excitation-contraction coupling of mammalian heart. In: Fozzard HA, Haber E, Jennings RB, Katz AM, Morgan HE, eds. *The heart and cardiovascular disease.* New York: Raven Press, 1992; 1223–48.
8. DiFrancesco D, Noble D. A model of cardiac electrical activity incorporating ionic pumps and concentration changes. *Philos Trans R Soc Lond* [*Biol*] 1985; 307:353–98.
9. Rasmusson RL, Clark JW, Giles WR, Shibata EF, Campbell DL. A mathematical model of a bullfrog cardiac pacemaker cell. *Am J Physiol* 1990; 259:H352–69.
10. Rasmusson RL, Clark JW, Giles WR, et al. A mathematical model of electrophysiological activity in a bullfrog atrial cell. *Am J Physiol* 1990; 259:H370–89.
11. Brown HF, Kimura J, Noble D, Noble SJ, Taupignon A. The ionic currents underlying pacemaker activity in rabbit sino-atrial node: experimental results and computer simulations. *Proc R Soc Lond* [*Biol*] 1984; 222:305–47.
12. Tohse N, Kameyama M, Irisawa H. Intracellular Ca and protein kinase C modulate K current in guinea pig heart cells. *Am J Physiol* 1987; 253:H1321–4.
13. Hagiwara N, Irisawa H, Kameyama M. Contribution of two types of calcium currents to the pacemaker potentials of rabbit sino-atrial node cells. *J Physiol* [Lond] 1988; 359:233–53.
14. Pelzer D, Pelzer S, McDonald TF. Calcium channels in heart. In: Fozzard HA, Haber E, Jennings RB, Katz AM, Morgan HE, eds. *The heart and cardiovascular disease.* New York: Raven Press, 1992, 1049–90.
15. January CT, Riddle JM, Salata JJ. A model for early afterdepolarizations: induction with Ca^{2+} channel agonist Bay K8644. *Circ Res* 1988; 62:563–71.
16. January CT, Fozzard HA. Delayed afterdepolarizations in heart muscle: mechanisms and relevance. *Pharmacol Rev* 1988; 40:219–27.

17. Robertson SP, Johnson JD, Potter JD. The time-course of Ca^{2+} exchange with calmodulin, troponin, paravalbumin, and myosin in response to transient increase in Ca^{2+}. *Biophys J* 1981; 34:559–69.
18. Campbell DL, Giles WR, Robinson K, Shibata EF. Studies of the sodium-calcium exchanger in bull-frog atrial myocytes. *J Physiol* [Lond] 1988; 403:317–40.
19. Inesi G. Characterization of partial reactions in the catalytic and transport cycle of sarcoplasmic reticulum ATPase. In: Hille B, Frambrough DM, eds. *Proteins of excitable membranes*. New York: John Wiley & Sons, 1987; 231–55.
20. Fabiato A. Calcium-induced release of calcium from the cardiac sarcoplasmic reticulum. *Am J Physiol* 1983; 245:C1–14.
21. Fabiato A. Time and calcium dependence of activation and inactivation of calcium-induced release of calcium from the sarcoplasmic reticulum of a skinned canine cardiac Purkinje cell. *J Gen Physiol* 1985; 85:247–90.
22. Fabiato A. Simulated calcium current can both cause calcium loading in and trigger calcium release from the sarcoplasmic reticulum of a skinned canine cardiac Purkinje cell. *J Gen Physiol* 1985; 85:291–320.
23. Beuckelmann DJ, Wier WG. Mechanism of release of calcium from sarcoplasmic reticulum of guinea-pig cardiac cells. *J Physiol* [Lond] 1988; 405:233–55.
24. Niggli E, Lederer WJ. Voltage-independent calcium release in heart muscle. *Science* 1990; 250:565–8.
25. Sipido KR, Wier WG. Flux of Ca^{2+} across the sarcoplasmic reticulum of guinea-pig cardiac cells during excitation-contraction coupling. *J Physiol* [Lond] 1991; 435:605–30.
26. Ringer S. A further contribution regarding the influence of the different constituents of the blood on the contraction of the heart. *J Physiol* [Lond] 1883; 4:29–42.
27. Pelzer D, Pelzer S, McDonald TF. Properties and regulation of calcium channels in muscle cells. *Rev Physiol Biochem Pharmacol* 1990; 114:107–206.
28. Powell T, Twist VW. A rapid technique for the isolation and purification of adult cardiac muscle cells having respiratory control and a tolerance to calcium. *Biochem Biophys Res Commun* 1976; 72:327–33.
29. Isenberg G, Klockner U. Glycocalyx is not required for slow inward calcium current in isolated rat heart myocytes. *Nature* 1980; 284:358–60.
30. Hamill OP, Marty A, Neher E, Sakmann B, Sigworth FJ. Improved patch-clamp techniques for high-resolution current recording from cells and cell-free membrane patches. *Pflügers Arch* 1981; 391:85–100.
31. Catterall WA. Structure and function of voltage-sensitive ion channels. *Science* 1988; 242:50–61.
32. Tanabe T, Takeshima H, Mikami A, et al. Primary structure of the receptor for calcium channel blockers from skeletal muscle. *Nature* 1987; 328:313–8.
33. Beam KG, Tanabe T, Numa S. Structure, function, and regulation of the skeletal muscle dihydropyridine receptor. *Ann N Y Acad Sci* 1989; 560:127–37.
34. Mikami A, Imoto K, Tanabe T, et al. Primary structure and functional expression of the cardiac dihydropyridine-sensitive calcium channel. *Nature* 1989; 340:230–3.
35. Grynkiewicz G, Poenie M, Tsien RY. A new generation of Ca^{2+} indicators with greatly improved fluorescence properties. *J Biol Chem* 1985; 260:3440–50.
36. Hagiwara S, Ozawa S, Sand O. Voltage clamp analysis of two inward current mechanisms in the egg cell membrane of a starfish. *J Gen Physiol* 1975; 63:617–44.
37. Nowycky MC, Fox AP, Tsien RW. Three types of neuronal calcium channels with different calcium agonist sensitivity. *Nature* 1985; 316:440–3.
38. Bean BP. Two kinds of calcium channels in canine atrial cells. Differences in kinetics, selectivity, and pharmacology. *J Gen Physiol* 1985; 86:1–30.
39. Bean BP. Multiple types of calcium channels in heart muscle and neurons. Modulation by drugs and neurotransmitters. *Ann N Y Acad Sci* 1989; 560:334–45.

40. Nilius B, Hess P, Lansman JB, Tsien RW. A novel type of cardiac calcium channel in ventricular muscle. *Nature* 1985; 316:440–6.
41. Balke CW, Rose WC, Marban E, Wier WG. Macroscopic and unitary properties of physiological ion flux through T-type Ca^{2+} channels in guinea-pig heart cells. *J Physiol* [Lond] 1992; 456: 247–265.
42. Rose WC, Balke CW, Wier WG, Marban E. Macroscopic and unitary properties of physiological ion flux through L-type Ca^{2+} channels in guniea-pig heart cells. *J Physiol* [Lond] 1992; 456: 267–284.
43. Mitra R, Morad M: Two types of calcium channels in guinea-pig ventricular myocytes. *Proc Natl Acad Sci U S A* 1986; 83:5340–4.
44. Tseng GN, Boyden PA. Multiple types of Ca^{2+} currents in single canine Purkinje cells. *Circ Res* 1989; 65:1735–50.
45. Tytgat J, Nilius B, Vereeke J, Carmeliet E. The T-type Ca channel in guinea-pig ventricular myocytes is insensitive to isoproterenol. *Pflügers Arch* 1988; 411:704–6.
46. Hirano Y, Fozzard HA, January CT. Characteristics of L- and T-type Ca^{2+} currents in canine cardiac Purkinje cells. *Am J Physiol* 1989; 256:H1478–92.
47. Eckert R, Chad JE. Inactivation of Ca channels. *Prog Biophys Mol Biol* 1984; 44:215–67.
48. Kass RS, Sanguinetti MC. Inactivation of calcium channel current in the calf cardiac Purkinje fiber: evidence for voltage- and calcium-mediated mechanisms. *J Gen Physiol* 1984; 84:705–26.
49. Lee KS, Marban E, Tsien RW. Inactivation of calcium channels in mammalian heart cells; joint dependence on membrane potential and intracellular calcium. *J Physiol* [Lond] 1985; 364:395–411.
50. Droogmans HC, Nilius B. Kinetic properties of the cardiac T-type calcium channel in the guinea-pig. *J Physiol* [Lond] 1989; 419:627–50.
51. Chen CF, Hess P. Mechanism of gating of T-type calcium channels. *J Gen Physiol* 1990; 96:603–30.
52. Fox AP, Nowycky MC, Tsien RW. Kinetic and pharmacological properties distinguishing three types of calcium current in chick sensory neurones. *J Physiol* [Lond] 1987; 394:149–204.
53. Yue DT, Marban E. Permeation in the dihydropyridine-sensitive calcium channel. Multi-ion occupancy but no anomalous mole-fraction effect between Ba^{2+} and Ca^{2+}. *J Gen Physiol* 1990; 95:911–39.
54. Balke CW, Rose WC, O'Rourke B, Mejia-Alvarez R, Backx P, Marban E. Biophysics and physiology of cardiac calcium channels. *Circulation;* in press.
55. Yue DT, Backx PH, Imredy JI. Calcium-sensitive inactivation in the gating of single calcium channels. *Science* 1990; 250:1735–8.
56. Hodgkin AL, Huxley AF. A quantitative description of membrane currents and its application to conduction and excitation in nerve. *J Physiol* [Lond] 1952; 117:500–44.
57. Aldrich RW, Corey DP, Stevens CF. A reinterpretation of mammalian sodium channel gating based on single channel recording. *Nature* 1983; 306:436–41.
58. Zagotta WN, Aldrich RW. Voltage-dependent gating of *Shaker* A-type potassium channels in *Drosophila* muscle. *J Gen Physiol* 1990; 95:29–60.
59. Hess P, Lansman JB, Tsien RW. Calcium channel selectivity for divalent and monovalent cations. *J Gen Physiol* 1986; 88:293–319.
60. Mazzanti M, DeFelice LJ. Ca gating during cardiac action potentials. *Biophys J* 1990; 58:1059–65.
61. Cavalié A, Pelzer D, Trautwein W. Fast and slow gating behavior of single cardiac channels in cardiac cells: relation to activation and inactivation of calcium-channel current. *Pflügers Arch* 1986; 406:241–58.
62. Plummer MR, Hess P. Reversible uncoupling of inactivation in N-type calcium channels. *Nature* 1991; 351:657–9.

63. Hess P, Tsien RW. Mechanism of ion permeation through calcium channels. *Nature* 1984; 309:453–6.
64. Almers W, McCleskey EW. Non-selective conductance in calcium channels of frog muscle: calcium selectivity in a single-file pore. *J Physiol* [Lond] 1984; 353:585–608.
65. Rosenberg RL, Hess P, Tsien RW. Cardiac calcium channels in planar lipid bilayers. *J Gen Physiol* 1988; 92:27–54.
66. Tang CM, Presser F, Morad M. Amiloride selectively blocks the low threshold (T) calcium channel. *Science* 1988; 240:213–5.
67. Carbone E, Lux HD. Na^+ currents through low-voltage-activated Ca^{2+} channels of chick sensory neurons: block by external Ca^{2+} and Mg^{2+}. *J Physiol* [Lond] 1990; 430:159–88.
68. Perez-Reyes E, Kim HS, Lacerda AE, et al. Induction of calcium currents by the expression of the alpha-1-subunit of the dihydropyridine receptor from skeletal muscle. *Nature* 1989; 340:233–6.
69. Bean BP. Nitrendipine block of cardiac calcium channels: high affinity binding to the inactivated state. *Proc Natl Acad Sci* U S A 1984; 81:6388–92.
70. Kameyama M, Hofmann F, Trautwein W. On the mechanism of α-adrenergic regulation of the Ca channel in the guinea pig heart. *Pflügers Arch* 1985; 405:285–93.
71. Trautwein W, Hescheler J. Regulation of cardiac L-type calcium current by phosphorylation and G proteins. *Ann Rev Physiol* 1990; 52:257–74.
72. Yatani A, Brown AM. Rapid β-adrenergic modulation of cardiac calcium channel currents by a fast G protein pathway. *Nature* 1989; 245:71–4.
73. Hartzell HC, Méry PF, Fischmeister R, Szabo G. Sympathetic regulation of cardiac calcium current is due exclusively to cAMP-dependent phosphorylation. *Nature* 1991; 351:573–6.
74. Curtis BM, Catterall WA. Purification of the calcium antagonist receptor of the voltage-sensitive calcium channel from skeletal muscle transverse tubules. *Biochemistry* 1984; 23:2113–8.
75. Vaghy PL, Striessnig J, Miwa K, et al. Identification of a novel 1,4-dihydropyridine- and phenylalkylamine polypeptide in calcium channel preparations. *J Biol Chem* 1987; 262:14337–42.
76. Streissnig J, Scheffauer F, Mitterdorfer J, Schirmer M, Glossmann H. Identification of the benzothiazepine-binding polypeptide of skeletal muscle calcium channels with (+)-cis-azidodiltiazem and anti-ligand antibodies. *J Biol Chem* 1990; 265:363–70.
77. Curtis BM, Catterall WA. Phosphorylation of the calcium antagonist receptor of the voltage-sensitive calcium channel by cAMP-dependent protein kinase. *Proc Natl Acad Sci U S A* 1985; 82:2528–32.
78. Pelzer D, Grant AO, Cavalié A, et al. Calcium channels reconstituted from the skeletal muscle dihydropyridine receptor protein complex and its α_1 peptide subunit in lipid bilayers. Ann N Y Acad Sci 1989; 560:138–54.
79. Noda M, Simizu S, Tanabe T, et al. Primary structure of *Electrophorus electricus* sodium channel deduced from cDNA sequence. *Nature* 1984; 312:121–7.
80. Noda M, Ikeda T, Kayano T, et al. Existence of distinct sodium channel messenger RNAs in rat brain. *Nature* 1986; 320:188–92.
81. Tanabe T, Mikami A, Numa S, Beam KG. Cardiac-type excitation-contraction coupling in dysgenic skeletal muscle injected with cardiac dihydropyridine receptor cDNA. Nature 1990; 344:451–3.
82. Beam KG, Knudson CM, Powell JA. A lethal mutation in mice eliminates the slow calcium current in skeletal muscle cells. Nature 1986; 320:168–70.
83. Irisawa H, Yanagihara K. The slow inward current of the rabbit sino-atrial nodal cells. In: Zipes DP, Bailey JC, Elharrar V, eds. *The slow inward current and cardiac arrhythmias*. Boston: Martinus Nijhoff, 1980; 265–84.

84. Méndez C. The slow inward current and AV nodal propagation. In: Zipes DP, Bailey JC, Elharrar V, eds. *The slow inward current and cardiac arrhythmias.* Boston: Martinus Nijhoff, 1980; 285–94.
85. Tsien RW, Hess P. Excitable tissues: the heart. In: Andreoli TE, Hoffman JF, Fanestil DD, Schultz SG, eds. *Physiology of membrane disorders.* New York: Plenum, 1986; 469–90.
86. Carmeliet E. The slow inward current: non-voltage clamp studies. In: Zipes DP, Bailey JC, Elharrar V, eds. *The slow inward current and cardiac arrhythmias.* Boston: Martinus Nijhoff, 1980; 97–110.
87. Gilmour RF Jr, Zipes DP. Basic electrophysiology of the slow inward current. In: Antman E, Stone PH, eds. *Calcium blocking agents in the treatment of cardiovascular disorders.* Mt. Kisco, NY: Futura, 1983; 1–37.
88. Bers DM. *Excitation-contraction coupling and cardiac contractile force.* Boston: Kluwer Academic, 1991; 129–41.
89. Cannell MB, Berlin JR, Lederer WJ. Effect of membrane potential changes on the calcium transient in single rat cardiac muscle cells. *Science* 1987; 238:1419–23.
90. Callewaert G, Cleeman L, Morad M. Epinephrine enhances Ca^{2+} current-regulated Ca^{2+} release and Ca^{2+} reuptake in rat ventricular myocytes. *Proc Natl Acad Sci U S A* 1988; 85:2009–13.
91. Näbauer M, Callewaert G, Cleeman L, Morad M. Regulation of calcium release is gated by calcium current, not gating charge, in cardiac myocytes. *Science* 1989; 244:800–3.
92. Schwarz LM, McCleskey WE, Almers W. Dihydropyridine receptors in muscle are voltage-dependent but most are not functional calcium channels. *Nature* 1985; 314: 747–51.
93. Morad M. Cleeman L. Role of Ca^{2+} channel in development of tension in heart muscle. *J Mol Cell Cardiol* 1987; 19:527–53.
94. Llinas R. The intrinsic electrophysiological properties of mammalian neurons: insights into the central nervous system function. *Science* 1988; 242:1654–64.
95. Bonvallet R. A low threshold calcium current recorded at physiological Ca concentrations in single frog atrial cells. *Pflügers Arch* 1987; 408:540–2.
96. Singh BN. Control of cardiac arrhythmias by modulation of the slow myocardial channel. In: Hurwitz L, Partridge LD, Leach JK, eds. *Calcium channels: their properties, functions, regulation, and clinical significance.* Boston: CRC Press, 1991; 335.
97. Shen AC, Jennings, RB. Myocardial calcium and magnesium in acute ischemic injury. *Am J Pathol* 1972; 67:417–440.
98. Jennings RB, Hawkins HK, Lowe JE, Hill ML, Klotman S, Reimer KA. Relation between high energy phosphate and lethal injury in myocardial ischemia in the dog. *Am J Pathol* 1978; 92:187–214.
99. Jennings RB, Reimer KA. Factors involved in salvaging ischemic myocardium: effect of reperfusion of arterial blood. *Circulation* 1983; 68I:I25–36.
100. Chien KR, Engler R. Calcium and ischemic myocardial injury. In: Langer GA, ed. *Calcium and the heart.* New York: Raven Press, 1990; 333–54.
101. Zimmermann ANE, Hulsmann WC. Paradoxical influence of calcium ions on the permeability of the cell membranes of the isolated rat heart. *Nature* 1966; 211:646–7.
102. Fleckenstein A. Specific inhibitors and promoters of calcium action in the excitation-contraction coupling of heart muscle and their role in the prevention of production of myocardial lesions. In: Harris P, Opie L, eds. *Calcium and the heart.* Proceedings of the Meeting of the European Section of the International Study Group for Research in Cardiac Metabolism, London, September 1970. London: Academic Press, 1971; 135–88.
103. Naylor WG, Perry SE, Elz JS, Daly MJ. Calcium, sodium and the calcium paradox. *Circ Res* 1984; 55:227–37.

104. Factor SM, Cho S, Scheuer J, Sonnenblick EH, Malhotra A. Prevention of hereditary cardiomyopathy in the Syrian hamster with chronic verapamil therapy. *J Am Coll Cardiol* 1988; 12:1599–64.
105. Steenbergen C, Murphy E, Levy L, London RE. Elevation in cytosolic free calcium concentration early in the myocardial ischemia in perfused rat heart. *Circ Res* 1987; 60:700–7.
106. Lee H-C, Smith N, Mohabir R, Clusin WT. Cytosolic calcium transients from the beating heart. *Proc Natl Acad Sci U S A* 1987; 84:7793–7.
107. Marban E, Kitakase M, Kusuoka H, Porterfield JK, Yue DT, Chacko VP. Intracellular free calcium concentration measured with ^{19}F NMR spectroscopy in intact ferret hearts. *Proc Natl Acad Sci U S A* 1987: 84:6005–9.
108. Reimer KA, Lowe JE, Jennings RB. Effect of the calcium antagonist verapamil on necrosis following temporary coronary occlusion in dogs. *Circulation* 1977; 55:581–7.
109. Bersohn MM, Shine KI. Verapamil protection of ischemic isolated rabbit heart: dependence on pretreatment. *J Mol Cell Cardiol* 1983; 15:659–71.
110. Mori H, Nagata M, Miyazaki T, et al. Protection of hypoxic myocardium by intracoronary administration of verapamil in open-chest dogs. *Circulation* 1984; 70:742–7.
111. Murphy JG, Smith TW, Marsh JD. Mechanism of reoxygenation-induced calcium overload in cultured chick embryo heart cells. *Am J Physiol* 1988; 254:H1133–41.
112. Boveris A. Mitochondrial production of superoxide radical and hydrogen peroxide. *Adv Exp Biol Med* 1977; 78:707–16.
113. Ito BR, Tate H, Kobayashi M, Schaper W. Reversibly injured post-ischemic canine myocardium retains normal contractile reserve. *Circ Res* 1987; 61:834–46.
114. Post JA, Lamers PD, Verdouw FJ, ten Cate WJ, van der Giessen WJ, Verkleij AJ. Sarcolemmal destabilization and destruction after ischemia and reperfusion and its relation with long-term recovery of regional left ventricular function in pigs. *Eur Heart J* 1987; 8:423–30.
115. Hearse DJ, Humphrey SM, Chain EB. Abrupt reoxygenation of the anoxic potassium arrested perfused rat heart: a study of myocardial enzyme release. *J Mol Cell Cardiol* 1973; 5:395–407.
116. McCord JM. Oxygen derived free radicals in postischemic tissue injury. *N Engl J Med* 1985; 312:159–63.
117. Baker JE, Felix CC, Olinger GN, Kalyanaraman B. Myocardial ischemia and reperfusion: direct evidence for free radical generation by electron spin resonance spectroscopy. *Proc Natl Acad Sci U S A* 1988; 85:2786–9.
118. Burton KP. Evidence of direct toxic effects of free radicals on the myocardium. *Free Radic Biol Med* 1988; 4:15–24.
119. Katz AM. Cardiomyopathy of overload: a major determinant of prognosis in conjestive heart failure. *N Engl J Med* 1990; 322:100–10.
120. Morgan JP, Erny RE, Allen PD, Grossman W, Gwathmey JK. Abnormal intracellular calcium handling, a major cause of systolic and diastolic dysfunction in ventricular myocardium from patients with heart failure. *Circulation* 1990; 81:III-21–32.
121. Morgan JP. Abnormal intracellular modulation of calcium as a major cause of cardiac contractile dysfunction. *N Engl J Med* 1991; 325:625–32.
122. Gwathmey JK, Copelas L, MacKinnon R, et al. Abnormal intracellular calcium handling in myocardium from patients with end-stage heart failure. *Circ Res* 1987; 61:70–6.
123. Gwathmey JK, Slawsky MT, Briggs GM, Morgan JP. Role of intracellular sodium in the regulation of intracellular calcium and contractility. *J Clin Invest* 1988; 82:1592–605.
124. Gwathmey JK, Slawsky MT, Hajjar RJ, Briggs GM, Morgan JP. Role of intracellular calcium handling in force-interval relationships of human ventricular myocardium. *J Clin Invest* 1990; 85:1599–613.

125. Kuo TH, Johnson DF, Tsang W, Weiner J. Photoaffinity labeling of the calcium channel antagonist receptor in the heart of the cardiomyopathic hamster. *Biochem Biophys Res Commun* 1987; 148:926–33.
126. Dixon IMC, Lee S-L, Dhalla NS: Nitrendipine binding in congestive heart failure due to myocardial infarction. *Circ Res* 1990; 66:782–8.
127. Rasmussen PR, Minobe W, Bristow MR. Calcium antagonist binding sites in failing and nonfailing human ventricular myocardium. *Biochem Pharmacol* 1990; 39:691–6.
128. Beuckelmann DJ, Näbauer M, Erdmann E. Characteristics of calcium-current in isolated human ventricular myocytes from patients with terminal heart failure. *J Mol Cell Cardiol* 1991; 23:929–37.
129. Beuckelmann DJ, Näbauer M, Erdmann E. Intracellular calcium handling in isolated ventricular myocytes from patients with terminal heart failure. *Circulation* 1992; 85:1046–55.

26

Calcium Channel Blockers in Cardiovascular Diseases: A Clinical Approach

HANS-REINER FIGULLA

Medizinische Universitäts Kliniken
Göttingen, Germany

More than 23 years ago, the pharmacologic principle behind a new group of agents that mimicked the effect of Ca^{2+} withdrawal in heart and smooth muscle was discovered. These agents were consequently named Ca^{2+} antagonists (1). Their discovery occurred before the detection of the electrochemistry of the calcium channel (2), which makes up the core of the transsarcolemmal inflow of calcium. In 1972, it was found that Ca^{2+} antagonists selectively block this calcium channel (3), and thus the term *calcium channel blocker* was introduced.

This was the beginning of one of the most remarkable developments in cardiovascular drug therapy. The search for the application of calcium channel blockade has continued and been expanded since then, in particular for the treatment of the following diseases: cardiac arrhythmias; coronary heart disease; cardiomyopathies; pulmonary and systemic hypertension; arteriosclerosis; neurologic disorders such as epilepsy, migraine, and vertigo; gastrointestinal diseases such as spastic disorders of the esophagus (achalasia), small and large bowels, and bile tract; respiratory disorders such as asthma bronchiale and chronic obstructive lung disease; and congenital disorders such as chronic renal failure, ureter spasm, dysmenorrhea, and toxolysis.

This chapter is devoted to the clinical application of calcium channel blockers in cardiovascular diseases (Table 1).

I. MODE OF ACTION AND CLASSIFICATION

In cardiac tissue, because of the inhibition of Ca^{2+} transients, calcium channel blockers have negative chronotropic, negative inotropic, and negative dromotropic effects. They reduce smooth muscle tone in muscular arteries and arterioles, gastrointestinal and urogenital tracts, may decrease cerebral electric activity, and also may prevent tissue destruction due to enhanced calcium inflow.

Table 1 Calcium Channel Blockers in the Treatment of Cardiovascular Diseases

Arrhythmias
a Caused by abnormal impulse conduction (supraventricular tachycardia, Wolff-Parkinson-White syndrome, atrial fibrillation and flutter)
b Caused by abnormal impulse initiation (depolarization-induced automaticity, afterdepolarizations)
Ischemic heart disease
a Stable angina
b Prinzmetal's angina
c Unstable angina
d Non-Q-wave myocardial infarction
e Q-wave infarction
f Silent ischemia
Coronary sclerosis
Heart failure
Hypertrophic cardiomyopathy
Idiopathic dilated cardiomyopathy
Systemic hypertension
Pulmonary hypertension
Organ protection

The organic calcium channel blockers have been classified into 6 subgroups by the World Health Organization (4); at the time of writing, 12 diverse generics are on the market in Germany. Group I is represented by the benzothiazepines such as verapamil or gallopamil. Group II contains the 1,4 dihydropyridines such as nifedipine, nimodipine, and nitrendipine. Group III contains diltiazem: Groups IV–VI contain the phenylalkylamines such as flunarizine, cinnarizine (group IV), prenylamine, fendiline (group V), and perhexiline and etafenone (group VI).

Substances of groups I–III are water soluble and specifically block voltage-sensitive calcium L channels (4–6). Specific binding receptors have been identified (7). These substances can inhibit almost completely the Ca^{2+}-dependent excitation–contraction coupling in mammalian ventricular myocardium before the fast Na^+ influx is affected.

Group IV–VI agents are lipophilic and exhibit physicochemical stabilization of the membrane lipids (8). These calcium channel blocker are somewhat less potent and specific than those of groups I, II, and III. Under their influence, a concomitant inhibition of I_{Na} can be seen when contractile tension development of isolated papillary muscles has been reduced by 50–70% (9).

II. CARDIAC ARRHYTHMIAS

Cardiac arrhythmias can be organized into two major classes: those caused by abnormal impulse conduction and those caused by abnormal impulse initiation.

It is well known that the fundamental process of sinoatrial (SA) and atrioventricular (AV) mode automaticity is predominantly produced by the inflow of Ca^{2+} ions as electric charge carriers through the slow membrane channel. The effects of the calcium channel blocker verapamil parallel those of reduced external Ca^{2+} concentration: decrease of upstroke velocity and overshoot. Isoproterenol does not neu-

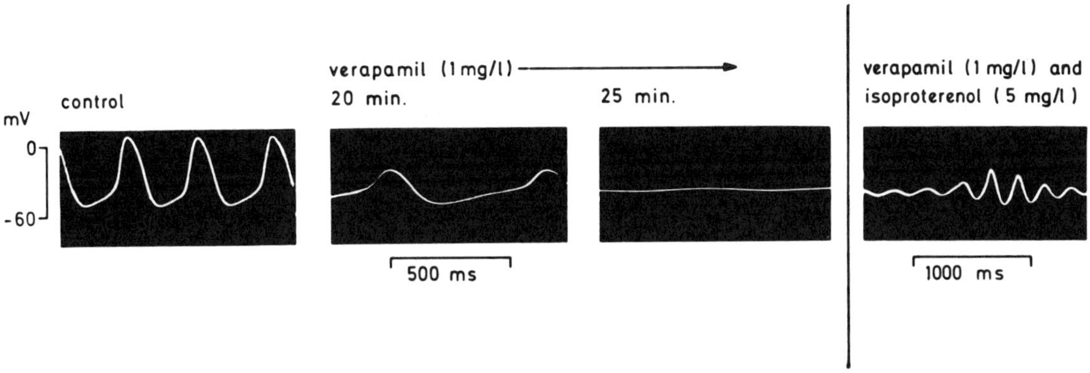

Figure 1 Blocking effect of verapamil (1 mg/liter) on the upstroke of the sinoatrial pacemaker action potential and on the rate of spontaneous diastolic depolarization. Isoproterenol (5 mg/liter) failed to neutralize the inhibitory verapamil effects (last record to the right). (Ref. 10.)

tralize these inhibitory effects (10,11) (Fig. 1). In addition, the rate of spontaneous diastolic depolarization is reduced. Consequently, it could be found in experimental models and human myocardium that calcium channel blockers reduce heart rate and prolong the atrio-His interval, the functional and effective refractory period of the AV node.

It thus became evident very early in the history of calcium channel blockers that the application of verapamil and diltiazem in supraventricular reentry tachycardia and tachyarrhythmia due to atrial fibrillation can be beneficial (12). Injection of 5–10 mg verapamil or 10–20 mg diltiazem in patients with supraventricular paroxysmal tachycardia very often terminates the tachycardia and, in patients with frequent supraventricular tachycardial episodes, oral verapamil or diltiazem can prevent further attacks.

In the case of patients with Wolff-Parkinson-White syndrome with accessory pathway conduction, calcium channel blockers can even accelerate tachycardia. Since calcium channel blockers are ineffective on the accessory pathway (due to reflex sympathetic activation) the impulse conduction velocity in the accessory pathway can even be enhanced (13).

Calcium channel blockers are ineffective in the conversion of atrial fibrilliation or flutter to sinus rhythm (14). A summary of the effects of verapamil on atrial arrhythmias is given in Table 2.

The role of calcium channel blockers in the management of abnormal impulse initiation is controversial. Calcium channel blockers may be involved in two mechanisms: depolarization-induced automaticity and afterdepolarization (15). In ischemic cells and in cells otherwise injured, the resting membrane potential is less negative. During the excitation process the upstroke velocity and overshoot are less than in normal cells. The differences in the membrane potentials between injured cells and normal cells are responsible for a current of injury. The injury current will reduce the resting membrane potential of normal myocardial cells attached to the injured cells. If normal cells are partly depolarized, the cells can develop automaticity and induce ectopic beats (16). Calcium channel blockers can reduce or

Table 2 Effects of Verapamil on Atrial Arrhythmias

Arrhythmia	Response
Sinus tachycardia	Slowing
Paroxysmal supraventricular tachycardia	
Reentry	Conversion in 95% of patients
Ectopic	Conversion in 65% of patients
With atrioventricular block	Conversion in 65% of patients
Atrial fibrillation	Ventricular slowing
	Ventricular "regularization"
	Conversion to normal sinus rhythm (rare)
Associated with Wolff-Parkinson-White syndrome	Ineffective
Atrial flutter	Conversion to atrial fibrillation, then normal sinus rhythm

Source: Ref. 38.

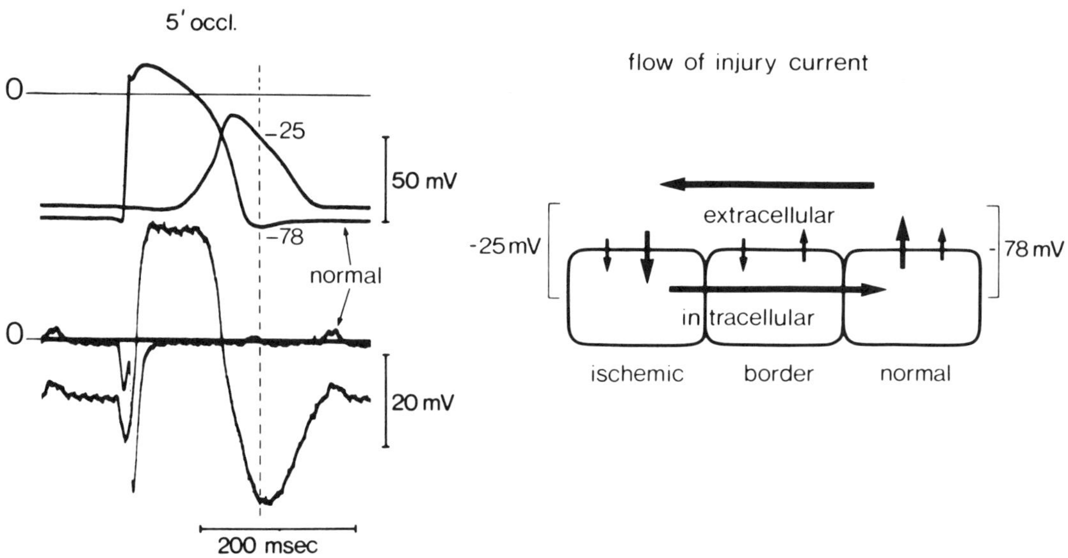

Figure 2 Current of injury between ischemic and normal zones of heart. A. Recordings of transmembrane (upper tracings) and extracellular (lower tracings) potentials from normal and ischemic regions of dog heart in situ. Maximum negativity (denoted by vertical dashed line) of extracellular potential recorded from ischemic occurs after cells in normal zone have fully depolarized. B. Diagram indicates flow of injury current between normal and ischemic zones at time denoted by vertical dashed line in A. (From Janse MJ, Kléber AG. Electrophysiological changes and ventricular arrhythmias in the early phase of regional myocardial ischemia. Circ Res 1981; 49:1049–81; with permission of the American Heart Association, Inc.)

abolish the ectopic firing caused by a current of injury by diminishing the Ca^{2+} current in normal cells (17) (Fig. 2).

The oscillatory instability in myocardial cells, which follows the action potential, is termed *afterdepolarization.* If the charge in membrane potential attains threshold, it may trigger action potentials. The essential initiating factor for such afterdepolarizations that trigger ectopic beats is a substantial increase in intracellular Ca^{2+} concentrations (15,18–20). Microinjections of EGTA, which chelates Ca^{2+} ions, inhibit afterdepolarizations in myocardial tissue (21).

Calcium channel blockers inhibit transsarcolemmal Ca^{2+} inflow (1,3) and thus should inhibit abnormal impulse initiation. However, in the clinical setting, calcium channel blockers have been used exploratorily in patients with premature ventricular contractions (PVCs) (22,23). Diltiazem was less effective than class I antiarrhythmic agents, but was just as effective as propranolol. Conclusive trials on the application of calcium channel blocker and sudden cardiac death are lacking.

III. ISCHEMIC HEART DISEASE

A. General Hemodynamic Effects

The calcium channel blockers nifedipine, diltiazem, and verapamil are at present used almost exclusively. These substances exhibit some differences in their chronotropic, inotropic, and vasodilatory actions.

In respect to coronary flow rate, nifedipine is the most effective substance, followed by verapamil and diltiazem. Peripheral vasodilation is most pronounced in nifedipine, followed by verapamil and diltiazem. The peripheral vasodilation reduces afterload of the left ventricle, thus counterbalancing (together with increased reflex adrenergic activity elicited by the baroreceptor system) the genuinely negative inotropic action of these three calcium channel blockers. However, in a study using combined autonomic blockade with atropine and propranolol performed in conscious dogs, reflex tachycardia was reversed to bradycardia and consistent negative inotropic effects were exhibited by all three calcium channel blockers (24).

A conclusive summary of the hemodynamic effects of nifedipine, verapamil, and diltiazem is given in Table 3.

Table 3 Hemodynamic Response to Calcium Channel Blockers

	Nifedipine	Verapamil	Diltiazem
Heart rate	↑	→ ↓	↓
Contractility	→	↓	→ ↓
Cardiac output	↑	→ ↓	↑
Peripheral resistance	↓ ↓	↓	↓
Coronary blood flow	↑ ↑	↑	↑
Arterial pressure	↓ ↓	↓	↓
LVEDP	→ ↓	→ ↓	→ ↓

LVEDP, left ventricular end-diastolic pressure, ↑ ↑, great increase; ↑, increase; →, no change; ↓, decrease; ↓ ↓, great decrease
Source: Ref. 25.

Since all calcium channel blockers inhibit the voltage-sensitive L calcium channel, what is the reason for the preferential vascular action of the 1,4 dihydropyridines? Three mechanisms may be considered (26): a higher affinity for Ca^{2+} channels, which may be attributed to the less negative resting membrane potential of vascular smooth muscle cells (−40−−60 mV compared to −80−−90 mV in cardiac myocytes); the longer duration of activating stimuli to which vascular smooth muscle cells are submitted; under pathologic conditions, the sensitivity to calcium antagonists may increase as a result of alterations of these parameters. Smooth muscle cells may become slightly depolarized in the vicinity of endothelial lesions, for instance in atheromatous arteries, which should enhance their preferential response to 1,4 dihydropyridines (27).

B. Mode of Action

Ischemic heart disease is due to compromised coronary circulation. As early as 1960, the coronary dilating potency of prenylamine (28) and, in 1962 (29), of verapamil, was discovered. This was prior to the detection of a common mode of action by Fleckenstein in 1967 (1). Thus, it became evident very early that calcium channel blockers may be used in ischemic heart disease to improve the oxygen supply/demand ratio.

All calcium channel blockers exhibit vasodilation actions on epicardial muscular coronary arteries and on the intramyocardial arterioles. However, simple vasodilation may result in shunting of coronary flow away from stunned myocardium (coronary steal), as in the case of "malignant" coronary vasodilators such as dipyridamol. In addition, the increase of luminal diameters in normal coronary arteries with calcium channel blockers is only 0–15% (30). What is the difference between calcium channel blockers and these malignant agents? By which mechanisms can calcium channel blockers increase blood flow and oxygen supply to the poststenotic area in ischemic heart disease? Two mechanisms are effective (31): In areas of pathologic narrowing during isometric and ergometric exercise, there is a further decrease in luminal cross-sectional area that can be prevented under treatment with calcium channel blockers: second, myocardial blood flow is normally controlled by vasomotor activity of the coronary resistance vessels, with a gradient favoring blood flow to the subendocardium. In coronary heart disease, reactive hyperemia follows short periods of ischemia. However, the vasomotor regulation maintaining a normal distribution of perfusion is lost, and thus subendocardial areas will remain ischemic after short ischemic periods following exercise. Calcium channel blockers can decrease postischemic hyperemia by antagonizing vasodilation in response to endogenous vasodilators such as adenosine. When flow was limited by a stenosis, both diltiazem and nifedipine blunted the hyperemia in the subendocardium and enhanced delivery of blood to the subendocardium (32,33) (Fig. 3).

During brief periods of ischemia, early diastolic relaxation is impaired. This impairment is attributed to an immediate gain of cytosolic-free Ca^{2+}, demonstrated recently by means of ^{19}F nuclear magnetic resonance spectroscopy (34,35). Multiple clinical investigations have shown improvement of diastolic filling in patients with ischemic heart disease when treated with calcium channel blockers (37). Conclusive data that calcium channel blockers reduce ischemia-induced cystosolic-free Ca^{2+} increase is still lacking (37).

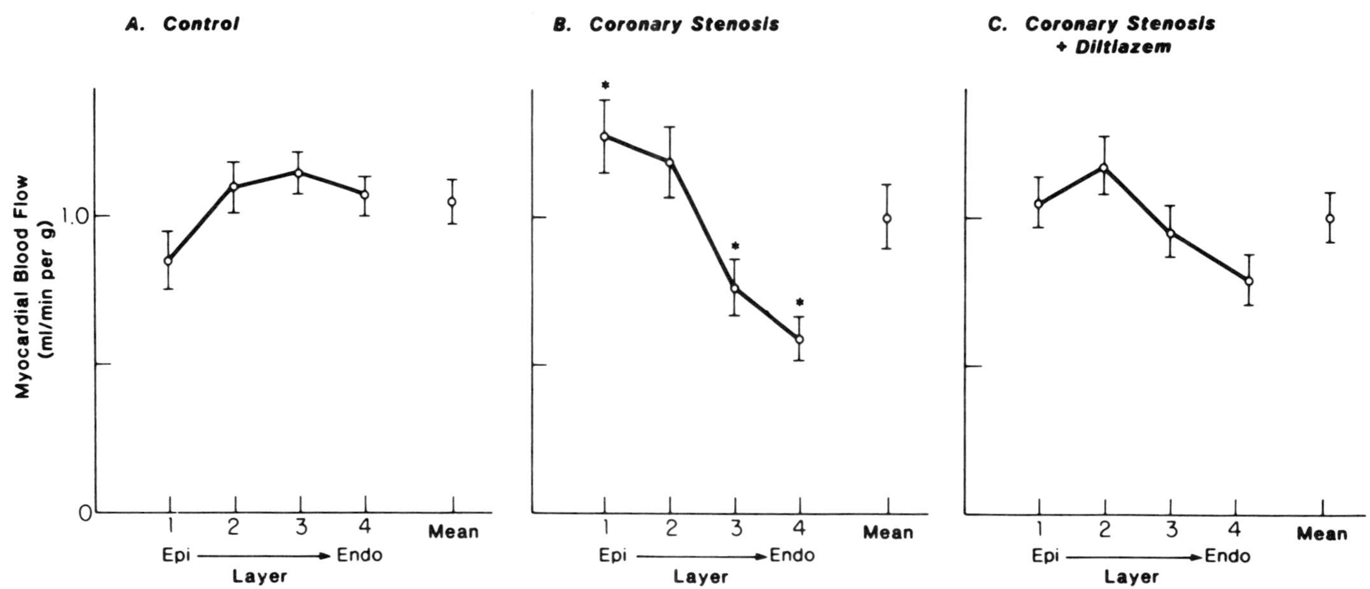

Figure 3 Graph of myocardial blood flow (mean ± SEM) to four transmural layers from epicardium to endocardium in eight chronically instrumented dogs. A. Myocardial blood flow during resting control conditions. B. Myocardial blood flow measured when coronary stenosis prevented arterial inflow from increasing above preocclusion control level after 10 sec coronary occlusion had resulted in ischemic vasodilation of coronary resistance vessels. C. Myocardial blood flow 30 min after diltiazem (0.30 mg/kg i.v.), when coronary stenosis prevented arterial inflow from increasing above preocclusion control level after 10-second coronary occlusion. *$p < 0.05$ compared with flow during control conditions. (Ref. 33.)

In conclusion, it can be stated that the predominant mechanism of action of calcium channel blockers in ischemic heart disease can be attributed to (38):

1. Increased myocardial oxygen supply
   a. Epicardial segment dilatation during isometric and ergometric exercise
   b. Improved subendocardial perfusion
2. Decreased myocardial oxygen demand
   a. Afterload reduction
   b. Heart rate reduction (diltiazem)
   c. Contractility reduction.

C. Stable Angina Pectoris

In the clinical setting, calcium channel blockers can abolish stable angina attacks in 29% of all patients treated with nifedipine and in 50–70% of all patients given diltiazem or verapamil. In the ergometric stress test, the time required to produce 1 mm S-T segment displacement improved with both verapamil and diltiazem treatment by 64% and 62%, respectively. Nifedipine improved this variable by 49% (39).

There is some controversy as to whether a calcium channel blocker or a β-blocker should be used first in the treatment of chronic stable angina pectoris. Multiple studies demonstrated that both classes of agents appear almost equally effective. In patients with severe angina, a combination of β-blocker, calcium channel blocker, and a long-acting nitrate may be employed. A number of studies have shown that the combination of a β-blocker with a calcium channel blocker is superior to either drug along (40,41); however, a combination of verapamil with a β-blocker should be avoided since this can produce significant negative inotropic and chronotropic effects (42).

D. Prinzmetal's Variant Angina

Prinzmetal's angina is a variant myocardial ischemic syndrome with preserved exercise capacity, characterized by episodic thoracic pain in combination with S-T elevation or S-T segment depression due to an intermittent brief period of vasospasm of the epicardial artery with inadequate coronary flow. In 65% of all cases the vasospasm is adjacent to coronary lesions. However, in several studies (for review, see (43)) it could be shown that calcium channel blockers are highly effective in reducing the frequency of angina attacks, nitroglycerin consumption, and electrocardiographic (ECG) changes. The average success rate in the treatment of Prinzmetal's variant angina in a compiled data survey is 83% for nifedipine, 80% for diltiazem, and 83% for verapamil (43). Thus, all calcium channel blockers seem to form an ideal therapy in this disorder; if they remain uneffective as monotherapy, they can be used in combination with nitroglycerin (44).

E. Unstable Angina Pectoris

Disorders of vasomotor tone were once considered to be responsible for unstable angina pectoris. It was proposed recently that the pathologic event responsible for all acute ischemic syndromes (e.g., myocardial infarct, non-Q-wave infarction, unstable angina) are predominantly due to the development of atherosclerotic plaque fissuring, fracture, or ulceration (45). Plaque disruption exposes collagen beneath the plaque to platelets. Platelets aggregate and release vasoactive substances such as thromboxane, serotonin, and platelet-derived growth factor. In many atherosclerotic lesions, there is an area of relatively normal vessel wall capable of vasoconstriction in response to the released vasoconstrictors. Thus, in unstable angina pectoris, calcium channel blockers have some beneficial effect; the predominant therapeutic aim is, however, antithrombotic management. In patients with unstable angina pectoris, calcium channel blockers should be combined with β-blockers. Calcium channel blocker monotherapy has been proven to have little effect (46,47). According to a survey by Held (48) in six trials addressing this question, the number of patients who developed myocardial infarction was 110 of 561 in patients treated with calcium channel blockers compared to 104 of 591 in the control group. The corresponding number of deaths was 14 of 591 and 9 of 578, respectively.

F. Non-Q-Wave Myocardial Infarction

From the anatomical point of view, myocardial infarcts are differentiated into transmural and nontransmural infarcts or intramural infarcts. The classic ECG criteria for both kinds are the exhibition of Q-waves and R-wave reduction for the former and the absence of Q-wave and persistent S-T segment depression and/or T-wave inversion in the latter. However, there is some overlap between anatomical criteria and ECG. Despite this, it could be demonstrated by perfusion and metabolic imaging studies that patients with non-Q-wave infarcts have a larger residual mass of viable but jeopardized myocardium than patients with Q-wave infarction (49,50). This is probably due to early reperfusion, nonocclusive coronary thrombosis, or effective collateral flow. Non-Q-wave infarction is associated with less initial damage, and thus the hospital mortality rate is lower. However, the pooled data of 22 long-term studies (51) indicate an even higher mortality rate in the non-Q-wave as opposed to in the Q-wave group (31.2% vs. 26.3%, $p < 0.001$). The unexpectedly high rate of mortality is most likely due to ongoing ischemia, leading to reinfarction.

The only study that has addressed the very specific problem of non-Q-wave infarction and calcium channel blocker treatment is the diltiazem reinfarction study (DRS) (52) and a subgroup analysis of the multicenter diltiazem postinfarction trial (MDPIT) that evaluated the effects of diltiazem (240 mg/day) on mortality and cardiac events (53) (death from cardiac causes or nonfatal reinfarction).

A total of 2466 patients were included in the MDPIT double-blind, placebo-controlled trial. The subset of 634 patients with non-Q-wave infarction was analyzed by Boden (54). The cumulative incidence of cardiac death and nonfatal reinfarction at 1 year was 15% in the placebo group vs. 9% in the diltiazem group, a reduction of 40% ($p=0.03$).

In the DRS trial, the effect of diltiazem (360 mg/day) vs. placebo on the prevention of early recurrent infarction between 24 and 72 hr after the onset of non-Q-wave infarction and 14 days was addressed. Diltiazem was documented as reducing the recurrent infarct rate from 9.3% to 5.2% ($p<0.05$).

In these two studies, the calcium channel blocker diltiazem was shown to be effective. However, those with non-Q-wave myocardial infarction are a very special subgroup of myocardial infarct patients. Whether these patients parallel those after therapeutically early thrombolysis who have a high incidence of reinfarction is unknown. A trial addressing the issue of diltiazem treatment in patients after thrombolysis therapy in myocardial infarction is currently underway (55).

G. Q-Wave Myocardial Infarction

Twenty-two clinical trials have reported the effects of calcium channel blockers in acute and postinfarction patients. The rationale for investigating the efficacy of these drugs in these patients is the well-recognized anti-ischemic properties, the possible cytoprotective properties (56), and the probable occurrence of changes in vasomotor tone following myocardial infarctions. There are two excellent reviews of the literature (48,57).

A total of about 18,000 patients have been studied and the number of patients in the individual trials varied from 20 to 450. Thirteen of these trials evaluated the effects of nifedipine, three of verapamil, four of diltiazem, one of tiapamil, and one of lidoflazine. In 19 of these trials, treatment was begun within a few hours after the onset of symptoms and in three trials, treatment began some days to weeks after the infarction. The following three aspects were studied in these trials: mortality, infarct size (based on creatine kinase levels), and reinfarction.

In summary, 9990 patients in the nifedipine trials showed no evidence of a beneficial treatment-related effect with respect to infarct size, mortality, or reinfarction rates. Moreover, several trials showed harmful effects, which were significant ($p=0.018$) in the nifidipine angina myocardial infarction study (NAMIS) (58).

In the trials with verapamil or diltiazem, no beneficial effect on mortality, reinfarction, or infarct size could be detected. However, a retrospective subgroup analysis and a new prospective trial (David II) have shown some beneficial effects in respect to reinfarction and mortality if treatment with verapamil began on days 7–21 after the myocardial infarct (59,60) or if diltiazem was given exclusively to patients with preserved left ventricular function (no pulmonary rales, left ventricular ejection fraction ≥ 0.40) (53).

In conclusion, it can be stated that the trials could not demonstrate any strong evidence for a beneficial effect of calcium channel blockers on mortality, infarct size, or rate of reinfarction in Q-wave myocardial infarction (48,57) (Fig. 4).

H. Silent Ischemia

Silent ischemia is defined as a myocardial ischemia insult without symptoms. The prevalence in middle-aged men without a history of coronary heart disease is about 4%. The ischemic episodes are caused by coronary artery disease; however, for reasons unknown these episodes have no clinical expression. Ischemia is detected by means of exercise tests, Holter monitoring and/or thallium scintiagraphy.

Patients with silent ischemia exhibit an adverse prognosis, as has been shown in several longitudinal studies. The mean cardiac event rate averaged 4.5% per year or increased by the factor 3.6 in a very recent study compared with 0.63% per year in subjects with a negative stress test (62). Patients after myocardial infarction showed a 27% yearly mortality rate if ischemia could be detected, whereas there was only a 2% mortality rate in patients with no evidence of exercise-induced angina after myocardial infarction (63).

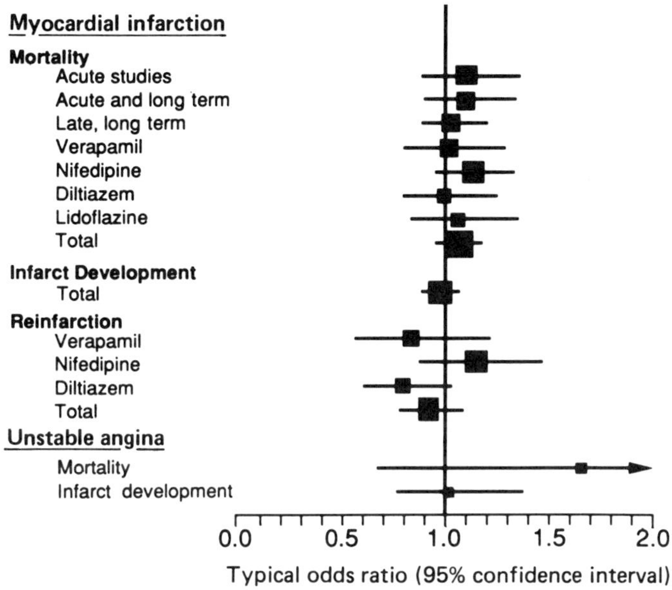

Figure 4 Typical odds of death, infarct development, and reinfarction by disease, types of trials, and drug used. Areas of squares proportional to number of patients. Bars indicate 95% confidence intervals. Portions left of vertical line (corresponding to odds ratio <1) indicate reduced risk with treatment; portions right of vertical line indicate increased risk with treatment. Note that treatment does not seem to reduce risk of any event. (Ref. 48.)

These data strongly suggest that it is important to detect silent ischemic episodes and, probably, to treat them. Since it is impossible to improve the general state of patients with asymptomatic ischemia, it is important not to worsen their condition by therapy (64). For this reason and also because of cost-efficacy, the well-tolerated calcium channel blocker diltiazem seems to accomplish this goal best. Diltiazem was reported to be more effective in controlling episodes of significant S-T segment depression (detected with Holter monitoring) than nifedipine. However, it is unclear whether therapy of asymptomatic ischemia will alter the prognosis (64).

IV. ANTISCLEROTIC AGENTS

Studies on several types of animal models, especially cholesterol-fed rabbits and vitamin D_3-intoxicated rats, showed that calcium competitors, calcium chelators, anticalcifying agents, and calcium antagonists can reduce the accumulation of atherogenic lesion components and may modify the progression of atherosclerosis (for review, see 65–67). However, the precise mechanisms of action of calcium channel blockers in relation to antiatherogenic function are unclear. Several of the reported mechanisms are shown in Table 4. Encouraged by these animal experiments, three clinical trials were launched (International Nifedipine Trial on Antiatherosclerotic Therapy [INTACT]; Frankfurt Isoptin Progression Study [FIPS], study from the Montreal Heart Institute). INTACT was completed in 1989; 425 patients were included in the trial and were treated for 3 years with 80 mg

Table 4 Reported Mechanisms of Action of Calcium Antagonists in Relation to Potential Antiatherogenic Function

Prevent intracellular calcium overload
Inhibit proliferation of smooth muscle cells
Inhibit chemotaxis of neutrophils, macrophages
Inhibit polymorphonuclear leukocyte function
Stimulate LDL receptor synthesis
Enhance receptor-mediated lipoprotein uptake
Inhibit lysosomal hydrolysis of lipoproteins
Inhibit cholesterol ester synthesis
Increase cholesteryl ester hydrolysis
Inhibit synthesis of matrix components
Inhibit VLDL secretion by hepatocytes

LDL, low-density lipoproteins; VLDL, very-low-density lipoproteins.
Source: Ref. 66.

nifedipine. A total of 282 patients finished the study. Coronary angiograms at entry and at the end of the study demonstrated 118 new lesions (stenoses > 20%) in the placebo group vs. 55 new lesions in the nifedipine group. A slowing of the progression of existing stenosis could not be detected. In addition, the mortality in the nifedipine group was higher (12 vs. 2 patients). The authors' conclusion that nifedipine should be given very early in the course of coronary heart disease (68) cannot yet be substantiated due to the enchanced mortality in the nifedipine group as well as the unexpected slight therapeutic benefit.

V. CHRONIC HEART FAILURE

"The systemic vasodilator action of calcium channel blockers make them potentially attractive as afterload-reducing agents in patients with left ventricular failure" (38).

"Although the vasodilator and anti-ischemic actions of calcium channel blocking drugs might be expected to produce hemodynamic benefits in chronic heart failure, none of these agents has been shown to exert favorable clinical effects in these patients" (69).

These controversial summarizing statements illustrate the dilemma: calcium channel blockers in patients with heart failure are a double-edged sword. They are powerful vasodilators, thus reducing afterload of the left ventricle, and they exhibit anti-ischemic properties and are perhaps cytoprotective. The overall acute hemodynamic response is thus beneficial (70,71) (Table 5). However, calcium channel blockers exhibit negative inotropic actions and further increase neuroendocrine secretion of catecholamines and renin (for review, see 69,72). Enhanced neuroendocrine secretion in chronic congestive heart failure is correlated with an adverse prognosis (73) and is attributable to many of the symptoms such as fluid retention and enhanced backward failure due to increased filling pressures and forward failure due to increased afterload (74).

Thus, after the use of a calcium channel blocker in a patient with congestive heart failure, there is usually a dissociation between the beneficial short-term

Table 5 Effects of Verapamil (0.25 mg/kg 30 m i.v.), Diltiazem (0.5 mg/kg 30 m i.v.), and Nifedipin (20 mg sublingual) on Hemodynamics in Patients with Idiopathic Dilated Cardiomyopathy and Severe LV Dysfunction

	Patients	Ejection fraction			Stroke volume index			Heart rate			Pressure rate product		
	n	K	M	p	K	M	p	K	M	p	K	M	p
Verapamil	8	0.29	0.31	n.s.	35	37	n.s.	92	81	n.s.	11,656	8,989	<0.02
Diltiazem	8	0.28	0.33	<0.05	33	39	<0.05	90	81	<0.05	9,844	8,073	<0.005
Nifedipine	8	0.32	0.39	<0.05	34	41	<0.05	91	90	n.s.	11,370	10,425	n.s.
P			n.s.			n.s.			n.s.			n.s.	
	Patients	PWP (mmHg)			PSP/ESVI (mmHg/mL/m^2)			PFR (s^{-1})			SVR (dyn/s/cm^{-3})		
	n	K	M	p	K	M	p	K	M	p	K	M	p
Verapamil	8	19	19	n.s.	1.65	1.46	n.s.	1.74	2.14	n.s.	1219	1160	n.s.
Diltiazem	8	11	13	n.s.	1.36	1.47	n.s.	1.73	1.92	n.s.	1329	1124	n.s.
Nifedipine	8	13	10	n.w.	1.83	1.87	n.s.	1.83	1.87	n.s.	1382	1008	<0.05
P		n.s.			n.s.			n.s.			n.s.		

K, control; M, after 30 min of medication; PWP, mean pulmonary wedge pressure; PSP/ESVI, peak systolic pressure/end-systolic volume index; PFR, peak filling rate; SVR, systemic vascular resistance.

hemodynamic effects (increase of ejection fraction, stroke volume) and the long-term effects (fluid retention, decreased endurance) (72,75). For the short term, calcium channel blockers may be applied in patients with left ventricular dysfunction if it is otherwise indicated (e.g., supraventricular tachycardia, severe angina pectoris), while in the long term, calcium channel blockers seem to be detrimental in patients with ischemic heart disease with impaired left ventricular function (53). In the longer course, angiotensin-converting enzyme inhibitors are superior in congestive heart failure. These substances suppress neuroendocrine secretion (69,74), abolish further left ventricular enlargement after anteroseptal myocardial infarcts (76), and improve survival in patients with severe congestive heart failure (77).

In the case of idiopathic dilated cardiomyopathy, a combination of both substances may be ideal. Such a combination would have the advantage of the specific cytoprotective mode of action of calcium channel blockers in this disease (78) (see below) and also inhibit neuroendocrine secretion by means of angiotensin-converting enzyme inhibitors.

VI. HYPERTROPHIC AND IDIOPATHIC DILATED CARDIOMYOPATHY

A. Hypertrophic Cardiomyopathy

Hypertrophic cardiomyopathy is a disorder characterized by a nondilated, hypertrophied left ventricle in the absence of any overt cause. The disease is characterized hemodynamically by increased contractility, outflow tract obstruction (exclusively in the case of hypertrophic obstructive cardiomyopathy) and delayed relaxation with decreased diastolic distensibility. The cause of the disease is unknown. Approximately 50% of the patients exhibit an autosomal dominant trait. Very recently, two laboratory observations were published indicating that abnormal calcium handling might be the pathophysiological link between inheritance and the above mentioned hemodynamic features: abnormal increased Ca^{2+} transients in human myocardium could be detected by means of the aequorin luminescence technique (79) and increased 1,4 dihydropyridine binding, suggesting an increased density of voltage-sensitive Ca^{2+} channels (80).

These findings may be the rationale for the beneficial effects of calcium channel blocker treatment, especially verapamil, in hypertrophic cardiomyopathy. Verapamil reduces hypercontractility and decreases the outflow pressure gradient concomitantly with an improvement in diastolic function (81,82).

In a longitudinal study comparing the effects of 2 years of verapamil with propranolol treatment, verapamil was superior to propranolol (83). In a 10 year trial (mean 52 months), 84 patients were treated with a mean daily dosage of 515 mg verapamil. They exhibited a reduction of left atrial diameter and ECG-derived indices for left ventricular hypertrophy (84). Thus, due to abnormal Ca^{2+} handling in hypertrophic cardiomyopathy, treatment with calcium channel blockers (mainly verapamil) seems to be indicated. The efficacy of this therapy and the beneficial long-term results make verapamil a first-line agent.

B. Idiopathic Dilated Cardiomyopathy

Knowledge of the cause of human idiopathic dilated cardiomyopathy (IDC) remains limited. Numerous possible factors might affect systolic function in DCM; on the cellular level, however, only a few pathogenic mechanisms may be taken into consideration:

1. Quantitative or qualitative abnormalities of the contractile proteins
2. Disorders of energy production due to mitochondrial failure
3. Abnormalities of energy utilization due to β-receptor modifications and coupling
4. Structural or functional disintegrity of the sarcolemmal membrane

In reference to mechanism 1, the contractile proteins in IDC were investigated and it was found that a structural alteration or functional defect of myofibrils does not seem to be primarily involved in the pathogenesis of reduced contractility (85). For 2, mitochondrial dysfunction in IDC seems possible. With respect to 3, an increase in the inhibitory component or decrease of the stimulatory subunits of the g-protein adenylate cyclase complex are possible. However, the results so far are varied (86–88).

With respect to 4, disorders of the sarcolemmal membrane are most likely. They may be due to virus infection, toxic effects (e.g., ethanol), catecholamines, ischemia induced by microcirculatory disorders, or unknown mechanisms such as binding of autoantibodies (89).

Membrane disruption in IDC can be determined using a new method, the antimyosin imaging technique. Indium 111-labeled antimyosin images myocardium if the cell membranes are disrupted (90). About half of all patients with IDC had a positive antimyosin scan (91).

Viral infection can cause membrane permeabilization due to integration of virus proteins in the sarcoplasmic bilayer. The latter might activate an autoimmunogenic response due to mimicry of viral proteins within the human sarcolemma (92). Recently, enterovirus replication was detected within myocardial tissue in 12–27% of patients with IDC using Coxsackie B cDNA hybridization techniques (93,94).

Ethanol is also held to be a risk factor in the development of IDC. Long-term administration of ethanol in animals is known to produce myocardial changes such as enlargement of the sarcoplasmic reticulum, swelling of mitochondria, and lipid deposition. By means of nuclear magnetic resonance spectroscopy in isolated hearts on ethanol-induced cardiac depression and in Syrian hamster cardiomyopathy, Wu and co-workers (95,96) showed that the phosphorylation potential decreases. The latter could be prevented by concomitant verapamil ingestion, probably due to prevention of an excessive mitochondrial calcium loading (95). It is hypothesized that alcohol produces membrane abnormalities that lead to adverse ion flux, and that these are largely prevented by concurrent administration of verapamil (95).

Increased adrenergic stimulation through both local neural and circulating catecholamines may lead to myopathic effects by two mechanisms (97): first, the mitochondria become overloaded with calcium due to excess phosphorylation of the slow inward membrane channels, and, second, the increased calcium influx activates membrane-bound phospholipases and proteases, which subsequently begin to autodigest surrounding sarcolemmal membranes (98). In human heart tissue obtained during heart transplantation of IDC patients, intracellular Ca^{2+} transients recorded during isometric contractions exhibited two distinct components: increased Ca^{2+} entry via voltage-dependent channels and slowed restoration to low diastolic Ca^{2+} concentration (79).

Microcirculatory disorders can be prevented, as shown in the cardiomyopathic Syrian hamster, with pretreatment of verapamil (99). Thus, the results described thus far underline the importance of investigating calcium antagonists in IDC more closely (100,101) (Fig. 5).

In a recent open trial, 22 patients were treated with diltiazem and compared to a historical control group of 25 patients. The aim of this study was to determine mortality, hemodynamic course, and clinical complaints. At the beginning of the trial, the patient groups were not different with respect to age, sex, or duration of symptoms, hemodynamic indices, ethanol consumption, and concomitant therapy. However, the mortality varied strikingly: mean survival was 29 months in the control group, whereas *no* patient in the diltiazem group died over a mean follow-up period of 15.4 months ($p < 0.001$). Mean left ventricular ejection fraction (LVEF) increased from 0.34 to 0.44 ($p < 0.001$), and functional classification according to the New York Heart Association improved significantly in the diltiazem treated group and in the crossover patients during the diltiazem period; these deteriorated, however, in the control group (78).

In conclusion, on the basis of these theoretical considerations, calcium antagonists seem to have several important effects in IDC. Therefore, a double-blind, multicenter, placebo-controlled trial (DiDi trial) is now underway in Germany.

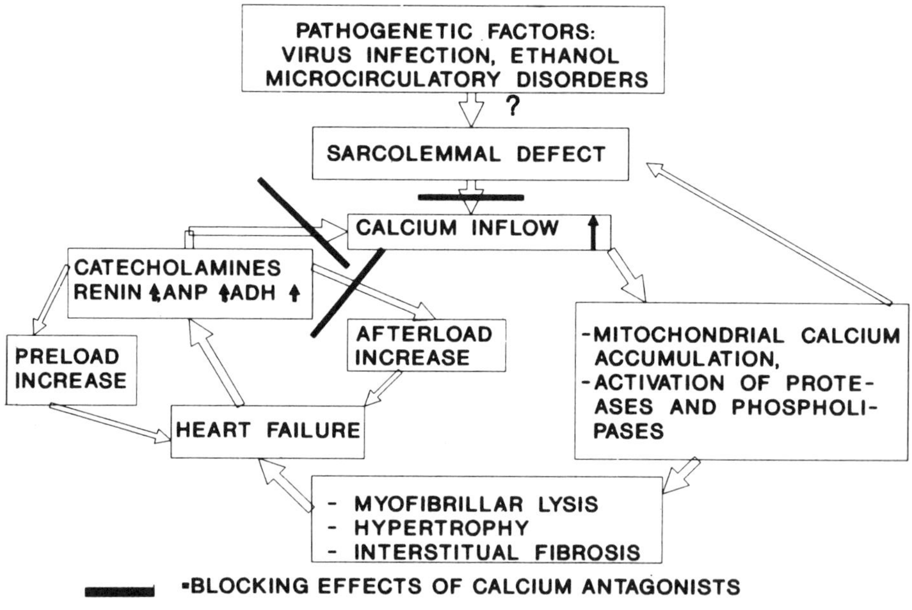

Figure 5 Rationale for the use of calcium antagonists in idiopathic dilated cardiomyopathy. Unknown pathogenetic factors might induce a sarcolemmal defect with concomitant increased calcium inflow, mitochondrial calcium accumulation, and activation of proteases and phospholipases. The latter could induce myocardial destruction leading to LV dysfunction, with compensatory neuroendocrine secretion and further calcium inflow via β-receptor stimulation. Calcium channel blockers could possibly lower elevated calcium inflow due to sarcolemmal destruction and neuroendocrine secretion and reduce elevated afterload. (Ref. 101.)

VII. SYSTEMIC HYPERTENSION

The main hemodynamic derangement in established essential systemic hypertension is increased systemic vascular resistance. The precise reason for this is unknown; however, it may be attributed to a genetically determined increase of the renal alpha-receptor density (102), which will lead to increased water and sodium resorption. Diminished sodium clearance induces intracellular sodium elevation. Sodium is eliminated through the sodium–Ca^{2+} exchange, leading to elevated intracellular Ca^{2+} activity in the vascular smooth muscle cell (103). Evidence for abnormal Ca^{2+} handling in essential hypertension was derived from two observations.

First regional (e.g., arteria brachialis) infusion of diverse calcium channel blockers caused a greater increase in forearm bloodflow than in normotensive subjects. The response to sodium nitroprusside, however, was similar. The similar response to the noncalcium-dependent vasodilator nitroprusside and the difference with respect to calcium channel blockers suggests a greater dependency of vascular resistance to calcium influx in hypertensive than normotensive subjects (104).

Second, in azygous vein cells harvested from spontaneously hypertensive rats, calcium inflow was increased through L-type slow channels (105) and, in the same animals, abnormal Ca^{2+} regulation could be restored with calcium channel blockers (106).

Although the affinity of the 1,4 dihydropyridines for the vascular smooth muscle cells is enhanced compared with the calcium channel blockers of groups I and II (verapamil, diltiazem), this difference could be overcome by the use of increased dosages of group I and II agents (104). Thus, in clinical practice, all calcium channel blockers lower blood pressure, if applied as monotherapy, in 40–70% of all patients (107,108). Monotherapy with calcium channel blockers was compared with several drugs and was found to be as effective as propranolol (an nonselective β-blocker), hydrochlorothiazide- and labetolol (104).

Nifidepine given sublingually has frequently been used for hypertensive crisis or the rapid control of severe hypertension. Decreases in blood pressure do not exceed normal values, and therefore, because of the efficacy, ease of administration as sublingual capsules, and because there is no need for invasive monitoring, nifedipine has become a first-line agent in these situations.

Since calcium channel blockers lack detrimental effects on lipid and carbohydrate metabolism, and have antianginal and antisclerotic effects, they have become an ideal therapy in the elderly hypertensive patient with or without coronary heart disease, diabetes mellitus, peripheral vascular disease, and beginning renal failure (109). These elderly hypertensive patients are characterized by an increased peripheral vascular resistance in combination with a diminished cardiac output, low plasma volume and impaired baroreceptor function (110). In these patient groups, and probably also in black patients, calcium channel blockers are effective (Fig. 6) and superior to β-blockers.

Therefore, calcium channel blockers have been incorporated into the latest proposal of the Joint National Committee on Detection, Evaluation and Treatment of High Blood Pressure (JNC), together with diuretics, β-blockers, and angiotensin-converting enzyme inhibitors, as step one treatment (111) until the Veterans Administration Cooperative Study Groups trial provides further information. This study will compare placebo, ochlorothiazide, atenolol, elonidine, prazosin, captopril, and diltiazem monotherapy for hypertension. It is scheduled to be completed at the end of 1990.

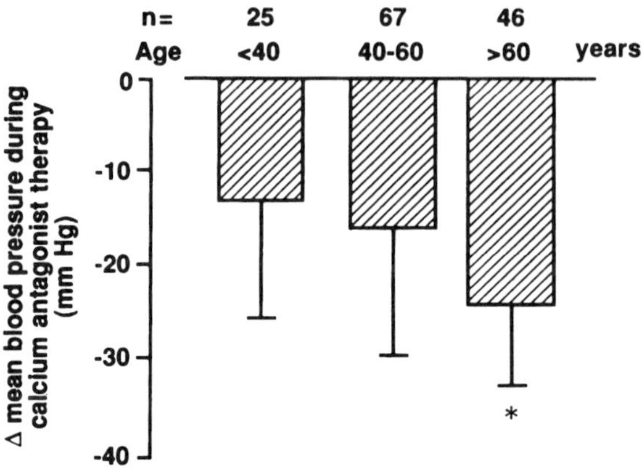

Figure 6 Bar graph shows mean blood pressure response to calcium antagonists in three age groups of patients after an average of 3 months of monotherapy. Patients older than 60 years, on average, had a significantly (*$p < 0.05$) greater reduction of blood pressure than patients aged less than 40 years. Values are mean ± SD. (Ref. 104.)

VIII. PRIMARY PULMONARY HYPERTENSION

In primary pulmonary hypertension (PPH), pathologic findings show intimal thickening of nonmuscular pulmonary arteries; medial hyperplasia; and, plexiform lesions (i.e., dilated thin-walled side branches, probably resulting from endothelial proliferation). Although there are severe structural and functional alterations in the pulmonary circulation, calcium channel blockers result in some reduction of pulmonary vascular resistance and improved survival (for review, see 112). However, conclusions derived from small trials are conflicting; in some cases, verapamil or nifedipine induced further deterioration of right ventricular function.

Thus, at present calcium channel blockers cannot be recommended for routine therapy in primary pulmonary hypertension since only a minority will respond to this treatment it remains to be proven whether they are superior to other vasodilators.

IX. MYOCARDIAL PROTECTION

In the resting myocyte the Ca^{2+} concentration outside of the cell is about 10,000 times higher than inside. The maintenance of this concentration gradient is dependent on an intact cell membrane with its ion-selective channels as well as proper functioning of energy-dependent ion pumps. According to our present knowledge, calcium enters the cell during depolarization through voltage-dependent channels whose functional capacity is regulated by cyclic AMP. A major mechanism to extrude calcium depends on the electrochemical gradient for Na^+ through a Na^+-Ca^{2+} exchange (113).

Due to the higher electrochemical gradient for Ca^{2+} ions with any irregularity of the Na^+-Ca^{2+} exchange, cyclic AMP generation and degeneration, Ca^{2+} will readily enter the cell. This could be shown during brief periods of ischemia (34,35). This increase in cytosolic calcium is thought to result in myocardial cell death (114), possibly due to an activation of Ca^{2+}-dependent ATPases, as well as lipases, proteases, and loss of mitochrondrial membrane integrity.

Calcium channel blockers selectively block the slow calcium-type channel. According to Kowalchuk and Nesto (56), there are several reasons to doubt that Ca^{2+} transients through the slow-inward channel are the predominant source of calcium inflow during ischemia. In experimental models measuring calcium uptake after a short period of myocardial ischemia, calcium channel blockers could not reliably delay calcium uptake. Despite these observations, numerous studies investigated the effect of reperfusion injury (for review, see 115) and consequently showed variable results.

During cardiopulmonary bypass, global ischemia occurs in the myocardium. To minimize myocellular injury during cardiac surgery, cardioplegia is initiated. In trials investigating the effects of the addition of nifedipine in the cardioplegic solution, a better postoperative recovery was demonstrated concomitant with serum creatine kinase and serum aspertate aminotransferase levels significantly lower than in the absence of nifedipine (116).

During percutaneous transluminal coronary angioplasty, regional coronary ischemia is unavoidable during balloon inflation. Various calcium channel blockers administered prior to or during occlusion increased ischemia tolerance time, accelerated diastolic and systolic recovery, and decreased coronary sinus lactate levels, probably due to a regional cardioplegic effect (117).

Table 6 Indications for Treatment with Calcium Channel Blockers in Cardiovascular Diseases

	Nifedipine	Diltiazem	Verapamil	Remarks
Arrhythmias				
Atrial	i	e	e	
Accesory bundle	i	i	i	
Ventricular	i	u	u	
Ischemic heart disease				
Prinzmetal's angina	e	e	e	
Unstable angina	i	i	i	Effective in combination with β-blocker, predominantly verapamil and diltiazem
Stable angina	e	e	e	
Non-Q-wave infarct	u	e	(e)	
Q-wave infarct	i	i	(e)	Verapamil is effective in the later course with preserved LV function
Silent angina	(e)	e	e	
Coronary sclerosis	(i)	u	u	
Heart failure				
Acute	(e)	(e)	i	
Chronic	i	i	i	
Hypertrophic cardiomyopathy	(e)	(e)	e	
Idiopathic dilated cardiomyopathy	u	(e)	u	
Systemic hypertension	e	e	e	Especially in the elderly and black patients
Pulmonary hypertension	(e)	(e)	i	
Organ protection	(i)	(e)	(e)	

i, Ineffective; e, effective; u, unknown; (), not well documented.

X. CONCLUSIONS

Due to the important function of intracellular calcium ion activity as a regulator of pacemaker activity, conduction velocity, contractility, and smooth muscle vascular tone, the inhibition of these ion transients by the application of calcium channel blockers will induce a wide variety of beneficial, therapeutic, and detrimental effects. This chapter has attempted to update the several thousands of studies on these agents in the treatment of cardiovascular diseases. Several questions remain unresolved. Table 6 provides a summary of treatment with calcium channel blockers at the time of writing in 1990.

REFERENCES

1. Fleckenstein A, Kammermeier H, Döring HJ, Freund HJ. Zum Wirkungsmechanismus neuartiger Koronardilatoren mit gleichzeitig Sauerstoff-einsparenden Myokardeffekten. Z Kreislaufforsch 1967; 56:716–44.
2. Reuter H, Beeler GW. Calcium current and activation of contraction in ventricular myocardial fibres. Science 1964; 163:399–401.
3. Kohlhardt M, Bauer B, Krause H, Fleckenstein A. Differentiation of the transmembrane Na and Ca channel in mammalian cardiac fibres by the use of specific inhibitors. Pflügers Arch Ges Physiol 1972; 335:309–22.
4. Vanhoutte PM, Paoletti R. The WHO classification of calcium antagonists. Trends Pharmacol Sci 1987; 8:4–5.
5. Zelis R, Moor R. Recent insights into calcium channels. Circulation 1989; 80 (Suppl IV): 14–6.
6. Nowycky MC, Fox AP, Tsien RW. Three types of neuronal calcium channels with different calcium antagonist sensitivity. Nature 1985; 316:440–3.
7. Glossmann H, Ferry DR, Goll A, Striesnig J, Zernig Y. Calcium channels and calcium channel drugs: recent biochemical and biophysical findings. Arzneim Forsch (Drug Res) 1985; 35:1917–35.
8. Boddeke E, Hugtenburg J, Jap W, Heynis J, van Zwieten P. New anti-ischaemic drugs: cytoprotective action with no primary haemodynamic effects. Trends Pharmacol Sci 1984; 10:397–400.
9. Fleckenstein A. The calcium channel of the heart. Ann NY Acad Sci 1988; 522:1–15.
10. Kohlhardt M, Figulla HR, Tripathi O. The slow membrane channel as the predominant mediator of the excitation process of the sinoatrial pacemaker cell. Basic Res Cardiol 1976; 71:17–26.
11. Okada T, Konishi T. Effect of verapamil on SA and AV nodal action potentials in the isolated rabbit heart. Jpn Circ J 1975; 39:913–17.
12. Krikler D, Spurrell AJ. Verapamil in the treatment of paroxsymal supraventricular tachycardia. Postgrad Med J 1974; 50:447–53.
13. Akhtar M, Tchou P, Jazayeri M. Use of calcium channel entry blockers in the treatment of cardiac arrhythmias. Circulation 1989; 80 (Suppl IV): 31–9.
14. Ochs HR, Anda L, Eichelbaum M, Greenblatt DJ. Diltiazem, verapamil and quinidine in patients with chronic atrial fibrillation. J Clin Pharmacol 1985; 25:204–9.
15. Levy MN. Role of calcium in arrhythmogenesis. 1989; Circulation 80 (Suppl IV): 23–30.
16. Katzung BG. Effects of extracellular calcium and sodium on depolarization-induced automaticity in guinea pig papillary muscle. Circ Res 1975; 37:118–27.
17. Katzung BG, Morgenstern JA. Effects of extracellular potassium on ventricular automaticity and evidence for a pacemaker current in mammalian ventricular myocardium. Circ Res 1977; 40:105–11.

18. Nordin C, Gilet E, Aronson R. Delayed after depolarizations and triggered activity in ventricular muscle with streptozytocin-induced diabetes. Circ Res 1985; 57:28–34.
19. Ferrier G, Moe G. Effect of calcium on acethyl strophantidin-induced transient depolarizations in canine Purkinje tissue. Circ Res 1973; 33:508–15.
20. Nordin C. Basic relationships between congestive heart failure and ventricular arrhythmias. Heart Failure 1986; 1:256–70.
21. Matsuda H, Noma K, Kurachi Y, et al. Transient depolarizations and spontaneous voltage fluctuations in isolated single cells from guinea pig ventricles. Calcium mediated potential fluctuations. Circ Res 1982; 51:142–51.
22. Tanabe T, Yoshikawa H, Tagawa R, Furuya H, Ide M, Yoto Y. Evaluation of antiarrhythmic drug efficacy using Holter electrographic technique. Jpn Circ J 1985; 49:337–44.
23. Massuni RA, Marin J, Vdhojc VN. Verapamil in parasystolic ventricular tachycardia and other wide QRS rhythms. Am Heart J 1986; 111:400–5.
24. Millard RW, Grupp G, Grupp IL, Disako J, Dopover A, Schwartz A. Chronotropic, inotropic and vasodilator actions of diltiazem, nifedipine and verapamil. Circ Res 1983; (Suppl I):29–39.
25. Hugenholtz PG. Calcium antagonists. In: Abshagen LV, ed. Clinical pharmacology of antianginal drugs. Berlin: Springer, 1985: 499–538.
26. Wibo M. Mode of action of calcium antagonists, voltage-dependence and kinetics of drug receptor interaction. Pharmacol Toxicol 1989; 65:1–8.
27. Taylor SG, Weston H. Endothelium-derived hyperpolarizing factor: a new endogenous inhibitor from the vascular endothelium. Trends Pharmacol Sci 1988; 9:272–4.
28. Lindner E. Phenyl-propyl-diphenyl-propyl-amin, eine neue Substanz mit coronargefäßerweiternder Wirkung. Arzneimittelforsch (Drug Res) 1969; 10:569.
29. Haas H, Härtfelder Y. Alpha-isoprophyl (N-methylhomoveratryl)-aminopropyl-34,-dimethoxyphenylacetonitrol, eine Substanz mit coronargefäßerweiternden Eigenschaften. Arzneimittelforsch (Drug Res) 1962; 12:549.
30. Chew CYC, Brown BG, Singh BM, et al. Mechanism of action of verapamil in ischemic heart disease: observations on changes in systemic and coronary hemodynamics and coronary vasomobility. Clin Invest Med 1980; 3:151–8.
31. Bache RJ. Effects of calcium entry blockade on myocardial blood flow. Circulation 1989; 80 (Suppl IV):40–6.
32. Bache RJ, Tockman BA. Effect of nitroglycerin and nifedipine on subendocardial perfusion in the presence of a flow-limiting coronary stensosis in the awake dog. Circ Res 1982; 50:678–87.
33. Bache RJ, Dymek DJ. Effect of diltiazem on myocardial blood flow. Circulation 1982; 65 (Suppl I): 19–26.
34. Steenbergen C, Murphy E, Levy L, London RE. Elevation in cytosolic free calcium concentration early in myocardial ischemia in perfused rat heart. Circ Res 1987; 60:700–171.
35. Marban E, Kitakaze M, Kusoka H, Porterfield JK, Yue DT, Chacko VP. Intracellular free calcium concentration measured with 19F NMR spectroscopy in intact ferret hearts. Proc Natl Acad Sci USA 1987; 84:6005–7.
36. Lahiri A, Rodrigues EA, Carboni GP, Raftery EB. Effects of long-term treatment with calcium antagonists on left ventricular diastolic function in stable angina and heart failure. Circulation 1990; 81 (Suppl III): 130–8.
37. Walsh RA. The effect of calcium entry blockade on normal and ischemic ventricular diastolic function. Circulation 1989; 80 (Suppl IV):52–28.
38. Braunwald E. Mechanisms of action of calcium channel blocking agents. N Engl J Med 1982; 307:1618–27.
39. Subramanian VB. Calcium channel blockers in chronic stable angina. A review. Herz 1982; 7:211–20.

40. Johnston DC, Lesoway R, Humen DP, Kostuk WJ. Clinical and hemodynamic evaluation of propranolol in combination with verapamil, nifedipine and diltiazem in exertional angina pectoris: a placebo-controlled, double-blind, randomized cross-over study. Am J Cardiol 1985; 55:680–7.
41. Subramanian VB. Combined therapy with calcium channel and beta-blockers: facts, fiction and practical aspects. Cardiovasc Rev Rep 1986; 7:259–74.
42. Packer M, Meller J, Medina N, et al. Hemodynamic consequences of combined beta-adrenergic and slow calcium channel blockade in man. Circulation 1982; 65:660–8.
43. Belber GA. Calcium antagonists in the treatment of Prinzmetal's angina and unstable angina pectoris. Circulation 1989; 80 (Suppl IV):78–87.
44. Winniford MD, Gabliami G, Johnson SM, et al. Concomitant calcium antagonist plus isosorbide dinitrate therapy for markedly active variant angina. Am Heart J 1984; 108:1269–73.
45. Fuster V, Badimon L, Cohen M, Ambrose JA, Badimon JJ, Chesebr Y. Insight into the pathogenesis of acute ischemic syndrome. Circulation 1988; 77:1213–20.
46. Muller JE, Turi ZG, Parle DL, et al. Nifedipin and conventional therapy for unstable angina pectoris. A randomized double-blind comparison. Circulation 1984; 69:728–39.
47. Lubsen J, Tijissen JGP, Kerkamp HJJ. Early treatment of unstable angina in the coronary care unit. Br Heart J 1984; 56:400–13.
48. Held PH, Yusuf S, Furberg CD. Calcium channel blockers in acute myocardial infarction and unstable angina: an overview. Br Med J 1989; 299:1187–92.
49. Bisset JK, Matts J, Sharma B. The program on surgical control for hyperlipidemia study group: residual myocardial jeopardy in patients with Q-wave and non-Q-wave infarctions. Br Heart J 1987; 58:460–4.
50. Hoshimato T, Kambara H, Fudo T, et al. Non-Q-wave versus Q-wave myocardial infarction: regional myocardial metabolism and bloodflow assessed by positron emission tomography. J Am Coll Cardiol 1988; 12:88–93.
51. Gibson RS. Non-Q-wave myocardial infarction: diagnosis, prognosis and management. Curr Probl Cardiol 1988; 13:9–72.
52. Gibson RS, Boden WE, Theroux P, et al. Diltiazem and reinfarction in patients with non-Q-wave myocardial infarction. Results of a double-blind, randomized, multicenter trial. N Engl J Med 1986; 315:423–9.
53. The Multicenter Diltiazem Postinfarction Trial Research Group. The effect of diltiazem on mortality and reinfarction after myocardial infarction. N Engl J Med 1988; 319:385–92.
54. Boden WE, Krone RJ, Kleiger RE, et al. Diltiazem reduces long-term cardiac event rate after non-Q-wave infarction. Multicenter Diltiazem Post Infarction Trial (MDPIT). Circulation 1988; 78 (Suppl II):96.
55. Roberts R. Thrombolysis and its sequelae. Calcium antagonists as potential adjunctive therapy. Circulation 1989; 80 (Suppl IV):93–101.
56. Kowalchuk GJ, Nesto RW. Calcium antagonists and myocardial protection. Am J Cardiol 1989; 64:10–7F.
57. Gibson RS. Current status of calcium channel-blocking drugs after Q-wave and non-Q-wave myocardial infarction. Circulation 1989; 80 (Suppl IV):107–19.
58. Muller JE, Morrison J, Stone PH, et al. Nifedipine therapy for patients with threatened and acute myocardial infarction: a randomized double-blind, placebo-controlled comparison. Circulation 1984; 69:740–7.
59. The Danish Study Group on Verapamil in Myocardial Infarction. Verapamil in acute myocardial infarction. Eur Heart J 5:516–528, 1984
60. The Danish Study Group on Verapamil in Myocardial Infarctions. Effects of verapamil on mortality and major events after acute myocardial infarction (The Danish verapamil infarction trial II—DAViT II). Am J Cardiol 1990; 66:779–785.

61. Fleg JL, Gerstenblith G, Zonderman AB, et al. Prevalence and prognostic significance of exercise-induced silent myocardial ischemia detected by thallium scintigraphy and electrocardiography in asymtomatic volunteers. Circulation 1990; 81:428–36.
62. Rozanski A, Berman DS. Silent myocardial ischemia. Am Heart J 1987; 114:615–38.
63. Theroux P, Waters DD, Halpher C, DeBaisieux JC, Mizgala HF. Prognostic value of exercise testing soon after myocardial infarction. N Engl J Med 1979; 301:341–5.
64. Crawford HM. Theoretical considerations in the use of calcium entry blockers in silent myocardial ischemia. Circulation 1989; 80 (Suppl IV):74–7.
65. Frey M, Zorn J, Fleckenstein A, Fleckenstein-Grün G. Protection of arterial and arterolar wall structure by specific calcium antagonists. NY Acad Sci 1988; 522:420–32.
66. Weinstein DB, Heider JG. Antiatherogenic properties of calcium antagonists. Am J Med 1989; 86 (Suppl 4A):27–32.
67. Henry PD. Calcium antagonists as antiatherogenic agents. NY Acad Sci 1988; 522: 411–9.
68. Lichtlen PR, Hugenholtz P, Rafflenbeul W, Jost T, Hecker H. Intact study group: retardation of the progression of coronary artery disease with nifedipine. Results of Intact. Circulation 1989; 80 (Suppl II):382.
69. Packer M. Pathophysiologic mechanisms underlying the adverse effects of calcium-blocking drugs in patients with chronic heart failure. Circulation 1989; 80 (Suppl IV): 59–67.
70. Figulla HR, Kreuzer H, Luig H. Verpamil, diltiazem and nifedipin bei schwerer links-ventrikulärer Funktionsstörung. Eine Vergleichsstudie der hämodynamischen Akut-wirkungen. Dtsch Med Wochenschr 1986; 111:11–4.
71. Walsh RW, Porter CB, Starling MR, O'Rourke RA. Beneficial hemodynamic effects of intravenous and oral diltiazem in severe congestive heart failure. J Am Coll Cardiol 1984; 3:1044–50.
72. Barjon JN, Rouleau JL, Bichet D, Jeneau C, de Champlain J. Chronic renal and neurohumeral effects of the calcium entry blocker nisoldipine in patients with congestive heart failure. J Am Coll Cardiol 1987; 9:622–30.
73. Cohn JN, Levine TB, Olivare MT, et al. Plasma norepinephrine as a guide to prognosis in patients with chronic congestive heart failure. N Engl J Med 1984; 311:819–23.
74. Packer M. Neurohormonal interactions and adaptations in congestive heart failure. Circulation 1988; 77:721–30.
75. Figulla HR, Luig H, Nieschlag F, Kreuzer H. Klinische und hämodynamische Wirkungen von Nisoldipin und Captopril bei der Herzinsuffizienz. Eine doppelblinde Vergleichsstudie der Kurz- und Langzeitwirkungen. Z Kardiol 1987; 76:167–74.
76. Pfeffer MA, Lamas GA, Vaughn DE, Parisi AF, Braunwald E. Effect of captopril on progressive ventricular dilatation after anterior myocardial infarcts. N Engl J Med 1988; 319:80–6.
77. The CONSENSUS Trial Study Group. Effect of enalapril on mortality in severe congestive heart failure. N Engl J Med 1987; 316:1429–35.
78. Figulla HR, von Rechenberg J, Wiegand V, Soballa R, Kreuzer H. Beneficial effects of long-term diltiazem treatment in dilated cardiomyopathy. J Am Coll Cardiol 1989; 13:653–8.
79. Gwathmey JK, Copelas L, MacKinnon R, Schoen FJ, Feldman MD, Grossmann W, Morgan JP. Abnormal intracellular calcium handling in myocardium from patients with endstage heart failure. Circ Res 1987; 61:70–6.
80. Wagner JA, Sax FL, Weisman HF, et al. Calcium antagonist receptors in the atrial tissue of patients with hypertrophic cardiomyopathy. N Engl J Med 1984; 320:755–61.
81. Wigle ED. Hypertrophic cardiomyopathy: a 1987 viewpoint. Circulation 1987; 75: 311–22.
82. Rosing DR, Kint KM, Bover JS, Seides SF, Maron BJ, Epstein SE. Verapamil therapy:

a new approach to the pharmacologic treatment of hypertrophic cardiomyopathy. I. Hemodynamic effects. Circulation 1979; 60:1201–7.

83. Kober G, Hopf R, Biamino G, Bubenheimer P, Förster K, Kuck KH, Hanrath P, von Olshausen KE, Schlepper M, Kaltenbach M. Long-term treatment of hypertrophic cardiomyopathy with verapamil or propranolol in matched pairs of patients: results of a multicenter study. In: Kaltenbach M, Hopf R, Kunkel B, eds. New aspects of hypertrophic cardiomyopathy. Darmstadt: Steinkopff; New York: Springer, 1988: 191–201.
84. Hopf R, Kaltenbach M. 10 year results and survival of patients with hypertrophic cardiomyopathy treated with calcium antagonists. Z Kardiol 1987; 76 (Suppl 3):137–144.
85. Wiegand V, Ebecke M, Figulla HR, Schüler S, Kreuzer H. Structure and function of contractile proteins in human dilated cardiomyopathy. Clin Cardiol 1989; 12:656–60.
86. Neumann J, Schmitz W, Scholz H, Meyerinck VL, Döring V, Kalamar P. Increase in myocardial g_i. Lancet 1988; 22:936–7.
87. Horn EM, Corvin SJ, Steinberg SF, Chow YK, Neuberg GW, Cannon PJ, Powers ER, Bilezikian JP. Reduced lymphocyte stimulatory guanine nucleotide regulatory protein and β-adrenergic receptors in congestive heart failure and reversal with angiotensin-converting enzyme inhibitor therapy. Circulation 1988; 78:1373–9.
88. Bristow MR, Port JD, Sandovel AB, Rasmussen R, Ginsburg R, Feldmann AM. β-adrenergic receptor pathways in the failing human heart. Heart Failure 1989; 5:77–90.
89. Katz AM, Freston JW, Messineo FC, Herbette LG. Membrane damage and the pathogenesis of cardiomyopathies. J Mol Cell Cardiol 1985; 17 (Suppl 2):11–20.
90. Johnson LL, Lerrick KS, Coromilas J, et al. Measurement of infarct size and percentage myocardium infarcted in a dog preparation with single photon-emission computed tomography, thallium 201, and indium 111 monoclonal antimyosin Fab. Circulation 1987; 76:181–90.
91. Figulla HR, Munz DL, Bardosi A, Wiegand V. Myocardial imaging using indium 111 monoclonal antimyosin Fab in dilated cardiomyopathy. Circulation 1989; 80 (Suppl II):666.
92. Maisch B, Deeg P, Liebau G, Kochsiek K. Diagnostic relevance of humoral and cytotoxic immune reactions in primary and secondary cardiomyopathy. Am J Cardiol 1983; 52:1072–8.
93. Kandolf R, Hofschneider PH. Viral heart disease. Semin Immunopathol 1989; 11:1–13.
94. Bowles NE, Rose ML, Taylor P, et al. Endstage dilated cardiomyopathy: persistence of enterovirus RNA in myocardium at cardiac transplantation and lack of immune response. Circulation 1989; 80:1128–36.
95. Wu S, White R, Wikman-Coffelt J, et al. The preventive effect of verapamil on ethanol-induced cardiac depression: phosphorus-31 nuclear magnetic resonance and high pressure liquid chromatographic studies of hamsters. Circulation 1987; 75:1058–64.
96. Markiewicz W, Wu SS, Parmley WW, et al. Evaluation of the hereditary Syrian hamster cardiomyopathy by ^{31}P nuclear magnetic resonance spectroscopy: improvement after acute verapamil therapy. Circ Res 1986; 59:597–604.
97. Mann DL, Cooper G. Neurohumor activation in congestive heart failure: a doubled-edged sword? Clin Cardiol 1989; 12:485–90.
98. Nayler WG. Calcium and cell death. Eur Heart J 1983; 4 (Suppl C):33–8.
99. Figulla HR, Vetterlein F, Glaubitz M, Kreuzer H. Inhomogenous capillary flow and its prevention by verapamil and hydralazine in the cardiomyopathic Syrian hamster. Circulation 1987; 76:208–16.
100. Opie LH, Walpoth B, Barsacchi R. Calcium and catecholamines. Relevance to cardiomyopathies and significance in therapeutic strategies. J Moll Cell Cardiol 1985; 17 (Suppl 2):21–34.
101. Figulla HR, Kreuzer H. Arguments supporting the use of calcium antagonists in

idiopathic dilated cardiomyopathy. Theoretical considerations and clinical results. J Cardiovasc Pharmacol 1990; 16 (Suppl. 6):45–49.
102. Michel MC, Insel PA, Brodde OE. Renal alpha-adrenergic receptor alterations. A cause of essential hypertension. FASEB J 1989; 3:139.
103. Blaustein MP. Sodium ions, calcium ions, blood pressure regulation and hypertension. A reassement and a hypothesis. Am J Physiol 1989; 232:C165–73.
104. Kiowski W, Bolli P, Erne P, Müller FB, Hulthein UL, Bühler FR. Mechanisms of action and clinical use of calcium antagonists in hypertension. Circulation 1989; 80 (Suppl IV):136–44.
105. Rusch NJ, Hermsmeyer K. Calcium currents are altered in the vascular muscle cell membranes of spontaneously hypertensive rats. Circ Res 1988; 63:997–1002.
106. Erne P, Hermsmeyer K. Intracellular vascular muscle Ca^{2+} modulation in genetic hypertension. Hypertension 1989; 14:145–151.
107. Midtbo K, Heds O, von der Meer J. Verapamil compared with nifedipine in the treatment of essential hypertension. J Cardiovasc Pharmacol 1982; 4 (Suppl 3):36–8.
108. Klein W, Brand D, Vreck O, Harringer M. Role of calcium antagonists in the treatment of essential hypertension. Circ Res 1982; 52 (Suppl 1):174–81.
109. Busse JC, Matersen BJ. Geriatric hypertension: the growing use of calcium channel blockers. Geriatrics 1988; 43:51–9.
110. Messerli FH, Sungaard-Riise K, Ventura HO, Dunn FG, Glade LB, Frohlich ED. Essential hypertension in the elderly: hemodynamics, intravascular volume, plasma renin activity and circulating catecholamine levels. Lancet 1983; 2:983–6.
111. 1988 Joint National Committee. The 1988 report of the Joint National Committee on detection, evaluation and treatment of high blood pressure. Arch Intern Med 1988; 148:1023–38.
112. Packer M. Vasodilator therapy for primary pulmonary hypertension. Ann Intern Med 1985; 103:258–70.
113. Reiter M. Calcium mobilisation and cardiac inotropic mechanisms. Pharmacol Rev 1984; 40:189–217.
114. Katz AM, Reuter H. Cellular calcium and cardiac cell death. Am J Cardiol 1979; 44:188–90.
115. Kloner RA, Braunwald E. Effects of calcium antagonists on infarcting myocardium. Am J Cardiol 1987; 59:84B–94B.
116. Hicks GL Jr, Salley RK, de Weese JA. Calcium channel blockers: an intraoperative and postoperative trial in women. Ann Thorac Surg 1984; 37:319–23.
117. Schlant RC, King III SB. Usefulness of calcium entry blockers during and after percutaneous transluminal coronary artery angioplasty. Circulation 1989; 80 (Suppl IV):88–92.

27

Role of the Sodium Channel on the Development of Force in Myocardium

G. MAURICE BRIGGS

Sterling Winthrop Pharmaceuticals Research Division, Rensselaer, New York

JUDITH K. GWATHMEY

Harvard Medical School, Boston, Massachusetts

Cardiac contraction follows depolarization of the sarcolemma by the action potential and the coupled release of calcium from the sarcoplasmic reticulum. The action potential is the coordinating event for contraction of the heart and is generated by voltage-dependent ion channels in the membrane. Sodium and calcium channels depolarize the sarcolemma and trigger calcium release while potassium channels repolarize the membrane. These channels are coupled with ionic pumps, sodium/potassium ATPase and the sodium/calcium exchanger in the membrane to maintain ionic homeostasis. These pumps also generate current, which contributes to the action potential. Alterations of channel function will affect not only the excitation contraction cycle but also ionic concentrations. The intracellular calcium concentration is sensitive to the sodium gradient across the membrane since sodium/calcium exchange is a major determinant of intracellular calcium concentrations. It follows that alterations of sodium channel function will affect the contraction of the heart and there are now several lines of evidence to support this hypothesis. Several pharmacologic agents have been developed that modify sodium flux through sodium channels that also affect contraction.

I. BIOPHYSICAL DESCRIPTION OF THE SODIUM CHANNEL

Ion channels are thought of as pores across biological membranes. Since an open pathway across the membrane would allow ions to flow across the membrane, there must be a mechanism to regulate this flux. Channels are further characterized by their preference or selectivity for ionic species (i.e., sodium vs. potassium). Original investigations of nerve electrical activity were performed primarily using biophysical techniques. The most significant was the development of the voltage clamp. This allowed, for the first time, direct measurement of the ionic currents (conductance) that underlie the nerve action potential. The work of Hodgkin and colleagues in 1952 (1) is a milestone in this field. They arrived at a description of sodium channel function that continues to influence the interpretation of ion channel data today. They described a channel that was selective for sodium and controlled by two sets of "gates." There were three activation gates (m) and an inactivation gate (h). When the activation gates opened, sodium ions flowed through the channel until the inactivation gate closed. This characterization was based on an analysis of sodium current kinetics. The voltage-dependent activation gates opened faster than the inactivation gates closed. This is described by the equation:

$$I_{Na} = m^3 \, h \, g_{Na}(E\text{-}E_{Na})$$

where I_{Na} is the current; m and h represent the activation and inactivation gates, respectively; g_{Na} is the conductance; E is the membrane potential; and E_{Na} is the equilibrium potential for sodium. Thus a current was produced while the channel was transiently open. The biophysical approach to defining ion channel function was advanced in the 1950s by increased sophistication of the voltage clamp technique, which aided kinetic characterization. Radioisotopic techniques were also applied to investigate ion permeation. From these studies the structure of the channel was conceptualized as a pore across the membrane with a selectivity filter located within the pore. At the extracellular surface were the activation gates, while the inactivation gate was located at the intracellular surface.

In the 1960s further biochemical characterization of the sodium channel was achieved (2,3). The discovery of toxins that covalently bound to the channel facilitated isolation and purification of the channel protein. Sodium channels can be solubilized and then assayed by high-affinity binding to tetrodotoxin (TTX) or to saxitoxin (STX). The channel protein can then be purified. The rat brain sodium channel is composed of three subunits (260 kDa α , a 36 kDa β_1, and a 33 kDa β_2 subunit). However, sodium channels purified from the eel electroplax contain only an α subunit. The β_1 subunit is covalently attached to the α subunit while the β_2 subunit is linked to the α subunit by disulfide bonds. Both the α and the β_1 are covalently labeled by toxins and are heavily glycosylated. Reconstitution of these proteins into phospholipid vesicles was found to have selective sodium conductance by radiosotopic flux measurements. Purified sodium channels were activated and inactivated by the appropriate toxins. Thus these proteins provide selectivity, flux rates, and pharmacologic binding similar to those of in situ sodium channels.

The development of the patch clamp and lipid bilayer clamp techniques in the 1970s greatly enhanced the biophysical characterization of the sodium channel (4,5). We will consider the influence of the patch clamp technique on sodium channel function in the next section. Here we will concentrate on the structural details revealed by the bilayer reconstitution technique. Reconstitution of the purified protein from rat brain responded as a sodium channel with appropriate conductances, voltage dependence, and gating charge movement (6). The β subunits can be removed from the α subunit. Removal of the β_2 subunit does not affect the function of the reconstituted channel. However, removal of the β_1 subunit abolishes function. Reconstitution of the channel from eel electroplax (α only) provides a functional channel. The mammalian α subunit can be forced into a functional channel by the formation of intramolecular isopeptide bonds. The β_1 subunit would seem to play a role in stabilizing the functional α subunit (7).

II. STRUCTURE OF THE VOLTAGE-SENSITIVE SODIUM CHANNEL

Molecular biology arrived in the 1980s and provided a powerful new tool for the study of ion channels. We will briefly review the advances in channel structure (for more detailed information see several recent reviews, 8–12). Determination of the protein primary structure was facilitated as a result of purification of the channel protein. In 1984 Noda *et al.* (13) reported the primary structure of the eel electoplax channel, which consisted of 1832 amino acids. It was subsequently found that the sodium channel α subunit from rat brain is encoded by three genes (14,15). These channel proteins contain 2008–2012 amino acids. All of the α subunit proteins contain four repeated domains of 300–400 amino acids that are highly conserved.

Several models have been proposed for the secondary structure of the channel (11, 16–19). A model of the general transmembrane organization is illustrated in Figure 1, which is supported by several lines of evidence. Each of the repeated domains contain six to eight hydrophobic segments that can be arranged as transmembrane α helices (18). This is analogous to the nicotinic acetylcholine channel subunits, which also form a pore (20). The segments consist of 20 amino acid residues with a length of ~30 Å. This length is sufficient to span the membrane.

The voltage dependence of activation requires that there be a region of strong dipole or charged amino acid residues within the membrane electric field. The S4 segment contains both hydrophobic and high charge residues. This S4 segment is highly conserved in all cloned voltage-sensitive channels. This may be the voltage sensor (11). Proposed models provide the expected amount of charge movement for gating.

Inactivation is thought to be a weakly voltage-dependent process that is apparently voltage dependent due to coupling to highly voltage-dependent activation (21,22). The portion of the protein that controls inactivation is thought to be intracellular since it is removed by intracellular proteases. Antibodies to the segment between domains III and IV slow inactivation (23). Furthermore, there is a weak voltage dependence of antibody binding with greater binding at more negative potentials. This segment is also highly conserved.

Intracellular phosphorylation is known to affect sodium channel function. The α subunit is rapidly phosphorylated by cAMP-dependent protein kinase at 5 sites between domains I and II (11). STX is known to bind extracellularly and was found

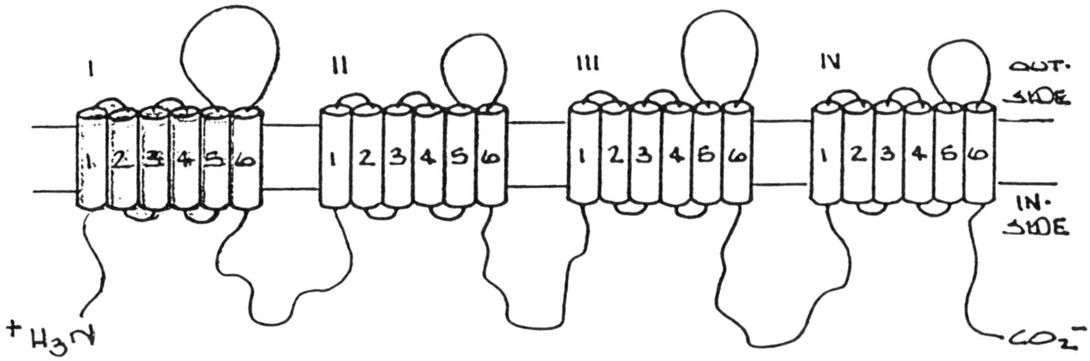

Figure 1 Schematic diagram of the architectural features of the α subunit primary sequence of the sodium channel.

to bind between segments S5 and S6. These segments are also found to be glycosylated, indicating an extracellular orientation. Binding of an antibody to the C terminus and to the segment between domain II and III has been found to be intracellular by electron microscopic evaluation.

The pore size formed by this model would be approximately 3 × 5 Å, which is consistent with that obtained from permeability size data (11). Furthermore, the selectivity of the sodium channel can be explained on the basis of aspartate and glutamate residues in the conserved sequence of the pore (9).

Functional sodium channels can be obtained by injecting frog oocytes with α subunit mRNA (15, 24–27). This implies that the β subunits are not necessary for channel function. However, the inactivation rates of these channels are different from those expressed from whole mRNA from rat brain (28,29). The inactivation rate of the α subunit channel can also be returned to normal by coexpression of a low-molecular-weight mRNA from rat brain (29). This indicates that the β subunits could act to modify channel function. It has recently been demonstrated that two separate types of gating responses can be encoded in a single primary structure of the channel protein (30). The human cardiac sodium channel has now been expressed from total RNA (31).

III. SODIUM CHANNEL FUNCTION

We have previously noted that the classic Hodgkin Huxley (1,32) characterization of function was that activation was fast and inactivation was slow. This interpretation has come under question (33) since the advent of single-channel recordings using the patch clamp technique (4,5). It is readily observable from such recordings that channel openings are discrete events. Each channel opens rapidly, remains open for a period, and then closes rapidly. This revelation required a new formulation to describe the sodium current. The current recorded from the whole cell (macroscopic current, I_{Na}) is related to the conductance (microscopic current, i_{Na}) of each channel, the probability (P_o) it will be open, and the number of channels (N) in the membrane:

$$I_{Na} = P_o * i_{Na} * N$$
$$i_{Na} = E\text{-}E_{Na}$$

The macroscopic current is therefore the summation (ensemble) of all the discrete single-channel events. Sodium channels have a higher density (N) relative to the calcium channel (34,35) in cardiac tissue.

While the classic interpretation from the macroscopic current is functionally correct it cannot be translated into molecular mechanisms. If inactivation is fast, why does it appear to be slow? The answer is that activation is actually slow. This has been demonstrated for neuroblastoma cells in which a channel will only open once for a voltage clamp step (33,36). It was observed that channels would open throughout the time course of the macroscopic current. Some channels would open early, while others opened later. Thus, macroscopic inactivation rate was the result of the latency or time until a channel would open. This is described by the latency function, which was determined to be voltage dependent. Inactivation is addressed by determining the mean open time of the channel. This is the reciprocal of the inactivation rate constant and is independent of membrane potential. There is an implicit assumption in this model that after a channel opens it is not available to reopen and a open channel has a single conductance level. Thus the time course of I_{Na} in neuroblastoma cells is primarily determined by the activation of new channels. The sodium channel can then be modeled with three states, a closed state (C) from which the channel can open, and the open state (O) from which the channel then inactivates (I) and can not reopen.

Before the development of the patch clamp technique, accurate determinations of ionic currents in cardiac tissue were extremely difficult to make. The maximal upstroke velocity (V_{max}) was used extensively as a substitute for direct measurements of I_{Na} (37,38). This is a convenient method but it is only qualitative due to the nonlinear relationship between V_{max} and I_{Na} (39–41). Sodium currents have now been investigated by several laboratories in cardiac muscle both macroscopically and microscopically (16,17,42–46). The description presented above for neuroblastoma cells of I_{Na} does not accurately describe the data from cardiac cells. In cardiac cells there are at least three areas in which differences have been reported. There are multiple conductance states (47,48), inactivation is voltage dependent (18,49–51), and channels can close and reopen before inactivating (47,49,51). Similar differences have been reported for other neural tissues (52) and skeletal muscle (17). These differences may be related to the primary function of the tissue source. Thus, where the need is for rapid conduction and sure firing all available channels open at one time and then close off. However, where the need is also for control of intracellular events, longer channel openings or reopenings may be needed. This conceptualization would fit the case in cardiac tissue, where both rapid conduction of the action potential and coordination with intracellular events are important. The concept can be extended to those neural tissues that must integrate signals from several sources. It is important to note that channels from different tissues have a similar primary structure (main) but slight modifications give specific new functions for particular tissues. These differences may reflect the subtle structural differences now known to exist in rat brain sodium channels. It has been argued that for cardiac sodium channels the functional differences can arise from a single channel. However, there is evidence for at least two separate channels (47). These questions are currently being addressed since cloning of cardiac sodium channels is currently underway. Much information is yet to be gained by the combination of molecular biological and electrophysiological techniques.

The observation that a channel can reopen means that a three-state model as presented above may not suffice. This has led to the formulation of a model in which there are several closed states (50,53). However, this more complicated view has been challenged (51).

The relatively long cardiac action potential duration is primarily maintained by the calcium current. However, pharmacologic agents that affect only the sodium channel also affect action potential duration (45). Prolonged channel openings, reopenings, or long latency periods for some channels can account for this. These processes could also be important in determining the refractory period, especially the voltage dependence of inactivation.

IV. PHYSIOLOGICAL ROLE OF SODIUM CHANNELS IN CONTRACTION

The question now arises as to what importance can be attributed to sodium channel function and cardiac muscle contraction. The remainder of this chapter will deal with the positive and negative influences of sodium channel function on cardiac contraction.

In 1871 Bowditch reported that the contractile force of the heart depended on heart rate. It was subsequently demonstrated that an increase in intracellular calcium was associated with this positive force-frequency effect (54). The mechanism for the increased calcium is now recognized as an increase in intracellular sodium (40,55–59). Intracellular sodium concentration is a balance between influx via sodium channels and efflux via the sodium/potassium ATPase. As is described in other chapters in this book, intracellular sodium is important in the activity of sodium/calcium exchange, which, in turn, is important in regulating intracellular calcium concentration.

Regulation of intracellular sodium can also explain the observed frequency and postrest contraction differences observed between rat and rabbit cardiac muscle. Rats demonstrate a negative force-frequency relationship and have a greater postrest contraction. Intracellular sodium levels are elevated in rats relative to rabbits (60). The explanation is that in rats the combination of a short plateau phase of the action potential and an elevated intracellular sodium level promote Ca^{++} efflux via sodium/calcium exchange during the contraction. At rest in rat cardiac muscle calcium influx is promoted, whereas the opposite would be expected in rabbits.

The influence of intracellular sodium concentration has been examined in several pathologic conditions in which there is altered cardiac function. Intracellular sodium was measured and found to be equal in normal and hypertrophied ferrets. However, hypertrophied muscle demonstrated a decreased time constant for sodium concentration equilibration with altered extracellular sodium (61). This indicates that in noncontracting hypertrophied muscle sodium concentration is the same, but there is an altered regulation. This may potentially affect muscle contractile force and time course. However, experiments to test this hypothesis have not been performed.

The phenomenon, known as the "calcium paradox," shows that after exposure of a cardiac muscle preparation to calcium-free solution followed by reperfusion with a calcium-containing solution there is a loss of function (62–65). There is a loss of intracellular content and loss of electrical activity followed by a massive rise in intracellular calcium and a strong contracture. The rise in intracellular calcium is responsible for the resultant damage. It has been demonstrated that the rise in intracellular calcium is the result of a rise in intracellular sodium. Upon removal of extracellular calcium, the calcium channel-lose selectivity and conduct sodium ions. Depolarization of the membrane activates these channels and sodium enters via the noninactivating channels. The resulting sodium influx leads to a rise in intracellular calcium via sodium/calcium exchange. However, the role of intracellular sodium in the calcium paradox has been refuted by van Echteld *et al.* (66).

Intracellular sodium levels have been demonstrated to be elevated (25 mM) during ischemia and reperfusion (66). This would lead to an increased intracellular calcium concentration, which underlies the loss of contractile function associated with ischemia and reperfusion. Takeo et al. (67) examined the role of intracellular sodium in the alterations in cardiac function during hypoxia and reoxygenation. The loss of cardiac function and the increase in diastolic tension were attenuated by concentrations of yohimbine that block sodium channels. They reported an increase in tissue sodium that was reversed by yohimbine. Meng and Pierce (68) have also reported a major role of intracellular sodium in the dysfunction associated with ischemia and reperfusion. They demonstrated a normalization of both function and sodium content after exposure to dimethyl-amiloride, which blocks sodium/hydrogen exchange.

A role for intracellular sodium in regulating the response of ion channels to cAMP has recently been put forward (69). Harvey et al. (69) report a decreased sensitivity of channels to phosphorylation-dependent regulation when intracellular sodium is decreased. The reverse could also exist: an increase in intracellular sodium would increase sensitivity. This could be important during treatment of heart failure with agents that increase intracellular sodium. These agents would also increase the responsiveness of the heart to adrenergic stimulation and promote arrhythmogenesis.

V. PHARMACOLOGY OF THE SODIUM CHANNEL

A. Toxin-Binding Sites

Much of the sodium channel purification was facilitated by specific binding of toxins. Five toxin-binding sites have been identified on the channel. 1. Site **I** binds tetrodotoxin, saxitoxin, and u-conotoxins (10,70). The latter toxin is a polypeptide believed to bind via multiple arginine residues. This binding site is located on the extracellular surface near the opening of the channel. Binding to this site is associated with inhibition of the channel. 2. Site **II** binds veratridine, batrachotoxin, aconitine, and grayanotoxin (10). These toxins are lipophilic and easily enter the membrane. Binding at site **II** results in a loss of inactivation and a negative voltage shift of activation. This site is associated with the portion of the channel that controls activation and inactivation. 3. Site **III** binds polypeptide α-scorpion toxins and sea anemone toxins (10). Binding to site **III** is affected by membrane potential, which indicates that the binding site is located on a portion of the channel involved in conformation changes. 4. Site **IV** binds b-scorpion toxins (71). There is a shift of the voltage dependence of activation produced by binding of these toxins. These are distinct from α-scorpion toxins. 5. Site **V** binds the polyether toxins brevetoxins and siguatoxins (72). These toxins produce a repetitive firing associated with decreased inactivation.

B. Influence on Contractility

1. Positive Inotropic Effect

Pharmacologic agents that affect the sodium channel also affect contractile force development. The plant alkaloid veratridine has been reported to prolong action potential duration and to increase developed force (73). This effect was prevented by substituting Li^+ for Na^+ or TTX, indicating a role of sodium channels in the inotropic effect. It was subsequently demonstrated that veratridine prevents inactivation of sodium channels (74) and increased intracellular sodium (75). Germitrine acts in a similar fashion (76). By prolonging the influx of sodium via sodium channels, there is an increase in intracellular calcium via sodium/calcium exchange. The effectiveness of vertridine on increasing ventricular contractility in human myocardium has been demonstrated (77).

DPI 201-106 is an agent developed as a positive inotrope and to which a separate chapter in this book is dedicated (78). DPI 201-106 has been demonstrated to act by preventing inactivation of sodium channels (49,79). We evaluated DPI 201-106 in human ventricular muscle from normal and myopathic hearts. There was a concentration-related effect on intracellular calcium and the contraction. The effects were similar to those produced by veratridine but dissimilar to BayK 8644 or increases in extracellular calcium. Figure 2 illustrates these effects on the contraction

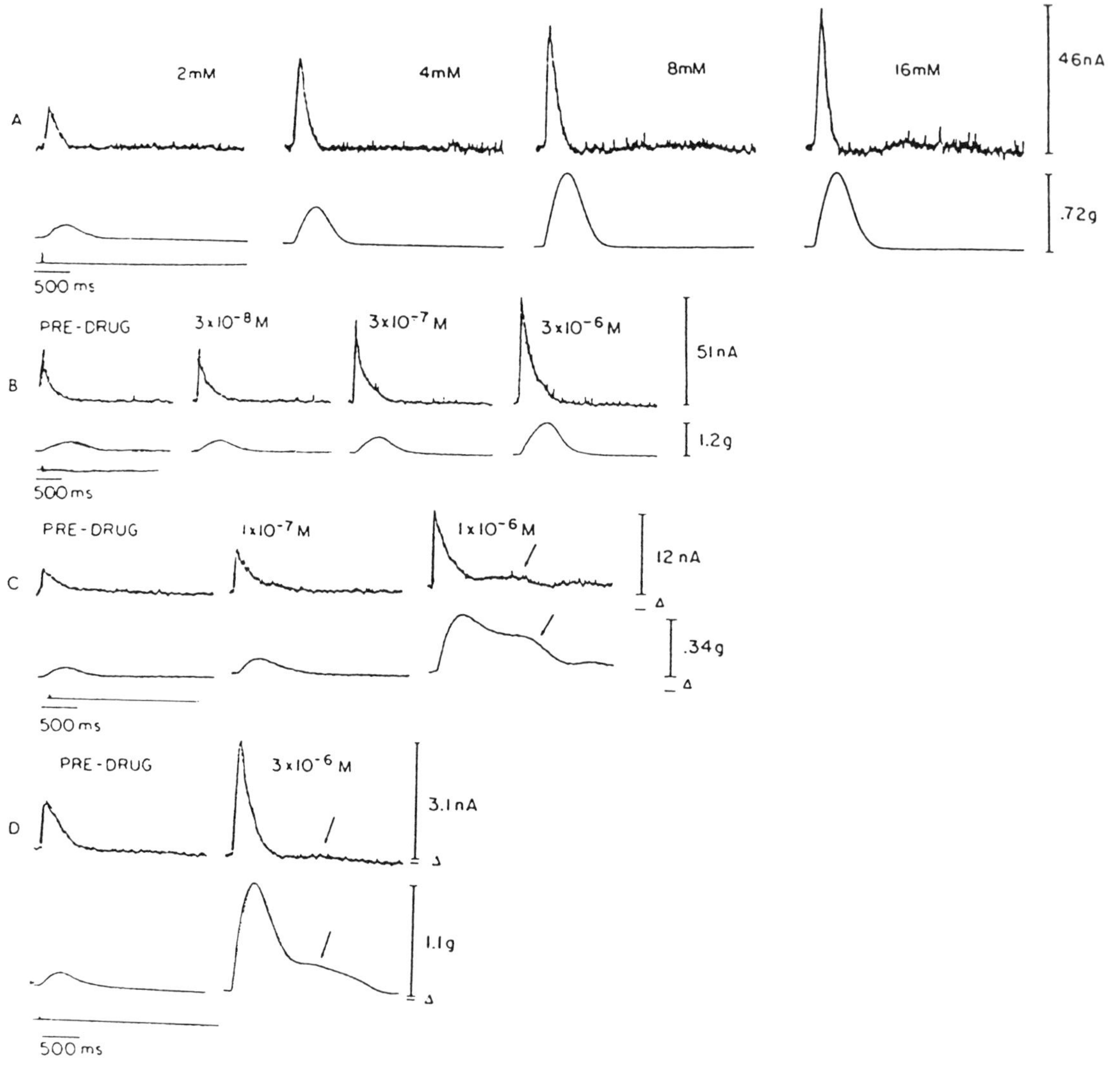

Figure 2 Intracellular calcium transient (aequorin light) and tension recorded from human ventricular trabeculae in the presence of positive inotropic agents with different mechanism of action. A. Increasing extracellular calcium. B. Bay K 8644. C. DPI 201-106. D. Veratridine. Upper trace is the aequorin light signal illustrated as the current recorded from the photomultiplier tube. Lower trace is isometric tension response illustrated in grams. △ indicates change from resting tension or calcium from predrug control. Each illustration is the average of 20–100 responses. Arrow denotes L′ in the calcium response and second component of relaxation in tension response. In all experiments stimulus frequency was 0.33 Hz and the temperature was 30 °C. (From Ref. 77.)

and intracellular calcium transient. It is clear that only DPI 201-106 and veratridine increased the resting calcium level and that a second component developed in both the calcium transient and tension response. This second component in cases of elevated extracellular calcium would exceed the primary calcium transient. The effects were antagonized by agents that block the sodium channel as illustrated in Figure 3. When the sodium channels were blocked with yohimbine there was a decline in the resting calcium and elimination of the second component of the calcium transient. This resulted in a decrease in resting tension and an increase in active force.

We investigated the source of the second component of the calcium transient. Inhibition of sarcoplasmic reticular calcium release and elevation of extracellular calcium coupled with a prolonged action potential resulted in a slowly developing calcium transient and tension response. Figure 4 illustrates the developed tension and action potential recorded under these conditions. The intracellular calcium

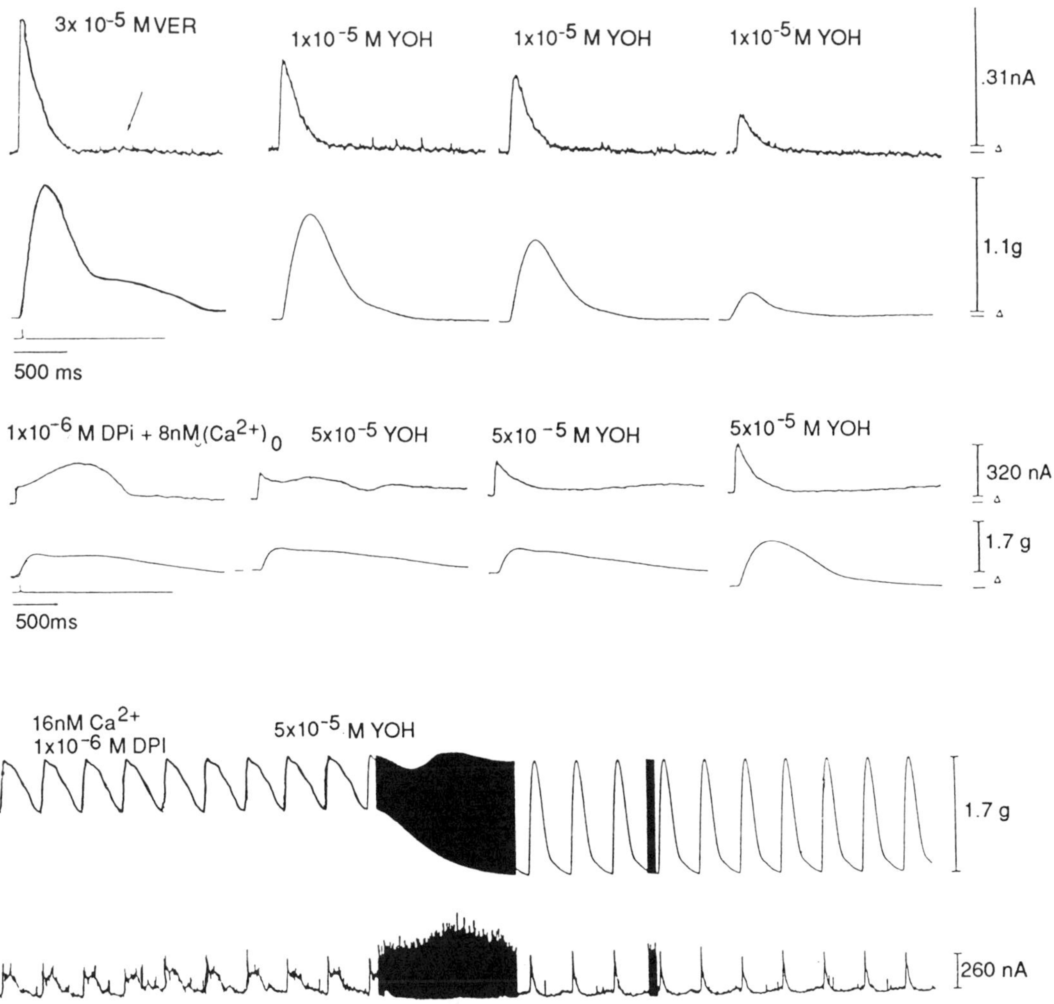

Figure 3 Reversal of the effects of veratridine (VER) and DPI 201-106 (DPI) by yohimbine (YOH) at concentrations that block sodium channels. (From Ref. 77.)

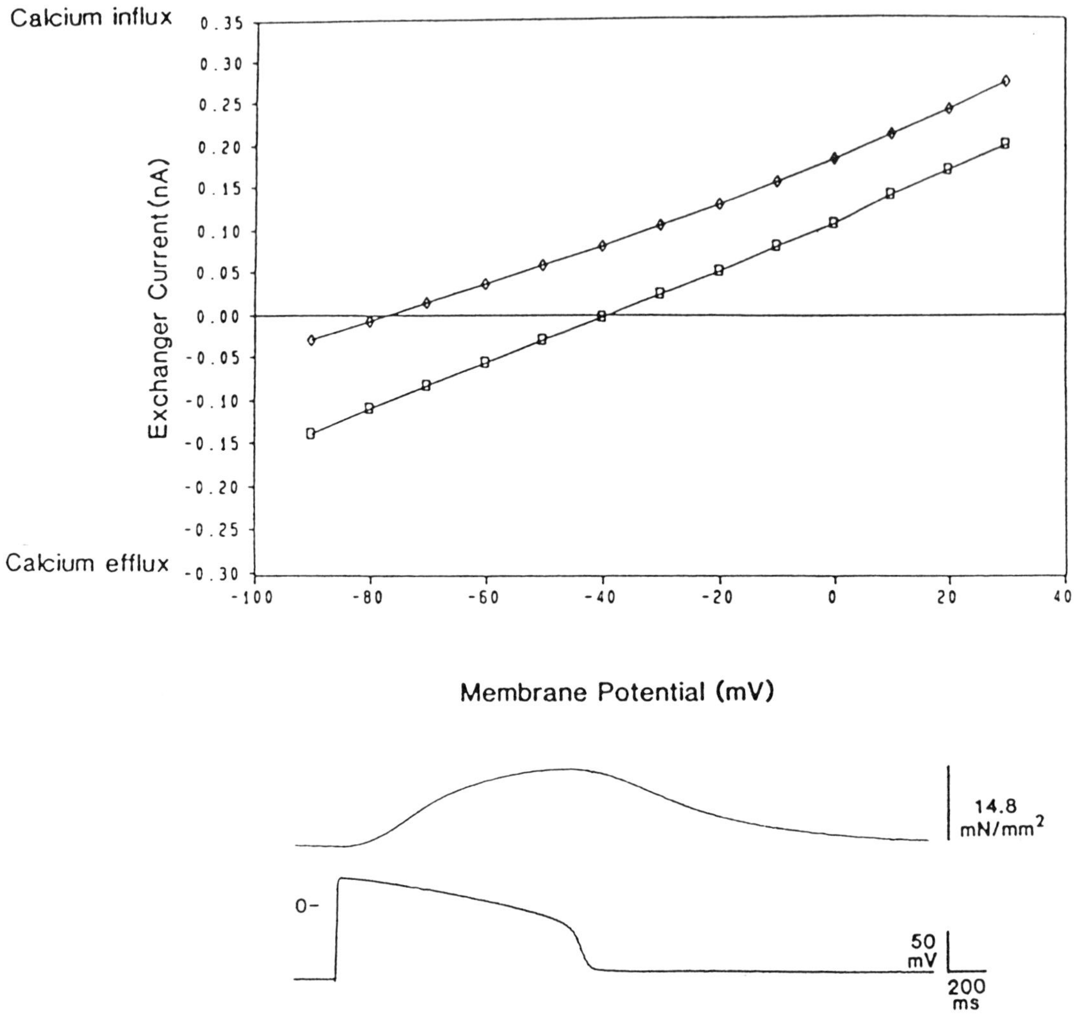

Figure 4 Calculated current–voltage relationship for sodium / calcium exchange (top) from the resting ionic concentrations (◇) and the ionic concentrations at the peak intracellular calcium concentration (□) from the experiment illustrated (bottom). A positive current (hyperpolarizing) results in calcium influx, whereas a negative current (depolarizing) results in calcium efflux. Conditions of experiment were 8 mM extracellular calcium, 1 μM DPI 201-106, and 3 μM ryanodine. (From Ref. 77.)

transient mimicked the developed tension (77). The analysis indicates that the activator calcium was provided completely by sodium/calcium exchange. The modeling of the flux indicates that at the resting potential there is no transport of calcium. The depolarization associated with the upstroke of the action potential results in calcium influx. While depolarized, the potential is in the range that yields calcium influx. The intracellular calcium rises, which shifts the gradients driving the exchanger. As the action potential repolarizes below −40 mV, calcium is removed from the cell and relaxation of the contraction follows.

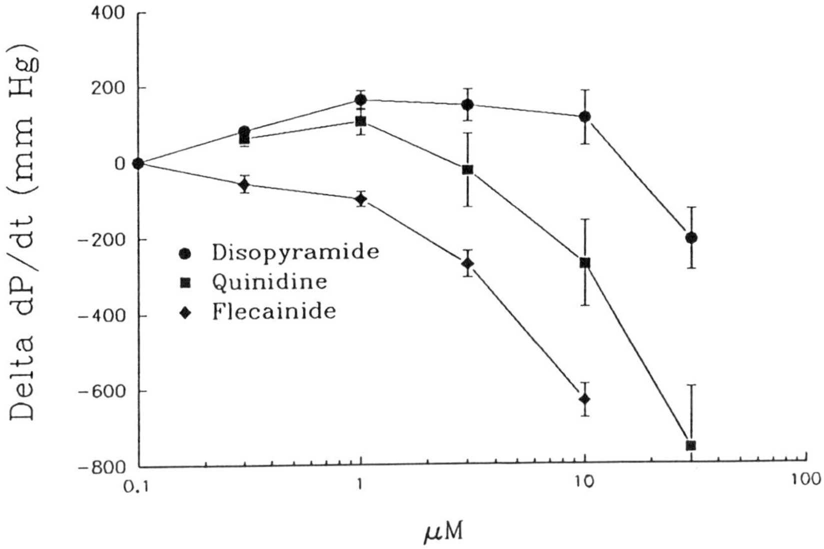

Figure 5 Negative effect of class I antiarrhythmic agents on the contractility of isolated Langendorf perfused rabbit hearts.

Schwinger et al. (80) investigated the effects of another sodium channel inactivator BDF 9148 on increasing active force in myopathic human ventricle. This compound produced similar effects as DPI 210-106 with similar potenciecs. Hearts from patients with NYHA class IV failure were more responsive than those from patients with class III failure. BDF 9148 has a similar effect and potency in guinea pig papillary muscle to that we reported for DPI 201-206 (81). The dihydropyridine compound PD 122860 has both sodium channel inactivating properties and calcium channel blocking properties in rat heart (82).

2. Negative Inotropic Response

If increasing sodium influx via sodium channels can increase contractility, inhibiting sodium influx via sodium channels would decrease contractility. This is the case for class I antiarrhythmics, which act by blocking sodium channels. Figure 5 illustrates the effect of three class I antiarrhythmics on contractility measured in isolated isovolumic contracting rabbit hearts. The concentration-dependent reduction in contractility is primarily due to decreased sodium influx via sodium channel blockade. In this study stimulus strength was controlled to prevent any effect due to reduced excitation. Another possible mechanism related to this negative inotropic response is related to the reported inhibition of calcium channels by this class of compounds. The negative inotropic effects of the class IC antiarrhythmics investigated in the CAST study may be a significant component of the reported negative effect of these agents on survival (83). Agents that block sodium channels have been demonstrated to reduce intracellular sodium concentration (84).

VI. CONCLUSION

There is a great amount of new information regarding sodium channel structure and function. Alterations in intracellular sodium have a direct effect on intracellular calcium and contractility. These effects are mediated by effects on the sodium/calcium exchange mechanism and possibly by a cAMP-dependent pathway. Pharmacologic agents that modify sodium channel flux will also affect contractility and therefore might be used as positive inotropic agents in the treatment of heart failure.

REFERENCES

1. Hodgkin, A L, Huxley A F, Katz B. Measurements of current-voltage relations in the membrane of the giant axon of Loligo. J Physiol (Lond) 1952; 108:37–77.
2. Agnew W S. Voltage-regulated sodium channel molecules. Annu Rev Physiol 1984; 46:517–30.
3. Barchi R L. Voltage-sensitive sodium ion channels. Molecular properties and functional reconstitution. Trends Biochem Sci 1984; 9:358–61.
4. Sakmann B, Neher E. Single channel recording. New York: Plenum, 1983.
5. Hamill O P, Marty A, Neher E, Sakmann, B, Sigworth F J. Improved patch clamp techniques for high resolution current recording from cells and cell-free membrane patches. Pflugers Arch 1981; 391:85–100.
6. Kraner S, Tanaka J, Barchi R. Purification and functional reconstitution of the voltage-sensitive sodium channel from rabbit T-tubular membranes. J Biol Chem 1985; 260:6341–7.
7. Messner D J, Feller D J, Scheuer T, Catterall W. A. Functional properties of rat brain sodium channels lacking the $beta_1$ or $beta_2$ subunit. J Biol Chem 1986; 261:14882–90.
8. Miller C. Genetic manipulation of ion channels: a new approach to structure and mechanism. Neuron 1989; 2:1195–1205.
9. Montal M. Molecular anatomy and molecular design of channel proteins. FASEB J 1990; 4:2623–35.
10. Catterall W A. Neurotoxins that act on voltage sensitive sodium channels in excitable membranes. Annu Rev Pharmacol Toxicol 1980; 20:15–43.
11. Catterall W A. Structure and function of voltage-sensitive ion channels. Science 1988; 242:50–61.
12. Kreger B K. Toward an understanding of structure and function of ion channels. FASEB J 1989; 3:1906–14.
13. Noda M, Shimizu S, Tanabe T, Takai T, Kayano T, Ikeda T, Takahashi H, Nakayama H, Kanaoka Y, Minamino N, Kangawa K, Matsuo H, Raftery M A, Hirose T, Inayama S, Hayashida H, Miyata T, Numa S. Primary structure of *Electrophorus electricus* sodium channel deduced from cDNA sequence. Nature (London) 1984; 312:121–7.
14. Noda M, Ikeda T, Kayano T, Suzuki H, Takeshima H, Kurasaki M, Takahashi H, Numa S. Existence of distinct sodium channel messenger RNAs in rat brain. Nature (London) 1986; 320:188–92.
15. Noda M, Ikeda T, Kanyano T, Suzuki H, Takashima H, Takahashi H, Kuno M, Numa S. Expression of functional sodium channels from cloned cDNA Nature 1986; 322:826–8.
16. Cachelin A B, De Peyer J E, Kokubun S, Reuter H. Sodium channels in cultured cardiac cells. J Physiol (Lond) 1983; 340:389–401.
17. a. Patlak J B, Ortiz M. Slow current through single channels of the adult rat heart. J Gen Physiol 1985; 86:89–104.
    b. Patlak J B, Ortiz M. Two modes of gating during the Na channel currents in frog sartorius muscle. J Gen Physiol 1986; 87:305–26.
18. Ellis S B, Williams M E, Ways N R, Brenner R, Sharp A H, Leung A T, Campbell K P, McKenna E, Koch W J, Hui A, et al. Sequence and expression of mRNA encoding the $alpha_1$ and $alpha_2$ subunits of the DHP sensitive Ca channel. Science 1988; 241:1661–4.

19. Kayano T, Noda M, Flockerzi V, Takahashi H, Numa S. Primary structure of rat brain sodium channel III deduced from the cDNA sequence. FEBS Letts 1988; 228:187–94.
20. Karlin A, Kao P N, DiPola M. Molecular pharmacology of the nicotinic acetylcholine receptor. Trends Pharmacol Sci 1986; 7:304–308.
21. Armstrong R W, Stevens C F. Inactivation of the sodium channel. II. Gating current experiments. J Gen Physiol 1977; 70:567–90.
22. Bezanilia F, Armstrong C M. Inactivation of the sodium channel. I. Sodium current experiments. J Gen Physiol 1977; 70:549–66.
23. Vassilev P, Scheuer T, Catterall W. Inhibition of inactivation of single sodium channels by a site-directed antibody. Proc Natl Acad Sci USA 1989; 86:8147–51.
24. Sumikawa K, Parker I, Miledi R. Partial purification and functional expression of brain mRNAs coding for neurotransmitter receptors and voltage operated channels. Proc Nat Acad Sci USA 1984; 81:7994–8.
25. Hirono C, Yamagishi S, Ohara R, Hisanage Y, et al. Characterization of functional sodium channels in *Xenopus* oocytes. Brain Res 1985; 359:57–64.
26. Stuhmer W, Methfessel C, Sakmann B, Noda M, Numa S. Patch clamp characterization of sodium channels expressed from rat brain cDNA. Eur Biophys J 1987; 14:131–8.
27. Stuhmer W. Structure function studies of voltage gated ion channels. Annu Rev Biophys Chem 1991; 20:65–78.
28. Krafte D S, Snutxch T P, Leonard J P, Davidson N, Lester H A. Evidence for the involvment of more than one mRNA species in controlling the inactivation process of rat and rabbit brain Na Channels expressed in *Xenopus* ooyctes. J Neurosci 1988; 8:2859–68.
29. Auld V J H, Goldin A L, Krafte D S, Marshall J, Dunnb J M, Catterall W A, Lester H A, Davidson N, Dunn R J. A rat brain Na channel α subunit with novel gating properties. Neuron 1988; 1:449–61.
30. Moorman J R, Kirsch G E, VanDongen A M J, Joho R H, Brown A M. Fast and Slow gating of sodium channels encoded by a single mRNA. Science 1990; 250:688–91.
31. Tomaselli G F, Feldman A M, Yellen G, Marban E. Human cardiac sodium channels expressed in *Xenopus* oocytes, Am J Physiol 1990; 2587:H903–6.
32. a. Hodgkin, A L, Huxley A F. Currents carried by sodium and potassium ions through the membrane of the giant axon of Loligo. J Physiol (Lond) 1952; 116:449–72.
b. Hodgkin A L, Huxley A F. The components of membrane conductance in the giant axon of Loligo. J Physiol (Lond) 1952; 116:473–96.
c. Hodgkin A L, Huxley A F. The dual effect of membrane potential on sodium conductance in the giant axon of Loligo. J Physiol (Lond) 1952; 116:497–506.
d. Hodgkin A L, Huxley A F. A quantitative description of membrane current and its application to conductance and excitation in nerve. J Physiol (Lond) 1952; 117:500–44.
33. Aldrich R W, Corey D P, Stevans C F. A reinterpretation of mammalian sodium channel gating based on single channel recording. Nature 1983; 306:436–41.
34. Bean B P, Rios E. Nonlinear charge movement in mammalian cardiac ventricular cells. Components from Na and Ca channel gating. J Gen Physiol 1989; 94:65–93.
35. Hank D A, Sheets M F, Fozzard H A. Gating current associated with Na channels in canine cardiac purkinje cells J. Gen Physiol 1990; 95:439–57.
36. French R J, Horn R. Sodium channel gating: models, mimics and modifiers Annu Rev Biophys Bioeng 1983; 12:319–56.
37. Weidmann S. The effect of the cardiac membrane potential on the rapid availability of the sodium-carrying system J Physiol 1955; 127:213–24.
38. Hondeghem L M, Katzung B G. Time and voltage-dependent interactions of antiarrhythmic drugs with cardiac sodium channels. Biochim Biophys Acta 1977; 472:373–98.
39. Sheets M F, Hanck D A, Fozzard H A. Nonlinear relation between V_{max} and I_{Na} in Canine cardiac purkinje cells. 1988; 63:386–98.

40. Cohen C J, Fozzard H A, Sheu S-S. Increase in intracellular sodium ion activity during stimulation in mammalian cardiac muscle. Circ Res 1982; 50:651–62.
41. Cohen C J, Bean B P, Tsien R W. Maximal upstroke velocity as an index of available sodium conductance: comparison of V_{max} and voltage clamp measurments of I_{Na} in rabbit purkinje fibers Circ Res 1984; 54:636–51.
42. Grant A O, Starmer C F. Mechanism of closure of cardiac sodium channels in rabbit ventricular myocytes: single channel analysis. Circ Res 1987; 60:897–913.
43. Greenblatt R, Blatt Y, Montal M. The structure of the voltage-sensitive sodium channel. FEBS Letts 1985; 193:125–34.
44. Fozzard H A, Hanck D A, Makielski J C, Scanley B E, Sheets M F. Sodium channels in cardiac Purkinje cells. Experimentia 1987; 43:1162–8.
45. Kiyosue, T, Arita M. Late sodium current and its contribution to action potential configuration in guinea pig ventricular myocytes. Circ Res 1989; 64:389–97.
46. Murray K T, Anno T, Bennett P B, Hondeghem L M. Voltage clamp of the cardiac sodium current at 37°C in physiological solutions. Biophys J 1990; 57:607–13.
47. Nilius B, Vereecke J, Carmeliet E. Different conductance states of the bursting Na channel in guinea-pig ventricular myocytes. Pflugers Arch 1989; 413:242–8.
48. Follmer C H, Ten Eick R E, Yeh J Z. Sodium current kinetics in cat atrial myocytes J Physiol 1987; 384:169–97.
49. Kolhardt M, Frobe U, Herzig J W. Properties of normal and non-inactivating single cardiac Na channels. Proc R Soc Lond B 1987; 232:71–93.
50. Scanley B E, Hanck D A, Chay T, Fozzard H A. Kinetic analysis of single sodium channels from cardiac purkinje cells. J Gen physiol 1990; 95:411–37.
51. Yue D T, Lawerence J H, Marban E. Two molecular transitions influence cardiac sodium channel gating. Science 1989; 244:349–52.
52. Vandenberg C A, Horn R. Inactivation viewed through single sodium channels. J Gen Physiol 1984; 84:535–64.
53. Berman M F, Camardo J S, Robinson R B, Siegelbaum S A. Single sodium channels from canine ventricular myocytes: voltage dependence and relative rates of activation and inactivation. J Physiol (Lond) 1989; 415:503–31.
54. Allen D G, Blinks J R. Calcium transients in aequorin injected frog cardiac muscle. Nature Lond 1978; 273:509–13.
55. Boyett M R, Hart G, Levi A J, Roberts A. Effects of repetitive activity on developed force and intracellular sodium in isolated sheep and dog Purkinje fibers. J Physiol Lond 1987; 388:295–322.
56. Lee C O, Vassalle M. Modulation of intracellular Na activity and cardiac force by norepinephrine and Ca. Am J Physiol 1983; 244:C110–4.
57. Wang D Y, Chae S W, Gong Q Y, Lee C O. Role of a^i_{na} in positive force-frequency staircase in guinea pig papillary muscle. Am J Physiol 1988; 255:C798–807.
58. Ruch S, Kennedy R H, Seifen E. Effect of stimulation frequency on inracellular Na activity in rat atrial muscle. Can J Physiol Pharmacol 1989; 66:1565–9.
59. Buckley N M. The role of intracellular sodium ions in the regulation of cardiac contractility. J Mol Cell Cardiol 1982; 14:189–92.
60. Shattock M J, Bers D M. Rat vs Rabbit ventricle: Ca flux and intracellular Na assessed by ion-selective microelectrodes. Am J Physiol 1989; 256:C813–22.
61. Baudet S, Norieaud J, Leoty. Intracellular Na activity measurements in the control and hypertrophied heart of ferret: an ion-sensitive micro-electrode study. Pflugers Arch 1991; 418:313–8.
62. Chapman R A, Rodrigo G C, Tunstall J, Yates R J, Busselen P. Calcium paradox of the heart: a role for intracellular sodium ions. Am J Physiol 1984; 247:H874–9.
63. Chapman R A. A rise in intracellular sodium would seem to predispose the heart to the calcium paradox. J. Mol Cell Cardiol 1991; 22:503–5.

64. Bhojani I H, Chapman R A. The effects of bathing sodium ions upon the intracellular sodium activity in calcium free media and the calcium paradox of isolated ferret ventricular muscle. J Mol Cell Cardiol 1990; 22:507–22.
65. Rodrigo G C, Chapman R A. The calcium paradox in isolated guinea-pig ventricular myocytes: effects of membrane potential and intracellular sodium. J Physiol Lond 1991; 434:627–645.
66. van Echteld, C J A, Kirkels J H, Eijgelshoven M H J, van der Meer P, Ruigrok T J C. Intracellular sodium during ischemia and calcium-free perfusion: a ^{23}Na NMR study. J Mol Cell Cardiol 1991; 23:297–307.
67. Takeo S, Hayashi M, Tanonaka K, Yamamoto K. Beneficial effects of yohimbine on posthypoxic recovery of cardiac function and myocardial metabolism in isolated perfused rabbit hearts. J Pharmacol Exp Ther 1991; 258:94–102.
68. Meng H, Pierce G N. Involvement of sodium in the protective effect of 5-(n,n-dimethyl)-amiloride on ischemia-reperfusion injury in isolated rat ventricular wall. J Pharmacol Exp Ther 1991; 256:1094–1100.
69. Harvey R D, Jurevicius J A, Hume J R. Intracellular Na modulates the cAMP-dependent regulation of ion channel in the heart. Proc Natl Acad Sci USA 1991; 88:6946–50.
70. Ohizumi Y, Nakamura H, Kobayashi J, Catterall W A. Geographutoxin II, a peptide Na Channel blocker that selectively inhibits [^{3}H] saxitoxin binding to muscle and nerve Na channels. J Biol Chem 1986; 261:6149–52.
71. Strichartz G, Rando T, Wang GK. An integrated view of the molecular toxicology of sodium channel gating in excitable cells. Annu Re Neurotoxicol 1987; 10:237–67.
72. Lombet A, Bidard J-N, Lazdunski M. Ciguatoxin and brevetoxins share a common receptor site on the neuronal voltage dependent Na channel. FEBS Lett 1987; 219:355–9.
73. Horackova M, Vassort G. Transmembrane sodium movement and regulation of contraction in frog atrial muscle during the inotropic effect of veratridine. In Fleckenstein A, Dhalla N S, eds. Recent advances in studies on cardiac structure and metabolism. Vol. 5. Basic functions of cations in myocardial activity. Baltimore: University Park Press, 1975.
74. Honerjager P. Cardioactive substances that prolong the open state of sodium channels. Rev Physiol Biochem Pharmacol 1982; 20:1–74.
75. Brill D M, Wasserstrom A. Intracellular sodium and the positive inotropic effect of veratridine and cardiac glycoside in sheep purkinje fibers. Circ Res 1986; 58:109–19.
76. Honerjager P, Reiter M. Sarcolemmal sodium permeability and contractile force of guinea pig papillary muscle. Circ Res 1977; 40:90–98.
77. Gwathmey J K, Slawsky M T, Briggs G M, Morgan J P. Role of intracellular sodium in the regulation of intracellular calcium and contractility. Effects of DPI 201-106 on excitation contraction coupling in human ventricular myocardium. J Clin Invest 1988; 82:1592–605.
78. Scholtysik G. Cardiac Na channel activation as a positive inotropic principle. J Cardiovasc Pharmacol 1989; 14 (Suppl. 3):S24–9.
79. Buggish D, Isenberg G, Ravens U, Scholtysik G. The role of sodium channels in the effects of the cardiotonic compound DPI 201-106 on contractility and membrane potentials in isolated mammalian heart preparations. Eur J Pharmacol 1985; 118:303–11.
80. Schwinger R H G, Bohm M, Mittmann C, LaRosee K, Erdmann E. Evidence for a sustained effectiveness of sodium channel activators in falling human myocardium. J Mol Cell Cardiol 1991; 23:461–71.
81. Brasch H, Iven H. Inotropic and electrophysiological effects of BDF 9148, a congener of DPI 201-106, a guinea-pig atria and papillary muscles. Br J Pharmacol 1991; 103:1939–45.

82. Haleen S J, Steffen R P, Sircar L A, Major T C, Taylor M D, Pugsley T A, Weisharr R E. PD 122860: a novel dihyropyridine with sodium channel stimulating and calcium channel blocking properties. J Pharmacol Exp Ther 1989; 250:22–30.
83. Pfisterer, M. Negative inotropic effects of antiarrhythmic drugs: a clinical point of view. J Cardiovasc Pharmacol 1991; 17 (suppl 6):S44–7.
84. Deitmer J W, Ellis D. The intracellular sodium activity of sheep heart purkinje fibers: effects of local anesthetics and tetrodotoxin. J Physiol 1980; 300:269–82.

28

Control of Cardiac Contractility by K^+ Channel Modulators

MICHAEL C. SANGUINETTI and PETER K. S. SIEGL

Merck Research Laboratories
West Point, Pennsylvania

At least seven distinct K^+ channels have been characterized in cardiac cells, although not all types have been recorded from a single type of cardiac cell. Table 1 lists these K^+ channels and their proposed function, as well as the possible influence of channel activity on the inotropic state of cardiac muscle. The two major roles of cardiac K^+ channels are to maintain the resting membrane potential during diastole and to repolarize the membrane potential following depolarization. In general, agents and interventions that increase K^+ conductance (gK) shorten action potential duration (APD) and tend to have negative inotropic effects, whereas agents that decrease K^+ current lengthen APD and may have positive inotropic effects. The relationship between APD and contractile force in amphibian and mammalian muscle is reviewed elsewhere (1,2). In general, peak tension is directly related to APD in frog ventricle (Fig. 1), whereas in mammalian cardiac tissue short action potentials can lead to disproportionately large effects (relative to the frog) on contractile activity when the sarcoplasmic reticulum is adequately loaded with Ca^{2+} (3). This difference between frog and mammalian heart can be explained by the relative importance of Ca^{2+} entry through sarcolemmal Ca^{2+} channels for excitation–contraction coupling in these two classes. Contraction of amphibian cardiac muscle is dependent solely upon extracellular Ca^{2+} as a source of activator Ca^{2+} (1). In contrast, extracellular Ca^{2+} is more important as the "trigger" signal in mammalian cardiac muscle, causing Ca^{2+}-induced release of intracellular stores (sarcoplasmic reticulum) of activator Ca^{2+} (4). The relationship between APD and tension is more complicated in mammalian cardiac muscle because of the beat-dependent interplay between intracellular stores of Ca^{2+} and Ca^{2+} current (I_{Ca}). Voltage clamp experiments allow a more quantitative measure of the relationship between the duration of depolarization of the membrane potential and resulting tension. The voltage clamp protocol greatly influences the effect of pulse duration on the tension response (5). For example, steady-state pulsing of canine cardiac Purkinje fibers at 0.4

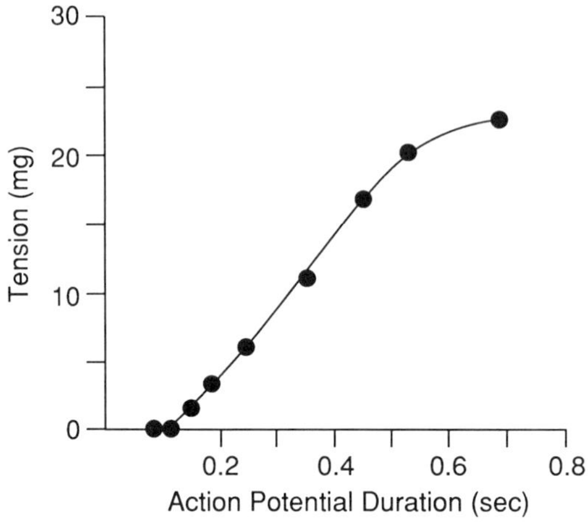

Figure 1 Relationship between developed tension and action potential duration of frog (*Rana pipiens*) ventricular strip. Stimulation rate was 12/min. (Redrawn, with permission from Ref. 82.)

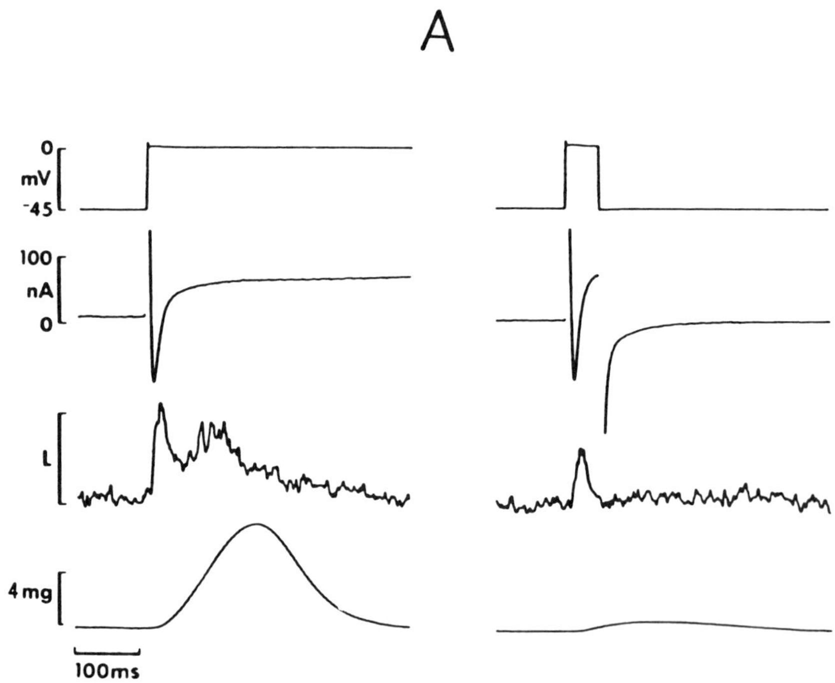

Figure 2 Effect of voltage pulse duration on current, Ca^{2+} transient, and tension in an isolated canine Purkinje fiber. A. Duration of clamp step was either 500 msec (left traces) or 50 msec (right traces). Voltage step protocol, current, aequorin light signal, and tension are shown in descending order. B. Effect of pulse protocol on resulting light signal (L) and tension. Pulses were applied at 0.4 Hz for 500 msec (a), 50 msec (b), or were alternated between 50 and 500 msec (c and d). (With permission from Ref. 5.)

Hz with 500 msec pulses results in much greater developed tension than that achieved using 50 msec pulses (Fig. 2A). However, if short and long pulses are alternated, there is little dependency between the measured force of contraction and pulse duration (Fig. 2B). The results of these types of experiments are explained by loading or depletion of releasable stores of Ca^{2+} from the sarcoplasmic reticulum, which is dependent upon pulse duration and pulsing rate. The relationship between pulse duration and force is also influenced by the voltage of the test pulse. Steady-state tension is enhanced by increasing depolarizations over a limited range of voltage (Fig. 3), limited in part by the voltage dependence of inward I_{Ca} (6).

For the remainder of this chapter we will limit our discussion to the inotropic effects of K^+ channel modulation in mammalian cardiac muscle. The reader will be referred to several excellent reviews that adequately cover the biophysical characterization of cardiac K^+ channels.

Many positive inotropic agents act either directly or indirectly on cardiac Ca^{2+} channels (e.g., catecholamines, Bay K 8644, CGP 28392, OPC 8212) or Na^+channels (e.g., DPI 201-106, veratrine alkaloids). Some of these drugs and natural products also affect cardiac K^+ channels, although most often this occurs at higher concentrations and the effects are not usually responsible for the desired positive inotropic effects. For example, isoproterenol and other beta-adrenergic agonists increase the conductance of delayed rectifier K^+ current (I_K) as well as I_{Ca} (for review, see Ref. 7). The increase in I_{Ca} is in part responsible for the increase in force of contraction, but the increase in gK acts to shorten the duration of the action potential. This decreases the time during which Ca^{2+} enters the cell through L-type Ca^{2+} channels and via Na^+/Ca^{2+} exchange, and might therefore be expected to limit the inotropic response to these agents.

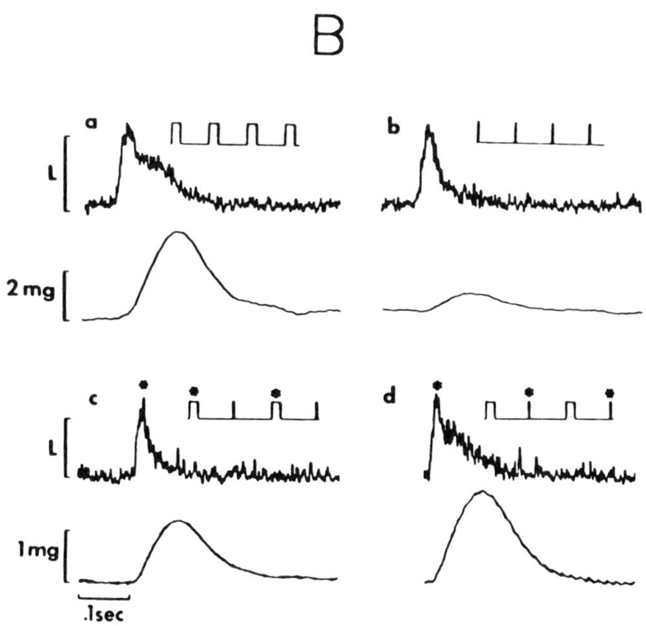

Figure 2 Continued

Table 1 Cardiac K^+ Channels

Cardiac K^+ current	Name	Proposed function	Role in modulation of cardiac contraction
I_K	Delayed rectifier (multiple types)	Repolarization of AP (especially phase 2)	Activation shortens APD and ↓ force Block by class III antiarrhythmic agents lengthens APD, ↑ force
I_{K1}	Inward rectifier	Maintain resting potential; terminal repolarization (phase 3) of AP.	Unknown
I_{KACh}	Acetylcholine-activated	Mediates vagal slowing of nodal pacemaker cells	Decreases atrial APD and contractility during vagal stimulation
I_{KNa}	Na^+-activated	Shortens APD during ischemia (?)	Indirect activation by cardiac glycosides or ischemia shortens APD and ↓ force
I_{KCa}	Ca^{2+}-activated (multiple types?)	Initial repolarization (phase 1) of AP	Unknown
I_{to}	Voltage-dependent transient outward	Initial repolarization (phase 1) of AP	Rate-dependent inactivation results in shorter APDs at slow pacing rates. Activation of α_1-adrenoceptors ↓ I_{to}, ↓ force.
I_{KATP}	ATP_i-sensitive	shortens APD during ischemia, hypoxia	Activation during hypoxia or exposure to specific agonists (eg, cromakalim) ↓ APD and ↓ force.

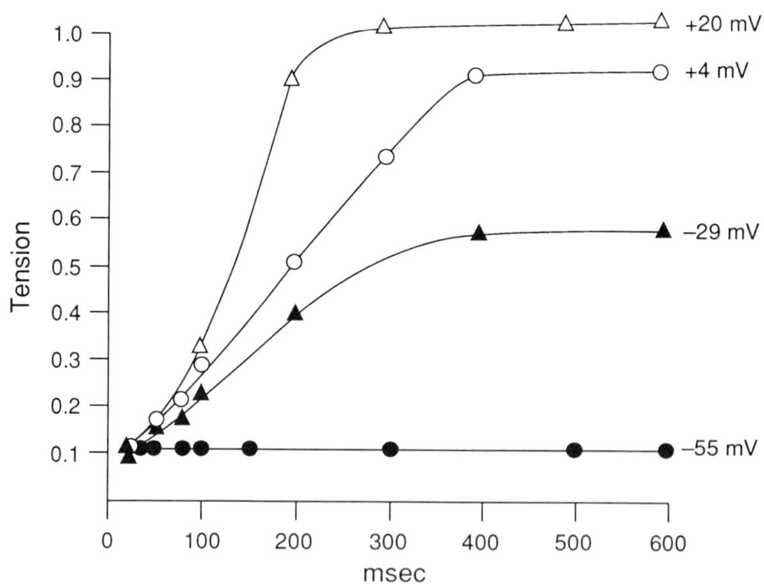

Figure 3 Effect of clamp duration (abscissa) and test potential (in mV) on steady-state tension recorded from dog ventricular trabecula. (Redrawn, with permission from Ref. 6.)

I. POSITIVE INOTROPIC EFFECTS OF K^+ CHANNEL BLOCKERS

A decrease in gK, either by block of specific channels or by control of intracellular modulators of channel activity, often results in an increase in contractility. It is often assumed that agents that prolong APD will have positive inotropic effects (84), a correlation expected from the known relationship between APD and tension cited above. Comparative studies with a specific group of antiarrhythmic drugs ("class III" agents) suggest that this assumption is not always valid.

A. Class III Antiarrhythmic Agents

Class III antiarrhythmic agents prevent sustained ventricular tachycardia by prolonging the APD of cardiac cells. ICS 205-930 (Fig. 4) is a 5-HT_3 receptor antagonist and Class III antiarrhythmic agent (8). This drug prolongs APD and refractory period, but also decreases the force of contraction of isolated guinea pig left atria. ICS 205-930 (100 μM) increased the refractory period 75%, but depressed contractile force by 50% (8). Voltage clamp of guinea pig ventricular cells revealed that ICS 205-930 blocks I_{K1} and I_K with IC_{50} values of 20 μM and 37 μM, respectively (9). The resulting decrease in gK is responsible for the observed APD prolongation. The mechanism of its negative inotropic effect is unexplained. This drug also blocks I_{Ca}, but only 20% at 100 μM (8). This weak block of I_{Ca} does not adequately explain

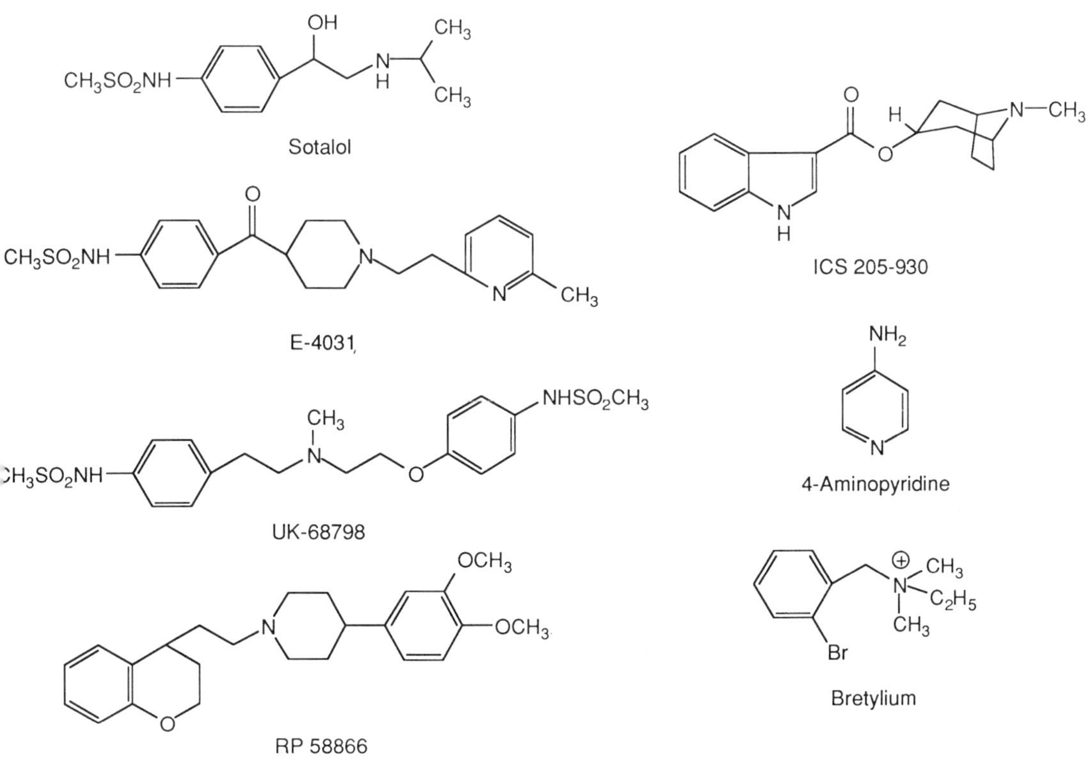

Figure 4 Structures of K^+ current blockers discussed in this chapter.

the extent of its negative inotropic activity. Thus, ICS 205-930 is an example of a compound that prolongs APD without having a positive inotropic effect.

Sotalol, a racemic drug, is a class III antiarrhythmic and beta-adrenergic blocker. Depending upon the type of assay, the l-isomer is 19–46 times more potent as a beta-blocker than the d-isomer (10). There is no difference in the potency of the two isomers with respect to APD prolongation in guinea pig papillary muscles (11), but d-sotalol is about three times more potent than l-sotalol in canine Purkinje strands (12). Both isomers produce increases in developed tension in canine trabecular muscle and Purkinje strands. The effect on force is rate-dependent in the Purkinje strands, having no effect at 2 Hz, but producing large increases at the slower rates of 0.33–0.5 Hz (12). Sotalol increases contractile activity of isolated cardiac tissue preparations, but decreases left ventricular $+(dP/dt)_{max}$ in anesthetized dogs due to its beta-adrenoceptor blocking activity (13). D-Sotalol has been reported to depress $+(dP/dt)_{max}$ and peak left ventricular pressure markedly in rats after global myocardial ischemia at a dosage that had no effect on these parameters in normal rats (14). The mechanism for this altered activity during ischemia is not understood. Many of the newer class III antiarrhythmic agents are structural analogs of sotalol that lack beta-blocking activity. Several of these agents, including UK-68,798 (86), UK-66,914 (85), and E-4031 (15) increase left ventricular $+(dP/dt)_{max}$ (maximum of approximately 35%) without any effect on $-(dP/dt)_{max}$ in chloralose-anesthetized dogs (16). E-4031 increases developed tension in isolated rabbit papillary muscles by a maximum of 26%. This effect was associated with a 38% increase in the maximal velocity of contraction but only a small change in the rate of relaxation (17), consistent with effects of this drug on $(dP/dt)_{max}$ in the aforementioned anesthetized dog study. Bretylium is a class III antiarrhythmic agent that prolongs APD by blocking I_K (18). It also has a marked positive inotropic effect, but this arises entirely from drug-induced release of endogenous norepinephrine, since the increase in tension is prevented by administration of beta-adrenoceptor blockers (19).

The mechanism of action of most class III agents is believed to be block of I_K (20). In guinea pig ventricular myocytes I_K is the sum of two distinct delayed rectifier K^+ currents. In these cells two class III antiarrhythmic agents, E-4031 and d-sotalol, inhibit only one type of delayed rectifier (a relatively small, rapidly activating component, I_{Kr}), without having any effect on the larger, slowly activating component of I_K, I_{Ks} (21).

Another class III agent, RP 58866, is reported to be a specific blocker of inward rectifier K^+ current, I_{Kl} (22). In halothane-anesthetized dogs, this class III agent was devoid of effects on hemodynamics at dosages that prolonged QT_c intervals (23).

B. Modulators of Transient Outward K^+ Current

Aminopyridines, especially 4-aminopyridine (4-AP), are K^+ channel blockers that are also strong positive inotropes. For example, 4-AP more than doubles the magnitude of twitches in electrically driven guinea pig atria (24). However, several studies have demonstrated that a large part of this augmentation of force results from a stimulated release of catecholamines from sympathetic axon terminals (25). Despite the certain role of catecholamine release in the mechanism of inotropy exerted by 4-AP, a direct positive inotropic effect also occurs when tissues are exposed to beta-adrenoceptor blockers, probably a result of prolonged APD.

4-AP is a more potent blocker of transient outward K^+ current (I_{to}) than of other cardiac K^+ currents (26). I_{to} is characterized by a very rapid onset of activation and inactivation and therefore is the major outward current during the initial repolarization (phase 1) of the action potential in many cardiac cell types. I_{to} is especially prominent in atrial cells of rabbits (27) and humans (28), and ventricular cells of the rat (29), which are all characterized by relatively short APDs. Rapid pulsing inactives I_{to}, resulting in a disappearance of the repolarization notch (phase 1) characteristic of action potentials observed during slow stimulation rates in these cells.

Stimulation of alpha-adrenergic receptors leads to a marked increase in refractory period and force of contraction in the same types of cardiac tissues that are most affected by 4-AP. Voltage clamp studies have revealed that alpha-adrenoceptor agonists such as methoxamine and phenylephrine decrease the magnitude of I_{to} in rabbit atrial cells (30) and rat ventricular cells (31). Alpha-adrenoceptor stimulation with norepinephrine (in the presence of propranolol to block beta-receptors) also reduces I_{to} in isolated rat ventricular cells (32). 4-AP appears to block I_{to} channels directly, whereas alpha-adrenoceptor agonists act indirectly to decrease I_{to}, via an unidentified second messenger (83). The inotropic response to alpha-adrenergic receptor stimulation is very modest in some cardiac preparations such as guinea pig papillary muscles. In this tissue alpha-adrenoceptor agonists have almost no effect on APD (33), which suggests that the inotropic and action potential effects are related. This is consistent with the finding that I_{to} is very small in guinea pig ventricular cells (Sanguinetti, unpublished). Finally, the positive inotropic action of methoxamine in rabbit papillary muscles is very rate-dependent (34), similar to the rate dependence of I_{to} magnitude and the slow recovery from inactivation following depolarization observed in several cardiac cell types (27,35,36). Thus, in cardiac tissues in which repolarization of action potentials is largely dependent on I_{to}, drugs and neurohormones that decrease the conductance of this current will augment contractility, especially at low heart rates. These findings raise the interesting question of whether alpha-adrenerigc receptor stimulation causes a gradient of inotropic effects across the ventricular wall in species (such as the dog) where I_{to} is more important for repolarization of epicardial cells than of endocardial cells (37).

C. Block of K^+ Currents by Cardiotonic Agents

Several new positive inotropic agents block K^+ current and prolong APD of cardiac muscle in addition to their more well-known mechanism(s) of action. For example, OPC 8212, a phosphodiesterase inhibitor, decreases I_K and I_{Kl} at the same concentrations used to achieve positive inotropic effects in isolated cardiac muscle (38). Most phosphodiesterase inhibitors increase heart rate and relax vascular smooth muscle. It is not clear whether block of K^+ currents contributes to the positive inotropic actions of OPC 8212, but this activity may explain the lack of chronotropic and vascular effects of this agent.

MCI-154 is a pyridazinone with cardiotonic activity that has been attributed to an increase in Ca^{2+} sensitivity of cardiac contractile proteins (39). MCI-154 has no effect on APD of guinea pig papillary muscles under normal conditions, but markedly prolongs APD of slow response action potentials at a concentration of 1 μM (40). The lengthening of slow-response APD was associated with a block of I_{Kl}

without effects on I_K or I_{Ca} in voltage clamp experiments (40). Since MCI-154 did not alter the configuration of normal action potentials, it is doubtful that the block of I_{Kl} contributes to the positive inotropic effects of this drug.

II. NEGATIVE INOTROPIC EFFECTS OF K^+ CHANNEL ACTIVATION

Shortening of cardiac action potentials by activation of any of the identified K^+ channels can lead to a decrease in contractile force. The most likely mechanism is a decrease in Ca^{2+} entry via L-type Ca^{2+} channels and Na^+/Ca^{2+} exchange that results secondary to an abbreviated APD. The most significant changes in APD occur with activation of I_{KACh} channels in atrial muscle or I_{KATP} channels in all types of cardiac muscle. When fully activated, either of these currents can essentially eliminate the plateau phase and transform the relatively long cardiac action potential into a nerve cell-like spike. The role of I_{KNa}, a current activated by abnormally high intracellular $[Na^+]$, in repolarization of cardiac cells is just beginning to be explored.

A. Acetylcholine-Activated K^+ Current

I_{KACh} is an inwardly rectifying K^+ current present in atrial and cardiac Purkinje cells. The current–voltage relationship and single channel conductance of I_{KACh} channels are similar to the inward rectifier K^+ current (I_{Kl}) of ventricular cells. Both types of channels are present in atrioventricular nodal (AVN), sinoatrial nodal (SAN) (41), and Purkinje cells (42), and are responsible for maintaining the resting membrane potential near E_K, the equilibrium potential for K^+. I_{KACh} is activated by acetylcholine (41,43,44) as well as adenosine (45) and somatostatin (46); each agonist is mediated by distinct receptors. Vagal stimulation releases acetylcholine from parasympathetic nerve endings that innervate the SAN and AVN. Nerve endings are also dispersed throughout the atrium and to some extent in the ventricle (47). Binding of acetylcholine to muscarinic receptors (blocked by atropine) activates a pertussis toxin-sensitive, GTP-binding protein (G_k, 48). Both the $\beta\gamma-$ (49) and the $\alpha-$ (50–52) subunits of G_k have been shown to activate I_{KACh} channels directly in excised patches from atrial cells. The α-subunit is 1000 times more potent than the $\beta\gamma$-subunits in activation of these channels (55), thus the α-subunit probably modulates the I_{KACh} channel in vivo. Activation of I_{KACh} leads to hyperpolarization and shortening of APD. The shortening of APD in atrial tissue is in part responsible for the negative inotropic effects reported for acetylcholine, adenosine, and somatostatin. The inhibition of contractile activity by acetylcholine and adenosine is most pronounced in muscle that has been treated with beta-adrenoceptor agonists. This effect is probably mediated through an increase in cGMP and a decrease in cAMP activity (54), and not directly related to any simultaneous effect on K^+ channels.

B. ATP-Sensitive K^+ Current

A K^+ current activated by low intracellular [ATP] was first described in isolated cardiac cells by Noma (55). Under normal conditions, I_{KATP} channels are closed and therefore do not contribute to repolarization of cardiac action potentials. Intracellular ATP (ATP_i) normally blocks these channels; however, reduction of $[ATP]_i$ by any mechanism removes this block and results in I_{KATP} activation. In cardiac cells,

I_{KATP} activation and the resulting decrease in APD limit the entry of Ca^{2+} through Ca^{2+} channels. The shortening of the action potential limits contractility in cells where intracellular ATP levels are precariously low, thus sparing the limited metabolic reserve remaining in hypoxic or ischemic tissues. Thus, the physiological role of I_{KATP} channels might be to protect cardiac cells from Ca^{2+} overload that might otherwise occur during ischemia (55).

ATP_i can be lowered experimentally by exposing cells to uncouplers of oxidative phosphorylation (e.g., cyanide, 2,4-dinitrophenol, deoxyglucose) or to hypoxic solutions. These experimental manipulations activate I_{KATP} and decrease APD, I_{Ca}, and contractile force (20,56–58). Thus, the effect of I_{KATP} activation on contractile activity is difficult to assess using metabolic inhibitors. It has been questioned whether shortening of cardiac APD during ischemia and anoxia results from activation of I_{KATP} channels. Simultaneous measurement of APD, contractility and $[ATP]_i$ in isolated ferret hearts during metabolic blockade has shown that a rapid decrease in force and APD is not accompanied by a significant lowering in $[ATP]_i$ as measured by phosphorus NMR spectroscopy (59). In this study it was calculated that myoplasmic $[ATP]_i$ fell from 5.4 to 4.3 mM during which time APD was decreased by 44%. In guinea pig ventricular myocytes it has been estimated that the $[ATP]_i$ must fall to about 1 mM before sufficient activation of I_{KATP} occurs to account for a 50% reduction in APD (60). This corresponds to activation of less than 2% of peak I_{KATP} conductance in these cells. Much of the apparent discrepancy between the observed decrease in APD and activation of I_{KATP} may relate to poorly understood mechanisms of I_{KATP} modulation in intact cells. Most important is that changes in [ATP] in the immediate vicinity of I_{KATP} channels have not been accurately measured. Activation of I_{KATP} channels is affected more by changes in glycolysis than in oxidative phosphorylation, suggesting that glycolytic enzymes may be located near the sarcolemmal-bound channels and that glycolysis may be the physiologically relevant source of ATP that controls the conductance of I_{KATP} (61). Furthermore, the form of ATP (free-acid or divalent cation-bound) and $[ADP]_i$ influences the modulatory role of ATP on these channels in cardiac cells (62,63). These and other possible explanations of the apparent discrepancy between measured levels of myoplasmic [ATP] and concentrations needed to close I_{KATP} channels are reviewed by Ashcroft (64).

Activation of cardiac I_{KATP} channels can also be achieved with several so-called K^+ channel openers (Fig. 5), such as cromakalim (BRL 34915), pinacidil, RP 49356, or diazoxide (65–67). These agents are best known for their ability to hyperpolarize and relax vascular smooth muscle (68). The K^+ current activated by these agents in smooth muscle cells is controversial. Effects of chromakalim on ATP-regulated K^+ channels (69) and delayed rectifier K^+ current (70) have been demonstrated in vascular smooth muscle cells. These agents activate I_{KATP} channels in cardiac cells without having any measurable effect on other K^+ currents (67,71). Activation of I_{KATP} by these agents occurs in the presence of normal $[ATP]_i$, although the extent of activation is dependent upon $[ATP]_i$ (72). The decrease in APD caused by I_{KATP} activation by these drugs and the resulting negative inotropic response in vitro (73) and in vivo (74) are not complicated by the metabolic changes associated with possible I_{KATP} activation during ischemia and anoxia. With the use of these specific pharmacologic activators of the channel, there is a direct relationship between I_{KATP} activation and decreased force.

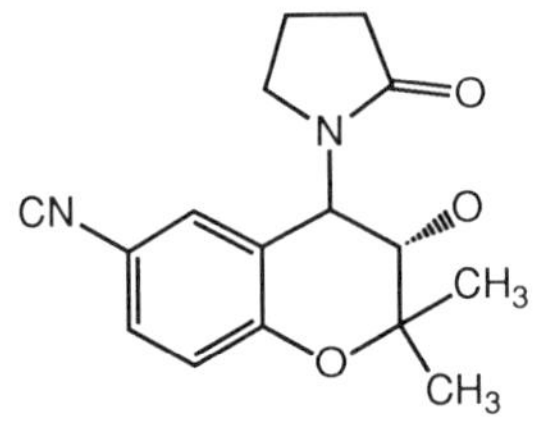

Cromakalim

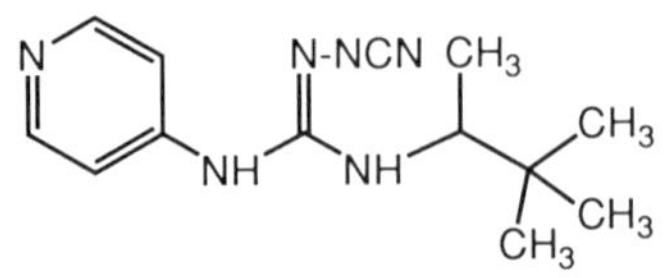

Pinacidil

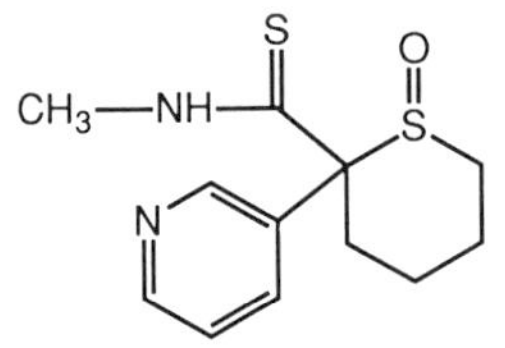

RP 49356

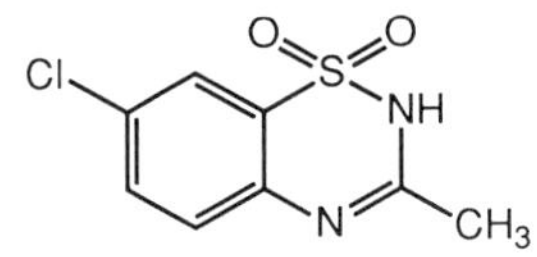

Diazoxide

Figure 5 K^+ channel openers. These compounds have all been reported to activate I_{KATP} in cardiac myocytes.

I_{KATP} channels of ventricular cells isolated from hypertrophied cat hearts appear to be more sensitive to changes in $[ATP]_i$ than are channels recorded from cells isolated from normal hearts (75). These data suggest that hypertrophied cardiac muscle may respond to hypoxia with a decrease in contractility during conditions insufficient to alter force in normal tissue. Other K^+ currents are also reported to be altered in cardiac hypertrophy. In cats, hypertrophy produced by pressure overload leads to a decrease in I_K, an increase in I_{K1}, a lengthening of APD, and a decrease in force (76). The decrease in contractility associated with hypertrophy is obviously not due simply to changes in K^+ currents.

C. Na^+-Activated K^+ Current

Inhibition of Na/K ATPase by cardiac glycosides increases $[Na^+]_i$ (77). It has been suggested that during ischemia, digitalis overdose, or any other condition that results in failure of active Na^+ pumping and raises $[Na^+]_i$ may activate I_{KNa} (78,79). Similar to activation of I_{KATP}, activation of I_{KNa} might protect cells from Ca^{2+} overload. An elevation of intracellular Na^+, either by treatment with ouabain or by dialysis of the cell during voltage clamp, leads to activation of I_{KNa} and shortening of APD (80,81). It remains to be determined if drugs such as DPI 201-106 and the veratrine-like alkaloids also activate I_{KNa} indirectly via their ability to increase $[Na^+]_i$. Perhaps both I_{KNa} and I_{KATP} channels are activated during ischemia in cardiac muscle and are partially responsible for the decrease in contractile force in this condition. The contribution of I_{KATP} and I_{KNa} to the net outward current responsible for repolarization of cardiac action potentials has not yet been determined in cells subjected to a variable degree of hypoxia, anoxia or metabolic stress.

III. SUMMARY

Modulation of Ca^{2+} channels directly influences excitation–contraction coupling in mammalian cardiac cells, whereas modulation of K^+ channels only indirectly alters cardiac contractility by shortening or lengthening APD. The most dramatic changes in the inotropic state of cardiac muscle occur when K^+ channel conductance is increased sufficiently to shorten APD and thus decrease force by limiting Ca^{2+} entry into the cell via Ca^{2+} channels and Na/Ca exchange. Specific K^+ channels (i.e., I_{KATP} and I_{KNa}) that are activated during conditions of metabolic stress may have evolved to protect muscle cells from the damaging effects of cytosolic Ca^{2+} overload. Therapeutically useful positive inotropy cannot be attained by pharmacologic modulation of cardiac K^+ channels as it can be with manipulation of Na^+ or Ca^{2+} channel function.

REFERENCES

1. Morad M, Goldman Y. Excitation–contraction coupling in heart muscle: membrane control of development of tension. Prog Biophys Mol Biol 1973; 27:257–313.
2. Winegrad S. Membrane control of force generation. In: Fozzard HA, et al, eds. The heart and cardiovascular system. New York: Raven Press, 1986; 703–30.
3. Morad M, Trautwein W. The effect of the duration of the action potential on contraction in the mammalian heart muscle. Pflugers Arch. 1968; 299:66–82.
4. Fabiato A. Calcium-induced release of calcium from the cardiac sarcoplasmic reticulum. Am J Physiol 1983; 245:Cl–C14.
5. Wier W G, Isenberg G. Intracellular [Ca^{2+}] transients in voltage clamped cardiac Purkinje fibers. Pfugers Arch. 1982; 392:284–90.
6. Beeler G W, Reuter H. The relation between membrane potential, membrane currents and activation of contraction in ventricular myocardial fibres. J Physiol 1970; 207:211–29.
7. Trautwein, W, Osterrieder W. Mechanisms of -adrenergic and cholinergic control of Ca and K currents in the heart. In: Nathan RD, ed. Cardiac muscle: the regulation of excitation and contraction. Orlando, FL: Academic Press, 1986; 87–128.
8. Scholtysik G. Evidence for inhibition by ICS 205-930 and stimulation by BRL 34915 of K^+ conductance in cardiac muscle. Naunyn-Schmiedeberg's Arch Pharmacol 1987; 335:692–6.
9. Scholtysik G, Imoto Y, Yatani A, Brown A. M. 5-hydroxytryptamine antagonist ICS 205-930 blocks cardiac potassium, sodium and calcium currents. J Pharmacol Exp Ther 1988; 245:773–8.
10. Gomoll A W, Bartek M J. Comparative B-blocking activities and electrophysiologic actions of racemic sotalol and its optical isomers in anesthetized dogs. Eur J Pharmacol 1986; 132:123–35.
11. Hafner D, Berger F, Borchard U, Kullmann A, Scherlitz A. Electrophysiological characterization of the Class III activity of sotalol and its enantiomers. Arzneim.-Forsch./ Drug Res. 1988;38:231–6.
12. Lathrop D A. Electromechanical characterization of the effects of racemic sotalol and its optical isomers on isolated canine ventricular trabecular muscles and Purkinje strands. Can J Physiol Pharmacol 1985; 63:1506–12.
13. Antonaccio M J, Gomoll A W. Sotalol—pharmacological and antiarrhythmic effects. Cardiovasc Drug Rev 1988; 6:239–63.
14. Hoffmeister H M, Muller S, Seipel L. Influence of the new class III antiarrhythmic drug d-sotalol on contractility of normal and postischemic myocardium. Circulation 1989; 80:II–326.

15. Katoh H, Nomoto K, Sawada K, Shoji T. Electrophysiologic, antiarrhythmic and hemodynamic effects of E-4031, a novel class III antiarrhythmic agent in intact and infarcted dogs. Eur Soc Cardiol 1988; 9:232.
16. Stupienski R, Wallace A, Brookes L, Claremon D, Selnick H, Stein R, Lynch J. Cardiac electrophysiologic and hemodynamic effects of class III antiarrhythmic agents in anesthetized dogs. Fed Proc 1990; 4:A455.
17. Lynch J J, Wiedmann R T, Baskin E P, Heaney L A, Stein R, B, and Cingolani H E. Contractile behavior of a novel class III antiarrhythmic agent. Circulation 1989; 80:II–16.
18. Bacaner M B, Clay J R, Shrier A, Brochu R M. Potassium channel blockade: a mechanism for suppressing ventricular fibrillation. Proc Natl Acad Sci 1986; 83:2223–7.
19. Markis J E, Koch-Weser J. Characteristics and mechanism of inotropic and chronotropic actions of bretylium tosylate. J Pharmacol Exp Ther 1971; 178:94–102.
20. Carmeliet E. Cardiac transmembrane potentials and metabolism. Circ Res 1978; 42:577–87.
21. Sanguinetti M C, Jurkiewicz N K. Two components of cardiac delayed rectifier K^+ current: differential sensitivity to block by class III antiarrhythmic agents. J Gen Physiol 1990; 96:195–215.
22. Escande D, Mestre M, Hardy J-C, Cavero I. RP 58866, a pure class III antiarrhythmic agent, specifically blocks the inwardly rectifying K^+ current in heart cells. 1989; Circulation 80:II–607.
23. Mestre M, Hardy J-C, Escande D, Cavero I. Pharmacological relevance in animal models of a pure class III antiarrhythmic agent. Circulation 1989; 80:II–139.
24. Savage A O. A comparison of the effects of 4-dimethylaminopyridine and 4-aminopyridine on isolated cardiac and skeletal muscle preparations. Arch Int Pharmacodyn 1985; 273:262–76.
25. Sugimori T, Nagashima H, Vizi E S, et al. Effect of mono- and diaminopyridines on release of [^{3}H]norepinephrine from isolated guinea-pig atrium. Neuropharmacology 1987; 26:621–6.
26. Kenyon J L, Gibbons W R. 4-Aminopyridine and the early outward current of sheep cardiac Purkinje fibers. J Gen Physiol 1979; 73:139–57.
27. Giles W R, Imaizumi Y. Comparison of potassium currents in rabbit atrial and ventricular cells. J Physiol 1988; 405:123–45.
28. Escande D, Coulombe A, Faivre J-F, Deroubaix E, Coraboeuf E. Two types of transient outward currents in adult human atrial cells. Am J Physiol 1987; 252:H142–8.
29. Josephson I R, Sanchez-Chapula J, Brown A M. Early outward current in rat single ventricular cells. Circ Res 1984; 54:157–62.
30. Fedida D, Shimoni Y, Giles W R. A novel effect of norepinephrine on cardiac cells is mediated by α_1-adrenoceptors. Am J Physiol 1989; 256:H1500–4.
31. Apkon M, Nerbonne J M. α_1-Adrenergic agonists selectively suppress voltage-dependent K^+ currents in rat ventricular myocytes. Proc Natl Acad Sci USA 1988; 85:8756–60.
32. Ravens U, Wang X-L, Wettwer E. Alpha adrenoceptor stimulation reduces outward currents in rat ventricular myocytes. J Pharmacol Exp Ther 1989; 250:364–70.
33. Sanchez-Chapula J. Multiple effects of putative -adrenoceptor agonists on the electrical and mechanical activity of guinea pig papillary muscle. Naunyn-Schmiedebergs Arch Pharmacol 1981; 316:108–11.
34. Endoh M, Schumann H J. Frequency-dependence of the positive inotropic effects of methoxamine and naphazoline mediated by α-adrenoceptors in the isolated rabbit papillary muscle. Naunyn-Schmiedebergs Arch Pharmacol 1975; 287:377–89.
35. Simurda J, Simurdova M, Cupera P. 4-aminopyridine sensitive transient outward current in dog ventricular fibres. Pflugers Arch 1988; 411:442–9.
36. Tseng G-N, Hoffman B F. Two components of transient outward current in ventricular myocytes. Circ Res 1989; 64:633–47.

37. Litovsky S H, C Antzelevitch Transient outward current prominent in canine ventricular epicardium but not epicardium. Circ Res 1988; 62:116–26.
38. Iijima T, Taira N. Membrane current changes responsible for the positive inotropic effect of OPC-8212, a new positive inotropic agent, in single ventricular cells of the guinea pig heart. J Pharmacol Exp Ther 1987; 240:657–62.
39. Kitada Y, Narimatsu A, Matsumura N, Endo M. Contractile proteins: possible targets for the cardiotonic action of MCI-154, a novel cardiotonic agent? Eur J Pharmacol 1987; 134:229–31.
40. Katayama S, Narimatsu A, Suzuki R, Iijima T, Taira N. Changes in membrane potentials and currents of ventricular cells of the guinea pig heart by a new cardiotonic drug, MCI-154. Jpn J Pharmacol 1987; 44:481–8.
41. Noma A, Trautwein W. Relaxation of the ACh-induced potassium current in the rabbit sinoatrial node cell. Pflugers Arch 1978; 377:193–200.
42. Carmeliet E, Mubagwa K. Characterization of the acetylcholine-induced potassium current in rabbit cardiac Purkinje fibres. J Phyisol 1986; 371:219–37.
43. Pfaffinger P J, Martin J M, Hunter D D, Hille B. GTP-binding proteins couple cardiac muscarinic receptors to a K^+ channel. Nature 1985; 317:536–8.
44. Soejima M, Noma A. Modes of regulation of the ACh-sensitive K-channel by the muscarinic receptor in rabbit atrial cells. Pflugers Arch 1984; 400:424–31.
45. Tawfik-Schlieper H, Klotz K-N, Kreye V A W, Schwabe U. Characterization of the K^+-channel-coupled adenosine receptor in guinea pig atria. Naunyn-Schmiedebergs Arch Pharmacol 1989; 340:684–688.
46. Lewis D L, Clapham D E. Somatostatin activates an inwardly rectifying K^+ channel in neonatal rat atrial cells. Pflugers Arch 1989; 414:492–4.
47. Yamauchi A. Ultrastructure of the inervation of the mammalian heart. In: Challice C E, Viragh S, eds. Ultrastructure of the mammalian heart. New York: Academic Press, 1973; 127–78.
48. Yatani A, Codina J, Brown A M, Birnbaumer L. Direct activation of mammalian atrial muscarinic potassium channels by GTP regulatory protein G_k. Science 1987; 235:207–11.
49. Logothetis D E, Kurachi Y, Galper J, Neer E J, Clapham D E. The $\beta\gamma$ subunits of GTP-binding proteins activate the muscarinic K^+ channel in heart. Nature 1987; 325:321–6.
50. Cerbai E, Klockner U, Isenberg G. The subunit of the GTP binding protein activates muscarinic potassium channels of the atrium. Science 1988; 240:1782–3.
51. Kirsch G E, Yatani A, Codina J, Birnbaumer L, Brown A M. α-Subunit of G_k activates atrial K^+ channels of chick, rat, and guinea pig. Am J Physiol 1988; 254:H1200–5.
52. Yatani A, Hamm H, Codina J, Mazzoni M R, Brinbaumer L, Brown A M. A monoclonal antibody to the subunit of G_k blocks muscarinic activation of atrial K^+ channels. Science 1988; 241:828–31.
53. Codina J, Yatani A, Grenet D, Brown A M, Birnbaumer L. The subunit of the GTP binding protein G_k opens atrial potassium channels. Science 1987; 236:442–5.
54. Watanabe A M, Besch H R Jr. Interaction between cyclic adenosine monophosphate and cyclic guanosine monophosphate in guinea pig ventricular myocardium. Circ Res 1975; 37:309–17.
55. Noma A. ATP-regulated K^+ channels in cardiac muscle. Nature 1983; 305:147–8.
56. Goldhaber J I, Ji S, Lamp S T, Weiss J N. Effects of exogenous free radicals on electromechanical function and metabolism in isolated rabbit and guinea pig ventricle. J Clin Invest 1989; 83:1800–9.
57. Isenberg G, Vereecke J, van der Heyden G, Carmeliet E. The shortening of the action potential by DNP in guinea-pig ventricular myocytes is mediated by an increase of a time-independent K conductance. Pflugers Arch. 1983; 397:251–9.
58. McDonald T F, MacLeod D P. Metabolism and the electrical activity of anoxic ventricular muscle. J Physiol 1973; 229:559–82.
59. Elliott A C, Smith G L, Allen D G. Simultaneous measurements of action potential

duration and intracellular ATP in isolated ferret hearts exposed to cyanide. Circ Res 1989; 64:583–91.
60. Nichols C G, Ripoll C, Lederer W J. How does [ATP] influence the duration of the cardiac action potential? Biophys J 1990; 57:133a.
61. Weiss J N, Lamp S T. Glycolysis preferentially inhibits ATP-sensitive K^+ channels in isolated guinea pig cardiac myocytes. Science 1987; 238:67–9.
62. Findlay I. ATP^{4-} and ATP-Mg inhibit the ATP-sensitive K^+ channel of rat ventricular myocytes. Pflugers Arch. 1988; 412:37–41.
63. Findlay I. Effects of ADP upon the ATP-sensitive K^+ channel in rat ventricular myocytes. J Membr Biol 1988; 101:83–92.
64. Ashcroft F M. Adenosine 5′-triphosphate-sensitive potassium channels. Annu Rev Neurosci 1988; 11:97–118.
65. Escande D, Thuringer D, Le Guern S, Cavero I. The potassium channel opener cromakalim (BRL 34915) activates ATP-dependent K^+ channels in isolated cardiac myocytes. Biochem Biophys Res Commun 1988; 154:620–5.
66. Escande D, Thuringer D, Le Guern S, Courteix J, Laville M, Cavero I. Potassium channel openers act through an activation of ATP-sensitive K^+ channels in guinea-pig cardiac myocytes. Pflugers Arch 1989; 414:669–75.
67. Sanguinetti M C, Scott A L, Zingaro G J, Siegl P K S. BRL 34915 (cromakalim) activates ATP-sensitive K^+ current in cardiac muscle. Proc Natl Acad Sci 1988; 85:8360–4.
68. Quast U, Cook N S. Moving together: K^+ channel openers and ATP-sensitive K^+ channels. Trends Pharmacol Sci 1989; 10:431–45.
69. Standen N B, Quayle J M, Davies N W, Brayden J E, Huang Y, Nelson M T. Hyperpolarizing vasodilators activate ATP-sensitive K^+ channels in arterial smooth muscle. Science 1989; 245:177–80.
70. Beech D J, Bolton T B. Properties of the cromakalim-induced potassium conductance in smooth muscle cells isolated from the rabbit portal vein. Br J Pharmacol 1989; 98:851–64.
71. Escande D, Thuringer D, Le Guern S, Cavero I. The potassium channel opener cromakalim (BRL 34915) activates ATP-dependent K^+ channels in isolated cardiac myocytes. Biochem Biophys Res Commun 1988; 154:620–5.
72. Arena J P, Kass R S. Activation of ATP-sensitive K channels in heart cells by pinacidil: dependence on ATP. Am J Physiol 1989; 257:H2092–6.
73. Liu B, Golyan F, McCullough J R, Vassalle M. Electrophysiological and antiarrhythmic effects of the K-channel opener, BRL 34915, in cardiac Purkinje fibers. Drug Dev Res 1988; 14:123–139.
74. Smallwood J K, Steinberg M I. Cardiac electrophysiological effects of pinacidil and related pyridylcyanoguanidines: relationship to antihypertensive activity. J Cardiovasc Pharmacol 1988; 12:102–9.
75. Cameron J S, Kimura S, Jackson-Burns D A, Smith D B, Bassett A L. ATP-sensitive K^+ channels are altered in hypertrophied ventricular myocytes. Am J Physiol 1988; 255:H1254–8.
76. Kleiman R B, Houser S R. Outward currents in normal and hypertrophied feline ventricular myocytes. Am J Physiol 1989; 256:H1450–H1461.
77. Lee C O, Kang D H, Sokol J H, Lee K S. Relation between intracellular Na iron activity and tension of sheep cardiac Purkinje fibers exposed to dihydro-ouabain. Biophys J 1980; 29:315–30.
78. Kameyama M, Kakei M, Sato R, Shibasaki T, Matsuda H, Irisawa H. Intracellular Na^+ activates a K^+ channel in mammalian cardiac cells. Nature 1984; 309:354–6.

79. Sanguinetti M C. Na^+-activated and ATP-sensitive K^+ channels in the heart. In: Colatsky TJ, ed. Potassium channels basic function and therapeutic aspects. New York: Wiley-Liss, 1990; 85–109.
80. Carmeliet E. Na^+ activated K^+ channel in cardiac myocytes: rectification, open probability and block. Biophys J 1990; 57:118a.
81. Luk H-N. Induction and block of Na^+ activated K^+ current in guinea-pig ventricular myocytes. Biophys J 1990; 57:118a.
82. Morad M, Orkand R. Excitation–contraction coupling in frog ventricle: evidence from voltage clamp studies. J Physiol 1971; 219:167–89.
83. Fedida D, Braun A P, Clark R B, Giles W R. Alpha$_1$-adrenergic modulation of a transient K^+ current in rabbit atrial myocytes is via a pertussis toxin insensitive G-protein and a diffusible second messenger. Biophys J 1990; 57:13a.
84. Farah A E, Alousi A A, Schwarz R P Jr. Positive inotropic agents. Ann. Rev. Pharmacol. Toxicol. 1984; 24:275–328.
85. Gwilt M, Dalrymple H W, Blackburn K J, Burges R A, Dickinson R P, Cross P E, Higgins A J. UK-68,914, a novel class III antiarrhythmic agent which blocks potassium channels. Circulation 1988; 78:II150.
86. Dalrymple H W, Butler P, Sutton M R, Dodd M G. Effects of UK-68,798, a novel class III antiarrhythmic agent, in conscious dogs. J. Mol. Cell. Cardiol. 1989; 21(Suppl. II):S10.

29

Na–Ca Exchange: Basic Science and Experimental Pharmacology

GREGORY J. KACZOROWSKI

Merck Research Laboratories
Rahway, New Jersey

I. THE Na–Ca EXCHANGE REACTION

Regulation of calcium homeostasis in electrically excitable cells is critical for the normal function of excitation–response coupling processes. A number of pathways have evolved to control flux of Ca^{2+} across the plasma membrane of cells and these are outlined schematically in Figure 1. Among the pathways that mediate Ca^{2+} influx directly are voltage-dependent and receptor-operated Ca^{2+} channels. K^+ channels also regulate Ca^{2+} influx, but do so in an indirect fashion by controlling repolarization of the plasma membrane. Once Ca^{2+} enters the cell and acts as a second messenger, elevated intracellular Ca^{2+} must be returned to resting levels. This can occur by sequestration of Ca^{2+} into intracellular organelles, or by the removal of Ca^{2+} using various Ca^{2+} efflux pathways. The two prominent mechanisms that carry out Ca^{2+} removal are the plasmalemmal Ca^{2+}-ATPase and Na–Ca exchange reactions. The Ca^{2+}-ATPase transport mechanism is a high-affinity, low-capacity system that utilizes the energy in ATP hydrolysis to pump Ca^{2+} from the cell, against a chemical concentration gradient approximately four orders in magnitude for this ion. Na–Ca exchange, on the other hand, is an antiport reaction that utilizes the energy present in the electrochemical potential of one ion as it passes down its concentration gradient to drive the movement of another ion against its concentration gradient (i.e., transport of the first ion is manditorily coupled to flux of the second ion). Because plasmalemmal Na–Ca exchange has been demonstrated to be a completely reversible, electrogenic (i.e., net charge movement occurs) transport reaction, the direction in which Ca^{2+} moves is controlled by the magnitude and orientation of transmembrane electrical and chemical concentration gradients. Therefore, Na–Ca exchange can either provide a Ca^{2+} efflux pathway or it can promote net influx of Ca^{2+}, depending on physiological conditions within the cell.

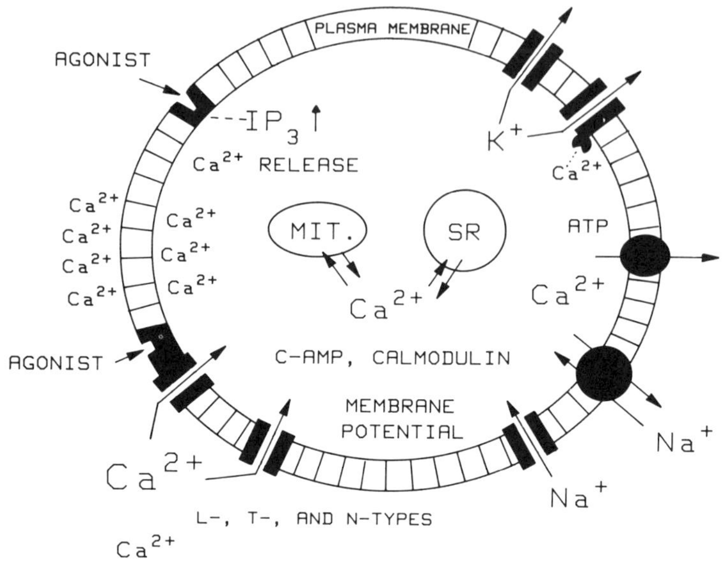

Figure 1 The processes that control Ca^{2+} homeostasis in electrically excitable cells are outlined schematically. Voltage-dependent and receptor-operated Ca^{2+} channels provide a pathway for Ca^{2+} influx. Membrane potential can be modulated by either voltage-dependent K^+ or Ca^{2+}-activated K^+ channels. Intracellular organelles (e.g., mitochondria, sarcoplasmic reticulum) can sequester Ca^{2+}, thereby lowering cytoplasmic Ca^{2+} levels. The Na–Ca exchange and Ca^{2+}–ATPase reactions provide efflux pathways to clear intracellular Ca^{2+}. Na–Ca exchange can also mediate Ca^{2+} influx. Together, these mechanisms regulate the movement of Ca^{2+} into and out of cells, and maintain resting cell Ca^{2+} levels at 100 nM.

Whether Na–Ca exchange is present in the plasma membrane had been a matter of considerable controversy. The first direct evidence for the existence of this transport system was provided by data obtained with squid axon (1). It was shown that certain movements of $^{45}Ca^{2+}$ across the axon plasmalemma were coupled directly to transport of Na^+ in the opposite direction. Subsequently, Na–Ca exchange reactions have been described in a variety of different cell types. These include excitable cells, such as those comprising muscular (e.g., cardiac, smooth, and skeletal), neural (e.g., brain and cell lines derived from neuronal sources), endocrine (e.g., pancreatic β cells, pituitary), and visual transducing (e.g., rod outer segments) tissues. The Na–Ca exchange system has also been detected in some nonexcitable cells (e.g., kidney, bladder, blood cells such as platelets, lymphocytes and neutrophils, and sperm). A different, nonelectrogenic, Na–Ca exchange reaction is present in mitochondria isolated from electrically excitable cells (e.g., heart and brain). Although the existence of Na–Ca exchange in a variety of cells is now well accepted, the precise physiological role of this mechanism in controlling Ca^{2+} homeostasis is still the subject of much debate. The highest levels of Na–Ca exchange are present in cardiac and vascular smooth muscle tissues. This review will concentrate on studies directed at determining the role of Na–Ca exchange in those tissues. For further information regarding the characteristics and physiological significance of the Na–Ca exchange reaction, the reader is directed to several other recent reviews in which these subjects are discussed (2–8).

Many different approaches have been used to elucidate the properties of the Na–Ca exchange system. The transport reaction has been monitored in whole cells either by direct measurements of $^{45}Ca^{2+}$ fluxes, or by recording currents that result from electrogenic flux of ions during carrier turnover. Na-dependent $^{45}Ca^{2+}$ fluxes have been characterized in atria (9), in embryonic myocytes (10), and in isolated vascular smooth muscle cells (11), while electrophysiological measurements have been used to demonstrate Na–Ca exchange activity in intact cardiac myocytes (12–15). Similar important studies have been carried out with squid axon and barnacle muscle preparations (16, 17).

Purified plasma membrane vesicles derived from the tissue of interest are perhaps the most convenient system for characterizing the properties of any transport system, including Na–Ca exchange. Such a preparation affords the opportunity of studying the transport reaction in isolation, under conditions in which other cellular mechanisms thought to be involved in Ca^{2+} transport, binding, and sequestration are not operable. With the use of this type of approach, Na–Ca exchange activity has been unequivocally demonstrated in heart and vascular smooth muscle sarcolemma.

The initial description of Na–Ca exchange in cardiac sarcolemmal membranes was made by Reeves and Sutko, who demonstrated that this vesicle preparation would transport Ca^{2+} in response to an imposed Na^+ gradient (18). A wealth of information regarding the cardiac transport system has since been obtained by studying sarcolemmal membranes. The Na–Ca exchange reaction has been shown to be electrogenic (19), to function in a bidirectional fashion (20), and to operate with a stoichiometry of 3 Na^+/Ca^{2+} (21). The kinetic parameters of the cardiac transport reaction have also been well characterized (22–24). These studies indicate that Na–Ca exchange is kinetically symmetrical, and that the specific activity of transport is highest in heart, as compared with the activity present in membranes from any other sources which have been investigated.

Data obtained by analyzing the kinetics of the cardiac sarcolemmal Na–Ca exchange transporter have been used to support a hypothetical model describing turnover of this protein (25). Based on flux measurements, two classes of ion binding sites have been detected on the transporter: a site common for Ca^{2+} and Na^+ (A-site), and another site to which only Na^+ binds (B-site). Binding two Na^+ at the A-site, and one Na^+ at the B-site, is required for transport of Ca^{2+} bound to an A-site on the opposite face of the membrane. This reaction is thought to occur by a concerted mechanism. When Ca^{2+} occupies A-sites on both faces of the carrier, the B-site exhibits broader substrate specificity, and it is presumed that this is where alkali metal ions bind that are known to stimulate the rate of Ca–Ca exchange, a nonproductive mode of carrier turnover. Binding sites for such monovalent cations apparently exist at both surfaces of the transporter, since rates of Ca–Ca exchange are highest when these ions are present simultaneously at both membrane surfaces. These stimulatory cations are not transported, however. The model proposed for cardiac Na–Ca exchange is similar in many of its details to a scheme put forth by Blaustein to describe the transport mechanism in squid axon and barnacle muscle (26).

The cardiac vesicle system has also been employed in attempts to identify and purify the cardiac Na–Ca exchange protein, but these approaches have met with limited success. Four different groups have published data regarding the molecular size of the Na–Ca exchange carrier. In the initial report (27), cardiac sarcolemmal vesicles were subjected to proteolysis with pronase, which digested most of the membraneous proteins but left Na–Ca exchange activity intact. Analysis of the resulting protein content suggested that the cardiac transporter exists as an 82 kDa glycoprotein. This group subsequently demonstrated that transport activity was not associated with that particular candidate protein. In another approach, the cardiac Na–Ca exchange carrier was partially purified using rate-zonal centrifugation, and was tentatively identified as a protein of 33 kDa (28). Moreover, in a second study employing antibodies against the 33 kDa protein, this group reported that the cardiac carrier was composed of a tetramer of 33 kDa subunits that display 33, 70, and 140 kDa bands on Western blots (29). In an independent study, another laboratory suggested that 70 and 120 kDa proteins are associated with the cardiac transporter based upon a different fractionation procedure they developed (30). However, since this preparation was not homogeneous, it has not been possible to assign a molecular mass to the Na–Ca exchange transporter with any degree of certainty. In a recent study, the cardiac carrier protein was identified as having a native molecular weight of at least 225 kDa (31). This postulate is based on three different experimental findings: data obtained from radiation inactivation analysis which gives some indication of the size of the transporter; molecular size determination using high-performance liquid chromatographic (HPLC) sieve fractionation techniques; and identification of Ca^{2+}-binding proteins of this molecular mass in cardiac sarcolemmal membrane extracts. No consensus opinion has been reached as to what protein is associated with Na–Ca exchange activity. Recent flux measurements obtained using a reconstitution-protein dilution technique have demonstrated that the cardiac carrier is most likely a low-density, high-turnover transport system (32). Therefore, it may be technically formidable to purify the cardiac Na–Ca exchange protein to homogeneity using conventional techniques. To circumvent this difficulty, several groups have tried to express the cardiac transporter in a *Xenopus* oocyte system as a first step in the cloning of the protein (33, 34). In initial attempts, the functional expression of Na–Ca exchange activity after injection of oocytes with cardiac mRNA was successful, although the level of expression was low (5-fold), and the results appeared highly variable. More recently, these techniques have been used to clone and functionally express the Na–Ca exchange protein from dog heart (34a). The isolated cDNA codes for a protein of 970 residues: the N-terminus is hydrophobic with 6 potential transmembrane spanning regions coupled to a hydrophilic cytoplasmic domain followed by another hydrophobic region at the C-terminus of the protein with an additional 6 transmembrane helices. A homology exists with the Na^+, K^+, ATPase. Interestingly, polyclonal antibodies produced against synthetic peptides derived from the deduced amino acid sequence recognize sarcolemmal proteins of 70, 120 and 160 kDa on immunoblots. The functional expression of the Na–Ca exchanger will lead to the production of significant quantities of this protein for biochemical studies, and may ultimately provide structural information with which to rationally design transport inhibitors.

II. PHYSIOLOGICAL IMPORTANCE AND PATHOPHYSIOLOGICAL ROLE OF Na–Ca EXCHANGE

Although biochemical studies of vesicular Na–Ca exchange have helped to define the properties of the transport reaction, the physiological role of Na–Ca exchange in heart and vascular smooth muscle is still controversial. Most investigators who have addressed this issue have done so by studying cardiac models. A major problem hampering these studies is determinating the relative contribution of Na–Ca exchange to that of other mechanisms that transport Ca^{2+}, sequester Ca^{2+}, or bind Ca^{2+} in the control of myocyte Ca^{2+} homeostasis. As one example of this dilemma, it has been postulated that both Na–Ca exchange and plasmalemmal Ca^{2+}-ATPase function in removing Ca^{2+} from the cell. However, because specific inhibitors do not exist for either of these systems, it is not possible to assess accurately the importance of either process as Ca^{2+} efflux pathways. In addition, most data generated regarding the relative contribution of Na–Ca exchange compared with other systems in regulating cell Ca^{2+} are highly dependent on experimental conditions, making extrapolation to physiological situations difficult. Theoretical arguments have also been used to predict the relative role of Na–Ca exchange in cardiac contractility. For example, it has been proposed on thermodynamic grounds that Na–Ca exchange functions primarily in the Ca^{2+} efflux mode in well-polarized cardiac cells (4, 35), while this process promotes net Ca^{2+} influx during the plateau phase of the cardiac action potential, when the cell is depolarized (6). However, because of uncertainties that arise in application of equilibrium thermodynamics to *in vivo* situations, where the intracellular ionic environment exists under steady-state rather than equilibrium conditions, it is not possible to quantitate the direction or amount of Ca^{2+} flux through the Na–Ca exchange pathway on a beat-to-beat basis in heart using these means. Thus, the physiological significance of Na–Ca exchange as a modulator of intracellular Ca^{2+}, either by acting directly, or by indirectly controlling total intracellular Ca^{2+} stores, needs to be clarified in cardiac as well as in other issues.

Regardless of these problems, a number of different experimental paradigms exist that appropriately illustrate a correlation between the operation of Na–Ca exchange and physiological responses in heart (for reviews, see 3–7). For example, intracellular Na^+ and Ca^{2+} activities have been measured by microelectrode recording techniques, and have been found to vary in response to alterations in extracellular Na^+ in a fashion consistent with the operation of a highly active Na–Ca exchange mechanism. Moreover, the positive inotropic effect that results when intracellular Na^+ is elevated suggests that Na–Ca exchange can affect contractility of cardiac tissue by modulating total intracellular Ca^+ stores. Baker et al. originally hypothesized that the mechanism by which cardiac glycosides increase contractility results from elevation of intracellular Na^+ due to Na^+, K^+-ATPase block, and subsequent influx of Ca^{2+} by the Na–Ca exchange reaction (36). It appears that a number of new positive inotropic agents (e.g., DPI 201-106) that promote elevation of intracellular Na^+ by slowing inactivation of voltage-dependent Na^+ channels also act in this way. Whether an inhibitor that directly affects activity of Na–Ca exchange will possess cardiotonic properties (37) remains to be determined.

Cardiac Na–Ca exchange has been implicated in a number of different pathophysiological conditions in which intracellular Na^+ concentration is elevated. During ouabain-induced arrhythmogenesis, the action of Na–Ca exchange is probably responsible for Ca^{2+} overloading of the sarcoplasmic reticulum. When the sarcoplasmic reticulum becomes overloaded, spontaneous and asynchronous release of Ca^{2+} occurs, which results in widely varying fluctuations in intracellular Ca^{2+} levels (38). Since intracellular Ca^{2+} not only regulates activity of various ion channels present in the sarcolemma but also controls muscle contractility, such variations could disrupt normal patterns of electrical activity and destroy synchronous contractility, leading to an arrhythmogenic situation. Under certain conditions of cardiac ischemia, it is known that Na^+ levels also become elevated (39). Some of the cellular damage and subsequent arrhythmias that arise during reperfusion may likewise be due to Ca^{2+} influx through Na–Ca exchange. Therefore, a selective inhibitor of the transport reaction might prove beneficial in treating ouabain toxicity, or ischemia and reperfusion injury.

Recent studies on reoxygenation-induced Ca^{2+} overload of hypoxic cultured myocytes support the idea that Ca^{2+} entry via Na–Ca exchange can occur during reperfusion (40). Although Ca^{2+} entry blockers were not effective in preventing Ca^{2+} gain when added upon reoxygenation, an inhibitor of Na–Ca exchange did ameliorate Ca^{2+} overloading under these conditions. In addition, agents acting as free radical scavengers were also cytoprotective in these protocols. Therefore, it is of interest that certain copper-containing cryptand complexes act both as O_2 free radical scavengers and as inhibitors of Na–Ca exchange in isolated cardiac sarcolemmal membranes (41). It may be possible to use similar agents during ischemia and reperfusion episodes to elicit cardioprotective behavior. When the effect of ischemic insult was monitored directly on Na–Ca exchange activity in sarcolemmal membranes isolated from damaged tissue, transport activity was reduced, but the consequences of ischemia caused less inhibition of Na–Ca exchange activity in newborns than in adult tissue (42). These results probably correlate with the observation that the newborn heart shows greater tolerance to ischemia than does adult cardiac tissue. It has also been noted that fatty acids are generated during ischemia (43), and that fatty acids enhance turnover of Na–Ca exchange by modifying the membrane environment surrounding the transporter (see below). To what extent fatty acid production modulates Na–Ca exchange activity or other sarcolemmal ion flux pathways *in vivo* under this pathophysiological state, has not been resolved. Nevertheless, taken together, these data suggest that a selective inhibitor of Na–Ca exchange would protect ischemic tissue during reperfusion by preventing any Ca^{2+} overload that occurs via action of this transport system.

The role of Na–Ca exchange in heart failure has been investigated by monitoring transport activity in vesicles isolated from tissues representing this pathophysiological condition. In one series of studies, membranes were prepared from animals of different ages and the specific activity of Na–Ca exchange was correlated with age of the heart. Although no differences were observed in the kinetics of the transport reaction in neonatal and adult rabbit heart membranes (44), another study found that Na–Ca exchange activity was attenuated in the aging myocardium (45). This could be associated with age-induced heart failure. Using the Syrian cardiomyopathic hamster as a model for congestive heart failure, another type of study demonstrated a relationship between levels of Na–Ca exchange activity and intracellular Ca^{2+} concentration (46). Ca^{2+} overload in aged animals is associated with an increase in voltage-dependent Ca^{2+} channels that occurs in the early necrotic stage of the disease. Na–Ca exchange activity is normal in the heart of young animals, but increases to 400% of control levels a month after birth. This time course suggests that augmentation in transport activity might be a secondary response to the increased level of Ca^{2+} channels present in myocytes. In elderly animals with heart failure, Na–Ca exchange was decreased by 50%, most likely due to the progressive cardiac damage that occurs with time. Correlating with these results is another study showing that Na–Ca exchange activity, but not other sarcolemmal processes, is decreased in membranes isolated from ventricles hypertrophied by pressure overload (47). Given these findings, it is difficult to predict how beneficial an inhibitor of Na–Ca exchange would be in heart failure in a situation in which cardiac cells are already Ca^{2+} overloaded. However, an appropriate inhibitor of this system that would block Ca^{2+} influx in damaged cells, while promoting a positive inotropic response in healthy myocytes, might elicit an overall positive therapeutic response.

It has been hypothesized that cardiac Na–Ca exchange may promote some of the cellular damage that occurs in endotoxin shock (48). This study suggested the interesting possibility that transport activity is decreased during endotoxemia by modification of the exchange reaction's stoichiometry from $3Na^+/Ca^{2+}$ to $2Na^+/Ca^{2+}$, thereby altering Ca^{2+} homeostasis through interference with endogenous regulation of carrier activity. Previous studies indicate the feasibility of accurately measuring the stoichiometry of Na–Ca exchange in cardiac sarcolemmal vesicles by employing a thermodynamic approach and using initial rate kinetic measurements (21). Upon applying these procedures, no alteration was detected in the stoichiometry of the transport reaction as a result of endotoxemia (49). Thus, currently little evidence exists to support the suggestion that Na–Ca exchange is a major target in the pathophysiology of endotoxic shock.

The other muscle tissue in which Na–Ca exchange has been postulated to play an important physiological role is vascular smooth muscle. Although tension development of vascular tissue under conditions that implicate the activity of an Na–Ca exchange mechanism had been reported in early studies (50), the existence of this transport reaction in smooth muscle has been debated (51). However, based on recent evidence obtained with whole cell and purified vesicle preparations, it is now well established that high levels of Na–Ca exchange exist in smooth muscle. In primary cultures of aortic smooth muscle cells, lowering extracellular Na^+ results in marked uptake of $^{45}Ca^{2+}$ into Na^+-loaded cells (52), extracellular Na^+ causes the efflux of intracellular Ca^{2+} released from the sarcoplasmic reticulum by treatment with the ionophore ionomycin (53), and Na^+-mediated transmembrane Ca^{2+} fluxes have been well characterized by Fura-2 fluorescence recording techniques (54). Taken together, these studies suggest that Na–Ca exchange functions in Ca^{2+} homeostasis of aortic smooth muscle, particularly under conditions of elevated intracellular Na^+, or when intracellular Ca^{2+} is increased following agonist stimulation of muscle tissue. Recent experiments with arterial smooth muscle rings derived from different tissues have also illustrated the participation of the Na–Ca exchange mechanism in tension development. With the use of thoracic aorta and tail artery, contractility data have been obtained that are consistent with the proposal that Na–Ca exchange can transport Ca^{2+} in either direction across the smooth muscle sarcolemmal membrane (55). It was also found that Na–Ca exchange can increase the Ca^{2+} load of the sarcoplasmic reticulum, so that under certain conditions muscle contractility can be markedly enhanced, even though the action of this transport system may cause less dramatic effects on basal muscle tone.

Experiments with membrane vesicles isolated from smooth muscle have confirmed and extended the cell and tissue studies. It was originally reported that Na–Ca exchange activity in aortic and other types of smooth muscle sarcolemmal membranes is very low, and that Ca^{2+}-ATPase is the predominant plasmalemmal Ca^{2+}

transport system (56, 57). However, recent evidence obtained with vesicles from mesenteric arteries (58, 59) and aorta (60) have yielded significantly different results. Indeed, data acquired with highly purified sarcolemmal preparations from either bovine or porcine aortic tissue demonstrate that the specific activity of Na–Ca exchange in these sources is comparable to that present in cardiac sarcolemmal membranes prepared from the same species (60). The reasons for discrepancies in the various studies are twofold: one pertains to the preparation of highly purified sarcolemmal membranes, which forms the basis for the flux measurements, and the other relates to the determination of vesicular Ca^{2+} fluxes under initial rate conditions. A procedure has been developed for the preparation of vesicles from aorta that are highly enriched in sarcolemmal marker activities (e.g., binding of Ca^{2+} entry blockers as markers for L-type Ca^{2+} channels, binding of cyanopindolol as a marker for β receptors, and binding of ouabain as a marker for Na^+,K^+-ATPase; 60). When Na-dependent Ca^{2+} uptake is monitored in this preparation, the membranes rapidly accumulate Ca^{2+} by a process that is completely reversible and dependent on the presence of a transmembrane Na^+ gradient (Fig. 2). The kinetics of Na–Ca exchange determined under initial velocity conditions (i.e., using 0.5 sec time points) indicate similar K_m values for Ca^{2+} and Na^+ as have been measured in the cardiac system, and the V_{max} for Ca^{2+} transport is typically fivefold lower than V_{max} values found in heart preparations. Similar to the transport reaction in heart, aortic Na–Ca exchange is electrogenic, and blocked by well-characterized mechanism-based or-

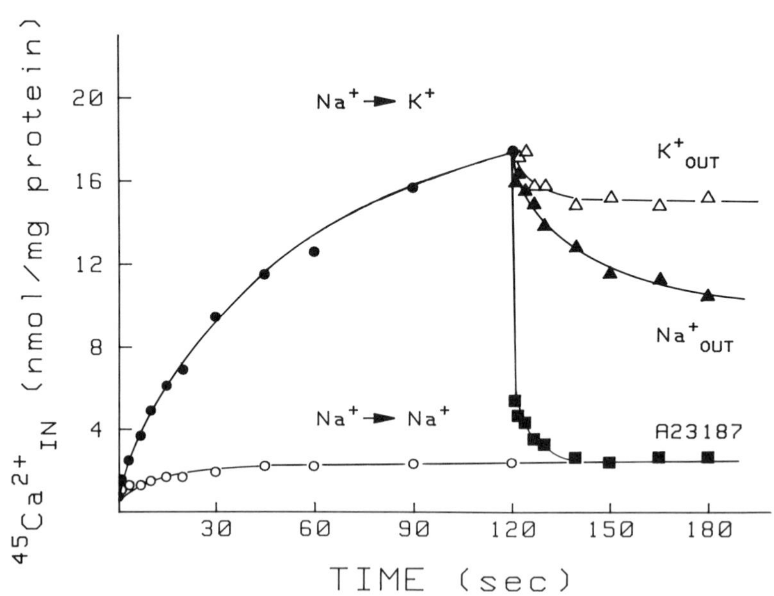

Figure 2 Purified sarcolemmal membrane vesicles derived from bovine aortic smooth muscle were passively loaded with 160 mM NaCl, 20 mM Mops-Tris, pH 7.4. Aliquots of membranes were diluted 100-fold into the same buffer containing either 160 mM NaCl (○), or 160 mM KCl (●), with 15 μM $^{45}CaCl_2$ also present at 37°C. At the time indicated, the reaction mixture was diluted fivefold into a solution containing 100 μM EGTA and 160 mM KCl (△), 50 mM NaCl and 110 mM KCl (▲), or 160 mM KCl and 2 μM A23187 (■). Uptake and efflux of $^{45}Ca^{2+}$ were determined using filtration techniques.

ganic inhibitors (see below). When Na–Ca exchange and Ca^{2+}-ATPase activities were compared in the same membrane preparation under similar experimental conditions, maximal transport activity of Na–Ca exchange was 5–10-fold greater than that of the Ca^{2+}-ATPase. Similar findings have been reported with isolated sarcolemmal membranes derived from airway smooth muscle (61). These results unequivocally demonstrate that Na–Ca exchange is a primary pathway for Ca^{2+} transport in smooth muscle, and imply that this transport reaction plays a major role in controlling Ca^{2+} homeostasis of vascular tissue.

Even before the verification of high levels of Na–Ca exchange in smooth muscle, the pathophysiology of essential hypertension had been linked to this transport reaction in vascular tissue (62, 63). It was hypothesized that an endogenous Na^+,K^+-ATPase inhibitor appeared in the circulatory system in response to excess Na^+ and water retention. This ouabain-like substance was postulated to inhibit Na^+ pump activity in vascular smooth muscle, thereby leading to an elevation of intracellular Na^+ and consequent Ca^{2+} influx through the Na–Ca exchange mechanism, to culminate ultimately in an increase in vascular tone and peripheral resistance. Although this scheme provides a mechanistic foundation for essential hypertension, the endogenous substance had not been purified, or its structure determined. However, these issues have recently been clarified by the detection and purification of a ouabain-like component of human plasma (64, 65). This material has been purified 10^{10}-fold with respect to endogenous plasma levels, and appears to be homogeneous. It has been shown to block Na^+, K^+-ATPase activity with greater potency than that displayed by ouabain, it displays selectivity in that it does not inhibit other types of ATPases, and it behaves as a strictly competitive inhibitor of ouabain binding in both equilibrium and kinetic binding protocols. Moreover, the level of this factor was shown to increase in mineralcorticoid-induced hypertension in a pig model (66). When considered together, these data provide strong support for the notion that an endogenous ouabain-like substance exists, and that this agent controls contractility of vascular smooth muscle via affecting the sarcolemmal Na–Ca exchange process. This relationship could form a basis for the pathophysiology of essential hypertension. Recently, one of the ouabain-like substances purified from human plasma was shown to be oubain, itself (66a).

As a corollary to investigations linking vascular Na–Ca exchange to a hypertensive response, several studies were carried out in which absolute levels of transport activity were measured in different animal modes of hypertension. Such studies have been performed with both tissues and sarcolemmal membrane preparations isolated from target organs of interest. With the use of the spontaneously hypertensive rat (SHR) as a model, increased Na–Ca exchange activity has been observed in sarcolemmal membranes prepared from mesenteric arteries when these data are compared with transport levels present in tissues from normotensive (WKY) rats (67). A similar conclusion was obtained from indirect measurements of Na–Ca exchange activity using mechanical responses of aortic rings isolated from the SHR (68). Other studies measuring electrical and mechanical responses in cardiac muscle preparations from SHR and normotensive animals have also suggested the possibility that Na–Ca exchange is altered in the SHR (69). In another animal model of hypertension, the stroke-prone spontaneously hypertensive rat (SP-SHR), it was observed that Na–Ca exchange was decreased in isolated tail artery rings compared to that present in tissues from WKY rats (70). It is likely that the absolute levels of transport activity present in hypertensive animals are a secondary consequence of the pathophysiological condition. For example, it has been observed that growth of cardiac myocytes in the presence of ouabain increases the level of Na–Ca exchange in the sarcolemma (71), while subjecting heart tissue to long-term Ca^{2+} overload results in a diminished transport capacity of this system (46). Therefore, it is not clear whether the specific activity of Na–Ca exchange in smooth muscle is more closely controlled by chronic exposure to an endogenous ouabain-like substance or by the absolute levels of intracellular Ca^{2+}. Nonetheless, if intracellular Na^+ levels do elevate in vascular tissue, and this in turn brings about a hypertensive crisis, it is exciting to speculate that a selective inhibitor of Na–Ca exchange would possess therapeutic utility in essential hypertension.

Studies directed at determining the physiological or pathophysiological roles of Na–Ca exchange in heart, vascular smooth muscle, or any other tissues in which this transport system is present have been hampered by the lack of potent, selective blockers with which to modulate activity of the transport reaction *in vivo*. Because of the fact that Na–Ca exchange is a bidirectional process, whose operation is governed by the physiological conditions within the cell, it is nearly impossible to predict the absolute contribution of Na–Ca exchange in controlling cellular Ca^{2+} homeostasis without the use of an inhibitor. Therefore, progress in this area is critically linked to the discovery of specific agents that can either inhibit or enhance turnover of the Na–Ca exchange carrier. The utility of such compounds in deciphering the physiological role of Na–Ca exchange, and in developing new therapies, cannot be disputed.

III. INHIBITORS AND STIMULATORS OF TRANSPORT ACTIVITY

It is very difficult to identify specific inhibitors of the Na–Ca exchange reaction. Since no natural product toxins have been discovered that will potently block this transport system, leads for inhibitors have been sought by testing agents with existing cardiovascular pharmacologic effects, compounds known to block other transport systems, or organic molecules selected by random screening. Inorganic cations have also been examined for their ability to inhibit the Na–Ca exchange reaction. In general, screening using these approaches has met with limited success, although a small number of transport inhibitors have been identified and characterized (Fig. 3).

As expected, metal ions that interact at the different binding sites on the carrier protein will inhibit Na–Ca exchange activity in either vesicles or whole cells. Cardiac sarcolemmal membranes have been used to determine the rank order of potency of various ions as inhibitors (72). Of the tri- and divalent cations investigated, La^{3+} was most potent, followed by Nd^{3+}, Tm^{3+}, Y^{3+}, Cd^{2+}, Sr^{2+}, Ba^{2+}, Mn^{2+}, and Mg^{2+}, in decreasing order of potency. Some of these ions serve as carrier substrates (e.g., Ba^{2+}, Sr^{2+}), and thereby inhibit Ca^{2+} movement by competing with the latter ion for binding at the A-site of the transporter (73). The most potent inorganic inhibitor of Na–Ca exchange in vesicles (18), whole cells (10), or intact tissues (9) is La^{3+}, but since this ion blocks most Ca^{2+} transporting proteins its utility as an inhibitor is limited. However, under prescribed experimental conditions in which Na–Ca exchange activity can be isolated, La^{3+} is an effective transport inhibitor (10). Other divalent cations have been used similarly to probe Na–Ca exchange activity in cultured smooth muscle cells, where these agents either serve as carrier

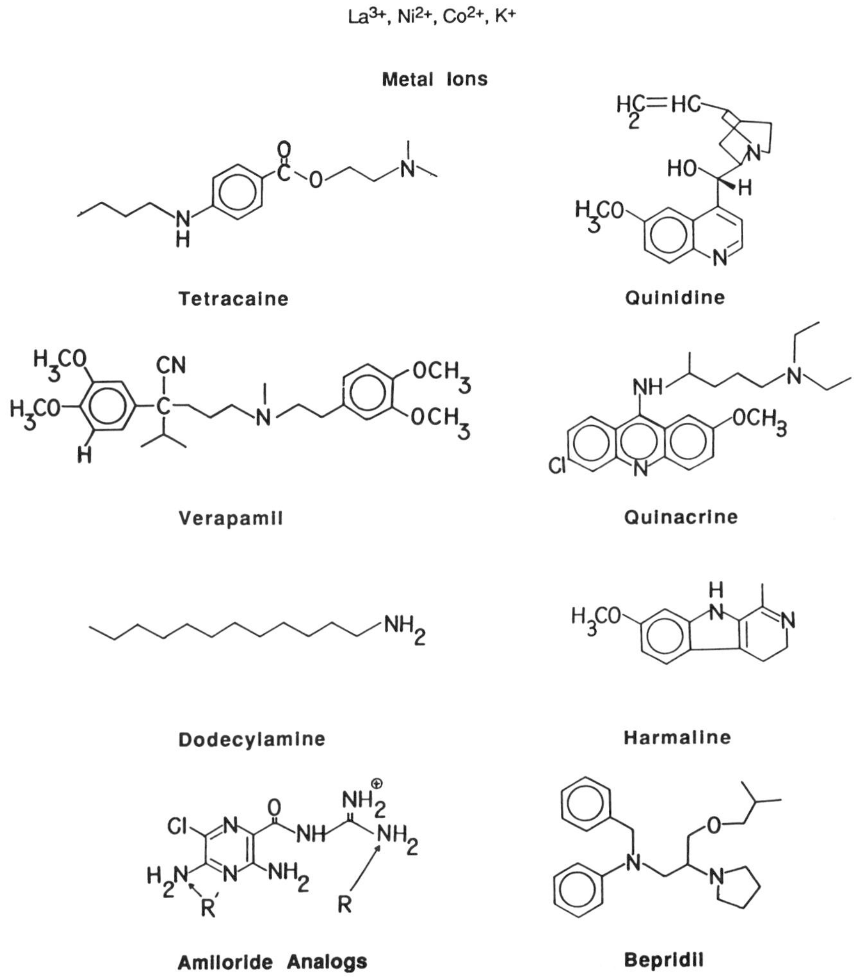

Figure 3 Various structural classes of sarcolemmal Na–Ca exchange inhibitors are illustrated. Amiloride analogs derivatized at the terminal guanidino-nitrogen (R), the 5 pyrazinoyl-nitrogen (R′), or at both of these positions are more potent Na–Ca exchange inhibitors than amiloride itself. Amiloride analogs, bepridil, and metal ions are mechanism-based inhibitors.

substrates (e.g., Sr^{2+}), or compete with Ca^{2+} for binding at the A-site as non-transportable substrates (Mg^{2+}; 74). Likewise, Ni^{2+}, Mn^{2+}, and Co^{2+}, can be used to block both influx and efflux modes of carrier turnover in squid axon (75). Several monovalent cations (Li^{+}, K^{+}, Rb^{+}, choline, and, of course, Na^{+}), have also been demonstrated to block Na–Ca exchange in membrane preparations derived from heart and smooth muscle, with a wide range of potencies (22, 60).

Many different organic compounds that have lipophilic properties will inhibit Na–Ca exchange, but these agents do so without selectivity. Indeed, in most cases, exceptionally high concentrations are required to achieve blocking activity. Among these weak inhibitors are local anesthetics such as tetracaine, dibucaine, and ethanol (75–77), neuroleptic agents such as chlorpromazine (78), very hydrophobic Ca^{2+} entry blockers such as verapamil (79), antiarrhythmic agents such as quinidine (80), and the membrane-active antibiotic polymyxin B (81). It is unlikely that any of these agents interact in a specific fashion with the Na–Ca exchange carrier, given the high concentrations required to achieve inhibition. Instead, block of carrier function could simply result from perturbation of lipid-protein interactions.

Other membrane active agents inhibit Na–Ca exchange by more interesting mechanisms. Quinacrine is an effective blocker of Na–Ca exchange in cardiac sarcolemmal membranes (82) and myocytes (83). Quinacrine blocks all modes of carrier turnover (i.e., Na–Ca, Ca–Ca, and Na–Na exchange reactions) with an IC_{50} of 50 μM. A kinetic analysis of the resulting inhibitory patterns reveals that block is noncompetitive *vs.* Ca^{2+} but competitive *vs.* Na^+. Similar patterns have also been observed with classes of Na–Ca exchange blockers termed mechanism-based inhibitors that interact at discrete substrate-binding sites on the carrier (see below). However, subsequent experiments have revealed that quinacrine does not bind to either the well-defined A- or B-sites on the transporter (84, J. Reeves, personal communication). Nevertheless, quinacrine interacts directly with the transport protein because the alkylating agent, quinacrine mustard, causes irreversible inactivation of carrier activity, a property maintained following solubilization and reconstitution procedures (85). In addition, under some experimental conditions, quinacrine stimulates Na–Ca exchange activity (82). Stimulation is due to a decrease in the K_m for Ca^{2+} and appears to be related to an electrostatic interaction between quinacrine and the carrier protein at the inner membrane surface causing acceleration of the rate-determining step of the transport reaction. This is a unique effect that is not observed with other inhibitors of Na–Ca exchange. Therefore, these data suggest that quinacrine recognizes a previously undescribed site on the transporter. The utility of quinacrine as an effective probe of Na–Ca exchange is limited, however, because of the numerous other membrane processes that have been shown to be affected by this agent.

A number of other membrane agents are potent inhibitors of Na–Ca exchange, but apparently do not interact directly with the transporter. Examples of this type of agent are a series of amphiphilic cations, of which dodeclyamine is a representative member (86). These lipophilic cations block Na–Ca exchange activity in cardiac sarcolemmal membranes at lower concentrations (e.g., the IC_{50} of dodecylamine is 20 μM) than those at which they disrupt the osmotic integrity of the membrane. Although these agents have been demonstrated to affect contractility of isolated cardiac muscle preparations in a fashion consistent with block of Na–Ca exchange (87), they are also potent inhibitors of voltage-dependent Ca^{2+} and K^+ channels in heart (83). In addition, a kinetic analysis of dodecylamine action indicates that this compound does not interact at any of the known substrate-binding sites on the carrier (84). More likely, it functions by disrupting the membrane environment surrounding the transport protein. This hypothesis is consistent with the finding that a number of different amphiphilic molecules (e.g., phospholipids, fatty acids, and other structurally similar agents) affect Na–Ca exchange in membrane vesicles (see below). Therefore, it is unlikely that amphiphilic cations like dodecylamine are leads for specific inhibitors of Na–Ca exchange, since not only do they interact indirectly with the transport protein but they also affect a number of other membrane-associated processes.

Another type of Na–Ca exchange inhibitor are those molecules that chelate intracellular Ca^{2+}. Typical of such agents is the fluorescent Ca^{2+} indicator quin 2, which blocks this transport reaction in squid axon (88). Inhibition of Na–Ca exchange is specific for the Na_i-dependent Ca^{2+} influx mode, with no effect on the back reaction. This behavior is not unexpected given that Na–Ca exchange in this preparation requires the presence of intracellular Ca^{2+} to activate the carrier. Similar activation of Na–Ca exchange by internal Ca^{2+} exists in intact myocytes (for a discussion, see 89). Therefore, use of Ca^{2+}-chelating dyes to monitor cellular Ca^{2+} homeostasis could generate misleading information in cells where intracellular Ca^{2+} regulates activity of the Na–Ca exchange mechanism.

A number of drugs possessing known cardiovascular pharmacology have been tested to determine whether they will inhibit the Na–Ca exchange reaction. It might be expected that the positive inotropic activity of some cardiotonic agents would be related to inhibition of sarcolemmal Na–Ca exchange. However, none of the various classes of compounds thus far investigated (e.g., cardiotonic agents such as DPI 201-106, milrinone, dobutamine, digitalis analogs) have any effect on this transport reaction. It was reported that the positive inotrope, amrinone, inhibits Na–Ca exchange in cardiac membranes, albeit very high concentrations were required to achieve partial inhibition (90). This finding has not been confirmed by other investigators (91). Another agent with a cardiovascular profile suggesting that it might inhibit Na–Ca exchange is the antimetastatic anthracycline drug adriamycin (doxorubicin). This agent, which is cardiotoxic, has been reported to inhibit Na–Ca exchange in cardiac sarcolemmal vesicles with high potency (92). This observation has not been confirmed by other investigators who have monitored the effect of adriamycin on Na–Ca exchange in pituitary (93) or cardiac (4) membrane vesicles. Moreover, adriamycin does not inhibit currents related to Na–Ca exchange in myocytes (80), or affect Na–Ca exchange in squid axon (75).

Investigators have inquired whether various structural classes of organic Ca^{2+} entry blockers, clinically used vasodilators that are known inhibitors of L-type Ca^{2+} channels, will block Na–Ca exchange. In general, none of the Ca^{2+} entry blockers tested, representing benzothiazepine-, dihydropyridine-, aralkylamine-, or diphenylbutylpiperidine-type agents, affect cardiac Na–Ca exchange (84, 94). Of these different structural types, only one class has been shown to block a related transport system present in mitochondria isolated from some electrically excitable cells (i.e., the electroneutral Na–Ca exchange system present in the inner mitochondrial membrane). The benzothiazepine diltiazem is a relatively potent inhibitor of heart and brain mitochondrial Na–Ca exchange (95), despite it not displaying any effect on the plasmalemmal transporter. A number of different benzothiazepines and benzodiazepines inhibit Na–Ca exchange in cardiac mitochondria with K_i values in the low μM range (96). Although benzothiazepines are effective inhibitors of the L-type Ca^{2+} channel, some benzodiazepine blockers of mitochondrial Na–Ca exchange, such as clonezapam, are void of this activity (97). In addition, a complete structure-activity relationship has been developed for benzodiazepine-like agents as inhibitors of the mitochondrial transport reaction (98). Moreover, comparison of the effectiveness of diltiazem stereoisomers as blockers of L-type Ca^{2+} channels and mitochondrial Na–Ca exchange reveals different stereochemical requirements for inhibition of these two systems (99). These results suggest two possible uses for this structural class as a means of probing mitochondrial Na–Ca exchange. Since diltiazem is completely without effect in blocking sarcolemmal Na–Ca exchange, this agent can be used as a convenient way of determining the contamination level of cardiac sarcolemmal preparations with membranes derived from mitochondria. Moreover, certain benzodiazepines that do not inhibit L-type Ca^{2+} channels may be useful for assessing the physiological role of mitochondrial Na–Ca exchange in intact cardiac tissue.

Hydrophobic representatives of the aralkylamine and diphenylbutylpiperidine Ca^{2+} entry blocker classes are known to inhibit, at high concentration, a number of different ion transport pathways besides L-type Ca^{2+} channels (e.g., Na^+, K^+, and T-type Ca^{2+} channels, as well as Ca^{2+}-ATPase activities) because of their local anesthetic-like properties. Despite this pharmacologic profile, these agents are not usually effective inhibitors of sarcolemmal Na–Ca exchange. For example, verapamil, a member of the aralkylamine family, is a weak inhibitor of transport in cardiac membranes with an IC_{50} of ca. 250 μM (100). This is not clinically significant because inhibition occurs at much higher concentrations than those used therapeutically to achieve antihypertensive or antiarrhythmic activity. When a number of other members of these structural classes were investigated for their ability to block Na–Ca exchange in cardiac membranes, including WB 4101, D-600 (methoxyverapamil), desmethoxyverapamil, AQA 39, TMB 8, lidoflazine, cinnarizine, flunarizine, cyproheptadine, prenylamine, fluspiriline, pimozide, chlopimozide, and penfluridol, none were found to be active in the 1–10 μM range (84; unpublished observations). Thus, none of the Ca^{2+} entry blocker activity of the compounds listed above can be ascribed to inhibition of sarcolemmal Na–Ca exchange. The only structurally similar agent with moderately potent inhibitory activity identified to date is the mechanism-based inhibitor, bepridil (see below).

Some reports have claimed that dihydropyridine Ca^{2+} entry blockers inhibit sarcolemmal Na–Ca exchange (75, 101, 102), although most common examples of this structural type (e.g., nitrendipine, nimodipine, nifedipine) have no effect on the transport reaction (100; unpublished observations). In those instances in which dihydropyridines block transport activity, either very high concentrations were used or the inhibitory profile displayed peculiar properties. For example, nicardipine inhibits Na_i-dependent Ca^{2+} uptake into cardiac membranes, but has either no effect on, or causes slight stimulation of, Na_o-dependent Ca^{2+} efflux in this preparation (101). Because of the symmetrical nature of Na–Ca exchange in cardiac vesicles, it is not clear what this type of interaction indicates. Such a phenomenon could be related to diminished intravesicular Ca^{2+} binding capacity in the presence of drug. Other types of compounds (e.g., certain lipophilic cations) appear to be inhibitors of Na_i-dependent Ca^{2+} uptake, but do not block transport in a bidirectional fashion. It has been determined that these compounds decrease net Ca^{2+} uptake, when measurements are made over an extended period of time, by occluding intravesicular Ca^{2+} binding sites, thereby decreasing the total vesicular capacity for Ca^{2+} accumulation. These data demonstrate that inhibitors displaying this property represent false positives. Whether this is the case with nicardipine is not known, although recent electrophysiological experiments indicate that the dihydropyridine may have some efficacy as an Na–Ca exchange inhibitor in the μM concentration range (103).

A logical source of putative Na–Ca exchange inhibitors would be compounds known to block membrane transport processes in which movement of Na^+ occurs.

An example of such an agent is the alkaloid harmaline, which inhibits a variety of Na-dependent transport mechanisms (104). It was initially hypothesized from pharmacologic experiments with smooth muscle that harmaline blocks Na–Ca exchange (105). This was substantiated by demonstrating harmaline inhibition of Na–Ca exchange in cardiac membranes (IC_{50} of 250 μM; 106). The utility of harmaline as a cardiac Na–Ca exchange inhibitor is limited because, in addition to blocking a number of other Na-dependent transport reactions, it also displays significant Ca^{2+} entry blocker activity (107).

Another Na^+ transport inhibitor is the acylguanidine diuretic amiloride, which blocks epithelial Na^+ channels, Na-H exchange, and a number of other Na^+ transport reactions (for a review, see 108). Amiloride is a weak inhibitor of Na–Ca exchange in cells (109), and in membrane vesicles isolated from heart (110), brain (111, 112), kidney (113), and pituitary (93). In all cases, amiloride functions at mM concentration to inhibit transport activity. Since amiloride affects other cellular processes in the same concentration range, the lack of selectivity illustrates the limited use of this drug as a probe for Na–Ca exchange. However, amiloride analogs have been identified that do block Na–Ca exchange more potently (114, 115). These agents have been invaluable in exploring the mechanism of the antiport reaction (see below). In addition to blocking the sarcolemmal transport system, amiloride and amiloride derivatives also inhibit mitochondrial Na–Ca exchange by a different mechanism of action (116–118). Since both transport reactions are affected, it is difficult to differentiate between block of these systems in intact cell experiments, although the structure–activity relationship for inhibition of the two processes appears different.

It is possible to inhibit Na–Ca exchange in cardiac membranes by using chemical reagents that irreversibly modify either amino acid residues on the carrier protein or phospholipid residues in the membrane surrounding the transporter. For example, amino acid-specific alkylating agents alter Na–Ca exchange activity in sarcolemmal vesicles. Derivitization of free sulfhydryl groups with N-ethylmaleimide inhibits transport activity in this preparation (119). In fact, alkylating or reducing sulfhydryl residues produces a range of effects on Na–Ca exchange activity (120). The alteration in transport activity is highly dependent on the ionic composition of the incubation medium. Reducing agents inhibit Na–Ca exchange when vesicles are treated in the presence of K^+, whereas when the experiment is repeated in the presence of Na^+, no effect is manifested. Alkylation of protein sulfhydryl groups by N-ethylmaleimide is enhanced in the presence of Na^+. Other types of sulfhydryl alkylating reagents stimulate Na–Ca exchange through a mechanism blocked by the presence of Na^+. When considered together, these data suggest that a critical sulfhydryl residue(s) is located in close proximity to one of the substrate-binding sites on the carrier where Na^+ interacts. Reagents that modify other amino acid residues such as hydroxyl, amino, imidazole, guanidino, carboxyl, phenol, or indole groups, also modify carrier activity, but do not require the presence of Na^+ to have an effect (120). Chemical modification of phospholipid residues will also affect Na–Ca exchange activity in sarcolemmal membranes (121). Methylation of the phosphatidylethanolamine amino groups results in a diminution of transport activity, correlating with the hypothesis that transporter activity is regulated by the membrane environment. Part of the loss of Na–Ca exchange activity after treatment of membranes in this fashion may be due to direct methylation of the carrier (122).

Attempts have been made to prepare antibodies directed against the cardiac Na–Ca exchange protein to aid in identification and purification of the carrier, as well as to help assess the physiological role of this transport mechanism. Three separate laboratories have reported antibody production. Initially, it was noted that certain monoclonal antibodies that elevate intracellular Ca^{2+} in parathyroid cells will cause inhibition of Na–Ca exchange in cardiac membranes by directly interacting with the carricr protein (123). Three independent laboratories have been unable to confirm this observation (J. Reeves, and K. Philipson, personal communications, and unpublished observations from this laboratory). Most likely, this discrepancy is due to inaccurate measurements of Na–Ca exchange activity in the original investigation. It was also reported that polyclonal antibodies raised against cardiac sarcolemmal proteins isolated by preparative sodium dodecyl sulfate–polyacrylamide gel electrophoresis (SDS-PAGE) will inhibit Na–Ca exchange in heart membranes (29). Maximum inhibition of transport activity by this antibody preparation was 50%, suggesting that the antibodies that block function recognize epitopes exposed in only half of the membrane preparation. This is consistent with independent observations that sarcolemmal vesicles consist of 50% right-side-out and 50% inside-out membranes. However, the titer of active antibodies is not very high because excess IgG over sarcolemmal protein was required to elicit inhibitory activity. Because of low potency, such antibody preparations probably have little use in intact tissue studies, but do suggest the possibility for future preparation of antibodies that will block carrier function. There have been no further reports of experiments with these antibodies. It was reported more recently that antibodies raised against a partially purified sarcolemmal protein preparation displaying Na–Ca exchange activity would immunoprecipitate carrier activity (30). Although the precipitate contains a number of different sarcolemmal proteins, these results confirm that the transporter is a viable substrate for antibody production. With the use of similar approaches, antibodies were raised against the Na–Ca exchange carrier from brain, and they immunoprecipitate transport activity from detergent extracts of membranes (124). In neither case, however, do the antibodies block Na–Ca exchange in vesicles. Thus, such antibody preparations would be primarily indicated for identification and purification of the Na–Ca exchange protein.

In addition to inhibitors, a number of agents have been identified that stimulate Na–Ca exchange activity. These compounds can be classified into two categories: hydrophobic membrane components and redox active molecules. The first structural group shown to stimulate transport consists of negatively charged hydrophobic molecules that perturb the membrane environment and enhance turnover of the carrier. Examples of this type of agent include anionic phospholipids (125, 126), negatively charged amphiphilic molecules (86), fatty acids (127), and fatty acid derivatives (128). All of these stimulate transport activity in cardiac sarcolemmal vesicles. Perhaps the production of fatty acids during cardiac ischemia modulates Na–Ca exchange activity, although the quantity of fatty acids produced under pathophysiological conditions may not be great enough to achieve the type of stimulation observed in in vitro experiments (43). Neutral membrane constituents such as cholesterol also stimulate Na–Ca exchange (129 130). Incorporation of cholesterol into cardiac membranes by fusion with cholesterol-containing liposomes causes stimulation of transport activity due to an increase in the affinity for Ca^{2+}. Other membrane transport systems (e.g., Ca^{2+}-ATPase and Na^+, K^+-ATPase activities) were depressed by enrichment of membranes with cholesterol (129). In a separate study in which phospholipid composition was controlled by reconstitution, cholesterol incorporation into artificial liposomes also increased Na–Ca exchange activity (130). Using appropriate mixtures of anionic and neutral lipid components, it was possible to achieve maximal activation of carrier activity. Therefore, the Na–Ca exchange reaction appears to be more sensitive to its membrane environment than are other sarcolemmal-based transport systems. It was recently reported that Na–Ca exchange is also modulated by phosphatidylinositol metabolites (131). Hydrolysis of membrane phosphatidylinositol by phospholipase C results in stimulation of transport activity in cardiac membranes. It was suggested that this lipid either inhibits the transporter directly or modulates carrier activity by anchoring an endogenous regulatory protein to the sarcolemmal membrane. Phosphatidylinositol breakdown could stimulate Na–Ca exchange-mediated Ca^{2+} influx into specific target cells. Besides being sensitive to membrane components, Na–Ca exchange is stimulated by the lectin concanavalin A (132). It has been speculated that lectin-like substances may play a regulatory role in controlling transsarcolemmal Ca^{2+} flux.

The other general class of agents that stimulate Na–Ca exchange in cardiac vesicles are those that do so by direct redox modification of the carrier protein (133). The presence of both an oxidizing agent (e.g., O_2, H_2O_2, oxidized glutathione) and a reducing agent (e.g., O_2^- Fe^{2+}, dithiothreitol, reduced glutathione) is required for the stimulatory effect. Carrier substrates control the activation process, since Ca^{2+} blocks stimulation, but Na^+ is required to enhance transport activity. Under certain pathophysiological conditions such as ischemia, regulation of Na–Ca exchange by a redox mechanism could be important. This pathway might also be involved in controlling transport activity under normal conditions. Since no physiological studies have addressed these issues, it is impossible to speculate further as to the consequences of regulating Na–Ca exchange by redox active agents.

IV. DEVELOPMENT OF MECHANISM-BASED INHIBITORS OF Na–Ca EXCHANGE

Mechanism-based inhibitors of Na–Ca exchange are those agents that interact directly with the carrier at discrete substrate-binding sites, and whose inhibitory activity is dictated by conditions that control turnover of the transporter (134, 135). Two structural classes of molecules have been identified that inhibit Na–Ca exchange in this fashion. The first group is represented by amiloride analogs that are widely used probes of Na-coupled transport systems. The second structural class is typified by the Ca^{2+} entry blocker and antiarrhythmic agent bepridil. These two inhibitor classes behave differently in their interaction with the transporter, and consequently produce distinct inhibitory patterns. Despite these differences, both classes bind at discrete sites on the carrier. Investigation of these compounds has established mechanistic criteria by which to evaluate other types of Na–Ca exchange inhibitors. These studies also delineate certain criteria by which to develop more selective Na–Ca exchange inhibitors.

Even though amiloride is a weak inhibitor of Na–Ca exchange, various derivatives have been identified that block transport with significantly greater potency than the parent compound (110, 114). Three analog series are active in inhibiting this reaction: terminal guanidino-nitrogen-substituted analogs, derivatives substituted at the 5-position pyrazinoyl-nitrogen, and molecules derivatized at both of these positions. Members of each structural class inhibit Na–Ca exchange in cardiac membranes with a defined rank order of potency. For example, of the many different acyl-guanidine derivatives investigated, increasing hydrophobicity of substituents within defined structural constraints results in compounds 100-fold more potent than amiloride at blocking the transport reaction (114). The most potent inhibitors in this series are the result of addition of aryl groups to the terminal guanidino-nitrogen. Strict increases in hydrophobicity are not the only requirement for enhanced activity because many hydrophobic alkyl derivatives are no more potent than amiloride itself. No stereochemical restrictions are associated with guanidino-nitrogen substituents since the two stereoisomers of N-1-naphthylethylamiloride are equipotent inhibitors, demonstrating the lack of interaction at a chiral site on the transporter. The cationic form of amiloride is required for an interaction with the carrier, since deletion of the guanidino-group, or substitution to lower the pK_a of the guanidinium nitrogen from 9.0, results in loss of activity. These observations are consistent with the idea that amiloride analogs mimic Na^+ in their interaction with Na–Ca exchange, as has been shown with many different amiloride-sensitive transport systems. The hypothesis that a positively charged molecule is necessary for blocking the Na–Ca exchange reaction was recently confirmed (136). In this case, the degree of inhibition was found to correlate with the extent of protonation of amiloride's acylguanidinium group, and Na^+ protected against inhibition. Na^+ blocked amilorde action when it was present at the same membrane surface as drug, but it promoted amiloride inhibition when present on the opposite side of the sarcolemma. Perhaps occupation of Na^+ binding sites by substrate on one carrier face promotes binding of amiloride to sites on the opposite surface.

Another class of amiloride analogs shown to possess Na–Ca exchange inhibitory activity is the 5-pyrazinoyl-nitrogen-substituted derivative (114). In this series, potency is enhanced by increasing hydrophobicity of the substituent group, aryl and alkyl moieties are equally effective, and potency correlates strictly with the hydrophobic index of the substituent. Inhibitors have been identified that are 50–100-fold more potent than amiloride at blocking cardiac Na–Ca exchange. Regardless of these structural differences, mechanisms by which terminal guanidino-nitrogen and pyrazinoyl-nitrogen-substituted analogs block Na–Ca exchange are identical (114).

Amiloride derivatives containing both N^5- and guanidinium substitutions have been synthesized. These compounds are the most effective inhibitors of Na–Ca exchange of all analogs analyzed to date, with the best agents displaying almost 1000-fold better potency than amiloride at blocking carrier activity (84). However, most of these molecules are markedly insoluble in aqueous buffers, making their utility limited. As expected, the disubstituted compounds are mechanistically indistinguishable from the other amiloride inhibitor classes in blocking Na–Ca exchange activity.

A variety of other amiloride derivatives have been studied, but none of these is a potent inhibitor of Na–Ca exchange, and in most cases they are less active than the parent compound. Some nonpyrazine-containing acylguanidines still maintain the ability to inhibit Na–Ca exchange, although not all guanidines examined display this activity (84). This structure–activity relationship is noteworthy because the interaction of amiloride with epithelial Na^+ channels, the basis for its diuretic activity, requires a pyrazine functionality (108). Since amiloride blocks Na^+ channels with an affinity of at least 3 orders of magnitude greater than that at which it inhibits Na–Ca exchange, these results suggest that the structural requirements for inhibiting the two transport systems are likely to be different.

The specificity with which amiloride derivatives inhibit Na–Ca exchange is an important question. Although these compounds are mechanism-based inhibitors, they cannot be used in physiological experiments because they possess too many other activities. This lack of selectivity does not compromise their use in vesicle flux experiments, but their use in *in vitro* or *in vivo* tissue studies as specific Na–Ca exchange inhibitors is unwarranted. For example (108), amiloride analogs inhibit Na–H exchange, Na^+, K^+-ATPase, epithelial Na^+ channels, many other types of Na–coupled transport systems, voltage-gated Na^+, K^+, and Ca^{2+} channels, various receptor systems (including nicotinic, muscarinic, α and β receptors), different enzymatic reactions, and gross cellular metabolic processes (such as protein, RNA and DNA synthesis). This multiplicity of activities is probably related to the hydrophobic and cationic properties of these molecules. Thus, with the exception of epithelial Na^+ channels, no significant window of specificity exists for inhibition of one system over another. One important finding arguing against the use of amiloride analogs in intact tissue studies is that most possess significant Ca^{2+} entry blocker activity through their inhibition of L-, T-, and N-type Ca^{2+} channels (137–139). Indeed, the same amiloride analogs that are widely used to block Na–Ca and Na-H exchange act more potently as Ca^{2+} entry blockers (139). Therefore, although it is possible to use amiloride derivatives in some cellular studies in which Na–Ca exchange activity can be isolated through specialized experimental paradigms, general use of these compounds to study the physiological role of Na–Ca exchange is inappropriate.

A representative of the other structural class of mechanism-based inhibitors is the substituted pyrrolidineethanamine, bepridil, which is a Ca^{2+} entry blocker and antiarrrhythmic agent (140). The mechanism by which bepridil blocks Na–Ca exchange in cardiac membranes has been extensively investigated (135). Unfortunately, this compound, like amiloride analogs, lacks the selectivity required for it to be a specific probe of Na–Ca exchange. Bepridil interferes with many different cellular ion transport systems including L-type Ca^{2+} channels (141), T-type Ca^{2+} channels (C. Cohen, personal communication), the sarcolemmal Ca^{2+}-ATPase (142), K^+ channel activity in heart (143), and myosin light-chain kinase activity through its calmodulin antagonist pharmacology (144). In addition, bepridil inhibits several mitochondrial functions (145). However, because bepridil is one of the more potent inhibitors of Na–Ca exchange thus far identified (K_i of 20 μM), and because bepridil displays interesting kinetic properties as a Na-Ca exchange inhibitor, its action has been characterized in detail.

The mechanisms by which amiloride analogs and bepridil inhibit Na–Ca exchange in cardiac sarcolemmal vesicles have been thoroughly investigated (134, 135). Quantitatively similar data have been obtained with membranes prepared from vascular (60) and respiratory (84) smooth muscle, as well as with plasma membranes derived from brain and pituitary tissues (114). In all of these preparations, the respective mechanisms of action of amiloride analogs and bepridil are identical. Amiloride derivatives block completely Na_i-mediated Ca^{2+} uptake and Na_o-mediated Ca^{2+} efflux reactions in concentration-dependent fashions. Inhibitory potencies for blocking both transport modes are identical, and the efficacies displayed by these agents against Na–Ca exchange in heart, smooth muscle, brain, and pituitary plasma membranes are nearly equivalent. The mechanism by which bepridil functions produces a different inhibitory pattern in these preparations. Bepridil elicits maximally 50% inhibition of Na_i-dependent Ca^{2+} uptake, and does so with an IC_{50} of 20 μM. On the other hand, either preincubation of vesicles with inhibitor before initiating the transport reaction or addition of extravesicular bepridil during Na_o-dependent Ca^{2+} efflux results in complete inhibition of transport activity. This phenomenon is not a reflection of some physical property of bepridil, but instead correlates with the manner in which bepridil blocks the Na–Ca exchange transporter (see below).

To determine how amiloride analogs and bepridil interact with the carrier protein, the kinetics of inhibition *vs.* Ca^{2+} or Na^+ concentration were determined (134, 135). Amiloride blocks Na–Ca exchange with noncompetitive kinetics *vs.* Ca^{2+} concentration in normal physiological saline. In contrast, if the experiment is repeated in media of low ionic strength, amiloride analogs generate mixed kinetic patterns of inhibition *vs.* Ca^{2+} concentration. Further studies have shown that K^+ shifts the inhibition by amiloride from displaying both competitive and noncompetitive components, to strictly noncompetitive behavior *vs.* Ca^{2+}. Bepridil, on the other hand, produces only noncompetitive inhibition kinetics *vs.* Ca^{2+} concentration, regardless of the ionic conditions employed. The kinetics of inhibition *vs.* Na^+ concentration by either amiloride or bepridil is competitive. In each case, Na^+ effectively reverses inhibition of Na_o-dependent Ca^{2+} efflux, and does so with a concentration dependence suggestive of a strictly competitive interaction. These results are in marked contrast to those obtained with non-mechanism-based inhibitors (e.g., dodecylamine, quinacrine) in which reversal of inhibition by Na^+ is incomplete, and the concentration dependence is very broad (84). The inhibitory patterns *vs.* Ca^{2+} and Na^+ suggest that amiloride analogs and bepridil are mechanism-based agents that interact at defined substrate-binding sites on the carrier. Given that amiloride derivatives display either noncompetitive or mixed inhibition *vs.* Ca^{2+}, that bepridil is strictly noncompetitive with Ca^{2+}, and that both types of inhibitors are competitive with Na^+, together this profile is a preliminary indication that bepridil might interact at only the B-site, while amiloride derivatives might recognize both A- and B-sites of the transporter.

It is possible to gain some insight into the amiloride mechanism by reviewing the effects of K^+ on Na–Ca and Ca–Ca exchange modes of carrier turnover (84). Increasing extravesicular K^+ concentration causes a correspondingly linear increase in the K_m of Ca^{2+} as a substrate in either Na_i-dependent Ca^{2+} uptake or in Ca^{2+} transport mediated by Ca–Ca exchange. K^+ does not effect the V_{max} of Na–Ca exchange but, as previously noted, K^+ and other alkali metal ions increase the V_{max} of the Ca–Ca exchange reaction. Competition data between K^+ and Ca^{2+} indicate that these two ions interact simultaneously at the same binding site (A-site) on the carrier. Thus, K^+ might decrease binding of amiloride derivatives at that site, thereby shifting their interaction primarily to the B-site. This hypothesis is consistent with the kinetic results observed for amiloride inhibition of Na–Ca exchange. The presence of K^+ limits access of inhibitor to the A-site, resulting in mainly noncompetitive kinetics of inhibition *vs.* Ca^{2+} concentration. In the absence of K^+, amiloride analogs bind at both A- and B-sites, causing mixed kinetic patterns of inhibition *vs.* Ca^{2+}. Therefore, the way in which amiloride derivatives bind to the carrier is dependent on the ionic composition of the extravesicular medium.

Bepridil, however, appears to bind only at the B-site since its kinetics of inhibition *vs.* Ca^{2+} concentration is always noncompetitive, and K^+ itself has no marked effect on the inhibitory profile of bepridil.

If Ca–Ca exchange is monitored in the presence of either type of inhibitor, both agents block carrier turnover (134, 135). This occurs no matter whether transport is monitored in sucrose or in the presence of monovalent stimulatory cations such as K^+. The kinetics of amiloride inhibition *vs.* Ca^{2+} is mixed in sucrose, but displays a more noncompetitive profile in the presence of K^+. In marked contrast, bepridil elicits strictly noncompetitive inhibition kinetics *vs.* Ca^{2+}, regardless of the ionic composition of the medium. These observations support the hypothesis that amiloride derivatives bind at both A- and B-sites on the carrier in the absence of K^+, but interact primarily at the B-site with K^+ present, while binding of bepridil to the transporter is exclusive for the B-site under all conditions. As expected, increasing K^+ concentration decreases the potency of amiloride analogs as Ca–Ca exchange inhibitors. This is not related to ionic strength, because choline, which is not a monovalent cation stimulator of Ca–Ca exchange, does not affect the ability of amiloride analogs to block the transporter. These data have been used to suggest that the monovalent cation regulatory site and the B-site of the carrier are the same entity (25). K^+ modulates bepridil inhibition of Ca–Ca exchange in a different manner; it not only lowers the potency of bepridil but also limits the maximal extent of inhibition possible. Bepridil achieves total block of Ca–Ca exchange in sucrose, but produces only 65% maximum inhibition when 160 mM K^+ bathes both membrane surfaces (135). These latter results suggest that K^+ enhances Ca–Ca exchange by binding at some other monovalent regulatory site besides the B-site.

A prediction of the schemes outlined above is that amiloride derivatives and bepridil must block the Na–Na exchange reaction. This postulate was confirmed by examining Na_i-dependent $^{22}Na^+$ fluxes in cardiac membranes (134). Such fluxes have been shown to reflect action of the Na–Ca exchange carrier because saturation behaviors for Na^+ in Na–Na and Na–Ca exchange are very similar (4). Amiloride derivatives inhibit Na–Na exchange at low extravesicular Na^+, but inhibition is reversed by increasing the concentration of Na^+ in the medium. Similar findings have been noted with bepridil. These results confirm the idea that amiloride analogs and bepridil interact competitively at Na^+-binding sites on the transporter.

As another way of demonstrating that amiloride derivatives bind at both carrier A- and B-sites, while the interaction of bepridil is restricted to the B-site, inhibition of Na–Ca exchange was subjected to a Dixon analysis (134, 135). It is predicted that if amiloride analogs bind at a single site, the ability of one derivative to block Na–Ca exchange in the presence of varying concentrations of a second structurally similar molecule will result in parallel line kinetics in a Dixon plot. The Dixon plot of inhibition produced by a single analog does not display linear behavior. Moreover, repetition of the experiment with increasing concentrations of a second analog generates a series of curves that intersect on the X-axis and deflect upward as inhibitor concentration is elevated. Analysis of these data as a second-order function of inhibitor concentration yields linear plots. This kinetic behavior suggests that amiloride analogs interact at two distinct sites on the Na–Ca exchange transporter. That hypothesis was confirmed by analyzing Na–Ca exchange inhibition in Hill representations (134). The Hill plot of inhibition by a single amiloride analog is biphasic, with Hill coefficients of 1 and 2 at low and high inhibitor concentrations, respectively. This behavior corroborates the view that amiloride derivatives interact at two domains on the carrier. Consistent with the postulate that one of these is the A-site is the observation that the inflection point in the biphasic plot can be shifted by changing the Ca^{2+} concentration in the experiment; this value is raised to a higher inhibitor concentration by increasing extravesicular Ca^{2+}. When Hill plots of Na–Ca exchange inhibition are generated with two amiloride derivatives, monophasic behavior is observed, and the Hill coefficient is 2. Taken together, these data strongly suggest that amiloride analogs bind at both A- and B-sites of the carrier but that they have a preference for the B-site at low inhibitor concentrations.

The inhibitory effects of bepridil, and combinations of bepridil and amiloride analogs, were also analyzed in Dixon plots (84, 135). As expected for two agents that share a common site, a Dixon analysis of joint bepridil and amiloride inhibition displays parallel line kinetics when the concentration of amiloride is low. This kinetic behavior is not only consistent with a competitive interaction between the two inhibitors but also confirms that bepridil binds at the B-site of the carrier, where amiloride analogs preferentially interact. This hypothesis was substantiated by monitoring bepridil block of Na–Ca and Ca–Ca exchange reactions using Hill representations. In all cases, bepridil produces monophasic Hill plots with Hill coefficients of 1. These data demonstrate that bepridil binds at a single site on the Na–Ca exchange carrier.

A model (Fig. 4) has been proposed to explain the inhibitory action of amiloride derivatives and bepridil, and this mechanism is based on the kinetic behavior outlined above (135). In this scheme, the protonated acyl guanidinium-group of amiloride mimics Na^+ in binding to both A- and B-sites of the transporter. It has a stronger preference for the B-site, however. Occupation of the carrier by amiloride blocks turnover in either Na–Ca, Ca–Ca, or Na–Na exchange modes through for-

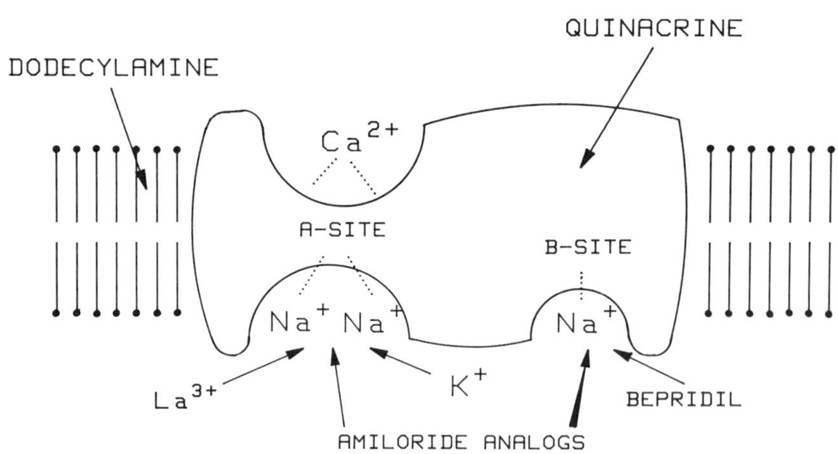

Figure 4 The model depicts schematically the action of various classes of Na–Ca exchange inhibitors. Of the mechanism-based inhibitors shown, La^{3+} interacts at the A-site, amiloride analogs bind at both A- and B-sites, with a preference for the B-site, while bepridil recognizes exclusively the B-site of the carrier. Also shown are quinacrine, which binds at a unique site on the transporter, and dodecylamine, which inhibits Na–Ca exchange activity by disrupting the membrane environment surrounding the carrier protein.

mation of a nonproductive complex. Bepridil, which is also protonated at physiological pH, binds only to the B-site to block turnover of the transporter. In neither case do these agents modify the membrane environment surrounding the transporter. Despite similarities in the action of amiloride derivatives and bepridil, these agents possess markedly different inhibitory patterns. The most striking difference is the fact that bepridil produces either partial or complete inhibition of transport activity, depending on experimental conditions, while amiloride always completely blocks carrier function. The extent of bepridil inhibition elicited under different conditions can be understood by considering the following observations. If bepridil is added at zero-time with Na^+ (e.g., as in Na_o-dependent Ca^{2+} efflux), or if vesicles are preincubated with inhibitor to allow equilibrium with the intravesicular space before initiating Na_i-dependent Ca^{2+} influx, complete inhibition of Na–Ca exchange activity occurs. However, if bepridil is added to the extravesicular buffer upon initiation of Na_i-dependent Ca^{2+} uptake, a maximum inhibition of 50% is noted. This pattern could be related to the finding that bepridil binds exclusively at the B-site. If Na^+ is released randomly from A- and B-sites in the Na_i-dependent Ca^{2+} uptake mode, and if bepridil binds solely at the external B-site under this condition, interaction between inhibitor and carrier may occur maximally only 50% of the time during turnover. Since bepridil inhibition is a completely reversible process, a kinetic scheme can be constructed depicting binding of inhibitor and recycling of the unloaded carrier in which partitioning takes place between blocked and free forms of the transporter to yield at most 50% inhibition. If bepridil and Na^+ are added simultaneously at the same surface of the transporter, the equilibrium between free and blocked forms of the carrier can be driven completely to the inhibitor occupied state by increasing bepridil concentration. This would result in complete block of Na–Ca exchange activity.

Data obtained from analyzing the inhibitory profiles of amiloride analogs and bepridil confirm and extend several aspects of the hypothetical model of cardiac Na–Ca exchange that was formerly proposed (4, 25). The findings that suggest preferential interaction of inhibitors with different types of Na^+ binding sites are consistent with a transport mechanism in which separate A- and B-sites exist. Given that hydrophobic amiloride analogs and bepridil bind more avidly at the B-site, it is probable that this domain is located either in a hydrophobic region on the protein or in close proximity to the membrane surface, so that agents partitioning into the membrane have access to the B-site through simple diffusion. On the other hand, it is likely that the A-site is exposed to the aqueous medium. The structure–activity relationships for Na–Ca exchange inhibition by terminal guanidino-nitrogen derivatives, N^5-pyrazinoyl-nitrogen derivatives, and disubstituted molecules support this idea because inhibitory activity correlates with hydrophobicity of the test compound. Moreover, the kinetics of Na–Ca exchange inhibition by less lipophilic amiloride analogs displays a greater competitive component *vs.* Ca^{2+} concentration than is observed with more hydrophobic molecules (85). This indicates that if partitioning of amiloride derivatives into the membranes is reduced, an interaction at the B-site might be diminished. Binding of radiolabeled amiloride derivatives to cardiac sarcolemmal membranes was used to explore this point (85). The compound investigated, $[^3H]N^5$-(methyl,isobutyl)amiloride, binds to membranes with an apparent affinity equivalent to its K_i as a Na–Ca exchange inhibitor (i.e., 35 μM). This phenomenon reflects partitioning into the membrane rather than a specific interaction with a protein component. That this is so was shown by experiments with protein-free liposomes, where the radiolabeled amiloride among displayed identical behavior. Moreover, many different Na–Ca exchange inhibitors (both amiloride derivatives and structurally distinct molecules) block binding of the radiolabeled probe with the same rank order of potency as they inhibit Na–Ca exchange. These findings suggest that amiloride analogs are effective inhibitors because they easily partition into the membrane via hydrophobic interactions, diffuse along the membrane surface into the B-site, and generate a high local concentration of cationic inhibitor that effectively prevents Na^+ from occupying this site. Data obtained with bepridil also substantiate this claim since it is also a very lipophilic agent that blocks a number of different membraneous systems, and it recognizes only the B-site. Furthermore, the effectiveness of amiloride analogs as inhibitors of Na–Ca exchange is related to the lipid composition of the membrane. In reconstituted vesicle systems, amiloride derivatives display an identical mechanism for block of Na–Ca exchange, but their absolute potency depends on lipid content (85). Therefore, the structure–activity relationship exhibited by the currently available Na–Ca exchange inhibitors reveals little about the substrate-binding sites on the transporter. Instead, these relationships simply reflect the ability of various compounds to partition into the membrane. Thus, it is not surprising that the present inhibitors display little selectivity as blockers of Na–Ca exchange because they interact with cation binding sites present on many different membrane associated proteins.

V. PHARMACOLOGIC PROPERTIES OF Na–Ca EXCHANGE INHIBITORS

It is clear from investigations with intact preparations that Na–Ca exchange inhibitors identified in vesicle studies will block the transport reaction in whole cells. For example, Na-dependent Ca^{2+} fluxes measured in embryonic myocytes are effectively blocked by amiloride derivatives with K_i values displaying greater potency than those measured in cardiac membranes (146). The difference in potencies in cells compared with vesicles is misleading, however, because of vastly different protocols used to determine inhibition constants in the two preparations. The limitations in calculating K_i values in vesicle experiments are related to knowing exact solution concentrations of inhibitors that easily partition into the membrane. In contrast, in cell transport studies initial rate measurements are not usually employed so that K_i values may appear to be more potent than they really are. Amiloride analogs also inhibit Na-dependent Ca^{2+} fluxes in cultured aortic smooth muscle cells, where they block both influx and efflux modes of the carrier (53, 74). Electrical currents in cardiac cells that result from the electrogenic operation of the carrier would be expected to be blocked by Na–Ca exchange inhibitors. Amiloride analogs inhibit a "creep current" due to Na–Ca exchange in Na-loaded frog atrial cells (83). Dodecylamine and quinacrine also inhibit this current. The analog 3,4-dichlorobenzylamiloride inhibits a transient inward current, and an outwardly rectifying background current associated with Na–Ca exchange in guinea pig atrial cells (147). In addition, other amiloride analogs inhibit a spontaneous inward current due to Na–Ca exchange in Na-loaded guinea pig myocytes (148). Therefore, several types of Na–Ca exchange inhibitors detected in vesicle transport studies have proven effective at inhibiting this system in intact cells.

Given the observation that the currently available Na–Ca exchange inhibitors do function in intact tissues, these compounds have been used in several pharmacologic investigations, despite their lack of selectivity. Two different sorts of investigations have been performed: monitoring Na–Ca exchange under normal physiological conditions, and in experimental settings where operation of this transport system is thought to be enhanced. In early studies, amiloride was shown to exhibit both positive inotropic and negative chronotropic effects in isolated guinea pig atrial muscle (149). This has been explored in further detail (150, 151). The effects of amiloride on contractility of guinea pig and rat atrial muscle are affected by frequency of stimulation and by the concentration ratio of extracellular Ca^{2+} and Na^+ present in the medium. The pharmacologic properties of amiloride in these studies were attributed directly to inhibition of Na–Ca exchange. Unfortunately, amiloride blocks a number of other ion flux pathways in heart, including delayed rectifying K^+ channels (83, 152), and Na^+, K^+-ATPase (108), whose inhibition would yield the same pharmacologic profile. Some amiloride analogs (e.g., 3,4-dichlorobenzylamiloride) cause a positive inotropic effect in atria (153), while eliciting a negative inotropic effect in papillary muscles (110). Other amiloride analogs (e.g., 2-chlorobenzylamiloride) produce positive inotropic effects in both of these cardiac preparations (154). Since all amiloride derivatives investigated are potent Na–Ca exchange inhibitors, the reason for such a discrepancy is not clear, but probably is related to the numerous other effects of these compounds. Dissimilar structural classes of Na–Ca exchange inhibitors (e.g., amphiphilic cations) also cause negative inotropic behavior in papillary muscle, while stimulators of Na–Ca exchange (e.g., amphiphilic anions) produce the opposite effect on contractility (87). Since amiloride analogs inhibit both L- and T-type Ca^{2+} channels (83, 91, 92), while amphiphilic cations inhibit L-type Ca^{2+} channels (83), it is not obvious whether the negative inotropic effects in papillary muscle are due to block of Ca^{2+} influx through the Na–Ca exchange pathway, to inhibition of voltage-dependent Ca^{2+} channels, or to a combination of both activities. Although there are theoretical grounds for arguing that Na–Ca exchange would drive net Ca^{2+} influx in papillary muscle, while promoting efflux of Ca^{2+} in atria (6), and that Na–Ca exchange inhibitors could therefore produce both positive and negative inotropism, because of poor selectivity of these agents caution should be exercised in the overinterpretation of data. Given that some blockers of Na–Ca exchange generate positive inotropic activity, arguments can be made that selective inhibitors would form a new class of therapeutically useful cardiotonic agents (37).

Na–Ca exchange inhibitors have also been used to address the importance of this transport system in other preparations besides cardiac muscle. It was postulated from an investigation of excitation–contraction coupling responses in frog skeletal muscle with amiloride analogs that Na–Ca exchange is involved in supplying trigger Ca^{2+} and in repriming the muscle for contraction (155). In smooth muscle, amiloride analogs cause endothelium-dependent relaxation of arteries (156), and they also block endothelin-induced contraction of aorta (157). The role of Na–Ca exchange in these processes, however, is obscured because amiloride analogs act directly on the Ca^{2+}-induced activation of myofilaments in smooth muscle. These latter results speak to the lack of selectivity of amiloride derivatives, and are examples of the difficulty encountered with these agents in correlating physiological responses with inhibition of Na–Ca exchange.

Of the various experimental paradigms that have been investigated, a good correlation exists between pharmacologic activity of Na–Ca exchange inhibitors and responses of tissues that have been Na^+ loaded. For example, treatment of cardiac muscle to raise intracellular Na^+ (e.g., by inhibition of the Na^+ pump, by prevention of Na^+ channel inactivation, or by increasing the frequency of muscle stimulation) results in a positive inotropic effect. Amiloride analogs block the responses resulting from such treatments (110, 154). Cardiac arrhythmias elicited by toxic concentrations of ouabain presumably result from overloading Ca^{2+} stores by Ca^{2+} influx through the Na–Ca exchange pathway. Spontaneous release of Ca^{2+} from overloaded sarcoplasmic reticulum results in inhomogeneity of cardiac electrical patterns because intracellular Ca^{2+} regulates the activity of various ion channels, and fluctuations in intracellular Ca^{2+} will interfere with the normal function of these channels (158). Amiloride analogs block ouabain-induced arrhythmogenesis in both isolated tissue preparations and *in vivo* animal models (154, 159). These inhibitors also block Ca^{2+} overload of cells in experimental models of cardiac ischemia (40). In addition, amiloride blocks tension development of vascular smooth muscle induced by elevation of intracellular Na^+ (160). Taken together, these data are consistent with the hypothesis that if intracellular Na^+ is elevated in cardiac or vascular tissue, influx of Ca^{2+} will occur through the Na–Ca exchange mechanism. It is important to note that the pharmacologic consequences of amiloride action under these various conditions are not mimicked by either Ca^{2+} entry blockers or Na^+ channel inhibitors, which suggests that Na–Ca exchange most likely is mediating Ca^{2+} movement in these cases.

There are other instances in which Na–Ca exchange is not easily studied in intact tissues with the nonselective Na–Ca exchange inhibitors currently available. In Ca^{2+} paradox, exposure of cardiac cells to Ca^{2+} free medium, followed by reperfusion with Ca^{2+}, causes Ca^{2+} overload, contracture, loss of excitability, and significant intracellular damage (161, 162). The major pathway for Ca^{2+} influx during this series of events is postulated to be Na–Ca exchange. Intracellular Na^+ is elevated during an exposure to Ca^{2+}-free medium due to Na^+ entering cells through L-type Ca^{2+} channels (163). Amiloride analogs are quite effective at blocking the Ca^{2+} paradox in frog atrial muscle (164). However, the activity of these agents correlates not with inhibition of Na–Ca exchange but with block of Ca^{2+} channels, which prevents Na^+ entry into myocytes. In other studies, the unexpected observation was made that amiloride analogs failed to inhibit contractions of cardiac tissue or isolated myocytes in Na^+-free medium, although these responses have traditionally been associated with operation of Na–Ca exchange (164, 165). Investigations into the processes that control cytoplasmic Ca^{2+} during Na^+-free exposure indicate that a number of different mechanisms are involved (165). Given the complicated physiology that exists in this experimental situation, little is learned from use of the existing Na–Ca exchange inhibitors.

The pharmacologic profile of the currently available Na–Ca exchange inhibitors is summarized in Table 1. When considered together, data from pharmacologic studies indicate that these inhibitors are useful in limited situations, under experimental conditions in which Na–Ca exchange activity is clearly expressed. Nevertheless, even in these paradigms, results obtained with the nonselective inhibitors must be interpreted with extreme caution.

Table 1 Pharmacologic Actions of Vesicular Na–Ca Exchange Inhibitors

Inhibit fluxes or currents related to Na–Ca exchange in intact cardiac and smooth muscle cells
Elicit either positive or negative inotropic effects in cardiac tissue depending on the type of tissue and compound studied
Block positive inotropic effects in cardiac tissue produced by ouabain or veratridine treatment, or elicited by a treppe response
Display antiarrhythmic activity in *in vitro* or *in vivo* models of arrhythmias associated with ouabain toxicity
Block Ca^{2+} overload in isolated myocytes produced by conditions of ischemia and reoxygenation
Inhibit contracture of smooth muscle due to elevation of intracellular Na^+
Abolish Ca^{2+} paradox in cardiac tissue by a mechanism unrelated to Na–Ca exchange inhibition (L-type Ca^{2+} channel block)
Do not inhibit Na-withdrawal contractures of cardiac tissue
Display a variety of other pharmacologic effects in different tissues that may or may not be related to inhibition of Na–Ca exchange activity

VI. POTENTIAL CARDIOTONIC UTILITY OF Na–Ca EXCHANGE MODULATORS

Congestive heart failure is traditionally managed by using agents that increase myocardial contractility, decrease peripheral resistance, and/or promote diuresis (166, 167). However, despite the use of digitalis glycosides, vasodilators, and diuretics, this condition continues to be a leading cause of cardiac mortality. New therapies have been envisioned that will promote an increase in myocardial contractility without having the narrow therapeutic index characteristic of cardiac glycosides. To this end, several strategies have been proposed to bring about beneficial Ca^{2+} loading of myocytes. These pharmacologic interventions fall into two main categories: enhancement of Ca^{2+} influx through L-type Ca^{2+} channels (e.g., elevation of intracellular c-AMP via either phosphodiesterase inhibition, stimulation of cardiac adenoreceptors, or activation of membrane-bound adenylate cyclase [168]; direct activation of the Ca^{2+} channel with an agonist), or increasing intracellular Ca^{2+} concentration through modulation of Na–Ca exchange activity. In its current form, the latter mechanism requires some means of raising intracellular Na^+ concentration to modify turnover of the Na–Ca exchange carrier. Although it is not resolved whether cardiac Na–Ca exchange acts primarily to clear Ca^{2+} from the cell or to direct Ca^{2+} influx, Na^+ loading in either case will decrease Ca^{2+} efflux under polarized conditions, and promote Ca^{2+} uptake when the membrane is depolarized. The net physiological response is the same: under equilibrium conditions intracellular Ca^{2+} stores increase, which results in the manifestation of a positive inotropic effect. This series of events accounts for the mode of action of Na^+, K^+-ATPase inhibitors. Supporting this conclusion is the observation that application of intracellular Na^+ in cardiac myocytes mimics the effects of ouabain-like agents (169). In addition, other mechanisms that elevate intracellular Na^+, such as agonism of voltage-dependent Na^+ channels (170), are expected to produce similar enhancement of myocardial contractility, and this has been demonstrated with a number of different pharmacologic agents. Thus, some investigators have hypothesized that small molecules that could directly affect Na–Ca exchange activity should achieve the same positive inotropic response without Na^+ loading (37, 171).

Since it has not been possible to identify specific inhibitors of Na–Ca exchange, the ability of such compounds to modulate myocardial contractility in a beneficial manner remains hypothetical. However, the ideal agent must do more than just selectively block Na–Ca exchange activity. It is hoped that inhibition of this transport system in healthy myocytes (i.e., in cells that are well polarized and have a normal inwardly directed Na^+ gradient) will increase contractility through moderate Ca^{2+} loading of the sarcoplasmic reticulum. This should occur if the physiological role of Na–Ca exchange in cardiac tissue is to drive Ca^{2+} efflux. At the same time, the inhibitor should prevent deleterious, Na–Ca exchange-dependent, Ca^{2+} loading in damaged myocytes (i.e., cells that are depolarized or Na-loaded) and thereby protect injured tissue. It is presumed that by preventing Ca^{2+} overload the agent would also abort subsequent arrhythmogenic responses. In addition, to the extent that Na^+ loading of vascular smooth muscle contributes to a hypertensive response, an inhibitor of Na–Ca exchange might decrease peripheral resistance, and, therefore, decrease the pressure load on the heart. In this fashion, blockers of Na–Ca exchange might provide a novel route to achieving a positive inotropic response in tissues that can tolerate extra work, while producing a cytoprotective effect, and also decreasing the work load on the heart, itself. Among the potential benefits of this approach, over other means of eliciting a positive inotropic response, is that the activity of a major Ca^{2+} flux pathway could be controlled directly in the target issue of interest, and the therapeutic index for the cardiotonic response may be greater than that of currently used pharmacologic agents. There are very few pharmacologic data available to support the above speculation. It is true that some of the identified inhibitors of Na–Ca exchange, notably amiloride and several amiloride derivatives, have been found to produce a positive inotropic effect in some isolated cardiac muscle preparations. However, these agents display multiple activities at the level of the sarcolemmal membrane, which limits their utility as potential drug development candidates in the cardiotonic area.

VII. CONCLUSIONS

To define the precise physiological role of Na–Ca exchange in cardiac and vascular tissue, and to determine whether this system is a target for therapeutic drug development, more selective inhibitors and/or stimulators of Na–Ca exchange must be discovered. The specificity of currently available agents is not sufficient for these purposes. Studies with known Na–Ca exchange blockers have provided a mechanistic basis by which to evaluate future inhibitors, and have yielded insight into which structural classes might provide leads for the design of selective transport modulators. Specificity will not be attained through the use of hydrophobic cations that mimic metal ions in binding to substrate sites on the carrier, because these same molecules can block any number of other ion-transporting systems. It is also unlikely that a selective inhibitor will be discovered by random screening. In work from this laboratory, more than 20,000 synthetic and natural product extracts have been tested for Na–Ca exchange inhibitory activity. While various structural classes of inhibitors have been identified, all positives are hydrophobic cations of limited potency that block carrier function either by interacting at substrate-binding sites or by perturbing membrane environment. Future directions in inhibitor development must be focused on the recently obtained data concerning the molecular structure of the carrier, so that specific agents can be rationally designed that will interfere with transporter activity by binding at unique sites on the protein. Some progress has been made in this regard with synthetic peptides based on a portion of the exchange protein that may have an autoinhibitory role (172). Further inhibitor development awaits either studies of this type, or the discovery of a natural product toxin.

REFERENCES

1. Baker PF, Blaustein MP, Hodgkin AL, Steinhardt RA. The effect of sodium concentrations on calcium movements in giant axons. *J Physiol* 1967; 192:43–44P.
2. Baker PF, Dipolo R. Axonal calcium and magnesium homeostasis. *Curr Top Membr Transp* 1984; 22:195–247.
3. Allen T J A, Nobel D, Reuter HA. *Sodium–calcium exchange*. London: Oxford University Press, 1989.
4. Reeves J P. The sarcolemmal sodium-calcium exchange system. *Curr Top Membr Trans* 1985; 25:77–127.
5. Sheu S-S, Blaustein M P. Sodium-calcium exchange and the regulation of cell calcium and contractility in cardiac muscle, with a note about vascular smooth muscle. In: Fozzard H A, Haber E, Jennings R B, Katz A M, Morgan H E, eds. The heart and cardiovascular system. 1986; New York: Raven Press, 509–35.
6. Mullins L J. *Ion transport in the heart*. New York: Raven Press, 1981.
7. Blaustein M P. Sodium–calcium exchange and the control of contractility in cardiac muscle and vascular smooth muscle. *J Cardiovasc Pharmacol* 1988; 12:56–68.
8. Hilgemann D W. Numerical approximations of sodium–calcium exchange. *Prog Biophys* 1988; 51:1–45.
9. Reuter H, Seitz N. The dependence of calcium efflux from cardiac muscle on temperature and external ion composition. *J Physiol (London)* 1968; 195:451–70.
10. Barry W H, Smith T W. Mechanisms of transmembrane calcium movement in cultured chick embryo ventricular cells. *J Physiol (London)* 1982; 325:243–260.
11. Smith J B, Smith L. Extracellular Na^+ dependence of changes in free Ca^{2+}, $^{45}Ca^{2+}$ efflux, and total cell Ca^{2+} produced by angiotensin II in cultured arterial smooth muscle cells. *J Biol Chem* 1987; 262:17455–60.
12. Hume J R, Uehara A. 'Creep currents' in single frog atrial cells may be generated by electrogenic sodium–calcium exchange. *J Gen Physiol* 1986; 87:857–84.
13. Kimura J, Noma A, Irisawa H. Sodium–calcium exchange currents in mammalian heart cells. *Nature* 1986; 319:596–7.
14. Mechmann S, Pott L. Identification of sodium–calcium exchange current in single cardiac myocytes. *Nature* 1986; 319:597–9.
15. Miura Y, Kimura J. Sodium–calcium exchange currrent dependence on internal calcium and sodium and competitive binding of external sodium and calcium. *J Gen Physiol* 1989; 93:1129–46.
16. DiPolo R, Bezanilla F, Caputo C, Rojas H. Voltage dependence of the Na–Ca exchange in voltage clamped, dialyzed squid axons. *J Gen Physiol* 1985; 86:457–78.
17. Rasgado-Flores H, Santiago E M, Blaustein M P. Kinetics and stoichiometry of coupled Na^+ flux and Ca^{2+} influx (Na–Ca exchange) in barnacle muscle cells. *J Gen Physiol* 1989; 93:1219–42.
18. Reeves J P, Sutko J L. Sodium–calcium ion exchange in cardiac membrane vesicles. *Proc Natl Acad Sci USA* 1979; 76:590–4.

19. Reeves J P, Sutko J L. Sodium–calcium exchange activity generates a current in cardiac membrane vesicles. *Science* 1980; 208:1461–4.
20. Philipson K D, Nishimoto A Y. Na–Ca exchange in inside-out cardiac sarcolemmal vesicles. *J Biol Chem* 1982; 257:5111–7.
21. Reeves J P, Hale C C. The stoichiometry of the cardiac sodium–calcium exchange system. *J Biol Chem* 1984; 259:7733–9.
22. Reeves J P, Sutko J L. Competitive interactions of sodium and calcium with the sodium–calcium exchange system of cardiac sarcolemmal vesicles. *J Biol Chem* 1983; 258:3178–82.
23. Kadoma M, Froehlich J, Reeves J P, Sutko J. Kinetics of sodium ion induced calcium ion release in calcium-loaded cardiac sarcolemmal vesicles: determination of initial velocities by stopped-flow spectrophotometry. *Biochemistry* 1982; 21:1914–8.
24. Philipson K D. Symmetry properties of the sodium–calcium exchange mechanism in cardiac sarcolemmal vesicles. *Biochem Biophys Acta* 1985; 821:367–76.
25. Reeves J P, Hale C C, de la Pena P, Slaughter R S, Boulware T, Froehlich J, Kaczorowski G J, Cragoe E J. A model for the cardiac sodium–calcium exchange carrier. In: Bronner F, Peterlik M, eds. *Epithelial calcium and phosphate transport; molecular and cellular aspects*. 1984; New York: Alan R. Liss, 77–82.
26. Blaustein M P. Effects of internal and external cations and of ATP on sodium–calcium exchange and calcium–calcium exchange in squid axons. *Biophys J* 1977; 20:79–111.
27. Hale C C, Slaughter R S, Ahrens D C, Reeves J P. Identification and partial purification of the cardiac sodium–calcium exchange protein. *Proc Natl Acad Sci USA* 1984; 81:6569–73.
28. Soldati L, Longoni S, Carafoli E. Solubilization and reconstitution of the Na–Ca exchanger of cardiac sarcolemma. *J Biol Chem* 1985; 260:13321–7.
29. Longoni S, Carafoli E. Identification of the Na–Ca exchanger of calf heart sarcolemma with the help of specific antibodies. *Biochem Biophys Res Commun* 1986; 145:1059–1063.
30. Philipson K D, Longoni S, Ward R. Purification of the cardiac Na–Ca exchange protein. *Biochim Biophys Acta* 1988; 945:298–306.
31. Hale C C, Kleiboeker S B, Carlton C G, Rovetto M J, Jung C, Kim H D. Evidence for high molecular weight Na–Ca exchange in cardiac sarcolemmal vesicles, *J Membr Biol* 1988; 106:211–8.
32. Reeves J P, Cheon J. Site density of the sodium–calcium exchange carrier in reconstituted vesicles from bovine cardiac sarcolemma. *J Biol Chem* 1988; 263:2309–15.
33. Sigel E, Baur R, Porzig H, Reuter H. mRNA-induced expression of the cardiac Na–Ca exchanger in *Xenopus* oocytes. *J Biol Chem* 1988; 263:14614–6.
34. Longoni S, Coady M J, Ikeda T, Philipson K D. Expression of cardiac sarcolemmal Na–Ca exchange activity in *Xenopus laevis* oocytes. *Am J Physiol* 1988; 255:C870–3.
34a. Nicoll DA, Longoni S, Philipson KD. Molecular cloning and functional expression of the cardiac sarcolemmal Na^+—Ca^{2+} exchanger. *Science* 1990; 250:562–5.
35. Chapman R A. Control of cardiac contractility at the cellular level. *Am J Physiol* 1983; 245:H535–52.
36. Baker P F, Blaustein M P, Hodgkin A L, Steinhardt R A. The influence of calcium on sodium efflux in squid axons, *J Physiol* 1969; 200:431–58.
37. Luciani S, Floreani M. Sodium–calcium exchange as a target for inotropic drugs. *Trends Pharmacol Sci* 1985; 6:316.
38. Orchard C H, Eisner D A, Allen D G. Oscillations of intra-cellular calcium in mammalian cardiac muscle. *Nature* 1983; 304:735–8.
39. Dixon I M, Eyolfson D A, Dhalla N S. Sarcolemmal Na–Ca exchange activity in hearts subjected to hypoxia reoxygenation. *Am J Physiol* 1987; 253:H1026–34.
40. Murphy J G, Smith T W, Marsh J D. Mechanisms of reoxygenation-induced calcium overload in cultured chick embryo heart cells. *Am J Physiol* 1988; 254:1133–41.

41. Vongai V G, Nazarov E I, Tsymbal I P, Savenki T A. Inhibition of Na^+- Ca^{2+}-exchange and superoxide dismutase activity by copper-containing cryptand complexes. *Ukr Biokhim Zh* 1988; 60:52–5.
42. Meno H, Jarmakani J M, Philipson K D. Effects of ischemia on sarcolemmal sodium–calcium exchange in neonatal hearts. *Am J Physiol* 1989; 256:H1615–20.
43. Ashavaid T F, Colvin R A, Messineo F C, MacAlister T, Katz A M. Effects of fatty acids on sodium–calcium exchange in cardiac sarcolemmal membranes. *J Mol Cell Cardiol* 1985; 17:851–62.
44. Meno H, Jarmakani J M, Philipson K D. Sarcolemmal calcium kinetics in the neonatal heart, *J Mol Cell Cardiol* 1988; 20:585–92.
45. Heyliger C E, Prakash A R, McNeil J H. Alterations in membrane sodium–calcium exchange in the aging myocardium, *Age* 1988; 11:1–6.
46. Wagner J A, Weisman H F, Snowman A M, Reynolds I J, Weisfeldt M L, Snyder S H. Alterations in calcium antagonist receptors and sodium–calcium exchange in cardiomyopathic hamster tissues. *Circ Res* 1989; 65:205–14.
47. Hanf R, Drubaix I, Marotte F, Lelievre L G. Rat cardiac hypertrophy: altered sodium–calcium exchange activity in sarcolemmal vesicles. *FEBS Lett* 1988; 236:145–49.
48. Liu M, Xuan Y. Mechanisms of endotoxin-induced impairment in Na–Ca exchange in canine myocardium. *Am J Physiol* 1986; 251:R1078–85.
49. Hale C C, Parker J L, Keller R S, Allert J A, Adams H R. Gram negative endotoxemia: effects on cardiac Na–Ca exchange and stoichiometry, *Circ Shock* 1989; 29:133–42.
50. Reuter H, Blaustein M P, Haeusler G. Na–Ca exchange and tension development in arterial smooth muscle. *Philos Trans R Soc Lond B* 1973; 265:87–94.
51. Aakjaer C, Mulvany M J. Effect of ouabain on tone, membrane potential and sodium efflux compared with [^{3}H]ouabain binding in rat resistance vessels. *J Physiol* 1985; 362:215–31.
52. Smith J B, Zheng T, Smith L. Relationship between cytosolic free calcium and sodium–calcium exchange in aortic muscle cells. *Am J Physiol* 1989; 256:C147–54.
53. Smith J B, Zheng T, Lyu R-M. Ionomycin releases calcium from the sarcoplasmic reticulum and activates sodium–calcium exchange in vascular smooth muscle cells. *Cell Calcium* 1989; 10:125–34.
54. Nabel E G, Berk B C, Brock T A, Smith T W. Sodium–calcium exchange in cultured vascular smooth muscle cells, *Circ Res* 1988; 62:486–93.
55. Ashida T, Blaustein M P. Regulation of cell calcium and contractility in mammalian arterial smooth muscle: the role of sodium–calcium exchange. *J Physiol* (*Lond*) 1987; 392:617–35.
56. Grover A K, Kwan C Y, Rangachari P K, Daniel E E. Na–Ca exchange in smooth muscle plasma membrane enriched fraction. *Am J Physiol* 1983; 244:C158–65.
57. Morel N, Godfraind T. Sodium–calcium exchange in smooth muscle microsomal fraction. *Biochem J* 1984; 281:421–7.
58. Matlib M A. Sodium–calcium exchange in sarcolemmal membrane vesicles of dog mesenteric artery. *Am J Physiol* 1988; 255:C323–30.
59. Kahn A M, Allen J C, Shelat H. Sodium–calcium exchange in sarcolemmal vesicles from bovine superior mesenteric artery. *Am J Physiol* 1988; 254:C441–9.
60. Slaughter R S, Shevell J L, Felix J P, Garcia M L, Kaczorowski G J. High levels of sodium–calcium exchange in vascular smooth muscle sarcolemmal membrane vesicles. *Biochemistry* 1989; 28:3995–4002.
61. Slaughter R S, Welton A F, Morgan D W. Sodium–calcium exchange in sarcolemmal vesicles from tracheal smooth muscle. *Biochem Biophys Acta* 1987; 904:92–104.
62. Blaustein M P, Hamlyn J M. Sodium transport inhibition, cell calcium, and hypertension. The natriuretic hormone-Na^+/Ca^{2+} exchange-hypertension hypothesis, *Am J Med* 1984; 77:45–49.

63. Blaustein M P, Ashida T, Hamlyn J M. Sodium metabolism and hypertension: how are they linked? *Klin Wochenschr* 1987; 65:21–32.
64. Hamlyn J M, Harris D W, Ludens J H. Digitalis-like activity in human plasma. *J Biol Chem* 1989; 264:7395–404.
65. Hamlyn J M, Harris D W, Clark M A, Rogowski A C, White R J, Ludens J H. Isolated and characterization of a sodium pump inhibitor from human plasma. *Hypertension* 1989; 13:681–9.
66. Hamlyn J M. Increased levels of a humoral digitalis-like factor in deoxycorticosterone acetate-induced hypertension in the pig. *J Endocrin* 1989; 122:409–20.
66a. Hamlyn J M, Blaustein M P, Bova S, DuCharme D W, Harris B W, Mandel F, Mathews W R, and Ludens J H. Identification and characterization of a ouabain-like compound from human plasma Proc Natl Acad Sci USA 1991; 88:6259–6263.
67. Lee S W, Lee J S, Park Y J, Park I S. Increase in sodium–calcium exchange activity in sarcolemma isolated from mesenteric arteries of spontaneously hypertensive rats. *Arch Pharmacol Res* 1989; 2:128–34.
68. Ashida T, Kuramochi M, Omae T. Increased sodium–calcium exchange in arterial smooth muscle of spontaneously hypertensive rats. *Hypertension* 1989; 13:890–5.
69. Hopp H H. Possible relationship between mechanical response, action potential repolarization and Na/Ca exchange in myocardium of normotensive (NWR) and spontaneously hypertensive rats (SHR). *Biomed Biochim Acta* 1987; 46:407–11.
70. Thompson L E, Rinaldi G J, Bohr D F. Sodium–calcium exchange in vascular smooth muscle of Wistar-Kyoto and stroke-prone spontaneously hypertensive rats. *J Hypertens* 1988; 4:160–2.
71. Vemuri R F, Longoni S, Philipson K D. Ouabain treatment of cardiac cells induces enhanced sodium–calcium exchange activity. *Am J Physiol* 1989; 256:C1273–6.
72. Trosper T L, Philipson K D. Effects of divalent and trivalent cations on sodium–calcium exchange in cardiac sarcolemmal vesicles. *Biochim Biophys Acta* 1983; 731:63–8.
73. Philipson K D. Sodium–calcium exchange in plasma membrane vesicles. *Annu Rev Physiol* 1985; 47:561–71.
74. Smith J B, Cragoe E J, Smith L. Sodium–calcium antiport in cultured arterial smooth muscle cells. *J Biol Chem* 1987; 262:11988–94.
75. Allen T J A and Baker P F. The effects of some putative calcium antagonists on sodium–calcium exchange in the squid axon. *Mol Pharmacol* (in press).
76. Michaelis M L, Michaelis E K. Alcohol and local anesthetic effects on sodium-dependent calcium fluxes in brain synaptic membrane vesicles. *Biochem Pharmacol* 1983; 32:963–9.
77. Michaelis M L, Michaelis E K, Nunley E W, Galton N. Effects of chronic alcohol administration on synaptic membrane sodium–calcium exchange activity, *Brain Res* 1987; 414:239–44.
78. Caroni P, Reinlib L, Carafoli E. Charge movements during the sodium–calcium exchange in heart sarcolemmal vesicles. *Proc Natl Acad Sci USA* 1980; 77:6354–8.
79. Erdreich A, Spanier R, Rahamimoff H. The inhibition of sodium-dependent calcium uptake by verapamil in synaptic plasma membrane vesicles. *Eur J Pharmacol* 1983; 90:193–202.
80. Mentrard D, Vassort G, Fischmeister R. Changes in external sodium induce a membrane current related to the sodium–calcium exchange in cesium-loaded frog heart cells. *J Gen Physiol* 1984; 84:201–20.
81. Philipson K D, Nishimoto A Y. Stimulation of sodium–calcium exchange in cardiac sarcolemmal vesicles by proteinase treatment. *Am J Physiol* 1982; 243:C191–5.
82. de la Pena P, Reeves J P. Inhibition and activation of sodium–calcium exchange activity in cardiac sarcolemmal vesicles by quinacrine. *Am J Physiol* 1987; 252:C24–9.

83. Bielefeld D R, Hadley R W, Vassilev P M, Hume J R. Membrane electrical properties of vesicular sodium–calcium exchange inhibitors in single atrial myocytes. *Circ Res* 1986; 59:381–9.
84. Kaczorowski G J, Garcia M L, King V F, Slaughter R S. Development and use of inhibitors to study sodium–calcium exchange. In: Allen T J A, Nobel D, Reuter H A, eds. Sodium–calcium exchange. London: Oxford University Press, 1989; 66–101.
85. de la Pena P, Reeves J P. Inactivation of the cardiac sodium–calcium exchange system with quinacrine mustard. *Biophys J* 1984; 45:81a.
86. Philipson K D. Interaction of charged amphiphiles with sodium–calcium exchange in cardiac sarcolemmal vesicles. *J Biol Chem* 1984; 259:13999–4002.
87. Philipson K D, Langer G A, Rich T L. Regulation of myocardial contractility and sarcolemmal calcium binding and transport by charged amphiphiles. *Am J Physiol* 1985; 248:H147–50.
88. Allen T J A, and Baker P F. Intracellular calcium indicator quin2 inhibits calcium influx via sodium–calcium exchange in squid axon. *Nature* 1985; 315:755–6.
89. Reeves J P, Poronnik P. Modulation of Na–Ca exchange in sarcolemmal vesicles by intravesicular Ca^{2+}. *Am J Physiol* 1987; 252:C17–23.
90. Mallov S. Effect of amrinone on sodium–calcium exchange in cardiac sarcolemmal vesicles. *Res Commun Chem Pathol Pharmacol* 1983; 41:197–210.
91. Sutko J L, Kenyon J L, Reeves J P. Effects of amrinone and milrinone on calcium influx into the myocardium. *Circulation* 1986; 73:III 52–8.
92. Caroni P, Villani F, Carafoli E. The cardiotoxic antibiotic doxorubicin inhibits the sodium–calcium exchange of dog heart sarcolemmal vesicles. *FEBS Lett* 1981; 130:184–6.
93. Kaczorowski G J, Costello L, Dethmers J, Trumble M J, Vandlen R L. Mechanisms of calcium tranport in plasma membrane vesicles prepared from cultured pituitary cells: I. Characterization of sodium–calcium exchange activity. *J Biol Chem* 1984; 259:9395–403.
94. Johansson B, Hellstrand P. Contractures induced by reversed sodium–calcium exchange in rat portal vein: effects of calcium antagonists. *J Cardiovasc Pharmacol* 1987; 10:575–81.
95. Vaghy P L, Johnson J D, Matlib M A, Wang T, Schwartz A. Selective inhibition of sodium-induced calcium release from heart mitochondria by diltiazem and certain other calcium antagonist drugs. *J Biol Chem* 1982; 257:6000–2.
96. Matlib M A, Lee S W, Depover A, Schwartz A. A specific inhibitory action of certain benzothiazepines and benzodiazepines on the sodium–calcium exchange process of heart and brain mitochondria. *Eur J Pharmacol* 1983; 89:327–8.
97. Matlib M A, Doane K D, Sperelakis N, Riccippo-Neto F. Clonazepam and diltiazem both inhibit sodium–calcium exchange of mitochondria, but only diltiazem inhibits the slow action potentials of cardiac muscle. *Biochem Biophys Res Commun* 1985; 128:290–6.
98. Chiesi M, Schwaller R, Eichenberger K. Structural dependency of the inhibitory action of benzodiazepines and related compounds on the mitochondrial sodium–calcium exchanger. *Biochem Pharmacol* 1988; 37:4393–403.
99. Chiesi M, Rogg H, Eichenberger K, Gazzotti P, Carafoli E. Stereospecific action of diltiazem on the mitochondrial sodium–calcium exchange system and on sarcolemmal calcium channels. *Biochem Pharmacol* 1987; 36:2735–40.
100. Van Amsterdam F T H M, Zaagsma J. Modulation of ATP-dependent calcium extrusion and sodium–calcium exchange across rat cardiac sarcolemma by calcium antagonists. *Eur J Pharmacol* 1986; 123:441–9.
101. Takeo S, Adachi K, Sakanashi M. A possible action of nicardipine on the cardiac sarcolemmal sodium–calcium exchange. *Biochem Pharmacol* 1985; 34:2303–8.

102. Takeo S, Elimban V, Dhalla N S. Modification of cardiac sarcolemmal Na–Ca exchange by diltiazem and verapamil. *Exp Cardiol* 1985; 1:131–8.
103. Richard S, Charnet P, Ouadid H, Tiaho F, Nargeot J. Effects of the Ca-antagonist nicardipine on K^+ currents and Na^+-Ca^{2+} exchange in frog atrial fibers. *J Mol Cell Cardiol* 1988; 20:1133–40.
104. Young J D, Mason D K, Fincham D A. Topographical similarities between harmaline inhibition sites on sodium-dependent amino acid transport system ASC in human erythrocytes and sodium-independent system ASC in horse erythrocytes. *J Biol Chem* 1988; 263:140–3.
105. Suleiman M S and Hider R C. The influence of harmaline on the movements of sodium ions in smooth muscle of the guinea pig ileum. *Mol Cell Biochem* 1985; 67:145–50.
106. Suleiman M S, Reeves J P. Inhibition of sodium–calcium exchange mechanism by harmaline. *Comp Biochem Physiol C Comp Pharmacol Toxicol* 1987; 88:197–200.
107. Karaki H, Kishimoto T, Ozaki H, Sakata K, Umeno H, Urakawa N. Inhibition of calcium channels by harmaline and other harmala alkaloids in vascular and intestinal smooth muscle. *Br J Pharmacol* 1986; 89:367–75.
108. Kleyman T R, Cragoe E J. Amiloride and its analogs as tools in the study of ion transport. *J Membr Biol* 1988; 105:1–21.
109. Smith R L, Macara I G, Levenson R, Housman D, Cantley L. Evidence that a sodium–calcium antiport system regulates murine erythroleukemia cell differentiation, *J Biol Chem* 1982; 257:773–80.
110. Seigl P K S, Cragoe E J, Trumble M J, Kaczorowski G J. Inhibition of sodium–calcium exchange in membrane vesicle and papillary muscle preparations from guinea pig heart by analogs of amiloride. *Proc Natl Acad Sci USA* 1984; 81:3238–42.
111. Schellenberg G D, Anderson L, Swanson P D. Inhibition of sodium–calcium exchange in rat brain by amiloride. *Mol Pharmacol* 1983; 24:251–8.
112. Gill D L, Chueh S H, Whitlow C L. Functional importance of the synaptic plasma membrane calcium pump and sodium–calcium exchanger. *J Biol Chem* 1984; 259:10807–13.
113. Scobel J E, Cragoe E J, Hruska K A. Sodium–calcium exchange and calcium permeability in canine basolateral membrane vesicles; the effects of dibutyryl cyclic AMP and specific inhibitors, *Biochim Biophys Acta* 1988; 944:233–41.
114. Kaczorowski G J, Barros F, Dethmers J K, Trumble M J, Cragoe E J. Inhibition of sodium–calcium exchange in pituitary plasma membrane vesicles by analogs of amiloride. *Biochemistry* 1985; 24:1394–403.
115. Schellenberg G D, Anderson L, Cragoe E J, Swanson P D. Inhibition of synaptosomal membrane sodium–calcium exchange transport by amiloride and amiloride analogs, *Mol Pharmacol* 1985; 27:537–43.
116. Jurkowitz M S, Altschuld R A, Brierley G P, Cragoe E J. Inhibition of sodium-dependent calcium efflux from heart mitochondria by amiloride analogs, *FEBS Lett* 1983; 162:262–5.
117. Sordahl L A, LaBelle E F, Rex K A. Amiloride and diltiazem inhibition of microsomal and mitochondrial sodium and calcium transport. *Am J Physiol* 1984; 246:C172–6.
118. Schellenberg G D, Anderson L, Cragoe E J, Swanson P D. Inhibition of brain mitochondrial calcium transport by amiloride analogs. *Cell Calcium* 1985; 6:431–47.
119. Hazama S, Hattori Y, Kanno M. Influence of N-ethylmaleimide on sodium–calcium exchange across cardiac sarcolemma. *Asia Pacific J Pharmacol* 1987; 2:1–6.
120. Pierce G N, Ward R, Philipson K D. Role for sulfur-containing groups in the sodium–calcium exchange of cardiac sarcolemmal vesicles. *J Membr Biol* 1986; 94:217–26.
121. Panagia V, Makino N, Ganguly P K, Dhalla N S. Inhibition of sodium–calcium exchange in heart sarcolemmal vesicles by phosphatidylethanolamine N-methylation, *Eur J Biochem* 1987; 166:597–604.

122. Vermuri R, Philipson K D. Protein methylation inhibits Na–Ca exchange activity in cardiac sarcolemmal vesices. *Biochim Biophys Acta* 1988; 939:503–8.
123. Michalak M, Quackenbush E J, Letarte M. Inhibition of sodium–calcium exchanger activity in cardiac and skeletal muscle sarcolemmal vesicles by monoclonal antibody 44D7. *J Biol Chem* 1986; 261:92–5.
124. Barzilai A, Spanier R, Rahamimoff H. Immunological identification of the synaptic plasma membrane sodium–calcium exchanger. *J Biol Chem* 1987; 262:10315–20.
125. Philipson K D, Frank J S, Nishimoto A Y. Effects of phospholipase C on the sodium–calcium exchange and calcium permeability of cardiac sarcolemmal vesicles. *J Biol Chem* 1983; 258:5905–10.
126. Philipson K D, Nishimoto A Y. Stimulation of sodium–calcium exchange in cardiac sarcolemmal vesicles by phospholipase D. *J Biol Chem* 1984; 259:16–9.
127. Philipson K D, Ward R. Effects of fatty acids on sodium–calcium exchange and calcium permeability of cardiac sarcolemmal vesicles. *J Biol Chem* 1985; 260:9666–71.
128. Philipson K D, Ward R. Modulation of sodium–calcium exchange and calcium permeability in cardiac sarcolemmal vesicles by doxylstearic acids. Biochim Biophys Acta 1987; 897:152–8.
129. Kutryk M J, Pierce G N. Stimulation of sodium–calcium exchange by cholesterol incorporation into isolated cardiac sarcolemmal vesicles. *J Biol Chem* 1988; 263: 13167–72.
130. Vemuri R, Philipson K D. Phospholipid composition modulates the Na–Ca exchange activity of cardiac sarcolemma in reconstituted vesicles. *Biochim Biophys Acta* 1988; 937:258–68.
131. Pierce G N, Vincenzo P. Role of phosphatidylinositol in cardiac sarcolemmal membrane sodium–calcium exchange. *J Biol Chem* 1989; 26:15344–50.
132. Makino N, Zhao D, Dhalla N S. Stimulation of heart sarcolemmal sodium–calcium exchange by concanavalin A. *Biochem Biophys Res Commun* 1988; 154:245–51.
133. Reeves J P, Bailey C A, Hale C C. Redox modification of sodium–calcium exchange activity in cardiac sarcolemmal vesicles. *J Biol Chem* 1986; 261:4948–55.
134. Slaughter R S, Garcia M L, Cragoe E J, Reeves J P, Kaczorowski G J. Inhibition of sodium–calcium exchange in cardiac sarcolemmal membrane vesicles: I. Mechanism of inhibition by amiloride analogs, *Biochemistry* 1988; 27:2403–9.
135. Garcia M L, Slaughter R S, King V F, Kaczorowski G J. Inhibition of sodium–calcium exchange in cardiac sarcolemmal membrane vesicles: II. Mechanisms of inhibition by bepridil. *Biochemistry* 1988; 27:2410–5.
136. DeBetto P, Luciani S, Tessari M, Floreani M, Carpenedo R. Inhibition of sodium–calcium exchange by amiloride acting from opposite sides of cardiac sarcolemma. *Biochem Pharmacol* 1989; 38:1137–46.
137. Feigenbaum P, Garcia M L, Kaczorowski G J. Evidence for distinct sites coupled to high affinity omega-conotoxin receptors in rat brain synaptic plasma membrane vesicles. *Biochem Biophys Res Commun* 1988; 154:298–305.
138. Suarez-Kurtz G, Kaczorowski G J. Effects of dichlorobenzamil on calcium currents in clonal GH_3 pituitary cells. *J Pharmacol Exp Ther* 1988; 247:248–53.
139. Garcia M L, King V F, Shevell J L, Slaughter R S, Suarez-Kurtz G, Winquist R J, Kaczorowski G J. Amiloride analogs inhibit L-type calcium channels and possess calcium entry blocker activity. *J Biol Chem* 1990; 265:3763–3771.
140. Flaim S F, Cummings D M. Bepridil hydrochloride—A review of its pharmacologic properties. *Curr Ther Res* 1986; 39:568–97.
141. Galizzi J P, Borsotto M, Barhanin J, Fosset M, Lazdunski M. Characterization and photoaffinity labeling of receptor sites for the Ca^{2+} channel inhibitors d-*cis*-diltiazem, (+/−)-bepridil, desmethoxyverapamil, and (+)-PN-200-110 in skeletal muscle transverse tubule membranes. *J Biol Chem* 1986; 261:1393–7.

142. Lamers J M J, Cysouw K J, Verdouw P D. Slow calcium channel blockers and calmodulin. Effect of felodipine, nifedipine, prenylamine and bepridil on cardiac sarcolemmal calcium pumping ATPase. *Biochem Pharmacol* 1985; 34:3837–42.
143. Reiser H J, Sullivan M E. Anti-arrhythmic drug therapy: new drugs and changing concepts. *Fed Proc* 1986; 45:2206–12.
144. Itoh H, Tanaka T, Mitani Y, Hidaka H. The binding of the calcium channel blocker, bepridil, to calmodulin. *Biochem Pharmacol* 1986; 35:217–20.
145. Matlib M A. Action of bepridil, a new calcium channel blocker, on oxidative phosphorylation, oligomycin-sensitive adenosine triphosphatase activity, swelling, Ca^{2+} uptake and Na^{+}-induced Ca^{2+} release processes of rabbit heart mitochondria *in vitro*. *J Pharmacol Exp Ther* 1985; 233:376–81.
146. Kim D, Smith T W. Inhibition of multiple trans-sarcolemmal cation flux pathways by dichlorobenzamil in cultured chick heart cells. *Mol Pharmacol* 1986; 30:164–70.
147. Lipp P, Pott L. Voltage dependence of sodium–calcium exchange current in guinea-pig atrial myocytes determined by means of an inhibitor. *J Physiol (Lond)*, 1988; 403:355–66.
148. Cragoe E, Ravens U, Wettwer E. Amiloride derivatives that block sodium–calcium exchange inhibit spontaneous inward currents in sodium-loaded myocytes. *Eur J Pharmacol* 1987; 140:113–6.
149. Pousti A, Khoyi M A. Effect of amiloride on isolated guinea-pig atrium. *Arch Int Pharmacodyn* 1979; 242:222–9.
150. Floreani M, Luciani S. Amiloride: relationship between cardiac effects and inhibition of sodium–calcium exchange. *Eur J Pharmacol* 1984; 105:317–22.
151. Cargnelli G, Bova S, Luciani S. Effects of amiloride in guinea-pig and rat left atrial contraction as affected by frequency of stimulation and initial calcium concentration–initial sodium concentration ratio; role of sodium–calcium exchange. *Br J Pharmacol* 1989; 97:533–41.
152. Yamashita S, Motomura S, Taira N. Cardiac effects of amiloride in the dog. *J Cardiovasc Pharmacol* 1981; 3:704–15.
153. Siegl P K S, Kaczorowski G J, Trumble M J, Cragoe E J. Inhibition of sodium–calcium exchange in guinea pig heart sarcolemmal vesicles and mechanical response by isolated atria and papillary muscle to 3,4-dichlorobenzamil (DCB). *J Mol Cell Cardiol* 1983; 14:363a.
154. Floreani M, Tessari M, Debetto P, Luciani S, Carpenedo F. Effects of N-chlorobenzyl analogues of amiloride on myocardial contractility, Na–Ca exchange carrier and other cardiac enzymatic activities. *Naunyn Schmiedebergs Arch Pharmacol* 1988; 336:661–9.
155. Curtis B A. Na–Ca exchange and excitation-contraction coupling in frog fast fibres. *J Muscle Res Cell Motil* 1988; 9:415–27.
156. Cocks T M, Little P J, Angus J A, Cragoe E J. Amiloride analogs cause endothelium-dependent relaxation in the canine coronary artery *in vitro:* possible role of sodium–calcium exchange, *Br J Pharmacol* 1988; 95:67–76.
157. Criscione L, Thomann H, Rodriguez C, Egleme C, Chiesi M. Blockade of endothelin-induced contractions by dichlorobenzamil: mechanism of action, *Biochem Biophys Res Commun* 1989; 163:247–54.
158. ter Keurs H E D J, Schouten V J A, Bucx J J, Mulder B M, de Tombe P P. Excitation–contraction coupling in myocardium: implications of calcium release and sodium–calcium exchange, *Can J Physiol Pharmacol* 1987; 65:619–26.
159. Bush L R, Kaczorowski G J, Siegl P K S. Anti-arrhythmic properties of dichlorobenzamil, a sodium–calcium exchange inhibitor. *Circulation* 1985; 72–III:313.
160. Bova S, Cargnelli G, Luciani S. Sodium–calcium exchange and tension development in vascular smooth muscle; effect of amiloride. *Br J Pharmacol* 1988; 93:601–8.

161. Nayler W G, Perry S E, Elz J S, Daly M J. Calcium, sodium, and the calcium paradox, *Circ Res* 1984; 55:227–37.
162. Chapman R A. Calcium channels, the sodium–calcium exchange and intracellular sodium in the predisposition of the heart to the calcium paradox. *Biomed Biochim Acta* 1987; 46:512–22.
163. Chapman R A, Rodrigo G C, Tunstall J, Yates R J, Busselen P. Calcium paradox of the heart: a role for intracellular sodium ions, *Am J Physiol* 1984; 247:H874–9.
164. Suarez-Kurtz G, Sollero T, Leal-Cardoso J H, Kaczorowski G J. Effects of dichlorobenzamil, a sodium–calcium exchange inhibitor, on the calcium paradox and the sodium withdrawal contractures of frog atrial muscle. *Braz J Med Biol Res* 1988; 21:1197–211.
165. Kim D, Okada A, Smith T W. Control of cytosolic calcium activity during low sodium exposure in cultured chick heart cells. *Circ Res* 1987; 61:29–41.
166. Smith T W, Braunwald E, Kelley R A. The management of heart failure. In: Braunwald E, ed. *Heart disease—a textbook of cardiovascular medicine, vol 1.* Philadelphia: W B Saunders, 1988; 485–543.
167. Taylor S H. Therapeutic targets and expectations for the treatment of heart failure. *Eur Heart J* 1989; 10 (Supplement C): 19–24.
168. v der Leyen H. Phosphodiesterase inhibition by new cardiotonic agents: mechanism of action and possible clinical relevance in the therapy of congestive heart failure. *Klin Wochenschr* 1989; 67: 605–15.
169. Borchard M, Ravens U. Intracellularly applied sodium mimics the effects of ouabain in single cardiac myocytes. *Eur J Pharmacol* 1986; 131: 269–72.
170. Scholtysik G. Cardiac Na^+ channel activation as a positive inotropic principle. *J Cardiovasc Pharmacol* 1989; 14 (Supplement 3): S24–9.
171. Ravens U, Wettwer E. Modulation of sodium–calcium exchange: a hypothetical positive inotropic mechanism. *J Cardiovasc Pharmacol* 1989; 14 (Suppl 3): S30–5.
172. Li Z, Nicoll DA, Collins A, Hilgemann DW, Filoteo AG, Penniston JT, Weiss JN, Tomich JM, and Philipson KD. Identification of a peptide inhibitor of the cardiac sarcolemmal Na^+-Ca^{2+} exchanger. J Biol Chem 1991; 266: 1014–1020.

30

Heart Failure: Is the Pathology Due to Calcium Overload or to Mismatch in Energy Supply and Demand?

JOANNE S. INGWALL, LUIGINO NASCIMBEN, and JUDITH K. GWATHMEY

Harvard Medical School
Boston, Massachusetts

I. INTRODUCTION

Heart failure has many causes, which complicates our understanding of the mechanisms underlying this disease. Many causes of reduced pump function have been suggested, including changes in the extracellular matrix and cell necrosis. Although these processes must contribute, it is most likely that the primary defect(s) leading to failure occurs within the myocyte. The two most widely held hypotheses are that heart failure is due to abnormal Ca^{2+} metabolism and to a mismatch in the critical balance between energy supply and utilization. Aspects of Ca^{2+} metabolism that could lead to pump failure include inadequate supply of Ca^{2+} to the myofibril or altered sensitivity of the myofilaments to Ca^{2+}. Mismatch in energy supply and utilization could be due to inadequate oxygen or substrate supply needed to support normal oxidative metabolism leading to ATP synthesis, inadequate energy reserves needed to support increased load on the heart, or abnormal energy utilization by the myofibril. Other defects in myofibrillar cross-bridge formation could also occur.

It has been difficult to test the hypothesis that the transition from normal or compensated hypertrophic myocardium to failure is caused by either of these two hypotheses, for several reasons. One is that the experimental models of human heart failure are imperfect. Another reason, integrally related to the first, is that we do not yet know the characteristics or markers of failure that would allow us to analyze the onset or progression of heart failure. Differentiating between cause and effect is a daunting problem. Thus, we are faced with using imperfect experimental models of human heart failure and using information obtained from biopsies of human myocardium at only one time. Another reason is that, until recently, techniques capable of addressing these issues directly were not available. Now new technologies allow us to gain new insights into this important problem.

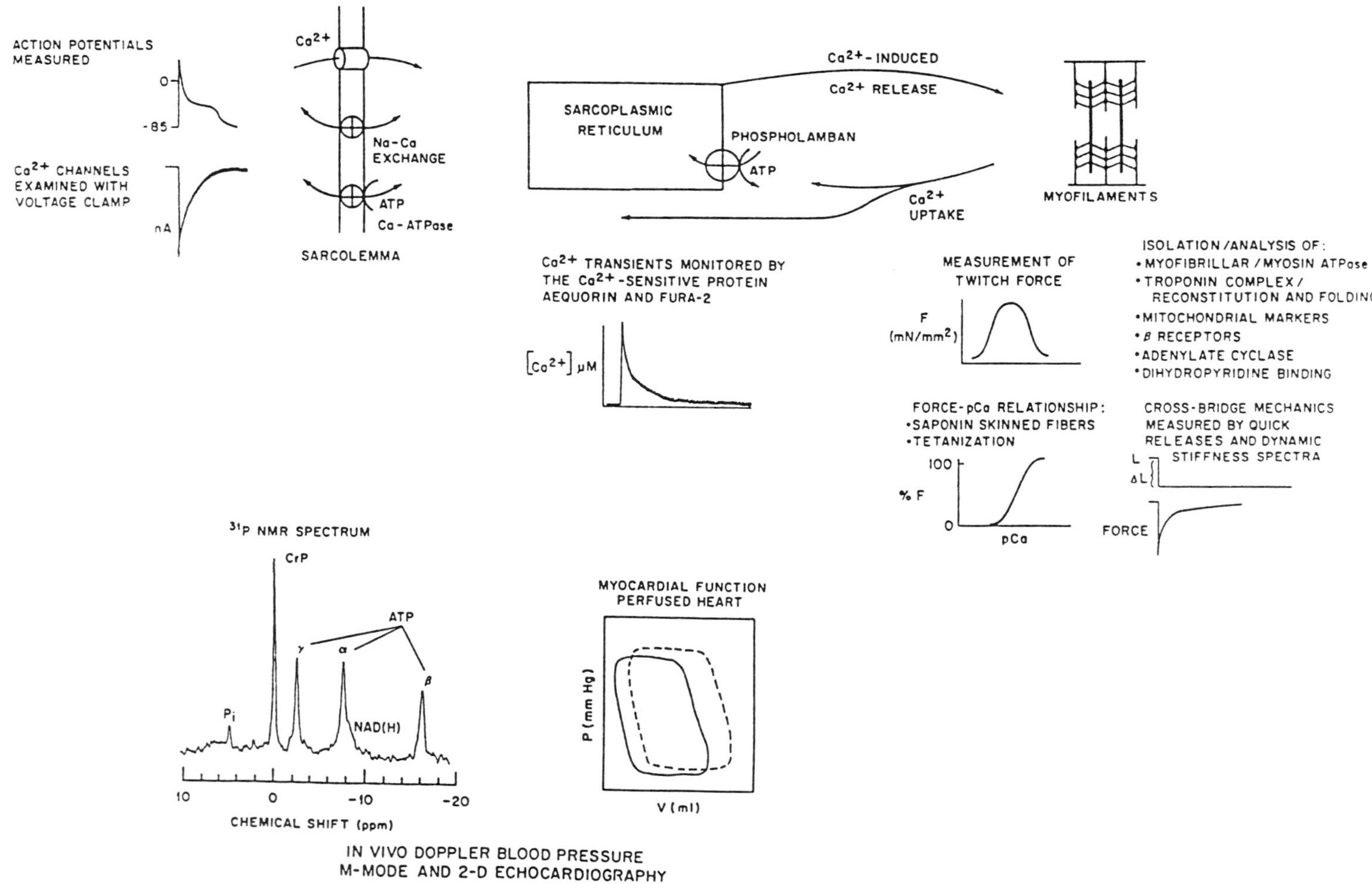

Figure 1 Techniques currently being used to study excitation–contraction coupling in normal and diseased myocardium. See text for details.

Figure 1 illustrates the techniques now being used by us as well as others to study heart failure. Sarcolemmal function has been assessed by measuring the action potential, Ca^{2+} currents (voltage clamp), dihydropyridine receptor binding, and β-receptor number (adenylate cyclase α_1 transmembrane signaling pathway). Sarcoplasmic reticular function has been assessed using aequorin and Fura-2 to measure the intracellular calcium concentration, $[Ca^{2+}]_i$, directly. Myofibrillar function has been assessed by twitch force, tetanus force, and force-Ca^{2+} relations using skinned fibers. Classic biochemical measures of myofibrillar and myosin ATPase activities and analysis of the thin filament protein composition have also been performed. Cross-bridge kinetics have been assessed by quick-release and dynamic stiffness spectra. Energy supply determined by high-energy phosphate content and the amount of those enzymes needed for ATP synthesis have been assesed biochemically. Using the biophysical tool of NMR spectroscopy, turnover of the dominant high-energy phosphate containing compounds, the energy reserve compound phosphocreatine (PCr), and the primary high-energy phosphate compound ATP have been measured using ^{31}P magnetization transfer.

Here we will review information now available relevant to the Ca^{2+} hypothesis in human myocardium. We will then discuss several aspects of energy supply and demand, focusing on what can be learned from measurements of high-energy phosphate contents and from activities of certain enzymes important in maintaining normal high-energy phosphate content in human myocardium. Results obtained from animal studies will be used for their interpretation. We will organize these results by considering normal physiology and biochemistry, changes in hypertrophy, and, finally, changes in failure. We will conclude by posing the hypothesis that these two hypotheses may not be independent since Ca^{2+}-dependent ATPases in the sarcolemma, sarcoplasmic reticulum, and myofibril all use ATP and are inhibited by products of ATP hydrolysis, namely ADP, inorganic phosphate (P_i), and H^+. Finally, we will compare and contrast results obtained for human failing myocardium with those obtained for two animal models of failure: cardiomyopathic hamster and the furazolidine-treated turkey poult.

II. HYPOTHESIS: PUMP FAILURE IS DUE TO ABNORMAL Ca^{2+} METABOLISM

A. Calcium–Force Relationship

1. Excitation–Contraction Coupling

The original observation by Ringer (1) that free ionized Ca^{2+} was required for contractile function in the heart initiated an era of investigation of the role of intracellular Ca^{2+} on force production. In cardiac tissue, depolarization of the sarcolemma results in an influx of Ca^{2+} from outside of the cell. It is currently believed that this small amount of Ca^{2+} results in the release of a much larger amount of Ca^{2+} from an intracellular store, specifically the sarcoplasmic reticulum. This phenomenon has been called Ca^{2+}-induced/Ca^{2+}-release and is quite different from excitation–contraction coupling in skeletal muscle, in which nearly all the Ca^{2+} used for contraction comes from the extracellular space. The landmark demonstration that Ca^{2+} is released from the sarcoplasmic reticulum in response to changes in the amount and rate of Ca^{2+} flux across the sarcolemma was first clearly shown by Alexandre Fabiato (2).

The Ca^{2+} released from the sarcoplasmic reticulum elevates the free ionized intracellular concentration from nM to μM, thereby activating the myofilaments. Relaxation occurs with the dissociation of Ca^{2+} from troponin C Ca^{2+} binding sites and sequestration of Ca^{2+} by the sarcoplasmic reticulum. Resting $[Ca^{2+}]_i$ is restored to the nM range by at least three mechanisms. Ca^{2+} is resequestered via the Ca^{2+}-ATPase pump in the sarcoplasmic reticulum requiring the splitting of 1 ATP for every two Ca^{2+} removed from the cytosol. Another Ca^{2+}-ATPase in the sarcolemma pumps Ca^{2+} to the outside of the cell, acting in concert with Na^+/Ca^{2+} exchange to further lower $[Ca^{2+}]_i$. The sarcolemmal Ca^{2+} ATPase pump has high affinity but low capacity for Ca^{2+} mobilization, as opposed to the electrogenic Na^+/Ca^{2+} exchanger (ratio 3:1), which has low affinity but high capacity and does not require direct ATP hydrolysis.

2. *Measuring* $[Ca^{2+}]_i$

The changes in $[Ca^{2+}]_i$ that accompany physiological twitches are complex. $[Ca^{2+}]_i$ varies rapidly and inhomogeneously throughout the cell. To investigate the relationship of force to $[Ca^{2+}]_i$ one needs to address the limitations of the techniques used to measure $[Ca^{2+}]_i$ and their implications on the force–$[Ca^{2+}]_i$ relationship. Because of the characteristics of the relationship between contractile force and $[Ca^{2+}]_i$, it is ideal to measure both parameters in the same preparation.

The techniques most widely used to measure $[Ca^{2+}]_i$ rely on the bioluminescent protein aequorin and fluorescent indicators Fura-2 and Indo-1. Aequorin is loaded into cells by diffusion across a transiently permeabilized sarcolemma or by microinjection. Indo-1 and Fura-2 can be used as an acetoxymethylester that crosses the sarcolemma by diffusion and then is hydrolyzed, or the pentasodium salts can be supplied via a micropipette (3). Bioluminescence or fluorescence occurs only when Ca^{2+} is bound to the receptor molecule. The primary limitation using aequorin is that the light signal is nonlinear over most of its range of $[Ca^{2+}]_i$. Problems inherent in fluorescent indicators include buffering, slow kinetics, probable underestimation of $[Ca^{2+}]_i$, the need to use multiple wavelengths for the measurement, and sequestration of the indicator in intracellular organelles. Photobleaching and diffusion from the cell make quantitative measurements difficult; they also preclude obtaining multiple recordings over a long period of time.

When spatial inhomogeneities in $[Ca^{2+}]_i$ are present, the estimates from spatially averaged signals may differ from the true spatial average $[Ca^{2+}]_i$, particularly if the indicator is nonlinear, as is the case with aequorin. Aequorin gives a signal proportional to $[Ca^{2+}]^{2.5}$. The rate constant for the rise of light intensity is about 100 s^{-1} at 20°C and is independent of $[Ca^{2+}]$. The steepness of the time-dependent change in $[Ca^{2+}]$ during a twitch means that local regions of high $[Ca^{2+}]$ will tend to dominate patterns of light emission. Cannel and Allen (4) have shown that spatial inhomogeneities of $[Ca^{2+}]_i$ become negligible shortly after the peak of the $[Ca^{2+}]_i$. Analysis indicates that spatial inhomogeneities of $[Ca^{2+}]_i$ throughout contraction are so small that estimates of $[Ca^{2+}]_i$ derived from aequorin luminescence provide an accurate estimate of spatially average $[Ca^{2+}]_i$ (4,5). The advantage of a linear response is that quantitative interpretation of results in terms of the spatial average $[Ca^{2+}]$ is possible even when gradients of $[Ca^{2+}]$ exist. It has been demonstrated using fluorescent linear indicators such as Fura-2 and Indo-1 that the time course of the isometric twitch and of $[Ca^{2+}]_i$ signals are closer than obtained with aequorin. However, if the light signal detected with aequorin is corrected for aequorin kinetics, the $[Ca^{2+}]_i$

returns to baseline only shortly before tension returns to baseline and thus more precisely tracks diastole (6).

3. *Calcium–Force Relationships*

Troponin is the regulatory contractile protein on the thin myofilament that binds Ca^{2+}. It consists of three subunits: troponin C is the Ca^{2+} binding protein; troponin I is the inhibitory subunit that, along with tropomyosin, blocks the interaction between myosin and actin; and troponin T is the tropomyosin-binding protein. It was originally proposed that Ca^{2+} binding to the regulatory proteins should fit a first-order chemical reaction scheme with a slope reflecting the number of Ca^{2+} binding sites according to the equation:

$$F = F_{max} \frac{[Ca^{2+}]}{[Ca^{2+}]_{50\%} + [Ca^{2+}]}$$

where F is developed force at a given $[Ca^{2+}]$, F_{max} is the maximal force attainable at saturating $[Ca^{2+}]$, and $[Ca^{2+}]_{50\%}$ is the $[Ca^{2+}]$ required for 50% activation of the myofilaments. However, skinned fiber preparations yielded Hill coefficients with values greater than 3, suggesting that this assumption might not be valid. Analysis of empirically derived data revealed that the Ca^{2+}–force relationship could best be described by the modified Hill equation:

$$F = F_{max} \frac{[Ca^{2+}]}{[Ca^{2+}]^n{}_{50\%} + [Ca^{2+}]^n}$$

This Ca^{2+}–force relationship results in an exponential function in which the Hill coefficient is thought to reflect cooperatively between the thick and thin myofilament as opposed to the number of Ca^{2+} binding sites on troponin C.

Errors in the estimate of $[Ca^{2+}]_i$ using aequorin could arise from possible differences between *in vivo* conditions and conditions used to obtain the calibration curve used to estimate the ratio of light to maximal light obtained in lysed cells, L/L_{max}. The limitations introduced by such errors in the aequorin signal would affect only the absolute values of the Hill parameters in the $[Ca^{2+}]$–force relationship, not the qualitative relationship. In the case of skinned fiber experiments, assumptions used to set ion concentrations and calculated binding constants may be in error. The use of skinned fiber preparations in conjunction with steady-state force determinations (tetanizations) in aequorin-loaded intact muscle preparations has allowed Ca^{2+}–force relationships to be compared in these two settings. Steady-state measurements in tetanus avoid the issue of inhomogeneities in $[Ca^{2+}]_i$ that may occur throughout force production.

Comparison of the Hill parameters for $[Ca^{2+}]_i$–force relations from intact and skinned preparations from human and ferret myocardium showed that there are differences in F_{max}, $[Ca^{2+}]_{50\%}$, $[Ca^{2+}]_{95\%}$, and n (Table 1). It is important to note that the Hill coefficient and $[Ca^{2+}]_{50\%}$ obtained from the Hill equation are less reliable than the $[Ca^{2+}]_{95\%}$ because of the few data points in the critical steep portion of the $[Ca^{2+}]$-force curve (7). At 95% Ca^{2+} activation, it is likely that all the cells in multicellular preparations are close to maximal activation, unlike at 50% activation, at which different cells can have different levels of activation averaging 50%. As shown in Table 1, maximal Ca^{2+}-activated force is higher in intact tetanized muscles than in skinned fiber preparations. Because skinning with saponin causes

Table 1 Comparisons of Hill Parameters Between Skinned Fiber Preparations and Tetanizations in Control and Myopathic Muscles

Preparation and group	$[Ca^{2}{}_{+}]_{50\%}$ (μM)	$[Ca^{2}{}_{+}]_{95\%}$ (μM)	n_h	F_{max} (g/mm^2)
Ferret skinned				
Control	1.84 ± 0.21	6.97 ± 0.80	2.21 ± 0.09	
POH	1.76 ± 0.30	5.97 ± 1.02	2.41 ± 0.13	
Human intact				
Control	0.56 ± 0.05	0.97 ± 0.05	5.21 ± 0.20	1.23 ± 0.49
Myopathic	0.54 ± 0.09	0.98 ± 0.03	5.61 ± 0.60	1.84 ± 0.74
Human skinned				
Control	1.56 ± 0.22	6.56 ± 0.93	2.05 ± 0.33	0.30 ± 0.09
Myopathic	1.44 ± 0.16	5.88 ± 0.67	2.30 ± 0.23	0.34 ± 0.08

Values are mean ± SEM.
$[Ca^{2+}]_{50\%}$, calcium concentration required for 50% activation; $[Ca^{2+}]_{95\%}$, calcium concentration required for 95% activation; n_h, Hill coefficient; F_{max}, maximal force developed; POH, right ventricle pressure-overload hypertrophy in the ferret.
Source: Refs. 10 and 33.

the fibers to swell, as shown in histologic stained specimens (8), it can be argued that the skinning procedure increases the intrafilament spacing and therefore decreases the developed force. Matsubara et al. (9) have recently shown that there is an optimal intrafilament spacing at which skinned fibers develop maximum force that correlates well with the intrafilament spacing in the intact tissue. Thus, this limitation can be overcome when tetanus is possible.

Steady-state $[Ca^{2+}]_i$–force relations from tetanized intact human muscles approach maximal force by 1 μM $[Ca^{2+}]_i$ (10), consistent with the results for ferret myocardium (7). However, skinned muscle preparations from the same human hearts exhibited a lower Ca^{2+} sensitivity (10). The discrepancy between $[Ca^{2+}]_{95\%}$ in intact versus skinned preparations from the same hearts may be due to depletion of membrane-bound phospholipids, peptides, amino acids, and soluble cofactors that determine the sensitivity of the myofilaments to Ca^{2+}. In support of this possibility, we have found that addition of the amino acid histidine to activating solutions in skinned fiber preparations results in a significant shift to lower $[Ca^{2+}]_i$, indicating increased myofilament Ca^{2+} sensitivity (Fig. 2).

We conclude that $[Ca^{2+}]$–force relations do not allow direct conclusions about affinity and cooperativity of Ca^{2+} binding to troponin C. A high Hill coefficient does not necessarily indicate long-range cooperativity among a large number of Ca^{2+} binding sites located along the thin filaments, but probably results from altered isometric cross-bridge turnover kinetics.

B. $[Ca^{2+}]_i$ in Normal Myocardium

All avian, reptilian, amphibian, and mammalian species studied to date demonstrate a monophasic Ca^{2+} transient (11). In avian and mammalian myocardium the Ca^{2+} transient as detected with aequorin reflects sarcoplasmic reticulum Ca^{2+} release and reuptake. This is demonstrated by addition of ryanodine (which prevents Ca^{2+} sequestration by the sarcoplasmic reticulum) to the aequorin-loaded preparation, with

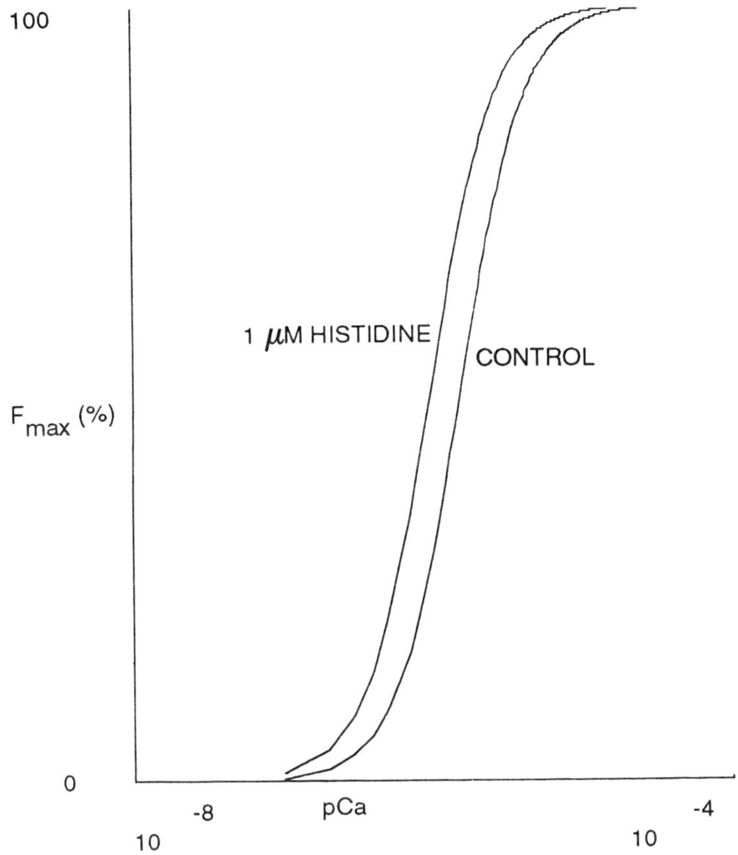

Figure 2 Addition of 1 μM histidine to a saponin-skinned fiber from a patient with known cardiac disease resulted in a shift of 0.2 pCa units to the left of the force–pCa relationship.

the resultant dissipation of the Ca^{2+} transient. In amphibian and reptilian myocardium, a portion of the Ca^{2+} transient appears to arise from transsarcolemmal Ca^{2+} flux. In most cases Ca^{2+} released from the sarcoplasmic reticulum activates the myofilaments. Increasing extracellular [Ca^{2+}] results in an increased sarcoplasmic reticulum loading and peak amplitude of the Ca^{2+} transient without a change in time course of the Ca^{2+} transient (Fig. 3). Associated with this observation is an increase in peak twitch force without a change in twitch duration. In ferret myocardium aequorin signals expressed as log L/L_{max} yield a resting value of -5.5 ± 0.1 with peak sarcoplasmic reticulum calcium release being -4.2 ± 0.2 in the presence of 2.5mM $[Ca^{2+}]_o$ (30°C, 0.33 Hz stimulation rate) (12). In normal human myocardium end-diastolic $[Ca^{2+}]_i$ at 0.33 Hz stimulation rate at 30°C is 250 ± 20 nM (13). With higher frequencies ($\geq$ 1Hz) of stimulation, resting $[Ca^{2+}]_i$ does not change significantly: 260 ± 10 nM. Peak sarcoplasmic reticulum Ca^{2+} release at 0.33 Hz and 1 Hz in the presence of 2.5 mM $[Ca^{2+}]_o$ was found to be 1.2 ± 0.4 μM and 2.36 ± 0.4 μM, respectively. These values for the $[Ca^{2+}]_i$ are similar to those reported for other mammalian species and correlate well with Ca^{2+}-specific microelectrode measurements (14).

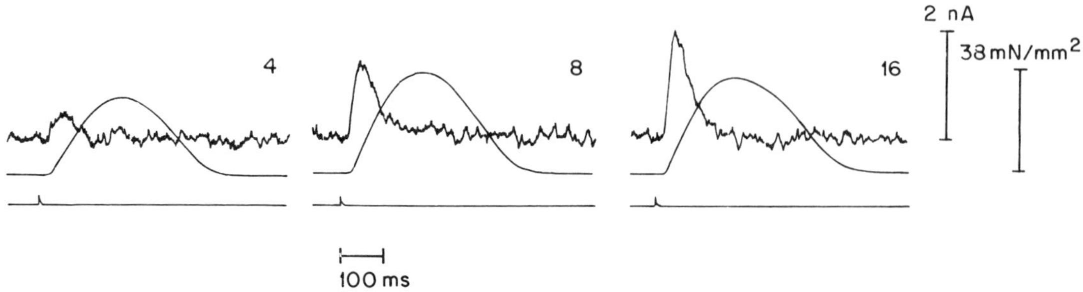

Figure 3 Effect of increasing $[Ca^{2+}]_o$ (4, 8 16 mM) on twitch force (smooth curve) and $[Ca^{2+}]_i$ as detected with aequorin in ferret papillary muscle. Scale for the aequorin signal is nA and for force, mNewtons/mm^2. (Data from Ref. 15.)

C. $[Ca^{2+}]_i$ in Hypertrophied Myocardium

The $Ca^{2+}{}_i$ transient is prolonged in papillary muscles isolated from ferrets with pressure-overload hypertrophy due to pulmonary artery banding (15). Resting $[Ca^{2+}]_i$ is not different from control age-matched animals (L/L_{max} -5.7 ± 0.06), nor is the peak sarcoplasmic reticulum Ca^{2+} release (L/L_{max} -4.2 ± 0.2) different (12). The observation that $[Ca^{2+}]_i$ was the same whether there was an increase or decrease in peak twitch force suggests that $[Ca^{2+}]_i$ is not the major determinant of twitch force in this model (12,15). Similar results have been observed in a guinea pig model of pressure overload (16). Peak systolic $[Ca^{2+}]$ measured in isolated hypertrophied myocytes increased as drive rate was increased, but peak systolic and diastolic $[Ca^{2+}]_i$ were not different from that for control animals. Thus, in these two models of hypertrophy, changes in $[Ca^{2+}]_i$ do not explain differences in peak twitch force.

Myocytes in older patients without known cardiac disease are larger (17.4 ± 1.6 μm) than myocytes obtained from younger patients (11.5 ± 1.3 μm) (17, 18). These hypertrophied myocytes have a stiletto-like Ca^{2+} transient with a very brief duration. When challenged with high $[Ca^{2+}]_o$, a second slower component to the Ca^{2+} transient appears that is also related to release of Ca^{2+} by the sarcoplasmic reticulum. However, the time course of the isometric twitch is unchanged. These data suggest that changes in the time course of the isometric twitch in "moderately hypertrophied" muscles may be dissociated from changes in Ca^{2+} mobilization and involve other mechanisms such as cross-bridge kinetics and cycling rates.

D. $[Ca^{2+}]_i$ in Heart Failure

Here we will consider three Ca^{2+}-related hypotheses proposed to explain decreased contractile performance in human heart failure.

1. Downregulation of Adrenergic Receptors

One of the first biochemical changes observed for overt heart failure (19) was downregulation of β-adrenergic receptors. Because of the known relationship between β-receptor stimulation and myocardial contractility, this observation suggested a causal role for uncoupled or desensitized β-receptors. Furthermore, correlations were observed between serum norepinephrine (NE) content (which tends to be high) and myocardial catecholamine content (which tends to be low) in the setting of heart failure. Although the relationship of heart failure to β-receptor density and NE content stimulated the development of positive inotropes, this approach has not yielded convincing results. In clinical trials using the β-receptor antagonist metoprolol there is ~30% improvement in β-receptor density, as opposed to a doubling in cardiac performance (20). More important, depletion of NE content did not affect contractile force in isolated muscle (21).

2. *Downregulation of Ca^{2+} Channels*

It has been proposed that depressed contractility is due to decreased Ca^{2+} availability (22). In support of this hypothesis, it was reported that Ca^{2+} channel number is reduced in myocardium from patients with idiopathic cardiomyopathy (IDC) (23). This finding is, however, inconsistent with reported physiological responses in failing human myocardium (24). Furthermore, in myocardium from patients with hypertrophic cardiomyopathy, an increase in Ca^{2+} channel number measured as dihydrophyridine binding sites (DHP) has been reported (25). Therefore, the controversy remains.

3. *Changes in the Myofilament Ca^{2+} Responsiveness*

Yet another hypothesis is that heart failure is due to a change in myofilament Ca^{2+} responsiveness. Reduced Ca^{2+} sensitivity (i.e., Ca^{2+} required for 50% activation of the myofilaments) and/or cooperativity (slope of the Ca^{2+}-force relationship) could result in reduced contractile activation and force. Alterations of loading conditions of heart cells are associated with macromolecular remodeling that can alter cardiac energy transduction and dynamics of contraction/relaxation (26). Important questions with regard to the remodeling process are: Which isoforms exist? What leads to the reprogramming of these proteins? What is the functional significance of a particular isoform switch? It is well known that the distribution of isoforms of myosin heavy chain in animal hearts (and skeletal muscle) is altered by changes in cardiac workload. However, myosin isoenzyme population does not always correlate with function (26). This suggests that proteins in the thin filament might also be altered during chronic hemodynamic load. Important questions that must be addressed are: Are differences in functional properties between diseased and normal myocardium caused by isoform switches of thin filament proteins? Do isoform switches alter thin-filament-related Ca^{2+} regulation? Are these changes adaptive or maladaptive? Can specific pharmacologic interventions reverse or prevent these changes?

We will now discuss what is currently known about these issues in human myocardium.

4. *On $[Ca^{2+}]_i$ Availability*

The Ca^{2+} transient detected with aequorin in trabeculae muscles from patients with end-stage heart failure due to either idiopathic cardiomyopathy or hypertrophic cardiomyopathy has two components (24, 27). The fast component is similar to that seen in normal nonfailing myocardium and arises solely from sarcoplasmic reticulum Ca^{2+} release. The second, slower, component arises from sarcoplasmic reticulum Ca^{2+} release and enhanced transsarcolemmal Ca^{2+} flux (24). Two components have also been identified in Fura-2-loaded isolated human myocytes with isoproterenol stimulation (28). Increasing the $[Ca^{2+}]_o$ results in an increase in amplitude of both components. Because failing myocardium is unable to maintain normal Ca^{2+} homeostasis, there is a rise in both resting $[Ca^{2+}]_i$ and diastolic force (24, 27). Despite this apparent impaired $Ca^{2+}{}_i$ mobilization, peak $[Ca^{2+}]_i$ was similar to that obtained in normal nonfailing myocardium at a time when there is reduced

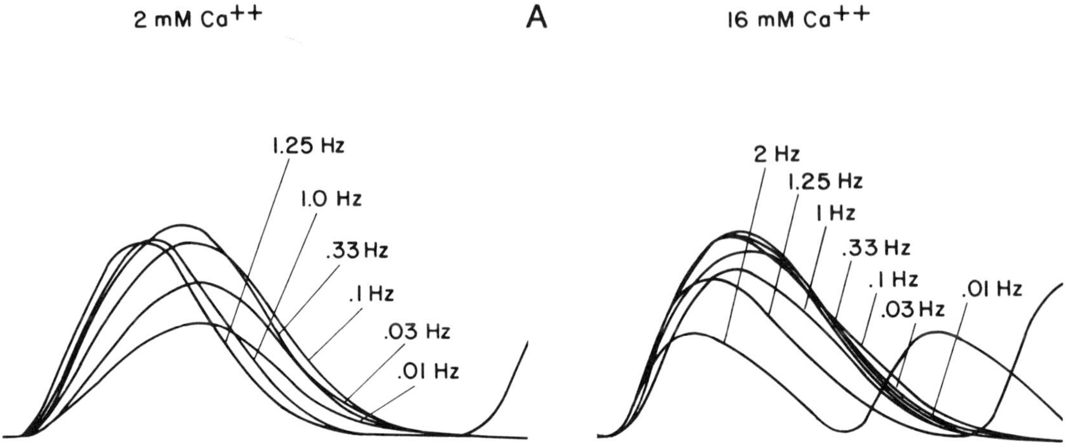

Figure 4 Isometric twitches in a trabeculae carneae from a patient with hypertrophic cardiomyopathy. A. The effects of increasing the frequency of stimulation on systolic function in the presence to 2 mM and 16 mM $[Ca^{2+}]_o$. As the frequency of stimulation is increased, there is a decrease in peak contractile force. Higher $[Ca^{2+}]_o$ results in exacerbation of the negative inotropic effect and blunted abbreviation of the twitch time course seen with increasing frequencies of stimulation. B. The effect of increasing stimulation rates on diastolic force in the presence of varying $[Ca^{2+}]_o$. Notice that passive tension increases as function of increasing $[Ca^{2+}]_o$ as well as with higher stimulation rates.

inotropy. These findings have been confirmed for $[Ca^{2+}]_i$ with steady-state tentani as a function of varying $[Ca^{2+}]_o$ and twitch. Data for control and myopathic muscles were fitted using the least-squares methods to yield simple regressions. Intercepts for tetani were 0.260 and 0.385 μM in the control and myopathic muscles, respectively, whereas slopes ($\times 10^3$) were 0.036 and 0.069. For the twitch the intercepts were 0.34 and 0.72 μM and the slopes ($\times 10^3$) were 0.062 and 0.034 for normal and myopathic muscle, respectively. These data indicate that contractile failure is not due to diminished intracellular Ca^{2+} availability.

It has been proposed that the negative treppe seen in human heart failure is due to diminished $Ca^{2+}{}_i$ availability. However, results using the Ca^{2+} indicator aequorin showed that the negative treppe seen in muscles from patients with end-stage heart failure was not due to diminished $[Ca^{2+}]_i$ (13). At 0.33 Hz end-diastolic $[Ca^{2+}]_i$ was 370 ± 10 nM and peak sarcoplasmic reticulum release was 1.26 ± 0.20 μM. In Indo-loaded isolated myocytes, $[Ca^{2+}]$ was 290 nM at rest and peak sarcoplasmic reticulum Ca^{2+} release was ~1 μM (29); with repetitive stimulation end-diastolic $[Ca^{2+}]$ was ~375 nM (29). At high rates of stimulation, where a negative force–interval relationship was seen, peak sarcoplasmic reticulum Ca^{2+} release was similar between control and myopathic muscles (1Hz, 2.36 ± 0.4 vs. 2.43 ± 0.28 μM for control vs. myopathic). Finally and most compelling, there was a significant increase, not decrease, in resting $[Ca^{2+}]_i$ in failing human myocardium (690 nM).

These results suggest that failing human myocardium has sufficient free ionized $[Ca^{2+}]_i$ to support contractile activation, but abnormal Ca^{2+} metabolism may result in negative treppe. Others have described an increase in end-diastolic $[Ca^{2+}]$ and a decrease in peak sarcoplasmic reticulum Ca^{2+} release in myocytes isolated from failing hearts (123). However, the time-averaged $[Ca^{2+}]_i$ was similar to the $[Ca^{2+}]_i$ seen in control myocytes. Thus, four different approaches all fail to show that

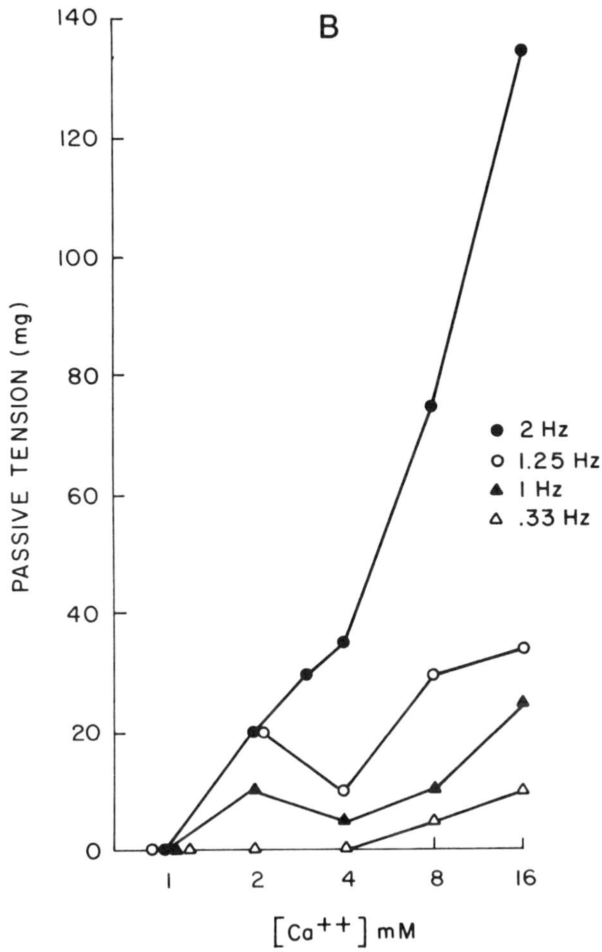

Figure 4 Continued

decreased contractility is due to decreased $[Ca^{2+}]_i$. Instead they suggest that the defect must be elsewhere.

Ca^{2+}–force relations have been obtained in an animal model of failure using Fura2-AM. There was no difference in diastolic $[Ca^{2+}]_i$ between control myocytes and myocytes isolated from guinea pig hearts exposed to a gradual pressure overload (16). The frequency-dependent increase in peak systolic $[Ca^{2+}]_i$ was most depressed with failure; intermediate values were obtained with hypertrophy. Peak $[Ca^{2+}]_i$ at 1 Hz was 600 ± 197 for normal myocytes and 303 ± 60 nM for failure myocytes. Although increasing $[Ca^{2+}]_o$ resulted in an increase in peak systolic $[Ca^{2+}]_i$, nevertheless the systolic $[Ca^{2+}]$ remained depressed. It is interesting to note that addition of norepinephrine (NE) normalized the peak systolic $[Ca^{2+}]_i$ in myocytes from the heart failure group. The different responses to $[Ca^{2+}]_o$ and NE remain to be explained.

The effects of diastolic dysfunction on systolic performance in human myocardium from patients with hypertrophic cardiomyopathy have been demonstrated (27). Increased $[Ca^{2+}]_o$ resulted in exacerbation of both systolic and diastolic dysfunction (Fig. 4). These data suggest that failing myocardium requires additional

$Ca^{2+}{}_i$ to generate the same level of force or fails to resequester $Ca^{2+}{}_i$ after the twitch. This hypothesis is supported by improved diastolic and systolic function in the presence of forskolin, an agent that results in improved sarcoplasmic reticulum Ca^{2+} uptake (13, 27).

5. Myofibrillar Ca^{2+} Sensitivity

In failing human, rat, and guinea pig myocardium force–pCa (log [Ca^{2+}]) relations were the same as for control (30–32). However, agents that change myofibrillar Ca^{2+} sensitivity affect myofilaments from control and myopathic human muscles differently. The relationship between force and free Ca^{2+} was not altered by addition of 1μM of the Ca^{2+} sensitizing agent DPI 201-106 in control muscles, but in myopathic muscles the $[Ca^{2+}]_{50\%}$ was shifted to the left by 0.2 pCa units in the presence of DPI (30). These data suggest that the composition of the thin myofilaments was changed in myopathic myocardium. Similar observations have also been observed in hypertrophied ferret myocardium by two laboratories (31, 33).

Protein kinase C phosphorylates both cardiac troponin I (TnI) and troponin T, (TnT). In the presence of DPBA, which activates protein kinase C, the [Ca^{2+}]–force relationship was shifted to the right in both control and myopathic human myocardium, indicating a decreased sensitivity of the myofilaments to Ca^{2+} activation (34). This is predominantly due to TnI phosphorylation, which results in a decreased calcium sensitivity of the myofilaments. However, in myopathic myocardium the slope of the [Ca^{2+}]–force relationship (i.e., cooperativity) was increased whereas it was decreased in control myocardium (34). It is possible that this is due not to TnI but to TnT phosphorylation. Myopathic human myocardium has been shown to express different troponin T isoforms that affect not only the myofilament Ca^{2+} sensitivity but also cooperativity (35, 36). Thus, different troponin T isoforms and/or levels of phosphorylation may affect the Ca^{2+}–force relationship. Altered thick and thin myofilament interaction and dynamics might contribute to the systolic and diastolic dysfunction seen in heart failure (37). These hypotheses merit further study.

6. Altered Cross-Bridge Kinetics in Heart Failure

Hasenfuss et al. (22) have suggested that diminished contractile performance in failing myocardium is due to a reduced number of cross-bridges. To investigate whether altered cross-bridge kinetics contribute to the systolic and diastolic abnormalities of heart failure, the mechanical properties of cardiac muscle from control and idiopathic dilated cardiomyopathic human heart (38) have been studied. Unloaded shortening velocity (V_0) was 0.72 ± 0.09 L_0/sec in control vs 0.41 ± 0.06 L_0/sec in myopathic muscle. Although no myosin isoforms have been reported in human ventricular myocardium (predominantly V_3), the slower cross-bridge cycling rate was associated with decreased myosin ATPase activity.

Muscle length was changed sinusoidally at frequencies ranging between 0.01 and 100 Hz. Dynamic stiffness was calculated from the ratio of force response amplitude to length oscillation amplitude. At low frequencies (below 0.2 Hz) the stiffness was constant but was slightly larger in myopathic muscle (1.38 ± 0.23 vs. 1.87 ± 0.28 g/mm, $p < 0.005$). In the range of 0.2–1 Hz there was a decrease in the magnitude of the dynamic stiffness. This range reflects cross-bridge turnover kinetics. The frequency of minimum stiffness was 0.78 ± 0.06 Hz in control muscle and 0.42 ± 0.07

Hz in myopathic muscles. At higher frequencies the dynamic stiffness increased and reached a plateau at 30 Hz. There were no differences in the plateau reached between control and myopathic muscles (5.97 ± 0.21 vs. 5.81 ± 0.33 g/mm). These results indicate that the number of force-generating cross-bridges are similar for control and myopathic hearts. Thus, although relaxation abnormalities seen in heart failure reflect in part changes at the level of the cross-bridge, myopathic myocardium has the potential for generating normal levels of force.

In summary, using results from many biophysical techniques, we conclude that failing myocardium has the potential to generate force comparable to normal myocardium and that decreased contractile performance cannot be explained by decreased systolic $[Ca^{2+}]_i$ (Fig. 5).

III. HYPOTHESIS: PUMP FAILURE IS DUE TO A MISMATCH IN ENERGY SUPPLY AND DEMAND

A. Energetics of the Normal Myocardium

1. *High-Energy Phosphate Content and Turnover in Heart*

ATP concentration in fetal, neonatal, and adult ventricular myocardium of mouse, rat, rabbit, ferret, dog, lamb, and humans is remarkably constant: ~30 nmoles/mg total cardiac protein or ~11 nM in the cytosol. In contrast, the rate at which ATP is made and used is not constant but is a dynamic property of muscle. Our understanding of this concept is based on measurements of myocardial oxygen consumption. Oxygen consumption, which is directly proportional to the rate of oxygen used for ATP synthesis by oxidative phosphorylation, changes with workload (energy utilization). Thus, ATP content remains the same but its synthesis rate matches metabolic demand.

In the 1930s Cain and Davies (39) showed that phosphocreatine (PCr) was the primary high-energy phosphate reservoir in striated muscle:

$$\text{PCr} + \text{ADP} + \text{H}^+ \rightleftharpoons \text{ATP} + \text{creatine}$$

In contrast to the constancy of the ATP concentration, the total creatine pool, and hence the PCr and free creatine concentrations, are not constant but change with age, substrate, and workload. Creatine is not made in the myocardium but must be transported against a concentration gradient from the blood into the myocyte. Phosphorylation effectivcly traps two-thirds of the creatine pool. The mechanism by which unphosphorylated creatine, a low-molecular-weight zwitterion, stays in the cell is unknown. Accumulation of creatine is developmentally regulated and increases when the MM and mitochondrial creatine kinase isoforms accumulate. This occurs during late fetal and early neonatal development in small animals and during fetal development in large animals and humans. Accumulation is less in atrial than in ventricular myocardium. In isolated hearts of adult small animals (rat, rabbit, guinea pig) supplied with glucose, total creatine content is ~90 nmoles/mg cardiac protein and the PCr content is 1.4–1.6 times greater than ATP. In hearts supplied with glucose plus insulin, pyruvate, or acetate, the ratio is close to 2.0. In blood-perfused isolated hearts and in hearts *in situ,* the ratio is also close to 2.0. In animal hearts such as ferret and dog, the total creatine content is ~140 nmol/mg cardiac protein, and the ratio is ~2 regardless of substrate (40). Recently Weiss et al. (41)

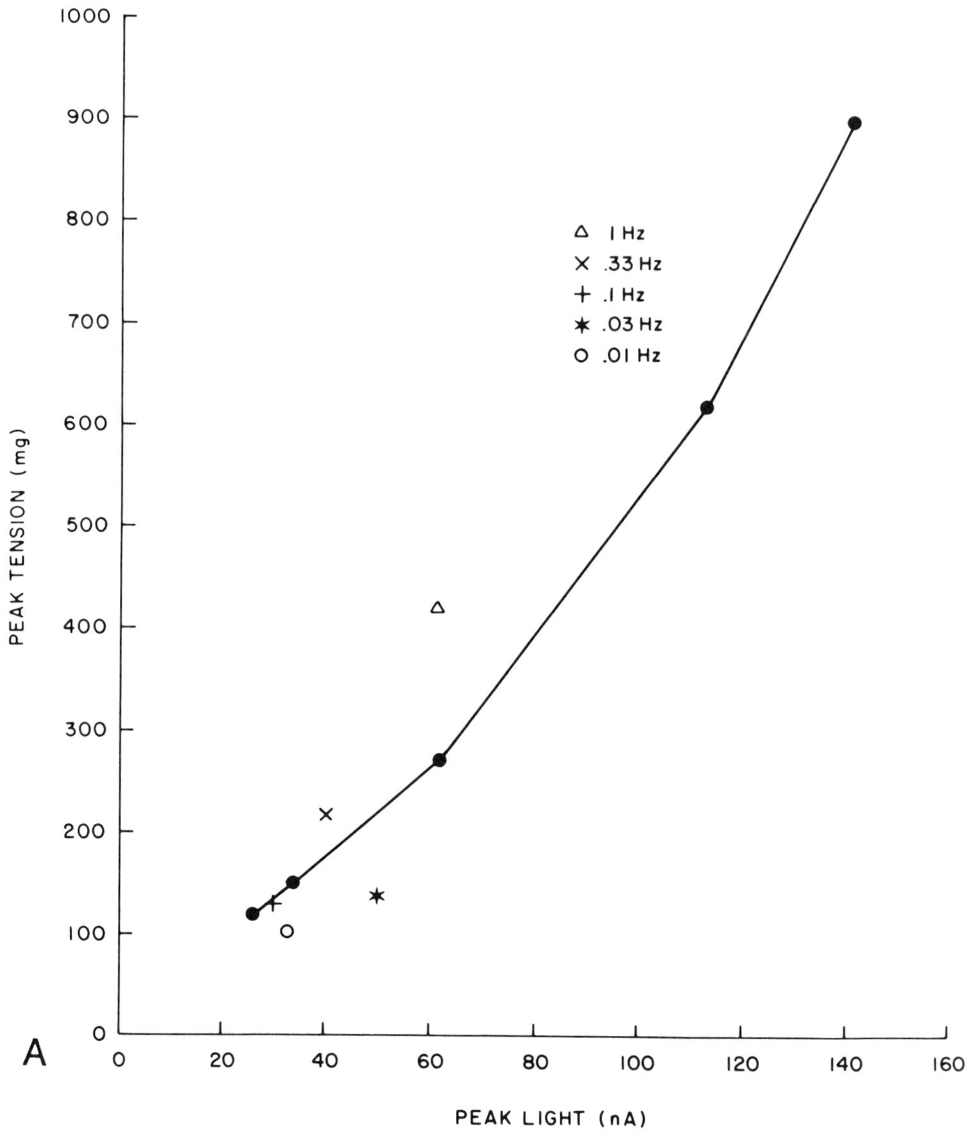

Figure 5 Relation of tension (mg) vs. light (nAmps). Solid lines were generated by increasing the $[Ca^{2+}]_o$ in the superfusate (stimulation ratio, 0.33 Hz). Frequency relationships were obtained in the same muscle preparation in the presence of 2 mM $[Ca^{2+}]_o$. A. Closed circles represent points generated by increasing the $[Ca^{2+}]_o$ in the superfusate for a trabeculae carneae from a patient without known cardiac disease. B. The same relationship is demonstrated in a muscle from a patient with hypertrophic cardiomyopathy. It is interesting to note that in the case of hypertrophic cardiomyopathy at 1 Hz stimulation rate, the point is shifted to the right and down. This indicates that despite relatively high $[Ca^{2+}]_i$ (similar to that obtained with 8mM $[Ca^{2+}]_o$), there is reduced peak twitch force (similar to 1–2 mM $[Ca^{2+}]_o$). Also note the steepness of the concentration response to varying $[Ca^{2+}]_o$ in the muscle from the patient with hypertrophic cardiomyopathy.

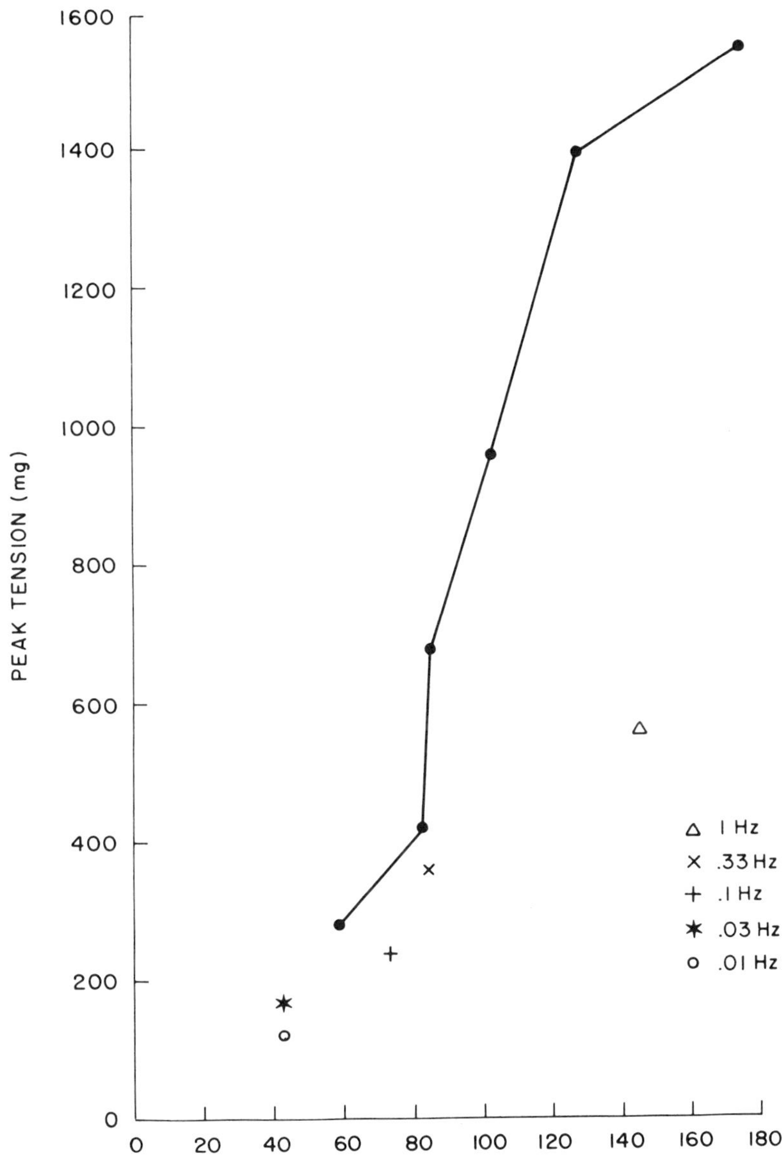

B

Figure 5 Continued

using ^{1}H image-aided [41]P nuclear magnetic resonance (NMR) spectroscopy showed that the PCr to ATP ratio for normal human myocardium was also close to 2.

Some, but not all, species demonstrate workload-dependent changes in the myocardial PCr content and hence the PCr/ATP ratio. In small animals such as rat, rabbit, and guinea pig, hearts display an inverse relationship between PCr and work over a broad range of cardiac performance (42, 43), whereas this relationship is weak for large animals such as ferret (44) and dog *in situ* (45). These species differences in PCr metabolism correlate with creatine kinase isoform diversity and total creatine content. Large animal hearts with low heart rates have low isoform diversity and high total creatine content, whereas small animal hearts with high heart rates have high isoform diversity and low total creatine content.

The metabolic machinery maintaining the balance between ATP supply and demand can establish new steady states. Using a dog model of chronic partial stenosis, Ross and colleagues (46) demonstrated that cardiac function decreased in response to reduced blood supply and that this new steady state persisted throughout the 5 hr period of partial stenosis. The biochemical analog of this experiment has also been performed (47). Although ATP and PCr levels decreased in response to the onset of stenosis, their contents remained nearly constant for the 5 hr period of stenosis. Thus a new steady state in both metabolism and function had been achieved. It is not known whether this new steady state can be maintained indefinitely.

Until recently, ATP turnover could be inferred only from changes in the physiological measurements of oxygen consumption and workload. Changes in PCr turnover could be inferred only from changes in its concentration measured using classical techniques and freeze-clamped tissue. Now, through the use of ^{31}P magnetization transfer techniques, several important aspects of high-energy phosphate turnover can be measured in the intact beating heart. These include the velocity of the creatine kinase reaction that catalyzes phosphoryl transfer between ATP and PCr (42–44) and rate of net ATP synthesis from oxidative phosphorylation and glycolysis (48). Recent developments using ^{13}C NMR show that flux through the tricarboxylic acid cycle can also be measured (49–51).

One important principle learned from NMR measurements of the creatine kinase reaction velocity is that the rate of this phosphoryl exchange in excitable tissue (heart, skeletal muscle, and brain) is at least 10 times faster than ATP synthesis from other pathways (Table 2) (52). This means that the creatine kinase reaction velocity is a good measure of high-energy phosphate turnover. This may be best illustrated by the following experiment (53, 54). Figure 6 shows two ^{31}P NMR spectra obtained from the same rat heart *in situ*. The spectrum on the top was obtained for the heart operating at a normal workload (rate pressure product of 29,000 mmHg/sec); the rate of phosphoryl transfer between ATP and PCr measured using ^{31}P magnetization transfer was 24 μmol/g dry weight/sec. The spectrum on the bottom shows the same amount of ATP and PCr in the myocardium, but was obtained when the heart was made hypoxic. The resultant workload was 14,700 mmHg/sec and the creatine kinase reaction velocity was 6 μmol/g dry weight/sec.

Table 2: Creatine Kinase Activity, Total Creatine Content, Creatine Kinase Reaction Velocity, and Oxygen Consumption in Excitable Tissues of the Living Rat

	CK Activity (mM/sec)	Total Cr (mM)	CK Velocity (mM/sec)	MVO_2 (mM/sec)
Brain	24±3	15±2	4.1±1.1	0.59
Heart	62±4	20±2	5.0±1.6	0.49
Skeletal muscle	224±16	55±6	18±1.7	0.02

Abbreviations: CK, creatine kinase; Cr, creatine; MVO_2, myocardial oxygen consumption. Data are taken from Bittl et al. (52).

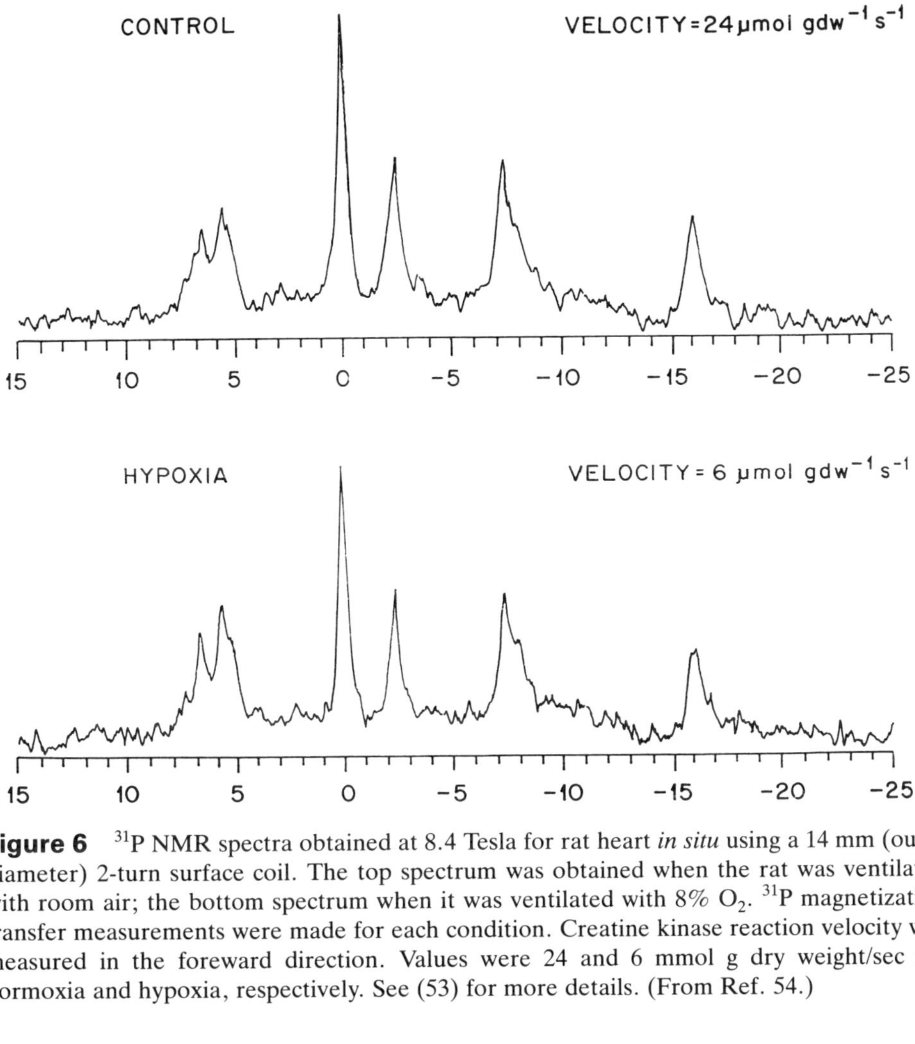

Figure 6 ^{31}P NMR spectra obtained at 8.4 Tesla for rat heart *in situ* using a 14 mm (outer diameter) 2-turn surface coil. The top spectrum was obtained when the rat was ventilated with room air; the bottom spectrum when it was ventilated with 8% O_2. ^{31}P magnetization transfer measurements were made for each condition. Creatine kinase reaction velocity was measured in the foreward direction. Values were 24 and 6 mmol g dry weight/sec for normoxia and hypoxia, respectively. See (53) for more details. (From Ref. 54.)

Several lessons can be learned from this experiment. First, phosphoryl turnover differed even though PCr and ATP contents were unchanged. This result illustrates the important principle that energy utilization and synthesis rates cannot be deduced from PCr or ATP content. Second, high-energy phosphate turnover assessed in this way changed with workload. Thus, the "downregulation" of energy supply and demand includes "downregulation" of the primary energy reserve system as well. The mechanism for this coupling is unknown. However, since changes in the concentrations of the creatine kinase reactants calculated for hypoxic heart predict that the creatine kinase reaction velocity should have increased (not decreased), we can rule out substrate regulation as the mechanism.

2. *Pathways of ATP Utilization and Synthesis*

The number of ways of making ATP in a cell is redundant: phosphoryl transfer from PCr catalyzed by creatine kinase; substrate-level phosphorylation of ADP via oxidative phosphorylation and glycolysis; use of preformed purine nucleobases, nucleosides, and nucleotides via salvage pathways; and *de novo* synthesis. The existence of many pathways for ATP synthesis ensures that normal ATP levels are maintained. ATP is utilized, either directly through ATPase activity or indirectly through cation gradients maintained by ATPases, for all steps in excitation–contraction.

There are species- and age-related differences in isoform composition of many proteins involved in ATP utilization and synthesis in mammalian myocardium. Based on differences in kinetic properties of these isoforms, differences in function have been inferred. Age-related changes in thick- (myosin) and thin- (tropomyosin and troponin) filament composition are well known. Differences in myosin isoforms correlate well with speed of muscle contraction, at least in most settings.

There are also many isoform families in the ATP-producing pathways. The glycolytic enzyme lactate dehydrogenase is a classic example. Lactate dehydrogenase contains five isoforms, some of which are predominant in anaerobic muscle while others are predominant in aerobic muscle including heart. The anaerobic skeletal muscle type is also the dominant form in the fetal myocardium. During cardiac maturation the aerobic forms preferentially accumulate. The functional significance assigned to this distribution is based on the differences in affinity of these isoforms for pyruvate. Anaerobic isoenzymes are more efficient in reoxidizing NADH with pyruvate to produce NAD and lactate whereas aerobic isoenzymes allow more NADH to be reoxidized by oxidative phosphorylation. In this way, the aerobic isoenzymes support high rates of oxidative phosphorylation.

Creatine kinase isoenzyme distribution in heart is also developmentally regulated and differs with species. Fetal myocardium contains low levels of total creatine kinase activity and is primarily the BB isoform. Depending on the species, either during mid or late fetal development, the genes encoding M creatine kinase are activated and MM creatine kinase accumulates. Later during terminal differentiation another isoform, mitochondrial creatine kinase, accumulates. This occurs during neonatal development in small animals and during midfetal development in large animals. Mitochondrial creatine kinase is located on the outside of the inner mitochondrial membrane (55). In addition to localization of MM in the M-band of the sarcomere, a significant fraction of the MM may be localized in the myofibril. BB and the hybrid MB isoforms are not localized to any organelle.

The schematic diagram of a myocyte in Figure 7 shows the integration of ATP-synthesizing and -utilizing pathways. Excitation–contraction coupling is supported by ATP hydrolysis by myofibrils and ion pumps in the sarcolemma and sarcoplasmic reticulum (here illustrated by the Ca^{2+}-pumps, but ATP-dependent Na^+ and K^+ movements should not be ignored). Resynthesis of ATP occurs via oxidative phosphorylation and, to a lesser extent, glycolysis. In normal myocardium, glycolysis, contributes 5–15% of the total ATP pool. Because of its location mitochondrial creatine kinase must operate unidirectionally, synthesizing PCr from ATP produced by oxidative phosphorylation. Calculations suggest that as much as 90% of the high-energy phosphate produced by mitochondria is converted to PCr (56). The cytosolic creatine kinase reaction, which must be in equilibrium (i.e., is strictly substrate driven), reports the rate of phosphoryl exchange between PCr and ATP (i.e., high-energy phosphate turnover). PCr content decreases only under conditions of supply–demand mismatch such as high workload, hypoxia, and ischemia; ATP content decreases only during prolonged hypoxia and ischemia.

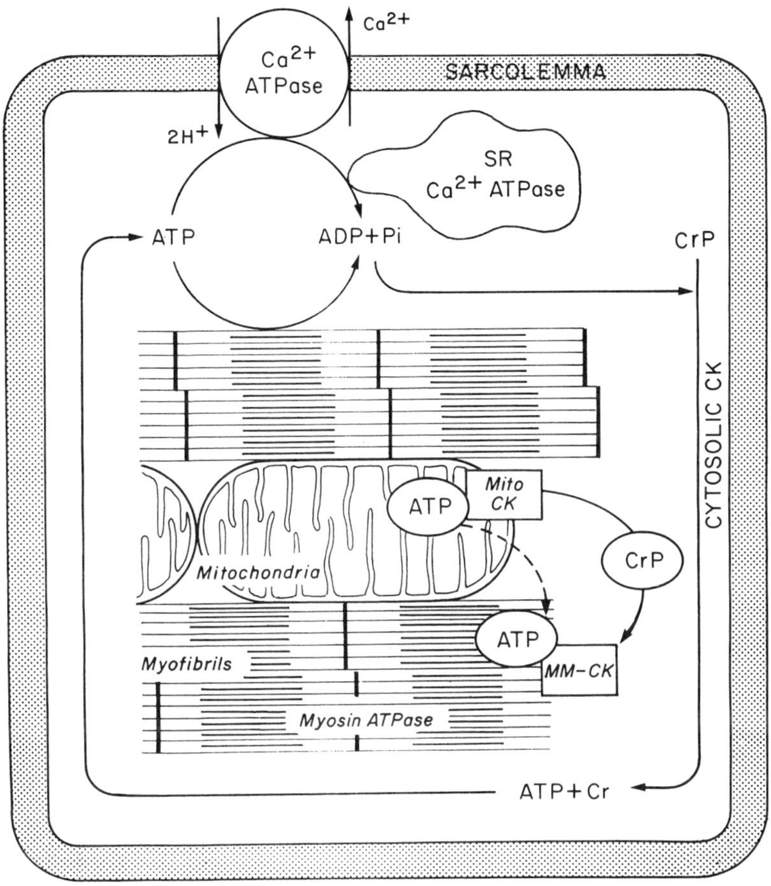

Figure 7 Schematic diagram of a myocardial cell shows some of the major sites of ATP utilization (Ca^{2+} ATPases in the sarcolemma and sarcoplasmic reticulum and myofibrillar ATPase) and ATP synthesis (oxidative phosphorylation in the mitochondria and via cytosolic and mitochondrial creatine kinase). CK, creatine kinase; mito CK, mitochondrial creatine kinase; CrP, phosphorylcreatine; SR, sarcoplasmic reticulum.

B. Energetics of the Hypertrophied Myocardium

1. High-Energy Phosphate Content

Analysis of ATP and PCr contents in nonfailing hypertrophied myocardium provides no consistent evidence for decreased ATP content but it seems likely that PCr content decreases. For example, measurements of total creatine content, which is proportional to PCr content, show that this energy reserve compound is decreased in pressure overload human myocardium (57).

2. Pathways of ATP Synthesis and Utilization

The earliest reports of protein isoform changes in hypertrophy were made for the lactate dehydrogenase system. In the early 1970s, Sobel et al. (58), Bishop and Altschuld (59), and Fox (60) reported a shift from the aerobic to the anaerobic lactate dehydrogenase isoforms in hypertrophied myocardium. In 1976, the first observation that B-creatine kinase also accumulated in the hypertrophied myocardium was made in volume overload hypertrophy in the dog (61). Since both the B creatine kinase and anaerobic-type lactate dehydrogenase accumulate in hypertrophied myocardium, these results suggested that an important characteristic of the hypertrophied myocardium may be accumulation of fetal-type isoforms. With the subsequent discovery by Swynghedauw and colleagues (62) in 1979 that the fetal-type myosin (V_3) also accumulates in the hypertrophied myocardium, this concept became widely accepted. Myosin isoform redistribution in hypertrophy occurs in species that contain primarily the V_1 or fast myosin isoform. In species in which ventricular myosin is the V_3 isoform or slow myosin isoform, such as humans, no change can occur. In these species, changes in the creatine kinase system do occur (57). It is now known that many isoforms switches occur in hypertrophied myocardium, especially rapid-onset hypertrophy.

The creatine kinase isoenzyme distribution has now been defined for hearts of many species hypertrophied in response to both physiological and pathologic stimuli (12, 61, 63–66) (Table 3). Given this large data base, some generalization about reprogramming of the creatine kinase system can now be made.

First, total creatine kinase activity normalized to cardiac protein is usually unchanged in compensated hypertrophied myocardium. Exceptions are the volume-overload hypertrophy in the dog heart (61) and hypertrophy secondary to hypertension (Goldblatt model) in the rat heart (63). In both of these cases, creatine kinase

Table 3: Total Creatine Kinase Activity and % (BB and MB) Creatine Kinase Activity in Normal and Hypertrophied Mammalian Myocardium

Species	Stimulus to hypertrophy	Sample analyzed	CK Activity	%(BB & MB)	Reference
Rat	none	LV, RV	1.12	12	64
	aortic banding	LV	1.04	**19**	66
	pulmonary banding	RV	**0.50**	**25**	64
	thyroxine supply	LV	0.97	**17**	64
	spontaneously hypertensive	LV	1.20	**19**	64
	swimming	LV	1.10	13	68
	none	LV myocytes	5.26	11	63
	renal hypertension	LV myocytes	**4.17**	**27**	63
Dog	none	LV, RV	1.93	<2	64
	arterio-venus fistula	LV	**1.35**	**5**	61
	renal hypertension	LV	1.94	**5**	64
	aortic banding	LV	1.93	**14**	65
	pulmonary banding	RV	1.86	**8**	65
Baboon	none	LV	1.63	17	67
	hypertension	LV	1.34	14	67
Man	none	LV	2.04	<2	57
	aortic stenosis	LV	**1.07**	**15**	57

IU/mg wet weight except for myocytes, where units are IU/mg protein; bolded numbers are significantly different from their controls.
Abbreviations: CK, creatine kinase; LV, left ventricle; RV, right ventricle.
This table and discussion is reproduced from Ref. 122.

activity is "diluted," that is, total amount of creatine kinase per unit total cardiac protein is less than in control myocardium.

Second, an increase in B-creatine kinase with a concomitant decrease in M-creatine kinase has now been observed in several species: rat, dog, and human. This observation applies both to species for which normal B creatine kinase activity is ≤2% of the total, as in dog and human, and to species in which B creatine kinase activity is as high as 13%, as occurs in the rat. It also applies to both left and right ventricles. The sole unexplained exception found to date is for the baboon, which has high percentage MB in control and shows no consistent increase in response to pressure overload hypertrophy (67).

Third, the increase in B creatine kinase does not occur in physiological hypertrophy. B creatine kinase content was unchanged for mild hypertrophy caused by swimming in the rat heart (68) and for moderate hypertrophy in hearts of greyhounds (69). There are many differences between physiological and pathologic hypertrophy, including rate of onset of overload, frequency (intermittent vs. chronic stimuli), intensity, duration, and extent of compensation.

Fourth, the stimulus to increased B creatine kinase synthesis is most probably wall stress. This conclusion is based on two observations. The first is that B creatine kinase accumulation occurs primarily in the overloaded ventricle; changes in the unaffected contralateral ventricle were delayed and quantitatively smaller (63, 65). The second is based on comparison of creatine kinase isoenzyme distribution in myocytes obtained from different regions of the left and right ventricles of rats with the same amount of hypertrophy (determined as myocyte size) but with either normal or high blood pressures (63). This analysis showed that although B creatine kinase activity was higher in "nonhypertensive hypertrophy" than in control, more B creatine kinase accumulated in regions that underwent "hypertensive hypertrophy." Fifth, total creatine pool is lower in hypertrophied myocardium, thus limiting energy reserve.

The fundamental question raised by these results is: Do these changes have any functional significance? Based on measurements of heat production and force in normal and hypertrophied muscles containing predominantly V_1 or V_3 myosin, Alpert and colleagues (70) have proposed that accumulation of specific myosin isoenzymes changes the economy of the muscle. For example, hypertrophied rabbit hearts accumulate slow myosin. Although this change would be adaptive at low and moderate workloads, such reprogramming might impair ability of the remodeled myocardium to respond to abrupt overload. The accumulation of anaerobic lactate dehydrogenase isoforms has traditionally been interpreted to report a shift from aerobic to anaerobic pathways of ATP synthesis, but any functional advantage remains to be demonstrated.

Any physiological advantage for accumulating the B creatine kinase must also rely on the subtle kinetic differences among creatine kinase isoenzymes. The B-containing creatine kinase isoenzymes produce ATP more efficiently from PCr than the MM isoform. Thus, it is possible that the increase in MB creatine kinase (which is as large as 10-fold) is adaptive, compensating for decreased energy reserve caused by decreased PCr content. With the use of ^{31}P magnetization transfer, creatine kinase reaction velocity was directly measured in hearts of 12-month-old spontaneously hypertensive rats with 225 mIU (BB + MB)/mg wet weight and age-matched normotensive rats with 150 mIU (BB +

MB)/mg wet weight. No difference was found (71). There are at least three possible interpretations of these results. The first is that accumulation of B creatine kinase has no effect. The second is that B for M replacement is compensatory, maintaining normal reaction velocity. The third, and most likely, is that a much larger change in isoenzyme redistribution (as occur in the dog and human) is required to test the hypothesis. The physiological conditions tested (workload and susceptibility to hypoxic or ischemic stress) must also be considered in future experiments.

C. Energetics of the Failing Myocardium

The hypothesis that the balance between ATP supply and demand is abnormal in failing myocardium is based in part on observations that PCr, and sometimes ATP, contents are lower in failing myocardium. The imbalance could be due to increased demand. More cross-bridge attachment in response to increase stress would lead to increased ATP turnover, as shown by increased oxygen consumption and ATP depletion. In 1974 Meerson (72) proposed that increased ATP (and also PCr) hydrolysis would decrease the phosphorylation potential, $\frac{[ATP]}{[ADP][Pi]}$, which would inhibit myofibrillar ATPase. Arguments against this hypothesis invoke the presence of many redundant systems for ATP resynthesis in the heart. The presence of high activity of creatine kinase and the large size of the energy reserve pool of PCr are also cited.

The imbalance could also be due to reduced supply. One way to limit ATP supply is to reduce oxygen. Increased myocyte mass may outstrip oxygen supply. Results measuring relative capillary density in hypertrophy and failure are conflicting, suggesting that the result depends on species and stimulus to hypertrophy (73). A critical issue is whether capillaries can be recruited during stress (74). Few data are available to define the relation between pO_2 and ATP content, but results using acute hypoxic models suggest that pO_2 must be greatly reduced to cause ATP depletion (75). Observations that ATP and PCr contents were reduced during a 5 hr period of partial stenosis (blood flow reduced ~50%) are consistent with the hypothesis that reduced O_2 supply limits high-energy phosphate synthesis (47). However, these experiments are acute; nothing is known about this relation for chronic hypoxia. Regional analyses of ATP content and turnover should be performed to evaluate this hypothesis more carefully.

A related hypothesis is that the myofibrillar mass outstrips the mitochondrial mass, again producing a mismatch in supply and demand. In this case, ATP supply to the myofibrils and ion transport sites is limited by increased diffusion distances within the myocyte. The possibility that there is a diffusion limitation of either ATP movement from the mitochondria to the myofibril or, more likely, for ADP return to the mitochondria, is difficult to test experimentally.

A third way to limit ATP supply is to deplete energy reserves, primarily PCr. Since the creatine kinase reaction velocity is directly proportional to the amount of enzyme activity (V_{max}) and to the concentration of the guanidino substrate, decreases in either of these parameters should result in decreased capacity to maintain normal ATP levels. Accordingly, the activity of creatine kinase, isozyme distribution and total creatine content were measured in left ventricular biopsies of patients who underwent cardiac transplantation for idiopathic dilated cardiomyopathy (IDC) and normal donor hearts (76). All values were normalized to total cardiac

(Lowry) protein, thereby eliminating possible confounding contributions of edema or differences in excellular matrix protein. There was a 32% reduction in total creatine kinase activity, redistribution of creatine kinase isoenzymes with a ninefold increase of MB-creatine kinase and 57% reduction in total creatine content. Similar changes have been observed in dog hearts failing due to chronic pacing (77). These results suggest that decreases in total Cr (and hence PCr) and total CK activity combine to limit energy reserve for contraction.

Are these changes in the energy reserve system sufficient to cause systolic dysfunction? Two strategies have been used to address this question. To test whether decreased creatine kinase activity limits ability of the heart to do work, creatine kinase activity was inhibited by supplying perfused rat hearts with iodoacetamide. Hearts were characterized biochemically and challenged to perform high levels of work (78). Creatine kinase activity measured by standard biochemical assay and by ^{31}P magnetization transfer was inhibited $\geq$90% but neither purified actomyosin activity nor respiratory rates (measured in isolated mitochondria) were affected. Thus supplying iodoacetamide to hearts specifically inhibited creatine kinase, leaving the major energy-consuming (actomyosin) and -supplying (mitochondria) organelles functionally intact. This conclusion was supported by the ability of iodacetamide-treated hearts to maintain normal work loads. Hearts were challenged by increasing work either by increasing $[Ca^{2+}]_o$ or by supplying NE before and after iodoacetamide supply. Hearts supply with iodoacetamide developed only 62% and 46% (Ca^{2+} and NE challenges, respectively) of peak left ventricular developed pressure. Thus, inhibiting creatine kinase activity acutely (decreasing energy reserve) resulted in decreased contractile reserve.

The second set of results that support the hypothesis that energy reserve is important to maintain ability of the heart to do work comes from ^{31}P magnetization transfer results from failing aged, spontaneously hypertensive rat hearts (71). In these hearts MM and mitochondrial creatine kinase activities and PCr content were decreased. As a result, creatine kinase reaction velocity was lower in failing spontaneously hypertensive rat hearts compared both to younger compensated hypertrophied rat hearts and to age-matched nonhypertensive rat hearts. Thyrotoxic rat hearts, which were 50% PCr depleted, performed less well than controls during hypoxic insult, failing to match either diastolic or systolic performance (79).

Taken together, these results support the hypothesis that decreased energy reserve limits the ability of the myocardium to perform work. All of these experiments were relatively acute. It seems likely that chronic depletion of PCr and/or decreased creatine kinase activity (V_{max}), as occurs in human IDC, could produce even more dramatic results.

IV. ANIMAL MODELS OF FAILURE

Identifying experimental animal models with both physiological and biochemical characteristics of human heart disease remains a major challenge. Models of cardiac dilatation can be created through surgical intervention (such as porta–cava vein shunt or high-frequency pacing) but have disadvantages related to the stress of the intervention and often to the unpredictable course of the disease. Animal models obtained through pharmacological intervention (such as adriamicin) or infection (such as encephalomyocarditis virus in kittens) have similar disadvantages. Moreover, the reproductibility of failure is often uncertain. Two animal models of heart failure reproduce many biochemical and physiological characteristics of failure in humans. They also allow study of the evolution of the disease and intervention: the cardiomyopathic hamster and furazolidone-supplied turkey poult. Comparison of physiological and biochemical parameters relevant to the subject of this chapter are shown in Figure 8.

	HUMAN DCM	TURKEY DCM (Fz & SCM)	HAMSTER DCM
FUNCTION			
EF	↓	↓	unknown
EDV	↑	↑	↑
GROSS MORPHOLOGY			
DILATED	yes	yes	yes
HISTOPATHOLOGY			
MYOCYTE SIZE	↑	↑	↑
NUCLEUS SIZE	↑	↑	↑
MUSCLE PHYSIOLOGY			
SLOWED RELAXATION	yes	yes	yes
ISO RESPONSE	↓	↓	↓
TREPPE	↓	↓	unknown
NOREPINEPHRINE			
CONTENT	↓	↓*	↓
TURNOVER	↑	↑*	↑
β RECEPTOR ADENYLATE CYCLASE SIGNALLING SYTEM			
↓ ADENYLATE CYCLASE RESPONSE	↓	↓*	↓
CALCIUM HANDLING			
$[Ca^{2+}]_i$	↔	unknown	↑
I_{si}	unknown	unknown	
Ca^{2+} CHANNEL NUMBER	↑↓	↑↓	↑↓
RESPONE TO Ca^{2+} SENSITIZERS	↑*	↑*	↑
MYOFILAMENTS			
Ca^{2+} RESPONSIVENESS	↔	↔*	↓
Tn INTERACTION	unknown	n/a	unknown
MYOFIBRILLAR PROTEIN CONTENT	↓	↓*	↓
ENERGY UTILIZATION			
MYOSIN ATPase	↓*	↓*	↓
MYOFIBRILLAR ATPase	↓*	↓*	↓
ENERGY SUPPLY			
CK, PCr, ATP	↓*	↓*	(CK only)
PFK, GAPdH, LDH			
CS	↔	↓*	unknown
ENERGY TRANSFER			
CK FLUX	unknown	↓*	unknown
BENEFICIAL EFFECTS OF β BLOCKADE	yes/no	yes*	yes
PHARMACOLOGIC AGENTS			
MACROMOLECULAR REMODELING	unknown	unknown	unknown

Figure 8 Comparative pathophysiology of heart failure. * Preliminary results obtained by one of the authors; CK, creatine kinase; CS, citrate synthase; DCM, dilated cardiomyopathy; EDV, end-diastolic volume; EF, ejection fraction; Fz, furazolidine; GAPdH, glyceraldehyde phosphate dehydrogenase; I_{si}, voltage-dependent Ca^{2+} current; ISO, isoproterenol; LDH, lactate dehydrogenase; PCr, phosphocreatine; PFK, phosphofructokinase; SCM, spontaneously cardiomyopathy; Tn, troponin.

A. Cardiomyopathic Hamster

The Syrian cardiomyopathic hamster is a spontaneous, reproducible model of failure with many characteristics that resemble human heart failure. It is available in large numbers at a relatively low cost. The first strain of cardiomyopathic hamster (CMH), named BIO 1.5, was obtained in 1956 (80) from inbred lines of *Mesocricetus auratus*. Since then additional strains have been developed to conserve the phenotype of the disease. The genetic defect, still unknown, appears to be an autosomal recessive trait. The disease is a polymyopathy that affects both skeletal and heart muscle. Strains now available have been modified to set the progression of the disease and extent of the focal characteristic lesions; nevertheless, the principal cause of death in these animals remains cardiac failure. In the BIO 14.6 strain, the disease course is divided into four distinct periods marked by different histologic or physiological characteristics: prenecrotic, necrotic or myolytic, hypertrophic, and heart failure (terminal).

1. Pathophysiology

Abelmann (81) showed that in CMH with heart failure the left ventricular peak systolic pressure was reduced and left ventricular end-diastolic pressure was increased; hence left ventricular performance was reduced. In addition, due to pulmonary hypertension, both peak systolic and end-diastolic pressures were increased in the right ventricle. Heart rate was reduced and circulation times and stroke volume were increased, resulting in a normal cardiac output. In isolated papillary muscles, Forman (82) found that the total developed force and the maximum rate of force development corrected for the cross-sectional area of the muscle are decreased in CMH compared to controls. He also demonstrated that the velocity of shortening is reduced in CMH in the early and failure stage but not during the hypertropic stage. However, the maximum force of contraction of muscle was reduced at all stages. If maximum force of contraction is proportional to the number of active sites that generate force and velocity of shortening is related to the rate at which cross-bridges are formed by the actomyosin complex (83), these results suggest that there is a reduction in the number of working contractile elements in hearts of CMH at all stages. Cross-bridge dysfunction occurs only during the prenecrotic and failure stages. These observations spurred investigations to identify qualitative and quantitative biochemical defects that might elucidate the pathogenesis of the disease. There are three different hypotheses relevant to the theme of this chapter.

2. Role of Ca^{2+}

In CMH myocytes many biochemical abnormalities have been described that support the hypothesis that impaired intracellular Ca^{2+} homeostasis contributes to the pathologic changes seen. The administration of Ca^{2+}-channel blockers reduced the number of myocardial lesions and preserved contractility in CMH (84). An increased number of Ca^{2+} voltage-dependent channels have been described by Wagner (85), but not confirmed by Howlet et al. (86). Decreased activity of the sarcolemmal Ca^{2+} ATPase (87) and Na^+/Ca^{2+} exchange (88) has also been reported. Intramitochondrial calcium overload with impaired energy production could also play a role (89, 90). A generalized Ca^{2+} overload has been disputed. However, since electron probe studies in freeze-dried cryosections recently demonstrated that only cells close to focal lesions have elevated Ca^{2+} content and that Ca^{2+} was confined to the mitochondrial compartment (91), these findings support the hypothesis that focal vasospasm of the microvasculature can be responsible for the myocyte damage that leads to a Ca^{2+} overload (92).

3. *Role of the Catecholamines*

During the necrotic phase, an elevation of urinary NE levels (93), increase NE uptake (94), and increased number of adrenergic nerve terminals (95) have been demonstrated. It has been postulated that young CMH are genetically predisposed to catecholamine damage, since small doses had no affect on normal hamsters but provoked acute contraction band necrosis similar to that observed for the spontaneous disease (96). Additional data support the idea that the lesions could be an indirect effect of microvasculature hypersensitivity to catecholamines (97). Thus, both vascular and muscular hypersensitivity contribute to the necrotic lesions.

CMH at all ages exhibit increased cardiac NE turnover and increased dopamine-β-hydroylase activity. Using radioligands and isolated CMH myocytes, an increased number of both α and β adrenergic receptors have been observed (94). The increased number of receptors could explain Ca^{2+} overload, since it would increase the slow inward Ca^{2+} current of myocytes (98). However, this observation has not been confirmed by other studies (99). Still other investigators have attributed the increased Ca^{2+} content to stimulation of α_1 receptors mediated by pertussis toxin-sensitive G protein (100). In hearts of CMH of all ages, decreased adenylate cyclase and phosphorylase activities coupled with an increase of cyclic nucleotide phosphodiesterase activity (101) and decreased activity of the guanine-nucleotide-binding protein that stimulates adenylate cyclase (102) have been observed. These findings are also compatible with a decreased catecholamine-sustained contractility.

4. *Pathways for ATP Synthesis and Utilization*

Alterations of structural or regulatory contractile proteins could also play a role in cardiac failure in CMH. Disarray of the myofilaments has been documented by many investigators (103). Myofilament composition also differs. The distribution of myosin isoenzymes in CMH heart is altered with a shift towards the slow form V_3 that, like rats, has a lower Ca^{2+}-activated ATPase activity (104). Troponin–tropomyosin (Tn-Tm) complex isolated from CMH hearts is also abnormal (105). Thus, both thick- and thin-filament regulation differs in CMH hearts. These modifications in the contractile proteins have been interpreted (104) as compensatory responses to increased workload or to decreased energy supply.

Results describing cardiac mitochondrial function have been contradictory (106–108), but evidence for changes in energy supply has been found. Consistent with observations made in the failing spontaneously hypertensive rat heart, decreased total creatine kinase activity and mitochondrial-creatine kinase activity in CMH hearts (109) suggests that energy reserve is impaired. The relation between energy production and mechanical work remains to be defined.

B. Cardiomyopathic Turkey

Spontaneous cardiomyopathy of unknown cause occurs in a small percentage of turkeys (10%). The first published report of the disease was by Magwood and Bray (110). Histopathologically, morphologically, and functionally it resembles the drug-induced (furazolidone) cardiomyopathy in turkey poults. Therefore, in an effort to simplify this discussion, we will discuss both spontaneous and furazolidone-induced cardiomyopathy with appropriate references to the literature (see review by Czarnecki, 111, 112).

Furazolidone is a nitrofuran used as a feed additive and growth promoter. Jankus et al. (113) found that administering this feed additive at therapeutic dosages induced an experimental condition mimicking spontaneous round heart disease. Low concentrations (110 ppm) have no effect on cardiac function; however, concentrations of 700 ppm resulted in significant cardiac dilatation and failure. Furazolidone-induced cardiomyopathy demonstrates biventricular dilatation with increased end-diastolic volumes and reduced ejection fraction (114). Blood pressures tend to be low in animals with cardiac failure.

It has been suggested that furazolidone acts via monoamine oxidase inhibition (115). However, there is no clear evidence for this hypothesis. Administration of tranylcypromine, a potent monoamine oxidase inhibitor, failed to induce cardiomyopathy in turkey poults (116). Furthermore, animals are not tachycardiac as would be expected if the cardiomyopathy was induced by catecholamine stimulation. On histopathologic examination, animals with furazolidone-induced cardiomyopathy do not demonstrate the myocytolysis or other associated light microscopic findings seen with catecholamine-induced cardiomyopathy (117, 118).

Many biochemical characteristics of the failing myocardium in turkey poults are similar to failing myocardium both in humans and CMH (Fig. 8). The β-adrenergic–adenylate cyclase system has been reported to be reduced in inbred turkeys with spontaneous cardiomyopathy (119). There is a decreased myocardial lipid peroxidation, suggesting that free radical injury is not involved in the cardiomyopathy (120). Compared to control, activities of many proteins were decreased: creatine kinase by 40%, glycolytic proteins by 30%, myofibrillar ATPase activity by 20%, Krebs' cycle enzymes by 20%, fatty acid oxidation by 15%, and total soluble protein by 10%. In contrast, calcium ATPase activity of the sarcoplasmic reticulum was increased by 60% (121).

Studies in our laboratories have found that myocardium from turkey poults is similar to mammalian myocardium with regard to several physiological and biochemical characteristics: β-adrenergic-adenylate cyclase system; calcium channel number assessed as dihydropyridine binding; force–pCa relationships in skinned fibers; activities of citrate synthase, lactate dehydrogense, and creatine kinase; NE content and turnover; positive force interval relationship; and whole heart and isolated muscle physiology.

V. CONCLUSIONS

With the use of new biophysical tools to measure $[Ca^{2+}]_i$ directly, the hypothesis that cardiac failure is due to decreased Ca^{2+} availability has been tested in both human and nonprimate mammalian myocardium. The results show that decreased contractile performance cannot be explained simply by decreased $[Ca^{2+}]_i$. The possibility remains that changes in myofilament composition and hence Ca^{2+} responsiveness contribute to contractile failure.

Also with the use of new biophysical techniques to measure ATP and PCr content and turnover in intact heart, some aspects of the hypothesis that contractile failure is due to a mismatch in energy supply and demand have been tested. Although molecular remodeling of ATP producing and utilizing pathways occurs, it is still unknown whether it is adaptive or maladaptive. Finally, new experiments showing that decreased energy reserve limits contractile reserve support the hypothesis that ATP supply is compromised in the failing myocardium.

We close by suggesting that the Ca^{2+} and energy hypotheses are interrelated. $[Ca^{2+}]_i$ is set by the combined actions of ATP-dependent Ca^{2+} pumps and specific Ca^{2+} exchangers in the sarcolemma and a Ca^{2+} pump in the sarcoplasmic reticulum. The rate of Ca^{2+} recycling is determined in part by the myofibrils. All of these ATPases are regulated by substrate (ATP) supply and, even in the presence of ATP, are inhibited by the products of ATP hydrolysis, namely, ADP, P_i, and H^+, as well as Ca^{2+}. Thus, a derangement in ATP supply with accumulation of P_i and H^+ would lead to impaired function of the Ca^{2+} pumps and myosin ATPase and hence contractile performance.

ACKNOWLEDGMENTS

We acknowledge support from National Institutes of Health grants HL38189 and 43170 to Joanne S. Ingwall; from Merck Sharp and Dohme, Italy, to Luigino Nascimben; and from National Institutes of Health grant HL 39091; and grants from Glaxco, Inc. and the Upjohn Company to Judith K. Gwathmey. Dr. Gwathmey is an Established Investigator of the American Heart Association.

REFERENCES

1. Ringer S. A further contribution regarding the influence of the blood on the contraction of the heart. *J Physiol* (London) 1883;4:29–42.
2. Fabiato A. Calcium-induced release of calcium from the sarcoplasmic reticulum. *J Gen Phys* 1985;85:189–320.
3. Beuckelmann DJ, Wier WG. Mechanism of release of calcium from sarcoplasmic reticulum of guinea pig cardiac cells. *J Physiol* 1988;405:233–55.
4. Cannel MB, Allen DG. Model of calcium movements during activation in the sarcomere of frog skeletal muscle. *Biophys J* 1984;45:913–25.
5. Yue DT, Wier W. Estimation of intracellular $[Ca^{2+}]$ by nonlinear indicators. *Biophys J* 1985;48:533–7.
6. MacKinnon R, Gwathmey JK, Allen PD, Briggs GM, Morgan JP. Modulation by the thyroid state of intracellular calcium and contractility in ferret ventricular muscle. *Circ Res* 1988;63:1080–9.
7. Yue DT, Marban E, Wier WG. Relationship between force and intracellular $[Ca^{2+}]$ in tetanized mammalian heart muscle. *J Gen Physiol* 1986;87:223–42.
8. Maughan D, Berman M. Radial compression of functionally skinned cardiac bundles abolishes calcium activated force. *Biophys J* 1981;30:27–40.
9. Matsubara I, Umazume Y, Yagi N. Lateral shrinkage of the myofilament lattice in chemically skinned muscles during contraction In: Pollack G, Sugi H, eds. *Contractile mechanisms in muscle.* New York: Plenum Publishing, 1984;711–20.
10. Gwathmey JK, Hajjar RJ. Relation between steady-state force and intracellular $[Ca^{2+}]$ in intact human myocardium. Index of myofibrillar responsiveness to Ca^{2+}. *Circulation* 1990;82:1266–78.
11. Gwathmey JK, Morgan JP. Calcium handling in myocardium from amphibian, avian, and mammalian species: the search for two components. *J Comp Physiol B* 1991; 161:19–25.

12. Gwathmey JK, Ingwall JS, Morgan JP. Is hypertrophy bad? Functional and biochemical assessment. *Circulation* 1990;82(4):III–111.
13. Gwathmey JK, Slawsky MT, Hajjar RJ, Briggs GM, Morgan JP. Role of intracellular calcium handling in force-interval relationships of human ventricular myocardium. *J Clin Invest* 1990;85:1599–613.
14. Blinks JR. Intracellular [Ca^{2+}] measurements. In: Fozzard HA, et al., eds. *The heart and cardiovascular system.* New York: Raven Press, 1986;671–701.
15. Gwathmey JK, Morgan JP. Altered calcium handling in experimental pressure overload hypertrophy in the ferret. *Circ Res* 1985;57:836–43.
16. Siri FM, Krueger J, Nordin C, Ming Z, Aronson RS. Depressed intracellular calcium transients and contraction in myocytes from hypertrophied and failing guinea pig hearts. *Am J Physiol* 1991;261:H514–30.
17. Gwathmey JK, Bentivegna LA, Ransil BJ, Grossman W, Morgan JP. Relationship of abnormal intracellular calcium mobilization to myocyte hypertrophy in human ventricular myocardium. *Cardivasc Res* 1993:27 in press.
18. Olivetti G, Melissari M, Capasso JM, Anversa P. Cardiomyopathy of the aging human heart. Myocyte loss and reactive cellular hypertrophy. *Circ Res* 1991;68:1560–8.
19. Bristow MR, Ginsburg R, Minobe W, Cubicciotti RS, Sageman WS, Lurie K, Billingham ME, Harrison DC, Stinson EB. Decreased calecholamine sensitivity and beta-adrenergic receptor density in failing human hearts. *N Engl J Med* 1982;307:205–11.
20. Waagstein F, Caidahl K, Wallentin I, Bergh C-H, Hjalmarson A. Long-term β-blockade in dilated cardiomyopathy. Effects of short and long-term metoprolol treatment followed by withdrawal and readministration of metoprolol. *Circulation* 1989;80:551–63.
21. Lakatta EG, Gerstenblith G, Angell CS, Shock NW, Weisfeldt ML. Prolonged contraction duration in aged myocardium. *J Clin Invest* 1975;55:61–8.
22. Hasenfuss G, Mulieri LA, Blanchard EM, Holubarsch C, Leavitt BJ, Ittleman F, Alpert NR. Energetics of isometric force development in control and volume-overload human myocardium. *Circ Res* 1991;68:836–46.
23. Marsh JD, Allen PD, Denniss AR. Decreased calcium channel expression in sarcolemmal membranes from human hearts with congestive heart failure. *J Mol Cell Cardiol* 1987;19(IV):533.
24. Gwathmey JK, Copelas L, MacKinnon R, Schoen FJ, Feldman MD, Grossman W, Morgan JP. Abnormal intracellular calcium handling in myocardium from patients with end-stage heart failure. *Circ Res* 1987;61:70–6.
25. Wagner JA, Sax FL, Weisman HF, Potterfield J, McIntosh C, Weisfeldt ML, Snyder SH, Epstein SE. Calcium-antagonist receptors in the atrial tissue of patients with hypertrophic cardiomyopathy. *N Engl J Med* 1989;320(12):755–61.
26. Solaro RJ, El-Saleh SC, Kentish J, Meyer A, Martin A. Transitions in isoform populations of thick and thin filament proteins and calcium activation of force and ATP hydrolysis by cardiac myofilaments. *Muscle Energ* 1989;487–502.
27. Gwathmey JK, Warren SE, Briggs GM, Copelas L, Feldman MD, Phillips PJ, Callahan M, Schoen FJ, Grossman W, Morgan JP. Diastolic dysfunction in hypertrophic cardiomyopathy. Effect on active force generation during systole. *J Clin Invest* 1991;87:1023–31.
28. Li Q, Biagi B, Starling R, Hohl C, Altschuld R, Stokes B. Characteristics of calcium transients and electrophysiology in human ventricular myocytes. *Biophys J* 1989; 55:486a.
29. Lederer WJ, Berlin JR, Cohen NM, Hadley RW, Bers DM, Cannel MB. Excitation–contraction coupling in heart cells. *Ann NY Acad Sci* 1990;588:190–206.
30. Hajjar RJ, Gwathmey JK, Briggs GM, Morgan JP. Differential effect of DPI 201-106 on the sensitivity of the myofilaments to Ca^{2+} in intact and skinned trabeculae from control and myopathic human hearts. *J Clin Invest* 1988;82:1578–84.

31. Baudet S, Ventura-Clapier R. Differential effects of caffeine on skinned fibers from control and hypertrophied ferret hearts. *Am J Physiol* 1990;259:H1803–8.
32. Ventura-Clapier R. Skinned fibers in cardiac overload. In Swynghedauw B, ed. *Research in cardiac hypertrophy and failure*. INSERM/John Libbey Eurotext, 1990; 161–8.
33. Hajjar RJ, Gwathmey JK. Modulation of calcium-activation in control and pressure-overload hypertrophied ferret hearts: Effect of DPI 201-106 on myofilament calcium responsiveness. *J Mol Cell Cardiol* 1991;23:65–75.
34. Gwathmey JK, Hajjar RJ. Effect of protein kinase C activation on sarcoplasmic reticulum function and apparent myofibrillar Ca^{2+} sensitivity in intact and skinned muscles from normal and diseased human myocardium. *Circ Res* 1990;67:744–52.
35. McAuliffe JJ, Gao L, Solaro RJ. Changes in myofibrillar activation and troponin C Ca^{2+} binding associated with troponin T isoform switching in developing rabbit heart. *Circ Res* 1990;66:1204–16.
36. Anderson PAW, Oakley A, Allen PD. Human troponin T expression in normal and end-stage heart failure patients. *Circulation* 1991;80(Suppl II):503.
37. Solaro RJ, Powers FM, Gaol L, Gwathmey JK. Control of myofilament activation in heart failure. *Circulation* 1993 in press.
38. Hajjar RJ, Gwathmey JK. Cross-bridge dynamics in human ventricular myocardium: Regulation of contractility in the failing heart. *Circulation* 1993;86 in press.
39. Cain DF, Davies RE. Breakdown of ATP during a single contraction of working muscle. *Biochem Biophys Res Commun* 1962;8:361.
40. Neubauer S, Ingwall JS. The isolated buffer-perfused ferret heart: a new model for the study of cardiac physiology and metabolism. *Lab Anim* 1991;25:348–53.
41. Weiss RG, Bottomley PA, Hardy CJ, Gerstenblith G. Regional myocardial high-energy phosphates during isometric exercise in patients with coronary artery disease. *N Engl J Med* 1990;323:1593–600.
42. Bittl JA, Ingwall JS. Reaction rates of creatine kinase and ATP synthesis in the isolated rat heart. A P-31 magnetization transfer study. *J Biol Chem* 1985;260:3512–7.
43. Perry SB, McAuliffe J, Balsch JA, Hickey PR, Ingwall JA. Velocity of the creatine kinase reaction in the neonatal rabbit heart: the role of mitochondrial creatine kinase. *Biochemistry* 1988;27:2165–72.
44. Neubauer S, Ingwall JS. In the ferret heart creatine kinase flux is not coupled to cardiac workload: a ^{31}P NMR saturation transfer study. *Proceedings of the Second European Congress of NMR in Medicine and Biology,* 1988, p. 80.
45. Balaban RS, Kantor HL, Katz LA, Briggs RW. Relation between work and phosphate metabolites in the in vivo paced mammalian heart. *Science* 1986;232:1121–3.
46. Matsuzaki M, Gallagher KP, Kemper WS, White F, Ross J Jr. Sustained regional dysfunction produced by prolonged coronary stenosis: gradual recovery after reperfusion. *Circulation* 1983;68:170–82.
47. Neill WA, Ingwall JS. Stabilization of a derangement in ATP metabolism during sustained, partial ischemia in the dog heart. *J Am Coll Cardiol* 1986;8:894–900.
48. Sako EY, Kingsley-Hickman PB, From AHL, Foker JE, Urgubil K. ATP synthesis kinetics and mitochondrial function in the postischemic myocardium as studied by ^{31}P NMR. *J Biol Chem* 1988;263(22):10600–7.
49. Weiss RG, Chacko VP, Glickson JB, Gerstenblith G. Comparative ^{13}C and ^{31}P NMR assessment of altered metabolism during graded reductions in coronary flow in intact hearts. *Proc Natl Acad Sci* (USA) 1989;86:6426–30.
50. Lewandowski ED, Johnson DL. Reduced substrate oxidation in postischemic myocardium: ^{13}C and ^{31}P NMR analyses. *Am J Physiol* 1990;258:H1357–65.
51. Malloy CR, Thompson JR, Jeffrey FMH, Sherry AD. Contribution of exogenous substrates to acetyl coenzyme. A measurement of ^{13}C NMR under non-steady-state conditions. *Biochemistry* 1990;29:6756–61.

52. Bittl JA, Delayre J, Ingwall JS. Rate equation for creatine kinase predicts the in vivo reaction velocity: ^{31}P NMR surface coil studies in brain, heart and skeletal muscle of the living rat. *Biochemistry* 1987;26:6083–90.
53. Bittl JA, Balschi JA, Ingwall JS. Contractile failure and high-energy phosphate turnover during hypoxia: ^{31}P-NMR surface coil studies in living rat. *Circ Res* 1987;60: 871–8.
54. Ingwall JS, Weiss RG. ^{31}P NMR spectroscopy: the non-invasive tool for the study of the biochemistry of the cardiovascular system. *Trends Cardiovasc Med* 1993; in press.
55. Jacobus WE, Lehninger AL. Creatine kinase of rat heart mitochondria. *J Biol Chem* 1973;248:4803–10.
56. Saks VA. Creatine kinase isozymes and the control of cardiac contraction. In: Jacobus WE, Ingwall JS, eds. *Heart creatine kinase.* Baltimore: Williams & Wilkins 1980;109–24.
57. Ingwall JS, Kramer MF, Fifer MA, Lorell BH, Shemin R, Grossman W, Allen PD. The creatine kinase system in normal and diseased human myocardium. *N Engl J Med* 1985;313:1050–4.
58. Sobel BE, Henry PD, Ehrlich BJ, Bloor CM. Altered myocardial lactic dehydrogenase isoenzymes in experimental cardiac hypertrophy. *Lab Invest* 1970;22:23–7.
59. Fox AC. High energy phosphate compounds and LDH isozymes in the hypertrophied right ventricle. In Alpert NR, ed. *Cardiac hypertrophy.* New York: Academic Press, 1971:203–12.
60. Bishop SP, Altschuld RA. Increased glycolytic metabolism in cardiac hypertrophy and congestive failure. *Am J Physiol* 1970;218:153–9.
61. Ingwall JS, Badke FR, Pavelec RS, Covell JW. Alterations in creatine phosphokinase activity and isoenzyme composition in the volume loaded, hypertrophied heart. *Circulation* 1979;54 (Suppl II):59.
62. Lompre AM, Schwartz K, d'Albis A, Lacombe G, Thiem NV, Swynghedauw B. Myosin isoenzyme redistribution in chronic heart overload. *Nature* 1979;282:105–7.
63. Smith SH, Kramer MF, Reis I, Bishop SP, Ingwall JS. Regional changes in creatine kinase and myocyte size in hypertensive and nonhypertensive cardiac hypertrophy. *Circ Res* 1990;67:1334–44.
64. Ingwall JS. The hypertrophied myocardium accumulates the MB-creatine kinase isozyme. *Eur Heart J* 1984;5 (Suppl F):129–39.
65. Vatner DE, Vatner SF, Sit SP, Ingwall JS. Selectivity of altered creatine kinase isozyme distribution in pressure overload ventricular hypertrophy. *Circulation* 1982;66:II–203.
66. Vatner DE, Ingwall JS. Effects of moderate pressure overload cardiac hypertrophy on the distribution of creatine kinase isozymes. *Proc Soc Exp Biol Med* 1984;175:5–9.
67. Ingwall JS, Walsh R. Unpublished results.
68. Spencer RS, Buttrick P, Scheuer J, Ingwall JS. Unpublished results.
69. Ingwall JS, Covell JW. Unpublished results.
70. Alpert NR, Mulieri LA. Heat mechanics and myosin ATPase in normal and hypertrophied heart muscle. *Fed Proc* 1982;41:192–8.
71. Bittl JA, Ingwall JS. Intracellular high-energy phosphate transfer in normal and hypertrophied myocardium. *Circulation* 1987;75(I):96–101.
72. Meerson FV. Development of modern components of the mechanism of cardiac hypertrophy. *Circ Res* 1974;(Suppl. II) 5:58–63.
73. Bache RJ. Effects on the coronary circulation. *Prog Cardiovasc Dis* 1988;31(6):403–40.
74. Honig CR, Gayeski TEJ. Capillary reserve and tissue O_2 transport in normal and hypertrophied hearts. In Tarzi RC, Dunbar JB Jr, eds. *Cardiac hypertrophy in hypertension.* New York: Raven Press, 1983; 249.
75. Clarke KC, Willis RJ. Energy metabolism and contractile function in rat heart during graded, isovolumic perfusion using 31P nuclear magnetic resonance spectroscopy. *J Mol Cell Cardiol* 1987;19:1153–60.

76. Nascimben L, Ingwall JS. Decreased energy reserve may cause pump failure in human dilated cardiomyopathy. *Circulation* 1991; II:563.
77. deTombe PP, Wolff MR, Kass DA, Hunter WC, Reis I, Ingwall JS. Creatine kinase isoenzyme expression is altered in experimental canine dilated cardiomyopathy without hypertrophy. *Circulation* 1991; II:280.
78. Hamman BL, Bittl JA, Jacobus WE, Ingwall JS. Inhibition of creatine kinase decreases the contractile reserve of the isolated rat heart. *Proceedings of the 5th Annual Meeting of the Society of Magnetic Resonance in Medicine,* 1986, P:133.
79. Ingwall JS, Atkinson DA, Clarke K, Fetters JA. Energetic correlates of cardiac failure: changes in the creatine kinase system in the failing myocardium. *Eur Heart J* 1990; 11(Suppl B):108–15.
80. Bajusz E, Baker JR, Nixon CW, Whitney R, Homburger F. Spontaneous hereditary myocardial degeneration and congestive failure in a strain of Syrian hamsters. *Ann NY Acad Sci* 1969;156:105–129.
81. Abelmann WH, Jeffrey FE, Wagner R. Circulatory dynamics in heart failure of Syrian hamsters. *Progr Exp Tumor Res* 1972;16:261–73.
82. Forman R, Parmley W, Sonnenblick EH. Myocardial contractility in relation to hypertrophy and failure in myopathic Syrian hamsters. *J Mol Cell Cardiol* 1972;4:203–11.
83. Ebashi S. Ca^{2+} and the contractile proteins. *J Mol Cell Cardiol* 1984;16:129–36.
84. Rouleau JL, Chuck LHS, Hollosi G, Kidd P, Sievers RE, Wilkman-Coffelt J, Parmley WW. Verapamil preserves myocardial contractility in the hereditary cardiomyopathy of the Syrian hamster. *Circ Res* 1982;50:405–12.
85. Wagner JA, Reynolds IJ, Weisman HF, Dudeck P, Weisfeldt ML, Snyder SH. Calcium antagonist receptors in cardiomyopathic hamster: selective increase in heart, muscle, brain. *Science* 1986;232:515–8.
86. Howlett SE, Gordon T. Calcium channels in normal and dystrophic hamster cardiac muscle. *Biochem Pharmacol* 1987;36(16):2653–9.
87. Kuo TH, Tsang W, Weiner J. Defective Ca^{2+} pumping ATPase of heart sarcolemma from cardiomyopathic hamster. *Biochem Biophys Acta* 1987;900:10–6.
88. Wagner JA, Weisman HF, Snowman AM, Reynolds IJ, Weisfeldt ML, Snyder SH. Alterations in calcium antagonist receptors and sodium–calcium exchange in cardiomyopathic hamsters tissues. *Circ Res* 1989;65(1):205–14.
89. Wrogeman K, Nylen EG. Mitochondrial calcium overload in cardiomyopathic hamsters. *J Mol Cell Cardiol* 1978;10:185–95.
90. Proschek L, Jasmin G. Hereditary polymyopathy and cardiomyopathy in the Syrian hamster: II. Development in the heart necrotic changes in relation to defective mitochondrial function. *Muscle Nerve* 1982;5:26–32.
91. Bond M, Jaraki AR, Disch CH, Healy BP. Subcellular calcium content in cardiomyopathic hamster hearts in vivo: an electron probe study. *Circ Res* 1989;64:1001–12.
92. Sonnenblick EH, Fein F, Capasso JM, Factor SM. Microvascular spasm as a cause of cardiomyopathies and the calcium blocking agent verapamil as a potential primary therapy. *Am J Cardiol* 1985;55:179–84B.
93. Kabara JJ, Riggin RM, Kissinger PT. Abnormal levels of urinary catecholamines in distrophic mice and hamsters. *Proc Soc Exp Biol Med* 1976;151:168.
94. Karliner JS, Alabaster C, Stephens H, Barnes B, Dollery C. Enhanced noradrenaline response in cardiomyopathic hamsters: possible relation to changes in adrenoceptors studied by radioligand binding. *Cardiovasc Res* 1981;15:296–304.
95. Jasmin G, Proschek L. The permissive role of catecholamines in the pathogenesis of hamster cardiomyopathy. *Adv Myocardiol* 1983;3:45–53.
96. Bajusz E, Homburger F, Baker JR, Bogdonoff P. Dissociation of factors influencing myocardial degeneration and generalized cardiocirculatory failure. *Ann NY Acad Sci* 1969;156:396–420.

97. Conway RS, Factor SM, Sonnenblick EH, Baez S. Microvascular reactivity of the myopathic Syrian hamster cremaster muscle. *Cardiovasc Res* 1987;21:796–803.
98. Buckner R, Scholz H. Effects of α adrenoceptor stimulation with phenylephrine in the presence of propranolol on force of contraction, slow inward current and cyclic AMP content in the bovine heart. *Br J Pharmacol* 1984;82:223–32.
99. Kobayashi A, Yamashita TM, Nishiyama T, Hayashi H, Yamazaki N. Effects of verapamil on experimental cardiomyopathy in Bio 14.6 Syrian hamster. *J Am Coll Cardiol* 1987;10:1128–34.
100. Sen L, Liang BT, Colucci WS, Smith TW. Enhanced alpha-1-adrenergic responsiveness in cardiomyopathic hamster cardiac myocytes. *Circ Res* 1990;67:1182–92.
101. Sulakhe SJ, Russel BL, Sulakhe PV. Adenylate cyclase, cyclic nucleotide phosphodiesterase and phosphorylase activity of cardiomyopathic hamster hearts. In: Kobayashi T, Ito Y, Rona G, eds. *Recent advances in studies on cardiac structure and metabolism,* vol 12, Cardiac adaptation. Baltimore: University Park Press. 1978.
102. Kessler PD, Cates AE, Van Dop C, Feldman AM. Decreased bioactivity of the guanine nucleotide-binding protein that stimulates adenylate cyclase in hearts from cardiomyopathic hamsters. *J Clin Invest* 1989;84(1):244–52.
103. Malhotra A, Karell M, Scheuer J. Multiple cardiac contractile protein abnormalities in myopathic Syrian hamsters. *J Mol Cell Cardiol* 1985;17:95–107.
104. Wiegand V, Stroh E, Henniges A, Lossnitzer K, Kreutzer H. Altered distribution of myosin isoenzymes in the cardiomyopathic Syrian hamster. *Basic Res Cardiol* 1983; 78(6):665–70.
105. Malhotra A, Scheuer J. Troponin-tropomyosin abnormalities in hamster cardiomyopathy. *J Clin Invest* 1990;86:286–92.
106. Lyndemayer GE, Harigaya S, Bajusz S, Swartz A. Oxidative phosphorylation and calcium transport of mitochondria isolated from cardiomyopathic hamsters hearts. *J Mol Cell Cardiol* 1970;1:249–59.
107. Lochner A, Opie LH, Brink AJ, Bosman AR. Defective oxidative phosphorylation in hereditary myocardiopathy in the Syrian hamster. *Cardiovasc Res* 1968(2):297–307.
108. Wrogemann K, Blanchaer MC, Thakar JH, Mezon BJ. On the role of mitochondria in the hereditary cardiomyopathy of the Syrian hamster. *Rec Adv Stud Cardiac Struct Metabol* 1975;6:231–41.
109. Khuchua ZA, Ventura-Clapier R, Kuznetzov RV, Grishin MN, Saks VA. Alterations in the creatine-kinase system in the myocardium of the cardiomyopathic hamsters. *Biochem Biophys Res Commun* 1989;165(2):748–57.
110. Magwood SE, Bray DF. Disease condition of turkey poults characterized by enlarged and rounded hearts. *Can J Comp Med Vet Sci* 1962;26:268–72.
111. Czarnecki CM. Animal models of drug-induced cardiomyopathy. *Comp Biochem Physiol* 1984;79C:9–14.
112. Czarnecki CM. Review: cardiomyopathy in turkeys. *Comp Biochem Physiol* 1984; 77:591–8.
113. Jankus EF, Noren GR, Staley NA. Furazolidone-induced cardiac dilatation in turkeys (research note). *Avian Dis* 1972;16:958–61.
114. Einzig S, Staley NA, Mettler E, Nicoloff DM, Noren GR. Regional myocardial blood flow and cardiac function in a naturally occurring congestive cardiomyopathy of turkeys. *Cardiovasc Res* 1980;14:396–407.
115. Stern IJ, Hollifield RD, Wilk S, Buzard JA. The antimonamine oxidase effects of furazolidone. *J Pharmacol Exp Ther* 1967;156:492–99.
116. Powers MD, Good AL, Czarnecki CM, Evanson OA. Monamine oxidase inhibition and furazolidone-induced cardiomyopathy in turkey poults. *Poultry Sci* 1983;62: 1850–5.
117. Gough AW, Pinn S, Hullan TJ, Thompson RG, de la Iglesia F. Spontaneous

cardiomyopathy: histopathologic and ultrastructural alterations of turkey heart tissue. *Am J Vet Res* 1981;42:1290–7.

118. Czarnecki CM, Grahn DA. A morphometric study of myocardial mitochondria and myofibrils in turkey poults during development of furazolidone-induced cardiomyopathy. *Avian Dis* 1980;24:955–70.
119. Staley NA, Einzig S, Noren GR, Surdy JE, Elsperger J. β-Adrenergic function in a congestive cardiomyopathy model. *Am J Physiol* 1987;252:H334–9.
120. Lax D, Zhang SL, Li Y, Williams L, Berry JM, Elsperger J, Staley NA, Noren GR, Einzig S. Reduced lipid peroxidation in dilated hearts of cardiomyopathic turkeys. *Cardiovasc Res* 1980;14:396–407.
121. Mirsalimi SM, Qureshi FS, Julian RJ, O'Brien PJ. Myocardial biochemical changes in furazolidone-induced cardiomyopathy of turkeys. *J Comp Pathol* 1990;102:139–46.
122. Ingwall JS. On the hypothesis: cardiac failure is a consequence of decreased energy reserve. *Circulation* 1993, in press.
123. Beuckelmann DJ, Nabaurer M, Erdmann E. Intracellular calcium handling in isolated ventricular myocytes from patients with terminal heart failure. *Circulation* 1992;85:1046–55.

Index

about the editors

Judith K. Gwathmey is Director of the Institute for Cardiovascular Disease and Muscle Research, Associate Professor of Cellular and Molecular Physiology in the Department of Medicine at Harvard Medical School, and Research Associate in Medicine in the Cardiovascular Division at Beth Israel Hospital, Boston, Massachusetts. The author or coauthor of over 70 professional papers and an invited reviewer for several scientific journals, Dr. Gwathmey is a Fellow of the American College of Cardiology and a member of the American Heart Association, the American Society for Pharmacology and Experimental Therapeutics, the Biophysical Society, and the International Society for Heart Research, among others. She received the B.A. degree (1972) in biology and the V.M.D. degree (1977) from the University of Pennsylvania, Philadelphia, and the Ph.D. degree (1983) in physiology and pharmacology from Ohio State University, Columbus.

G. Maurice Briggs is a Research Investigator in the Department of Cardiovascular Pharmacology at Sterling Winthrop Pharmaceuticals, Rensselaer, New York. The coauthor of over 20 professional papers, Dr. Briggs is a member of the American Heart Association, the Biophysical Society, and the International Society for Heart Research, among others. He received the B.S. degree (1978) in biology/chemistry from the University of Texas at Arlington, and the Ph.D. degree (1986) in pharmacology from the College of Medicine, University of Oklahoma Health Sciences Center, Oklahoma City.

Paul D. Allen is Associate Professor of Anesthesia at Harvard Medical School and an Anesthesiologist at Brigham and Women's Hospital, Boston, Massachusetts. The author or coauthor of over 60 professional papers, Dr. Allen is a member of the American Society of Anesthetists, the Biophysical Society, and the International Society of Heart Research, among others. He received the B.A. degree (1967) in medical science and the M.D. degree (1967) from Boston University, Massachusetts, and the Ph.D. degree (1973) in physiology from the University of Florida, Gainesville.